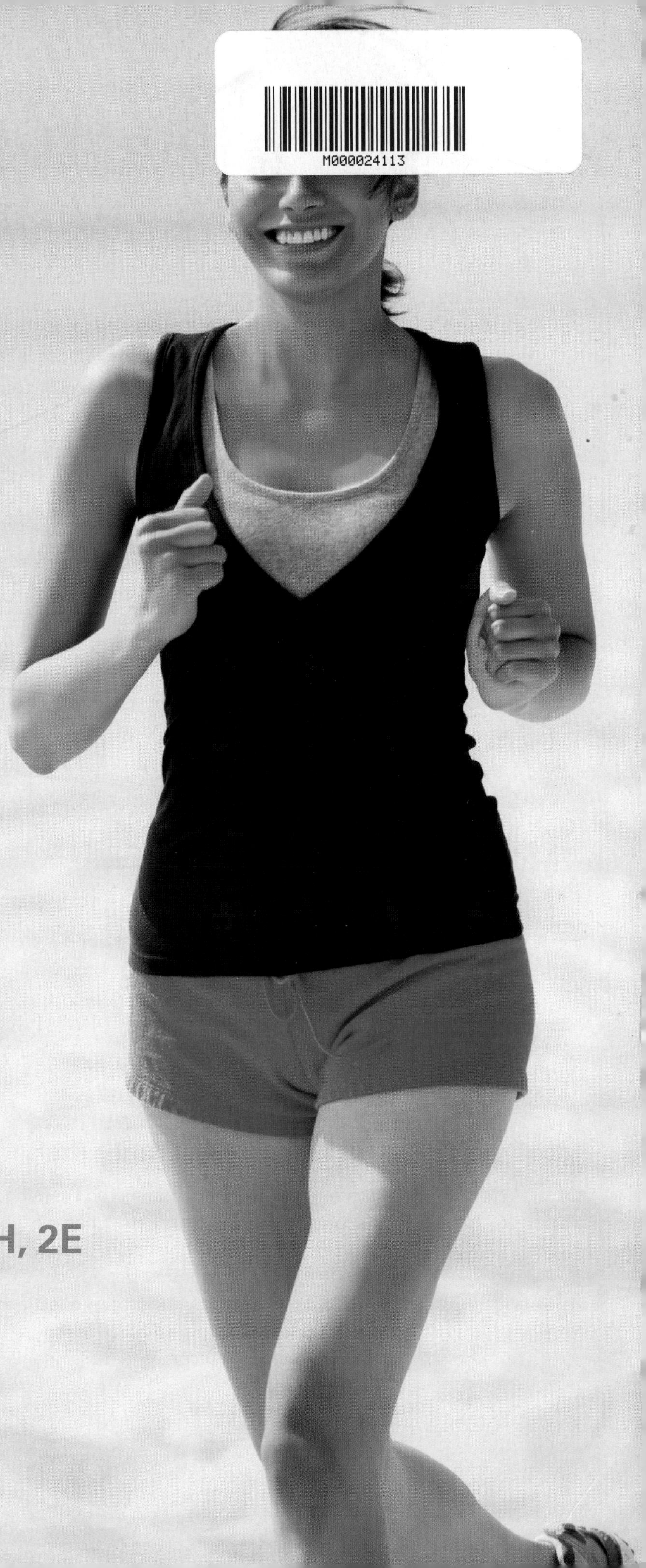

Ready, Set, GO!

WITH DONATELLE, MY HEALTH, 2E

The MasteringHealth Edition

Get Your **Students Ready!**

For today's students, text and media go hand in hand as study tools. The MasteringHealth Edition of *My Health* brings text and online practice together to meet students where they are, providing them with the tools that they need to effectively learn and master health concepts and to apply those concepts to their daily lives. The MasteringHealth Edition provides YOU, the instructor, with the ability to evaluate student comprehension and assign specific content from the text for extra practice, improving overall student performance.

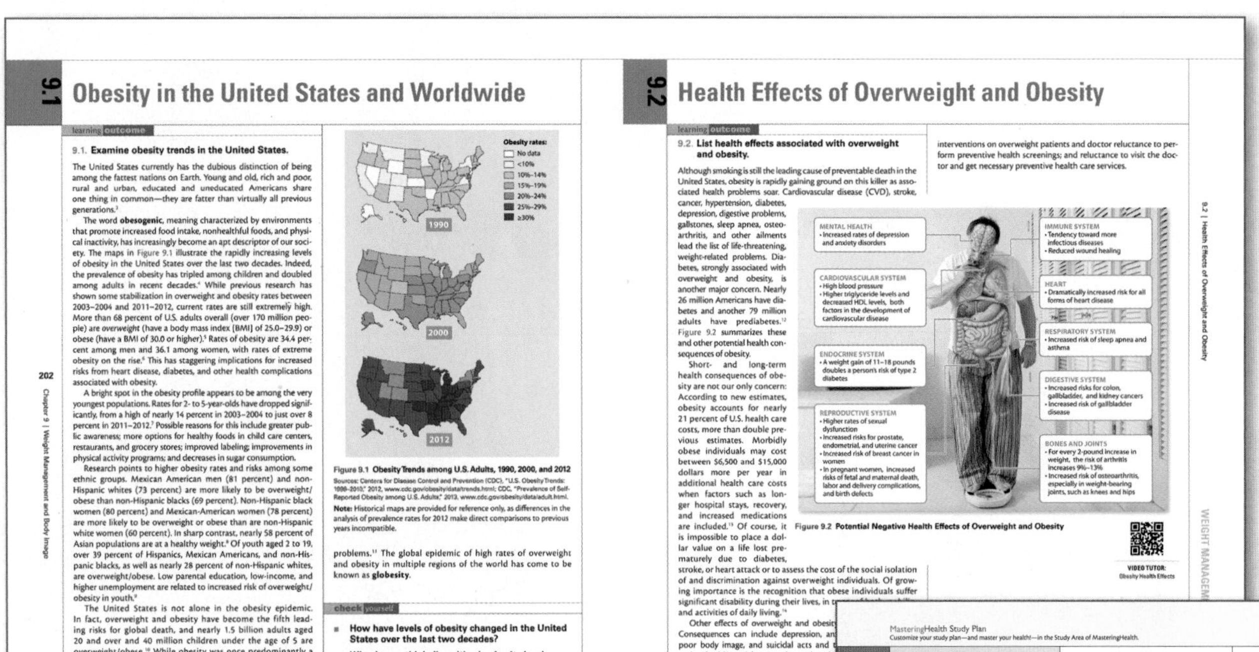

9.1 **Obesity in the United States and Worldwide**

learning outcome

9.1. **Examine obesity trends in the United States.**

Figure 9.1 **Obesity Trends among U.S. Adults, 1990, 2000, and 2012**

check yourself

- **How have levels of obesity changed in the United States over the last two decades?**
- **Why do you think disparities in obesity levels exist among certain populations in the United States?**

9.2 **Health Effects of Overweight and Obesity**

learning outcome

9.2. **List health effects associated with overweight and obesity.**

Figure 9.2 **Potential Negative Health Effects of Overweight and Obesity**

MasteringHealth Study Plan

Summary

Pop Quiz

NEW! Numbered Learning Outcomes and Study Plan

Each module now has a numbered Learning Outcome, giving students a roadmap for their reading. Every chapter concludes with a Study Plan, which summarizes key points of the chapter and provides review questions to check understanding, both tied to the chapter's learning outcomes and assignable in MasteringHealth.

NEW! QR Codes link to Video Tutors

Video tutors highlight a book figure in an engaging video, covering key concepts such as how drugs act on the brain, reading food labels, and the benefits of regular exercise. Using a QR code reader, students can easily access the Video Tutors on their mobile device—just scan the code and the Video Tutor loads instantly.

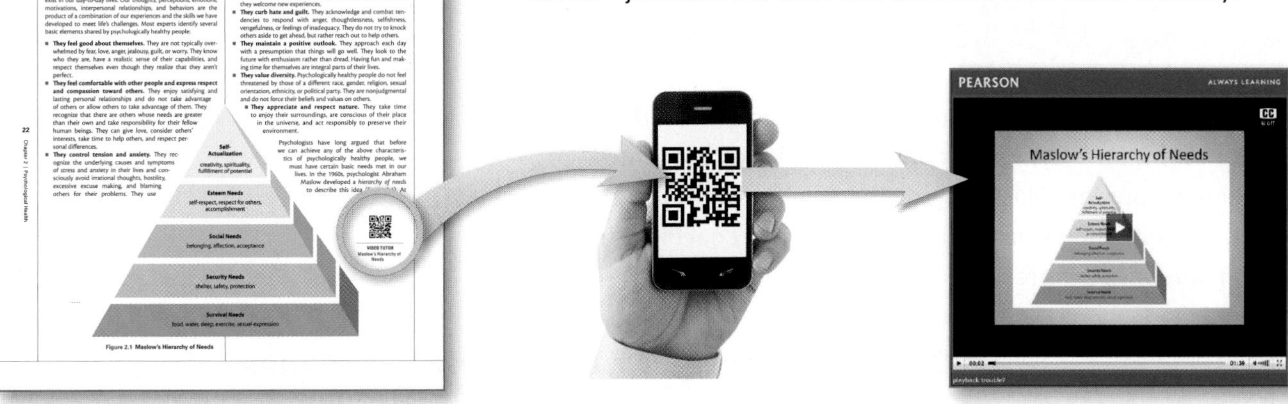

UPDATED! Modular organization for effective student learning

Each health concept is covered in a one-or two-page spread, allowing students to pace their learning. The text flows smoothly from the newly numbered learning outcome to questions without being interrupted by feature boxes or other distractions.

Learning Outcome gives students a clear and specific goal for what they should be able to accomplish after completing the module.

Striking photos and graphics capture student attention.

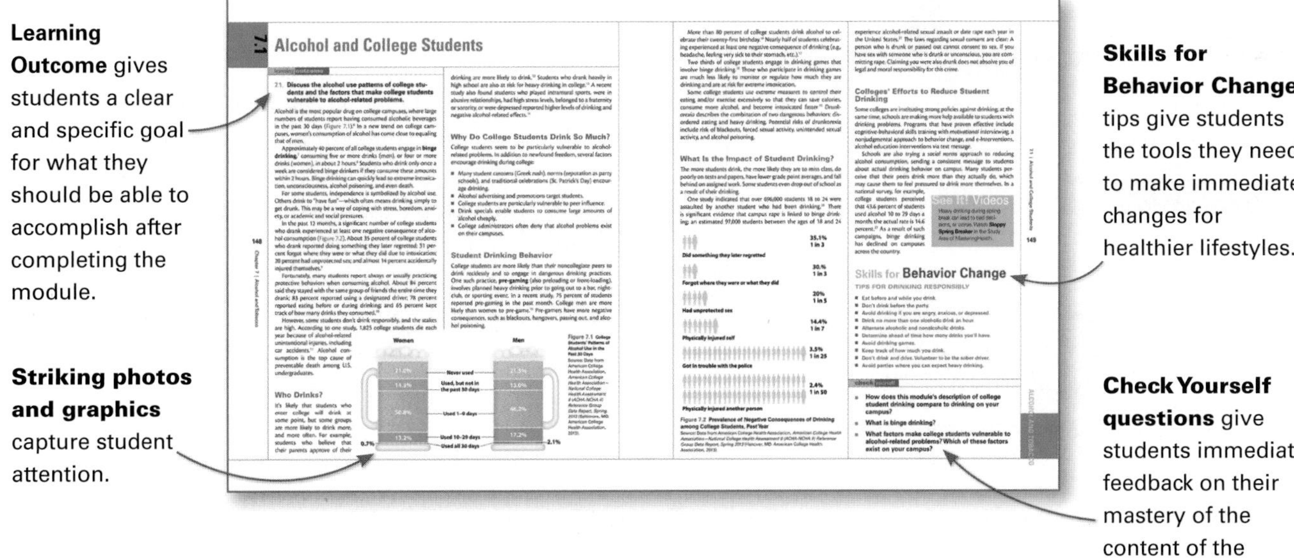

Skills for Behavior Change tips give students the tools they need to make immediate changes for healthier lifestyles.

Check Yourself questions give students immediate feedback on their mastery of the content of the module.

UPDATED! Cutting-edge coverage of hot topics

Current health issues are covered throughout the new edition, speaking to students' questions and concerns. New and updated material covers such areas as mindfulness, gender differences in responses to stress, social media and relationships, spiritual health, the Affordable Care Act, marijuana legalization, functional foods, e-cigarettes, campus violence, environmental health, and more.

Get Your ***Students Going*** with MasteringHealth™ Before, During & After Class

Mastering is the most effective and widely used online homework, tutorial, and assessment system for the sciences and now includes content specifically for health courses. Mastering delivers self-paced tutorials that focus on your course objectives, provides individualized coaching, and responds to each student's progress.

Before Class

Dynamic Study Modules and Pre-Class Assignments provide students with a preview of what's to come.

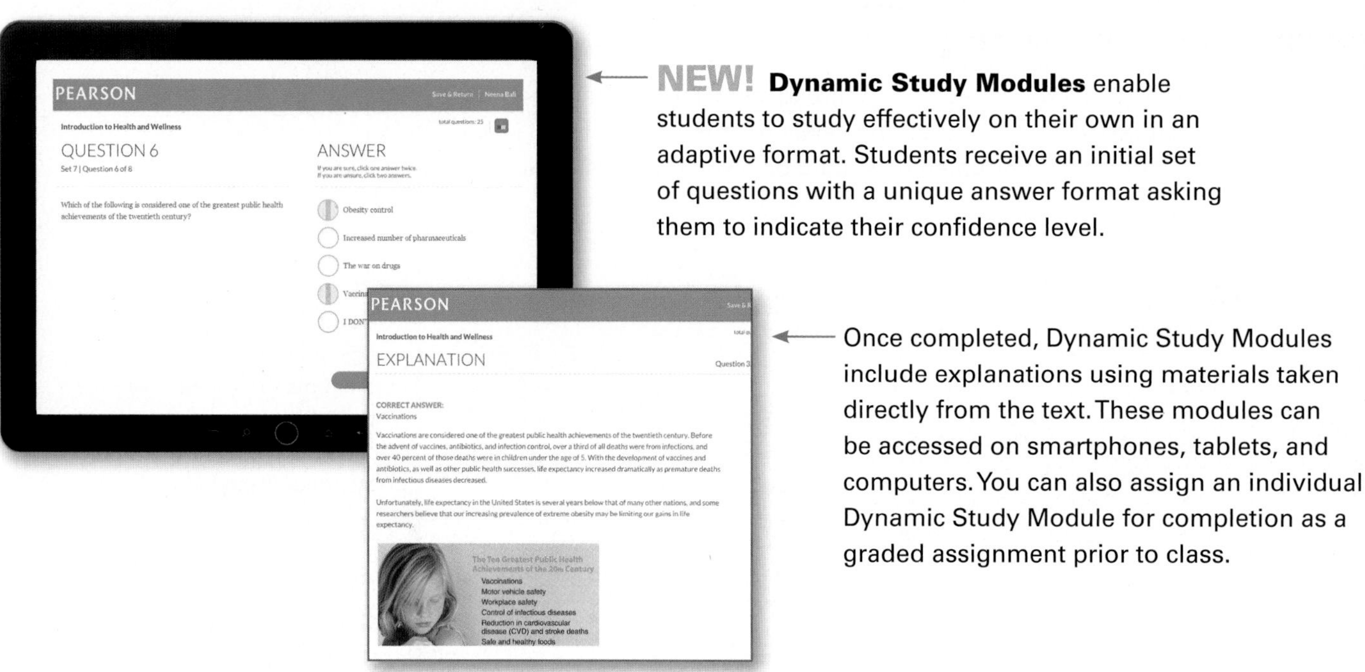

NEW! **Dynamic Study Modules** enable students to study effectively on their own in an adaptive format. Students receive an initial set of questions with a unique answer format asking them to indicate their confidence level.

Once completed, Dynamic Study Modules include explanations using materials taken directly from the text. These modules can be accessed on smartphones, tablets, and computers. You can also assign an individual Dynamic Study Module for completion as a graded assignment prior to class.

MasteringHealth offers Pre-Lecture Quiz Questions that are easy to customize and assign.

NEW! **Reading Questions** ensure that students complete the assigned reading before class and understand the reading material. Reading Questions are 100% mobile ready to give students extra flexibility for study time.

3.1 What Is Stress?

Reading Questions NEW — Chapter 3 Reading Question 1 — [[Bloom's Taxonomy: Knowledge/Comprehension]] (a) A series of mental and physiological res… a real or perceived threat to one's well-being is referred to as ________.

Reading Questions NEW — Chapter 3 Reading Question 2 — [[Bloom's Taxonomy: Knowledge/Comprehension]] (a) Positive stress that presents the opport… is known as ________.

Reading Questions — Chapter 3 Reading Question 3 — [[Bloom's Taxonomy: Application/Analysis]] (a) An example of an event that is likely to be asso…

During Class

Learning Catalytics™ and Engaging Media

What has professors and students so excited? Learning Catalytics, a "bring your own device" student engagement, assessment, and classroom intelligence system, allows students to use their smartphones, tablets, or laptops to respond to questions in class. With Learning Catalytics, you can:

- Assess students in real-time using open-ended question formats to uncover student misconceptions and adjust lectures accordingly.
- Automatically create groups for peer instruction based on student response patterns, to optimize discussion productivity.

My students are so busy and engaged answering Learning Catalytics questions during lecture that they don't have time for Facebook.

Declan De Paor
Old Dominion University

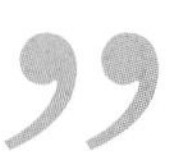

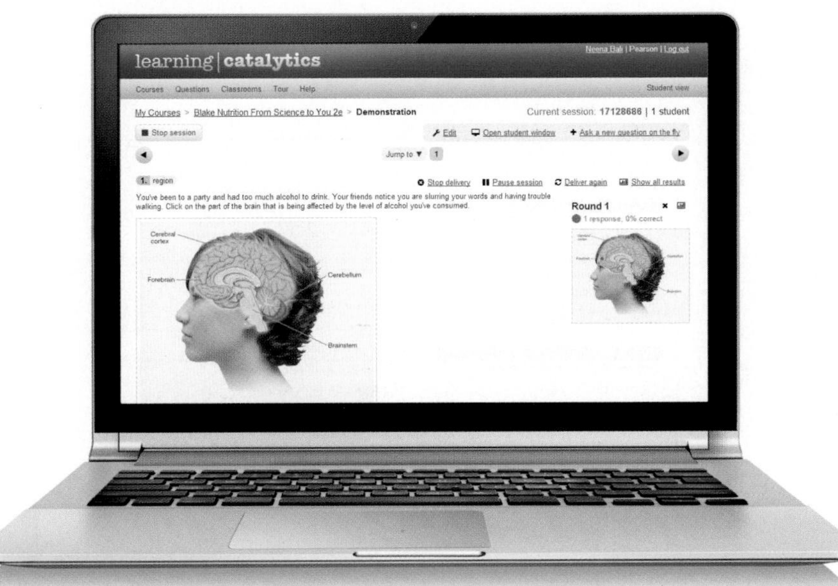

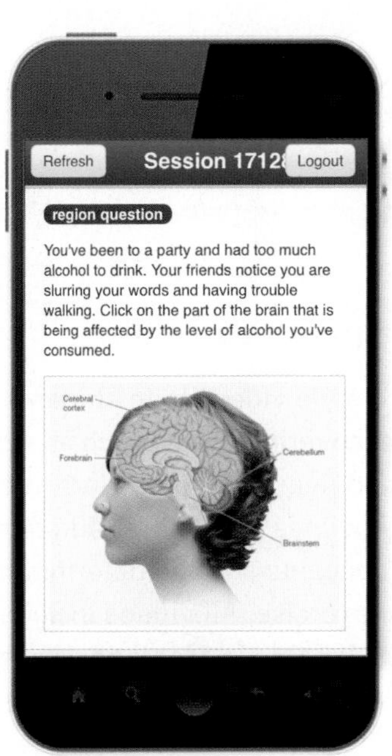

Engaging In-class Media

Instructors can also incorporate dynamic media from the **Teaching Toolkit** DVD into lecture and build class discussions and activities around *ABC News* Lecture Launchers, Video Tutors, and more. For more information, please see the last page of this walkthrough.

MasteringHealth™

After Class

Easy-to-Assign, Customizable, and Automatically Graded Assignments

The breadth and depth of content available to you to assign in MasteringHealth is unparalleled, allowing you to quickly and easily assign homework to reinforce key concepts.

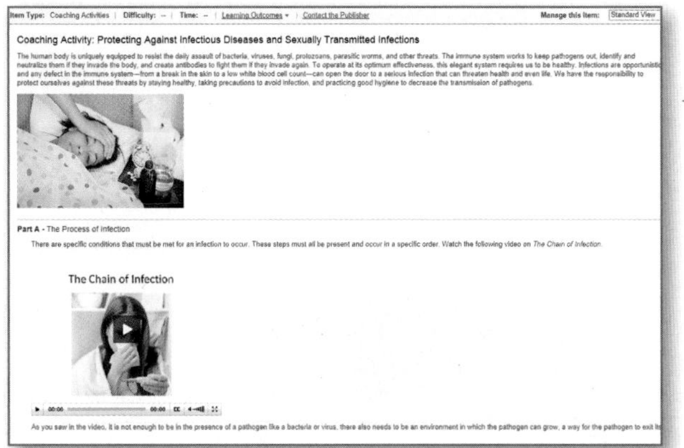

Health and Fitness Coaching Activities

Coaching activities guide students through key health and fitness concepts with interactive mini-lessons that provide hints and feedback.

Behavior Change Videos

Concise whiteboard-style videos help students with the steps of behavior change, covering topics such as setting SMART goals, identifying and overcoming barriers to change, planning realistic timelines, and more. Additional videos review key fitness concepts such as determining target heart rate range for exercise. All videos include assessment activities and are assignable in MasteringHealth.

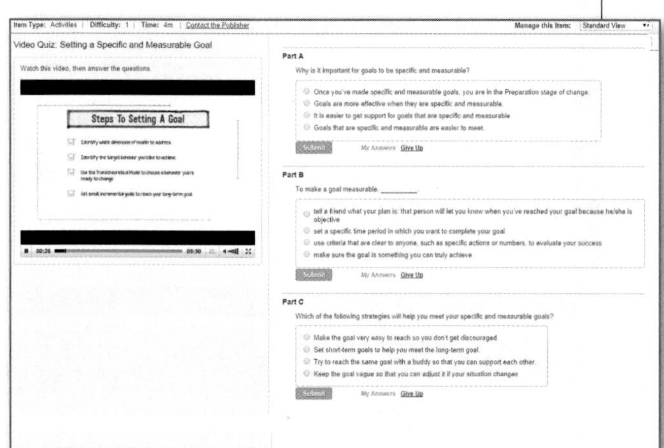

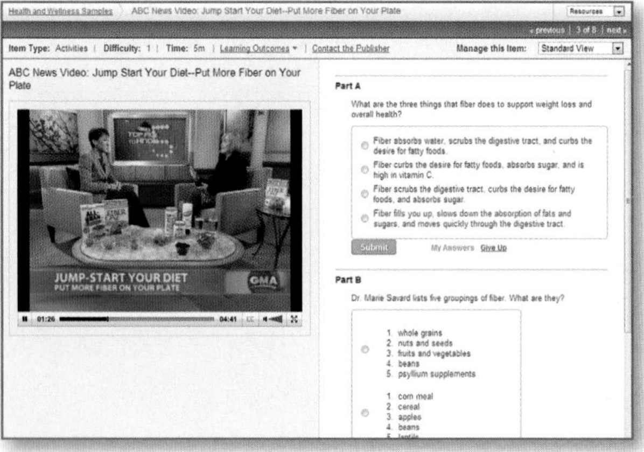

ABC News Videos

51 *ABC News* videos with assessment and feedback help health come to life and show how it's related to the real world.

Other automatically graded health and fitness activities include

- Health Video Tutors
- Chapter Reading Quizzes
- MP3 Tutor Sessions

Self-Assessments from the Text

Do you want your students to write a self-reflection piece on their self-assessment? Or would you like them to complete the self-assessment and have it automatically speak to the gradebook so that students will get credit for these activities? Self-assessments are assignable within MasteringHealth both in PDF format with a self-reflection section and as a multi-part activity.

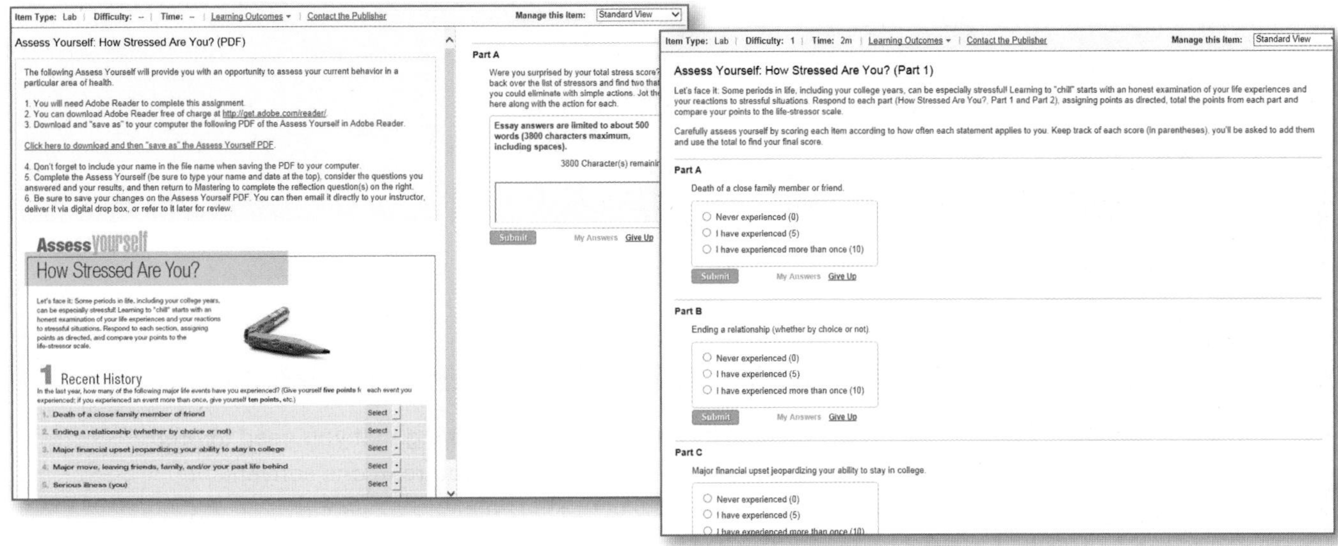

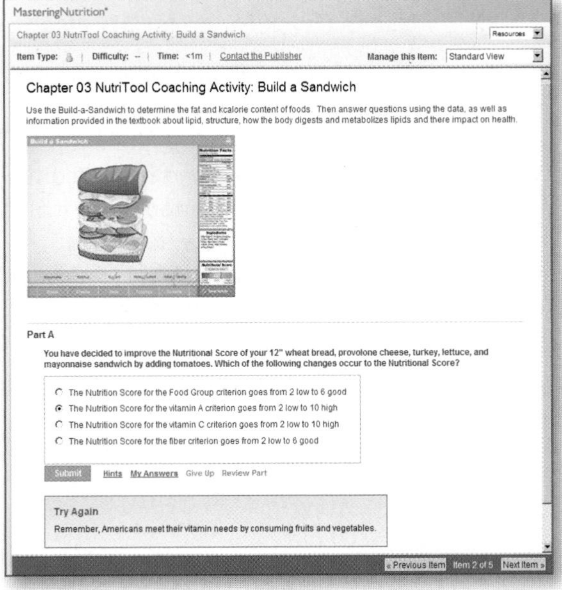

NutriTool Build-A-Meal Activities

These unique activities allow students to combine and experiment with different food options and learn first-hand how to build healthier meals.

Learning Outcomes

All of the MasteringHealth assignable content is tagged to book content and to Bloom's Taxonomy. You also have the ability to add your own outcomes, helping you track student performance against your learning outcomes. You can view class performance against the specified learning outcomes and share those results quickly and easily by exporting to a spreadsheet.

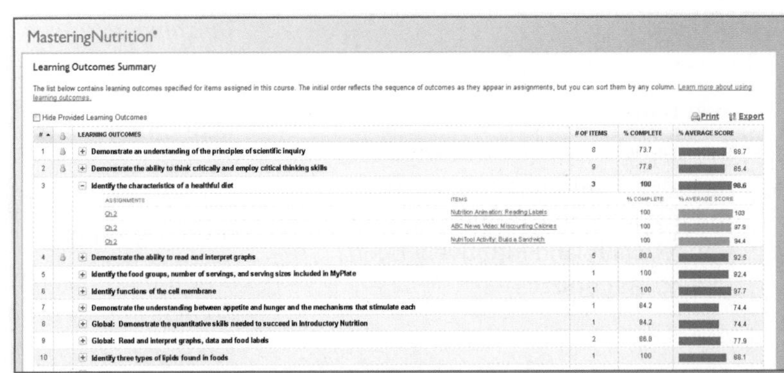

Everything You Need to Teach **In One Place**

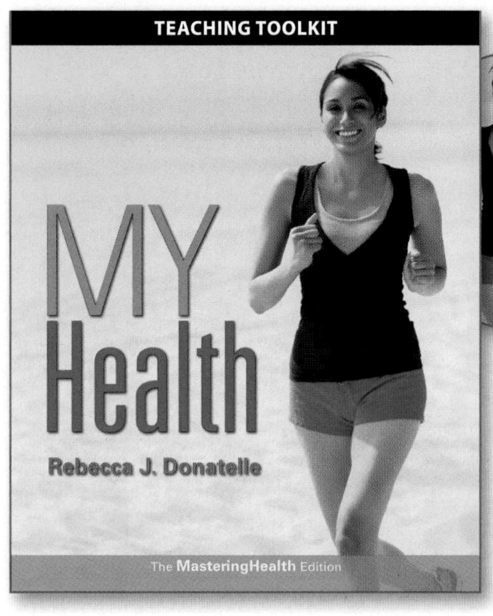

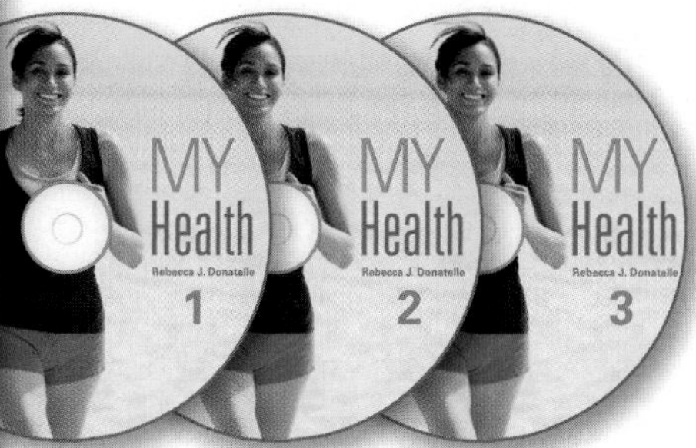

Teaching Toolkit DVD for *My Health*

The Teaching Toolkit DVD provides everything that you need to prep for your course and deliver a dynamic lecture in one convenient place. Included on 3 disks are these valuable resources:

DISK 1

Robust Media Assets for Each Chapter

- *51 ABC News* Lecture Launcher videos
- PowerPoint Lecture Outlines
- PowerPoint clicker questions and Jeopardy-style quiz show questions
- Files for all illustrations and tables and selected photos from the text

DISK 2

Comprehensive Test Bank

- Test Bank in Word and RTF formats
- Computerized Test Bank, which includes all of the questions from the test bank in a format that allows you to easily and intuitively build exams and quizzes

DISK 3

Additional Innovative Supplements for Instructors and Students

For Instructors

- Instructor's Resource Support Manual
- Introduction to MasteringHealth
- Introductory video for Learning Catalytics
- *Teaching with Student Learning Outcomes*
- *Teaching with Web 2.0*

For Students

- Take Charge of Your Health worksheets
- Behavior Change Log Book and Wellness Journal
- *Live Right! Beating Stress in College and Beyond*
- *Eat Right! Healthy Eating in College and Beyond*
- *Food Composition Table*

User's Quick Guide for *My Health*

This easy-to-use printed supplement accompanies the Teaching Toolkit and offers easy instructions for both experienced and new faculty members to get started with rich Toolkit content, how to access assignments within MasteringHealth, and how to "flip" the classroom with Learning Catalytics.

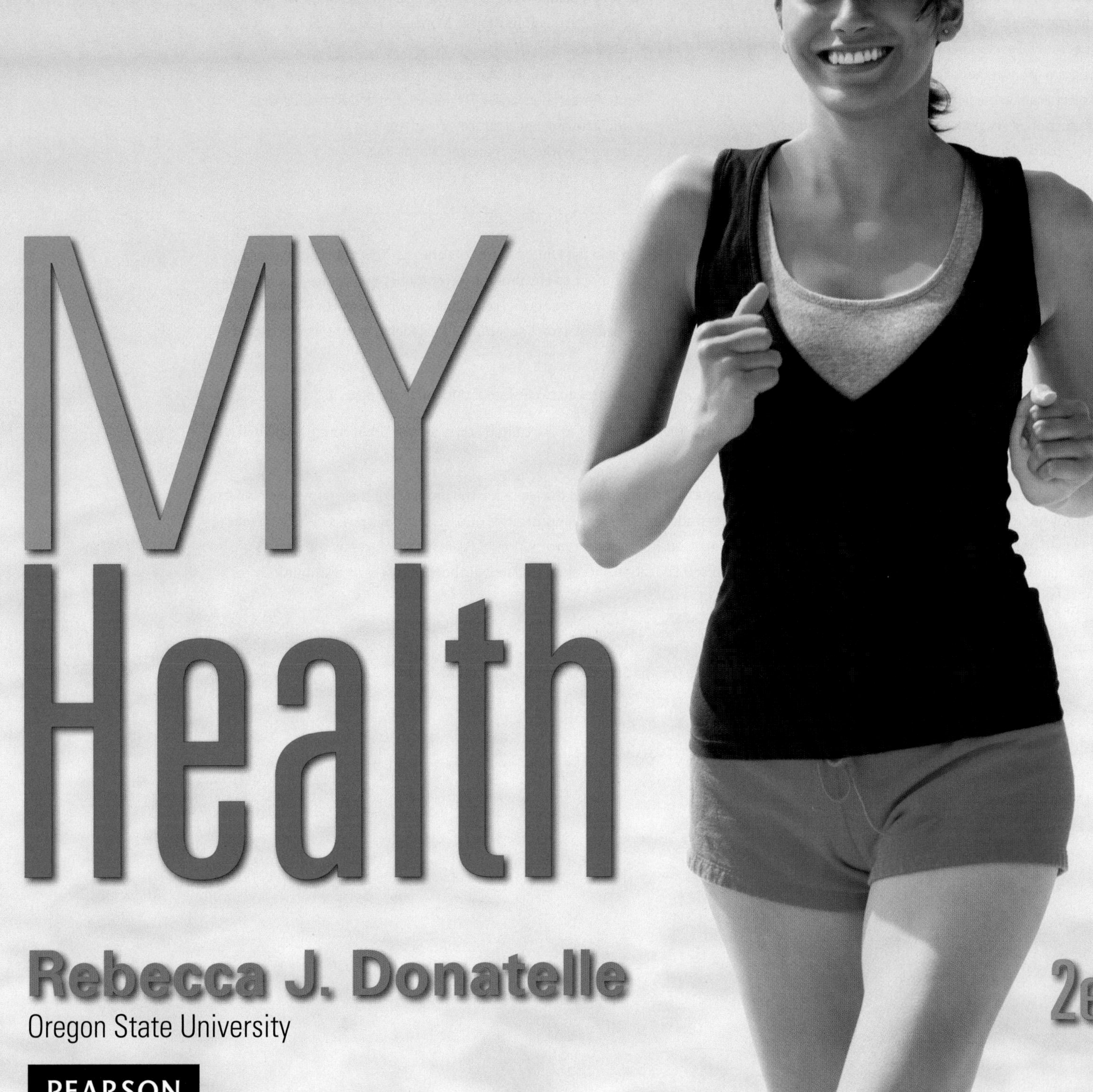

MY Health

Rebecca J. Donatelle
Oregon State University

2e

PEARSON

The **Mastering Health** Edition

Senior Acquisitions Editor: Michelle Cadden
Project Manager: Jessica Picone
Program Manager: Susan Malloy
Development Editor: Erin Schnair
Editorial Assistant: Leah Sherwood
Director of Development: Barbara Yien
Program Management Team Lead: Mike Early
Project Management Team Lead: Nancy Tabor
Production Management: Thistle Hill Publishing Services
Copy Editor: Jane Loftus
Compositor: Cenveo® Publisher Services
Cover and Interior Designer: Mark Ong
Illustrators: Precision Graphics
Rights & Permissions Project Manager–Image: Maya Gomez
Rights & Permissions Project Manager–Text: William Opaluch
Rights & Permissions Management: Rachel Youdelman
Photo Researcher: Jamey O'Quinn, Lumina Datamatics, Inc.
Manufacturing Buyer: Stacey Weinberger
Executive Marketing Manager: Neena Bali

Cover Photo Credit: Tetra Images/Corbis

Library of Congress Cataloging-in-Publication Data

Donatelle, Rebecca J., 1950–
My health : the masteringhealth edition / Rebecca J. Donatelle, Oregon State University. — Second edition.
pages cm
Includes bibliographical references and index.
ISBN 978-0-13-386564-6 — ISBN 0-13-386564-9
1. Health. 2. Health behavior. 3. Diseases—Prevention. I. Title.
RA776.D6635 2016
613—dc23

2014042092

ISBN 10: **0-13-386564-9**; ISBN 13: **978-0-13-386564-6** (Student Edition)
ISBN 10: **0-13-398079-0**; ISBN 13: **978-0-13-398079-0** (Instructor's Review Copy)

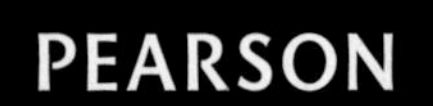

www.pearsonhighered.com

2 3 4 5 6 7 8 9 10—**V011**—18 17 16 15

About the Author

Rebecca J. Donatelle, Ph.D.

Oregon State University

Rebecca Donatelle has served as a faculty member in the Department of Public Health, College of Health and Human Sciences, at Oregon State University for the last two decades. In that role, she has chaired the department and been program coordinator for the Health Promotion and Health Behavior Program (bachelor's degree, master of public health, and Ph.D. degree programs), as well as served on over 50 national, state, regional, and university committees focused on improving student academic success and improving the public's health. Most importantly to her, she has also taught and mentored thousands of undergraduate and graduate students. She is proud of the many outstanding accomplishments of her students! Many of these students gained community-based intervention and research skills while working on Dr. Donatelle's funded projects, and those experiences have led to exciting career paths nationally and internationally. Others have gone on to receive advanced degrees in public health and have assumed leadership roles in a wide range of academic, community, and health care system positions. "I believe that my successes are measured in large part by the successes of the students I have worked with and their contributions to the improved health of others," says Donatelle.

Dr. Donatelle has a Ph.D. in community health/health promotion and health education, with specializations in health behaviors, aging, and chronic disease prevention, from the University of Oregon; a master of science degree in health education from the University of Wisconsin, La Crosse; and a bachelor of science degree from the University of Wisconsin, La Crosse, with majors in health/physical education and English. In recent years, Dr. Donatelle has received several professional awards for leadership, teaching, and service within the university and for her work on developing nationally ranked undergraduate and graduate programs in the health promotion/health behavior areas.

Her primary research and scholarship areas have focused on finding scientifically appropriate means of motivating behavior change among resistant populations. Specifically, her work uses incentives, social and community supports, and risk communication strategies in motivating diverse populations to change their risk behaviors. She has worked with pregnant women who smoke in an effort to motivate them to quit smoking, obese women of all ages who are at risk for cardiovascular disease and diabetes, prediabetic women at risk for progression to type 2 diabetes, and a wide range of other health issues and problems. Earlier research projects have focused on decision making and factors influencing the use of alternative and traditional health care providers for treatment of low back pain, illness and sick role behaviors, occupational stress and stress claims, and worksite health promotion.

Brief Contents

Contents

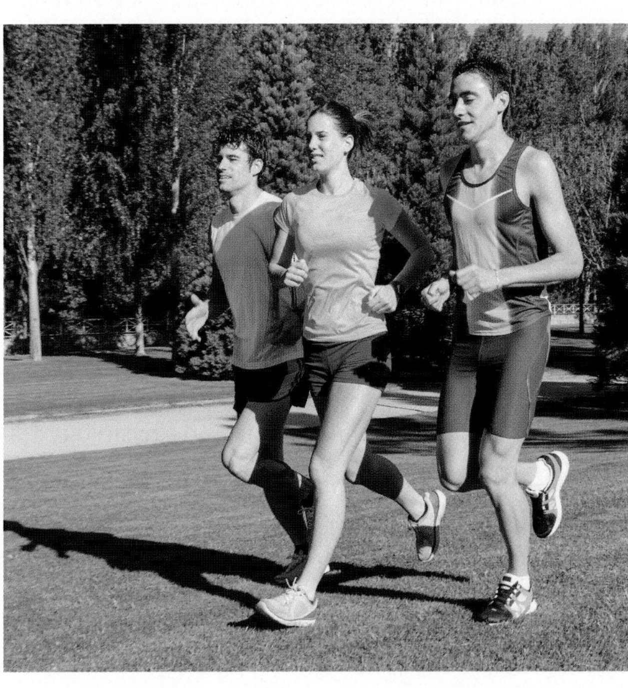

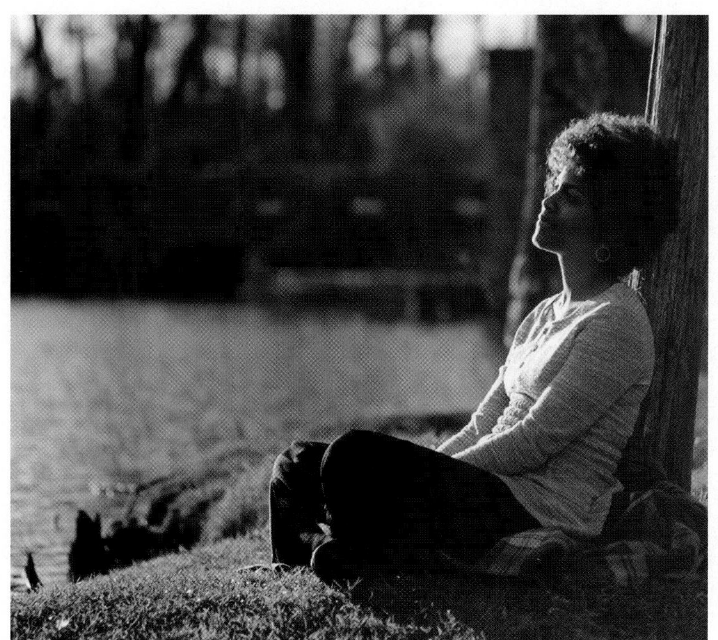

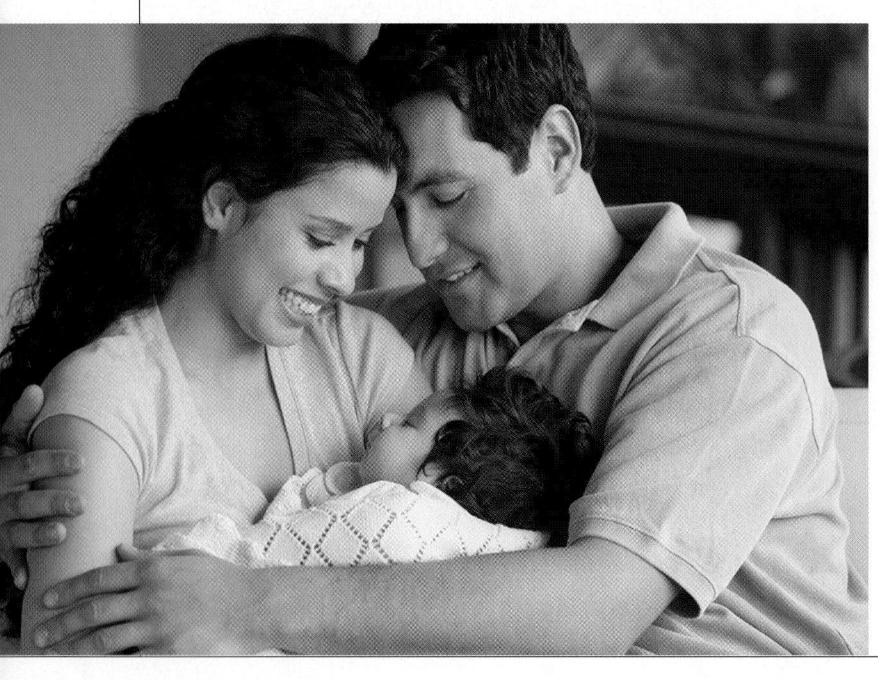

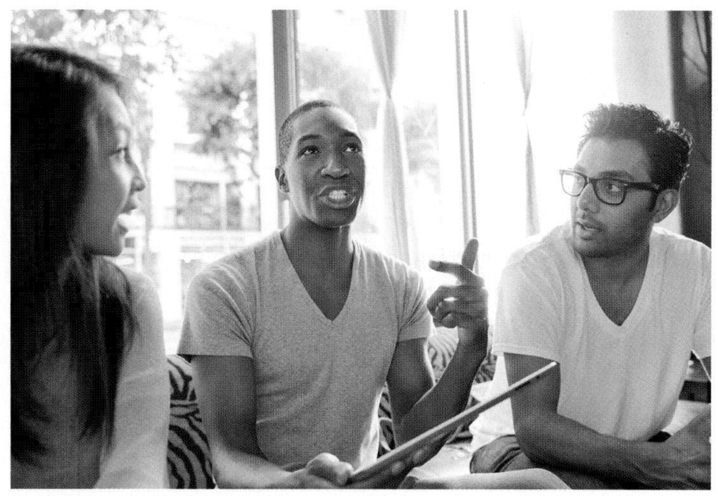

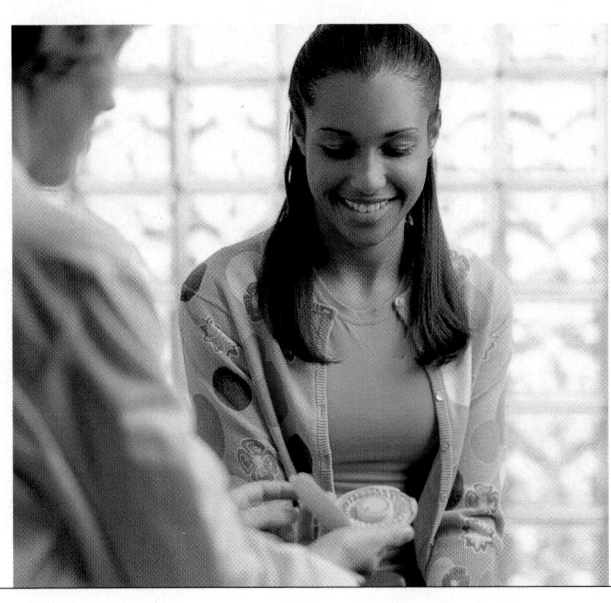

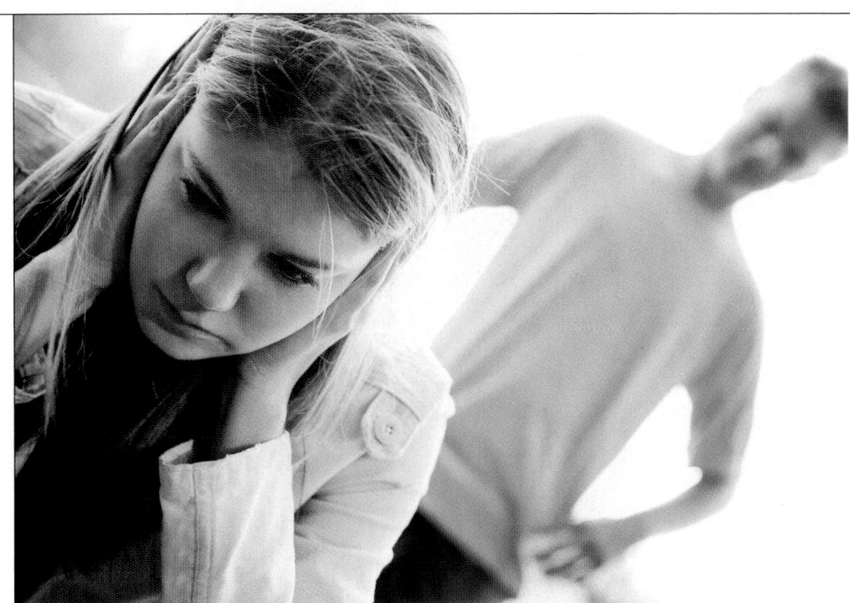

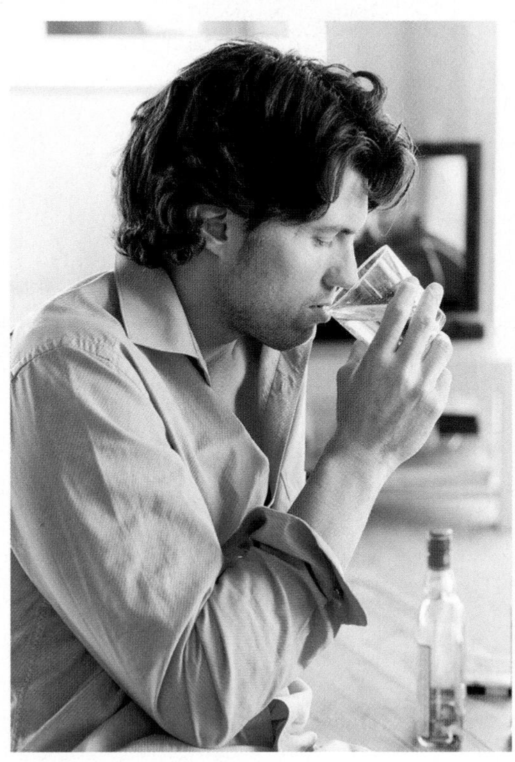

7 Alcohol and Tobacco 147

8 Nutrition 173

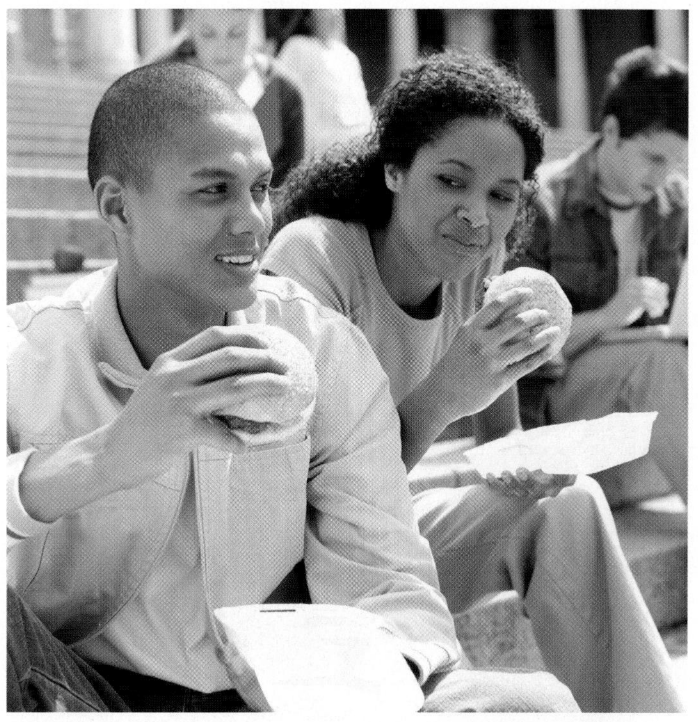

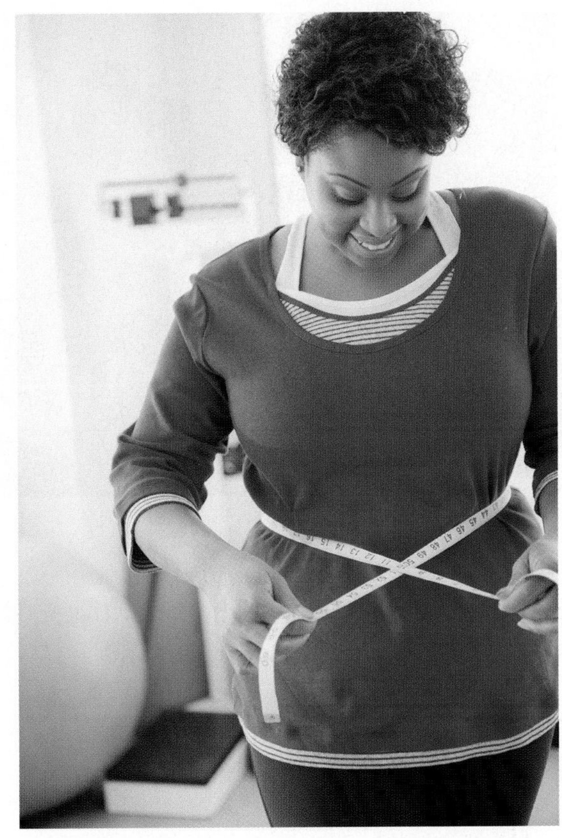

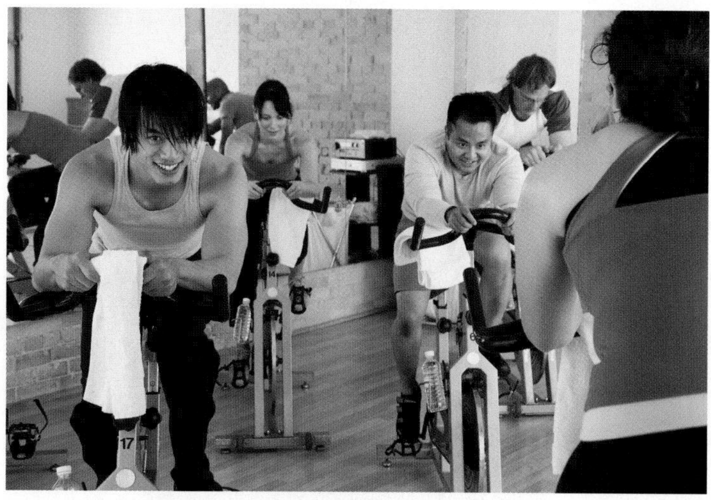

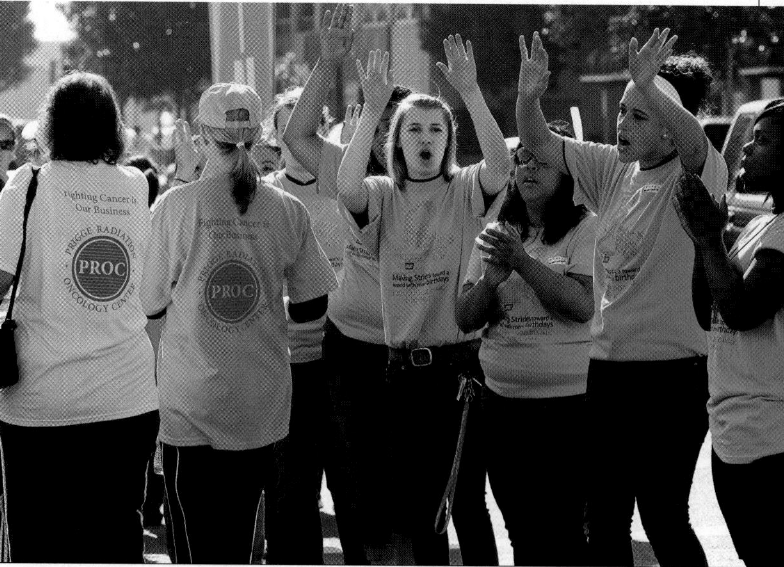

PROC

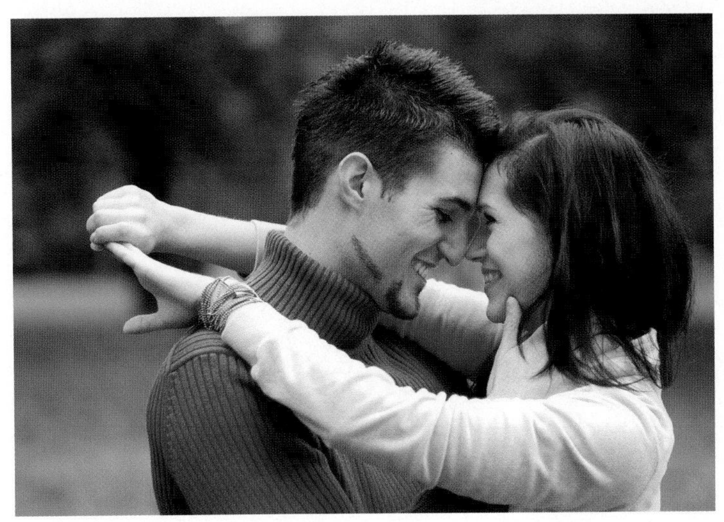

STAY
ALERT

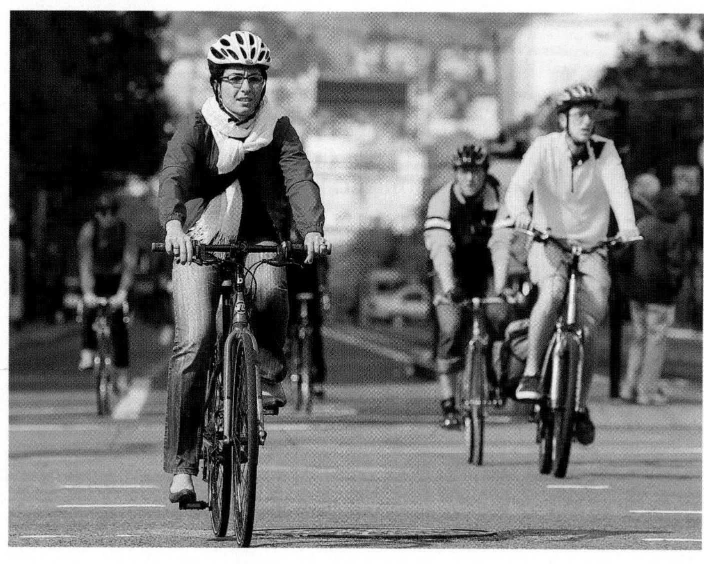

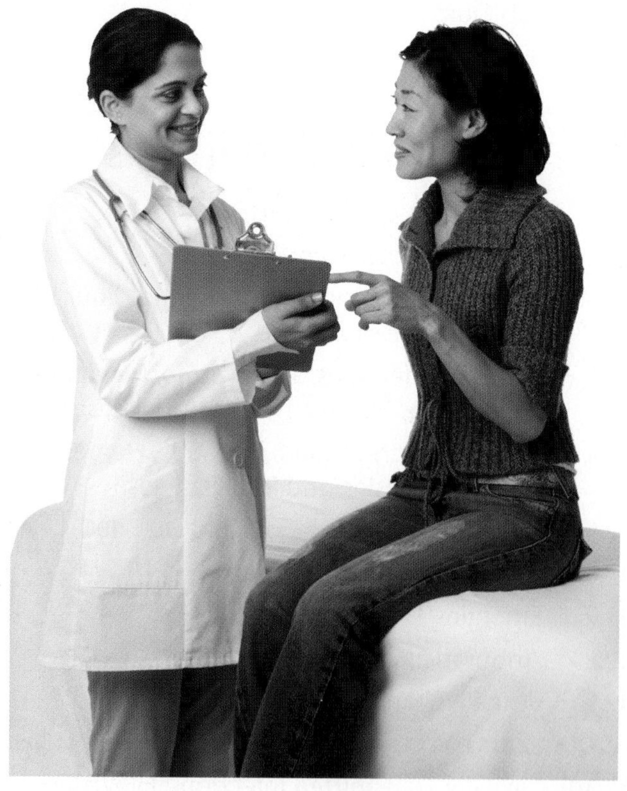

Preface

For students today, health is headline news. Whether it's the latest cases of life-threatening *E. coli* infections from eating infected produce, a deadly Ebola epidemic threatening to kill millions, a new environmental catastrophe brought on by global warming, or increasing rates of obesity and diabetes, the issues often seem overwhelming. However, although many things that influence our health are beyond our control, we are lucky that we do have control over many of the health risks we face. Health is multifaceted, and achieving it is a personal and societal responsibility.

As I have taught personal health courses over the past two decades, I have seen changes in students, especially regarding their health, their health concerns, and the way they assimilate information and make decisions about their health and the health of those around them. A new mode of instruction and a new approach to learning is required for instructors and textbook authors to present and relay scientifically valid information, create learning environments that meet diverse needs, and motivate students to engage in their own learning experiences. Students today want their information to be organized and concise. They want to know what they should be learning, see the relevance in knowing the information so that they can apply it to real world situations, and be able to test themselves to confirm that they understand the material. What's more, students and their instructors want to be able to demonstrate that they know more about their health, see things with a more critical eye, and have options for making changes to improve their health and the health of others as a result of a particular course or course sequence. When they want to delve more deeply into a given topic, they will have the skills and resources to get more information. For these reasons and more, I decided that the time had come to bring to fruition a new textbook that would change the health text marketplace. I decided to tap the creative minds of my colleagues and students and work with a great publishing company in writing *My Health: The MasteringHealth Edition*.

Key Features of This Text

My Health: The MasteringHealth Edition maintains many features that this text is known for, including the following:

- **The modular organization,** which presents information in one- and two-page spreads, helping students to pace their learning and highlighting the most essential, up-to-date information about each topic in a synthesized, easy-to-understand format.
- **Student learning outcomes**, which give instructors and students a measurable goal for each module and are matched specifically to the content in each module in the text. These take the guesswork out of the question that students inevitably ask: "What do I need to know for this exam or this performance outcome?"
- **Check Yourself questions** to help students confirm that they have mastered the content of each module.
- **Assess Yourself modules**, which provide opportunities for students to assess their current behaviors, with at least one Assess Yourself at the end of every chapter.
- **Skills for Behavior Change boxes**, which are featured in many modules and are designed to help students develop the skills necessary to use what they have learned in making practical and important improvements in their health behaviors.
- **Striking figures and photos** on every page to engage students and encourage learning.
- **A streamlined approach**, with feature-box material integrated into the text so that students can follow the narrative without interruptions, quickly navigate through the material, and apply what they have learned.

Student learning outcomes are a critical part of this book. Learning outcomes are a powerful tool to set clear expectations for students and to assess their level of mastery of a subject area. Outcomes for this text were developed based on foundational personal health content appropriate for college level learners. These outcomes were then revised and edited based on careful review and input from health instructors and other experts from representative colleges and universities throughout the country (their names are listed later in the Acknowledgments section). Each module has a specific outcome that students must try to achieve to be successful. This mastery approach helps students hone in on the relevant information and focus attention on achieving this learning outcome.

At the end of each module, students are challenged by Check Yourself questions. If students can successfully answer these questions, then they are ready to move on to the next module. If they have difficulty answering the questions, they are able to go back through the material and focus on key points until they have mastered the module content.

We know that students are often pressed for time and may only be able to read through a few pages of this book in one sitting. With the learning outcomes and the Check Yourself questions, students can learn the material in one or two modules, test themselves, and know that they have accomplished a measurable portion of their reading goal, even if they can only complete part of a reading assignment.

In addition to the modular organization, learning outcomes, and Check Yourself questions, you will notice Skills for Behavior Change boxes throughout the chapters. Using the skills learned from these boxes, students can engage in behaviors that will contribute to improved health. You will also see that these are the only feature boxes in the text. In order to keep the book streamlined and focused on essential points, the type of information that traditionally has been relegated to a feature box has been included in the text, if it is important for student understanding, or it has been omitted. I hope that you will agree that this provides students with a clear, concise presentation of the most important health information.

New to This Edition

Video Tutors

Video tutors highlight a book figure in an engaging video, covering key concepts such as how drugs act on the brain, reading food labels, and the benefits of regular exercise. Using a QR code reader, students can easily access the Video Tutors on their mobile device—just scan the code and the Video Tutor loads instantly.

Study Plan

Each module now has a numbered Learning Outcome, giving students a road map for their reading. Each chapter concludes with a Study Plan, which summarizes key points of the chapter and provides review questions to check understanding, both tied to the chapter's learning outcomes.

Chapter-by-Chapter Revisions

My Health: The MasteringHealth Edition has been thoroughly updated to reflect the most cutting-edge, scientifically valid, and relevant information available and includes additional references that will allow students to glean additional information from key sources in the area. Portions of modules have been reorganized to improve the flow of topics, while figures, tables, and photos have all been added, improved on, and updated. The following is a chapter-by-chapter listing of some of the most noteworthy changes, updates, and additions.

Chapter 1: Healthy Change

- Reorganized section on *Healthy People 2020*, including adding description of leading health indicators
- New coverage of the Affordable Care Act (ACA)

Chapter 2: Psychological Health

- New Skills for Behavior Change box on relationships
- New module on the importance of spiritual health
- New Assess Yourself on spiritual health
- Added coverage of Seligman's happiness theory (PERMA)

Chapter 3: Stress

- Increased coverage of mindfulness
- New section on happiness and flourishing
- New section named "Men and Women Respond to Stress Differently"
- New section on shift and persist

Chapter 4: Relationships and Sexuality

- New module on relationships and social media
- New module on using technology responsibly

Chapter 5: Reproductive Choices

- New section on abortions in the developing world
- New section on contingency planning for parents
- Expanded coverage of nutrition and exercise in prenatal care

Chapter 6: Addiction and Drug Abuse

- New figure on college students who use drugs and employment rates
- New information about medicinal and legal marijuana
- New content on harm reduction strategies

Chapter 7: Alcohol and Tobacco

- New content on e-cigarettes
- New content on different ethnicities and alcoholism

Chapter 8: Nutrition

- New module on the health benefits of functional foods
- New content on the Dietary Reference Intakes (DRIs)

Chapter 9: Weight Management and Body Image

- New Skills for Behavior Change box on portion distortion
- New figure showing an overview of methods to measure body composition
- Expanded coverage of treatment of anorexia and bulimia
- New table on popular diet programs

Chapter 10: Fitness

- Expanded coverage of SMART fitness goals and objectives
- New coverage of physical inactivity
- New coverage of alcohol and exercise

Chapter 11: CVD, Cancer, and Diabetes

- New table on the signs of a heart attack in men and women
- New Skills for Behavior Change box on recognizing the signs of a stroke
- Increased coverage on diabetes prevalence rates and risks
- New Skills for Behavior Change box on reducing your risk for diabetes
- New module on diabetes diagnosis and treatment

Chapter 12: Infectious Conditions

- New cold and flu module
- New sections on mumps, measles, and rubella
- Expanded discussion of other pathogens

Chapter 13: Violence and Unintentional Injuries

- New section on rape on U.S. campuses and government policies on violence
- New section on coping in the event of campus violence
- Added new statistics and information related to texting and driving

Chapter 14: Environmental Health

- Updated coverage of climate change
- New section on fracking
- New information on sustainable ways to use consumer electronics
- Expanded coverage related to green cities and campuses

Chapter 15: Consumerism and Complementary and Alternative Medicine

- New table on common nonherbal supplements
- New figure on where our health care dollars are spent

Supplementary Materials

Available with *My Health: The MasteringHealth Edition* is a comprehensive set of ancillary materials designed to enhance learning and to facilitate teaching.

Instructor Supplements

- **MasteringHealth.** MasteringHealth coaches students through the toughest health topics. Instructors can assign engaging tools to help students visualize, practice, and understand crucial content, from the basics of health to the fundamentals of behavior change. **Coaching Activities** guide students through key health concepts with interactive mini-lessons, complete with hints and wrong-answer feedback. **Reading Quizzes** (20 questions per chapter) ensure students have completed the assigned reading before class. ***ABC News* Videos** stimulate classroom discussions and include multiple-choice questions with feedback for students. **NutriTools Coaching Activities** in the nutrition chapter allow students to combine and experiment with different food options and learn firsthand how to build healthier meals. **MP3s** relate to chapter content and come with multiple-choice questions that provide wrong-answer feedback. **Learning Catalytics** provides open-ended questions students can answer in real time. Through targeted assessments, Learning Catalytics helps students develop the critical-thinking skills they need for lasting behavior change.
- **Teaching Toolkit DVD.** The Teaching Toolkit DVD includes everything instructors need to prepare for their course and deliver a dynamic lecture in one convenient place. Resources include the following: *ABC News* videos, Video Tutor videos, clicker questions, Quiz Show questions, PowerPoint lecture outlines, all figures and tables from the text, PDFs and Microsoft Word files of the *Instructor Resource and Support Manual* and the Test Bank, the Computerized Test Bank, the User's Quick Guide, *Teaching with Student Learning Outcomes, Teaching with Web 2.0, Behavior Change Log Book and Wellness Journal, Eat Right!, Live Right!,* and *Take Charge of Your Health* worksheets.
- ***ABC News* Videos** and **Video Tutors.** Fifty-one new *ABC News* videos, each 5 to 10 minutes long, and 22 brand-new brief videos accessible via QR codes in the text help instructors stimulate critical discussion in the classroom. Videos are provided already linked within PowerPoint lectures and are also available separately in large-screen format with optional closed captioning on the Teaching Toolkit DVD and through MasteringHealth.
- ***Instructor Resource and Support Manual.*** This teaching tool provides chapter summaries and outlines of each chapter. It includes information on available PowerPoint lectures, integrated *ABC News* video discussion questions, tips and strategies for managing large classrooms, ideas for in-class activities, and suggestions for integrating MasteringHealth and MyDietAnalysis into your classroom activities and homework assignments.
- **Test Bank.** The Test Bank incorporates Bloom's Taxonomy, or the higher order of learning, to help instructors create exams that encourage students to think analytically and critically, rather than simply to regurgitate information. Test Bank questions are tagged to global and book-specific student learning outcomes.
- **User's Quick Guide.** Newly redesigned to be even more useful, this valuable supplement acts as your road map to the Teaching Toolkit DVD.
- ***Teaching with Student Learning Outcomes.*** This publication contains essays from 11 instructors who are teaching using student learning outcomes. They share their goals in using outcomes and the processes that they follow to develop and refine them, and they provide many useful suggestions and examples for successfully incorporating outcomes into a personal health course.
- ***Teaching with Web 2.0.*** From Facebook to Twitter to blogs, students are using and interacting with Web 2.0 technologies. This handbook provides an introduction to these popular online tools and offers ideas for incorporating them into your personal health course. Written by personal health and health education instructors, each chapter examines the basics about each technology and ways to make it work for you and your students.
- ***Behavior Change Log Book and Wellness Journal.*** This assessment tool helps students track daily exercise and nutritional intake and create a long-term nutritional and fitness prescription plan. It also includes a Behavior Change Contract and topics for journal-based activities.

Student Supplements

- **The Study Area of MasteringHealth** is organized by learning areas. *Read It* houses the Pearson eText 2.0, with which users can create notes, highlight text in different colors, create bookmarks, zoom, click hyperlinked words for definitions, and change page view. Pearson eText 2.0 also links to associated media files. *See It* includes 51 *ABC News* videos on important health topics and the key concepts of each chapter. *Hear It* contains MP3 Study Tutor files and audio case studies. *Do It* contains critical-thinking questions and Web links. *Review It* contains study quizzes for each chapter. *Live It* helps jump-start students' behavior-change projects with assessments and resources to plan change; students can fill out a Behavior Change Contract, journal and log behaviors, and prepare a reflection piece.
- ***Behavior Change Log Book and Wellness Journal.*** This assessment tool helps students track daily exercise and nutritional intake and create a long-term nutrition and fitness prescription plan. It includes Behavior Change Contracts and topics for journal-based activities.
- ***Eat Right! Healthy Eating in College and Beyond.*** This booklet provides students with practical nutrition guidelines, shopper's guides, and recipes.

- ***Live Right! Beating Stress in College and Beyond.*** This booklet gives students useful tips for coping with stressful life challenges both during college and for the rest of their lives.
- **Digital 5-Step Pedometer** Take strides to better health with this pedometer, which measures steps, distance (miles), activity time, and calories, and provides a time clock.
- **MyDietAnalysis** (www.mydietanalysis.com). Powered by ESHA Research, Inc., MyDietAnalysis features a database of nearly 20,000 foods and multiple reports. It allows students to track their diet and activity using up to three profiles and to generate and submit reports electronically.

Flexible Options

My Health: The MasteringHealth Edition is also available in alternate print and electronic versions:

- **CourseSmart eTextbooks** are an exciting new choice for students looking to save money. As an alternative to purchasing the print textbook, students can subscribe to the same content online and save 40% off the suggested list price of the print text. Access the CourseSmart eText at www.coursesmart.com.
- **Books a la Carte** offers the exact same content as *My Health: The MasteringHealth Edition* in a convenient, three-hole-punched, loose-leaf version. Books a la Carte offers a great value for your students—this format costs 35% less than a new textbook!
- Creating a customized version of the book from the **Pearson Custom Library**, with only the chapters that you select, is also possible. Contact your Pearson sales representative for more details.

A Note on the Text

From my earliest years of college instruction, I have believed that in order to motivate students to focus on their health, they needed to understand the complex health world that people live in, to appreciate how the macroenvironment and culture influence health decision making, and to understand that there is no "best" recipe for health. Helping students access the best information available and motivating them to ask the right questions and be thoughtful in their analysis of issues, as well as mindful in their approach to healthy change, has been a part of my overall approach to teaching, learning, and writing.

Today's students have been raised on a steady dose of health information, some of which sounds good, but may be highly questionable in terms of accuracy. Helping them sift through the changing sands of health information, examine their own risks, and make positive changes that affect them, their loved ones, and others in the community is key to improving health. Writing a text such as this one has helped keep me current in my teaching and tuned in to the needs of twenty-first-century students and those who teach classes such as this one. This text, focused on a more technology-based, interactive, and challenging approach to learning, cuts to the chase in delivering essential information and thought-provoking questions. Consistent with an ever-evolving and "information at your fingertips" approach, this format is designed to help students navigate the seemingly endless world of health and bring it to life in a colorful and fresh format. In keeping with the times, this text is a "work in continual progress," and it will benefit greatly from your feedback and suggestions. As an author, I'd love to hear from you!

Acknowledgments

Writing and developing a textbook is truly a team effort. Each step along the way in planning, developing, and translating critical health information to students and instructors requires a tremendous amount of work from many dedicated professionals, including contributors who are at the top of their games in their knowledge of health science and behaviors and publishing professionals who personify all that is the absolute "best" in terms of qualities an author looks for in bringing a text to fruition. I cannot help but think how fortunate I have been to work with the gifted contributors to this text and the extraordinary publishing professionals at Pearson. Through time constraints, exhaustive searches for cutting-edge background research, and the writing process, these contributors were outstanding.

From painstaking efforts in development, design, editing, and editorial decision making to highly skilled marketing and dedicated sales efforts, the Pearson group handled every detail, every obstacle with patience, professionalism, and painstaking attention to detail. From this author's perspective, these personnel personify key aspects of what it takes to be successful in the publishing world: (1) drive and motivation; (2) commitment to excellence; (3) fantastic job and performance skills; (4) a vibrant, youthful, forward-thinking and enthusiastic approach; and (5) personalities that motivate an author to continually strive to produce market-leading texts. I have been amazed at the way that this team continually works to be well ahead of the curve in terms of cutting-edge information. Asking "what do students need to know" and "what will help instructors and students thrive in today's high-pressure academic settings" was at the heart of our efforts. I am deeply indebted to everyone who has played a role in making this book come alive for students and get into the hands of instructors.

In particular, credit goes to my development editor for this edition, Erin Schnair, who worked with Susan Malloy and Jessica Picone in painstakingly merging and synthesizing content and provided additional insight and expertise in making this new edition accessible to students. Erin did an extraordinary job of streamlining and revising material to fit within the constraints of the modular outline, while retaining accuracy and readability. Without her, this book would not exist—thank you!

Further praise and thanks go to the highly skilled and hardworking executive editor Sandra Lindelof, who was responsible for the conceptualization of this text and helped spearhead its initial development in the marketplace, doing the necessary work to procure the cutting-edge technology and skilled professionals that were key to its success. Her successor, Michelle Cadden, quickly took charge of the list after Sandy's departure and worked closely with Susan and Jessica to ensure that this text provided the necessary framework to meet the needs of an increasingly demanding group of instructors and students.

Although these women were key contributors to the finished work, there were many other people who worked on *My Health: The MasteringHealth Edition*. Thanks go to Angela Urquhart and Andrea Archer at Thistle Hill Publishing Services, who reliably kept us on track with flexibility and dedication. Design director Mark Ong refreshed the visually impactful design while keeping students and instructors in mind. We could not have created this book without his creativity and dedication. Mark also created the remarkable cover, which we feel perfectly conveys the unique qualities of the text. Denise Wright of Southern Editorial gets major kudos for overseeing the supplements package. Director of Media Development Laura Tommasi put together an innovative and comprehensive set of assets for *My Health: The MasteringHealth Edition*. Additional thanks go to the rest of the team at Pearson, especially Editorial Assistant Leah Sherwood, Program Manager Team Lead Mike Early, Project Manager Team Lead Nancy Tabor, and Director of Development Barbara Yien.

The editorial and production teams are critical to a book's success, but I would be remiss without thanking another key group who ultimately help determine a book's success: the textbook sales group and Executive Marketing Manager Neena Bali. With Neena's support, the Pearson sales representatives traverse the country, promoting the book, making sure that instructors know how it compares to the competition, and providing support to customers. From directing an outstanding marketing campaign to the everyday tasks of being responsive to instructor needs, Neena does a superb job of making sure that *My Health* gets into instructors' hands and that adopters receive the service they deserve. In keeping with my overall experiences with Pearson, the marketing and sales staff is among the best of the best. I am very lucky to have them working with me on this project and want to extend a special thanks to all of them!

This book was developed in part from material from my other textbooks, *Access to Health* and *Health: The Basics*. I would like to thank the contributors to those books, particularly Dr. Patricia Ketcham (Oregon State University and immediate past president of the American College Health Association); Dr. Susan Dobie, associate professor in the School of Health, Physical Education, and Leisure Services at the University of Northern Iowa; Dr. Kathy Munoz, professor in the Department of Kinesiology and Recreation Administration at Humboldt State University; Dr. Erica Jackson, associate professor in the Department of Public and Allied Health Sciences at Delaware State University; Dr. Karen Elliot, senior instructor in the Health Promotion and Health Behavior Program at Oregon State University; and Laura Bonazzoli, who has been instrumental in writing key Focus On chapters and updating material and content for several editions of these texts. A special thanks to Niloofar Bavarian (Oregon State University), who drafted the original student learning outcomes on which the book is based.

Thanks also to the talented people who contributed to the supplements package: Denise and her team at Southern Editorial who updated the *Instructor Resource and Support Manual*; Brent

Goff, who updated the Test Bank; and Melanie Healey (University of Washington-La Crosse), who updated the PowerPoint lecture slides and PowerPoint quiz show slides.

Reviewers

This book is the result of not only my efforts, but also the invaluable contributions of the many reviewers. From the initial idea to the fine-tuning of each and every learning outcome, the thoughtful comments from reviewers shaped this book in many ways. I am extremely grateful for your feedback.

I am forever grateful to all of those who contributed in large and small ways to the success of this text. It really does take a village to make things happen, and this village was extraordinary!

Rebecca J. Donatelle, PhD

Second Edition Reviewers

Debbie Allison
Guilford Technical Community College

Nicole Clark
Indiana University of Pennsylvania

Henry Counts
University of South Carolina

Teresa Dolan
Lincoln University

Kathy Finley
Indiana University Bloomington

Ari Fisher
Louisiana State University

Chris Isenbarth
Weber State University

Ellen Larson
Northern Arizona University

Cynthia Smith
Central Piedmont Community College

MasteringHealth Faculty Advisor Board Reviewers

Kris Jankovitz
California Polytechnic State University

Stasi Kasianchuk
Oregon State University

Lynn Long
University of North Carolina at Wilmington

Ayanna Lyles
California University of Pennsylvania

Steven Namanny
Utah Valley University

Healthy Change 1

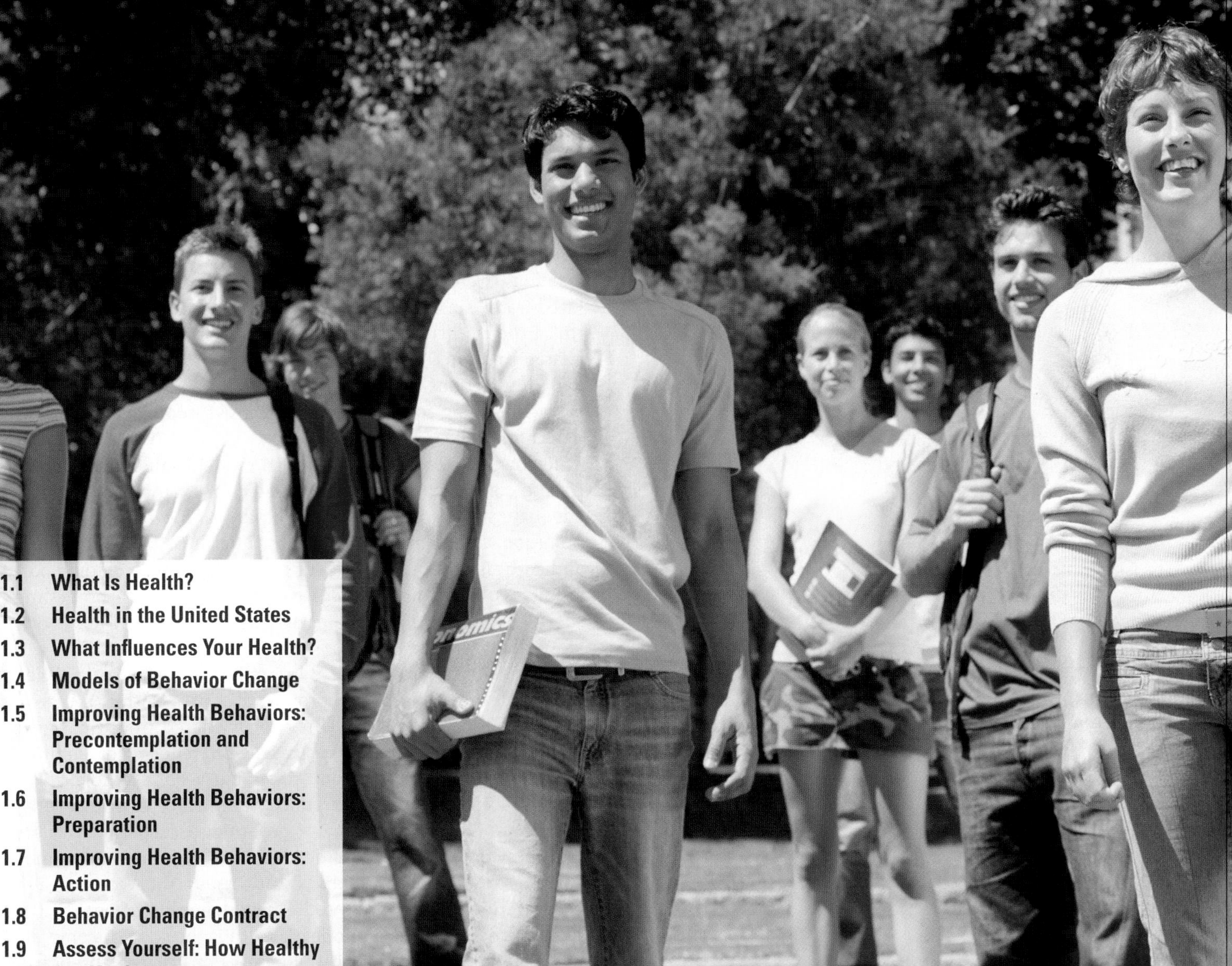

Got health? That may sound like a simple question, but it isn't; health is a process, not something we just "get." People who are healthy in their forties, fifties, sixties, and beyond aren't just lucky or the beneficiaries of hardy genes. In most cases, those who are healthy and thriving in their later years have set the stage for good health by making it a priority in their early years. You've probably heard others say that your college years are some of the best years of your life. Whether your story is filled with good health, happiness, great relationships, and fulfillment of your life goals is largely dependent on the health choices you make—beginning right now.

We aspire to be fit; we want to be more environmentally conscious; we search for relationships that are meaningful, loving, and lasting; and we want to live to a healthy, happy old age. How does what you do today influence you and those around you?

1.1 What Is Health?

learning **outcome**

1.1 Discuss definitions of health used throughout history, and distinguish among the dimensions of health and wellness.

Over the centuries, different ideals—or models—of human **health** have dominated. Our current model has broadened from a focus on the individual body to an understanding of health as a reflection of not only ourselves but also our communities. The choices we make about our health every day affect our lives in many ways. For instance, did you know that the amount of sleep that you get each night could affect your body weight, your ability to ward off colds, your mood, and your driving? What's more, inadequate sleep is one of the most commonly reported impediments to academic success (Figure 1.1).

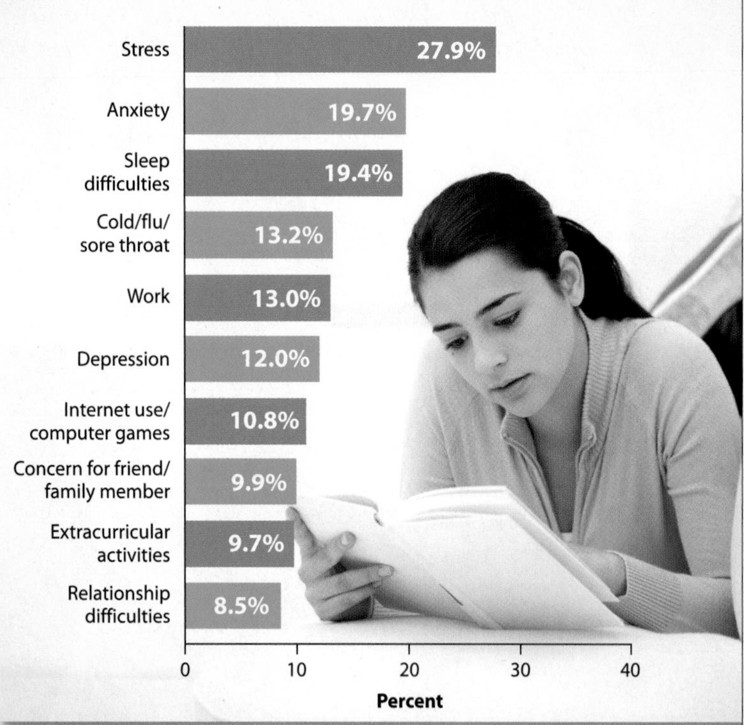

Figure 1.1 Top 10 Reported Impediments to Academic Performance—Past 12 Months

In a recent survey by the National College Health Association, students indicated that stress, poor sleep, recurrent minor illnesses, and anxiety, among other things, had prevented them from performing at their academic best.

Source: Data are from American College Health Association, *American College Health Association—National College Health Assessment II (ACHA-NCHA II) Reference Group Data Report, Fall 2013* (Hanover, MD: American College Health Association, 2014), Available at www.acha-ncha.org.

Models of Health

Before the twentieth century, if you made it to your fiftieth birthday, you were regarded as lucky. Survivors were believed to be of healthy stock—having what we might refer to today as "good genes." During this time, perceptions of health were dominated by the **medical model,** in which health status focused primarily on the individual and his or her tissues and organs. The surest way to improve health was to cure the individual's disease, either with medication to treat the disease-causing agent or through surgery to remove the diseased body part. Government resources focused on initiatives that led to disease treatment rather than prevention.

In the early 1900s, researchers begin to recognize that entire populations of poor people, particularly those living in certain locations, were victims of environmental factors—such as polluted water, air, and food—over which they often had little control. Experts then began to realize that disease and health are related to more than just physical factors. A field of study examining interactions between the social and physical environment evolved, leading to a more comprehensive **ecological** or **public health model.**

Recognition of the public health model enabled health officials to control contaminants in water, for example, by building adequate sewers and to control burning and other forms of air pollution. Over time, public health officials began to recognize and address other forces affecting human health, including hazardous work conditions, negative influences in the home and social environment, stress, unsafe behavior, diet, and sedentary lifestyle.

By the 1940s, progressive thinkers began calling for policies, programs, and services to improve individual health and that of the population as a whole. Their focus shifted from treatment of individual illness to **disease prevention,** reducing or eliminating the factors that cause illness and injury. For example, childhood vaccination programs reduced the incidence and severity of infectious disease, and laws governing occupational safety reduced worker injuries and deaths. In 1947, at an international conference focusing on global health issues, the World Health Organization (WHO) proposed a new definition of health that rejected the old medical model: "Health is the state of complete physical, mental, and social well-being, not just the absence of disease or infirmity."[1]

Alongside prevention, the public health model emphasized **health promotion**—policies and programs promoting behaviors known to support health. Such programs identify people engaging in **risk behaviors** (behaviors increasing susceptibility to negative health outcomes) and motivate them to change their actions by improving their knowledge, attitudes, and skills.

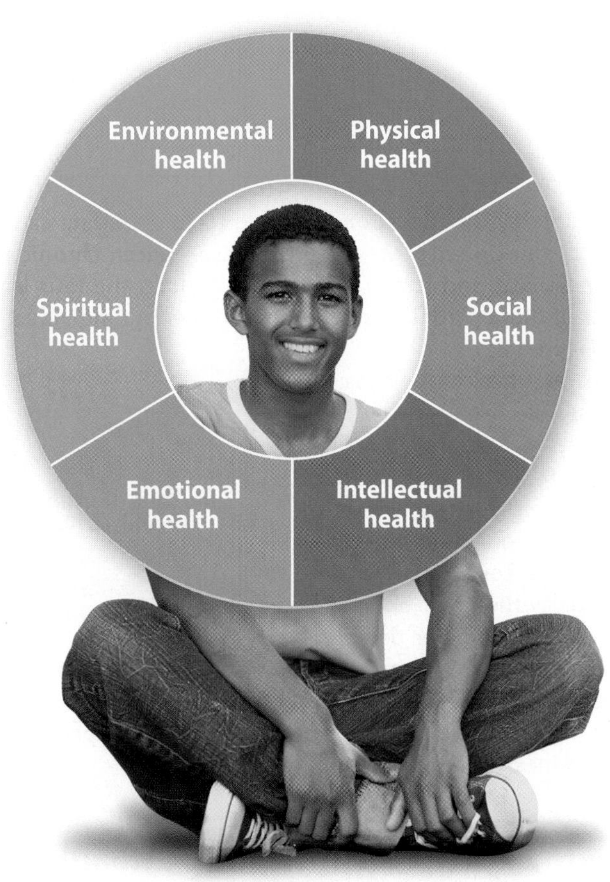

Figure 1.2 The Dimensions of Health

When all dimensions of health are in balance and well developed, they can support your active and thriving lifestyle.

VIDEO TUTOR
Dimensions of Health

Wellness and the Dimensions of Health

In 1968, René Dubos proposed an even broader definition of health. In his book, *So Human an Animal,* Dubos defined *health* as "a quality of life, involving social, emotional, mental, spiritual, and biological fitness on the part of the individual, which results from adaptations to the environment."[2] This concept of adaptability became a key element in our overall understanding of health.

Eventually the word **wellness** entered the popular vocabulary, further enlarging Dubos's definition of health by recognizing levels—or gradations—of health within each category. Today, the words *health* and *wellness* are often used interchangeably to mean the dynamic, ever-changing process of trying to achieve one's potential in each of six interrelated dimensions (Figure 1.2):

- **Physical health.** Physical health includes characteristics such as body size and shape, sensory acuity and responsiveness, susceptibility to disease and disorders, body functioning, physical fitness, and recuperative abilities. Newer definitions of physical health include our ability to perform normal *activities of daily living (ADLs),* or those tasks necessary to normal existence in society, such as getting up from a chair, bending to tie your shoes, or writing a check.
- **Social health.** The ability to have satisfying interpersonal relationships with friends, family members, and partners is a key part of overall wellness. This implies being able to give and receive love, to be nurturing and supportive in social interactions, and to interact and communicate with others.
- **Intellectual health.** The ability to think clearly, reason objectively, analyze critically, and use brainpower effectively to meet life's challenges are all part of this dimension. This includes learning from successes and mistakes; making sound, responsible decisions that consider all aspects of a situation; and having a healthy curiosity about life and an interest in learning new things.
- **Emotional health.** This is the feeling component—being able to express emotions when appropriate, and to control them when not. Self-esteem, self-confidence, self-efficacy, trust, and love are all part of emotional health.
- **Spiritual health.** This dimension involves having a sense of meaning and purpose in your life. This may include believing in a supreme being or following a particular religion's rules and customs. It may also include the ability to understand and express one's purpose in life; to feel part of a greater spectrum of existence; to experience peace, contentment, and wonder over life's experiences; and to care about and respect all living things.
- **Environmental health.** This dimension entails understanding how the health of the environments in which you live, work, and play can affect you; protecting yourself from hazards in your own environment; and working to protect and improve environmental conditions for everyone.

Achieving wellness means attaining the optimal level of well-being for your unique limitations and strengths. For example, a physically disabled person may function at his or her optimal level of performance; enjoy satisfying interpersonal relationships; work to maintain emotional, spiritual, and intellectual health; and have a strong interest in environmental concerns. In contrast, someone who spends hours lifting weights to perfect each muscle but pays little attention to social or emotional health may look healthy but may not maintain a balance in all dimensions. The perspective on wellness we need is *holistic,* emphasizing balanced integration of mind, body, and spirit.

check yourself

- **How have definitions of health changed over time?**
- **What are the dimensions of health? Explain the differences among them.**
- **When you think of someone as being "healthy," what comes to mind? Are your criteria consistent with modern definitions?**

1.2 Health in the United States

learning outcome

1.2 Specify major present-day health issues affecting the United States population, and explain the overall goals of Healthy People 2020.

Our health choices are not only personal; they affect the lives of others in many ways. For example, overeating and inadequate physical activity contribute to individual obesity, but obesity also burdens the U.S. health care system and economy. According to one report, nearly 21 percent of current medical spending in the United States is due to obesity.[3] Obesity also costs the public indirectly, for example, by increased disability payments and health insurance rates. Similarly, smoking, excessive consumption of alcohol, and use of illegal drugs place an economic burden on our communities and our society as a whole—not to mention social and emotional burdens on families and caregivers.

How Healthy Are We?

According to current **mortality** statistics—which reflect the proportion of deaths within a population—average **life expectancy** at birth in the United States is projected to be 78.7 years for a child born in 2011.[4] In other words, American infants born today will live to an average age of over 78 years, much longer than the 47-year life expectancy for people born in the early 1900s.

In the last century, with the development of vaccines, antibiotics, and other public health successes, as well as advances in medications, diagnostic technologies, surgery, and cancer treatments, life expectancy increased dramatically.[5] The leading cause of death shifted to **chronic diseases**, such as heart disease, cerebrovascular disease (which leads to strokes), cancer, and diabetes.

Unfortunately, life expectancy in the United States is several years below that of many other nations, and some researchers believe that our increasing prevalence of extreme obesity may be limiting our gains.[6] Others cite more complex issues, including poor access to health care, poor health behaviors, social inequality, and poverty.[7]

Lifestyle factors are strongly linked to four leading causes of death in the United States: heart disease, cancer, chronic respiratory disease, and stroke (Table 1.1).[8] In fact, the four leading causes of these chronic diseases are all under our individual control (Figure 1.3).

Clearly, healthful choices increase life expectancy. But they also increase **healthy life expectancy**—the years of full health a person enjoys without disability, chronic pain, or significant illness. For example, if we could delay the onset of diabetes until age 60 rather than 30, there would be a 30-year increase in that individual's healthy life expectancy. The prevalence of health issues affecting the U.S. population highlights the need to focus on healthy life expectancy as a cornerstone of public health.

See It! Videos

Why are women experiencing a decline in life expectancy? Watch **Women's Life Expectancy in Decline** in the Study Area of MasteringHealth.

Healthy People 2020: Setting Health Objectives

The Surgeon General's health promotion plan, *Healthy People*, has been published every 10 years since 1990 with the goal of improving quality of life and years of life for all Americans. Each plan consists of a series of long-term objectives for the decade to come. The overarching goals set out by the newest version, *Healthy People 2020*, are to (1) attain high-quality, longer lives free of preventable diseases; (2) achieve health equity, eliminate disparities, and improve health of all groups; (3) create social and physical environments that promote good health for all; and (4) promote quality of life, healthy development, and healthy behaviors across all life stages.[9] In recognition of the changing demographics of the U.S. population and vast differences in health status based on racial or ethnic background, *Healthy People 2020* included strong language about the importance of reducing disparities.

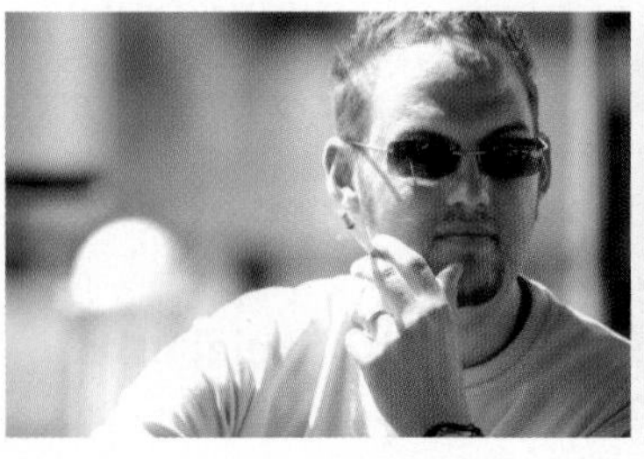
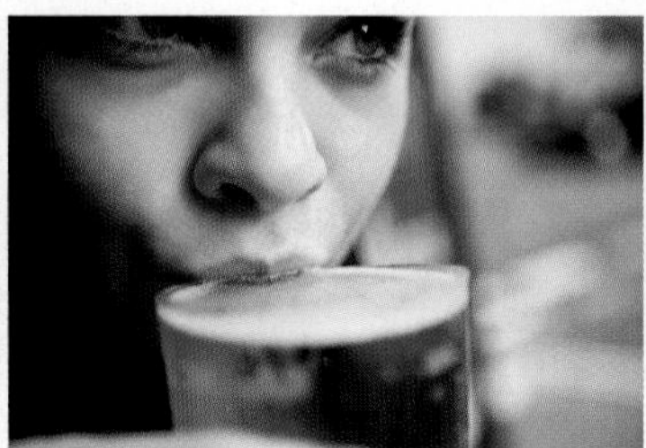
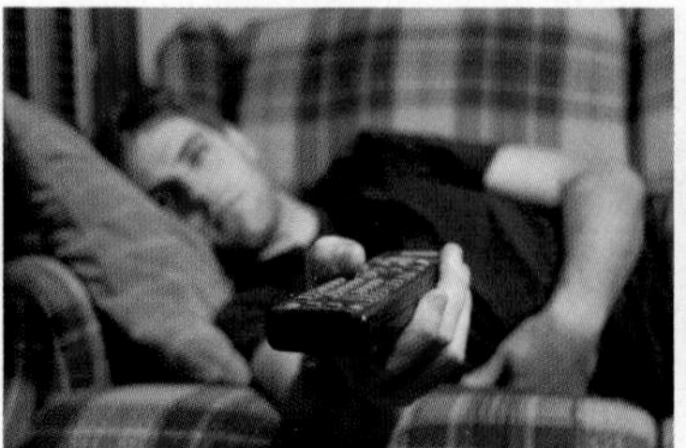
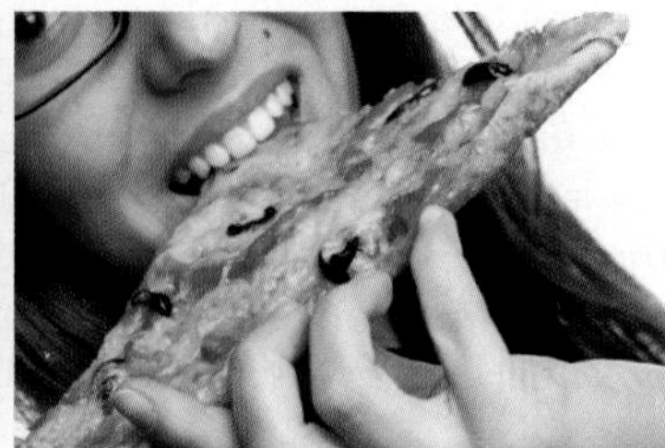

Figure 1.3 Four Leading Causes of Chronic Disease in the United States.
Tobacco use, excessive alcohol consumption, lack of physical activity, and poor nutrition—all modifiable health determinants— are the four most significant factors leading to chronic disease among Americans today.

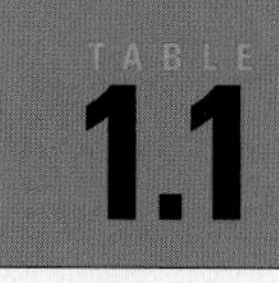

TABLE 1.1 Leading Causes of Death in the United States, 2010, Overall and by Age Group

All Ages	Number of Deaths
Diseases of the heart	597,680
Malignant neoplasms (cancer)	574,743
Chronic lower respiratory diseases	138,080
Cerebrovascular diseases	128,476
Accidents (unintentional injuries)	120,859
AGED 15–24	
Accidents (unintentional injuries)	12,341
Assault (homicide)	4,678
Suicide	4,600
Malignant neoplasms (cancer)	1,604
Diseases of the heart	1,028
AGED 25–44	
Accidents (unintentional injuries)	29,365
Malignant neoplasms (cancer)	15,428
Diseases of the heart	13,816
Suicide	12,306
Assault (homicide)	6,731

Source: Data from M. Heron, "Deaths: Leading Causes for 2010, Table 1," *National Vital Statistics Reports* 62, no. 6 (2013): 17–18, Available at www.cdc.gov.

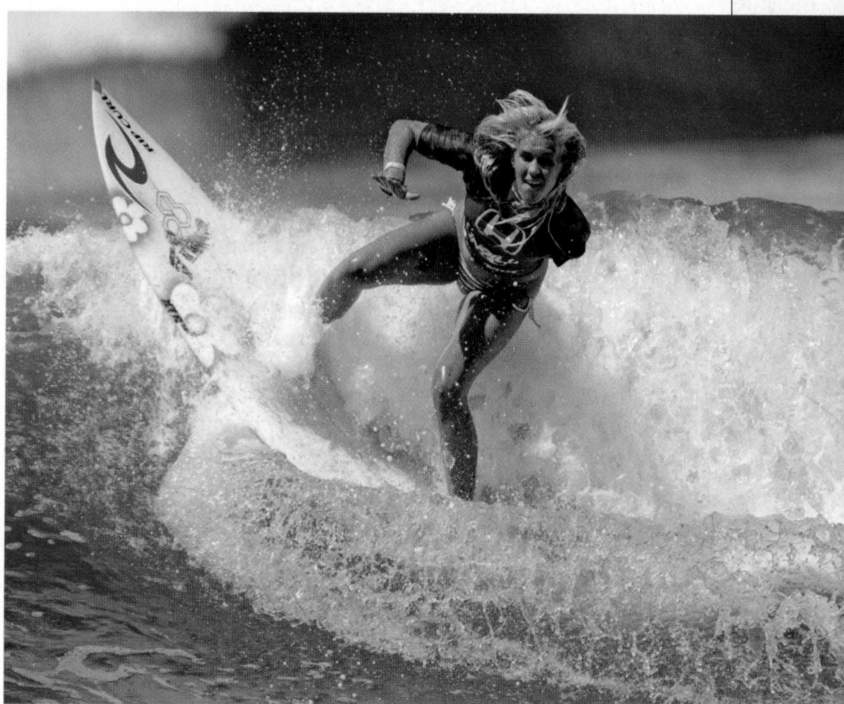

How are *health* and *quality of life* related?

Just because a person has a disability doesn't mean his or her quality of life is necessarily low. Surfer Bethany Hamilton lost her arm in a shark attack while surfing at age 13, but she returned to surfing just 1 month after the attack and has since traveled around the world competing professionally.

At the root of *Healthy People 2020* are "foundation health measures" designed to indicate progress toward reaching these four goals:

- Measures of *general health status,* including life expectancy, healthy life expectancy, and chronic disease prevalence
- Measures of *health-related quality of life and well-being,* including physical, mental, and social factors and participation in common activities
- *Determinants of health,* which are the personal, social, economic, and environmental factors that influence health status
- Measures of *disparities* and inequity, including differences in health status based on race/ethnicity, gender, physical and mental ability, and geography

At the heart of *Healthy People 2020* are 42 topic areas, each representing a public health priority, such as diabetes, physical activity, or substance abuse.[10] Under each area is an overview describing health issues within its scope, objectives for the nation to achieve during the decade to come, and resources for communities and individuals. For instance, objectives for the nutrition topic include "Increase the proportion of schools that offer nutritious foods and beverages outside of school meals" and "Increase the proportion of physician office visits that include counseling or education related to nutrition or weight." For each objective, the report lists baseline statistics and a target goal for the year 2020.

Within the 42 topic areas, a smaller set of topics, called *leading health indicators,* indicate high-priority health issues and actions. Topics include access to health services and reproductive and sexual health, among others.[11]

Perhaps one of the most revealing aspects of the report are the 13 topic areas newly added for this decade, which reflect concern over health disparities, the relationship of lifestyle and wellness, and issues affecting the young and the very old.[12] These include adolescent health; global health; lesbian, gay, bisexual, and transgender health; older adults' health; sleep health; and health-related quality of life and well-being. Health is a comprehensive system encompassing the individual and the society, with influences both intensely personal and broadly global in scope.

check yourself

- **What are four key health issues in the United States?**
- **How are national health objectives used to improve health among Americans?**

1.3

What Influences Your Health?

learning outcome

1.3 Describe the major factors affecting an individual's ability to attain optimal health, and explain the connection between lifestyle and health outcomes.

If you're lucky, aspects of your world promote health: Your family is active and fit; there are fresh apples on sale at the neighborhood farmers market; and a new walking trail opens along the river. If you're not so lucky, aspects of your world discourage health: Your family eats a high-fat diet; cigarettes, alcohol, and junk food dominate the corner market; and you wouldn't dare walk along the river for fear of being mugged. This variety of influences explains why seemingly personal choices aren't totally within an individual's control.

Public health experts refer to the factors that influence health as **determinants of health,** a term the U.S. Surgeon General defines as "the range of personal, social, economic, and environmental factors that influence health status" (Figure 1.4).[13]

Biology and Genetics

In the domain of health determinants, *biology* refers to an individual's genetics, ethnicity, age, and gender. Biological determinants—what health experts refer to as *nonmodifiable determinants*—are things you can't change or modify. Your sex is a key biological determinant: As compared to men, women have an increased risk for low bone density and autoimmune diseases (in which the body attacks its own cells), whereas men have an increased risk for heart disease compared to women. Biology also includes family history; for example, if your parents developed diabetes in their forties, that's a biological determinant for you. Your history of illness and injury factors in, too; a serious injury might influence your ability to participate in physical activity, which in turn may predispose you to weight gain.

Individual Behavior

In contrast to biological factors, *behaviors* are responses to internal and external conditions. By definition, behaviors are changeable; health experts refer to them as *modifiable determinants.* They significantly influence your risk for chronic disease, which is responsible for 7 out of 10 deaths in the United States.[14] Just four modifiable determinants are responsible for most illness and early death related to chronic diseases:[15]

- **Lack of physical activity.** Low levels of physical activity contribute to over 200,000 deaths in the United States annually.[16]
- **Poor nutrition.** Diets low in whole foods like fruits, vegetables, nuts, and seeds, but high in sodium, processed meats, and *trans* fats, are associated with the greatest burden of disease.[17]
- **Excessive alcohol consumption.** Alcohol causes 88,000 deaths in adults annually, through cardiovascular disease, liver disease, cancer, and other conditions, as well as traffic accidents and violence.[18]
- **Tobacco use.** Tobacco smoking and the high blood pressure it causes are responsible for about 1 in 5 deaths in American adults.[19]

Other modifiable determinants include use of vitamins and other supplements, caffeine, over-the-counter medications, and illegal drugs; sexual behaviors and use of contraceptives; sleep habits; and hand washing and other simple infection-control measures.

Social Factors

Social determinants of health refer to the social factors and physical conditions in the environment in which people are born or live. Your social environment includes your exposure to crime, mass media, technology, and poverty, as well as availability of healthful foods, transportation, living wages, social support, and educational or job opportunities.[20]

Among the most powerful determinants of health in the social environment are economic factors; even in affluent nations such as the United States, people in lower socioeconomic brackets have substantially shorter life expectancies and more illnesses than do people who are wealthy.[21] Economic disadvantages exert

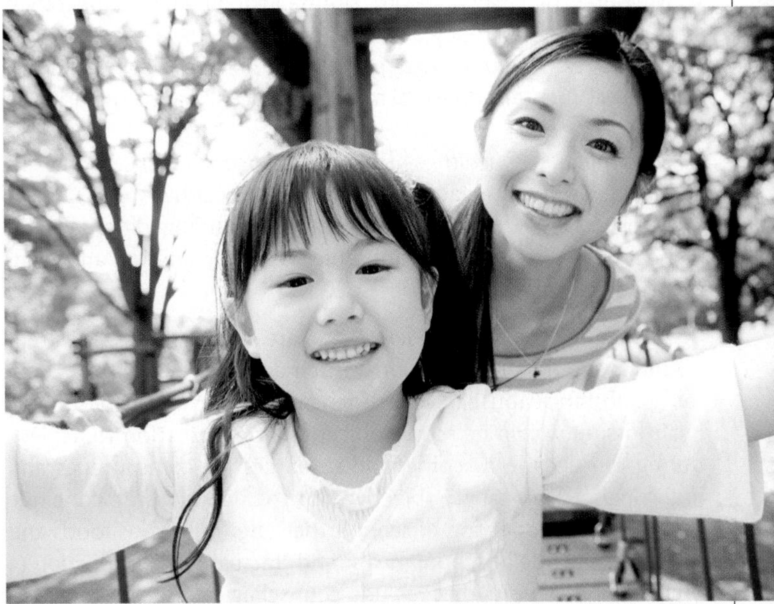

The effects of family on health can be both biological and environmental. Genetics determine some of your health status, but the actions and values of your family also have a strong influence on health.

their effects on health in areas such as access to quality education, safe housing, nourishing food, warm clothes, medication, and transportation.

The physical environment is anything—from skyscrapers to snowfall—that you can perceive with your senses. It also includes less tangible things such as radiation and air pollution. Individuals and communities exposed to toxins, radiation, irritants, and infectious agents can suffer significant harm. And the effects go beyond the local; the pollutants one region produces, or the diseases it harbors, can affect people worldwide. Examples include the burning of the South American rainforest, which is contributing to global warming, and the swift transmission of strains of severe influenza across populations.

One part of the physical environment that has garnered attention from public health officials is the built environment: anything created or modified by human beings, from buildings to transportation to electrical lines. Changes to the built environment can improve the health of community members.[22] These include construction of sidewalks, "open streets" free of motor traffic, bike paths, public transit systems, and supermarkets in inner-city neighborhoods to increase residents' access to fresh fruits and vegetables.[23]

Health Services

The health of individuals and communities is also determined by access to quality health care, not only provider services but also accurate information and products such as eyeglasses, medical supplies, and medications.

Policymaking

Public policies and interventions can have a powerful effect on the health of individuals and communities. Examples include campaigns to prevent smoking, laws mandating seatbelt use, vaccination programs, and public funding for mental health services.[24]

Policymaking also includes health insurance legislation. In 2010, President Obama signed into law the Affordable Care Act (ACA), a set of reforms intended to reduce the nation's health care costs while increasing Americans' access to quality care. In the first 6 months of open enrollment, over 7 million Americans signed up for coverage under the ACA.[25]

Health Disparities

Among the factors that can influence an individual's ability to attain optimal health are **health disparities**. Health disparities can arise from a variety of factors, including the following:[26]

- **Race and ethnicity.** Research indicates dramatic health disparities across racial and ethnic backgrounds. Socioeconomic differences, stigma based on "minority status," poor access to care, cultural barriers and beliefs, discrimination, and limited education and employment opportunities can all affect health.
- **Inadequate health insurance.** A large and growing number of the *uninsured* or *underinsured* face unaffordable payments or co-payments, high deductibles, or limited care in their area.

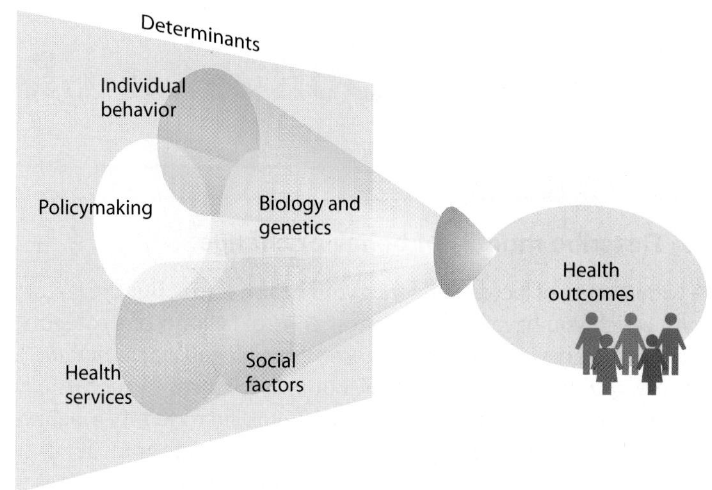

Figure 1.4 ***Healthy People 2020*** **Determinants of Health**
The determinants of health often overlap one another. Collectively, they impact the health of individuals and communities.

- **Sex and gender.** At all stages of life, men and women experience differences in rates of disease and disability. For instance, men smoke more than do women, but women who smoke have higher rates of lung disease. In contrast, men have much higher rates of drug-induced deaths and deaths from suicide and homicide. Overall, men have a lower healthy life expectancy than females.
- **Economics and education.** Poverty may make it difficult to afford healthy food, preventive medical visits, or medication. Economics also influences access to safe, affordable exercise. Moreover, poor Americans with a low level of education experience increased rates of illness, premature death, and risk-taking behaviors such as smoking and binge drinking.
- **Geographic location.** Whether you live in an urban or rural area and have access to public transportation or your own vehicle can have a huge impact on what you eat, your physical activity, and your ability to visit the doctor or dentist.
- **Sexual orientation.** Gay, lesbian, bisexual, or transgender individuals may lack social support, are often denied health benefits due to unrecognized marital status, and face unusually high stress levels and stigmatization by other groups.
- **Disability.** Disproportionate numbers of disabled individuals lack access to health care services, social support, and community resources.

See It! Videos

How can a community's cafe help fight hunger? Watch **Hunger at Home** in the Study Area of MasteringHealth.

check yourself

- **What are the determinants that affect health identified in this section?**
- **Give three examples of the connection between lifestyle and health outcomes.**

1.4 Models of Behavior Change

learning outcome

1.4 Describe models of behavior change.

A wide variety of factors influence your health status. But the factors over which you have by far the most control fall into one category: individual behaviors (otherwise known as *modifiable determinants*). Clearly, change is not always easy. But your chances of successfully changing negative habits improve when you first identify a behavior that you want to change, then develop a plan for gradual transformation—one that allows you time to unlearn negative patterns and substitute positive ones. Many experts advocate breaking any health behavior you want to change into small parts, then working on them one at a time in "baby steps."

In other words, to successfully change a behavior, you need to see change not as a singular *event* but instead as a *process*—one that requires preparation, consists of several stages, and takes time to succeed.

Over the years, social scientists and public health researchers have developed a variety of models to reflect the multifaceted process of behavior change. We explore three such models here.

The Health Belief Model

Many people see changing health behaviors as a straightforward process: When rational people realize that their behaviors put them at risk, they will change those behaviors and reduce that risk. But, for many (even most) of us, it's more complicated than that. Consider the number of health professionals who smoke, consume junk food, and act in other unhealthy ways. They surely know better, but "knowing" is disconnected from "doing." One classic model of behavior change proposes that our beliefs may help to explain why this occurs.

A **belief** is an appraisal of the relationship between some object, action, or idea (e.g., smoking) and some attribute of that object, action, or idea (e.g., "smoking is expensive, dirty, and causes cancer,"—or "smoking is sociable and relaxing"). Psychologists studying the relationship between beliefs and health behaviors have determined that although beliefs may subtly influence behavior, they may or may not cause people to actually behave differently. In 1966, psychologist I. Rosenstock developed a classic theory, the **health belief model (HBM),** to show when beliefs about health affect behavior change.[27] The HBM holds that, before change is likely to happen, our beliefs must reflect the following:

- **Perceived seriousness of the health problem.** The more serious the perceived effects, the more likely that action will be taken.
- **Perceived susceptibility to the health problem.** People who perceive themselves at high risk are more likely to take preventive action.
- **Perceived benefits.** People are more likely to take action if they believe that this action will benefit them.
- **Perceived barriers.** People who believe an action is too expensive, difficult, or inconvenient must overcome or acknowledge these barriers as less important than the perceived benefits.
- **Cues to action.** People who are reminded or alerted about a potential health problem are more likely to take action.

People follow the HBM many times every day. Take, for example, smokers. Older smokers are likely to know other smokers who have developed serious heart or lung problems. They are thus more likely to perceive tobacco as a threat to their health than are teenagers who have just begun smoking. The greater the perceived threat of health problems caused by smoking, the greater the chance a person will quit.

But many chronic smokers know the risks, yet continue to smoke. Why do they miss these cues to action? According to Rosenstock, some people do not believe that they, personally, are susceptible to a severe problem, and so act as though they are immune to it. Such people are unlikely to change their behavior.

The Social Cognitive Model

The **social cognitive model (SCM)** developed from the work of several researchers and their models over the years, though it is most closely associated with the work of psychologist Albert Bandura. Fundamentally, SCM proposes that three factors interact in a reciprocal fashion to promote and motivate change. These are

The top New Year's resolution for both 2012 and 2013 was to become more physically fit.

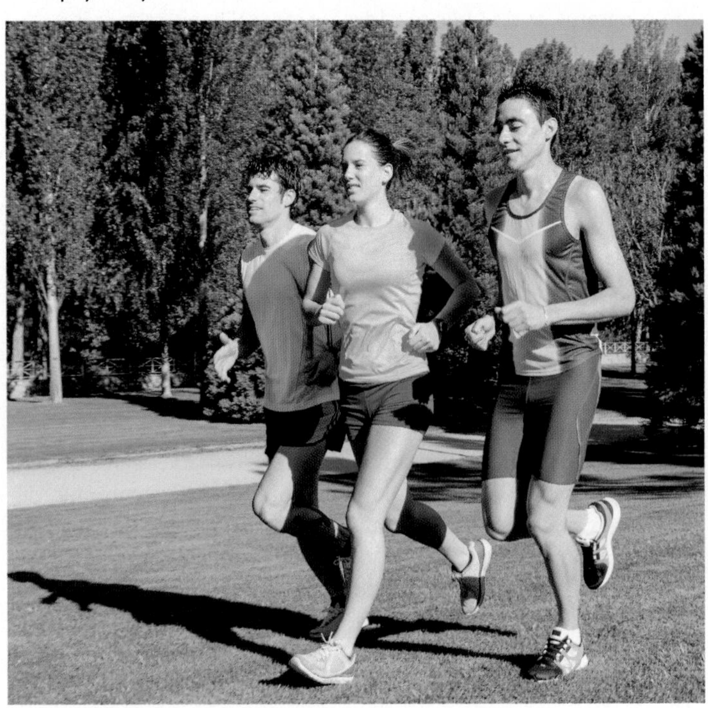

the social environment in which we live, our thoughts or cognition (including our values, perceptions, beliefs, expectations, and sense of self-efficacy), and our behaviors. We change our behavior, in part, by observing models in our environments—from childhood to the present moment—reflecting on our observations, and regulating ourselves accordingly.

For instance, if as a child you observed your mother successfully quitting smoking, you may be more apt to believe that you can quit, too. In addition, when we succeed in changing ourselves, we change our thoughts about ourselves. This in turn may promote further behavior change: After you've successfully quit smoking, you may feel empowered to increase your level of physical activity. Moreover, as we change ourselves, we change our world; in this case, you become a model of successful smoking cessation for others to observe. In this model, we are not just products of our environments, but also producers of it.

The Transtheoretical Model

Why do so many New Year's resolutions fail before Valentine's Day? According to Drs. James Prochaska and Carlos DiClemente, it's because most of us aren't really prepared to take action. Their research indicates that behavior changes usually do not succeed if they start with the change itself. Instead, we must go through a series of stages to adequately prepare ourselves for an eventual change.[28] According to Prochaska and DiClemente's **transtheoretical model** of behavior change (also called the *stages of change model*), our chances of keeping those New Year's resolutions will be greatly enhanced if we have proper reinforcement and help during each of the following stages:

1. **Precontemplation.** People in the precontemplation stage have no current intention of changing. They may have tried to change a behavior before and given up, or they may be in denial and unaware of any problem.
2. **Contemplation.** In this phase, people recognize that they have a problem and begin to contemplate the need to change. Despite this acknowledgment, people can languish in this stage for years, realizing a problem but lacking the time or energy to make the change.
3. **Preparation.** Most people at this point are close to taking action. They've thought about what they might do and may even have come up with a specific plan.
4. **Action.** In this stage, people begin to follow their action plans. Those who have prepared for change appropriately and made a plan of action are more ready for action than those who have given it little thought.
5. **Maintenance.** During the maintenance stage, a person continues the actions begun in the action stage and works toward making them a permanent part of his or her life. In this stage, it is important to be aware of the potential for relapses and to develop strategies for dealing with such challenges.
6. **Termination.** By this point, the change in behavior is so ingrained that constant vigilance may be unnecessary. The new behavior has become an essential part of daily living.

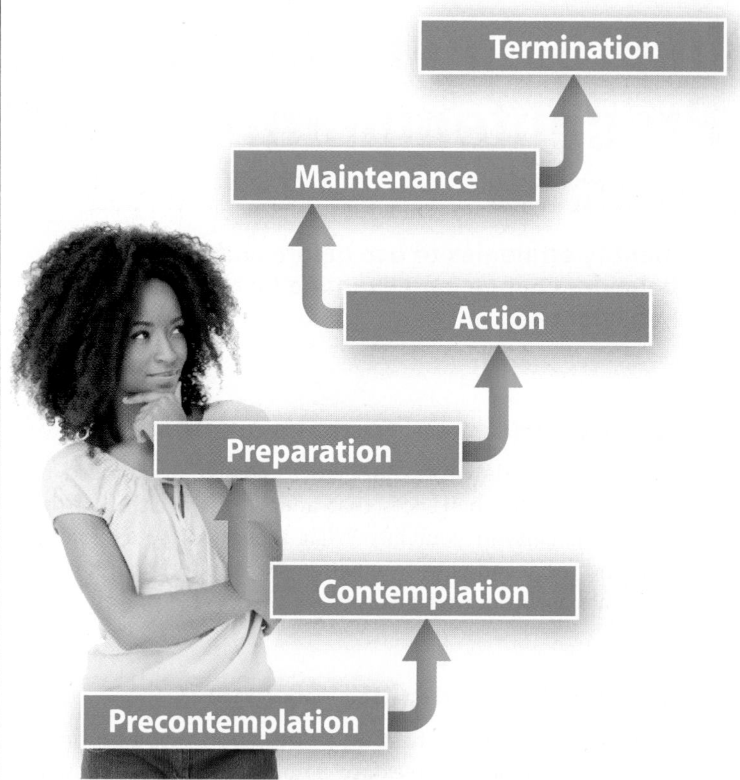

Figure 1.5 Transtheoretical Model
People don't move through the transtheoretical model stages in sequence. We may make progress in more than one stage at one time, or we may shuttle back and forth from one to another—say, contemplation to preparation, then back to contemplation—before we succeed in making a change.

We don't necessarily go through these stages sequentially. They may overlap, or we may shuttle back and forth from one to another—say, contemplation to preparation, then back to contemplation—for a while before we become truly committed to making the change (Figure 1.5). Still, it's useful to recognize where we are with a change, so we can consider the appropriate strategies to move us forward.

See It! Videos

How can you change your habits and stick with it? Watch **New Year's Resolutions** in the Study Area of MasteringHealth.

check yourself

- **Compare and contrast models of behavior change.**
- **Which model of behavior change reflects most accurately your experiences? Why?**

1.5 Improving Health Behaviors: Precontemplation and Contemplation

learning outcome

1.5 Identify strategies to use before and during behavior change, and examine factors that affect behavior change.

Step One: Increase Your Awareness

Before you can decide what you want to change, you'll need to learn about both the behaviors that affect your health and the health determinants in your life. What aspects of your biology, behavior, and social and physical environment support your health, and which are obstacles to overcome?

Step Two: Contemplate Change

Examine Your Health Habits and Patterns Do you routinely stop at Dunkin' Donuts for breakfast? Smoke when you're stressed? Party too much? Get to bed way past 2 A.M.? When considering habits, ask yourself the following:

- How long has this been going on?
- How often does it happen?
- How serious are its consequences?
- What are your reasons for the behavior?
- What situations trigger it?
- Are others involved? How?

Health behaviors involve personal choice, but are also influenced by determinants that make them more or less likely. Some are *predisposing factors*—for instance, if your parents smoke, you're more likely to start smoking than is a child of nonsmokers. Some are *enabling factors*—for example, peers who smoke enable one another's smoking.

Reinforcing factors can also contribute to habits. If you decide to stop smoking but your friends all smoke, you may lose your resolve. In such cases, it can be helpful to employ the social cognitive model and deliberately change your environment—spending more time with nonsmoking friends who model behavior you want to emulate.

Identify a Target Behavior Ask yourself these questions:

- **What do I want?** Is your ultimate goal to lose weight? Exercise more? Reduce stress? Have a lasting relationship? Get a clear picture of your outcome.
- **Which change is my priority now?** Suppose you're gaining unwanted weight. Rather than saying, "I need to eat less and start exercising," identify one specific behavior that contributes to your problem, and tackle that first.
- **Why is this important to me?** Do you want to change for your health? To improve academic performance? To look better? To win someone's approval? It's best to target a behavior because it's right for you rather than because you think it will please others.

Learn about the Target Behavior Get solid information from reliable sources (see the **Do Your Research** section on the following page). Look at the behavior, its effects, and aspects of your world that could hinder your success. Let's say you want to meditate daily. You need to learn what meditation is, how it's practiced, and its benefits. Consider what else might pose an obstacle: Do you think of yourself as hyper? Do you live in a noisy dorm? Are you afraid your friends might find meditating weird? To prepare for change, learn everything you can about your target behavior now.

Assess Your Motivation and Readiness To change, you need not just desire but also **motivation**—a social and cognitive force that directs your behavior. To understand motivation, think about the health belief model (HBM) and the social cognitive model (SCM).

According to the HBM, beliefs affect ability to change. Smokers may think, "I'll stop tomorrow" or "They'll have a cure for lung cancer before I get it." These beliefs allow

Find reliable health information at your fingertips!

them to continue smoking—they dampen motivation. Ask yourself the following:

- Do you believe your current pattern could lead to a serious problem? The more severe the consequences, the more motivation for change. For example, smoking can cause deadly diseases. But what if cancer and emphysema were just words to you? To increase your motivation, you could study these disorders and the suffering they cause.
- Do you see yourself as personally likely to experience the consequences of your behavior? Losing a loved one to lung cancer could motivate you to stop smoking.

If you're struggling to perceive a behavior as serious or its consequences as personal, use the SCM. You could interview people struggling with the consequences of the behavior and ask if when they were engaging in the behavior they believed it would harm them. And don't ignore the motivating potential of positive role models. Do you know people who have successfully lost weight, stopped drinking, or quit smoking? Hang out with them!

Motivation is powerful, but it must be combined with common sense, commitment, and a realistic understanding of how to move from A to B. *Readiness* precedes behavior change. People who are ready to change possess the knowledge, skills, and external and internal resources that make change possible.

Develop Self-Efficacy **Self-efficacy**—a belief that one is capable of achieving certain goals or of influencing events in life—is one of the greatest influences on health. People who exhibit high self-efficacy are confident that they can succeed and approach challenges positively. They may therefore be more likely to succeed. Conversely, someone with low self-efficacy may give up easily or never try to change. Such people tend to avoid challenges and are more likely to revert to old patterns. If you suspect you have low self-efficacy, a technique of cognitive-behavioral therapy called *cognitive restructuring* can help; find out more by visiting your campus counseling services.

Cultivate an Internal Locus of Control The conviction that you have the power and ability to change is a powerful motivator. People with a strong *internal* **locus of control** believe that they have power over their own actions. They are more likely to state their opinions and be true to their own beliefs. In contrast, individuals with an *external* locus of control feel that they have limited control over their lives; they may easily succumb to feelings of anxiety and disempowerment and give up.

Do Your Research The Internet is a wonderful resource for finding answers to your questions, but it can also be a source of *misinformation*. To ensure that the sites you visit are trustworthy, follow these tips:

- Look for websites sponsored by government agencies (identified by *.gov* extensions—e.g., the National Institute of Mental Health at www.nimh.nih.gov); universities or colleges (*.edu* extensions—e.g., Johns Hopkins University at www.jhu.edu); or hospitals/medical centers (often *.org*—e.g., the Mayo Clinic at www.mayoclinic.org). Major philanthropic foundations (such as the Robert Wood Johnson Foundation and the Kellogg Foundation) and national nonprofit organizations (such as the American Heart Association and the American Cancer Society) are good, authoritative sources. Most foundation and nonprofit sites have *.org* extensions.
- Search for peer-reviewed journals such as the *New England Journal of Medicine* (content.nejm.org) and *Journal of the American Medical Association* (JAMA; jama.ama-assn.org). Although some of these sites require an access fee, many colleges give students free access to them.
- Other reliable sites include the Centers for Disease Control and Prevention (www.cdc.gov), the World Health Organization (www.who.int/en), FamilyDoctor.org (familydoctor.org), MedlinePlus (www.nlm.nih.gov/medlineplus), Go Ask Alice! (www.goaskalice.columbia.edu), and WebMD (my.webmd.com).
- Don't believe everything you read. Cross-check information against reliable sources. Be wary of websites selling you something. When in doubt, check with your health care provider or health professor.

Skills for Behavior Change

MAINTAIN YOUR MOTIVATION

- **Pick one specific behavior you want to change.** Trying to change many things at once can be overwhelming and can cause you to lose motivation.
- **Assess the behavior you wish to change.** Why is it important to change? If you can't find a compelling reason to motivate yourself, you probably shouldn't address this behavior right now.
- **Set achievable and incremental goals.** Developing short- and long-term goals and taking small steps to meet them improves your chances of staying motivated.
- **Reward yourself.** Create a list of things you find rewarding; link each to a specific goal. Having something to look forward to can help you stay focused and motivated.
- **Avoid or anticipate barriers and temptations.** Control or eliminate the environmental cues that provoke the behavior you want to change.
- **Remind yourself why you're trying to change.** List the benefits you'll get from this change, both now and down the road, as well as the risks of doing nothing.
- **Enlist the support of others.** They can serve as role models, a cheering squad, or partners in change. Let the people you care about know your plans, and ask for help.
- **Don't be discouraged.** Everyone, no matter how committed, experiences setbacks. A brief lapse doesn't mean the cause is lost. Look for new strategies, set new short-term goals, and then get back on track.

check yourself

- **What should I do before undertaking a behavior change?**
- **What are some common behavior change strategies?**
- **Name important factors that influence behavior and behavior change decisions.**

1.6 Improving Health Behaviors: Preparation

learning outcome

1.6 Set a behavior change goal, and identify obstacles to behavior change.

Prepare for Change

You've contemplated change for long enough—now it's time to set a realistic goal, anticipate barriers, reach out to others, and commit.

Set a SMART Goal Unsuccessful goals are vague and open-ended—for instance, "Get into shape by exercising more." In contrast, successful goals are SMART:

- **S**pecific. "Attend the Tuesday/Thursday aerobics class at the YMCA."
- **M**easurable. "Reduce my alcohol intake on Saturday nights from three drinks to two."
- **A**ction-oriented. "Volunteer at the animal shelter on Friday afternoons."
- **R**ealistic. "Increase my daily walk from 15 to 20 minutes."
- **T**ime-oriented. "Stay in my strength-training class for the full 10-week session, then reassess."

A SMART goal is one that you truly can achieve—not someday, when things in your life change, but within the circumstances of your life right now. Knowing that your goal is attainable increases your motivation. This, in turn, leads to a better chance of success and to a greater sense of self-efficacy—which can in turn motivate you to succeed even more.

Use Shaping **Shaping** is a process of making a series of small changes. Suppose you want to start jogging 3 miles every other day, but right now you get tired and winded after half a mile. Shaping would dictate a process of slow, progressive steps, perhaps beginning with walking 1 hour every other day at a slow, relaxed pace for the first week; walking for an hour every other day but at a faster pace that covers more distance the second week; and speeding up to a slow run the third week.

Regardless of the change you plan, remember that your current habits didn't develop overnight, and they won't change overnight, either. Prepare your goals and your plan of action with these shaping points in mind:

- Start slowly to avoid hurting yourself or causing undue stress.
- Keep the steps of your program small and achievable.
- Be flexible and ready to change your original plan if it proves uncomfortable.
- Master one step before moving on to the next.

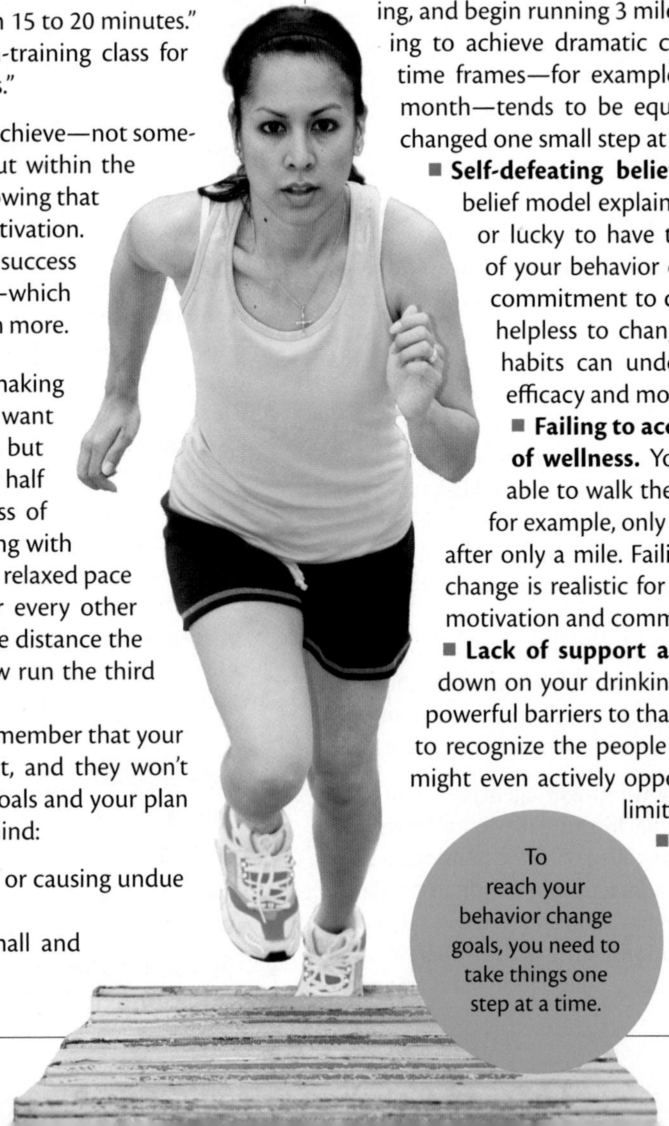

Anticipate Barriers to Change Anticipating *barriers to change*, or possible stumbling blocks, will help you prepare fully and adequately for change. For example, if you want to lose weight, you may face several barriers to change, including social determinants (your family members and friends are overweight), aspects of the built environment (the only food vendors on or near your campus are convenience stores and fast-food outlets), or lack of adequate health care (you have an inexpensive health insurance policy that doesn't cover treatment for weight loss). In addition to negative determinants, the following are a few general barriers to change that you may need to overcome:

- **Overambitious goals.** Remember the advice to set realistic goals? Even with the strongest motivation, overambitious goals can derail change. Most people cannot lose weight, stop smoking, and begin running 3 miles a day all at the same time. Wanting to achieve dramatic change within unrealistically short time frames—for example, aiming to lose 20 pounds in 1 month—tends to be equally unsuccessful. Habits are best changed one small step at a time.
- **Self-defeating beliefs and attitudes.** As the health belief model explains, believing you're too young or fit or lucky to have to worry about the consequences of your behavior can keep you from making a solid commitment to change. Likewise, seeing yourself as helpless to change your eating, smoking, or other habits can undermine your efforts. Greater self-efficacy and more positive expectations may help.
- **Failing to accurately assess your current state of wellness.** You might assume that you will be able to walk the 2 miles to campus each morning, for example, only to find yourself aching and winded after only a mile. Failing to make sure that the planned change is realistic for *you* can leave you with weakened motivation and commitment.
- **Lack of support and guidance.** If you want to cut down on your drinking, peers who drink heavily may be powerful barriers to that change. To succeed, you will need to recognize the people in your life who can't support, or might even actively oppose, your decision to change, then limit your interactions with them.
- **Emotions that sabotage your efforts and sap your will.** Sometimes the best laid plans go awry because you're having a bad day or are fighting with someone you

To reach your behavior change goals, you need to take things one step at a time.

care about. While emotional reactions to life's challenges aren't inherently bad, they can sabotage your efforts to change by distracting you and draining your reserves. Seek help for more severe psychological problems, and recognize that you may need to focus on those before you can effect significant change in other aspects of your health.

Enlist Others as Change Agents The social cognitive model recognizes the importance of our social contacts in successful change. Most of us are highly influenced by the approval or disapproval (real or imagined) of close friends, family members, and the social and cultural group to which we belong. In addition, watching others successfully change their behavior can give you ideas and encouragement for your own change. This **modeling**, or learning from role models, is a key component of the social cognitive model of change. Observing a friend who is a good conversationalist, for example, can help you improve your communication skills. Or find someone to share your plan for change! For instance, get your roommate to commit to taking a daily walk or run with you or sign a contract with a friend stipulating that you will never let each other drink and drive.

Family Members From the time of your birth, your parents and other family members have given you strong cues about which actions are and are not socially acceptable. Your family has also influenced your food choices, your activity patterns, your political beliefs, and many of your other values and actions. Strong and positive family units provide care, trust, and protection; are dedicated to the healthful development of all family members; and work together to reduce problems.

When a loving family unit does not exist or when it does not provide for basic human needs, a child can find it difficult to learn positive health behaviors. Healthy families provide the foundation for a clear and necessary understanding of what is right and wrong, what is positive and negative. Without this fundamental grounding, many young people have great difficulties.

Friends Just as your family influences your actions during your childhood, your friends and significant others influence your behaviors as you grow older. Most of us desire to fit the "norm." If you deviate from the actions expected in your hometown or among your friends, you may suffer ostracism, strange looks, and other negative social consequences. But if your friends offer encouragement, or even express interest in joining you in a behavior change, you are more likely to remain motivated. Cultivating and maintaining close friends who share your personal values can greatly affect your behaviors and improve your chances of success.

Professionals Sometimes the change you seek requires more than the help of well-meaning family members and friends. Depending on the type and severity of the problem, you may want to enlist support from professionals such as your health instructor, PE instructor, coach, health care provider, academic adviser, or religious adviser. As appropriate, consider counseling services offered on campus, as well as community services such as smoking cessation programs, Alcoholics Anonymous support groups, and your local YMCA.

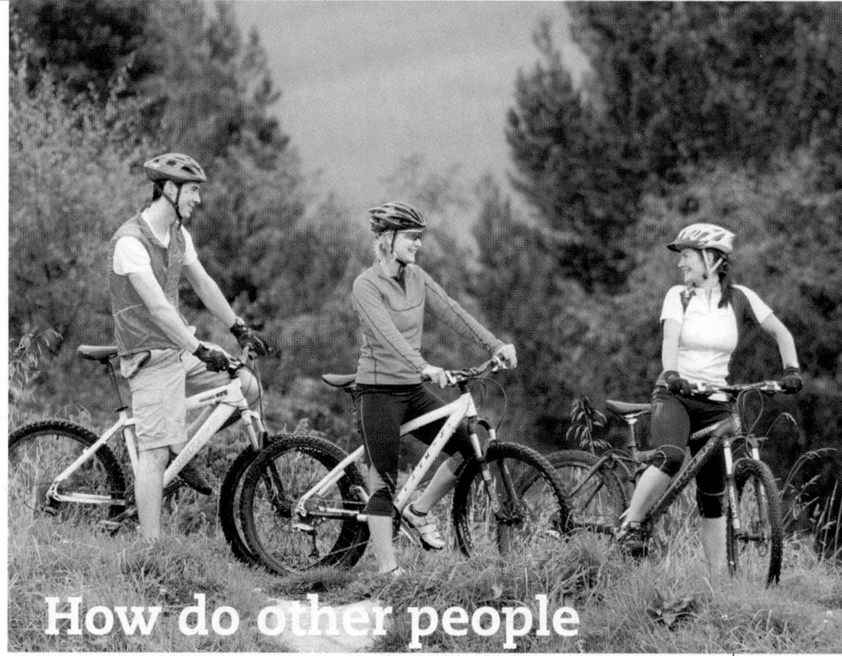

How do other people influence my health behaviors?

The people in your life, including family, friends, neighbors, coworkers, and society in general, can play a huge role—both positive and negative—in the health choices you make. The behaviors of those around you can predispose you to certain health habits, at the same time enabling and reinforcing them. Seeking out the support and encouragement of friends who have similar goals and interests will strengthen your commitment to develop and maintain positive health behaviors.

Sign a Contract It's time to get it in writing! A formal *behavior change contract* serves many powerful purposes. It functions as a promise to yourself, a public declaration of intent, an organized plan that lays out start and end dates and daily actions, a list of barriers you may encounter, a place to brainstorm strategies to overcome barriers, a list of sources of support, and a reminder of the benefits of sticking with the program.

Writing a behavior change contract will help you clarify your goals and make a commitment to change. In the next module, you will see an example of a completed behavior change contract, and later in the chapter, a blank behavior change contract. Fill out the blank contract to put your behavior change plan in writing.

check yourself

- **What is your behavior change goal? Does it fit the SMART system?**
- **What are some obstacles to change that you expect to face? What strategies will you employ to overcome them?**

1.7 Improving Health Behaviors: Action

learning outcome

1.7 Employ behavior change strategies to make a behavior change.

Take Action to Change

It's time to put your plan into action! Behavior change strategies include visualization, countering, controlling the situation, changing your self-talk, rewarding yourself, and journaling. The options don't stop here, but these are a good place to start.

Visualize New Behavior Mental practice can transform unhealthy behaviors into healthy ones. Using an **imagined rehearsal** to visualize an action ahead of time can help you reach your goals. Careful mental and verbal rehearsal of how you intend to act will help you anticipate problems and greatly improve the likelihood of success.

Learn to "Counter" Substituting a desired behavior for an undesirable one is called **countering**. You may want to stop eating junk food, but cutting out all the foods you crave at once isn't realistic. Instead, compile a list of substitute foods and where to get them—and have it ready before your mouth starts to water at the smell of a burger and fries.

Control the Situation Sometimes, the right setting or the right group of people will positively influence your behaviors. Any behavior has both antecedents and consequences. *Antecedents* are aspects of a situation that come beforehand, cueing or stimulating a person to act in certain ways. *Consequences*—the results of behavior—affect whether a person repeats an action. Both antecedents and consequences can be events, thoughts, emotions, or the actions of others.

Keeping a journal noting your undesirable behaviors and the settings in which they occur can be useful in helping you determine the antecedents and consequences. Once you have recognized the antecedents of a given behavior, use **situational inducement** to modify those that are working against you—consider which settings help and which hurt your effort to change. Identifying substitute antecedents that support a more positive result helps you control the situation further.

Change Your Self-Talk There is a close connection between what people say to themselves, known as **self-talk,** and how they feel. When we feel we have little control, it's tempting to engage in negative self-talk, which can sabotage our best intentions. According to psychologist Albert Ellis, most emotional problems and related behaviors stem from irrational statements that people make to themselves when events in their lives are different from what they would like them to be.[29]

For example, suppose you say to yourself, "I can't believe I flunked that exam. I'm so stupid." Changing such irrational, negative self-talk into rational, positive statements about what is really going on can increase the likelihood of positive change: "I didn't study enough for that exam. I'm not stupid; I just need to prepare better for the next test." Positive self-talk can help you recover from disappointment and take steps to correct problems.

Another technique for changing self-talk is to practice blocking and stopping negative thoughts. For example, suppose you're preoccupied with your ex-partner, who left you for someone else. By refusing to dwell on negative images and by forcing yourself to

Behavior Change Contract

My behavior change will be:
To snack less on junk food and more on healthy foods.

My long-term goal for this behavior change is:
Eat junk food snacks no more than once a week.

These are three obstacles to change (things that I am currently doing or situations that contribute to this behavior or make it harder to change):

1. The grocery store is closed by the time I come home from school.
2. I get hungry between classes, and the vending machines only carry candy bars.
3. It's easier to order pizza or other snacks than to make a snack at home.

The strategies I will use to overcome these obstacles are:

1. I'll leave early for school once a week so I can stock up on healthy snacks in the morning.
2. I'll bring a piece of fruit or other healthy snack to eat between classes.
3. I'll learn some easy recipes for snacks to make at home.

Resources I will use to help me change this behavior include:

a friend/partner/relative: my roommates: I'll ask them to buy healthier snacks instead of chips when they do the shopping.
a school-based resource: The dining hall: I'll ask the manager to provide healthy foods we can take to eat between classes.
a community-based resource: The library: I'll check out some cookbooks to find easy snack ideas
a book or reputable website: The USDA nutrient database at www.nal.usda.gov/fnic I'll use this site to make sure the foods I select are healthy choices.

In order to make my goal more attainable, I have devised these short-term goals:

short-term goal Eat a healthy snack 3 times per week target date September 15 reward new CD
short-term goal Learn to make a healthy snack target date October 15 reward concert tickets
short-term goal Eat a healthy snack 5 times per week target date November 15 reward new shoes

When I make the long-term behavior change described above, my reward will be:
ski lift tickets for winter break target date: December 15

I intend to make the behavior change described above. I will use the strategies and rewards to achieve the goals that will contribute to a healthy behavior change.

Signed: Elizabeth King Witness: Susan Bauer

Figure 1.6 Example of a Completed Behavior Change Contract

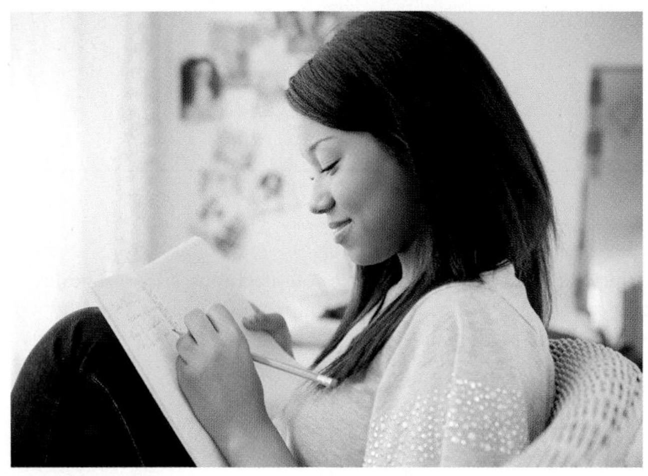

What can I do to change an unhealthy habit?

One of the best tools for helping you change your habits is journaling. Keeping track of your goals, behaviors, feelings, accomplishments, and setbacks can reinforce the healthy changes you are trying to make and provide motivation to continue. Other useful tools include shaping, enlisting supports, visualization, countering, controlling the situation, changing your self-talk, and rewarding yourself.

focus elsewhere, you can avoid wasting energy, time, and emotional resources and move on to positive change.

Reward Yourself Promote positive behavior change with **positive reinforcement**. Each of us is motivated by different positive reinforcers. Most of these fall into one of the following categories:

- *Consumable reinforcers* are edible items, such as a favorite fruit or snack mix.
- *Activity reinforcers* are opportunities to do something enjoyable, such as going on a hike or taking a trip.
- *Manipulative reinforcers* are incentives, such as reduced rent in exchange for mowing the lawn or the promise of a better grade for doing an extra-credit project.
- *Possessional reinforcers* are tangible rewards, such as a new gadget or car.
- *Social reinforcers* are signs of appreciation, approval, or love, such as hugs or praise.

Successful positive reinforcement often lies in choosing choosing an incentive that motivates you to change. Your reinforcers may initially come from others (*extrinsic* rewards), but as you see positive changes in yourself you will begin to reward and reinforce yourself (*intrinsic* rewards). Reinforcers should immediately follow a behavior, but beware of overkill; if you reward yourself with a movie every time you go jogging, the reinforcer will soon lose its power. It would be better to give yourself such a reward after, say, a full week of adherence to your jogging program.

Journal Writing down personal experiences, interpretations, and results in a journal is an important skill for behavior change. You can log your daily activities, monitor your progress, record your feelings, and note ideas for improvement.

Let's Get Started

Once you have the skills to support successful behavior change, you can apply them to your target behavior. Create a behavior change contract incorporating the goals and skills discussed here, and place it where you'll see it every day as a reminder that change doesn't "just happen." (See Figure 1.6 for an example.) Reviewing your contract helps you stay alert to potential problems, be aware of your alternatives, maintain a firm sense of your values, and stick to your goals under pressure.

Skills for Behavior Change

CHALLENGE THE THOUGHTS THAT SABOTAGE CHANGE

Are thought patterns and beliefs holding you back? Try these strategies:

- **"I don't have enough time!"** Chart your activities for 1 day. What are your highest priorities? What can you eliminate or reduce? Plan to make some time for a healthy change next week.
- **"I'm too stressed!"** Assess your major stressors right now. List those you can control and those you can change or avoid. Then identify two things you enjoy that can help you reduce stress now.
- **"I'm worried what others may think."** How much do others influence your decisions about drinking, sex, eating habits, and the like? What is most important to you? What actions can you take to act in line with your values?
- **"I don't think I can."** Just because you haven't done something before doesn't mean you can't do it now. To develop confidence, take baby steps and break tasks into small chunks of time.
- **"I can't break this habit!"** Habits are difficult to break, but not impossible. What triggers your behavior? List ways you can avoid triggers. Ask for support from friends and family.

check yourself

- **Describe the behavior change strategies that you used. What were the benefits and disadvantages of each strategy?**

1.8

Behavior Change Contract

learning **outcome**

1.8 Complete a behavior change contract.

Complete the Assess Yourself questionnaire. After reviewing your results and considering the various factors that influence your decisions, choose a health behavior that you would like to change, starting this quarter or semester. Sign the contract at the bottom to affirm your commitment to making a healthy change and ask a friend to witness it.

My behavior change will be:

____

My long-term goal for this behavior change is:

____

These are three obstacles to change (things that I am currently doing or situations that contribute to this behavior or make it harder to change):

1. ____
2. ____
3. ____

The strategies I will use to overcome these obstacles are:

1. ____
2. ____
3. ____

Resources I will use to help me change this behavior include:

a friend/partner/relative: ______________________________

a school-based resource: ______________________________

a community-based resource: ______________________________

a book or reputable website: ______________________________

In order to make my goal more attainable, I have devised these short-term goals:

short-term goal	target date	reward
short-term goal	target date	reward
short-term goal	target date	reward

When I make the long-term behavior change described above, my reward will be:

______________________________ target date: ______________

I intend to make the behavior change described above. I will use the strategies and rewards to achieve the goals that will contribute to a healthy behavior change.

Signed: ______________________ Witness: ______________________

check yourself

- **Do you think that completing the contract will make it more likely that you will succeed in your behavior change? Why or why not?**

How Healthy Are You?

An interactive version of this assessment is available online in MasteringHealth.

Although we all recognize the importance of being healthy, it can be a challenge to sort out which behaviors are most likely to cause problems or which ones pose the greatest risk. *Before* you decide where to start, it is important to look at your current health status.

By completing the following assessment, you will have a clearer picture of health areas in which you excel and those that could use some work. Taking this assessment will also help you to reflect on components of health that you may not have thought about.

Answer each question, then total your score for each section and fill it in on the Personal Checklist at the end of the assessment for a general sense of your health profile. Think about the behaviors that influenced your score in each category. Would you like to change any of them? Choose the area that you'd like to improve, and then complete the Behavior Change Contract on the previous page. Use the contract to think through and implement a behavior change over the course of this class.

Each of the categories in this questionnaire is an important aspect of the total dimensions of health, but this is not a substitute for the advice of a qualified health care provider. Consider scheduling a thorough physical examination by a licensed physician or setting up an appointment with a mental health counselor at your school if you need help making a behavior change.

For each of the following, indicate how often you think the statements describe you.

1 Physical Health

	Never	Rarely	Some of the time	Usually or Always
1. I am happy with my body size and weight.	1	2	3	4
2. I engage in vigorous exercises such as brisk walking, jogging, swimming, or running for at least 30 minutes per day, three to four times per week.	1	2	3	4
3. I get at least 7 to 8 hours of sleep each night.	1	2	3	4
4. My immune system is strong, and my body heals itself quickly when I get sick or injured.	1	2	3	4
5. I listen to my body; when there is something wrong, I try to make adjustments to heal it or seek professional advice.	1	2	3	4

Total score for this section: ______

2 Social Health

	Never	Rarely	Some of the time	Usually or Always
1. I am open, honest, and get along well with others.	1	2	3	4
2. I participate in a wide variety of social activities and enjoy being with people who are different from me.	1	2	3	4
3. I try to be a "better person" and decrease behaviors that have caused problems in my interactions with others.	1	2	3	4
4. I am open and accessible to a loving and responsible relationship.	1	2	3	4
5. I try to see the good in my friends and do whatever I can to support them and help them feel good about themselves.	1	2	3	4

Total score for this section: ______

3 Emotional Health

	Never	Rarely	Some of the time	Usually or Always
1. I find it easy to laugh, cry, and show emotions like love, fear, and anger, and try to express these in positive, constructive ways.	1	2	3	4
2. I avoid using alcohol or other drugs as a means of helping me forget my problems.	1	2	3	4
3. I recognize when I am stressed and take steps to relax through exercise, quiet time, or other calming activities.	1	2	3	4
4. I try not to be too critical or judgmental of others and try to understand differences or quirks that I note in others.	1	2	3	4
5. I am flexible and adapt or adjust to change in a positive way.	1	2	3	4

Total score for this section: ______

4 Environmental Health

	Never	Rarely	Some of the time	Usually or Always
1. I buy recycled paper and purchase biodegradable detergents and cleaning agents, or make my own cleaning products, whenever possible.	1	2	3	4
2. I recycle paper, plastic, and metals; purchase refillable containers when possible; and try to minimize the amount of paper and plastics that I use.	1	2	3	4
3. I try to wear my clothes for longer periods between washing to reduce water consumption and the amount of detergents in our water sources.	1	2	3	4
4. I vote for pro-environment candidates in elections.	1	2	3	4
5. I minimize the amount of time that I run the faucet when I brush my teeth, shave, or shower.	1	2	3	4

Total score for this section: ______

5 Spiritual Health

1. I take time alone to think about what's important in life—who I am, what I value, where I fit in, and where I'm going.	1	2	3	4
2. I have faith in a greater power, be it a supreme being, nature, or the connectedness of all living things.	1	2	3	4
3. I engage in acts of caring and goodwill without expecting something in return.	1	2	3	4
4. I sympathize and empathize with those who are suffering and try to help them through difficult times.	1	2	3	4
5. I go for the gusto and experience life to the fullest.	1	2	3	4

Total score for this section: ______

6 Intellectual Health

	Never	Rarely	Some of the time	Usually or Always
1. I carefully consider my options and possible consequences as I make choices in life.	1	2	3	4
2. I learn from my mistakes and try to act differently the next time.	1	2	3	4
3. I have at least one hobby, learning activity, or personal growth activity that I make time for each week, something that improves me as a person.	1	2	3	4
4. I manage my time well rather than let time manage me.	1	2	3	4
5. My friends and family trust my judgment.	1	2	3	4

Total score for this section: ______

Although each of these six aspects of health is important, there are some factors that don't readily fit in one category. As college students, you face some unique risks that others may not have. For this reason, we have added a section to this self-assessment that focuses on personal health promotion and disease prevention. Answer these questions and add your results to the Personal Checklist in the following section.

7 Personal Health Promotion/Disease Prevention

1. If I were to be sexually active, I would use protection such as latex condoms, dental dams, and other means of reducing my risk of sexually transmitted infections.	1	2	3	4
2. I can have a good time at parties or during happy hours without binge drinking.	1	2	3	4
3. I have eaten too much in the last month and have forced myself to vomit to avoid gaining weight.	4	3	2	1
4. If I were to get a tattoo or piercing, I would go to a reputable person who follows strict standards of sterilization and precautions against bloodborne disease transmission.	1	2	3	4
5. I engage in extreme sports and find that I enjoy the highs that come with risking bodily harm through physical performance.	4	3	2	1

Total score for this section: ______

Personal Checklist

Now, total your scores for each section on the next page and compare them to what would be considered optimal scores. Are you surprised by your scores in any areas? Which areas do you need to work on?

	Ideal Score	Your Score
Physical health	20	________
Social health	20	________
Emotional health	20	________
Environmental health	20	________
Spiritual health	20	________
Intellectual health	20	________
Personal health promotion/ disease prevention	20	________

What Your Scores in Each Category Mean

Scores of 15–20: Outstanding! Your answers show that you are aware of the importance of these behaviors in your overall health. More important, you are putting your knowledge to work by practicing good health habits that should reduce your overall risks. Although you received a very high score on this part of the test, you may want to consider areas in which your scores could be improved.

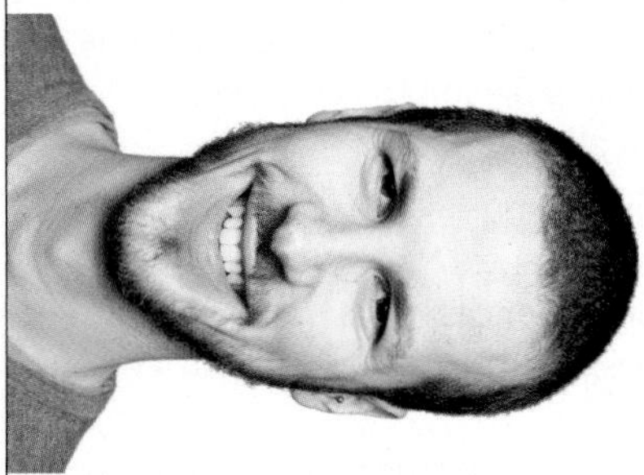

Scores of 10–14: Your health risks are showing! Find information about the risks you are facing and why it is important to change these behaviors. Perhaps you need help in deciding how to make the changes you desire. Assistance is available from this book, your professor, and student health services at your school.

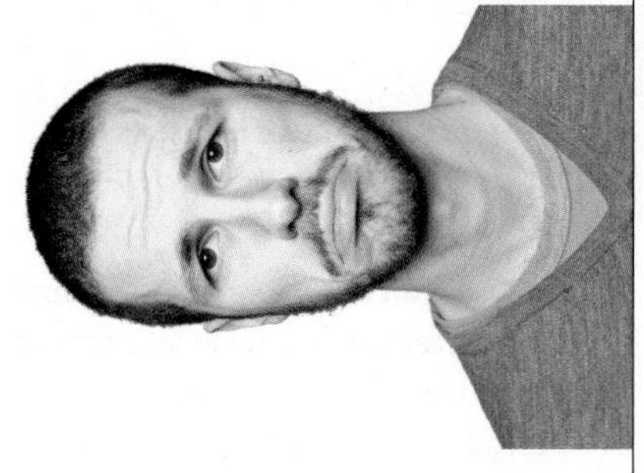

Scores below 10: You may be taking unnecessary risks with your health. Perhaps you are not aware of the risks and what to do about them. Identify each risk area and make a mental note as you read the associated chapter in this book. Whenever possible, seek additional resources, either on your campus or through your local community health resources, and make a serious commitment to behavior change. If any area is causing you to be less than functional in your class work or personal life, seek professional help. In this book you will find the information you need to help you improve your scores and your health. Remember that these scores are only indicators, not diagnostic tools.

Your Plan for Change

The Assess Yourself activity gave you the chance to look at the status of your health in several dimensions. Now that you have considered these results, you can take steps toward changing certain behaviors that may be detrimental to your health.

Today, you can:

◯ Evaluate your behavior and identify patterns and specific things you are doing.

◯ Select one pattern of behavior that you want to change.

◯ Fill out the Behavior Change Contract in this chapter. Be sure to include your long- and short-term goals for change, the rewards you'll give yourself for reaching these goals, the potential obstacles along the way, and your strategies for overcoming these obstacles. For each goal, list the small steps and specific actions that you will take.

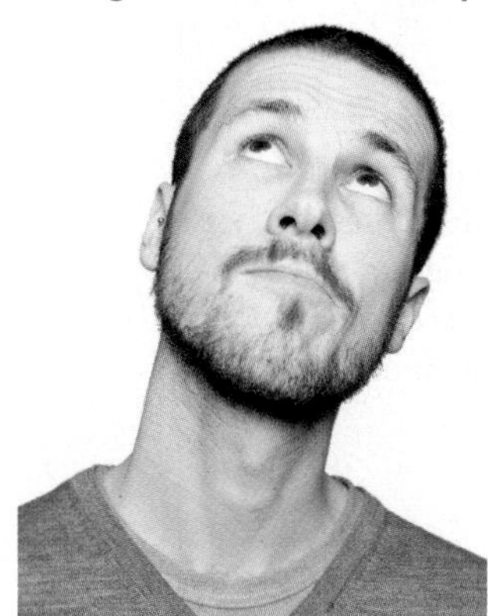

Within the next 2 weeks, you can:

◯ Start a journal and begin charting your progress toward your behavior change goal.

◯ Tell a friend or family member about your behavior change goal, and ask him or her to support you along the way.

◯ Reward yourself for reaching your short-term goals, and reevaluate your plan if you find that they are too ambitious.

By the end of the semester, you can:

◯ Review your journal entries and consider how successful you have been in following your plan. What helped you be successful? What made change more difficult? What will you do differently next week?

◯ Revise your plan as needed: Are the goals attainable? Are the rewards satisfying? Do you have enough support and motivation?

Summary

To hear an MP3 Tutor session, scan here or visit the Study Area in **MasteringHealth.**

LO 1.1 Health is the process of fulfilling one's potential in physical, social, emotional, spiritual, intellectual, and environmental dimensions of life. Wellness means achieving the best health possible in several dimensions.

LO 1.2 The goals of *Healthy People 2020* are to increase life span and the quality of life and to reduce and eliminate health disparities.

LO 1.3 Health is influenced by *determinants,* which the Surgeon General's health promotion plan, *Healthy People,* classifies as individual biology and behavior, the social environment, the physical environment, access to quality health care, and policies and interventions.

LO 1.4 Models of behavior change include health belief, social cognitive, and transtheoretical (stages of change) models. You can increase the chance of changing a behavior by viewing change as a process.

LO 1.5 When contemplating change, examine current habits, learn about a target behavior, and assess readiness.

LO 1.6 When preparing to change, set incremental goals, anticipate barriers to change, enlist support, and sign a behavior change contract.

LO 1.7 When taking action, visualize new behavior, practice countering, control the situation, change self-talk, reward yourself, and keep a log or journal.

Pop Quiz

Visit MasteringHealth to personalize your study plan with Chapter Review Quizzes and Dynamic Study Modules.

LO 1.1 1. Janice displays both high self-esteem and high self-efficacy. The dimension of health this relates to is the
a. social dimension.
b. emotional dimension.
c. spiritual dimension.
d. intellectual dimension.

LO 1.2 2. *Healthy People 2020 is*
a. a blueprint for actions designed to improve U.S. health.
b. a projection for life expectancy rates in the United States in the year 2020.
c. an international plan for achieving global health priorities for the environment by the year 2020.
d. a set of specific goals that states must achieve in order to receive federal funding for health.

LO 1.3 3. Which of the following is a *nonmodifiable* determinant for health?
a. Physical activity
b. Genetics
c. Nutrition
d. Tobacco use

LO 1.4 4. Cody has decided that he needs to improve his diet. He observes his roommates' healthy meal choices and decides to adopt some of their eating habits. This is an example of which model of behavior change?
a. Social cognitive
b. Health belief
c. Transtheoretical
d. Stages of change

LO 1.5 5. Jake is exhibiting *self-efficacy* when he
a. claims he will never be able to bench-press 125 pounds.
b. doubts he'll ever bench-press the weight he hopes for.
c. believes that he can and will be able to bench-press 125 pounds in his specified time frame.
d. does not believe he possesses personal control over this situation.

LO 1.5 6. Because Craig's parents smoked, he is 90 percent more likely to start smoking than someone whose parents didn't. This is an example of what factor influencing behavior change?
a. Circumstantial factor
b. Enabling factor
c. Reinforcing factor
d. Predisposing factor

LO 1.6 7. Suppose you want to lose 20 pounds. To reach your goal, you start by counting calories. After 2 weeks, you begin an exercise program and gradually build up to your desired fitness level. What behavior change strategy are you using?
a. Shaping
b. Visualization
c. Modeling
d. Reinforcement

LO 1.6 8. What strategy is advised for an individual in the preparation stage of change?
a. Seeking recommended readings
b. Finding ways to maintain positive behaviors
c. Setting realistic goals
d. Publicly stating the desire for change

LO 1.7 9. After Kirk and Tammy pay their bills, they reward themselves by watching TV together. This type of positive reinforcement is a(n)
a. activity reinforcer.
b. consumable reinforcer.
c. manipulative reinforcer.
d. possessional reinforcer.

LO 1.7 10. Aspects of a situation that cue or stimulate a person to act in certain ways are called
a. reinforcers.
b. antecedents.
c. consequences.
d. cues to action.

Answers to these questions can be found on page A-1. If you answered a question incorrectly, review the module identified by the Learning Outcome. For even more study tools, visit MasteringHealth.

Psychological Health

2

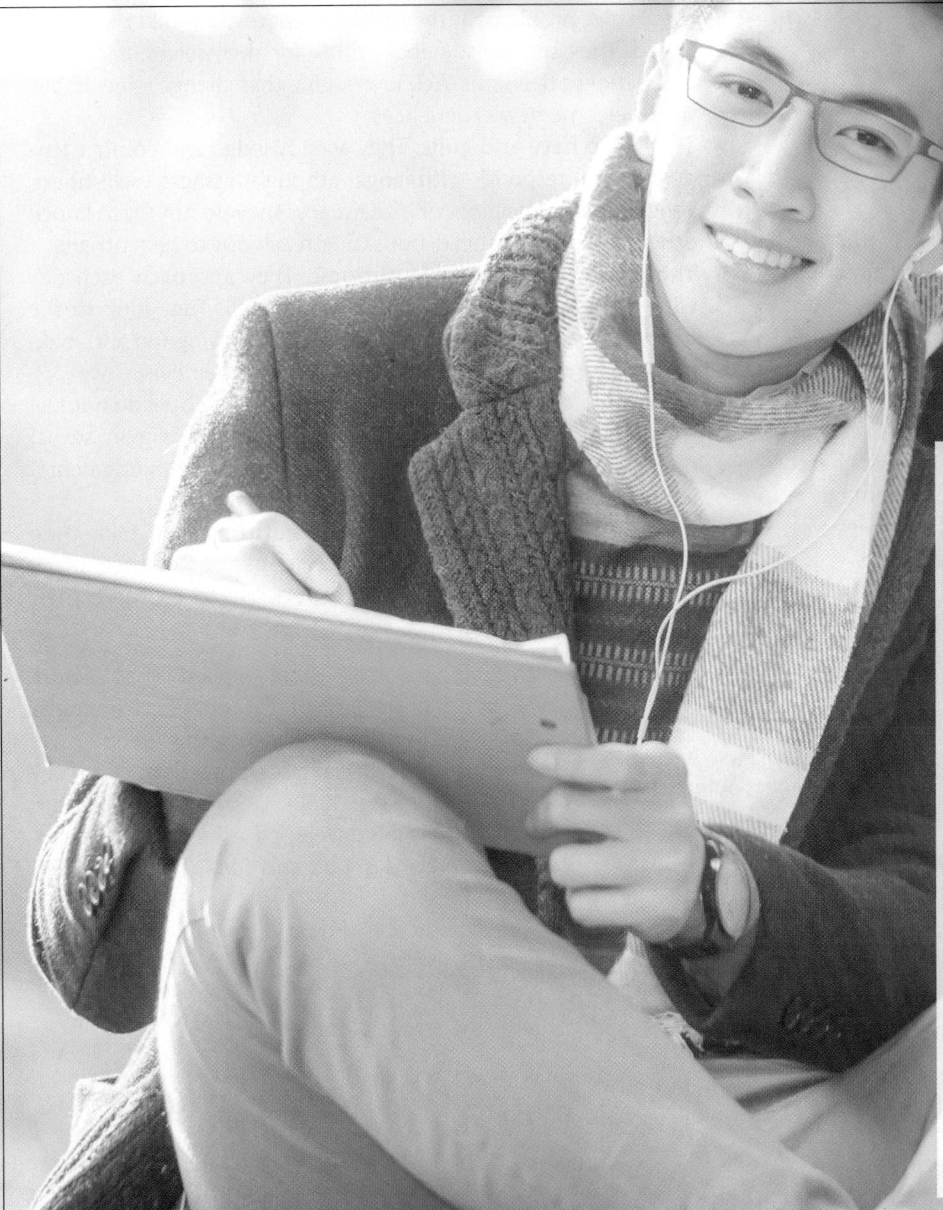

Although most college students describe their college years as among the best of their lives, many find the pressures of grades, finances, relationships, and the struggle to find themselves to be extraordinarily difficult. Psychological distress caused by relationship issues, family issues, academic competition, and adjusting to life as a college student is common. Many experts believe that the often anxiety-inducing campus environment is a major contributor to poor health decisions, such as high levels of alcohol consumption, and, in turn, to health problems that ultimately affect academic success and success in life.

Fortunately, even though we often face seemingly insurmountable pressures, human beings possess a **resiliency** that can enable us to cope, adapt, and even thrive in the face of life's challenges. How we feel and think about ourselves, those around us, and our environment can tell us a lot about our psychological health and whether we are healthy emotionally, socially, spiritually, and mentally.

2.1 What Is Psychological Health?

learning outcome

2.1 Describe basic characteristics shared by psychologically healthy people, and identify each level in Maslow's hierarchy of needs.

Psychological health is the sum of how we think, feel, relate, and exist in our day-to-day lives. Our thoughts, perceptions, emotions, motivations, interpersonal relationships, and behaviors are the product of a combination of our experiences and the skills we have developed to meet life's challenges. Most experts identify several basic elements shared by psychologically healthy people:

- **They feel good about themselves.** They are not typically overwhelmed by fear, love, anger, jealousy, guilt, or worry. They know who they are, have a realistic sense of their capabilities, and respect themselves even though they realize that they aren't perfect.
- **They feel comfortable with other people and express respect and compassion toward others.** They enjoy satisfying and lasting personal relationships and do not take advantage of others or allow others to take advantage of them. They recognize that there are others whose needs are greater than their own and take responsibility for their fellow human beings. They can give love, consider others' interests, take time to help others, and respect personal differences.
- **They control tension and anxiety.** They recognize the underlying causes and symptoms of stress and anxiety in their lives and consciously avoid irrational thoughts, hostility, excessive excuse making, and blaming others for their problems. They use resources and learn skills to control their reactions to stressful situations.
- **They meet the demands of life.** Psychologically healthy people try to solve problems as they arise, accept responsibility, and plan ahead. They set realistic goals, think for themselves, and make independent decisions. Acknowledging that change is inevitable, they welcome new experiences.
- **They curb hate and guilt.** They acknowledge and combat tendencies to respond with anger, thoughtlessness, selfishness, vengefulness, or feelings of inadequacy. They do not try to knock others aside to get ahead, but rather reach out to help others.
- **They maintain a positive outlook.** They approach each day with a presumption that things will go well. They look to the future with enthusiasm rather than dread. Having fun and making time for themselves are integral parts of their lives.
- **They value diversity.** Psychologically healthy people do not feel threatened by those of a different race, gender, religion, sexual orientation, ethnicity, or political party. They are nonjudgmental and do not force their beliefs and values on others.
- **They appreciate and respect nature.** They take time to enjoy their surroundings, are conscious of their place in the universe, and act responsibly to preserve their environment.

Psychologists have long argued that before we can achieve any of the above characteristics of psychologically healthy people, we must have certain basic needs met in our lives. In the 1960s, psychologist Abraham Maslow developed a *hierarchy of needs* to describe this idea (Figure 2.1). At

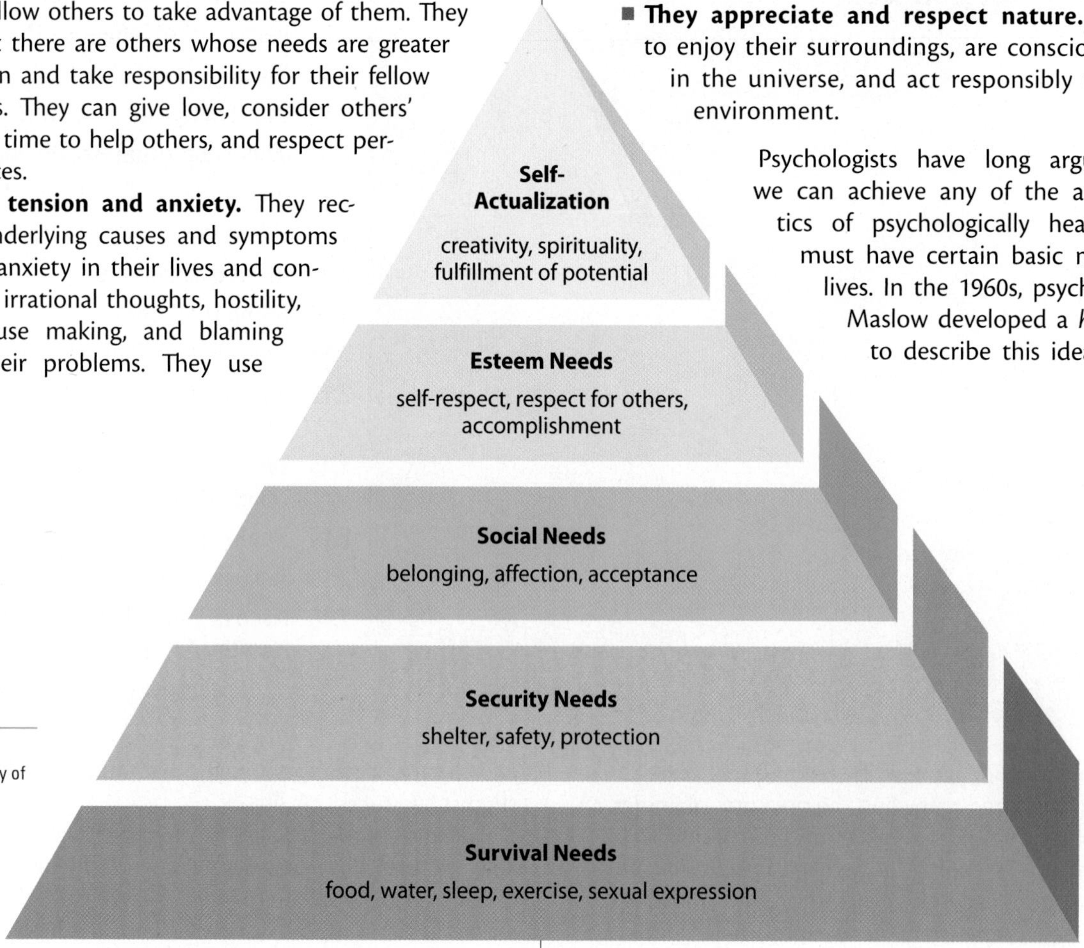

Figure 2.1 Maslow's Hierarchy of Needs

VIDEO TUTOR
Maslow's Hierarchy of Needs

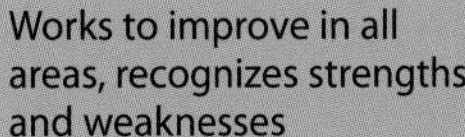

Psychologically unhealthy			Psychologically healthy
No zest for life; pessimistic/cynical most of the time; spiritually down	Shows poorer coping than most, often overwhelmed by circumstances	Works to improve in all areas, recognizes strengths and weaknesses	Possesses zest for life; spiritually healthy and intellectually thriving
Laughs, but usually at others, has little fun	Has regular relationship problems, finds that others often disappoint	Healthy relationships with family and friends, capable of giving and receiving love and affection	High energy, resilient, enjoys challenges, focused
Has serious bouts of depression, "down" and tired much of time; has suicidal thoughts	Tends to be cynical/critical of others; tends to have negative/critical friends	Has strong social support, may need to work on improving social skills but usually no major problems	Realistic sense of self and others, sound coping skills, open minded
A "challenge" to be around, socially isolated	Lacks focus much of the time, hard to keep intellectual acuity sharp	Has occasional emotional "dips" but overall good mental/emotional adaptors	Adapts to change easily, sensitive to others and environment
Experiences many illnesses, headaches, aches/pains, gets colds/infections easily	Quick to anger, sense of humor and fun evident less often		Has strong social support and healthy relationships with family and friends

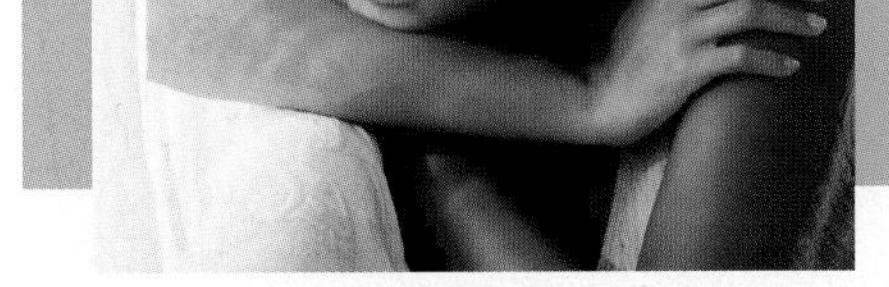

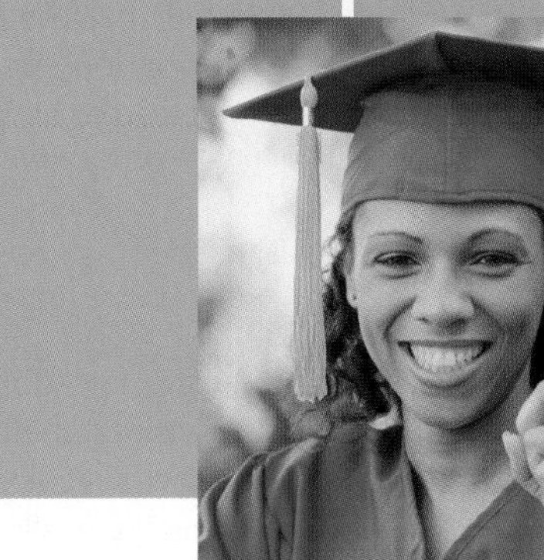

Figure 2.2 Characteristics of Psychologically Healthy and Unhealthy People
Where do you fall on this continuum?

the bottom of his hierarchy are basic *survival needs*, such as food, sleep, and water; at the next level are *security needs*, such as shelter and safety; at the third level—*social needs*—is a sense of belonging and affection; at the fourth level are *esteem needs*, self-respect and respect for others; and at the top are needs for *self-actualization* and self-transcendence.

According to Maslow's theory, a person's needs must be met at each of these levels before that person can ever truly be healthy. Failure to meet any of the lower levels of needs will interfere with a person's ability to address upper-level needs. For example, someone who is homeless or worried about threats of violence will be unable to focus on fulfilling social, esteem, or actualization needs.[1]

In sum, psychologically healthy people are emotionally, mentally, socially, and spiritually resilient. They most often respond to challenges and frustrations in appropriate ways, despite occasional slips (see Figure 2.2). When they do slip, they recognize that fact and take action to rectify the situation.

Attaining psychological well-being involves many complex processes. This chapter will help you understand not only what it means to be psychologically well, but also why we may run into problems in our psychological health. Learning how to assess your own health and take action to help yourself are important aspects of psychological health.

check yourself

- **What are the basic characteristics shared by psychologically healthy people?**
- **What are basic characteristics of psychologically unhealthy people?**
- **At which level of Maslow's hierarchy of needs do you face the most challenges?**

2.2 Dimensions of Psychological Health

learning outcome

2.2 List and define each dimension of psychological health.

Psychological health includes mental, emotional, social, and spiritual dimensions (see Figure 2.3).

Mental Health

The term **mental health** is used to describe the "thinking" or "rational" dimension of our health. A mentally healthy person perceives life in realistic ways, can adapt to change, can develop rational strategies to solve problems, and can carry out personal and professional responsibilities. In addition, a mentally healthy person has the intellectual ability to learn and use information effectively and strive for continued growth. This is often referred to as *intellectual health*, a subset of mental health.[2]

Emotional Health

The term **emotional health** refers to the feeling, or subjective, side of psychological health. **Emotions** are intensified feelings or complex patterns of feelings that we experience on a regular basis, including love, hate, frustration, anxiety, and joy. Typically, emotions are described as the interplay of four components: physiological arousal, feelings, cognitive (thought) processes, and behavioral reactions. As rational beings, we are responsible for evaluating our individual emotional responses, their causes, and the appropriateness of our actions.

Emotionally healthy people usually respond appropriately to upsetting events. Rather than reacting in an extreme fashion or behaving inconsistently or offensively, they can express their feelings, communicate with others, and show emotions in appropriate ways. Emotionally unhealthy people are much more likely to let their feelings overpower them. They may be highly volatile and prone to unpredictable emotional responses, which may be followed by inappropriate communication or actions.

Emotional intelligence is the ability to identify, use, understand, and manage one's emotions in positive and constructive ways. Emotional intelligence consists of four core abilities: self-awareness, self-management, relationship management, and social awareness. Developing your emotional intelligence can help you build strong relationships, succeed at work, and achieve your goals.[3]

Emotional health also affects social and intellectual health. People who feel hostile, withdrawn, or moody may become socially isolated. Because they are not much fun to be around, friends may avoid them at the very time they are most in need of emotional support. A concern for students is the impact of emotional trauma on academic performance. Have you ever tried to study for an exam after a fight with a close friend or family member? Emotional turmoil can seriously affect your ability to think, reason, and act rationally.

Social Health

Social health includes a person's interactions with others on an individual and group basis, the ability to use social resources and support in times of need, and the ability to adapt to a variety of social situations. Socially healthy individuals enjoy a wide range of interactions with family, friends, and acquaintances and are able to have healthy interactions with an intimate partner. Typically, socially healthy individuals can listen, express themselves,

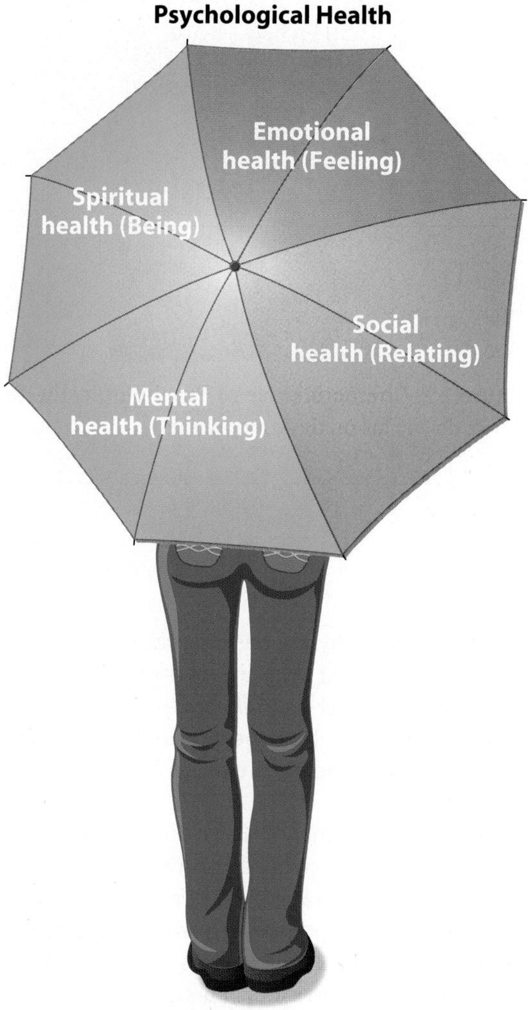

Figure 2.3 Psychological Health
Psychological health is a complex interaction of the mental, emotional, social, and spiritual dimensions of health. Possessing strength and resiliency in these dimensions can maintain your overall well-being and help you weather the storms of life.

How can I increase the **social support** in my life?

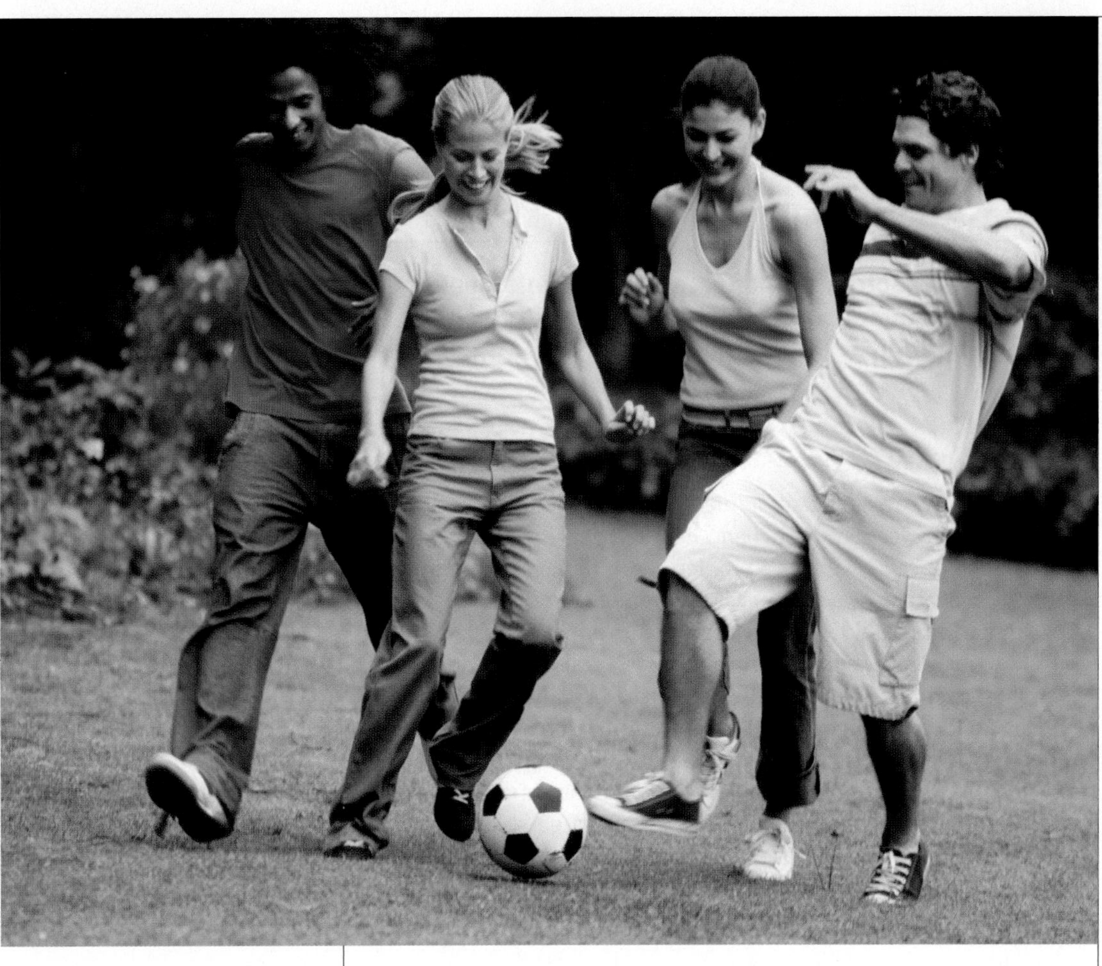

Fostering a solid social support group can be as simple as spending time playing a game with friends. Physical health affects mental health, so doing something active with others is doubly beneficial.

form healthy attachments, act in socially acceptable and responsible ways, and find the best fit for themselves in society. Numerous studies have documented the importance of positive relationships with family members, friends, and significant others in overall well-being and longevity.[4]

Social bonds, which reflect the level of closeness and attachment that we develop with other individuals, are the very foundation of human life. They provide intimacy, feelings of belonging, opportunities for giving and receiving nurturance, reassurance of one's worth, assistance and guidance, and advice. Social bonds take multiple forms, the most common of which are social support and community engagements.

The concept of **social support** is more complex than many people realize. In general, it refers to the networks of people and services with whom and which we interact and share social connections. These ties can provide *tangible support*, such as babysitting services or money to help pay the bills, or *intangible support*, such as encouraging you to share your concerns. Sometimes, support can just be the knowledge that someone would be there for you in a crisis. Generally, the closer and the higher the quality of the social bond with someone, the more likely one is to ask for and receive social support. For example, if your car broke down late at night, whom could you call for help—and know that the person would do everything possible to help you? Common descriptions of strong social support include the following:[5]

- Being cared for and loved, with shared intimacy
- Being esteemed and valued
- Sharing companionship, communication, and mutual obligations with others; having a sense of belonging
- Having "informational" support—access to information, advice, community services, and guidance from others

Spiritual Health

It is possible to be mentally, emotionally, and socially healthy and still not achieve optimal psychological well-being. What is missing? For many people, the difficult-to-describe element that gives purpose to life is the spiritual dimension.

Spirituality is broader in meaning than religion; it goes beyond material values and can be defined as an individual's sense of purpose and meaning in life and sense of peace and connection to others.[6] Spirituality may be practiced in many ways, including through religion; however, religion does not have to be part of a person's spiritual life. **Spiritual health** refers to the sense of belonging to something greater than the purely physical or personal dimensions of existence. For some, this unifying force is nature; for others, it is a feeling of connection to other people; for still others, the unifying force is a god or other higher power.

check yourself

- **When you think of someone as being "mentally healthy," what characteristics come to mind?**
- **What are the dimensions of psychological health?**
- **Assess your psychological health in each of the dimensions discussed here.**

2.3 Factors That Influence Psychological Health

learning outcome

2.3 Identify factors that affect your psychological health, and describe the interaction between psychological well-being and health.

The Family

Families have a significant influence on psychological development. Healthy families model and help develop the cognitive and social skills necessary to solve problems, communicate emotions in socially acceptable ways, manage stress, and develop a sense of self-worth and purpose. Children raised in nurturing homes are more likely to become well-adjusted, productive adults. In adulthood, family support is one of the best predictors of health and happiness.[7] Children brought up in **dysfunctional families**—in which there is violence; distrust; anger; deprivation; drug abuse; parental discord; or sexual, physical, or emotional abuse—may have a harder time adapting to life and run an increased risk of psychological problems. Yet not everyone raised in dysfunctional families becomes psychologically unhealthy, and not everyone from healthy environments becomes well adjusted.

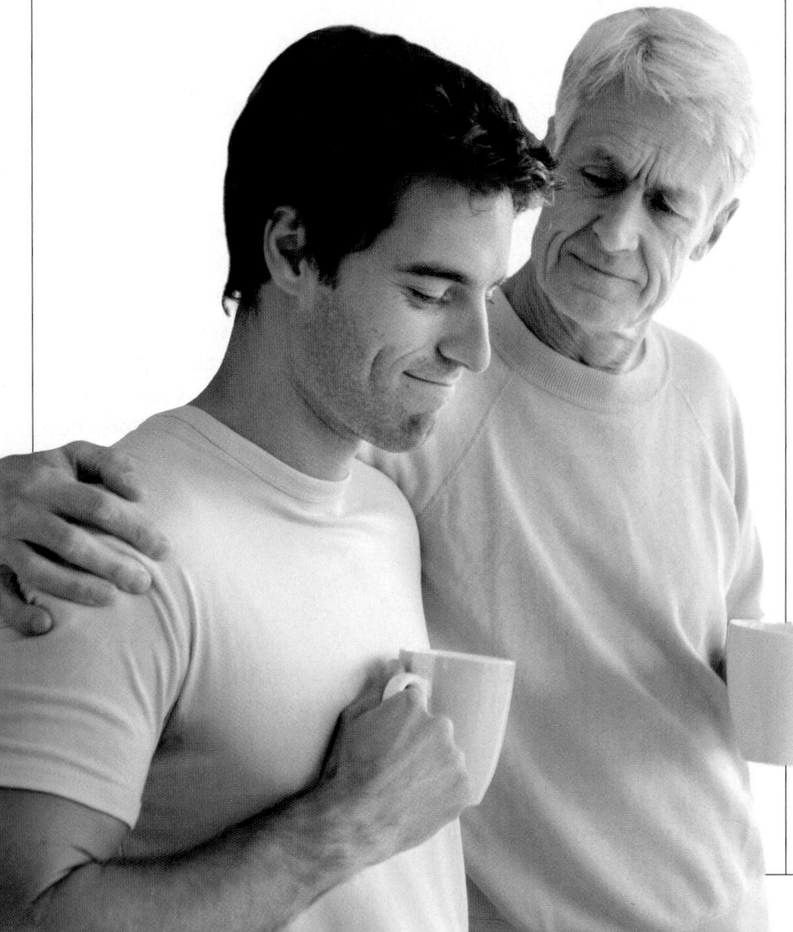

Support System

Initial social support may be provided by family, but as we develop, the support of peers becomes more and more important. We rely on friends to help us figure out who we are and what we want to do with our lives. We often bounce ideas off friends to see if they think we are being logical, smart, or fair. Research shows that college students with adequate social support have improved overall well-being, including higher GPAs, higher perceived ability in math and science courses, less peer pressure for binge drinking, lower rates of suicide, and higher overall life satisfaction.[8] Having people in our lives who provide positive support and whom we can rely on is important to our psychological health.

Community

Our communities can affect our psychological health through collective actions. For example, neighbors may come together to pick up trash, participate in a neighborhood watch, or initiate a community picnic. You are part of a campus community, which can support psychological health by creating a safe environment in which to develop your mental, emotional, social, and spiritual dimensions.

Self-Efficacy and Self-Esteem

During our formative years, successes and failures in school, athletics, friendships, relationships, jobs, and every other aspect of life subtly shape our beliefs about our personal worth and abilities. These beliefs in turn become influences on our psychosocial health.

Self-efficacy describes a person's belief about whether he or she can successfully engage in and execute a specific behavior. Self-efficacy is a result of life experiences, and our successes and failures. **Self-esteem** refers to one's sense of self-respect or self-worth. People with high levels of self-efficacy and self-esteem tend to express a positive outlook on life.

How do others influence my psychological well-being?

Your outlook on life is determined in part by your social and cultural surroundings, and your general sense of well-being can be strongly affected by the positive or negative nature of your social bonds.

In particular, family members shape your psychological health. As you were growing up, they modeled behaviors and skills that helped you develop cognitively and socially. Their love and support can give you a sense of self-worth and encourage you to treat others with compassion and care.

Self-esteem results from the relationships we have with our parents and family growing up; with our friends as we grow older; with our significant others as we form intimate relationships; and with our teachers, coworkers, and others throughout our lives.

Psychologist Martin Seligman proposed that people who continually experience failure may develop a pattern of responding known as **learned helplessness,** in which they give up and fail to take action to help themselves. Seligman ascribes this response in part to society's tendency toward *victimology*—blaming one's problems on other people and circumstances.[9] Although viewing ourselves as victims may make us feel better temporarily, it does not address the underlying causes of a problem. Ultimately, it can erode self-efficacy.

Many self-help programs use elements of Seligman's principle of **learned optimism**—the idea that by changing our self-talk, examining our reactions, and blocking negative thoughts, we can "unlearn" negative thought processes that have become habitual.

Personality

Your personality is the unique mix of characteristics that distinguishes you from others, as influenced by heredity, environment, culture, and experience. Personality determines how we react to the challenges of life, interpret our feelings, and resolve conflicts.

Recent psychological theories promote the idea that we have the power to understand and change our behavior, thus molding our own personalities.[10] A leading personality theory distills personality into five traits:[11]

- **Agreeableness**—People who score high are trusting, likable, and demonstrate friendly compliance and love, while low scorers are critical and suspicious.
- **Openness**—People who score high demonstrate curiosity, independence, and imagination, while low scorers are more conventional and down-to-earth.
- **Neuroticism**—People who score high are anxious and insecure, while those who score low show the ability to maintain emotional control.
- **Conscientiousness**—People who score high are dependable and demonstrate self-control, discipline, and a need to achieve, while low scorers are disorganized and impulsive.
- **Extroversion**—People who score high adapt well to social situations, demonstrate assertiveness, and draw enjoyment from the company of others, while low scorers are more reserved and passive.

Life Span and Maturity

Our temperaments change as we grow, and most of us learn to control our emotions as we age. The college years mark a transition period for young adults as they move away from families and become independent. This transition is easier for those who have accomplished earlier developmental tasks such as learning how to solve problems, to make and evaluate decisions, to define and adhere to personal values, and to establish both casual and intimate relationships. People who have not fulfilled these earlier tasks may find their lives interrupted by recurrent crises left over from earlier stages. For example, those who did not learn to trust others in childhood may have difficulty establishing intimate relationships as adults.

The Mind-Body Connection

Your emotional states can impact your overall health, especially in conditions of stress. At the core of this mind-body connection is the study of **psychoneuroimmunology (PNI)**, or how the brain and behavior affect the body's immune system.

Happiness—a collective term for positive states in which individuals actively embrace the world around them— appears to be particularly promising in enhancing physical health.[12] Happiness, and related psychological states such as hopefulness, optimism, and contentment, can have a profound impact on the body, appearing to reduce the risk or limit the severity of cardiovascular disease, diabetes, colds, and other infections.[13] Laughter can promote increases in heart and respiration rates and can reduce levels of stress hormones in much the same way as light exercise can. For this reason, it has been promoted as a possible risk reducer for people with hypertension and other forms of cardiovascular disease.[14]

Subjective well-being is that uplifting feeling of inner peace or an overall "feel-good" state, which includes happiness. It is defined by three components: satisfaction with present life, relative presence of positive emotions, and relative absence of negative emotions.[15] Everyone experiences disappointments, unhappiness, and times when life seems unfair. However, people with a high level of subjective well-being are typically resilient, able to look on the positive side, and less likely to fall into despair over setbacks.

Seligman suggests that we can develop well-being by practicing positive psychological actions. He describes five elements of well-being that help humans flourish:[16]

- **Positive emotion**—How happy and satisfied are you?
- **Engagement**—Can you get completely absorbed in a task?
- **Relationships**—Are there people in life who really care about you?
- **Meaning**—Are you working toward something bigger than yourself?
- **Accomplishment**—How hard will you work for something?

check yourself

- **What factors affect your psychological health?**
- **How does a person's psychological state affect his or her health?**
- **List three elements of well-being that help humans flourish.**

2.4 Strategies to Enhance Psychological Health

learning outcome

2.4 Describe behavior change strategies to improve psychological health.

As we have seen, psychological health involves four dimensions. Attaining self-fulfillment is a lifelong, conscious process that involves enhancing each of these components. Strategies include building self-efficacy and self-esteem, understanding and controlling emotions, maintaining support networks, and learning to solve problems and make decisions. Try the following strategies to support and improve your own psychological health:

- **Develop a support system.** One of the best ways to promote self-esteem is through a support system of peers and others who share your values. Members of your support system can help you feel good about yourself and force you to take an honest look at your actions and choices.

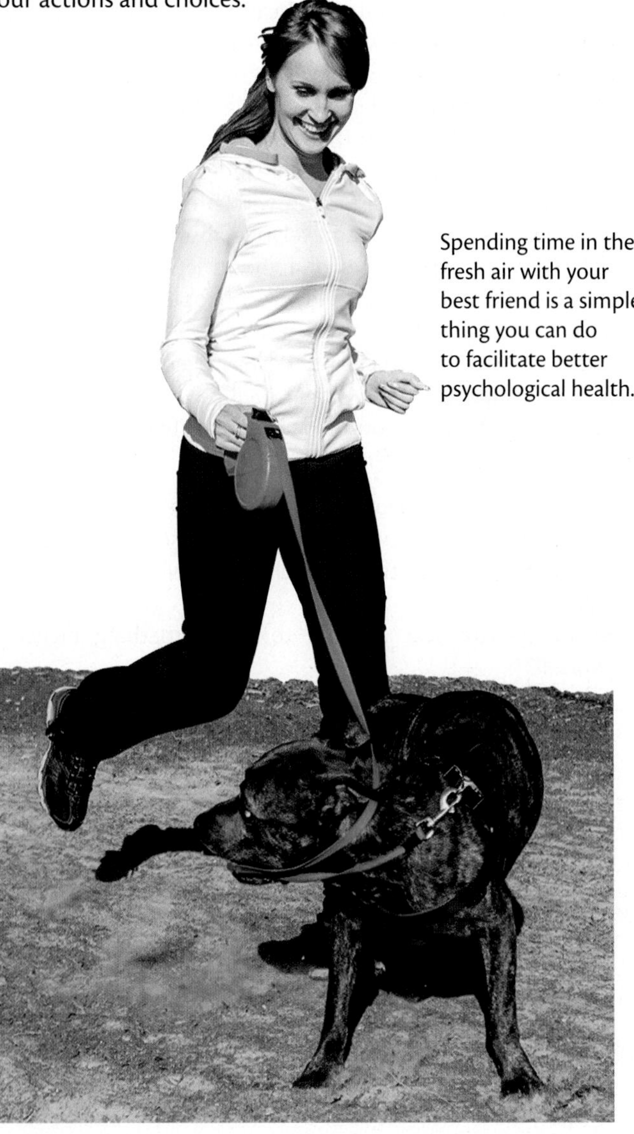

Spending time in the fresh air with your best friend is a simple thing you can do to facilitate better psychological health.

- **Complete required tasks to the best of your ability.** A good way to boost your sense of self-efficacy is to learn new skills and develop a history of success. Most college campuses provide study groups and learning centers that can help you manage time, develop study skills, and prepare for tests.
- **Form realistic expectations.** If you expect perfect grades, a steady stream of dates, and the perfect job, you may be setting yourself up for failure. Assess your current resources and the direction in which you are heading. Set small, incremental goals that you can actually meet.
- **Make time for you.** Taking time to enjoy your life is another way to boost your self-esteem and psychosocial health. View a new activity as something to look forward to and an opportunity to have fun.
- **Maintain physical health.** Regular exercise fosters a sense of well-being. More and more research supports the role of exercise in improved mental health.
- **Examine problems and seek help when necessary.** Knowing when to seek help from friends, support groups, family, or professionals is an important factor in boosting self-esteem. Sometimes you can handle life's problems alone; at other times you need assistance.
- **Get adequate sleep.** Getting enough sleep on a daily basis is a key factor in physical and psychological health. Not only do our bodies need to rest to conserve energy for our daily activities, but we also need to restore supplies of many of the neurotransmitters that we use up during our waking hours.

Skills for Behavior Change

TIPS TO ENHANCE YOUR SUPPORT NETWORK AND MAINTAIN POSITIVE RELATIONSHIPS

- **Keep in contact.** Call, e-mail, or visit those close to you. Old friends and important family members can provide a foundation of unconditional love that will help you through life transitions.
- **Lend a listening ear.** Pay attention to your friends' emotions, and be there for them when they're down. They'll be more likely to reciprocate for you when you're in a rough spot.
- **Make time for others.** Chatting with a classmate after class, sharing a story over coffee with a coworker, or inviting a new friend to hang out are all ways to foster lasting relationships.

check yourself

- **Which of these strategies do you think would be most effective for you?**
- **List five things you think would improve the psychological health of college students today.**

What Is Spiritual Health?

learning **outcome**

2.5 Define spirituality and describe how religion and values affect spirituality.

A majority of American college students share a desire to find a sense of purpose, meaning, and harmony in life. According to UCLA's Higher Education Research Institute (HERI), incoming undergraduate students have a wide spectrum of spiritual and ethical considerations.[17] Data from more than 192,912 students at 283 colleges and universities surveyed in 2012 found that, compared to their peers, 35.9 percent of incoming freshmen rated themselves above average in spirituality, 51.5 percent in emotional health, and 79.6 percent in being able to work with a diverse population.[18] Of those surveyed, 87.4 percent also reported volunteering in the past year, and 57.2 percent reported participating in community service as part of a class. Lastly, 73 percent of students reported high levels of being tolerant of diverse beliefs.[19]

What Is Spirituality?

Spirituality tends to defy the boundaries that strict definitions impose. The word's root, *spirit*, in many cultures refers to *breath*, or the force that animates life. When you're "inspired," your energy flows. You're not held back by doubts about the purpose or meaning of your work and life. Many definitions incorporate this sense of transcendence; the National Cancer Institute defines **spirituality** as an individual's sense of peace, purpose, and connection to others, and beliefs about the meaning of life.[20] Harold G. Koenig, MD, one of the foremost researchers of spirituality and health, defines spirituality as the personal quest for understanding answers to ultimate questions about life, meaning, and relationship with the sacred or transcendent.[21]

Spirituality may include participation in organized **religion**—a system of beliefs, practices, rituals, and symbols designed to facilitate closeness to the sacred or transcendent.[22] Most individuals consider spirituality to be important in their lives, but not necessarily in the form of religion: A global survey revealed that 1 in 6 people worldwide are religiously unaffiliated.[23] Even though they might not affiliate with a particular religion, they may still have certain religious or spiritual beliefs.[24]

Elements of Spirituality

Brian Luke Seaward, a professor at the University of Northern Colorado and author of several books on spirituality and mind-body healing, identifies the core of human spirituality as consisting of three elements: relationships, values, and purpose in life (Figure 2.4).[25]

Have you ever wondered if someone you were attracted to is right for you, or if you should break off a relationship? Have you wished you had more friends, or that you were a better friend to yourself? Such questions about relationships and yearnings are often triggers for spiritual growth.

Our **values** are our principles—the set of fundamental rules by which we conduct our lives. When we attempt to clarify our values and to live according to them, we're engaging in spiritual work.

What career do you plan to pursue? Do you hope to marry? Do you plan to have or adopt children? What things make you feel "complete"? Contemplating such questions about one's purpose in life fosters spiritual growth. People who are spiritually healthy are able to articulate their purpose, and to make choices that manifest that purpose.

Our relationships, values, and sense of purpose together contribute to our overall **spiritual intelligence (SI)**. This term was introduced by physicist and philosopher Danah Zohar, who defined it as "an ability to access higher meanings, values, abiding purposes, and unconscious aspects of the self."[26] Zohar includes self-awareness, spontaneity, and compassion in her definition, explaining that SI helps us use meanings, values, and purposes to live richer and more creative lives.

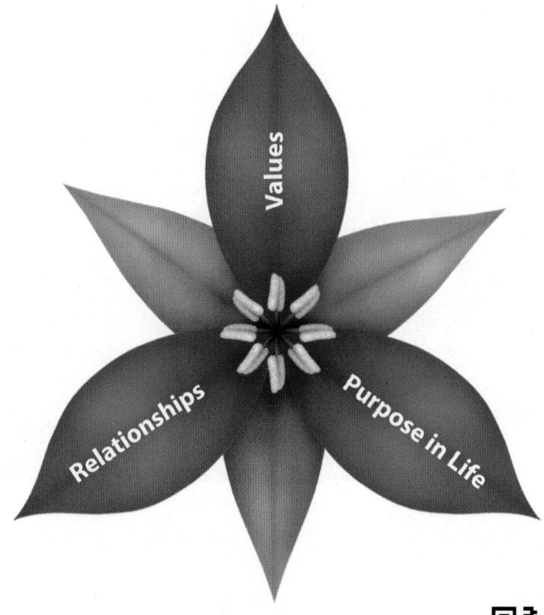

Figure 2.4 Three Facets of Spirituality
Most of us are prompted to explore our spirituality because of questions relating to our relationships, values, and purpose in life. At the same time, these three facets together constitute spiritual well-being.

VIDEO TUTOR
Facets of Spirituality

check yourself

- **What are some components of spirituality and spiritual intelligence?**

2.6 Why Is Spiritual Health Important?

learning outcome

2.6 Explain how spirituality contributes to physical and psychosocial health.

A broad range of large-scale surveys have documented the importance of the mind–body connection to human health and wellness.[27]

Physical Benefits

The emerging science of mind-body medicine is a research focus of the National Center for Complementary and Alternative Medicine (NCCAM) and an important objective of the organization's 2011–2015 Strategic Plan. One area under study is the association between spiritual health and general health. The NCCAM cites evidence that spirituality can have a positive influence on health and suggests that the connection may be due to improved immune function, cardiovascular function, or a combination of physiological changes.[28] Increasing numbers of studies are showing that certain spiritual practices, such as yoga, deep meditation, and prayer, can affect the mind, body, and behavior in ways that have potential to treat many health problems and promote healthy behavior. Ongoing research is investigating the role spirituality plays in treating insomnia, substance abuse, specific pain conditions, irritable bowel syndrome, obesity, and more.[29]

Some researchers believe that a key to understanding the improved health and longer life of spiritually healthy people is mindfulness training. In a recent study, participants who practiced mindfulness meditation showed notable changes in regions of the brain associated with stress and memory. These changes indicate that they may be more likely to cope better with stress on a daily basis.[30] Research also shows that mindfulness can increase memory, reduce emotional reactivity, and increase satisfaction with relationships, as well as improve fear modulation, intuition, and a sense of morality.[31]

Studies also suggest that meditation improves the brain's ability to process information; reduces stress, anxiety, and depression; improves concentration; and decreases blood pressure.[32] The physiological processes that produce these effects are only partially understood. One theory suggests meditation works by reducing the body's stress response. By practicing deep, calm contemplation, people who meditate seem to promote activity in the body's systems, leading to slower breathing, lower blood pressure, and easier digestion, along with the spiritual benefits.[33]

The National Cancer Institute (NCI) contends that when we get sick, spiritual or religious well-being may help restore health and improve quality of life because it does the following:[34]

- Decreases anxiety, depression, anger, discomfort, and feelings of isolation
- Decreases alcohol and drug abuse
- Decreases blood pressure and the risk of heart disease
- Increases the person's ability to cope with the effects of illness and with medical treatments
- Increases feelings of hope and optimism, freedom from regret, satisfaction with life, and inner peace

Several studies show an association between spiritual health and a person's ability to cope with a variety of physical illnesses, including cancer.[35] For example, a study of cardiac patients showed a benefit related to spiritual health and mind-body techniques.[36] Researchers have also looked into the overall association between spiritual practices and mortality, and a review of over a decade of

3 out of 5

entering first-year college students report that they are actively "searching for meaning and purpose in life."

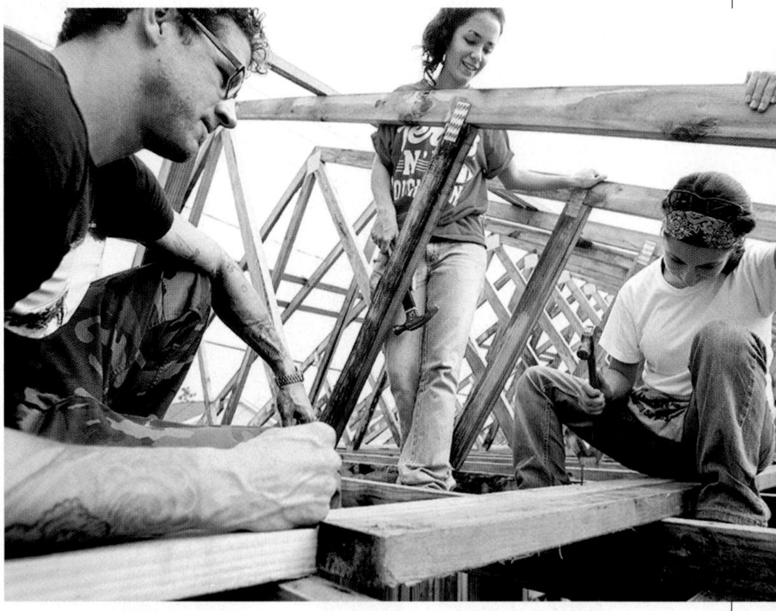

Can volunteers benefit from helping others?

Volunteering, and the associated "helpers high," can positively impact an individual's overall health. Many students contribute their time and skills to volunteer organizations, as these students are doing by working to build homes for Habitat for Humanity.

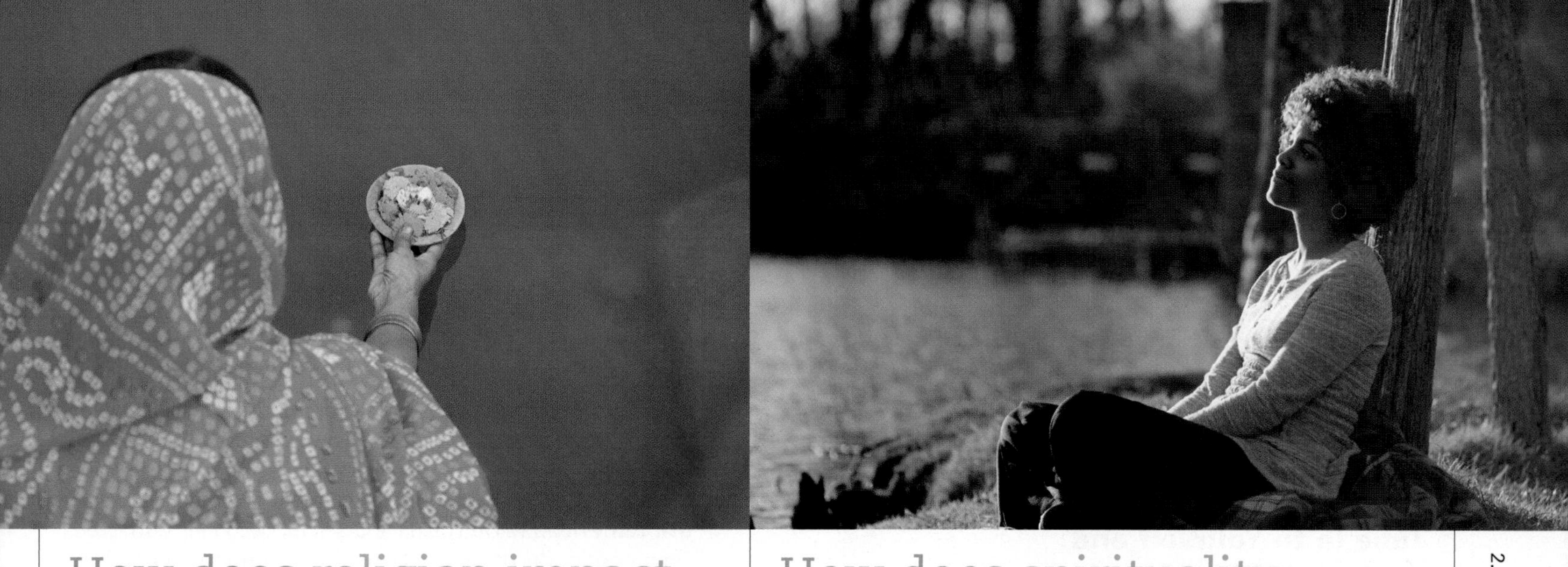

How does religion impact health?

Many people find that religious practices, such as the offerings this Hindu woman is preparing to place in the sacred Ganges River, help them to focus on their spirituality. Spiritual well-being, including the use of prayer, can increase the ability to cope and decrease stress.

How does spirituality influence health?

Spirituality is widely acknowledged to have a positive impact on health and wellness. The benefits range from reductions in overall morbidity and mortality to improved abilities to cope with illness and stress.

research studies indicated that individuals who incorporate spiritual practices regularly have a significant reduction in mortality and risk of cardiovascular events.[37]

Psychological Benefits

Current research also suggests that spiritual health contributes to psychological health. For instance, the NCI and independent studies have found that spirituality reduces levels of anxiety and depression.[38]

People who have found a spiritual community also benefit from increased social support. For instance, participation in religious services, charitable organizations, and social gatherings can help members avoid isolation. At such gatherings, clerics and others may offer spiritual support in regard to challenges that members may be facing. A community may include retired members who offer child care for working parents, meals for those with disabilities, or transportation to medical appointments. All such measures can contribute to members' overall feelings of security and belonging.

Meditation has been found to have specific benefits for psychological health. The NCCAM reports that researchers using brain-scanning techniques found experienced meditators to show a significantly increased level of *empathy*—the ability to understand and share another person's experience.[39] Similarly, a recent study found that participants who practiced a specific form of meditation, known as *compassion meditation*, further increased their levels of compassion toward others.[40]

Being genuinely concerned for others and lending a helping hand is a key aspect of a spiritually healthy lifestyle. Researchers have referred to the benefits of volunteering as a "helpers high," or a distinct sensation associated with helping. About half of participants in one study reported that they feel stronger and more energetic after helping others; many also reported feeling calmer and less depressed, with increased feelings of self-worth.[41]

Stress Reduction Benefits

The NCI cites stress reduction as one probable mechanism among spiritually healthy people for improved health and longevity and for better coping with illness.[42] In addition, several small studies support the contention that positive religious practices aid effective stress management.[43] Studies also suggest that increasing mindfulness through meditation reduces stress levels not only in people with physical and mental disorders, but also in healthy people as well.[44]

check yourself

- **List three benefits of spiritual health.**

2.7 Strategies for Cultivating Spiritual Health

learning outcome

2.7 Describe several strategies for improving spiritual health.

Cultivating your spiritual side takes just as much work as becoming physically fit. Here, we introduce some ways to develop your spiritual health by tuning in, training your body, expanding your mind, and reaching out.

Tune In to Yourself and Your Surroundings

Focusing on spiritual health has been likened to tuning in on a radio: Inner wisdom is available, but if we fail to tune our "receiver," we won't hear it for all the "static" of daily life. Four ancient practices used throughout the world can help you tune in: contemplation, mindfulness, meditation, and prayer.

In the domain of spirituality, **contemplation** usually refers to a practice of concentrating the mind on a spiritual or ethical subject, a view of the natural world, or an icon or other image representative of divinity. For instance, a Zen Buddhist might contemplate a riddle called a *koan*. A Sufi might contemplate the 99 names of God. A Catholic might contemplate an image of the Virgin Mary. Others might contemplate nature, a favorite poem, or an ethical question, or keep a gratitude journal. Many traditions advocate contemplating gratitude, forgiveness, and unconditional love.

A practice of focused, nonjudgmental observation, **mindfulness** is an awareness of present-moment reality—a holistic sensation of being totally involved in the moment rather than focused on some worry or being on "autopilot" (Figure 2.5).[45] If you've ever "forgotten yourself" while watching the sun set, listening to music, or performing challenging work, you've experienced mindfulness.

So how do you practice mindfulness? Living mindfully means allowing ourselves to become more deeply and completely aware of what we are sensing in each moment.[46] For instance, the next time you eat an orange, pay attention. What does it feel like to pierce the skin with your thumbnail? Do you smell the fragrance of the orange as you peel it? How does the juice splatter as you separate the segments? How does the taste change from the first bite to the last?

See It! Videos

Is meditation a key to happiness? Watch **Meditating to Happiness** in the Study Area of MasteringHealth.

Almost any endeavor that requires concentration can help you develop mindfulness. Consider arts such as sculpting, painting, writing, dancing, or playing a musical instrument. Even household activities such as cooking and cleaning can foster mindfulness—as long as you pay attention while you do them.

Meditation is a practice of cultivating a still or quiet mind. For thousands of years, many cultures have found that daily meditative stillness enhances spiritual health.

So how do you meditate? Most teachers advise sitting in a quiet place where you won't be interrupted. You may want to assume a modified lotus position, in which your legs are crossed in front of you. Lying down is not recommended because you may fall asleep. Beginners may find it easier to meditate with eyes closed. Now start quieting your mind; different schools of meditation teach different methods to achieve this:

- **Mantra meditation.** Focus on a *mantra*, a word such as *Om*, *Amen*, *Love*, or *God*, and repeat this word silently. When a distracting thought arises, simply set it aside. It may help to imagine the thought as a leaf, and mentally place it on a flowing stream that carries it away. Don't fault yourself for becoming distracted. Simply notice the thought, release it, and return to your mantra.
- **Breath meditation.** Count each breath: Pay attention to each inhalation, the brief pause that follows, and the exhalation; these equal one breath. When you have counted ten breaths, return to one. As distractions arise, release them and return to the breath.
- **Color meditation.** When your eyes are closed, you may perceive a field of color, such as a deep, restful blue. Focus on this color. Treat distractions as for other forms of meditation.
- **Candle meditation.** With your eyes open, focus on the flame of a candle. Allow your eyes to soften as you meditate on this object. Treat distractions as in the other forms of meditation.

After several minutes, with practice you may come to experience a sensation, sometimes described as "dropping down," in which you feel yourself release into the meditation. In this state, distracting thoughts are less likely and you may receive surprising insights.

When you're starting out, try meditating for just 10 to 20 minutes, once or twice a day. You may find yourself feeling more rested

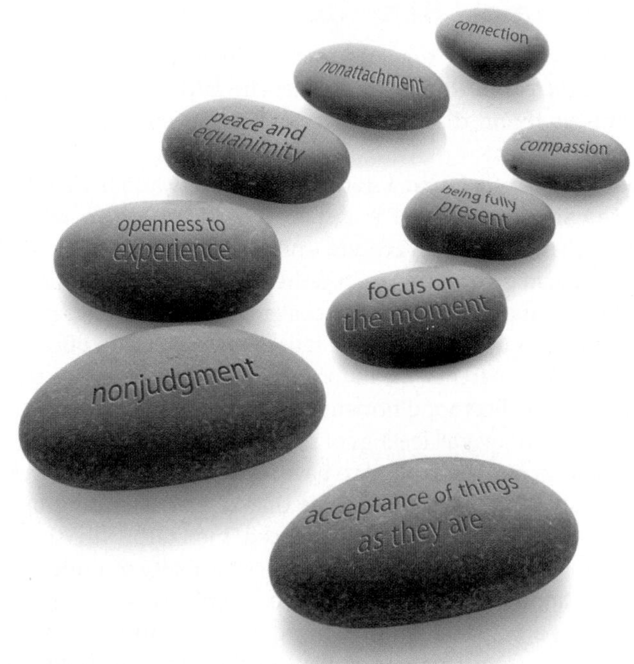

Figure 2.5 Qualities of Mindfulness

Source: M. Greenberg, "Nine Essential Qualities of Mindfulness," *Psychology Today*, February 22, 2012, www.psychologytoday.com.

and less stressed, and you may begin to experience increased empathy.

In **prayer**, rather than emptying the mind, an individual focuses it in communication with a transcendent Presence. For many, prayer offers a sense of comfort; a sense that we are not alone; and an avenue for expressing concern for others, admitting transgressions, seeking forgiveness, and renewing hope and purpose. Focusing on gratitude can provide strength in challenging times.

Train Your Body

For thousands of years, throughout the world, spiritual seekers have cultivated transcendence through physical means. A foremost example is the practice of **yoga**. Although in the West we think of yoga as involving controlled breathing and physical postures, traditional forms also emphasize meditation, chanting, and other practices believed to cultivate unity with the *Atman*, or spiritual life principle of the universe.

If you're interested in yoga, sign up for a class. Some forms, such as *hatha yoga*, focus on developing flexibility, deep breathing, and tranquility; others, such as *ashtanga yoga*, are fast paced and demanding. The instructor will likely lead you through warm-up poses; more challenging poses designed to align, stretch, and invigorate; and relaxation and deep-breathing exercises.

Training your body to improve spiritual health doesn't necessarily require a formal practice; any exercise can contribute to spiritual health. Begin by acknowledging gratitude for your body's strength and speed. Throughout the session, try to stay mindful of your breathing.

You can also cultivate spirituality through engaging or restricting your senses. Viewing artwork or listening to music can calm the mind and soothe the spirit. Alternatively, closing your eyes and sitting in silence removes visual and auditory distractions, helping you to focus. Try turning off your phone and taking a solitary walk or spending a weekend at a retreat center (for options, see www.SpiritSite.com).

Expand Your Mind

For many people, psychological counseling is a step toward spiritual health. Therapy helps you let go of past hurts, accept limitations, manage stress and anger, reduce anxiety and depression, and take control of your life—all steps toward spiritual growth.

You can also study the sacred texts of the world's major religions and spiritual practices, explore on-campus meditation groups, take classes in spirituality or comparative religions, attend religious meetings or services, attend public lectures, and check out the websites of spiritual and religious organizations.

Reach Out to Others

Altruism, the giving of oneself out of genuine concern for others, is a key aspect of a spiritually healthy life. Volunteering to help others, working for a nonprofit organization, donating money or other resources, picking up litter—all are ways to serve others and enhance your own spiritual health.

Community service can also take the form of **environmental stewardship**, which the Environmental Protection Agency (EPA) defines as the responsibility for environmental quality shared by all those whose actions affect the environment. Simple actions such as reducing and recycling packaging, turning off unused lights, and taking shorter showers are part of environmental stewardship.

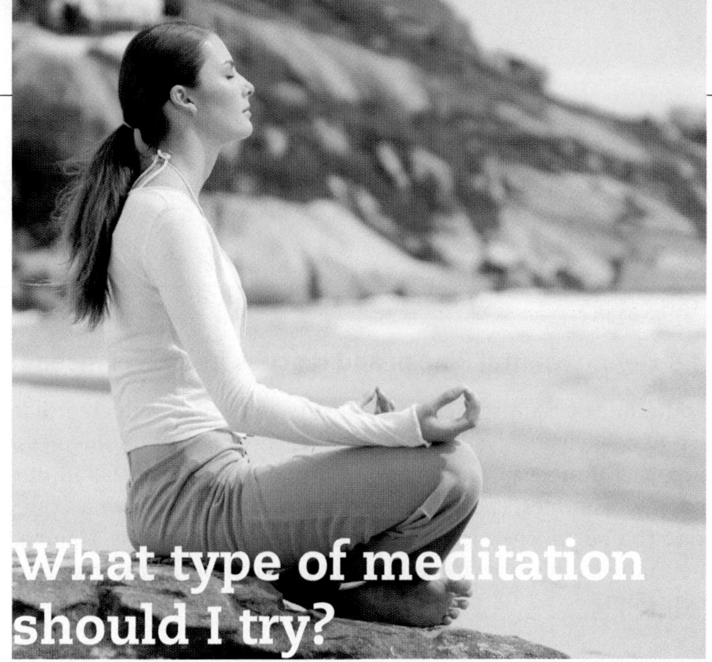

Experts suggest trying different meditation techniques and picking the one that works best for you.

Skills for Behavior Change

FINDING YOUR SPIRITUAL SIDE THROUGH SERVICE

Recognizing that we are all part of a greater system with responsibilities to and for others is a key part of spiritual growth. Volunteering your time and energy is a great way to connect with others and help make the world a better place while improving your own health. Here are a few ideas:

- Offer to help elderly neighbors with lawn care or simple household repairs.
- Volunteer with Meals on Wheels, a local soup kitchen, a food bank, or another program that helps people obtain adequate food.
- Organize or participate in an after-school or summertime activity for neighborhood children.
- Participate in a highway, beach, or neighborhood cleanup; restoration of park trails and waterways; or other environmental preservation projects.
- Volunteer at the local humane society.
- Apply to become a Big Brother or Big Sister and mentor a child who may face significant challenges or have poor role models.
- Join an organization working on a cause such as global warming or hunger, or start one yourself.
- Volunteer in a neighborhood challenged by poverty, low literacy levels, or a natural disaster. Or volunteer with an organization such as Habitat for Humanity to build homes or provide other aid to developing communities.

check yourself

- **How do physical, mental, and contemplative strategies affect spiritual health?**
- **What are some of the benefits of including spiritual health among the dimensions of health?**

2.8 When Psychological Health Deteriorates

learning outcome

2.8 Define mental illness and discuss its prevalence.

Sometimes circumstances overwhelm us to such a degree that we need help to get back on track. Stress, anxiety, loneliness, financial upheavals, and other traumatic events can derail our coping resources, causing us to turn inward or act in ways outside the norm; chemical imbalances, drug interactions, trauma, neurological disruptions, and other physical problems may also contribute.

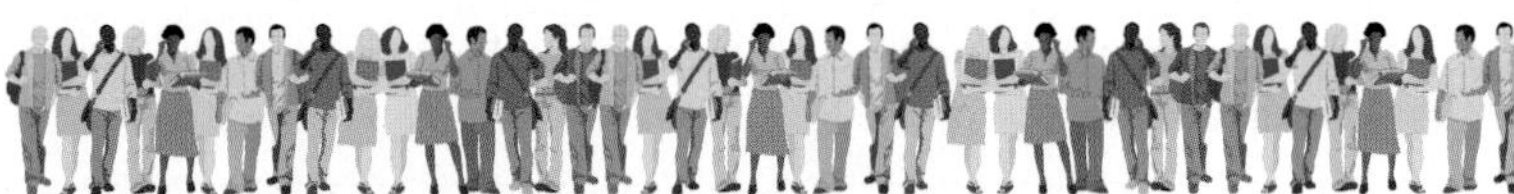

Felt overwhelmed by all they needed to do 84.4%

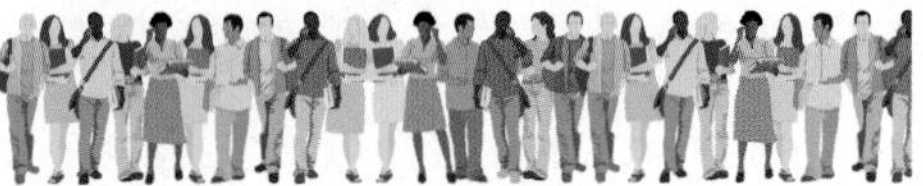

Felt overwhelming anxiety 51%

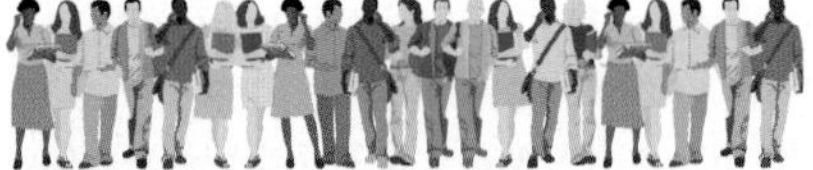

Felt things were hopeless 44.7%

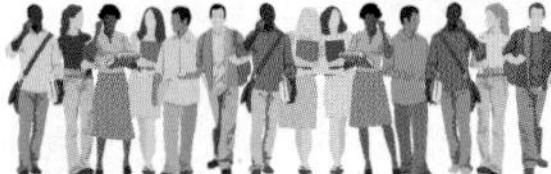

Felt so depressed that it was difficult to function 30.9%

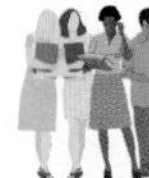

Seriously considered suicide 7.5%

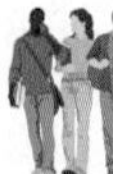

Intentionally injured themselves 5.9%

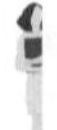

Attempted suicide 1.4%

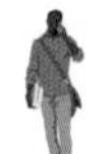

= 2%

Figure 2.6 Mental Health Concerns of American College Students, Past 12 Months

Source: Data are from American College Health Association, *American College Health Association—National College Health Assessment II (ACHA-NCHA II) Reference Group Data Report, Fall 2013* (Hanover, MD: ACHA, 2014).

Mental illnesses are disorders that disrupt thinking, feeling, moods, and behaviors, causing varying degrees of impaired functioning in daily living. They are believed to be caused by a variety of biochemical, genetic, and environmental factors.[47]

Risk factors for mental illness include having biological relatives with mental illness; malnutrition or exposure to viruses while in the womb; stressful situations such as financial problems, a loved one's death, or a divorce; chronic medical conditions; combat; taking psychoactive drugs during adolescence; childhood abuse or neglect; and lack of friendships or healthy relationships.[48]

As with physical disease, mental illnesses can range from mild to severe and can exact a heavy toll on quality of life, both for people with the illnesses and those in contact with them.

The basis for diagnosing mental disorders in the United States is the *Diagnostic and Statistical Manual of Mental Disorders*, Fifth Edition (*DSM-5*). An estimated 20 percent of Americans 18 and older—about 1 in 5 adults—suffer from a diagnosable mental disorder in a given year; nearly half of those have more than one mental illness at once.[49] About 5 percent, or 1 in 20, suffer from a serious mental illness requiring close monitoring, residential care in many instances, and medication.[50] Mental disorders are the leading cause of disability worldwide for people aged 15 to 44, costing more than $100 billion annually in the United States alone.[51]

Mental health problems are common among college students, and they appear to be increasing in number and severity.[52] According to experts in the field, this group has greater levels of stress and psychopathology than at any time in our nation's history. Last year, over 70 percent of college counseling center directors reported increases in severe psychological problems on their campuses.[53] The most recent National College Health Assessment survey found that approximately 1 in 3 undergraduates reported "feeling so depressed it was difficult to function" at least once in the past year, while 7.5 percent reported "seriously considering attempting suicide" in the past year.[54] Figure 2.6 shows more results from this survey. In all, more than 1 in 4 college students experience a mental health issue each year.[55] The survey found that 56.4% of women and 40.5% of men reported experiencing "overwhelming anxiety" episodes in the last year.[56] Although these data may appear alarming, increases in help-seeking behavior rather than actual increases in prevalence of disorders may be contributing to these trends.

check yourself

- **What is mental illness?**
- **Is mental illness more or less common than you expected?**

2.9

Anxiety Disorders

learning outcome

2.9 Describe common anxiety disorders and their causes.

Anxiety disorders, which are characterized by persistent feelings of threat and worry, are the number one mental health problem in the United States, affecting more than 21 percent of all adults ages 18 to 64.[57] Among U.S undergraduates, 13.2 percent report being diagnosed with or treated for anxiety in the past year.[58]

To be diagnosed with **generalized anxiety disorder (GAD)**, one must exhibit at least three of the following symptoms for more days than not during a 6-month period: restlessness or feeling on edge, being easily fatigued, difficulty concentrating or mind going blank, irritability, muscle tension, or sleep disturbances.[59] GAD often runs in families and is readily treatable.

Panic disorders are characterized by **panic attacks,** acute anxiety bringing on an intense physical reaction. Approximately 3 million Americans 18 and older experience panic attacks, usually in early adulthood.[60] Although highly treatable, panic attacks can become debilitating, particularly if they happen often and lead sufferers to avoid interacting with others. An attack typically starts abruptly, lasts about 30 minutes, and leaves the person tired and drained.[61] Symptoms include increased respiration, chills, hot flashes, shortness of breath, stomach cramps, chest pain, difficulty swallowing, and a sense of doom or impending death. Although researchers aren't sure what causes panic attacks, heredity, stress, and certain biochemical factors may play a role. Some researchers believe that sufferers are experiencing an overreactive fight-or-flight response.

Phobias, or phobic disorders, involve persistent and irrational fear of a specific object, activity, or situation, often out of proportion to circumstances. About 10 percent of American adults suffer from phobias such as fear of spiders, snakes, or public speaking.[62]

Another 8 percent suffer from **social phobia**, or social anxiety disorder,[63] characterized by persistent avoidance of social situations for fear of being humiliated, embarrassed, or even looked at. Some social phobias cause difficulty only in specific situations, such as speaking in front of a class. In extreme cases, sufferers avoid all contact with others.

People compelled to perform rituals over and over again; who are fearful of dirt or contamination; who have an unnatural concern about order and exactness; or who have persistent intrusive thoughts that they can't shake may suffer from **obsessive-compulsive disorder (OCD)**. Approximately 1 percent of Americans 18 and over have OCD.[64] Sufferers often see their behaviors as irrational, yet feel powerless to stop them. For a person to be diagnosed with OCD, the obsessions must consume more than 1 hour per day and interfere with normal life. The exact cause is unknown; genetics, biological abnormalities, learned behaviors, and environmental factors have been considered. Onset is usually in adolescence or early adulthood; median age of onset is 19.

People who have experienced or witnessed a natural disaster, violent assault, combat, or other traumatic event may develop **post-traumatic stress disorder (PTSD)**. PTSD is not rooted in weakness or an inability to cope; traumatic events can actually cause chemical changes in the brain that lead to PTSD.[65] About 4 percent of Americans suffer from PTSD each year, and 8 percent will experience PTSD in their lifetimes.[66] Fourteen percent of U.S. combat veterans who fought in Iraq and Afghanistan have experienced PTSD.[67]

Symptoms of PTSD include the following:

- Dissociation, or perceived detachment of the mind from the emotional state or even the body
- Intrusive recollections of the traumatic event—flashbacks, nightmares, or recurrent thoughts
- Acute anxiety or nervousness, in which the person is hyperaroused, may cry easily, or experience mood swings
- Insomnia and difficulty concentrating
- Intense physiological reactions, such as shaking or nausea, when reminded of the traumatic event

Although these are common initial responses to traumatic events, PTSD may be diagnosed if a person experiences them for at least 1 month following the event. In some cases, symptoms may not appear until months or years later.

See It! Videos

How can we help veterans who suffer from PTSD? Watch **Battling Post Traumatic Stress** in the Study Area of MasteringHealth.

Anxiety disorders vary in complexity and degree, and scientists have yet to find clear reasons why one person develops them and another doesn't. The following are cited as possible causes:[68]

- **Biology.** Positron-emission tomography (PET) scans can identify areas of the brain that react during anxiety-producing events. We may inherit tendencies toward anxiety disorders.
- **Environment.** Although genetic tendencies may exist, experiencing a repeated pattern of reaction to certain situations programs the brain to respond in a certain way. For example, if your sibling screamed whenever a large spider crept into view, you might be predisposed to react with anxiety to spiders later in life.
- **Social and cultural roles.** Because men and women are taught to assume different roles in society, women may find it more acceptable to express extreme anxiety. Men, in contrast, may have learned to repress such anxieties rather than act on them.

check yourself

- **What are the most common anxiety disorders?**

2.10 Mood Disorders

learning outcome

2.10 Describe common mood disorders and their causes.

Chronic mood disorders are disorders affecting how you feel. In any given year, approximately 10 percent of Americans 18 or older suffer from a mood disorder.[69]

Major Depression

Major depression, the most common mood disorder, affects approximately 8 percent of the American population[70]—though many are misdiagnosed or undiagnosed. Characterized by a combination of symptoms that interfere with work, study, sleep, appetite, relationships, and enjoyment of life, major depression is not just having a bad day or feeling down after a negative experience; it can't just be willed away. Symptoms can last for weeks, months, or years[71] and can include the following:

- Sadness and despair
- Loss of motivation or interest in pleasurable activities
- Preoccupation with failures and inadequacies
- Difficulty concentrating, indecisiveness, memory lapses
- Loss of sex drive or interest in close interactions with others
- Fatigue and loss of energy; slow reactions
- Sleeping too much or too little; insomnia
- Feeling agitated, worthless, or hopeless
- Withdrawal from friends and family
- Diminished or increased appetite
- Significant weight loss or gain
- Recurring thoughts that life isn't worth living; thoughts of death or suicide

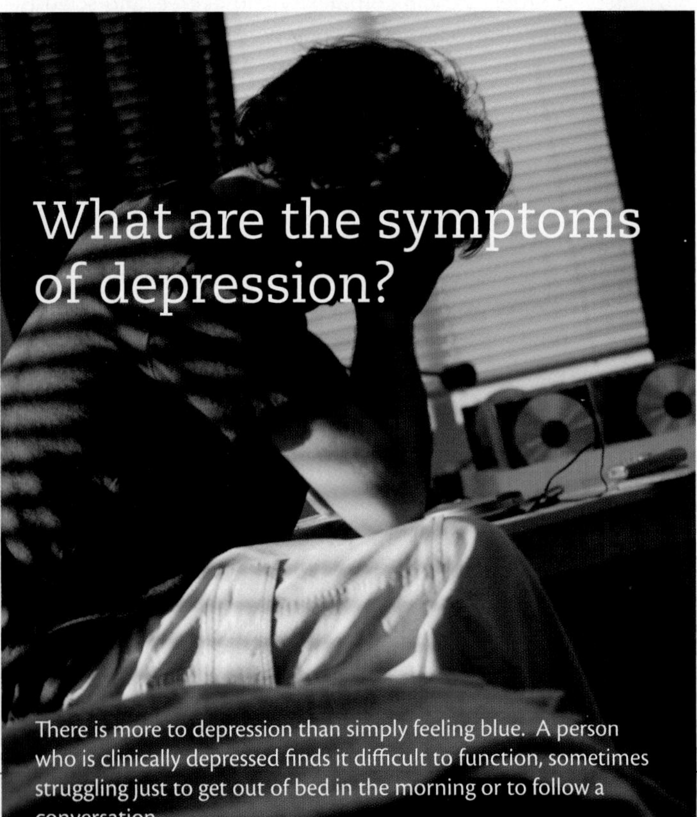

There is more to depression than simply feeling blue. A person who is clinically depressed finds it difficult to function, sometimes struggling just to get out of bed in the morning or to follow a conversation.

Depression in College Students Depression has gained increasing recognition as major obstacles to healthy adjustment and success in college. Stressors such as anxiety over relationships, pressure over grades and social acceptance, abuse of alcohol and other drugs, poor diet, and lack of sleep can overwhelm even resilient students. In a recent survey, 11 percent of students reported having been diagnosed with depression.[72]

Being far from home can exacerbate problems and make coping difficult; international students are particularly vulnerable to depression and other mental health concerns. Most campuses have counseling centers, cultural centers, and other services available, though many students do not use them because of persistent stigma.

Other Mood Disorders

Dysthymic disorder (dysthymia) is chronic, mild depression. Although dysthymic individuals may function acceptably, they may lack energy, be short-tempered and pessimistic, or not feel up to par without any overt symptoms. People with dysthymia may cycle into major depression over time. For a diagnosis, symptoms must persist for at least 2 years in adults (1 year in children). This disorder affects approximately 5 percent of the U.S. population in a given year.[73]

People with **bipolar disorder**, also called *manic depression*, often have severe mood swings, ranging from extreme highs (mania) to extreme lows (depression). Swings can be dramatic and rapid, or more gradual. When in the manic phase, people may be overactive, talkative, and have tons of energy; in the depressed phase, they may experience symptoms of major depression.

Although the cause of bipolar disorder is unknown, biological, genetic, and environmental factors, such as drug abuse and stressful or psychologically traumatic events, seem to be triggers. Once diagnosed, persons with bipolar disorder have several counseling and pharmaceutical options; most can live a healthy, functional life while being treated. Bipolar disorder affects approximately 2 percent of the adult population in the United States.[74]

Seasonal affective disorder (SAD) strikes during the winter and is associated with reduced exposure to sunlight. People with SAD suffer from irritability, apathy, carbohydrate craving and weight gain, increased sleep, and general sadness. Factors implicated in SAD include disruption in circadian rhythms and changes in levels of the hormone melatonin and the brain chemical serotonin.[75]

The most beneficial treatment for SAD is light therapy, using lamps that simulate sunlight. Other treatments include diet change, increased exercise, stress management, sleep restriction (limiting hours slept in a 24-hour period), psychotherapy, and prescription medications.

Causes of Mood Disorders

Mood disorders are caused by the interaction of factors including biological differences, hormones, inherited traits, life events, and trauma.[76] The biology of mood disorders is related to levels of brain chemicals called *neurotransmitters.* Several types of depression, including bipolar disorder, appear to have a genetic component. Depression can also be triggered by serious loss, difficult relationships, financial problems, and pressure to succeed. Early trauma, such as loss of a parent, may cause permanent changes in the brain, making one more prone to depression. Research has also shown that changes in physical health can be accompanied by mental changes, particularly depression. Stroke, heart attack, cancer, Parkinson's disease, chronic pain, diabetes, certain medications, alcohol, hormonal disorders, and a range of other afflictions can trigger depression.

Depression across Gender, Age, and Ethnicity

Although depression affects a wide range of people, it does not always manifest itself in the same way across populations. Women are almost twice as likely to experience depression as men are, possibly due to hormonal changes. Women often face stressors related to multiple responsibilities—work, child rearing, single parenthood, household work, and elder care—at rates higher than those of men. Researchers have observed gender differences in coping strategies (responses to certain events or stimuli) and proposed that some women's strategies make them more vulnerable to depression.[77]

Depression in men is often masked by alcohol or drug abuse, or by the socially acceptable habit of working excessively. Typically, depressed men present as irritable, angry, and discouraged. Men are less likely to admit they are depressed, and doctors are less likely to suspect it. Depression is associated with increased risk of heart disease in both men and women, but with a higher risk of *death* by heart disease in men.[78]

Depression in children is increasingly reported, with 1 in 10 children between ages 6 and 12 experiencing persistent feelings of sadness, the hallmark of depression. Depressed children may pretend to be sick, refuse to go to school or have a sudden drop in school performance, sleep incessantly, engage in self-mutilation, abuse drugs or alcohol, or attempt suicide. Before adolescence, girls and boys experience depression at about the same rate, but by adolescence and young adulthood, the rate among girls is higher. This may be due to biological and hormonal changes, girls' struggles with self-esteem and perceptions of success and approval, and an increase in girls' exposure to traumas such as childhood sexual abuse and poverty.[79]

As adults reach their middle and older years, most are emotionally stable and lead active and satisfying lives. However, when depression does occur, it is often undiagnosed or untreated, particularly in people in lower income groups or without access to resources. Depression is the most common mental disorder of people 65 and older. Rates are likely even higher than reported, as the symptoms of depression can be mistaken for dementia and thus be misdiagnosed.[80]

Rates of depression are higher among African Americans and Latinos than among Whites. However, true rates among minority populations are difficult to determine because members of these groups may have difficulty accessing mental health services because of economic barriers, social and cultural differences, language barriers, and lack of culturally competent providers. African American males specifically may avoid professional help due to stigma attached to mental illness in the African American community as well as greater distrust of physicians and poor patient-physician communication. Data indicate that when African Americans do report depression symptoms to a health care provider, they are significantly less likely to receive a depression diagnosis than are non-Hispanic Whites, and those who are diagnosed are less likely to be treated for depression.[81]

Skills for Behavior Change

DEALING WITH AND DEFEATING DEPRESSION

If you feel you have depression symptoms, make an appointment with a counselor. Depression is often a biological condition that you can't just "get over" on your own. You may need talk therapy, sometimes combined with antidepressant medication, to help you reach a place where you can play a greater role in getting well. Once you've started along a path of therapy and healing, these strategies may help you feel better faster:

- **Be realistic and responsible in setting appropriate personal goals.**
- **Break large tasks into small ones, set priorities, and do what you can as you can.**
- **Try to be with other people and to confide in someone.**
- **Mild exercise and religious or social activities may help.**
- **Try meditation, yoga, tai chi, or another mind-body practice. These disciplines can help you connect with your feelings, release tension, and clear your mind.**
- **Expect your mood to improve gradually, not immediately.**
- **Before deciding to make a significant transition, change jobs, or get married or divorced, discuss it with others who know you well.**
- **Let family and friends help you.**
- **Continue working with your counselor. If he or she isn't helpful, look for another.**

check yourself

- **What are the most common mood disorders?**
- **What are causes for mood disorders?**

2.11 Other Psychological Disorders

learning outcome

2.11 Describe personality disorders, schizophrenia, learning disabilities, and neurodevelopmental disorders.

Personality Disorders

A **personality disorder** is an "enduring pattern of inner experience and behavior that deviates markedly from the expectation of the individual's culture and is pervasive and inflexible."[82] About 10 percent of adults in the United States have some form of personality disorder.[83] People dealing with individuals suffering from personality disorders often find interactions with them challenging and destructive.

Paranoid personality disorder involves pervasive, unfounded mistrust of others, irrational jealousy, and secretiveness, often with delusions of being persecuted by everyone from family members to the government.

Narcissistic personality disorders involve an exaggerated sense of self-importance and self-absorption; sufferers are overly needy and demanding and feel "entitled" to nothing but the best.

Antisocial personality disorders involve a long-term pattern of manipulation and taking advantage of others. Symptoms include disregard for others' safety and lack of remorse, arrogance, and anger.

Borderline personality disorder (BPD) is characterized by risky behaviors such as gambling sprees, unsafe sex, use of illicit drugs, and daredevil driving.[84] Characteristics include mood swings and the tendency to see everything in black-and-white terms. Many people diagnosed with BPD engage in **self-injury**, or deliberately causing harm to one's own body—such as by cutting or burning—to cope with emotions.[85]

Researchers estimate that between 7 percent and 15 percent of college students engage in self-harm. Many people who inflict self-harm suffer from other mental health conditions and have experienced abuse as children or adults. If you or someone you know is engaging in self-injury, seek professional help. Not only must the behavior be stopped, but the sufferer must also learn to recognize and manage the feelings that triggered it.[86]

Previously, self-injury was thought to be more common in females, but recent research indicates that rates are generally the same for men and women.

Schizophrenia

Schizophrenia is a severe psychological disorder that affects about 1 percent of the U.S. population.[87] Schizophrenia is characterized by alterations of the senses (including auditory and visual hallucinations); the inability to sort out incoming stimuli and make appropriate responses; an altered sense of self; and radical changes in emotions, movements, and behaviors. Typical symptoms include delusional behavior, hallucinations, incoherent speech, inability to think logically, erratic movement, and difficulty with daily living.[88]

Schizophrenia is a biological disease, perhaps caused by brain damage that occurs as early as the second trimester of fetal development. Symptoms usually appear in men in their late teens and twenties and in women in their late twenties and early thirties.[89]

At present, schizophrenia is treatable but not curable. With proper medication, public understanding, support of loved ones, and access to therapy, many schizophrenics lead normal lives—though without such assistance, many have great difficulty.

Learning Disabilities and Neurodevelopmental Disorders

Learning disabilities and neurodevelopmental disorders are brain-based disorders that are not mental illnesses.

Attention-deficit/hyperactivity disorder (ADHD) is a learning disability usually associated with school-aged children, but symptoms may persist into adulthood. People with attention deficit disorder (ADD) and ADHD are distracted much of the time and find concentrating and organizing things difficult.

Dyslexia, a language-based learning disorder, can pose problems for reading, writing, and spelling. Lesser known, but equally challenging, are *dyscalculia* (a learning disability involving math) and *dysgraphia* (a learning disability involving writing).

Autism spectrum disorder (ASD) is a neurodevelopmental disorder (an impairment in brain development). People with ASD will continue to learn and grow intellectually throughout their lives, but struggle to master communication and social behavior skills, which impacts their performance in school and work.

check yourself

- **What are causes for personality disorders, schizophrenia, and learning disabilities and neurodevelopmental disorders?**

2.12 Psychological Health through the Lifespan: Successful Aging

learning outcome

2.12 Describe psychological conditions associated with aging, and explain the impact of loss on psychological health.

Most older adults lead healthy, fulfilling lives. However, some older people do suffer from mental and emotional disturbances. Depression is the most common psychological problem facing older adults—though the rate of major depression is lower among older than younger adults. Regardless of age, people who have a poor perception of their health, have multiple chronic illnesses, take many medications, abuse alcohol and other drugs, lack social support, and do not exercise face more challenges that may require emotional strength.

Memory failure, errors in judgment, disorientation, or erratic behavior can occur at any age and for various reasons. The term *dementing diseases*, or **dementias**, are used to describe either reversible symptoms or progressive forms of brain malfunctioning.

One of the most common dementias is **Alzheimer's disease (AD)**. Affecting an estimated 5.4 million Americans,[90] the disease first kills its victims through slow loss of personhood (memory loss, disorientation, personality changes, and eventual loss of independent functioning), and then through deterioration of body systems.

Patients with AD live for an average of 4 to 6 years after diagnosis, although the disease can last for up to 20 years.[91] Although often associated with the aged, AD has been diagnosed in people in their forties. In AD, areas of the brain that affect memory, speech, and personality develop "tangles" that impair nerve cell communication, causing cell death. It progresses in stages marked by increasingly impaired memory and judgment. In later stages, many patients become depressed, combative, and aggressive. In the final stage, the person becomes dependent on others; identity loss and speech problems are common. Eventually, control of bodily functions may be lost.

Researchers are investigating possible causes including genetic predisposition, immune malfunction, a slow-acting virus, chromosomal or genetic defects, chronic inflammation, uncontrolled hypertension, and neurotransmitter imbalance. No treatment can stop AD, but medications can slow or relieve some symptoms.[92]

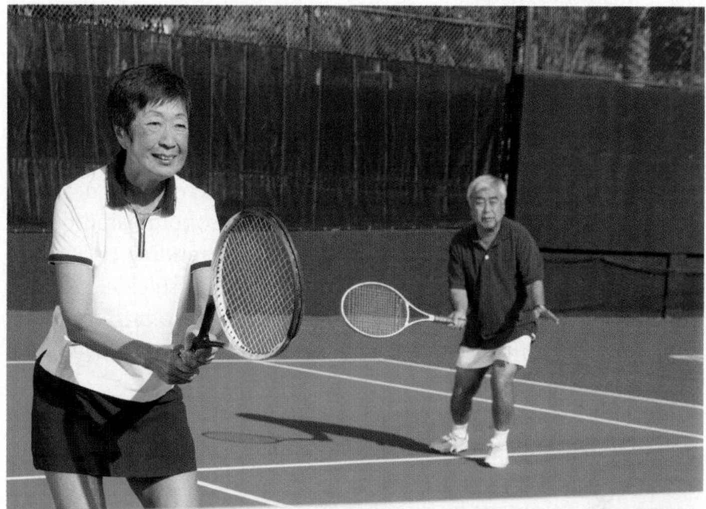

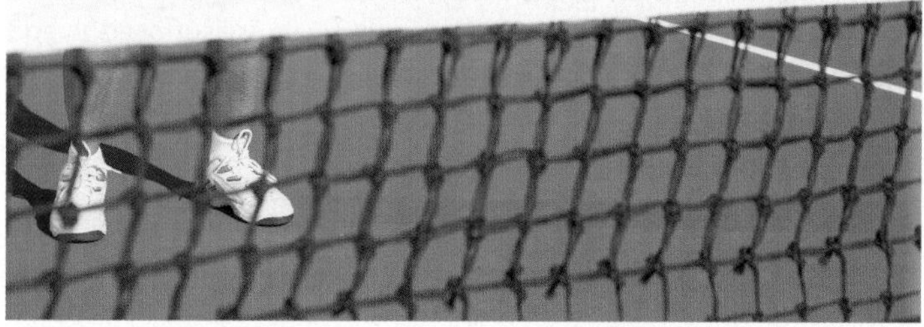

People who have aged successfully usually are resilient and able to cope well with physical, social, and emotional changes. They live independently and are actively engaged in mentally challenging and stimulating activities and in social and productive pursuits.

Coping with Loss

Coping with the loss of a loved one is extremely difficult. Understanding feelings and behaviors related to death can help you comprehend the emotional processes associated with it.

Bereavement is the loss or deprivation a survivor experiences when a loved one dies. In the lives of the bereaved or of close survivors, the loss of loved ones leaves "holes" and inevitable changes. Loneliness and despair may envelop survivors. Understanding of these normal reactions, time, patience, and support from loved ones can help the bereaved heal and move on.

Grief occurs in reaction to significant loss, including one's own impending death, the death of a loved one, or a loss (such as the end of a relationship or job) involving separation or change in identity. Grief may be a mental, physical, social, or emotional reaction, and often includes changes in eating, sleeping, working, and even thinking. Symptoms vary in severity and duration. However, the bereaved person can benefit from emotional and social support.

check yourself

- **What are three particular psychological issues associated with aging?**

2.13 When Psychological Problems Become Too Much: Suicide

learning outcome

2.13 Identify warning signs associated with suicide, and discuss strategies for suicide prevention.

Suicide is the fourth leading cause of death for 5- to 14-year-olds and the second leading cause of death for 15- to 24-year-olds in the United States.[93] It has recently become the leading cause of death on college campuses, now ranking higher than alcohol-related deaths or car crashes.[94] However, young adults not attending college are also at risk.[95] Risk factors include family history of suicide, previous suicide attempts, excessive drug and alcohol use, prolonged depression, financial difficulties, serious illness in oneself or a loved one, and loss of a loved one.

Suicide has become the leading cause of death by injury (both unintentional and intentional) among American adults.[96] Nearly four times as many men die by suicide than do women.[97] Firearms, suffocation, and poison are by far the most common methods of suicide. Men are almost twice as likely as women to use firearms, whereas younger women (10–24 years) are more likely to use suffocation and older women (25 and older) are more likely to use poisoning.[98]

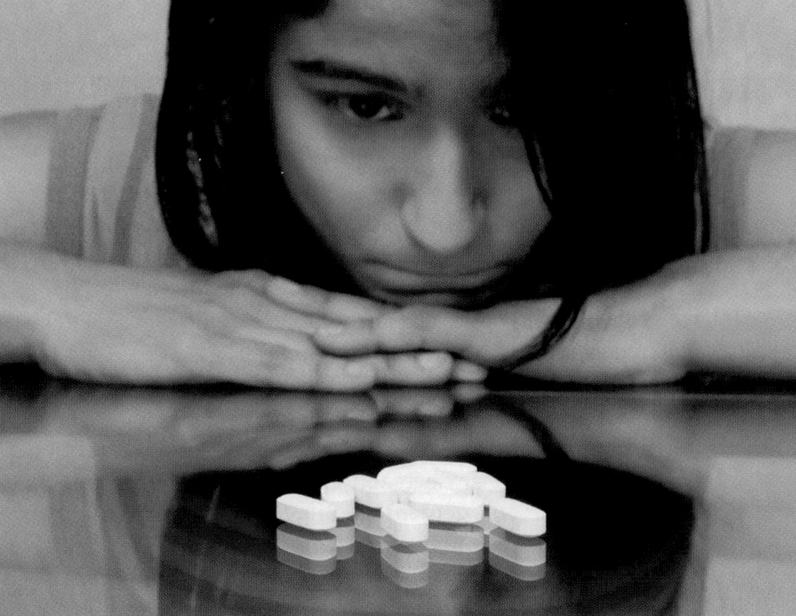

If you notice warning signs of suicide in someone you know, it is imperative that you take action.

Warning Signs

People who commit suicide usually indicate their intentions, although others do not always recognize their warnings.[99] Anyone expressing a desire to kill himself or herself or who has made an attempt is at risk. Signs that one may be contemplating suicide include the following:[100]

- Recent loss and a seeming inability to let go of grief
- History of depression
- Change in personality—withdrawal, irritability, anxiety, tiredness, apathy
- Change in behavior—inability to concentrate, loss of interest in classes or work, unexplained demonstration of happiness following a period of depression
- Sexual dysfunction (such as impotence) or diminished sexual interest
- Expressions of self-hatred and excessive risk-taking
- Change in sleep or eating habits or in appearance
- A direct statement such as "I might as well end it all"
- An indirect statement such as "You won't have to worry about me anymore"
- Final preparations such as writing a will or giving away prized possessions
- Preoccupation with themes of death

Preventing Suicide

Most people who attempt suicide want to live but see death as the only way out of an intolerable situation. Crisis counselors and suicide hotlines may help temporarily, but the best way to prevent suicide is to get rid of conditions and substances that may precipitate attempts, including alcohol, drugs, isolation, and access to guns.

If someone you know threatens suicide or displays warning signs of doing so, do the following:[101]

- **Monitor signals.** Ensure there is someone around the person as often as possible. Don't leave him or her alone.
- **Take threats seriously.** Don't brush them off as "just talk."
- **Let the person know how much you care.** Say you're there to help.
- **Ask directly,** "Are you thinking of hurting or killing yourself?"
- **Don't belittle feelings.** Don't tell the person he or she doesn't mean it or couldn't commit suicide. To some, such comments offer the challenge of proving you wrong.
- **Help think about alternatives.** Offer to go for help along with the person. Call a suicide hotline, and use all available community and campus resources.
- **Tell your friend's spouse, partner, parents, siblings, or counselor.** Don't keep your suspicions to yourself.

check yourself

- **What are five warning signs that someone may be contemplating suicide?**
- **What are five specific actions you can take to prevent suicide?**

2.14 Seeking Professional Help

learning **outcome**

2.14 Recognize feelings and behaviors that may warrant seeking help from a mental health professional, and describe possible treatment options for psychological problems.

A physical ailment will readily send most people to the nearest health professional, but many resist seeking help for psychological problems. Although estimates show that 20 percent of adults have some kind of mental disorder, only 6 to 7 percent of adults use mental health counseling services.[102] Consider seeking help if

- You feel you need help or feel out of control.
- You experience wild mood swings or inappropriate responses to normal stimuli.
- Your fears or feelings of guilt distract you.
- You have hallucinations.
- You feel worthless, or feel life is not worth living.
- Your life seems nothing but a series of crises.
- You're considering suicide.
- You turn to drugs or alcohol to escape.

Deciding to Seek Treatment

Common misconceptions about people with mental illness are that they're dangerous, irresponsible, or "need to get over it." The stigma of mental illness often leads to shame and isolation. Many people with mental illness report that the stigma was more disabling at times than the illness itself.[103] The group Active Minds (www.activeminds.org) works to end the stigma of mental illness on college campuses and encourage those at risk to seek care.

If you're considering treatment for a psychological problem, first see a health professional for an evaluation that should include the following:

1. A *physical checkup*, to rule out other issues that can result in depression-like symptoms
2. A *psychiatric history*, to trace the apparent disorder, genetic or family factors, and any past treatments
3. A *mental status examination*, including tests for other psychiatric symptoms

Type of Mental Health Professionals

The most common types of mental health professionals are psychiatrists, psychologists, social workers, counselors, psychoanalysts, and licensed marriage and family therapists. Which one you choose depends on your needs and goals. When choosing a therapist, the most important criterion is whether you feel you can work with him or her. The following are questions to ask the therapist and yourself:

- **Can you interview the therapist before starting treatment?** An initial meeting will help determine whether this person is a good fit for you.
- **Do you like the therapist?** Can you talk to him or her comfortably?
- **Does the therapist demonstrate professionalism?** Be concerned if your therapist frequently breaks appointments, suggests outside social interaction, talks inappropriately about himself or herself, has questionable billing practices, or resists releasing you from therapy.
- **Will the therapist help set goals?** A good professional should help you set small goals to work on between sessions.

What to Expect in Therapy

Before meeting, briefly explain your needs. Ask about the fee. Arrive on time and expect your visit to last about an hour. The therapist will ask about your history and what brought you to therapy. Answer honestly; it's critical that you trust this person enough to be open and honest.

Many types of counseling exist, including individual therapy and group therapy. *Cognitive therapy* focuses on the impact of thoughts on feelings and behavior. It helps a person correct habitually pessimistic or faulty thinking patterns. *Behavioral therapy* focuses on what we do, using the concepts of stimulus, response, and reinforcement to alter behavior patterns.

Pharmacological Treatment

Drug therapy can be important in the treatment of many psychological disorders. Such medications aren't, however, without side effects and contraindications. For example, the FDA requires warning labels on antidepressant medications about suicidal thinking and behavior in young adults aged 18 to 24.[104]

Talk to your health care provider to understand the risks and benefits of any medication prescribed; tell your doctor of any adverse effects. With some therapies, such as antidepressants, you may not feel effects for several weeks. Finally, compliance with your doctor's recommendations for beginning or ending a course of any medication is very important.

See It! Videos

Why are women more likely than men to take antidepressants? Watch **Antidepressant Use Increases Among Women** in the Study Area of MasteringHealth.

check yourself

- **Give four examples of feelings and behaviors that may warrant seeking help from a mental health professional.**
- **What are some advantages and disadvantages to the various treatment options described?**

Assessyourself

2.15

What's Your Spiritual IQ?

An interactive version of this assessment is available online in MasteringHealth.

Many tools are available for assessing your spiritual intelligence. Although each differs significantly according to its target audience (therapy clients, business executives, church members, etc.), most share certain underlying principles reflected in the questionnaire below. Answer each question as follows:

0 = not at all true for me
1 = somewhat true for me
2 = very true for me

_____ 1. I frequently feel gratitude for the many blessings of my life.

_____ 2. I am often moved by the beauty of Earth, music, poetry, or other aspects of my daily life.

_____ 3. I readily express forgiveness toward those whose missteps have affected me.

_____ 4. I recognize in others qualities that are more important than their appearance and behaviors.

_____ 5. When I do poorly on an exam, lose an important game, or am rejected in a relationship, I am able to know that the experience does not define who I am.

_____ 6. When fear arises, I am able to know that I am eternally safe and loved.

_____ 7. I meditate or pray daily.

_____ 8. I frequently and fearlessly ponder the possibility of an afterlife.

_____ 9. I accept total responsibility for the choices that I have made in building my life.

_____ 10. I feel that I am on Earth for a unique and sacred reason.

Scoring

The higher your score on this quiz, the higher your spiritual intelligence. To improve your score, apply the suggestions for spiritual practices from this chapter.

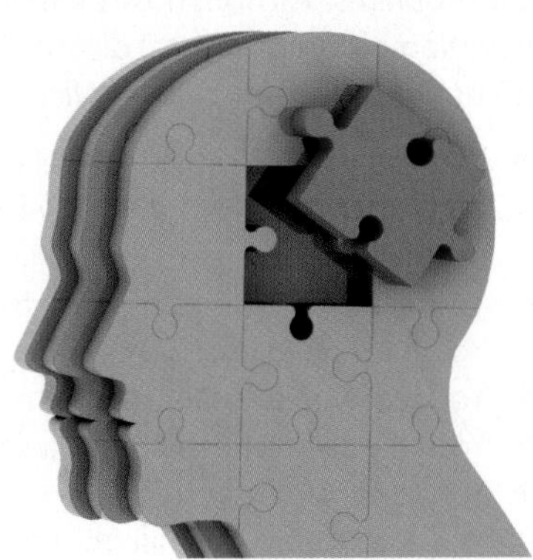

Your Plan for Change

The **Assess Yourself** activity gave you the chance to evaluate your spiritual intelligence. If you are interested in cultivating your own spirituality further, consider taking some of the small but significant steps listed below.

Today, you can:

◯ Find a quiet spot; turn off your cell phone; close your eyes; and contemplate, meditate, or pray for 10 minutes. Or spend 10 minutes in quiet mindfulness of your surroundings.

◯ In a journal or on your computer, begin a numbered list of things you are grateful for. Today, list at least ten things. Include people, pets, talents and abilities, achievements, favorite places, foods . . . whatever comes to mind!

Within the next 2 weeks, you can:

◯ Explore the options on campus for beginning psychotherapy, joining a spiritual or religious student group, or volunteering with a student organization working for positive change.

◯ Think of a person in your life with whom you have experienced conflict. Spend a few minutes contemplating forgiveness toward this person and then write him or her an e-mail or letter apologizing for any offense you may have given and offering your forgiveness in return. Wait for a day or two before deciding whether you are truly ready to send the message.

By the end of the semester, you can:

◯ Develop a list of several spiritual readings and books that you would like to read during your break.

◯ Begin exploring options for volunteer work next summer.

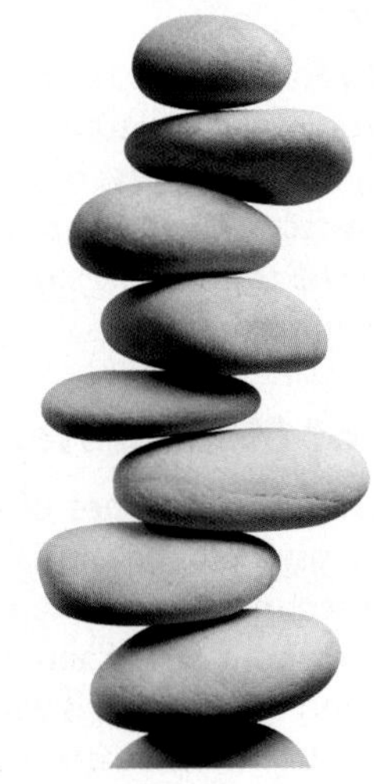

How Psychologically Healthy Are You?

An interactive version of this assessment is available online in MasteringHealth.

How do you stay psychologically healthy and well? There are many ways, but one particularly effective method is improving your coping skills. This assessment will help you identify how well you cope. It will also help you learn about some beneficial and healthy ways to cope, which will, in turn, help you stay psychologically healthy.

Carefully assess yourself by scoring each item according to how often each statement applies to you.

	Always	Often	Sometimes	Rarely	Never
1. I seek out emotional support from others.	1	2	3	4	5
2. In light of new developments, I am willing to change my opinions.	1	2	3	4	5
3. I find myself so overwhelmed that I completely shut down.	1	2	3	4	5
4. If I think there is some research or other information about a problem I have, I will seek it out.	1	2	3	4	5
5. I try to keep the situation in perspective.	1	2	3	4	5
6. I refuse to give up.	1	2	3	4	5
7. I remind myself that eventually things will get better.	1	2	3	4	5
8. It is difficult to forget about my problems and worries and just have fun.	1	2	3	4	5
9. I experience difficulty sleeping because my mind is racing.	1	2	3	4	5
10. I manage to find an outlet to express my emotions (writing a journal, drawing, exercising, etc.).	1	2	3	4	5

Interpreting Your Score

Add up your score for numbers 3, 8, and 9. A perfect score is 15. The higher your score, the stronger your coping skills.

Add up your score for numbers 1, 2, 4, 5, 6, 7, and 10. A perfect score is 7. The lower your score here, the greater your ability to cope with stress in an effective, healthy manner. The higher the score, the more you need to improve your coping skills. To see where you need the most improvement, look at your answers to these questions. For example, if your score for question 1 is "4, rarely," or "5, never," reaching out to others for emotional support will improve your psychological health.

Source: Psych Tests AIM Inc., "Coping and Stress Management Skills Test—Abridged/10 Questions, 5 Mins," http://testyourself.psychtests.com. Reprinted by permission.

Your Plan for Change

The Assess Yourself activity gave you the chance to assess your coping abilities. After considering the results, you can take steps to change behaviors that may be detrimental to your psychological health.

Today, you can:

◯ Evaluate your behavior and identify patterns and specific things you are doing that negatively affect your psychological health. What can you change now? What can you change in the near future?

◯ Start a journal and note changes in your mood. Look for trends and think about ways you can change your behavior to address them.

Within the next 2 weeks, you can:

◯ Visit your campus health center and find out about the counseling services they offer. If you are feeling overwhelmed, depressed, or anxious, make an appointment with a counselor.

◯ Pay attention to the negative thoughts that pop up throughout the day. Note times when you find yourself devaluing or undermining your abilities, and notice when you project negative attitudes on others. Bringing your awareness to these thoughts gives you an opportunity to stop and reevaluate them.

By the end of the semester, you can:

◯ Make a commitment to an ongoing therapeutic practice aimed at improving your psychological health. Depending on your current situation, this could mean anything from seeing a counselor or joining a support group to practicing meditation or attending religious services.

◯ Volunteer regularly with a local organization you care about. Focus your energy and gain satisfaction by helping to improve others' lives or the environment.

Summary

To hear an MP3 Tutor session, scan here or visit the Study Area in **MasteringHealth**.

LO 2.1 Psychological health is the sum of how we think, feel, relate, and exist in our daily lives.

LO 2.2 Mental, emotional, social, and spiritual dimensions are all components of psychological health.

LO 2.3 Many factors influence psychological health, including life experiences, family, the environment, other people, self-esteem, self-efficacy, and personality.

LO 2.3 The mind-body connection is an important link in overall health and well-being. Positive psychology emphasizes happiness as a key factor in determining overall reaction to life's challenges.

LO 2.4 Developing self-esteem and self-efficacy, making healthy connections, having a positive outlook, and maintaining physical health enhance psychological health.

LO 2.5–2.6 Spirituality is having a purpose and meaning in life that's guided by values. Spirituality is distinct from religion, and has numerous physical and psychological benefits.

LO 2.7 Practicing mindfulness, meditation, yoga, prayer, and altruism can all contribute to spiritual health.

LO 2.8, 2.9 Anxiety disorders include generalized anxiety disorder, panic disorders, phobic disorders, obsessive-compulsive disorder, and post-traumatic stress disorder.

LO 2.8, 2.10 Mood disorders include major depression, dysthymic disorder, bipolar disorder, and seasonal affective disorder. College is a high-risk time for developing depression or anxiety disorders because of high stress levels, pressures for grades, and financial problems, among others.

LO 2.11 Other psychological disorders include personality disorders, schizophrenia, and learning disabilities and neurodevelopmental disorders.

LO 2.12 Aging changes the mind in many ways. Potential mental problems include Alzheimer's disease.

LO 2.12 Grief is the state of distress felt after loss. People differ in their responses to grief.

LO 2.13 Suicide is a result of negative psychosocial reactions to life. People intending to commit suicide often give signs of their intentions. Such people can often be helped.

LO 2.14 Mental health professionals include psychiatrists, psychoanalysts, psychologists, social workers, and counselors. Many therapy methods exist, including group, individual, cognitive, and behavioral therapies.

Pop Quiz

Visit MasteringHealth to personalize your study plan with Chapter Review Quizzes and Dynamic Study Modules.

LO 2.2 **1.** The term that most accurately refers to the feeling or subjective side of psychological health is
- a. social health.
- b. mental health.
- c. emotional health.
- d. spiritual health.

LO 2.3 **2.** A person with high self-esteem
- a. possesses feelings of self-respect and self-worth.
- b. believes he or she can successfully engage in a specific behavior.
- c. believes external influences shape psychosocial health.
- d. has a high altruistic capacity.

LO 2.3 **3.** All the following traits have been identified as being related to psychological well-being *except*
- a. conscientiousness.
- b. introversion.
- c. openness to experience.
- d. agreeableness.

LO 2.3 **4.** Subjective well-being includes all the following components *except*
- a. spirituality.
- b. satisfaction with present life.
- c. relative presence of positive emotions.
- d. relative absence of negative emotions.

LO 2.3 **5.** People who have experienced repeated failures at the same task may eventually quit trying altogether. This pattern of behavior is termed
- a. post-traumatic stress disorder.
- b. learned helplessness.
- c. self-efficacy.
- d. introversion.

LO 2.7 **6.** Kayla is a diver who enjoys the deep concentration needed to jump from the board and land gracefully in the water. When Kayla dives, she is engaging in which aspect of spiritual health?
- a. altruism
- b. mindfulness
- c. meditation
- d. contemplation

LO 2.9 **7.** This disorder is characterized by a need to perform rituals over and over.
- a. Personality disorder
- b. Obsessive-compulsive disorder
- c. Phobic disorder
- d. Post-traumatic stress disorder

LO 2.9 **8.** What is the number one mental health problem in the United States?
- a. Depression
- b. Anxiety disorders
- c. Alcohol dependence
- d. Schizophrenia

LO 2.10 **9.** Every winter, Jose suffers from irritability, apathy, weight gain, and sadness. He most likely has
- a. panic disorder.
- b. generalized anxiety disorder.
- c. seasonal affective disorder.
- d. chronic mood disorder.

LO 2.12 **10.** What happens in the early stage of Alzheimer's disease?
- a. Depression and combativeness
- b. Loss of control of bodily functions
- c. Impaired memory and judgment
- d. Loss of eyesight and hearing

Answers to these questions can be found on page A-1. If you answered a question incorrectly, review the module identified by the Learning Outcome. For even more study tools, visit MasteringHealth.

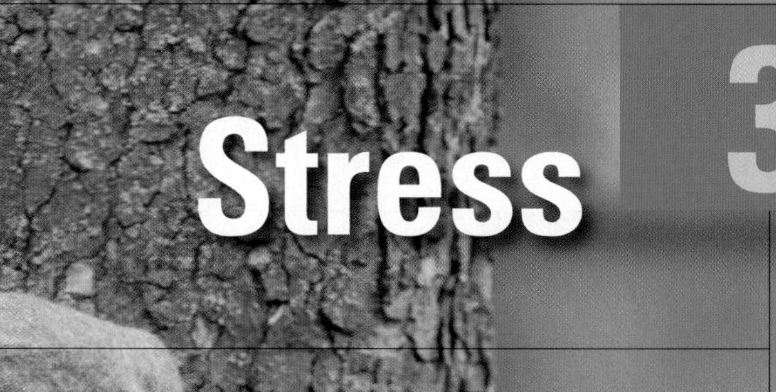

3 Stress

Rising tuition, difficult roommates, dating anxiety, grades, money, worries about what to do with your life—they all add up to STRESS. In today's 24/7 world, stress can lead us to feel overwhelmed. But it can also cause us to push ourselves to improve, bring excitement into an otherwise humdrum life, and leave us exhilarated. While we work, play, socialize, and sleep, stress affects us in myriad ways, many of which we may not even notice.

According to a recent American Psychological Association poll, Americans consistently report high stress levels, and 20 percent report extreme stress.[1] Adults ages 18–46 report the highest levels of stress and the greatest increases in stress levels.[2] The exact toll stress exerts on us during a lifetime of overload is unknown, but we do know that stress is a significant health hazard. It can affect virtually every system of the body, causing problems for us at work, in the home, and in our interactions with others. Even the youngest among us suffer from stress-related headaches, stomachaches, and difficulty sleeping, and stress seems to be particularly threatening to youth who are overweight.[3]

Is too much stress inevitable? Fortunately, the answer is no. To tame stress, we can learn to anticipate and recognize personal stressors—and develop skills to reduce or manage those we cannot avoid or control. First, we must understand what stress is and what effects it has on the body.

3.1 What Is Stress?

learning outcome

3.1 Define stress-related key terms.

Most current definitions state that **stress** is the mental and physical response and adaptation by our bodies to the real or perceived changes and challenges in our lives. A **stressor** is any real or perceived physical, social, environmental, or psychological event or stimulus that strains our abilities to cope. Several factors influence one's response to stressors, including the *characteristics of the stressor* (Can you control it? Is it predictable? Does it occur often?); *biological factors* (e.g., your age or gender); and *past experiences or fears* (e.g., things that have happened to you, their consequences, and how you responded). Stressors may be *tangible*, such as a failing grade on a test, or *intangible*, such as the angst associated with meeting your significant other's parents for the first time.

Distress, or negative stress, is more likely to occur when you are tired, under the influence of alcohol or other drugs, or coping with an illness, financial trouble, or relationship problems. In contrast, **eustress**, or positive stress, presents the opportunity for personal growth and satisfaction and can actually improve health. It can energize you, motivate you, and raise you up when you are down. Getting married or winning a major competition can give rise to the pleasurable rush associated with eustress.

There are several types of stress. **Acute stress** is typically intense, flares quickly, and disappears quickly. Seeing your crush could cause your heart to race and your muscles to tense while you appear cool, calm, and collected. Or anticipating a class presentation could cause shaking hands, nausea, headache, cramping, or diarrhea, along with a galloping heartbeat, stammering, and forgetfulness. **Episodic acute stress** is the state of *regularly* reacting with wild, acute stress to various situations. Individuals experiencing episodic acute stress may complain about all they have to do and focus on negative events that may or may not occur. These "awfulizers" are often reactive and anxious, but their thoughts and behaviors can be so habitual that to them they seem normal.

Although **chronic stress** may not feel as intense, it can linger indefinitely and wreak silent havoc on your body's systems. Caregivers are especially vulnerable to prolonged physiological stress as they watch a loved one struggle with a major disease or disability. Upon a loved one's eventual death, survivors may struggle to balance the need to process anger, grief, loneliness, and guilt with the need to stay caught up in classes, work, and everyday life. Another type of stress, **traumatic stress**, is often a result of witnessing or experiencing events like major accidents, war, shootings, assault, or natural disasters. Effects of traumatic stress may be felt for years after the event and cause significant disability, potentially leading to *post-traumatic stress disorder (PTSD)*.[4]

On any given day, we all experience both eustress and distress, each triggered by a wide range of both obvious and not-so-obvious

10.4%

of college students report experiencing "tremendous stress" over the past 12 months.

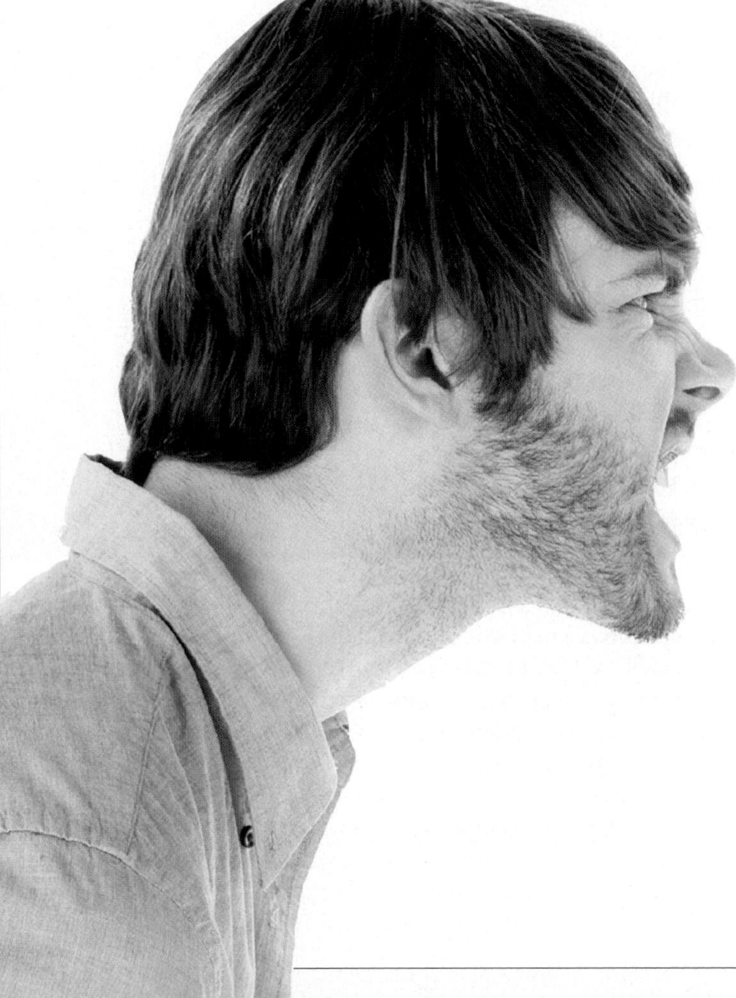

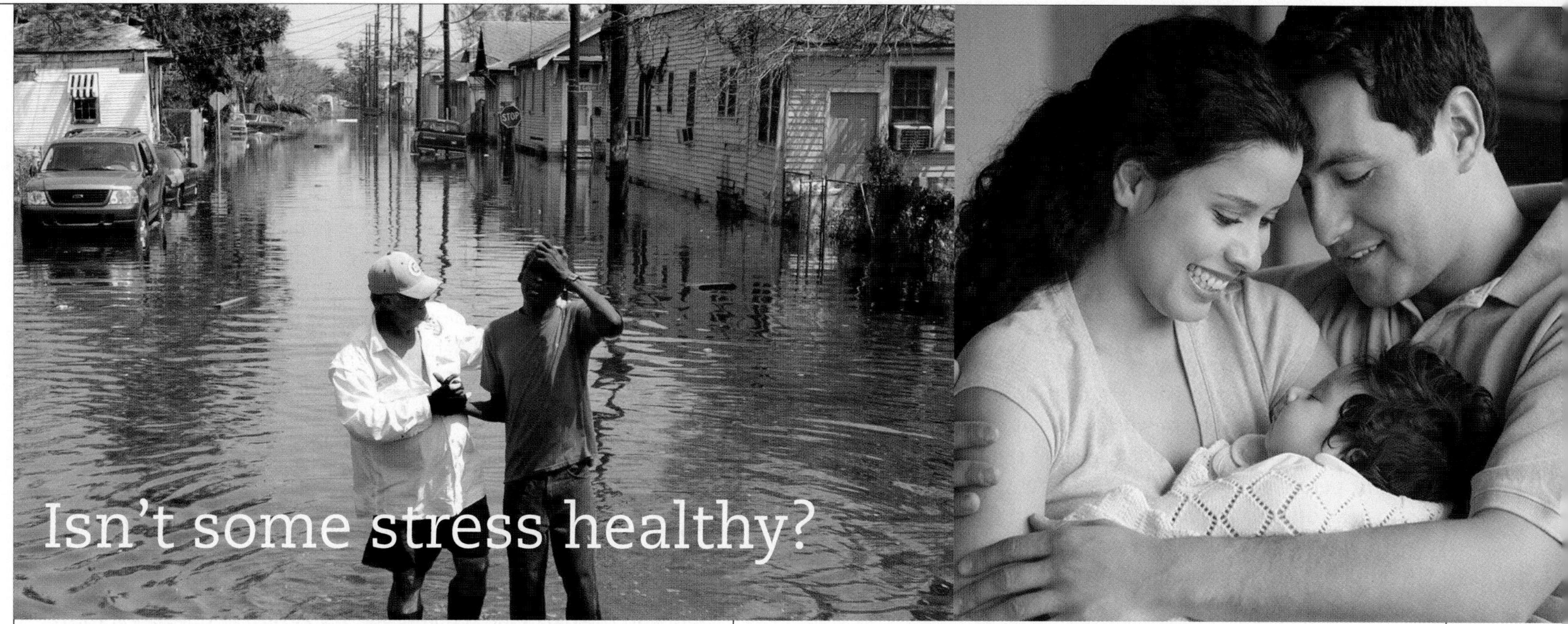

A moderate level of stress—especially eustress arising from new experiences—can actually help you live life to the fullest. Too much stress can affect your health for the worse, such as what is experienced by survivors of a natural disaster, but so can too little stress; we need change and challenge to keep us fulfilled and growing.

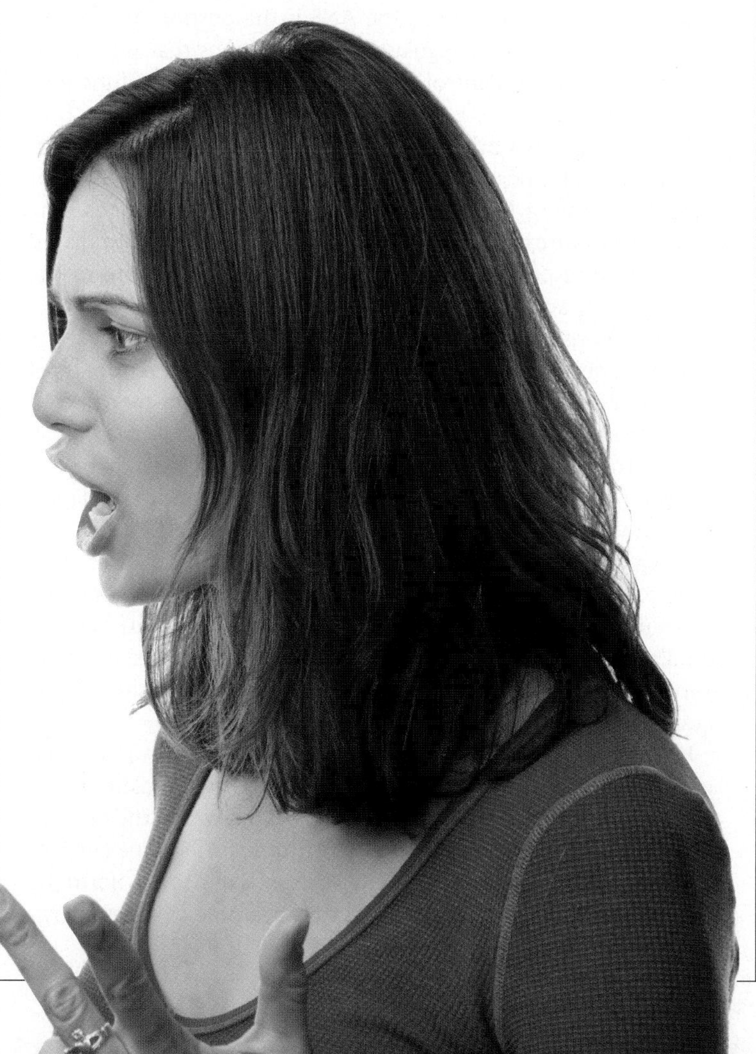

sources. Several studies in recent years have examined sources of stress among various populations in the United States and globally. One of the most comprehensive is conducted annually by the American Psychological Association; the 2013 survey found that the biggest sources of stress for adults ages 18–33 are work, money, and job stability, whereas individuals aged 67 and older were more likely to cite personal health concerns.[5] College students, in particular, face stressors that come from internal sources, as well as external pressures to succeed in a competitive environment that is often geographically far removed from the support of family and hometown friends.

While key sources of stress are similar for men and women (money, work, and the economy), huge gender differences exist in how people experience, report, and cope with stress. Both men and women report above average levels of stress, but women are more likely to report stress levels that are increasing and more extreme than those of their male counterparts.[6] Additionally, although men may recognize and report stress, they are much less likely to take action to reduce it.[7]

Awareness of the sources of the stress in your life can do much to help you develop a plan to avoid, prevent, and control the things that cause you stress.

check yourself

- **How do distress and eustress differ?**
- **Do you have more trouble managing acute stress or chronic stress? Why?**

3.2 Your Body's Response to Stress

learning outcome

3.2 Explain the purpose of the general adaptation syndrome, and the physiological changes that occur during each phase.

Our physiological responses evolved to protect us from harm. Thousands of years ago, if your ancestors didn't respond to stress by fighting or fleeing, they might have been eaten by a saber-toothed tiger or killed by a marauding enemy clan. Today when we face real or perceived threats, these same physiological responses kick into gear, but our instinctual reactions to fight, scream, or flee the enemy must be held in check. Restraining these responses rather than allowing them to run their course can make us physiologically charged for longer periods—sometimes chronically. Over time, a simmering stress response can wreak havoc on the body.

The General Adaptation Syndrome

When stress levels are low, the body is often in a state of **homeostasis**: All body systems are operating smoothly to maintain equilibrium. Stressors trigger a "crisis-mode" physiological response, after which the body attempts to return to homeostasis by means of an **adaptive response**. First characterized by Hans Selye in 1936, the internal fight to restore homeostasis in the face of a stressor is known as the **general adaptation syndrome (GAS)** (Figure 3.1). The GAS has three distinct phases: alarm, resistance, and exhaustion.[8]

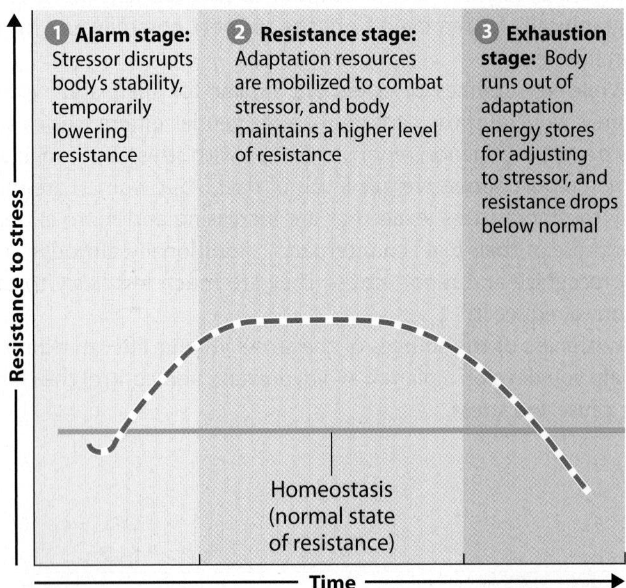

Figure 3.1 The General Adaptation Syndrome (GAS)
The GAS describes the body's method of coping with prolonged stress.

Regardless of whether you are experiencing distress or eustress, similar physiological changes occur.

Alarm Phase Suppose you are walking to your residence hall on a dimly lit campus after a night class. You hear someone cough behind you, and you sense someone approaching rapidly. You walk faster, only to hear the quickened footsteps of the other person. Your senses become increasingly alert, your breathing quickens, your heart races, and you begin to perspire. In desperation you stop, rip off your backpack, and prepare to fling it at your attacker to defend yourself. You turn around quickly and let out a blood-curdling yell. To your surprise, the only person you see is a classmate: She has been trying to stay close to you out of her own anxiety about walking alone in the dark. She screams and backs off the sidewalk into the bushes, and you both start laughing with startled embarrassment. You and your classmate have just experienced the alarm phase of the GAS. Also known as the **fight-or-flight response**, this physiological reaction is one of our most basic, innate survival instincts.[9]

When the mind perceives a real or imaginary stressor, the cerebral cortex, the region of the brain that interprets the nature of an event, triggers an **autonomic nervous system (ANS)** response that prepares the body for action. The ANS is the portion of the central nervous system that regulates body functions that we do not normally consciously control, such as heart and glandular functions and breathing.

The ANS has two branches: sympathetic and parasympathetic. The **sympathetic nervous system** energizes the body for fight or flight by signaling the release of several stress hormones. The **parasympathetic nervous system** slows all the systems stimulated by the stress response; in effect, it counteracts the actions of the sympathetic branch.

The responses of the sympathetic nervous system to stress involve a series of biochemical exchanges between different parts of the body. The brain's **hypothalamus** functions as the control center of the sympathetic nervous system and determines the overall reaction to stressors. When the hypothalamus perceives that extra energy is needed to fight a stressor, it stimulates the adrenal glands, which are located near the top of the kidneys, to release the hormone **epinephrine**, also called *adrenaline*. Epinephrine causes more blood to be pumped with each beat of the heart, dilates the airways in the lungs to increase oxygen intake, increases the breathing rate, stimulates the liver to release more glucose (which fuels muscular exertion), and dilates the pupils to improve visual sensitivity (see Figure 3.2).

In addition to the fight-or-flight response, the alarm phase can also trigger a longer-term reaction to stress. The hypothalamus uses chemical messages to trigger the pituitary gland within the brain to release a powerful hormone, *adrenocorticotropic hormone (ACTH)*. ACTH signals the adrenal glands to release **cortisol**, a hormone that makes stored nutrients more readily available to meet energy

More blood flows to brain; senses sharpen
Hearing ability increases
Perspiration increases
Respiration rate increases
Digestive system slows as blood supply is diverted to more critical areas
Blood-clotting ability increases
Immune system activity decreases
Pupils dilate to bring in more light and increase visual perception
Salivation decreases
Heart rate and blood pressure increase
Liver and fat tissues release energy-producing substances (such as glucose) into bloodstream
More blood flows to muscles; muscles tense
Urine production decreases

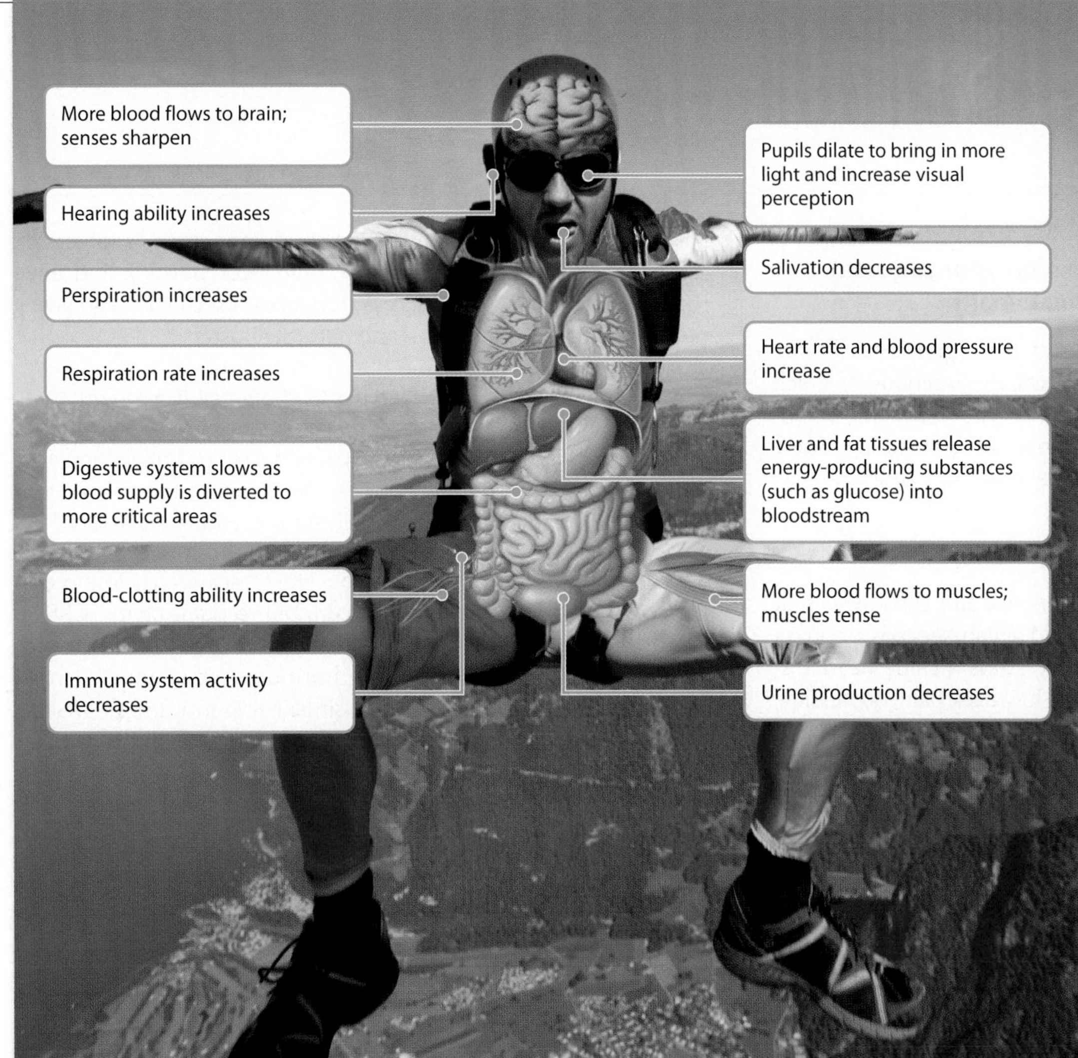

Figure 3.2 The Body's Acute Stress Response
Exposure to stress of any kind causes a complex series of involuntary physiological responses.

VIDEO TUTOR
Body's Stress Response

demands. Finally, other parts of the brain and body release endorphins, which relieve pain that a stressor may cause.

Resistance Phase In the resistance phase of the GAS, the body tries to return to homeostasis by resisting the alarm responses. However, because some perceived stressor still exists, the body does not achieve complete calm or rest. Instead, the body stays activated or aroused at a level that causes a higher metabolic rate in some organ tissues.

Exhaustion Phase In the exhaustion phase of the GAS, the hormones, chemicals, and systems that trigger and maintain the stress response are depleted, and the body returns to *allostasis*, or balance. You may feel tired or drained as your body returns to normal. In situations where stress is *chronic*, triggers may reverberate in the body, keeping body systems at a heightened arousal state. The prolonged effort to adapt to the stress response leads to **allostatic load**, or exhaustive wear and tear on the body. As the body adjusts to chronic unresolved stress, the adrenal glands continue to release cortisol, which remains in the bloodstream for longer periods of time as a result of slower metabolic responsiveness. Over time, cortisol can reduce **immunocompetence**, or the ability of the immune system to respond to attack. In turn, this increases the risk of diabetes, cardiovascular disease, and other chronic diseases.[10]

Men and Women Respond to Stress Differently

Ever since Walter Cannon's landmark studies in the 1930s, it's been thought that humans respond similarly to stressful events via the "fight-or-flight" response. However, several researchers now believe that men and women may respond differently to stressors. While men may be prone to fighting or fleeing, women may be more likely to "tend and befriend" by either trying to befriend the enemy or obtaining social support from others to ease stress-related reactions.[11] Additional studies point to the fact that one's mind-set may influence stress responses, and males and females may differ in their stress responses based on the way they perceive stressful events.[12]

check yourself

- **How does the general adaptation syndrome help us understand our reaction to stressors?**
- **How does the body react during each phase of the general adaptation syndrome?**
- **What are the differences between the *fight-or-flight* and the *tend-and-befriend* stress responses?**

3.3

Effects of Stress on Your Health

learning outcome

3.3 Describe the impact of stress on your physical, intellectual, and psychological health.

Stress is often described as a "disease of prolonged arousal" that leads to a cascade of negative health effects, the likelihood of which increases with ongoing stress. Nearly all body systems become potential targets, and the long-term effects may be devastating. Some warning symptoms of prolonged stress are shown in Figure 3.3.

Physical Effects of Stress

The higher the levels of stress you experience and the longer that stress continues, the greater the likelihood of damage to your physical health.[13] Ailments related to chronic stress include heart disease, diabetes, cancer, headaches, ulcers, low back pain, depression, and the common cold. Increases in rates of suicide, homicide, and domestic violence across the United States are additional symptoms of a nation under stress.

Stress and Cardiovascular Disease Perhaps the most documented health consequence of unresolved stress is cardiovascular disease (CVD). Research indicates that chronic stress plays a significant role in heart rate problems, high blood pressure, and atherosclerosis, as well as increased risk for a wide range of cardiovascular diseases.[14]

Chronic stress has been linked to increased arterial plaque buildup caused by elevated cholesterol, hardening of the arteries, increases in inflammatory responses in the body, alterations in heart rhythm, increased and fluctuating blood pressures, and other CVD risks.[15] Research has also shown direct links between CVD risks and social conditions, such as job strain, job instability, social isolation, discrimination, housing and environmental threats, lack of access to quality health care, caregiving responsibilities, bereavement, and natural disasters.[16]

Stress and Weight Gain You're not imagining it—you *are* more likely to gain weight when stressed. Higher stress levels may increase cortisol levels in the bloodstream, contributing to hunger and activating fat-storing enzymes; studies also support the theory that cortisol plays a role in increased belly fat and eating behaviors.[17]

Stress and Alcohol Dependence New research has found that a specific stress hormone, the *corticotropin-releasing factor* (CRF), is key to the development and maintenance of alcohol dependence in animals. CRF stimulates stress hormone secretion as part of the stress response. It may play a similar role in humans, making it harder for stressed alcoholics to abstain from alcohol. If proven, substances that diminish CRF receptor activity may help those dealing with the difficulties of abstaining from alcohol when stressed.[18]

Stress and Hair Loss The most common stress-induced hair loss is *telogen effluvium*. Often seen in individuals who have lost a loved one or experienced severe weight loss or other trauma, this condition pushes colonies of hair into a resting phase; over time, hair may begin to fall out. A similar condition, *alopecia areata*, occurs when stress triggers white blood cells to attack and destroy hair follicles.[19]

Stress and Diabetes Controlling stress is critical for preventing development of type 2 diabetes as well as for successful diabetes management.[20] People under severe stress often don't get enough sleep, don't eat well, and may drink or take other drugs. These behaviors can alter blood sugar levels and promote development of diabetes.

Stress and Digestive Problems Although stress may not directly cause digestive diseases or disorders, it is clearly related and may actually make

Why do I always get sick during finals week?

Prolonged stress can compromise your immune system, leaving you vulnerable to infection. If you spend exam week in a state of high stress—sleeping too little, studying too hard, and worrying a lot—chances are you'll reduce your body's ability to fight off any cold or flu bugs you may encounter.

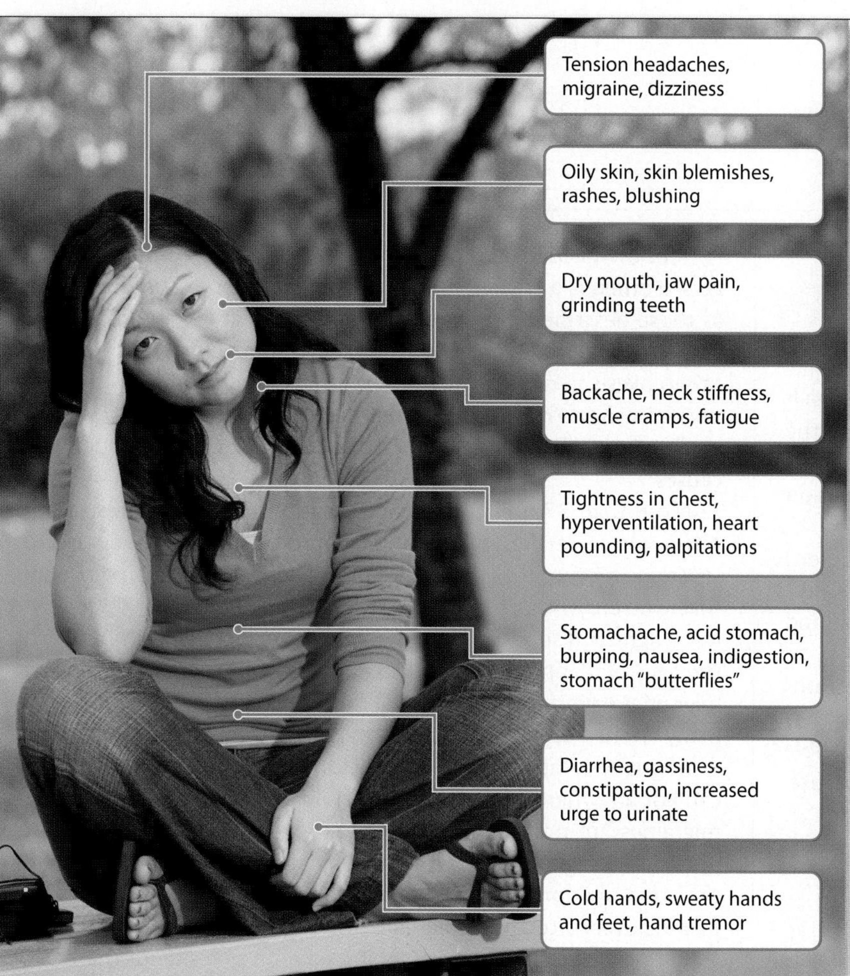

Figure 3.3 Common Physical Symptoms of Stress
You may not even notice how stressed you are until your body starts sending you signals. Do you frequently experience any of these physical symptoms of stress?

your risk of having symptoms worse.[21] Irritable bowel syndrome may be more likely, in part, because stress stimulates colon spasms by means of the nervous system. Relaxation techniques and mindfulness training may reduce the activity of the sympathetic nervous system, leading to decreases in heart rate, blood pressure, and other stress responses that trigger gastrointestinal tract flare-ups.[22]

Stress and Impaired Immunity A growing area of investigation known as **psychoneuroimmunology (PNI)** analyzes the relationship between stress and immune function. Research suggests that increased stress over time can affect cellular immune response. This increases risks for upper respiratory infections and certain chronic conditions, increases adverse birth outcomes and fetal development, and exacerbates problems for children and adults suffering from post-traumatic stress.[23]

Intellectual and Psychological Effects of Stress

In a recent national survey of college students, over half (51.8%) said they felt overwhelmed by all that they had to do within the past 2 weeks, with a similar number reporting they felt exhausted. Forty-two percent felt they had been under more than average stress in the past 12 months, with 10 percent reporting tremendous stress during that period. Not surprisingly, these same students rated stress as their number one impediment to academic performance, followed by anxiety and lack of sleep.[24] Stress can play a huge role in whether a student stays in school, gets good grades, and succeeds on a career path. It can also wreak havoc on a person's ability to concentrate, remember, and understand and retain complex information.

39% **of those ages 18–33 say their stress levels have increased in the last year, with 52 percent saying their stress levels keep them awake at night.**

Stress, Memory, and Concentration Animal studies provide compelling indicators of how *glucocorticoids*—stress hormones released from the adrenal cortex—affect memory. In humans, acute stress has been shown to impair memory—affecting the way we think, decide, and respond in stressful situations.[25] Prolonged exposure to *cortisol* (a key stress hormone) has been linked to shrinking of the hippocampus, the brain's major memory center.[26] Other research indicates that prolonged exposure to high levels of stress hormones may actually predispose women, in particular, to Alzheimer's disease.[27]

Stress and Mental Disorders Stress is an enormous contributor to mental disability and emotional dysfunction in industrialized nations. Studies have shown that the rates of mental disorders, particularly depression and anxiety, are associated with various environmental stressors from childhood through adulthood, including violence and abuse, marital and relationship conflict, poverty, and other stressful life events.[28]

See It! Videos
Can a test identify your risk for stress-related illnesses? Watch **Stress Can Damage Women's Health** in the Study Area of MasteringHealth.

check yourself

- **What are four possible effects of stress on your physical and psychological health?**
- **Give an example of an instance in which psychological stress had a physical effect on you.**

3.4 Stress and Headaches

learning **outcome**

3.4 Describe common types of headaches, and explain possible connections between stress and headaches.

Millions of people see their doctors for headaches each year; millions more put up with the pain or take pain relievers to blunt the symptoms. The good news: Most headaches are not a sign of serious diseases or underlying conditions. The vast majority are tension headaches and migraines.

Nearly 80 percent of adults (slightly more women than men) get the most common type of headache, a *tension-type headache*.[29] Symptoms may include dull pain; a sensation of tightness; and tender scalp, neck, and shoulder muscles.[30]

Tension headaches are generally caused by muscle contractions or tension and pain in the neck or head, forehead, or temples; they can last for as little as 30 minutes or as long as a week.[31] Possible triggers include red wine, lack of sleep, fasting, muscle overuse, stress, anger, and menstruation.

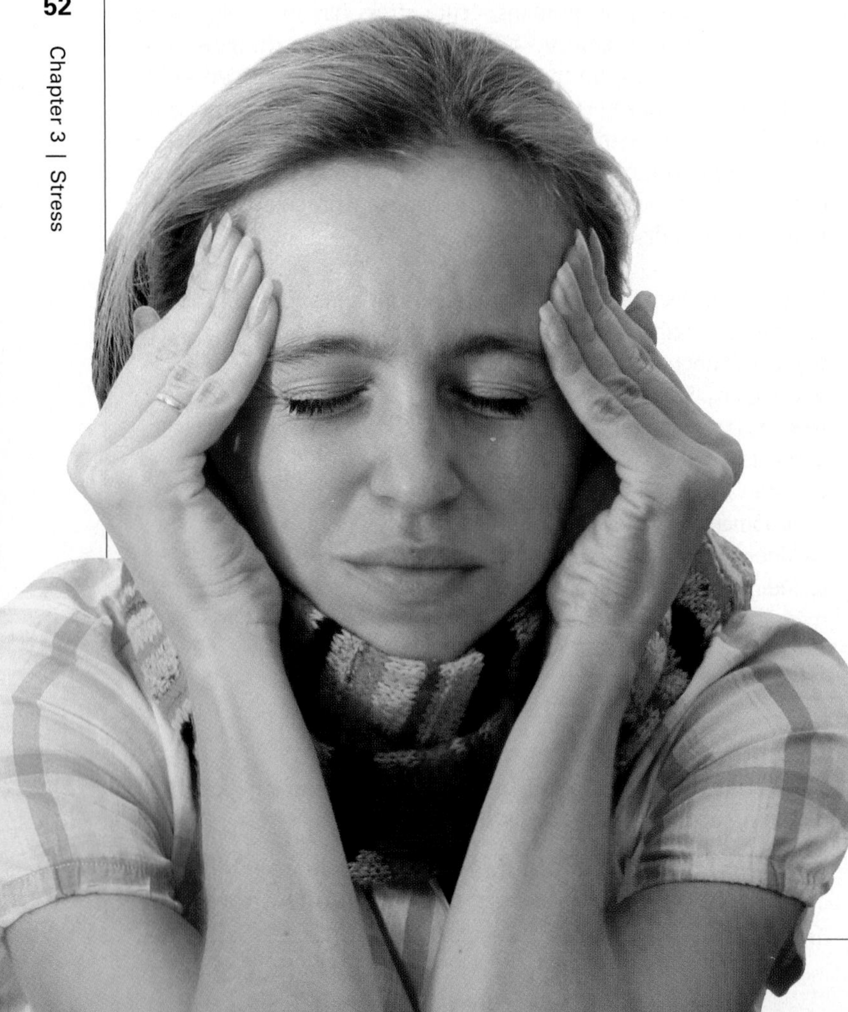

Tension headaches are most often helped by reducing triggers. If stress is a trigger, try a range of relaxation techniques, such as those described later in the module "Relaxation Techniques for Stress Management." Exercise can relieve some tension headaches, as can over-the-counter pain relievers. Frequent headaches that are unresponsive to over-the-counter medications are probably *chronic tension headaches*; these warrant a doctor visit to assess underlying causes.

More than 37 million Americans suffer from **migraines**, headaches whose severe, debilitating symptoms include moderate to severe pain on one or both sides of the head, throbbing pain, pain that worsens with or interferes with activity, nausea, and sensitivity to light and sound.[32] Usually, migraine incidence peaks between the ages of 15 and 55, and 70 to 80 percent of those experiencing migraines have a family history of these headaches.[33] Three times as many women as men suffer from migraines.[34]

Migraine symptoms vary greatly for each individual, and attacks can last anywhere from 4 to 72 hours. In about 20 percent of cases, migraines are preceded by a warning sign called an *aura*—most often flickering vision, blind spots, tingling in the arms or legs, or a sensation of odor or taste.[35] Prescription drugs and over-the-counter pain relievers often help migraine sufferers.

Cluster headaches cause stabbing pain on one side of the head, behind the eye, or in one defined spot. Fortunately, cluster headaches are among the more rare forms of headache, affecting less than 1 percent of people, usually men. Young adults in their twenties tend to be particularly susceptible.[36]

Cluster headaches can last for weeks and disappear quickly. More commonly, they last for 40 to 90 minutes during rapid eye movement (REM) sleep. Oxygen therapy, drugs, and even surgery have been used to treat severe cases.

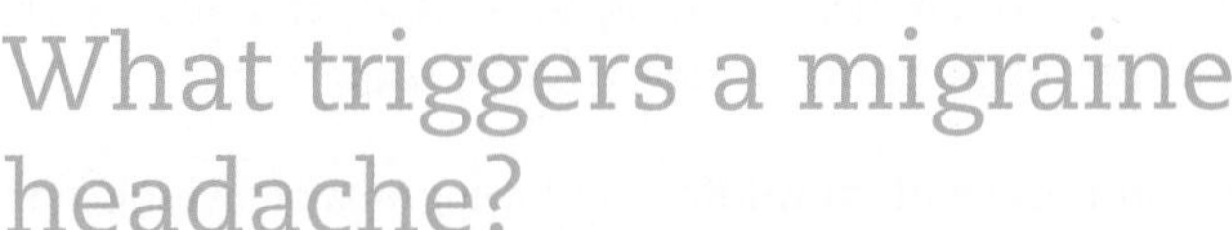

What triggers a migraine headache?

Patients report that migraines can be triggered by emotional stress, too much or not enough sleep, fasting, caffeine, alcohol, hormonal changes, altitude, weather, chocolate or other foods, and a litany of other causes. There is tremendous variability, and what triggers a migraine in one person may relieve it in another.

check yourself

- **What are three common types of headaches?**
- **How could effective stress management contribute to headache reduction?**

Stress and Sleep Problems

learning **outcome**

3.5 Describe the importance of sleep to good health, and list strategies for ensuring restful sleep.

In a recent survey, over 60 percent of students said they felt tired, dragged out, or sleepy for 3 or more days in the past week.[37] Sleep deficiencies have been linked to a host of student issues, including poor academic performance, weight gain, increased alcohol abuse, accidents, daytime drowsiness, relationship issues, depression, and other problems.[38]

Sleep is much more important than most people realize. Sleep conserves body energy and restores you physically and mentally. Sleep also contributes to healthy metabolism, which helps you maintain a healthy body weight.

Colds, flu, and many other ailments are more common when your immune system is depressed by lack of sleep. Recent studies found that poor sleep quality and shorter sleep duration increased susceptibility to the common cold.[39] Sleep disruption can also disrupt overall immune function.[40]

High blood pressure is more common in people who get fewer than 7 hours of sleep a night.[41] Short-duration sleep increases the risk of developing and/or dying from cardiovascular disease.[42]

Restricting sleep can cause attention lapses, slow or poor memory, reduced cognitive ability, and a tendency for thinking to get "stuck in a rut."[43] Your ability not only to remember facts but also to integrate those facts, make meaningful generalizations about them, and consolidate what you've learned requires adequate sleep.[44]

Sleep also has a restorative effect on motor function, affecting one's ability to perform tasks such as driving a car.[45] Researchers contend that a night without sleep impairs motor skills and reaction time as much as driving drunk.[46]

Certain brain regions, including the cerebral cortex (your "master mind"), achieve some form of essential rest only during sleep. You're also more likely to feel stressed out, worried, or sad when you're sleep deprived. Stress and sleep problems can reinforce or exacerbate each other.

Seven to 8 hours is considered "average" sleep time, and the vast majority of people need this much.[47] Individual variations do occur according to age (kids need more), gender (women need more), and other factors. In addition, when trying to figure out your sleep needs, you have to consider your body's physiological

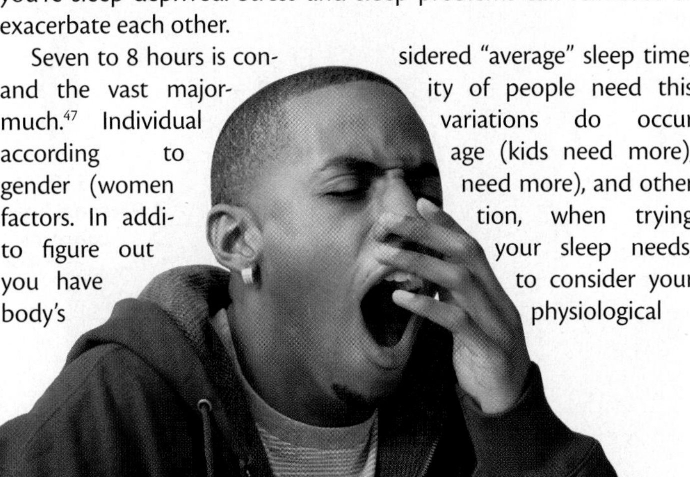

People aged

13 to 29

are the sleepiest members of the U.S. population.

need plus your **sleep debt**—the total hours of missed sleep you're carrying. The good news is that you can catch up, if you do it sensibly over time. Ways to ensure a good night's sleep include the following:

- **Let there be light.** Stay in sync with your circadian rhythm by spending time in the daylight.
- **Stay active.** Exercisers are much more likely to feel rested than those who are sedentary.
- **Sleep tight.** Comfortable pillows, bedding, and mattress can help you sleep more soundly.
- **Create a sleep "cave."** As bedtime approaches, keep your bedroom quiet, cool, dark, and free of technology.
- **Condition yourself into better sleep.** Go to bed and get up at the same time each day.
- **Avoid foods and drinks that keep you awake.** Large meals, nicotine, energy drinks, caffeine, and alcohol close to bedtime can affect your ability to fall asleep and stay asleep. It takes your body about 6 hours to clear just *half* of a caffeinated drink from your system.[48]
- **Don't drink large amounts of liquid before bed**. This prevents having to get up in the night to use the bathroom.
- **Don't toss and turn.** If you're not asleep after 20 minutes, read or listen to gentle music. Once you feel sleepy, go back to bed.
- **Don't nap in the late afternoon or evening**. Also, don't nap for longer than 30 minutes.
- **Don't read, study, watch TV, use your laptop, talk on the phone, eat, or smoke in bed.** Emotionally intense phone conversations can also make it hard to calm yourself enough to sleep.
- **Don't take sleeping pills.** Don't take sleep aids unless prescribed by your health care provider. Over-the-counter sleep aids can interfere with progression through the stages of sleep.

See It! Videos

What kind of sleep keeps your memory sharp? Watch **How Sleep Affects Your Memory** in the Study Area of MasteringHealth.

check yourself

- **Why is it important for your health to sleep well?**
- **What are three common reasons for poor sleep, and how can you overcome them?**

3.6 Psychosocial Causes of Stress

learning outcome

3.6 Discuss and classify psychosocial sources of stress.

Psychosocial stressors refer to the factors in our daily routines and in our social and physical environments that cause us to experience stress (Figure 3.4). Which of these are most common in your life?

Adjustment to Change Any change, whether good or bad, occurring in your normal routine can result in stress. The more changes you experience and the more adjustments you must make, the greater the chances are that stress will have an impact on your health. The enormous changes associated with starting college, while exciting, can also be among the most stressful you will face in your life. Moving away from home, trying to fit in and make new friends from diverse backgrounds, adjusting to a new schedule, learning to live with strangers in housing that is often lacking in the comforts of home—all of these things can cause sleeplessness and anxiety and keep your body in a continual fight-or-flight mode.

Hassles Some psychologists have proposed that little stressors, frustrations, and petty annoyances, known collectively as *hassles*, can be just as stressful as major life changes.[49] Listening to classmates who talk too much during lectures, being near people chatting on the phone and texting while you are trying to study, not finding parking on campus, and a host of other small but bothersome situations can trigger frustration, anger, and fight-or-flight responses.[50]

Technostress Technostress is stress created by a dependence on technology and the constant state of connection, which can include a perceived obligation to always respond or be ever present. Research supports the concept that being "wired" 24/7 can lead to anxiety, obsessive compulsive disorder, narcissism, sleep disorders, frustration, time pressures, and guilt—some of the negative consequences known as iDisorders.[51] According to a new study, college students who can't keep their hands off their mobile devices are reporting higher levels of anxiety, less satisfaction with life, and lower grades than peers who use their devices less often. The average student surveyed spent nearly 5 hours per day using his or her cell phone for everything from calling and texting to Facebook, e-mails, gaming, and more.[52]

To reduce technostress, set limits on your technology use, and make sure that you devote sufficient time to face-to-face interactions with people you care about, cultivating and nurturing your relationships. You don't always need to answer your phone or respond to a text or e-mail immediately. Leave your devices at home or turn them off when you are out with others or on vacation. Tune in to your surroundings, your loved ones and friends, your job, and your classes.

The Toll of Relationships Relationships can trigger enormous fight-or-flight reactions—whether we're talking about the exhilaration of new love or the pain of a breakup, the result is often lack of focus, lack of sleep, and an inability to focus on anything but the love interest. And although we may think first of love relationships, even relationships with friends, family members, and coworkers can be the sources of overwhelming struggles, just as they can be sources of strength and support. These relationships can make us strive to be the best that we can be and give us hope for the future, or they can diminish our self-esteem and leave us reeling from a destructive interaction.

69%
Money
61%
Economy
65%
Work
57% Family responsibilities
56%
Relationships
51%
Personal health concerns
52%
Family health problems

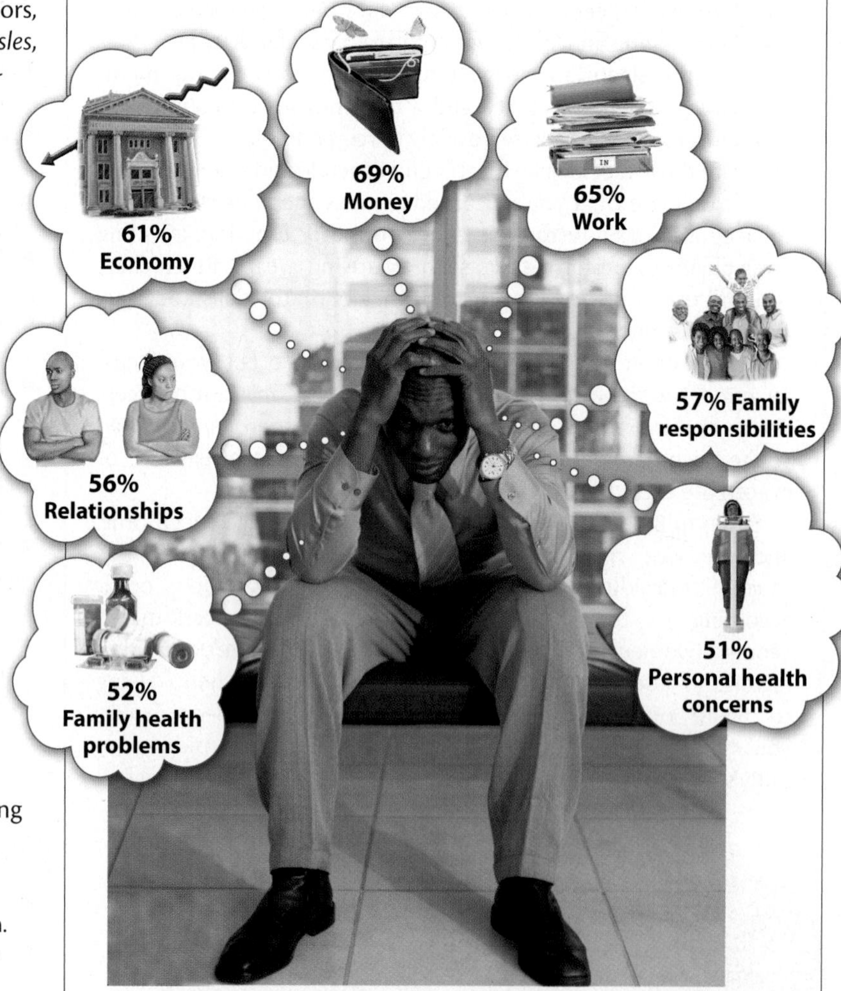

Figure 3.4 What Stresses Us?
Respondents indicated the events and issues that cause stress for them.
Source: Data are from the American Psychological Association, *2012 Stress in America, Key Findings*, 2013, www.apa.org.

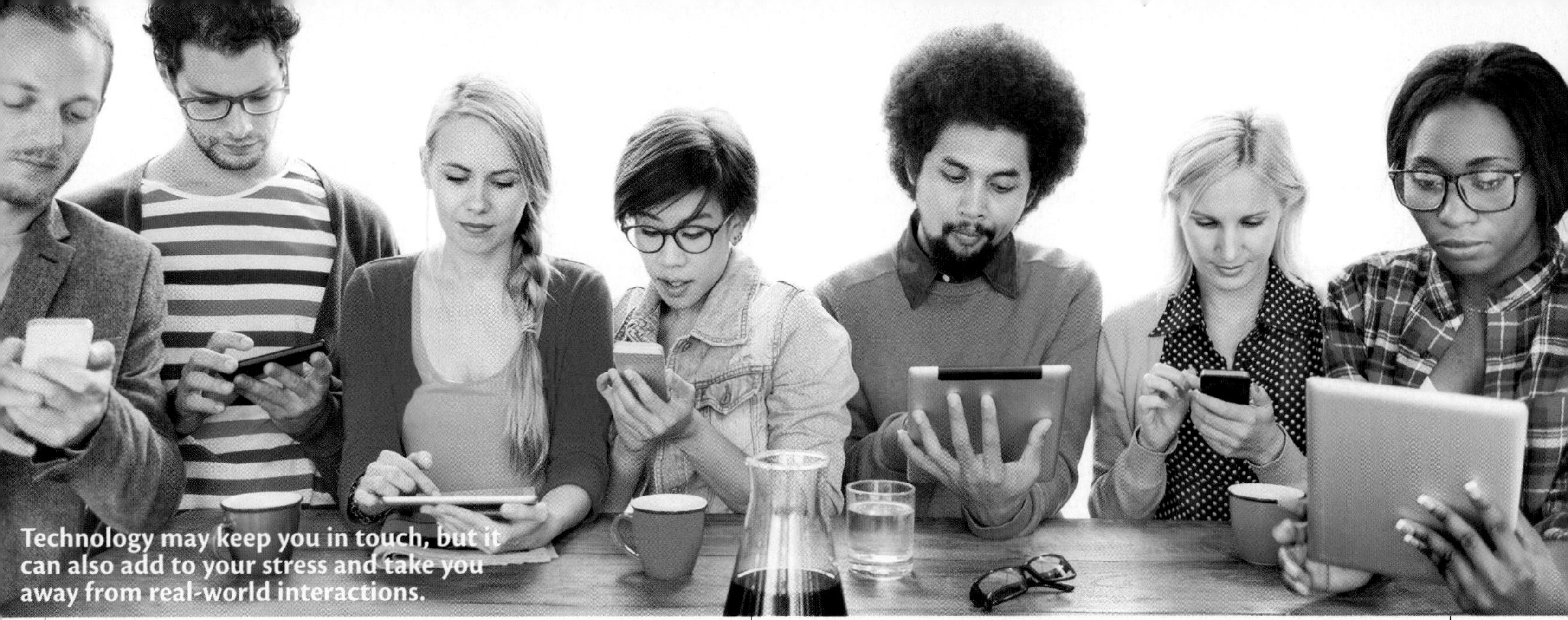
Technology may keep you in touch, but it can also add to your stress and take you away from real-world interactions.

Academic and Financial Pressure It isn't surprising that today's college and university students face mind-boggling amounts of pressure competing for grades, athletic positions, internships, and jobs. Challenging classes can be tough enough, but many students must also juggle work in order to pay bills. When economic conditions become strained, the effects on people with limited resources (particularly students) can be significant. An economic downturn can even make student dreams seem unattainable. Increasing reports of mental health problems on college campuses may be one of the results of too much stress.

Frustrations and Conflicts Disparity between our goals (what we hope to obtain in life) and our behaviors (actions that may or may not lead to these goals) can trigger frustration. Conflicts occur when we are forced to decide among competing motives, impulses, desires, and behaviors, or to face demands incompatible with our own values and sense of importance. College students away from their families and familiar communities for the first time may face conflicts among parental values, their own beliefs, and the beliefs of those different from themselves.

Overload We've all experienced times when the combined demands of work, responsibilities, and relationships seem to be pulling us under—and our physical, mental, and emotional reserves are insufficient to deal with it all. Students suffering from **overload** may experience depression, sleeplessness, mood swings, frustration, and anxiety. Unrelenting overload can lead to a state of physical and mental exhaustion known as *burnout*.

Stressful Environments For many students, the environment around them can cause significant stress. Perhaps you cannot afford safe, healthy housing, a bad roommate constantly makes life uncomfortable, or loud neighbors keep you up at night.

Unexpected natural disasters—such as flooding, earthquakes, hurricanes, blizzards, and tornadoes—can cause tremendous stress at the time and for years later. Often equally damaging are environmental **background distressors**—including noise, air, and water pollution; allergy-aggravating pollen and dust; and secondhand smoke—that trigger a constant resistance phase.

Bias and Discrimination Diversity of students, faculty members, and staff enriches everyone's educational experience. It also challenges us to examine our attitudes and biases. Those perceived as dissimilar due to race, ethnicity, religious affiliation, age, or sexual orientation—or differences in viewpoint, appearance, behavior, or background—may become victims of subtle and not-so-subtle bigotry, insensitivity, harassment, or hostility, or may simply be ignored.[53]

Evidence of the health effects of excessive stress in minority groups abounds. For example, African Americans suffer higher rates of hypertension, CVD, and most cancers than do whites.[54] Although poverty and socioeconomic status have been blamed for much of the spike in hypertension rates for African Americans and other marginalized groups, this chronic, physically debilitating stress may reflect real and perceived effects of institutional racism even more than it reflects poverty. While more research is necessary to show a direct link, racism may influence stress-related hypertension and make it difficult for those affected to engage in healthy lifestyle behaviors.[55]

International students experience unique adjustment issues such as language barriers, financial issues, cultural barriers, and a lack of social support. Academic stress may pose a particular problem for the more than 765,000 international students who have left family and friends in their native countries to study in the United States. Yet many international students refrain from seeking emotional support from others because of cultural norms, feelings of shame, or the belief that seeking support is a sign of weakness. These factors, coupled with language barriers, cultural conflicts, and other stressors, can lead international students to suffer significantly more stress-related illnesses than their American counterparts.[56]

check yourself

- **What are five sources of psychosocial stress?**
- **Which psychosocial sources of stress do you encounter most frequently?**

3.7 Internal Causes of Stress

learning outcome

3.7 Discuss and classify internal causes of stress.

Although stress can come from the environment and other external sources, it can result from internal factors as well. Internal stressors such as negative appraisal, low self-esteem, and low self-efficacy can cause unsettling thoughts or feelings and can ultimately affect your health. It is important to address and manage these internal stressors.

Appraisal and Stress Throughout life, we encounter many different demands and potential stressors—some biological, some psychological, and others sociological. In any case, it is our **appraisal** of these demands, rather than the demands themselves, that results in our experiencing stress. Appraisal is defined as the interpretation and evaluation of information provided to the brain by the senses. As new information becomes available, appraisal helps us recognize stressors, evaluate them on the basis of past experiences and emotions, and decide whether or not we have the ability to cope with them. When you feel that the stressors of life are overwhelming and you lack control, you are more likely to feel strain and distress.

Self-Esteem and Self-Efficacy *Self-esteem* refers to how you feel about yourself. Self-esteem varies; it can and does continually change.[57] When you feel good about yourself, you are less likely to view certain events as stressful and more likely to be able to cope.[58]

Of particular concern, research with high school and college students has found that low self-esteem and stressful life events significantly predict **suicidal ideation**, a desire to die and thoughts about suicide. On a more positive note, research has also indicated that it is possible to increase an individual's ability to cope with stress by increasing self-esteem.[59]

Self-efficacy, or confidence in one's skills and ability to cope with life's challenges, appears to be a key buffer in preventing negative stress effects. Research has shown that people with high levels of self-efficacy tend to feel more in control of stressful situations and, as such, report fewer stress effects.[60] Self-efficacy is considered one of the most important personality traits that influence psychological and physiological stress responses.[61]

Developing self-efficacy is also vital to coping with and overcoming academic pressures and worries. For example, by learning to handle anxiety around testing situations, you improve your chances of performing well; the more you feel yourself capable of handling testing situations, the greater will be your sense of academic self-efficacy.

Type A and Type B Personalities It should come as no surprise to you that personality can have an impact on whether you are happy and socially well-adjusted or sad and socially isolated. However, your personality may affect more than just your social interactions: It may be a critical factor in your stress level, as well as in your risk for CVD, cancer, and other chronic and infectious diseases.

In 1974, physicians Meyer Friedman and Ray Rosenman published a book indicating that type A individuals had a greatly increased risk of heart disease.[62] *Type A* personalities are defined as hard-driving, competitive, time-driven perfectionists. In contrast, *type B*

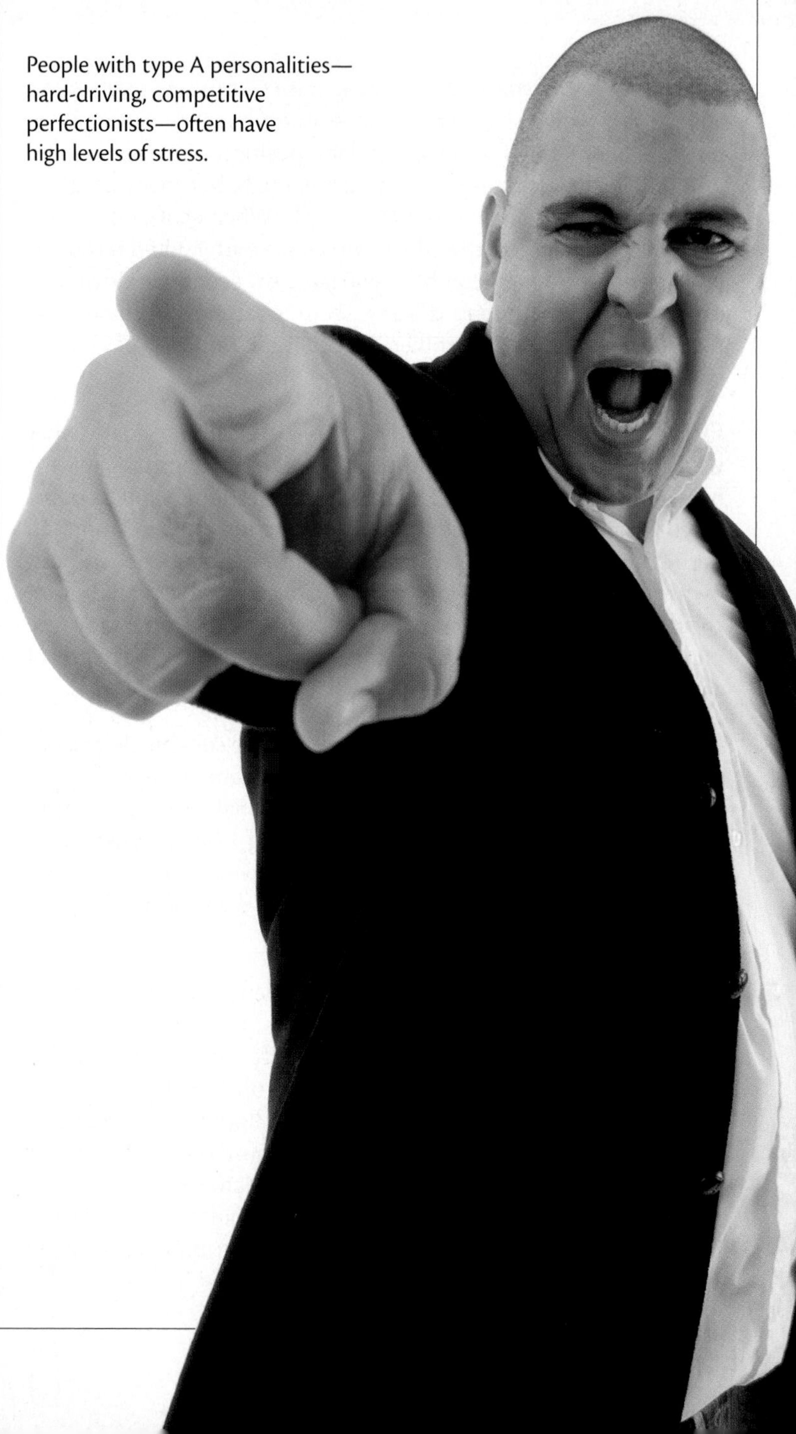

People with type A personalities—hard-driving, competitive perfectionists—often have high levels of stress.

personalities are described as being relaxed, noncompetitive, and more tolerant of others.

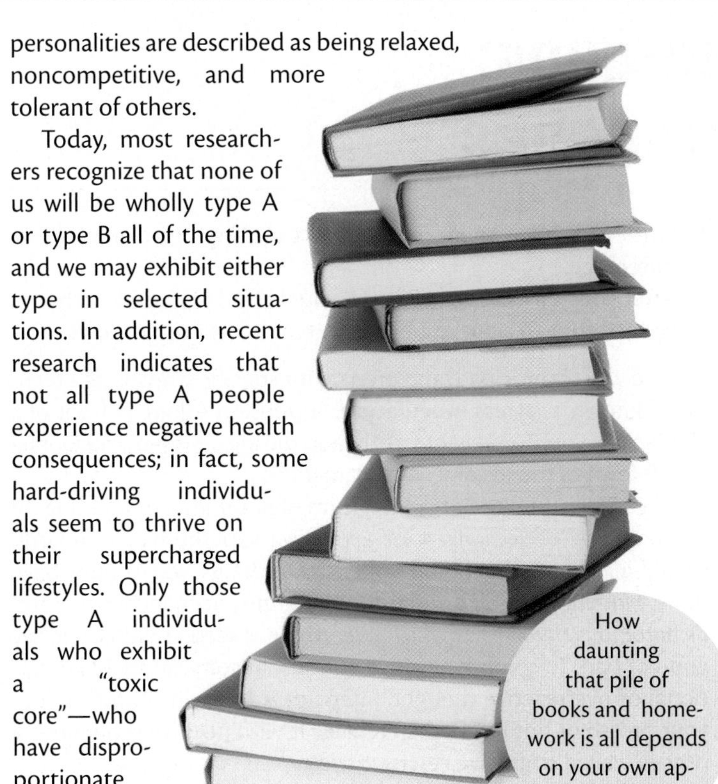
How daunting that pile of books and homework is all depends on your own appraisal of it.

Today, most researchers recognize that none of us will be wholly type A or type B all of the time, and we may exhibit either type in selected situations. In addition, recent research indicates that not all type A people experience negative health consequences; in fact, some hard-driving individuals seem to thrive on their supercharged lifestyles. Only those type A individuals who exhibit a "toxic core"—who have disproportionate amounts of anger, are distrustful of others, and have a cynical, glass-half-empty approach to life; in total, a set of characteristics referred to as **hostility**—are at increased risk for heart disease.[63]

Type C and Type D Personalities In addition to CVD risks, personality types have been linked to increased risk for a variety of illnesses ranging from asthma to cancer. *Type C* personality is one such type, characterized as stoic, with a tendency to stuff feelings down and conform to the wishes of others (or be "pleasers"). Preliminary research suggests that type C individuals may be more susceptible to illnesses such as asthma, multiple sclerosis, autoimmune disorders, and cancer; however, more research is necessary to support this relationship.[64]

A more recently identified personality type is *type D* (distressed), characterized by a tendency toward excessive negative worry, irritability, gloom, and social inhibition. Several recent studies have shown that type D people may be up to eight times more likely to die of a heart attack or sudden cardiac death.[65]

Psychological Hardiness and Resilience According to psychologist Susanne Kobasa, **psychological hardiness** may negate self-imposed stress associated with type A behavior. Psychologically hardy people are characterized by control, commitment, and willingness to embrace challenge.[66] People with a sense of control are able to accept responsibility for their behaviors and change those that they discover to be debilitating. People with a sense of commitment have good self-esteem and understand their purpose in life. Those who embrace challenge see change as a stimulating opportunity for personal growth. Today, the concept of hardiness has evolved to include a person's overall ability to cope with stress and adversity.[67] In recent years, it has become common for people to think of this general hardiness concept in terms of **psychological resilience**—our capacity to maintain or regain psychological well-being in the face of challenge.[68]

Shift and Persist An emerging body of research proposes that in the midst of extreme, persistent adversity, youth—often with the help of positive role models in their lives—are able to reframe appraisals of current stressors more positively (*shifting*), while *persisting* in focusing on a positive future. These youth are able to endure the present by adapting, holding on to meaningful things in their lives, and staying optimistic and positive. These "**shift-and-persist**" strategies are among the most recently identified factors that protect against the negative effects of too much stress in our lives.[69]

Skills for Behavior Change

OVERCOMING TEST-TAKING ANXIETY

Here are helpful hints to increase your self-efficacy and reduce your stress levels in a familiar situation: an academic exam.

Before the Exam

- **Manage your study time. Start studying at least a week before your test to reduce anxiety. Do a limited review the night before, get a good night's sleep, and arrive for the exam early.**
- **On an index card, write down three reasons you will pass the exam. Keep the card with you and review it whenever you study. When you get the test, write your three reasons on the test or on a piece of scrap paper.**
- **Eat a balanced meal before the exam. Avoid sugar and rich or heavy foods, as well as foods that might upset your stomach. You want to feel your best.**
- **Think about how much time you might need to answer different types of test questions. Make a general strategy before the test to efficiently use the time allotted. Wear a watch to class on the day of the test.**

During the Test

- **Manage your time during the test. Look at how many questions there are and what each is worth. Prioritize the high-point questions, allow a certain amount of time for each, and make sure that you leave some time for the rest. Hold to this schedule.**
- **Slow down and pay attention. Focus on one question at a time. Check off each part of multipart questions to make sure your answers are complete.**

check yourself

- **What are five causes of internal stress?**
- **Which internal causes of stress do you experience most frequently?**

3.8 Stress Management Techniques: Mental and Physical Approaches

learning outcome

3.8 Examine mental and physical approaches to stress management.

Being on your own in college may pose challenges, but it also lets you take control of and responsibility for your life and take steps to reduce negative stressors. **Coping** is the act of managing events or conditions to lessen the physical or psychological effects of excess stress.[70] One of the most effective ways to combat stressors is to build coping strategies and skills, known collectively as *stress-management techniques*.

Practicing Mental Work to Reduce Stress

Your perceptions often contribute to your stress, so assessing your "self-talk," beliefs, and actions are good first steps. Here's how:

- Make a list of things you're worried about.
- Examine the causes of your problems and worries.
- Consider the size of each problem. What are the consequences of doing nothing versus taking action?
- List your options, including ones you may not like much.
- Outline a plan, then act. Even little things can make a big difference.
- After you act, evaluate. How did you do? Do you need to change your actions to achieve a better outcome next time? How?

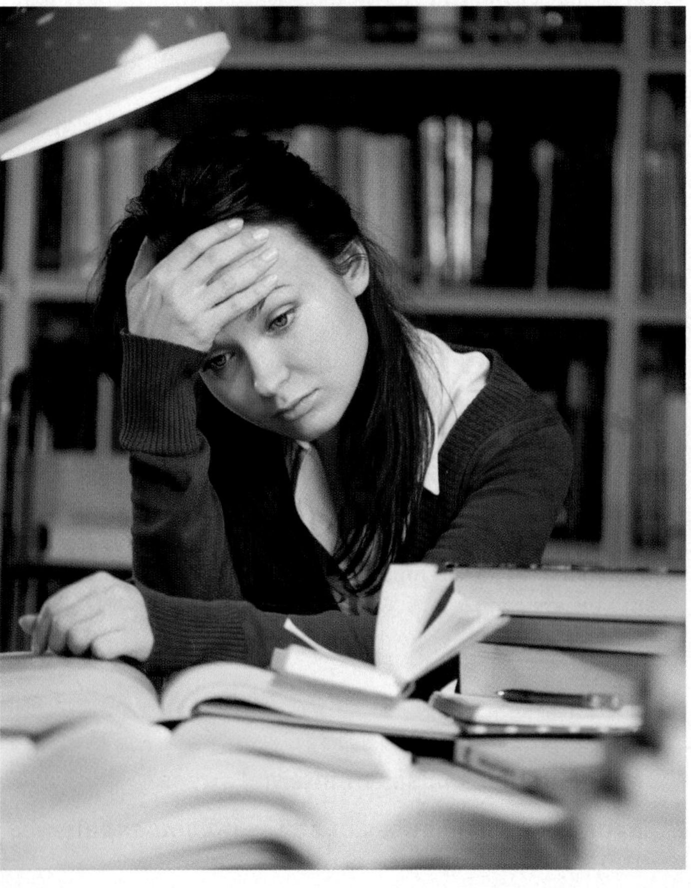

One way to anticipate and prepare for specific stressors is a technique known as **stress inoculation**. Suppose speaking in front of a class scares you. To prevent freezing up during a presentation, practice in front of friends or a video camera.

Negative self-talk can take the form of *pessimism*, or focusing on the negative; *perfectionism*, or expecting superhuman standards; *should-ing*, or reprimanding yourself for things you should have done; *blaming* yourself or others for circumstances and events; and *dichotomous thinking*, in which everything is seen as either entirely good or bad. To combat negative self-talk, become aware of an irrational or overreactive thought, interrupt it by saying "stop" (under your breath or out loud), then replace it with positive thoughts—a process called **cognitive restructuring**.

People fall into patterns and ways of thinking that can cause stress and increase their levels of anxiety. The fact is, your thought patterns can be your own worst enemy. If you can become aware of the internal messages you are giving yourself, you can recognize them and work to change them. Some strategies for doing this include the following:

- **Reframe a distressing event from a positive perspective.** For example, if you feel perpetually frustrated that you can't be the best in every class, reframe the issue to highlight your strengths.
- **Break the worry habit.** If you are preoccupied with "what if's" and worst case scenarios, doubts and fears can sap your strength and send your stress levels soaring.
  - If you must worry, create a "worry period"—a 20-minute time period each day when you can journal or talk about it. After that, move on.
  - Focus on the many things that are going right, rather than the one thing that might go wrong.
- **Look at life as being fluid.** If you accept that change is a natural part of living and growing, the jolt of changes will become less stressful.

Are college students more stressed out than other groups?

The combination of a new environment, peer and parental pressure, and the demands of course work, campus activities, and social life contribute to above average stress levels in college students.

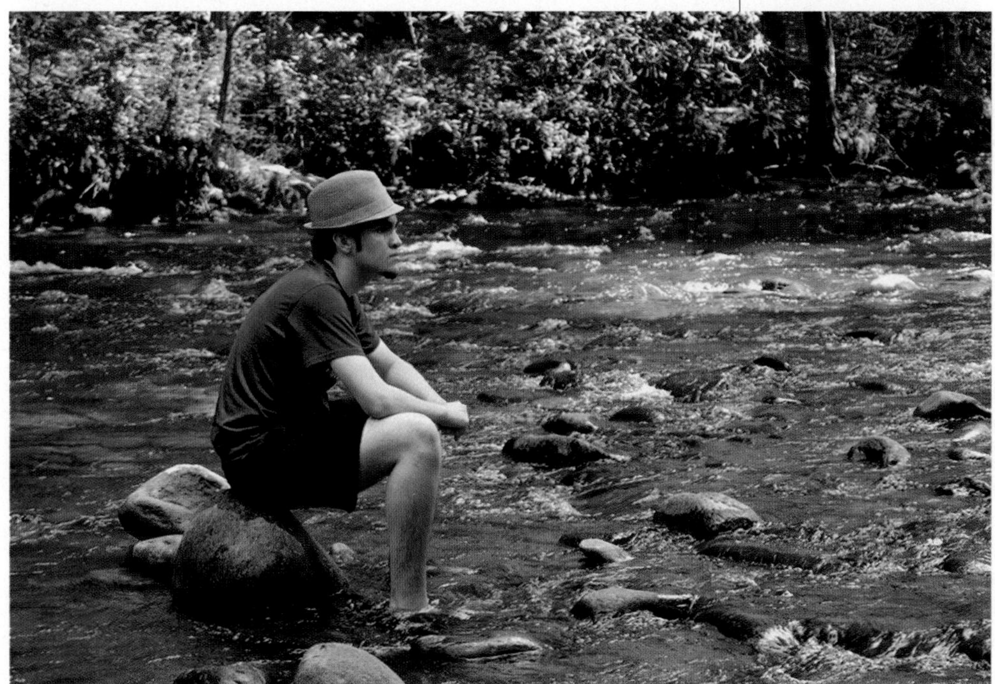

Practicing mindfulness means tuning in to the present, such as taking time to contemplate a scenic view. When you pay attention to the present, you can begin to let go of the stressful distractions in your life.

- **Moderate your expectations.** Aim high, but be realistic about your circumstances and motivation.
- **Weed out trivia.** Cardiologist Robert Eliot offers two rules for coping with life's challenges: "Don't sweat the small stuff," and remember, "It's all small stuff."
- **Tolerate mistakes by yourself and others.** Rather than getting angry or frustrated by mishaps, evaluate what happened and learn from it.

Mindfulness

Practicing *mindfulness*—by observing the present moment in a focused, nonjudgmental way—can help you increase awareness of your thinking patterns and refocus stressful thoughts. Try taking 10 minutes every day to pay focused attention to your senses and the world around you, without forming judgments. Rather than dwelling on the past or agonizing about the future, concentrate on the present. Recognize that your thoughts and emotions are fleeting, and they don't ultimately define who you are.

Cultivating Happiness

For decades, noted psychologist Martin Seligman has conducted research focused on positive psychology and authentic happiness. His work has been the framework for a new way of looking at life with a glass-half-full perspective. Research supports the idea that people who are optimistic and happier have fewer mental and physical problems.[71] Today, Seligman takes happiness a step further, focusing on the concept of *flourishing*. Flourishing consists of five elements, which positive psychologists believe will help you flourish in life, avoid stress, and be healthier:

- **Positive emotion.** Take time to get to know people's names. Share highs of the day rather than lows. Be active in complimenting others and verbalize their strengths.
- **Engagement.** Practice mindfulness: see, hear, touch, and feel the present moment. Make time to fully engage in the activities that bring you joy.
- **Relationships.** Listen to others and ask questions. Connect in person. Empower others to see their strengths, and check in to show that you care.
- **Meaning.** Think about how you want to be remembered. Read and explore new things. Learn about different cultures and history. Work to help others and to improve the world.
- **Achievement.** Consider the steps to achieve your goals in life, and view failure along the way as an opportunity. Celebrate accomplishments, both your own and those of others, and readily give praise.

Taking Physical Action

Physical activities can complement your strategies of stress management.

- **Exercise Regularly** The human stress response is intended to end in physical activity; exercise "burns off" stress hormones by directing them toward their intended metabolic function and can combat stress by raising levels of endorphins—mood-elevating, painkilling hormones—in the bloodstream.[72]
- **Get Enough Sleep** Adequate sleep allows you to cope with multiple stressors more effectively and to be more productive.
- **Practice Self-Nurturing** Find time each day for something fun—something that you enjoy and that calms you. Like exercise, relaxation can help you cope with stressful feelings, as well as preserve and refocus your energies.
- **Eat Healthfully** A balanced, healthy diet will help provide the stamina you need to get through problems while stress-proofing you in ways not yet fully understood. Undereating, overeating, and eating the wrong foods can create distress in the body. In particular, avoid **sympathomimetics**, foods that produce (or mimic) stresslike responses, such as caffeine.

check yourself

- **What are four effective mental or physical approaches to managing stress? Which might be best for you?**

3.9

Stress Management Techniques: Managing Emotional Responses

learning outcome

3.9 Explain how management of emotional responses contributes to stress management.

We often get upset not by realities, but by our faulty perceptions. Stress management requires examining your emotional responses to interactions with others—and remembering that you are responsible for the emotion and the resulting behaviors. Learning to identify emotions based on irrational beliefs, or expressed and interpreted in an over-the-top manner, can help you stop such emotions or express them in healthy and appropriate ways.

Learn to Laugh, Be Joyful, and Cry Smiling, laughing, and even crying can elevate mood, relieve stress, and improve relationships. In the moment, laughter and joy raise endorphin levels, increase blood oxygen, decrease stress, relieve pain, and enhance productivity. Additional evidence for long-term effects on immune function and protection against disease is only starting to be understood.[73]

Fight the Anger Urge Anger usually results when we feel we have lost control of a situation or are frustrated by events we can do little about. Major sources of anger include (1) perceived *threats* to self or others we care about; (2) *reactions to injustice*; (3) *fear*; (4) *faulty emotional reasoning* or misinterpretation of normal events; (5) *low frustration tolerance*, often fueled by stress, drugs, or lack of sleep; (6) *unreasonable expectations* for ourselves and others; and (7) *people rating*, or applying derogatory ratings to others.

To deal with anger, you can express, suppress, or calm it. Surprisingly, expressing anger is probably the healthiest option, if you do so assertively rather than aggressively. Several strategies can help redirect aggression into assertion:[74]

- **Recognize anger patterns and learn to de-escalate them.** Note what angers you. What thoughts or feelings led up to your boiling point? Try changing your self-talk or interrupting anger patterns by counting to ten or taking deep breaths.
- **Verbally de-escalate.** When conflict arises, be respectful and state your needs or feelings rather than shooting zingers. Avoid "you always" or "you never" and instead say, "I feel___ when you_____" or "I would really appreciate it if you could___."
- **Plan ahead.** Explore ways to minimize your exposure to anger triggers, such as traffic jams.
- **Vent to your friends.** Find a few close friends you trust and who can be honest with you about your situation. Allow them to listen to provide perspective. Don't wear down supporters with continual rants.
- **Develop realistic expectations.** Anger is often the result of unmet expectations, frustrations, resentments, and impatience. Are your expectations of yourself and others realistic?
- **Turn complaints into requests.** Try reworking a problem into a request. Instead of screaming because your neighbors' music woke you up at 2 A.M., talk with them. Try to reach an agreement.
- **Leave past anger in the past.** Learn to resolve issues that have caused pain, frustration, or stress. If necessary, seek professional counsel.

Invest in Loved Ones Too often, we don't make time for the people most important to us: friends and family. Cultivate and nurture relationships built on trust, mutual acceptance and understanding, honesty, and caring. Treating others empathically provides them with a measure of emotional security and reduces *their* anxiety.

Cultivate Your Spiritual Side Spiritual health and spiritual practice can link you to a community and offer perspective on the things that truly matter.

Spending time communicating and socializing can be an important part of building a support network and reducing your stress level.

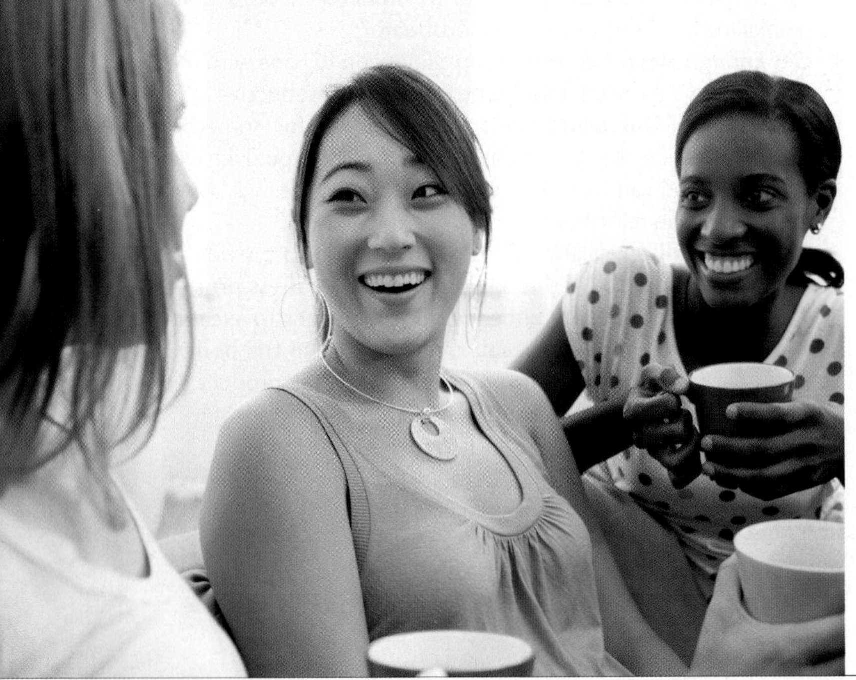

check yourself

- **How can emotions affect your stress levels?**
- **List three strategies to express anger assertively rather than aggressively.**

Stress Management Techniques: Managing Your Time and Your Finances

learning outcome

3.10 Describe strategies for managing your time and your finances.

Managing Your Time

Ever put off writing a paper until the night before it was due? We all **procrastinate**—voluntarily delay doing some task despite expecting to be worse off for it. Procrastination results in academic difficulties, financial problems, relationship problems, and stress-related ailments.

According to psychologist Peter Gollwitzer and colleagues, one key to beating procrastination is to set clear "implementation intentions."[75] Having a plan that includes specific deadlines (and rewards for meeting deadlines) can help you stay on task. Start with a simple plan and be flexible.

What else can you do to make better use of your time? Try logging your activities for 2 days—everything from going to class to doing laundry to texting friends—and the amount of time you spend doing each. Assess your results and make changes accordingly. Use these time-management tips to help you:

- **Do one thing at a time.** Don't try to watch television, wash clothes, and write your term paper all at once.
- **Clear your desk.** Toss unnecessary papers; file those you'll need later. Read your mail, recycle what you don't need, and file the rest for later action.
- **Prioritize tasks.** Make a daily "to do" list and stick to it. Categorize things you must do today, things you must do but not immediately, and "nice to dos" that you can take on if you finish the others or if they include something fun.
- **Find a clean, comfortable place to work, and avoid interruptions.** For a project that requires concentration, schedule uninterrupted time. Close your door and turn off your phone—or go to a quiet room in the library or student union.

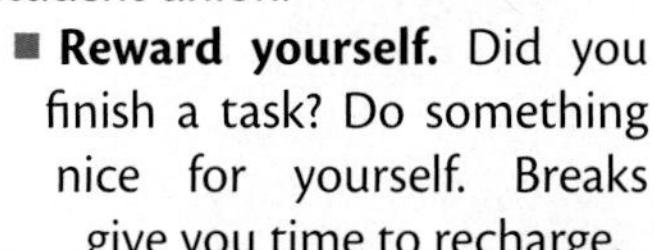

- **Reward yourself.** Did you finish a task? Do something nice for yourself. Breaks give you time to recharge.
- **Work when you're at your best.** If you're a morning person, study in the morning. Take breaks when you start to slow down.

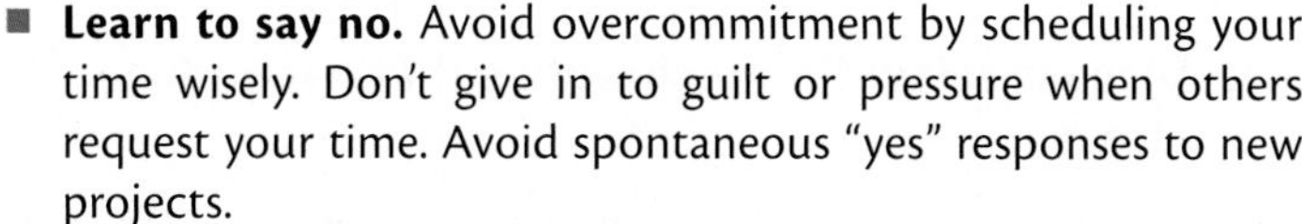

- **Learn to say no.** Avoid overcommitment by scheduling your time wisely. Don't give in to guilt or pressure when others request your time. Avoid spontaneous "yes" responses to new projects.

Managing Your Finances

Higher education can impose a huge financial burden on parents and students—and consequently become a major stressor. Over one-third of college students queried in a recent survey said finances have been "traumatic or very difficult to handle" in the past year.[76] These helpful tips can create a less stressful financial situation:

- **Create a budget**. Set a goal to avoid debt as much as possible. Track expenses such as tuition, books, rent, food, and entertainment. List your income to see if what you're spending is equitable to what you're earning or if it's putting you on the debt track.
- **Use credit cards wisely.** Resist credit card offers; racking up debt in school can affect your finances for years to come. Reserve credit cards you do have for less frequent, big-ticket buying, and carry cash whenever possible.
- **Complete a financial inventory.** How much money will you need to do the things you want to do in the future? Will you live alone or share costs with roommates? Do you need to buy a car, or can you rely on public transportation? Consider options for saving money; you need to prepare for emergencies and for future plans.

Consider Downshifting Many people, questioning whether "having it all" is worth it, are taking a step back and simplifying their lives. This trend has been labeled **downshifting**, or **voluntary simplicity**. Moving from a large urban area to a smaller town or leaving a high-stress job for one that makes you happy are examples of downshifting.

Downshifting involves a fundamental alteration in values and honest introspection about what is important in life. It means cutting down on shopping habits, buying only what you need to get by, and living within modest means. When you contemplate any form of downshift, move slowly by planning attainable goals to simplify your life.

check yourself

- **What are some time management strategies that could help reduce your stress levels?**
- **What are some strategies to improve your financial situation?**

3.11 Relaxation Techniques for Stress Management

learning **outcome**

3.11 Discuss relaxation techniques that can reduce stress.

Relaxation techniques to reduce stress have been practiced for centuries, and there is a wide array of practices from which to choose. Common techniques include yoga, qigong, tai chi, deep breathing, meditation, visualization, progressive muscle relaxation, massage therapy, biofeedback, and hypnosis.

Yoga Yoga is an ancient practice that combines meditation, stretching, and breathing exercises designed to relax, refresh, and rejuvenate. It began about 5,000 years ago in India and has been evolving ever since. In the United States today, some 20 million adults practice many versions of yoga.[77]

Classical yoga is the ancestor of nearly all modern forms of yoga. Breathing, poses, and verbal mantras are often part of classical yoga. Of the many branches of classical yoga, *Hatha yoga* is the most well known because it is the most body focused. This style of yoga involves the practice of breath control and *asanas*—held postures and choreographed movements that enhance strength and flexibility. Research shows increased evidence of benefits of Hatha yoga in reducing inflammation, boosting mood, increasing relaxation, and reducing stress among those who practice regularly.[78]

Qigong *Qigong* (pronounced "chee-kong"), one of the fastest-growing and most widely accepted forms of mind-body health exercises, is used by some of the country's largest health care organizations, particularly for people suffering from chronic pain or stress. Qigong is an ancient Chinese practice that involves becoming aware of and learning to control *qi* (or *chi*, pronounced "chee"), or vital energy in your body. According to Chinese medicine, a complex system of internal pathways called *meridians* carry *qi* throughout your body. If your *qi* becomes stagnant or blocked, you'll feel sluggish or powerless. Qigong incorporates a series of flowing movements, breath techniques, mental visualization exercises, and vocalizations of healing sounds designed to restore balance and integrate and refresh the mind and body.

Tai Chi *Tai chi* (pronounced "ty-chee") is sometimes described as "meditation in motion." Originally developed in China as a form of self-defense, this graceful form of exercise has existed for about 2,000 years. Tai chi is noncompetitive and self-paced. To do tai chi, you perform a defined series of postures or movements in a slow, graceful manner. Each movement or posture flows into the next without pause. Tai chi has been widely practiced in China for centuries and is becoming increasingly popular around the world, both as a basic exercise program and as a complement to other health

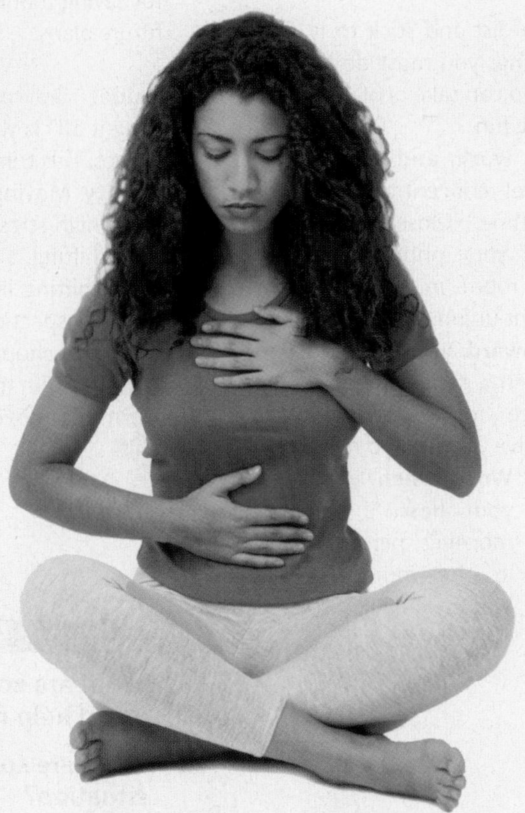

1. Assume a natural, comfortable position either sitting up straight with your head, neck, and shoulders relaxed, or lying on your back with your knees bent and your head supported. Close your eyes and loosen binding clothes.
2. In order to feel your abdomen moving as you breathe, place one hand on your upper chest and the other just below your rib cage.
3. Breathe in slowly and deeply through your nose. Feel your stomach expanding into your hand. The hand on your chest should move as little as possible.
4. Exhale slowly through your mouth. Feel the fall of your stomach away from your hand. Again, the hand on your chest should move as little as possible.
5. Concentrate on the act of breathing. Shut out external noise. Focus on inhaling and exhaling, the route the air is following, and the rise and fall of your stomach.

Figure 3.5 Diaphragmatic Breathing
This exercise will help you learn to breathe deeply as a way to relieve stress. Practice this for 5 to 10 minutes several times a day and soon diaphragmatic breathing will become natural for you.

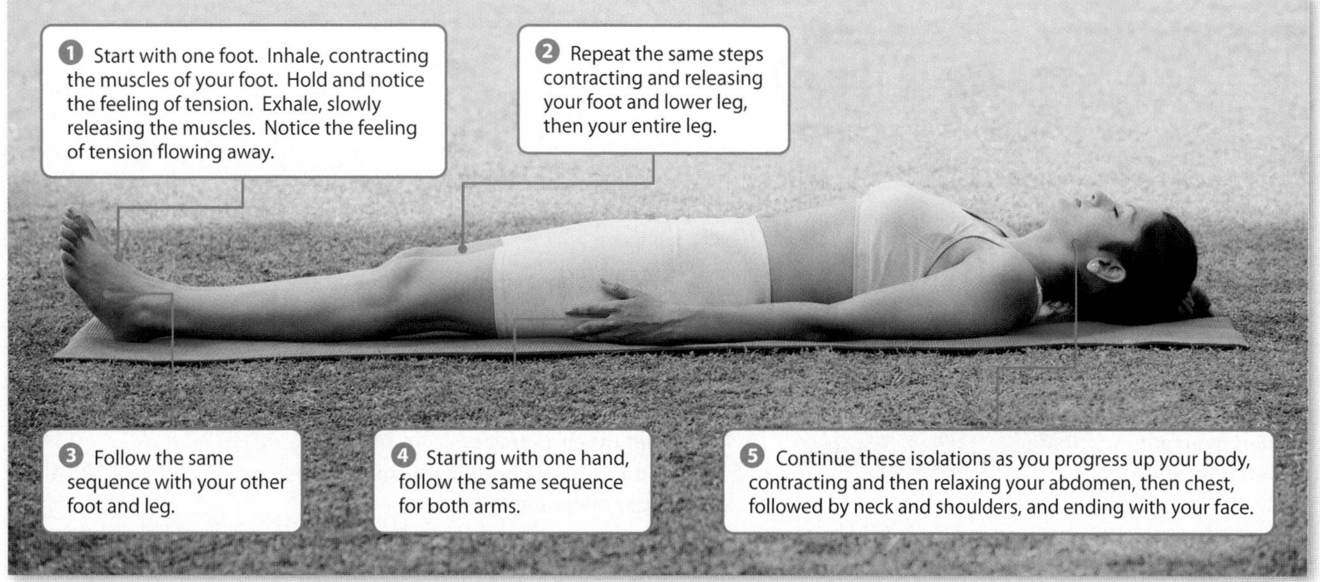

Figure 3.6 Progressive Muscle Relaxation
Sit or lie down in a comfortable position and follow the steps described to increase your awareness of tension in your body.

care methods. Health benefits include stress reduction, improved balance, and increased flexibility.

Diaphragmatic or Deep Breathing Typically, we breathe using only the upper chest and thoracic region rather than involving the abdominal region. Simply stated, diaphragmatic breathing is deep breathing that maximally fills the lungs by involving the movement of the diaphragm and lower abdomen. This technique is commonly used in yoga exercises and in other meditative practices. Try the diaphragmatic breathing exercise in Figure 3.5 right now and see if you feel more relaxed!

Meditation There are many different forms of **meditation**. Most involve sitting quietly for 15 minutes or longer, focusing on a particular word or symbol or observing one's thoughts, and controlling breathing. Practiced by Eastern religions for centuries, meditation is seen as an important form of introspection and personal renewal. Recent research found that one form of meditation, *transcendental meditation*, results in adults reducing their blood pressure as well as need for blood pressure medications.[79]

Visualization Often it is our own thoughts and imagination that provoke distress by conjuring up worst-case scenarios. Our imagination, however, can also be tapped to reduce stress. In **visualization**, you create mental scenes using your imagination. The choice of mental images is unlimited, but natural settings such as ocean beaches and mountain lakes are often used to represent stress-free environments. Recalling specific physical senses of sight, sound, smell, taste, and touch can replace stressful stimuli with peaceful or pleasurable thoughts.

Progressive Muscle Relaxation Progressive muscle relaxation involves systematically contracting and relaxing different muscle groups in your body. The standard pattern is to begin with the feet and work your way up your body, contracting and releasing as you go (Figure 3.6). The process is designed to teach awareness of the different feelings of muscle tension and muscle release. With practice, you can quickly identify tension in your body when you are facing stressful situations, then consciously release that tension to calm yourself.

Massage Therapy If you have ever had someone massage your stiff neck or aching feet, you know that massage is an excellent way to relax. Techniques vary from deep-tissue massage to gentler acupressure.

Biofeedback **Biofeedback** is a technique in which a person learns to use the mind to consciously control body functions like heart rate, body temperature, and breathing rate. Using machines from those as simple as stress dots that change color with body temperature variation to sophisticated electrical sensors, individuals learn to listen to their bodies and make necessary adjustments, such as relaxing certain muscles, changing breathing, or concentrating to slow heart rate and relax. Eventually, you develop the ability to recognize and lower stress responses without the help of the machine.

Hypnosis **Hypnosis** requires a person to focus on one thought, object, or voice, thereby freeing the right hemisphere of the brain to become more active. The person then becomes unusually responsive to suggestion. Whether self-induced or induced by someone else, hypnosis can reduce certain types of stress.

check yourself

- **What are three potential benefits to learning a variety of relaxation techniques?**
- **Which relaxation technique is the most effective for you? Why?**

Assessyourself

3.12

What's Your Stress Level?

An interactive version of this assessment is available online in MasteringHealth.

Let's face it: Some periods in life, including your college years, can be especially stressful! Learning to "chill" starts with an honest examination of your life experiences and your reactions to stressful situations. Respond to each section, assigning points as directed. Total the points from each section, then add them and compare to the life-stressor scale.

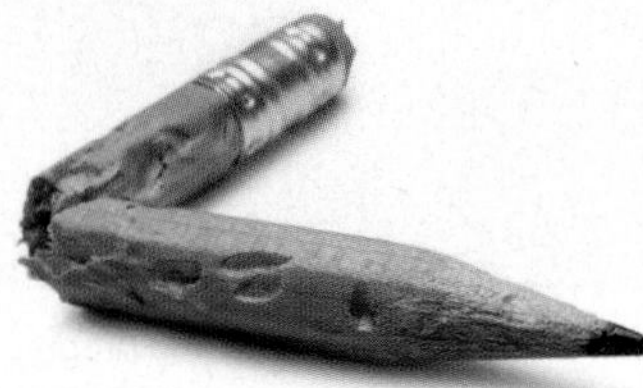

1 Recent History

In the last year, how many of the following major life events have you experienced? (Give yourself five points for each event you experienced; if you experienced an event more than once, give yourself ten points, etc.)

1. Death of a close family member or friend	_____
2. Ending a relationship (whether by choice or not)	_____
3. Major financial upset jeopardizing your ability to stay in college	_____
4. Major move, leaving friends, family, and/or your past life behind	_____
5. Serious illness (you)	_____
6. Serious illness (of someone you're close with)	_____
7. Marriage or entering a new relationship	_____
8. Loss of a beloved pet	_____
9. Involved in a legal dispute or issue	_____
10. Involved in a hostile, violent, or threatening relationship	_____
Total	_____

2 Self-Reflection

For each of the following, indicate where you are on the scale of 0 to 5.

	Strongly Disagree					Strongly Agree
1. I have a lot of worries at home and at school.	0	1	2	3	4	5
2. My friends and/or family put too much pressure on me.	0	1	2	3	4	5
3. I am often distracted and have trouble focusing on schoolwork.	0	1	2	3	4	5
4. I am highly disorganized and tend to do my schoolwork at the last minute.	0	1	2	3	4	5
5. My life seems to have far too many crisis situations.	0	1	2	3	4	5
6. Most of my time is spent sitting; I don't get much exercise.	0	1	2	3	4	5
7. I don't have enough control in decisions that affect my life.	0	1	2	3	4	5
8. I wake up most days feeling tired/like I need a lot more sleep.	0	1	2	3	4	5
9. I often have feelings that I am alone and that I don't fit in very well.	0	1	2	3	4	5
10. I don't have many friends or people I can share my feelings or thoughts with.	0	1	2	3	4	5
11. I am uncomfortable in my body, and I wish I could change how I look.	0	1	2	3	4	5
12. I am very anxious about my major and whether I will get a good job after I graduate.	0	1	2	3	4	5
13. If I have to wait in a restaurant or in lines, I quickly become irritated and upset.	0	1	2	3	4	5
14. I have to win or be the best in activities or in classes or I get upset with myself.	0	1	2	3	4	5
15. I am bothered by world events and am cynical and angry about how people behave.	0	1	2	3	4	5
16. I have too much to do, and there are never enough hours in the day.	0	1	2	3	4	5
17. I feel uneasy when I am caught up on my work and am relaxing or doing nothing.	0	1	2	3	4	5
18. I sleep with my cell phone near my bed and often check messages/tweets/texts during the night.	0	1	2	3	4	5
19. I enjoy time alone but find that I seldom get enough alone time each day.	0	1	2	3	4	5
20. I worry about whether or not others like me.	0	1	2	3	4	5
21. I am struggling in my classes and worry about failing.	0	1	2	3	4	5
22. My relationship with my family is not very loving and supportive.	0	1	2	3	4	5
23. When I watch people, I tend to be critical and think negatively about them.	0	1	2	3	4	5
24. I believe that people are inherently selfish and untrustworthy, and I am careful around them.	0	1	2	3	4	5
25. Life is basically unfair, and most of the time there is little I can do to change it.	0	1	2	3	4	5

	Strongly Disagree					Strongly Agree
26. I give more than I get in relationships with people.	0	1	2	3	4	5
27. I tend to believe that what I do is often not good enough or that I should do better.	0	1	2	3	4	5
28. My friends would describe me as highly stressed and quick to react with anger and/or frustration.	0	1	2	3	4	5
29. My friends are always telling me I "need a vacation to relax."	0	1	2	3	4	5
30. Overall, the quality of my life right now isn't all that great.	0	1	2	3	4	5
Total						______

Scoring: Total your points from Sections 1 and 2. ______

Although the following scores are not meant to be diagnostic, they do serve as an indicator of potential problem areas. If your scores are:

0–50, your stress levels are low, but it is worth examining areas where you did score points and taking action to reduce your stress levels.

51–100, you may need to reduce certain stresses in your life. Long-term stress and pressure from your stresses can be counter-productive. Consider what you can do to change your perceptions of things, your behaviors, or your environment.

100–150, you are probably pretty stressed. Examine what your major stressors are and come up with a plan for reducing your stress levels right now. Don't delay or blow this off because it could lead to significant stress-related problems, affecting your grades, your social life, and your future!

151–200, you are carrying high stress, and if you don't make changes, you could be heading for some serious difficulties. Find a counselor on campus to talk with about some of the major issues you identified above as causing stress. Try to get more sleep and exercise, and find time to relax. Surround yourself with people who are supportive of you and make you feel safe and competent.

Your Plan for Change

The Assess Yourself activity gave you the chance to look at your sources of chronic stress, identify major stressors in your life, and see how you typically respond to stress. Now that you are aware of these patterns, you can change behaviors that lead to increased stress.

Today, you can:

◯ Practice one new stress-management technique. For example, you could spend 10 minutes doing a deep-breathing exercise or find a good spot on campus to meditate.

◯ In a journal, write down stressful events or symptoms of stress that you experience.

Within the next 2 weeks, you can:

◯ Attend a class or workshop in yoga, tai chi, qigong, meditation, or some other stress-relieving activity. Look for beginner classes offered on campus or in your community.

◯ Make a list of the papers, projects, and tests that you have over the coming semester and create a schedule for them. Break projects and term papers into small, manageable tasks, and try to be realistic about how much time you'll need to get these tasks done.

By the end of the semester, you can:

◯ Keep track of the money you spend and where it goes. Establish a budget and follow it for at least a month.

◯ Find some form of exercise you can do regularly. You may consider joining a gym or just arranging regular "walk dates" or pickup basketball games with your friends. Try to exercise at least 30 minutes every day.

Summary

To hear an MP3 Tutor session, scan here or visit the Study Area in **MasteringHealth.**

LO 3.1 Stress is an inevitable part of our lives. *Eustress* refers to stress associated with positive events; *distress* refers to negative events.

LO 3.2 The alarm, resistance, and exhaustion phases of the general adaptation syndrome (GAS) involve physiological responses to both real and imagined stressors and cause complex hormonal reactions.

LO 3.3 Undue stress for extended periods of time can compromise the immune system. Stress has been linked to cardiovascular disease (CVD), weight gain, hair loss, diabetes, digestive problems, and increased susceptibility to infectious diseases. Psychoneuroimmunology is the science that analyzes the relationship between the mind's reaction to stress and immune function.

LO 3.3 Stress can affect intellectual and psychological health and contribute to depression and anxiety.

LO 3.4 The most common types of headaches are tension and migraine. Relaxation techniques can ease headaches triggered by stress.

LO 3.5 Sleep conserves body energy and restores physical and mental functioning.

LO 3.6 Psychosocial factors contributing to stress include change, hassles, relationships, pressure, conflict, overload, and environmental stressors. Persons subjected to discrimination or bias may face unusually high levels of stress.

LO 3.7 Some sources of stress are internal and related to appraisal, self-esteem, self-efficacy, personality, and psychological hardiness and resilience.

LO 3.8–3.11 College can be stressful. Recognizing the signs of stress is the first step toward better health. To manage stress, find coping skills that work for you—probably some combination of managing emotional responses, taking mental or physical action, downshifting, time management, managing finances, and relaxation techniques.

Pop Quiz

Visit MasteringHealth to personalize your study plan with Chapter Review Quizzes and Dynamic Study Modules.

LO 3.1 1. Even though Andre experienced stress when he graduated from college and moved to a new city, he viewed these changes as an opportunity for growth. What is Andre's stress called?
a. Strain
b. Distress
c. Eustress
d. Adaptive response

LO 3.1 2. Which of the following is an example of a chronic stressor?
a. Giving a talk in public
b. Meeting a deadline for a big project
c. Dealing with a permanent disability
d. Preparing for a job interview

LO 3.2 3. During what phase of the general adaptation syndrome has the physical and psychological energy used to fight the stressor been depleted?
a. Alarm phase
b. Resistance phase
c. Endurance phase
d. Exhaustion phase

LO 3.2 4. In which stage of the general adaptation syndrome does the fight-or-flight response occur?
a. Exhaustion stage
b. Alarm stage
c. Resistance stage
d. Response stage

LO 3.2 5. The branch of the autonomic nervous system that is responsible for energizing the body for either fight-or-flight and for triggering many other stress responses is the
a. central nervous system.
b. parasympathetic nervous system.
c. sympathetic nervous system.
d. endocrine system.

LO3.6 6. A state of physical and mental exhaustion caused by excessive stress is called
a. conflict.
b. overload.
c. hassles.
d. burnout.

LO3.6 7. Losing your keys is an example of what psychosocial source of stress?
a. Pressure
b. Inconsistent behaviors
c. Hassles
d. Conflict

LO3.7 8. Which of the following test-taking techniques is not recommended to reduce test-taking stress?
a. Plan ahead and study over a period of time for the test.
b. Eat a balanced meal before the exam.
c. Do all your studying the night before the exam so it is fresh in your mind.
d. Remind yourself of three reasons you will pass the exam.

LO3.10 9. After 5 years of 70-hour work-weeks, Tom decided to leave his high-paying, high-stress law firm and lead a simpler lifestyle. What is this trend called?
a. Adaptation
b. Conflict resolution
c. Burnout reduction
d. Downshifting

LO3.10 10. Which of the following is not an example of a time-management technique?
a. Doing one thing at a time
b. Rewarding yourself for finishing a task
c. Practicing procrastination in completing homework assignments
d. Breaking tasks into smaller pieces

Answers to these questions can be found on page A-1. If you answered a question incorrectly, review the module identified by the Learning Outcome. For even more study tools, visit MasteringHealth.

4 Relationships and Sexuality

Humans are social animals—we have a basic need to belong and to feel loved. We can't live without interacting with others in some way. We build "social capital," or networks of friends, family, and significant others, who help us feel connected and cope with life's challenges. Numerous studies have shown that supportive interpersonal relationships are beneficial to health.[1]

All relationships involve a degree of risk. However, only by taking these risks can we grow and experience all life has to offer. This chapter examines healthy relationships and the communication skills necessary to create and maintain them. Expressing ourselves well and knowing how to listen to and understand what others are saying are essential for healthy relationships.

Sexuality is a component of some of our most important relationships—and of our understanding of ourselves. How you experience yourself as a sexual person affects everything from your self-image to your identity, happiness, fertility, and health. Sexuality begins with our biological sex, gender, anatomy and physiology, and sexual functions, but it also encompasses values, beliefs, and attitudes about how we see ourselves as sexual beings and how we relate to others.

4.1 Characteristics and Types of Intimate Relationships

learning outcome

4.1 List characteristics of intimate relationships, and compare and contrast different theories of love.

Intimate relationships can be defined in terms of four characteristics: *behavioral interdependence, need fulfillment, emotional attachment*, and *emotional availability*.

Behavioral interdependence refers to the mutual impact that people have on each other as their lives intertwine. It may become stronger over time, to the point that each person would feel a great void if the other were gone.

Intimate relationships also provide *need fulfillment.* Through relationships with others, we fulfill our needs for *intimacy* (someone with whom we can share our feelings freely), *social integration* (someone with whom we can share worries and concerns), *nurturance* (someone we can take care of and who will take care of us), *assistance* (someone to help us in times of need), and *affirmation* (someone who will reassure us of our own worth and tell us that we matter).

Intimate relationships also involve strong bonds of *emotional attachment,* or feelings of love. When we hear the word *intimacy,* we often think of a sexual relationship. Although sex can play an important role in emotional attachment, a relationship can be very intimate and yet not sexual. Two people can be emotionally or spiritually intimate, or they can be intimate friends.

Does an intimate relationship have to be sexual?

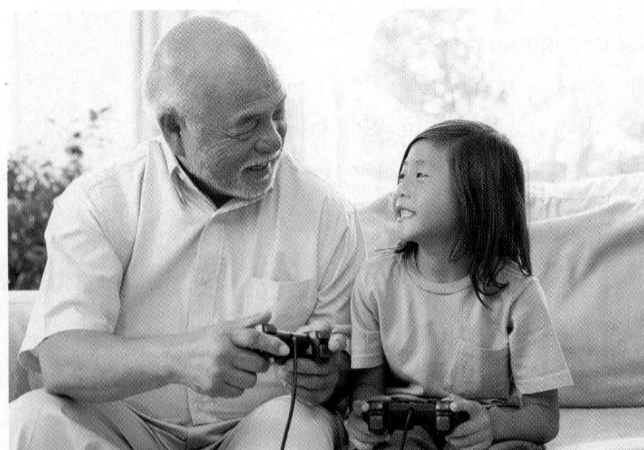

We may be accustomed to hearing *intimacy* used to describe romantic or sexual relationships, but intimate relationships can take many forms. The emotional bonds that characterize intimate relationships often span generations and give insight into each other's worlds.

Emotional availability is the ability to give to and receive from others emotionally without fear of being hurt or rejected. At times, we may limit our emotional availability—for example, after a painful breakup, holding back can offer time for healing. However, some people who have experienced intense trauma find it difficult to ever be available emotionally.

Relating to Yourself

You have probably heard that you must love yourself before you can honestly love someone else. But how do you learn to value and accept who you are? People with high self-esteem show respect for themselves by remaining true to their values and beliefs. They feel worthy of success in love, relationships, and life in general.

Two qualities important to any good relationship are *accountability* and *self-nurturance.* **Accountability** entails recognizing that you are responsible for your own decisions, choices, and actions. **Self-nurturance** means developing individual potential through a balanced and realistic appreciation of self-worth and ability. Individuals on a path of accountability and self-nurturance have a much better chance of maintaining satisfying relationships with others.

Self-Esteem and Self-Acceptance Factors that affect your ability to nurture yourself and maintain healthy relationships include how you define yourself (*self-concept*) and evaluate yourself (*self-esteem*).

Your perception of yourself influences your relationship choices. If you feel unattractive or inferior to others, you may choose not to interact with them. Or you may unconsciously seek out individuals who confirm your view of yourself by treating you poorly. Conversely, a positive self-concept makes it easier to form relationships with people who nurture you and to interact with others in a healthy, balanced way.

Family Relationships A family is a group whose central focus is to care for, love, and socialize with one another. The family is a dynamic institution that changes as society changes, and the definition of *family* changes over time. Historically, most families have been made up of people related by blood, marriage or long-term committed relationships, or adoption. Yet today, many other groups are recognized and functioning as family units. It is from our **family of origin**, those in our household during our first years, that we initially learn about feelings, problem solving, love, intimacy, and gender roles. We learn to negotiate relationships and have opportunities to communicate, develop attitudes and values, and explore spiritual beliefs. When we establish relationships outside the family, we often rely on experiences and skills modeled by our family of origin.

Friendships

Friendships are often the first relationships we form outside our immediate families, and they can be some of our most stable and enduring. Being able to establish and maintain strong friendships may be a good predictor of success in establishing love relationships because each requires shared interests and values, mutual acceptance, trust, and respect.

Developing meaningful friendships is more than merely "friending" someone on Facebook. Getting to know someone well requires time, effort, and commitment. A good friend can be an honest and trustworthy companion, someone who honors and respects your strengths and weaknesses, who can share your joys and sorrows, and whom you can count on for support.

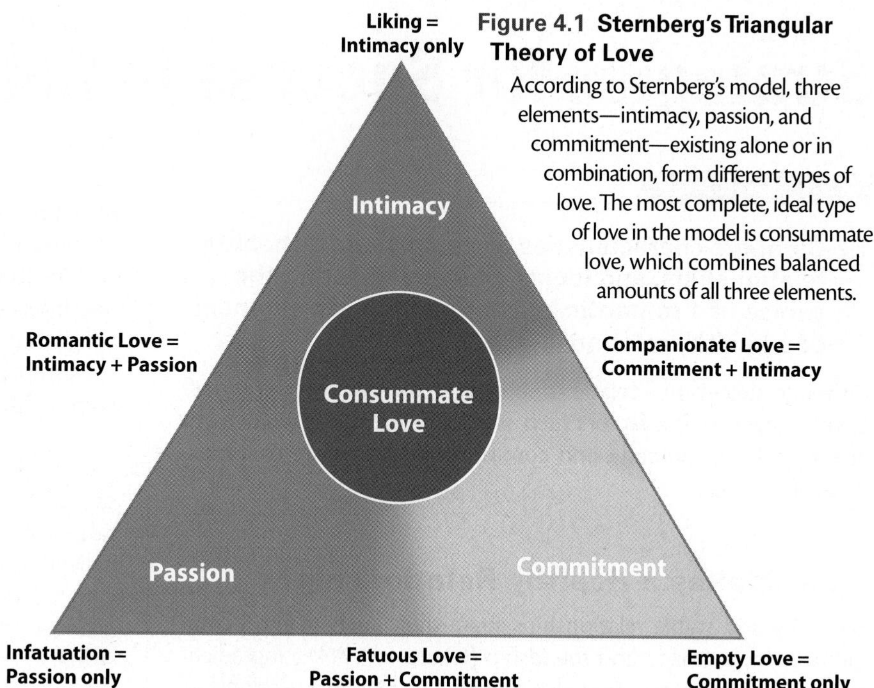

Figure 4.1 Sternberg's Triangular Theory of Love
According to Sternberg's model, three elements—intimacy, passion, and commitment—existing alone or in combination, form different types of love. The most complete, ideal type of love in the model is consummate love, which combines balanced amounts of all three elements.

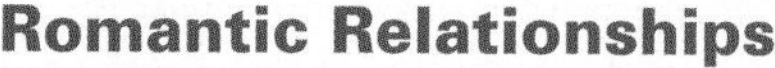

Romantic Relationships

Most people choose at some point to enter into an intimate romantic and sexual relationship with another person. Romantic relationships typically include all the characteristics of friendship as well as the following:

- **Fascination.** Lovers are often preoccupied by the other and want to think about, talk to, or be with the other.
- **Exclusiveness.** Lovers have a relationship that usually precludes having the same relationship with a third party. The love relationship often takes priority over all others.
- **Sexual desire.** Lovers desire physical intimacy and want to touch, hold, and engage in sexual activities with the other.
- **Giving the utmost.** Lovers care enough to give the utmost when the other is in need.
- **Being an advocate.** Lovers actively champion each other's interests and attempt to ensure that the other succeeds.

Theories of Love Love may mean different things to different people, depending on cultural values, age, gender, and situation. Although we may not know how to put our feelings into words, we know it when the "lightning bolt" of love strikes.

In his Triangular Theory of Love, psychologist Robert Sternberg proposes three key components to loving relationships (Figure 4.1):[2]

- **Intimacy.** The emotional component, which involves closeness, sharing, and mutual support.
- **Passion.** The motivational component, which includes lust, attraction, sexual arousal, and sharing.
- **Commitment.** The cognitive component, which includes the decision to be open to love in the short term and commitment to the relationship in the long term.

Sternberg uses the term **consummate love** to describe a combination of intimacy, passion, and commitment.

Quite different from Sternberg's approach are theories of love and attraction based on brain circuitry and chemistry. Anthropologist Helen Fisher, among others, has hypothesized that attraction and love follow a fairly predictable pattern based on (1) *imprinting*, in which our evolutionary patterns, genetic predispositions, and past experiences trigger a romantic reaction; (2) *attraction*, in which neurochemicals produce feelings of euphoria and elation; (3) *attachment*, in which endorphins—natural opiates—cause lovers to feel peaceful, secure, and calm; and (4) production of a *cuddle chemical*, in which the brain secretes the hormone oxytocin, stimulating sensations during lovemaking and eliciting feelings of satisfaction and attachment.[3]

A love-smitten person's endocrine system secretes chemical substances such as dopamine, norepinephrine, and phenylethylamine (PEA), which are chemical cousins of amphetamines.[4] Attraction may in fact be a "natural high." However, this passion "buzz" loses effectiveness over time as the body builds up a tolerance. Fisher suggests that the significant drop in PEA levels over a 3- to 4-year period leads to the "4-year itch" that manifests in peaking fourth-year divorce rates. Romances that last beyond the 4-year mark are influenced by endorphins that give lovers a sense of security, peace, and calm.[5]

check yourself

- **What are the common characteristics of intimate relationships?**
- **What are the most important characteristics you look for in a friend?**
- **What are the strengths and weaknesses of the proposed theories of love?**

4.2 Strategies for Success in Relationships

learning outcome

4.2 Compare characteristics of healthy and unhealthy relationships, and identify factors affecting the choice of a romantic partner and the achievement of a healthy relationship.

Although success in a relationship is often defined by the number of years together, it is factors such as respect, friendship, enjoyment of each other's company, and communication that are true measures of success.

What Makes a Healthy Relationship?

Satisfying and stable relationships share traits such as good communication, intimacy, and friendship (Figure 4.2). A key ingredient is trust, the degree of confidence each person feels in a relationship. Trust includes three fundamental elements:

1. **Predictability.** You can predict your partner's behavior based on past actions.
2. **Dependability.** You can rely on your partner for emotional support, particularly in situations where you feel threatened with hurt or rejection.
3. **Faith.** You feel certain about your partner's intentions and behavior.

How do you know whether you're in a healthy relationship? Answering some basic questions can help you determine if a relationship is working.

- Do you love and care for yourself to the same extent you did before the relationship? Can you be yourself in the relationship?
- Do you share interests, values, and opinions? Is there mutual respect for, and civil discussion of, differences?
- Is there genuine caring and goodwill? Is there mutual encouragement and emotional support?
- Do you trust each other? Are you honest with each other? Can you comfortably express feelings, needs, and desires?
- Is there room for growth as you both evolve and mature?

Choosing a Romantic Partner

The choice of partner is influenced by more than just chemical and psychological processes. One important factor is *proximity*—the more often you see someone, the more likely interaction will occur.

We often choose partners based on *similarities* (in attitudes, values, intellect, interests, education, and socioeconomic status); the adage that "opposites attract" usually isn't true.

Also playing a significant role is *physical attraction.* Attraction is complex and influenced by social, biological, and cultural factors.[6]

Hooking up Hooking up is a vague term often used to describe sexual encounters, from kissing to intercourse, without the expectation of commitment expected in a romantic relationship. While college students may feel that there is a new "hook up culture" on campus, research tells us that young adults' sexual behavior hasn't changed much in the past few decades in terms of the number of sexual encounters or the number of partners.[7]

Sternberg's Triangle of Love would place hooking up in the "infatuation" category, passion with no commitment or intimacy, far from Sternberg's picture of "ideal." Additionally, according to Fisher, attraction and sex create a chemical reaction in the brain that fosters an emotional response, even if we say "it's just about the sex."

It's important to understand the risks involved with hookups. In a recent study, students reported that they were more likely to hook up if they had been drinking alcohol.[8] Reduced inhibitions due to alcohol, plus a lack of communication with a new partner, increases the risk of unprotected sex and thus the risk for unintended pregnancy and sexually transmitted infections (STIs).

Confronting Couple Issues

Couples in long-term relationships must confront issues that can either enhance or diminish their chances of success.

Jealousy **Jealousy** is an unhappy or angry feeling caused by the belief that

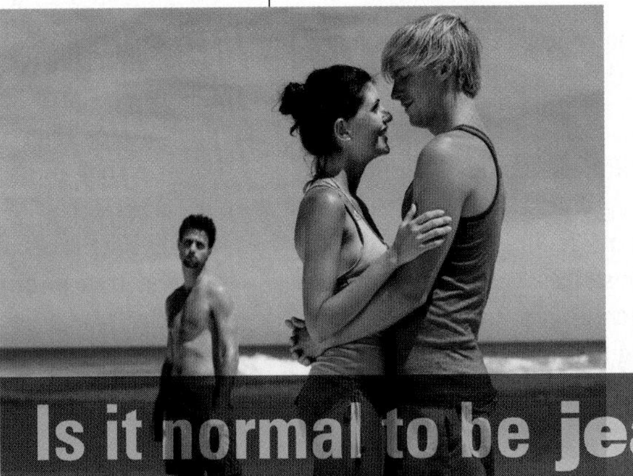

Is it normal to be jealous?

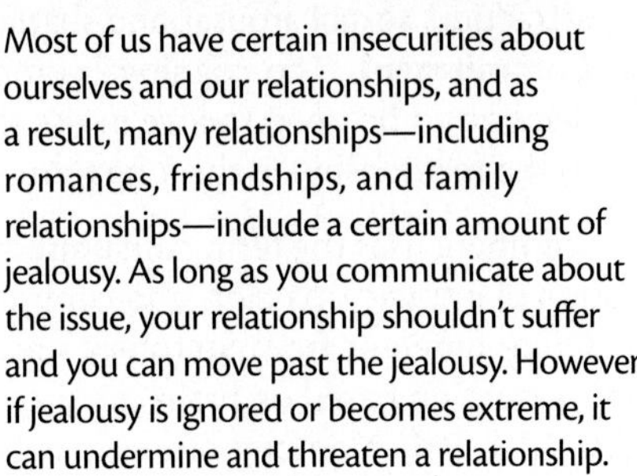

Most of us have certain insecurities about ourselves and our relationships, and as a result, many relationships—including romances, friendships, and family relationships—include a certain amount of jealousy. As long as you communicate about the issue, your relationship shouldn't suffer and you can move past the jealousy. However, if jealousy is ignored or becomes extreme, it can undermine and threaten a relationship.

In an unhealthy relationship...	In a healthy relationship...
You care for and focus on another person only and neglect yourself or you focus only on yourself and neglect the other person.	You both love and take care of yourselves before and while in a relationship
One of you feels pressure to change to meet the other person's standards and is afraid to disagree or voice ideas.	You respect each other's individuality, embrace your differences, and allow each other to "be yourselves."
One of you has to justify what you do, where you go, and whom you see.	You both do things with friends and family and have activities independent of each other.
One of you makes all the decisions and controls everything without listening to the other's input.	You discuss things with each other, allow for differences of opinion, and compromise equally.
One of you feels unheard and is unable to communicate what you want.	You express and listen to each other's feelings, needs, and desires.
You don't have any personal space and have to share everything with the other person.	You respect each other's need for privacy.
Your partner keeps his or her sexual history a secret or hides a sexually transmitted infection from you, or you do not disclose your history to your partner.	You share sexual histories and information about sexual health with each other.
You feel stifled, trapped, and stagnant. You are unable to escape the pressures of the relationship.	You both have room for positive growth, and you both learn more about each other as you develop and mature.

Figure 4.2 Healthy versus Unhealthy Relationships

Source: Adapted from Advocates for Youth, Washington, DC, www.advocatesforyouth.org. Copyright © 2000. Reprinted with permission.

someone you love likes or is liked by someone else. Jealousy often indicates underlying problems such as insecurity or possessiveness. Often, jealousy is rooted in past deception and loss. Other common causes include the following:

- **Overdependence.** People with few social ties who rely exclusively on their significant others tend to be fearful of losing them.
- **Severity of the threat.** People may feel uneasy if someone with stunning good looks and a great personality appears to be interested in their partner.
- **High value on sexual exclusivity.** People who believe that sexual exclusivity is a crucial indicator of love are more likely to become jealous.
- **Low self-esteem.** People who think poorly of themselves are more likely to fear someone will gain their partner's affection.
- **Fear of losing control.** Feeling one may lose attachment to or control over a partner can cause jealousy.

Although a certain amount of jealousy can be expected in any relationship, it doesn't have to threaten a relationship as long as partners communicate openly about it.[9]

Changing Gender Roles Throughout history, women and men have taken on various roles in relationships. Modern American society has very few gender-specific roles; many couples find it makes more sense to divide tasks based on convenience and preference. However, it rarely works out that the division is equal. Even when women work full time, they tend to bear heavy family and household responsibilities—and to become stressed and frustrated. Men may have expected a more traditional role for their partners. Over time, if couples can't communicate about this, the relationship may suffer.

Sharing Power **Power** can be defined as the ability to make and implement decisions. In traditional relationships, men were the wage earners and consequently had decision-making power. As women have become earners, the dynamics have shifted considerably. In general, successful couples share responsibilities, power, and control. If one partner always has the final say regarding social plans, for example, the unequal distribution of power may affect the relationship.

Unmet Expectations We all have expectations of ourselves and our partners—how we'll spend our time or money, express love, and grow as a couple. If we can't communicate our expectations, we set ourselves up for disappointment. Partners in healthy relationships can communicate wants and needs and have honest discussions when things aren't going as expected.

check yourself

- **What are three characteristics of a healthy relationship? Which do you consider most important?**
- **What factors are involved in the choice of a romantic partner?**
- **What are common obstacles to achieving a successful relationship?**

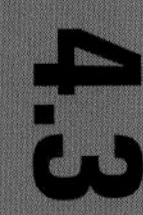

4.3 Relationships and Social Media

learning outcome

4.3 Discuss appropriate uses for social media in establishing and maintaining relationships.

Technology has revolutionized our access to information and the ways we communicate. Couples can meet on a site like Match.com, keep in constant contact via texting, and inform the world of their relationship highs and lows via Facebook and Twitter. With all these tools available, it can be easy to share TMI (too much information). Ilana Gershon, author of *The Breakup 2.0: Disconnecting over New Media*, suggests we lack standard etiquette for the use of new media in relationships.[10] At its best, social media can bring people closer together; at its worst, it can be used intentionally or unintentionally to embarrass or hurt.

Dating and Social Media

With the growing trend in online dating, you may be just as likely to meet your future life partner through a website or app than at school or work. According to a recent study, 35 percent of couples who married between 2005 and 2012 met online.[11] And according to a different survey, 11 percent of Americans have used an online dating website or mobile app at some point in their lives, with online dating most commonly reported by 25- to 34-year-olds (22%).[12]

When joining an online dating site or using social networks to meet others, it's important to be honest about yourself and your background. State your own interests and characteristics fairly, including things that you think might be less attractive than stereotypes and cultural norms dictate.

If you meet someone online and want to meet in person, put safety first! Plan something brief, preferably during daylight hours. Meet in a public place, like a coffee shop. Do not meet with anyone who wants to keep the time and location a secret. Tell a friend or family member the details of when and where you are meeting and any information you have on the person you are meeting (including his or her name and contact info).

Whether or not you meet romantic partners online, use social media responsibly while dating:

- Discuss limits with your partner on the type of info you each want shared online. Agree to share only within those limits.
- Be aware that your partner might not be as comfortable with posting information to social media as you are. Be mindful, and ask permission, before posting any pictures of you as a couple or information about your activities or whereabouts.
- Recognize that constant electronic updates throughout the day can leave little to share when you are together. Save some information for face-to-face talks!

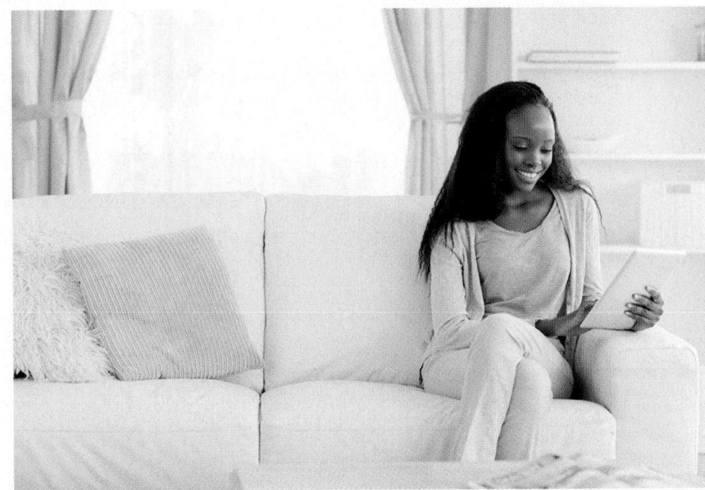

Chatting with potential romantic partners online? Be honest about yourself and your interests, and stay away from others who don't seem like they're being honest with you.

- Sober up before you click "submit." Things that seem funny under the influence may not seem funny the next morning.
- Remember that the Internet is forever. Once a picture or a post is sent, it can never be completely erased. Never post anything that would embarrass someone if it was seen by a family member or potential employer.
- Respect your partner's privacy. Logging on to his or her e-mail or Facebook account to look at private messages is a breach of trust.
- Know that the GPS in a phone can be used to track your location, and cell phone spyware can be installed that allows e-mail and texts to be read from another device. If you think you may be a victim of "cyberstalking" by a current (or former) partner, get a new phone or ask the phone company to reinstall the phone's operating system to wipe out the software.
- Do not break up with someone via text/e-mail/tweet/Facebook/chat. People deserve the respect of a more personal break up.
- Upon breaking up, be sure to change any passwords you may have confided in your partner. The temptation to use those for ill may be too strong to resist.

check yourself

- **What are three safety measures to take when dating online?**
- **How can social media be used responsibly when dating?**

Skills for Better Communication: Appropriate Self-Disclosure

learning outcome

4.4 Discuss the role of appropriate self-disclosure in good communication.

From the moment of birth, we struggle to be understood. We flail our arms, cry, scream, smile, frown, and make sounds and gestures to attract attention or to communicate what we want or need. By the time we enter adulthood, each of us has developed a unique way of communicating with gestures, words, expressions, and body language. No two people communicate in the exact same way or have the same need for connecting with others. Some of us are outgoing and quick to express our emotions and thoughts. Others are quiet and reluctant to talk about feelings.

Different cultures have different ways of expressing feelings and using body language. Men and women also tend to have different styles of communication, largely dictated by culture and socialization.

Although people differ in how they communicate, no one sex, culture, or group is better at it than another. We must be willing to accept differences and work to keep communication open and fluid. Remaining interested, engaged, and willing to exchange ideas and thoughts are skills typically learned with practice.

When two people begin a relationship, they bring their communication styles with them. How often have you heard someone say, "We just can't communicate" or "You're sending mixed messages"? Communication is a process; our every action, word, expression, gesture, and posture becomes part of our shared experience and part of the evolving impression we make on others. If we are angry in our responses, others will be reluctant to interact with us. If we bring "baggage" from past bad interactions to new relationships, we may be cynical, distrustful, and guarded. If we are positive, happy, and share openly, others will be more likely to communicate openly with us. This ability to communicate assertively is an important skill in relationships. Assertive communicators are in touch with their feelings and values and can communicate their needs directly and honestly.

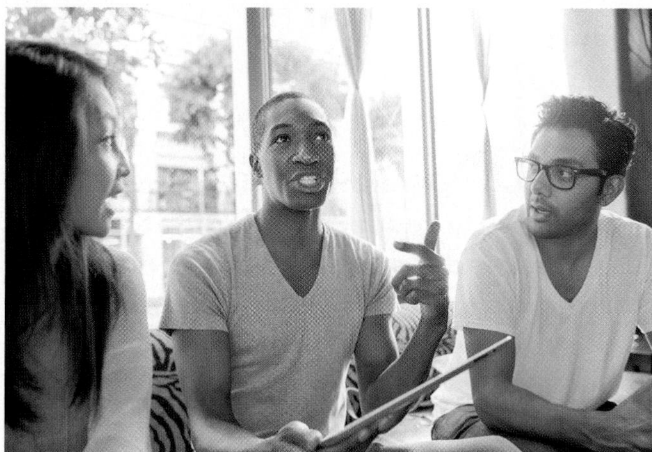

While everyone's communication style is unique, cultural norms have a big impact. Members of some cultures gesture broadly; others maintain a closed body posture. Some are offended by direct eye contact; others welcome a steady gaze.

Sharing personal information with others is called **self-disclosure**. If you want to learn more about someone, you have to be willing to share parts of yourself with that person. Self-disclosure is not storytelling or sharing secrets; rather, it is revealing how you are reacting to the present situation and giving any information about the past that is relevant to the other person's understanding of your current reactions.

If you sense that sharing feelings and thoughts will result in a closer relationship, you will likely take such a risk. But if you believe that the disclosure may result in rejection or alienation, you may not open up so easily. If the confidentiality of shared information has been violated, you may hesitate to disclose yourself in the future.

However, the risk in not disclosing yourself to others is that you will lack intimacy in relationships. Psychologist Carl Rogers believed that weak relationships were characterized by inhibited self-disclosure.[13]

If self-disclosure is such a key to creating healthy communication, but fear is a barrier to that process, what can we do? The following suggestions can help:

- **Get to know yourself.** The more you know about your feelings, beliefs, thoughts, and concerns, the more likely you'll be able to communicate with others about yourself.
- **Become more accepting of yourself.** No one is perfect, or has to be.
- **Be willing to discuss your sexual history.** The U.S. culture puts many taboos on discussions of sex, so it's no wonder we find it hard to disclose our sexual feelings. However, with the triple threat of unintended pregnancy, STIs, and HIV/AIDS, it is important to discuss sexual history with a partner.
- **Choose a safe context for self-disclosure.** When and where you make such disclosures and to whom may greatly influence the response. Choose a setting in which you feel safe to let yourself be known.

check yourself

- **How can appropriate self-disclosure contribute to healthy communication?**
- **Describe two ways to help get over fear of self-disclosure and create healthy communication.**

4.5 Skills for Better Communication: Using Technology Responsibly

learning outcome

4.5 Identify what is appropriate and inappropriate to share online.

Self-disclosure can be an effective method of building intimacy with another person, but not with large groups. While it may seem tempting or funny at the time, sharing information that is too personal via Facebook, Twitter, or other social networking sites can cause you to feel vulnerable or embarrassed later.

Headlines such as "*Prince Harry parties naked in Las Vegas*" and "*Gay students accidentally outed to parents via Facebook*"[14] remind us that we cannot expect privacy in a world where nearly everyone has a camera and an Internet connection. We are all a photo tag away from a family member or potential employer seeing us in less than flattering circumstances or knowing information we'd prefer kept secret.

"Social media screening," the practice of searching out all possible information on a prospective employee (sometimes to the point of asking for a Facebook password at an interview) is practiced by a third of employers.[15] Their biggest concerns: inappropriate photos, evidence of drug or alcohol use or abuse, and poor writing skills.

Posting negative comments online about employers, your peers, and anyone else you interact with can also spell trouble. It's not uncommon for employees to get fired for posting rants against their employers (or other inappropriate comments) on Facebook, blogs, and social networking sites. And while university administrators may not be regularly reading your social network feeds, your peers probably are—and any negative, damaging, or illegal information you post that gets reported can quickly escalate into an investigation by campus authorities. Increasing numbers of lawsuits for slander and defamation have been filed against people who post hateful, false, or damaging information about others online.

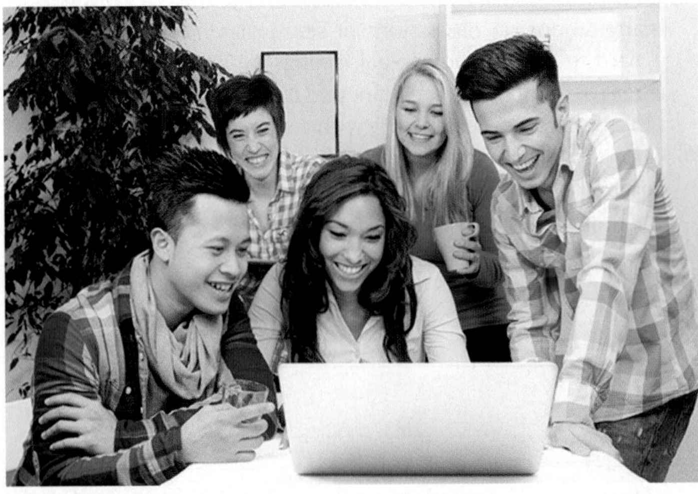

Avoid having your private life become the life of the party! Whenever you share information online—whether it's positive or negative—remember that it can easily be seen and shared beyond your intended audience.

Take measures to protect your privacy online and spare yourself from the damaging repercussions that can follow misuse of social media:

- Make sure your publicly available information is what you want prospective employers and family to see. Assume that potential employers will look you up on Facebook, Twitter, and other social media sites.
- Anything you posted in the past has the potential to resurface and damage your reputation now or in the future. Tighten your privacy settings and untag yourself in photos and videos you don't want others to see.
- Know your rights if someone posts photos or other information about you as a means of damaging your reputation.
- Don't post damaging or hurtful comments about anyone online, even if you feel you've been wronged or angered by that person. This includes employers, housemates, professors, and anyone else you're tempted to gripe about.
- Remember that even if you post comments on social networking sites "anonymously," it's still possible that someone determined enough could track you down. Be cautious even when you think you're incognito.

Furthermore, due to cached sites and reposts, you can't erase everything, so you may need to prepare an explanation for past posts, photos, and other information. As our "private" lives get more public all the time, we may have to accept Facebook founder Mark Zuckerberg's philosophy, that "privacy is no longer a social norm."[16]

In a survey, 34 percent of hiring managers who currently research candidates via social media said they have found information that has caused them not to hire a candidate.

check yourself

- **What types of information should you avoid sharing online?**
- **Do you think people have the right to say what they want about a person or a business online? Why or why not?**

4.6 Skills for Better Communication: Understanding Gender Differences

learning outcome

4.6 Describe differences and similarities in communication patterns between men and women.

According to Dr. Cynthia Burggraf Torppa at Ohio State University, differences in communication by gender are quite minor; what is important is how men and women interpret the same message.[17] She indicates that women are more sensitive to interpersonal meanings "between the lines," and men are more sensitive to subtle messages about status.

Within our society, some gender-specific communication patterns are obvious to the casual observer (Figure 4.3). Recognizing these differences and how they make us unique is a good step in avoiding unnecessary frustrations and irritations.

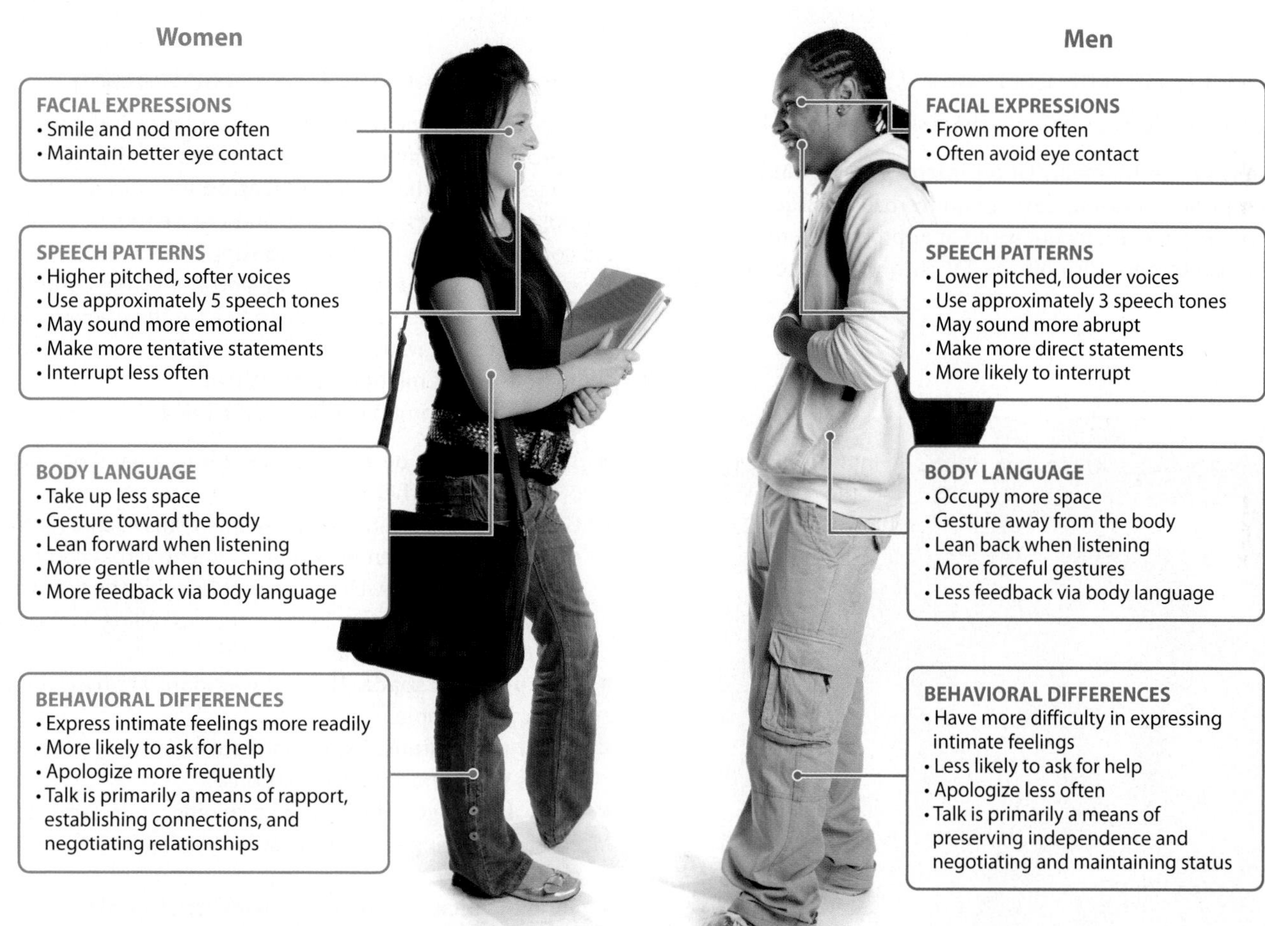

Figure 4.3 Differences in How Men and Women Communicate

VIDEO TUTOR
Gender Differences in Communication

check yourself

- **How would you describe communication patterns among men and women?**

4.7

Skills for Better Communication: Listening and Nonverbal Skills

learning outcome

4.7 Explain the importance of listening, and list and describe forms of nonverbal communication.

Listening allows us to share feelings, express concerns, communicate wants and needs, and make our thoughts and opinions known. Improving our speaking and listening skills can enhance our relationships. We listen best when (1) we believe that the message is important and relevant to us; (2) the speaker holds our attention through humor, dramatic effect, etc.; and (3) we are free of distractions and worries.

Becoming a Better Listener

To become a better listener, practice these skills on a daily basis:

- Be present in the moment. Good listeners acknowledge what the other person is saying through nonverbal cues such as nodding or smiling and asking questions at appropriate times.
- To avoid distractions, turn off the TV, shut your laptop lid, and put your phone away.
- Ask for clarification if you aren't sure what the speaker means, or paraphrase what you think you heard.
- Control the desire to interrupt. Try taking a deep breath, then holding it for another second and really listening to what is being said as you exhale.
- Avoid snap judgments based on what other people look like or say.
- Resist the temptation to "set the other person straight."
- Focus on the speaker. Hold back the temptation to launch into a story about your own experience in a similar situation.

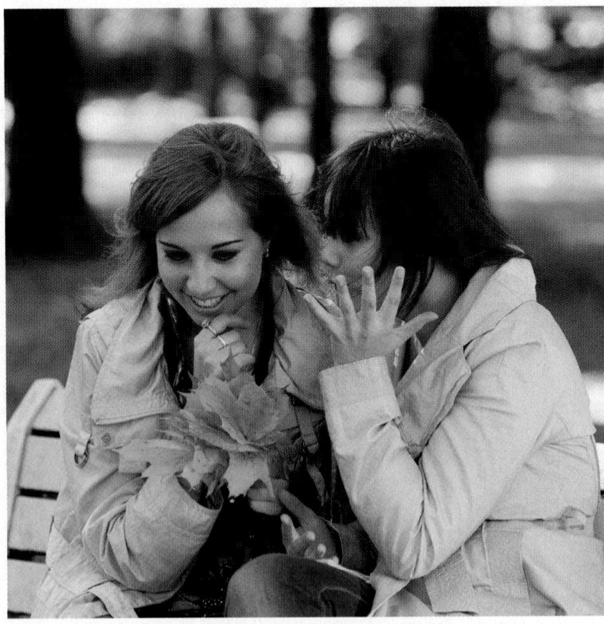

How can I communicate better?

One way to communicate better is to pay attention to your body language. Researchers have found that 93 percent of communication effectiveness is determined by nonverbal cues.

Using Nonverbal Communication

Smiling, eye contact or its lack, movements and gestures—these nonverbal clues influence how conversational partners interpret messages. **Nonverbal communication** includes all unwritten and unspoken messages, intentional and unintentional. Ideally, nonverbal communication matches and supports verbal communication. Research shows that when verbal and nonverbal communications don't match, we are more likely to believe the nonverbal cues.[18] It's important to be aware of the nonverbal cues we use and understand how others might interpret them.

Nonverbal communication can include the following:[19]

- **Touch.** This can be a handshake, a hug, a hand on the shoulder, or a kiss on the cheek.
- **Gestures.** These can include mannerisms such as a thumbs-up or a wave, or movements that augment verbal communication, such as indicating with your hands how big the fish was that got away. Gestures can also be rude, such as rolling one's eyes to indicate disdain for what has been said.
- **Interpersonal space.** This is the amount of physical space separating two people.
- **Facial expressions.** Expressions such as frowns, smiles, and grimaces signal moods and emotions.
- **Body language.** This includes folding your arms across your chest, indicating defensiveness, or leaning forward in your chair to show interest.
- **Tone of voice.** This refers to elements of speaking such as pitch, volume, and speed.

check yourself

- **Why is listening an important part of communication?**
- **How do nonverbal cues affect interactions?**

4.8

Skills for Better Communication: Managing Conflict

learning outcome

4.8 Identify strategies for managing and resolving conflict.

A **conflict** is an emotional state that arises when the behavior of one person interferes with that of another. Some conflict is inevitable, and not all conflict is bad; airing feelings and resolving differences can strengthen relationships. **Conflict resolution** and conflict management form a systematic approach to resolving differences fairly and constructively.

Prolonged conflict can destroy relationships unless the parties agree to resolve points of contention. As two people learn to negotiate and compromise, the number and intensity of conflicts should diminish.

During a heated conflict, try to pause before responding, consider the possible impact of your comments or actions, and state your point constructively. You can also say, "I can see we aren't going to resolve this right now. Let's talk when we've both cooled off."

E-mail messages are easily misunderstood because we can't see or hear the person talking. In general, when you're tempted to send a nasty response to an e-mail, stop. Observe the 24-hour rule—don't hit Send until the next day. Usually, you'll find it's better to hit Delete and move on, or to talk in person.

Rudeness or inconsiderate behavior usually develops when one person fails to recognize the feelings or rights of another. Try to see the other person's point of view, listen actively, avoid interrupting, and avoid gestures such as head-shaking or finger-pointing. Key elements of conflict management include validating others' opinions and treating others as you would like to be treated.

Here are some strategies for conflict resolution:

1. **Identify the problem.** Talk together to clarify the conflict or problem. Say what you want and listen to what the other person wants. Use "I" messages; avoid blaming "you" messages. Be an active listener—repeat what the other person has said and ask questions for clarification or information.
2. **Generate possible solutions.** Brainstorm ways to address the problem. Base your search on goals and interests identified in the first step. Come up with several alternatives, but avoid evaluating them for now.
3. **Evaluate solutions.** Review the possible solutions. Narrow your list to one or two that work for both parties. Focus on finding a solution you both feel is satisfactory.
4. **Decide on the best solution.** Choose an alternative acceptable to both parties. You must both commit to the decision for it to be effective.
5. **Implement the solution.** Discuss how the decision will be carried out. Establish who is responsible to do what and when.
6. **Follow up.** Check in and evaluate whether a solution is working. If it's not working as planned, or if circumstances have changed, revise your plan. Remember that both parties must agree to any changes to the original idea.

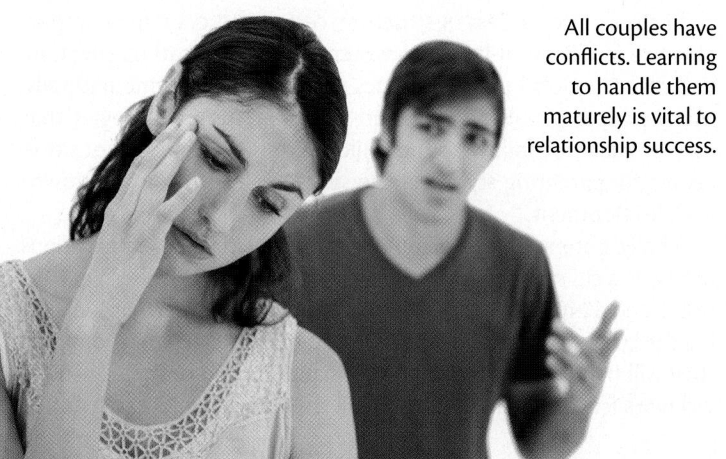

All couples have conflicts. Learning to handle them maturely is vital to relationship success.

Skills for Behavior Change

COMMUNICATING WHEN EMOTIONS RUN HIGH

These guidelines can help you express your feelings more effectively in an emotionally charged situation:

- **Try to be specific rather than general about how you feel.**
- **When expressing anger or irritation, describe the specific behavior you don't like, then your feelings.**
- **If you have mixed feelings, say so; express and explain each feeling.**
- **Use "I" messages, rather than "you" statements that can cast blame or imply fault. With "I" messages, the speaker takes responsibility for communicating his or her feelings, thoughts, and beliefs.**
- **When you ask for feedback, be prepared for an honest answer.**
- **Be careful when trying to communicate or interpret emotionally charged messages via e-mail or text. It can be hard to interpret their intended meaning without the nonverbal support of tone of voice and body language.**

check yourself

- **Which strategy for conflict resolution do you find most effective? Why?**

4.9

Committed Relationships

learning outcome

4.9 List different forms of committed relationships.

Commitment in a relationship means an intent to act over time in a way that perpetuates the well-being of the other person, oneself, and the relationship. Polls show that the vast majority of Americans strive to develop a committed relationship whether in the form of marriage, cohabitation, or partnerships.[20]

Marriage

In many societies, traditional committed relationships take the form of marriage. In the United States, marriage means entering into a legal agreement that includes shared finances and responsibility for raising children. Many Americans also view marriage as a religious commitment.

Nearly 90 percent of Americans marry at least once; at any given time, about 50 percent of U.S. adults are married (Figure 4.4). However, since 1960, annual marriages have steadily declined,[21] possibly due to factors including delay of first marriage, an increase in cohabitation, and fewer remarriages. In 1960, the median age for first marriage was 23 for men and 20 for women; by 2009, it had risen to 28.1 for men and 25.9 for women.[22]

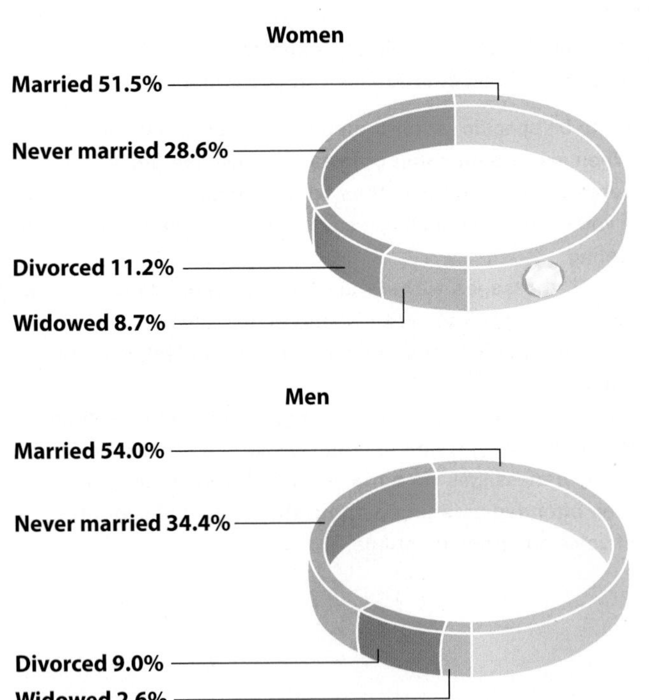

Figure 4.4 Marital Status of the U.S. Population by Sex

Note: The figure does not list the percentages for married men and women with a spouse absent and separated.

Source: U.S. Census Bureau, "Marital Status of People 15 Years and Over, by Age, Sex Personal Earnings, Race, and Hispanic Origin: 2013," Table A1, America's Families and Living Arrangements, 2013, www.census.gov.

Many Americans believe that marriage involves **monogamy**, or exclusive sexual involvement with one partner. In fact, the lifetime pattern for many Americans appears to be **serial monogamy**, where a person has a monogamous sexual relationship with one partner before moving on to another. Some people prefer **open relationships**, in which partners agree that each may be sexually involved with others outside their relationship.

Considerable research indicates that married people live longer, feel happier, remain mentally alert longer, and suffer fewer physical and mental health problems.[23] Healthy marriage contributes to less stress via financial stability, expanded support networks, and improved personal behaviors. Married adults are about half as likely to smoke as other adults.[24] They are also less likely to be heavy drinkers and more likely to get sufficient sleep compared to divorced adults.[25] The one negative health indicator for married people is body weight in men. Married men are far more likely than never-married men to be overweight.[26]

Choosing Whether to Have Children Choosing to raise children changes a marriage or other relationship. It can bring joy and meaning to your lives. However, it is also highly stressful: time, energy, and money are split many ways, and you will no longer be able to give each other undivided attention. Having a child does not save a bad relationship—in fact, it seems only to compound problems that already exist.

Changing patterns in family life affect the way children are raised. Now, either partner may choose to provide primary child care. Today, the blended family is the most common family unit, creating instant families for stepparents and stepchildren. In addition, many individuals have children in a family structure other than heterosexual marriage. Single women or lesbian couples can choose adoption or alternative insemination; single men or gay couples can choose to adopt or obtain the services of a surrogate mother. According to the U.S. Census Bureau, in 2012 over 28 percent of all children under age 18 were living in families headed by a man or woman raising a child alone.[27] Regardless of structure, certain factors remain important to a family's well-being: consistency, communication, affection, and respect. Good parenting does not necessarily come naturally. Many people parent as they were parented, using strategies that may or may not follow sound child-rearing principles. A positive, respectful parenting style sets the stage for healthy family growth and development.

Finally, potential parents must consider the financial implications of having a child. It is estimated that a family with a child born in 2012 will spend $240,000 on the child over the next 17 years, not including the cost of college.[28] Prospective parents should think about how they will handle child rearing both financially and practically—who will work less or not at all, or how will they pay for child care?

88%

of Americans list love as the most important reason to marry.

Cohabitation

Cohabitation is a relationship in which two unmarried people with an intimate connection live together. In some states, cohabitation lasting a designated number of years (usually 7) legally constitutes a **common-law marriage** for purposes of sharing many financial obligations.

Cohabitation can offer many of the same emotional benefits as marriage. Some people may also cohabit for financial reasons. The past 20 years have seen a large increase in the number of persons who have ever cohabited; cohabitation is increasingly the first coresidential partnership formed by young adults.[29]

Cohabitation before marriage has been a controversial issue for decades. While some voiced moral objections, other concerns were related to higher divorce rates among couples who cohabited before marriage. However, according to recent research, cohabitation before marriage is no longer a predictor for divorce.[30]

Cohabitation can be a prelude to marriage, but for some it is an alternative. It is more common among those of lower socioeconomic status, those who are less religious, those who have been divorced, and those who have experienced parental divorce or high parental conflict during childhood. Cohabitation has both advantages and drawbacks. Perhaps the greatest disadvantage is the lack of societal validation for the relationship, especially if the couple subsequently has children. Many cohabitants also deal with difficulties obtaining insurance and tax benefits and legal issues over property.

Gay and Lesbian Partnerships

Lesbians and gay men seek the same things in committed relationships that heterosexuals do: love, friendship, communication, validation, and stability. A 2011 survey identified an estimated 605,472 same-sex couples in the United States, 25 percent of whom are legally married.[31]

Challenges to successful lesbian and gay relationships often stem from discrimination and difficulties dealing with social, legal, and religious doctrines. For lesbian and gay couples, obtaining benefits such as tax deductions, power-of-attorney rights, partner health insurance, and child custody rights has been challenging.

In early 2014, the United States Justice Department extended the same rights in legal matters to married same-sex couples as married heterosexual couples receive under federal law. This announcement follows policy changes made in 2013, when the U.S. Supreme Court overturned a portion of the Defense of Marriage Act (DOMA) that prevented married homosexual couples from being legally recognized by the federal government.

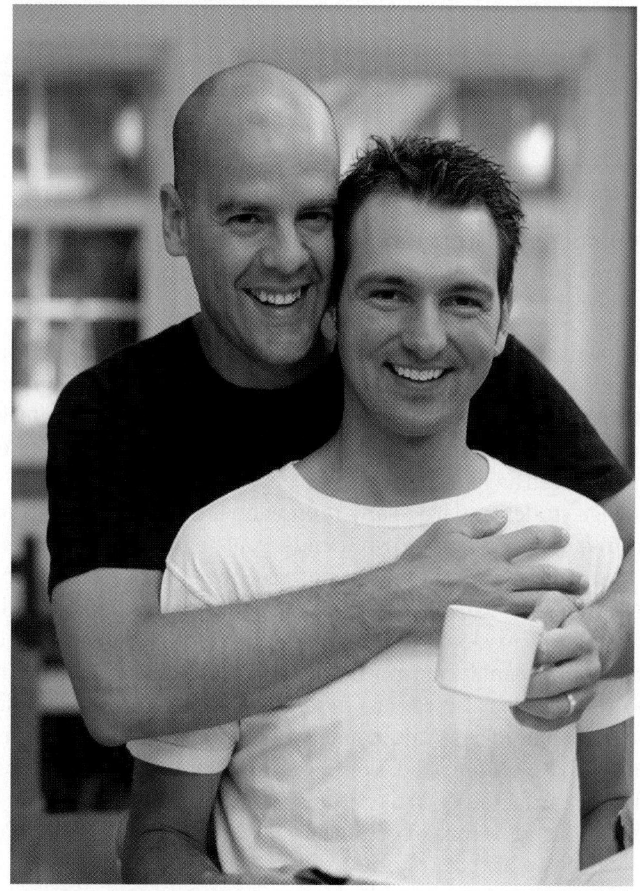

The desire to form lasting and committed intimate relationships is shared by most adults, regardless of sexual orientation.

As of 2014, California, Connecticut, Delaware, Hawaii, Illinois, Iowa, Maine, Maryland, Massachusetts, Minnesota, New Hampshire, New Jersey, New Mexico, New York, Oregon, Pennsylvania, Rhode Island, Vermont, Washington, and the District of Columbia grant same-sex couples full marriage equality. Three other states have broad relationship-recognition laws that extend to same-sex couples all, or nearly all, the state rights and responsibilities of married heterosexual couples.[32] As of 2014, 17 countries worldwide allow same-sex marriage.[33]

Staying Single

Increasing numbers of adults of all ages are electing to marry later or remain single altogether. According to data from the most recent census, 57 percent of women aged 20 to 34 had never been married.[34] Many singles live rewarding lives and maintain a network of close friends and families.

check yourself

- **What forms can committed relationships take?**

4.10 When Relationships Falter

learning outcome

4.10 Discuss common reasons that relationships end, and provide examples of how to cope with a failed relationship.

Breakdowns in relationships usually begin with a change in communication, however subtle. Either partner may stop listening and cease to be emotionally present for the other. In turn, the other feels ignored, unappreciated, or unwanted. Unresolved conflicts increase, and unresolved anger can cause problems in sexual relations.

College students, particularly those who are socially isolated or far from family and hometown friends, may be particularly vulnerable to staying in unhealthy relationships. They may become emotionally dependent on a partner for everything from sharing meals to spending recreational time. Mutual obligations, such as shared rental arrangements, transportation, and child care, can make it tough to leave. It's also easy to mistake sexual advances for physical attraction or love. Without a network of friends and supporters to talk with, to obtain validation for feelings, or to share concerns, a student may feel stuck in a relationship that is headed nowhere.

Honesty and verbal affection are usually positive aspects of a relationship. In a troubled relationship, however, they can be used to cover up irresponsible or hurtful behavior. "At least I was honest" is not an acceptable substitute for acting in a trustworthy way. "But I really do love you" is not a license for being inconsiderate or rude. Relationships that are lacking in mutual respect and consideration can become physically or emotionally abusive.

Recognizing a Potential Abuser

Is that new "item" in your life really what he or she appears to be? Your new love interest may appear sensitive, gentle, caring, respectful, and considerate in the beginning—all the things you've been looking for. It can be hard to tell what someone is really like early on, as that person tries to make a good impression on you. To avoid getting into a long-term relationship with an abuser, watch carefully and trust your instincts. Ask others about the person and find out about his or her history with partners, friends, and family. Be immediately wary if your partner demonstrates any of the following red flags:

- Gets extremely angry and swears at you or others.
- Hurts you by making fun of you or putting you down.
- Takes too much control. In a healthy relationship, partners share decision making.
- Displays excessive jealousy.
- Tries to shut out people you want to see, and wants to spend more and more time alone with you.
- Expresses continual negativity—sulks, angers easily, throws tantrums when things don't go his or her way.
- Pushes you verbally or physically to have unwanted sex or intimacy.
- Threatens you.
- Is often in trouble or fighting with someone.

The list above is not exhaustive, and there are degrees of seriousness for each. However, if someone you have known only for a short time displays any sign of physical anger or threatens you early on, it's time to walk away.

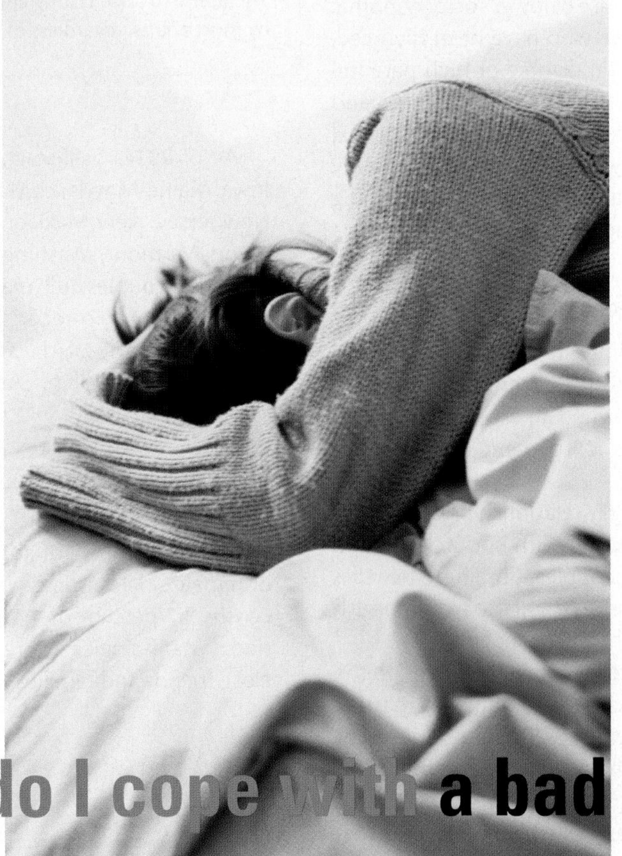

How do I cope with a bad breakup?

It may feel as if there is no end to the sorrow, anger, and guilt that often attend a difficult breakup, but time is a miraculous healer. Acknowledging your feelings, finding healthful ways to express them, spending time with friends, and allowing yourself to take as much time as you need to recover are all helpful strategies for dealing with the end of a romantic relationship.

When and Why Relationships End

Often we hear in the news that 50 percent of American marriages end in divorce. This number is based on comparing the annual marriage rate with the annual divorce rate. This is misleading, because in any given year, the people who are divorcing are not the same people who just got married.

It is more accurate to look at the total number of married people and calculate how many of them eventually divorce. Using this calculation, the divorce rate in the United States has never exceeded 40 percent.[35] The divorce rate in the United States shot up in the 1970s, peaked in the early 1980s, and has since declined to about 30 percent.[36] This decrease may be related to an increase in the age at which persons first marry as well as a higher level of education among those who are marrying—as both contribute to marital stability.[37] The risk of divorce is lower for college-educated people marrying for the first time and lower still for people who wait to marry until their mid-twenties and who haven't lived with multiple partners prior to marriage.[38]

Why do relationships end? There are many reasons and many factors, including illness, financial concerns, and career problems. Other breakups arise from unmet expectations. Many people enter a relationship with certain expectations about how they and their partner will behave. Failure to communicate these beliefs can lead to resentment and disappointment. Differences in sexual needs may also contribute to the demise of a relationship. Under stress, communication and cooperation between partners can break down. Conflict, negative interactions, and a general lack of respect between partners can erode even the most loving relationship.

What behaviors signal that trouble is coming? Based on 35 years of research and couples therapy, John Gottman has identified four behavior patterns in couples that predict future divorce with 85 percent or better accuracy.[39]

- **Criticism:** Phrasing complaints in terms of a partner's defect, for example: "You never talk about anyone but yourself. You are self-centered."
- **Defensiveness:** Righteous indignation as a form of self-protection, for example: "It's not my fault we missed the flight; you always make us late."
- **Stonewalling:** Withdrawing emotionally from a given interaction, for example: The listener seems to ignore the speaker as he or she speaks, giving no indication that the speaker was heard.
- **Contempt:** Talking down to a person; contempt is the biggest predictor of divorce, for example: "How could you be so stupid?"

While these behaviors do not guarantee that an individual couple will divorce, they are red flags for relationships that are at great risk for failure.

Coping with Failed Relationships

No relationship comes with a guarantee, no matter how many promises partners make to be together forever. Losing a love is as much a part of life as falling in love. That being said, the uncoupling process can be very painful. Whenever we risk getting close to another, we also risk being hurt if things don't work out. Remember that knowing, understanding, and feeling good about oneself before entering a relationship is very important. Consider these tips for coping with a failed relationship:

- **Acknowledge that you've gone through a rough spot.** You may feel grief, loneliness, rejection, anger, guilt, relief, and sadness. Seek out trusted friends and, if needed, professional help.
- **Let go of negative thought patterns and habits and engage in activities that make you happy.** Go for a walk, talk to friends, listen to music, work out at the gym, volunteer with a community organization, or write in a journal.
- **Spend time with current friends, or reconnect with old friends.** Get reacquainted with yourself, what you enjoy doing, and the people whose company you enjoy.
- **Don't rush into a "rebound" relationship.** You need time to resolve your past experience rather than escape from it. You can't be trusting and intimate in a new relationship if you are still working on getting over a past relationship.

Skills for Behavior Change

HOW DO YOU END IT?

Relationship endings are just as important as their beginnings. Healthy closure affords both parties the opportunity to move on without wondering or worrying about what went wrong and whose fault it was. If you need to end a relationship, do so in a manner that preserves and respects the dignity of both partners. If you are the person "breaking up," you have probably had time to think about the process and may be at a different stage from your partner.

Here are some tips for ending a relationship in a respectful and caring way:

- Arrange a time and quiet place where you can talk without interruption.
- Say in advance that there is something important you want to discuss.
- Accept that your partner may express strong feelings and be prepared to listen quietly.
- Consider in advance if you might also become upset and what support you might need.
- Communicate honestly using "I" messages and without personal attacks. Explain your reasons as much as you can without being cruel or insensitive.
- Don't let things escalate into a fight, even if you have very strong feelings.
- Provide another opportunity to talk about the end of the relationship when you both have had time to reflect.

check yourself

- **What are some common reasons that relationships end?**
- **What are three ways to cope with a failed relationship?**

4.11 Your Sexual Identity: More than Biology

learning outcome

4.11 Define and discuss the major components of sexual identity.

Sexual identity, the recognition and acknowledgment of oneself as a sexual being, is determined by the interaction of genetic, physiological, environmental, and social factors.

The beginning of sexual identity occurs at conception with the combining of chromosomes. All eggs (ova) carry an X chromosome; sperm may carry either an X or a Y chromosome, and thus determine sex. If a sperm carrying an X fertilizes an egg, the resulting combination of chromosomes (XX) produces a female. If a sperm carrying a Y fertilizes an egg, the XY combination produces a male.

The genetic instructions included in the sex chromosomes lead to the differential development of male and female **gonads** (reproductive organs). Once the male gonads (testes) and the female gonads (ovaries) develop, they play a key role in all future sexual development, being responsible for production of sex hormones. The primary female sex hormones are estrogen and progesterone; the primary male sex hormone is testosterone. The release of testosterone in a maturing fetus stimulates the development of a penis and other male genitals. If no testosterone is produced, female genitals form.

At the time of **puberty,** hormones released by the **pituitary gland**, the gonadotropins, stimulate the testes and ovaries to make appropriate sex hormones. The increase of estrogen production in females and testosterone production in males leads to the development of **secondary sex characteristics**, features that distinguish the sexes but that have no direct reproductive function. For males, these include deepening of the voice, development of facial and body hair, and growth of the skeleton and musculature. For females, they include growth of breasts, widening of hips, and development of pubic and underarm hair.

Another important component of sexual identity is **gender**, which refers to characteristics and actions typically associated with men or women (masculine or feminine) as defined by culture. Our sense of masculine and feminine traits is largely a result of **socialization** during childhood. **Gender roles** are the behaviors and activities we use to express maleness or femaleness in ways that conform to society's expectations. For example, you may learn to play with dolls or trucks, based on how your parents influence your actions. For some, gender roles can be confining when they lead to stereotyping. Boundaries established by **gender-role stereotypes** can make it difficult to express one's identity. In the United States, men are traditionally expected to be independent, aggressive, logical, and in control of emotions. Women are traditionally expected to be passive, nurturing, intuitive, and emotional. **Androgyny** refers to the combination of traditional masculine and feminine traits in a single person; each of us is in small or large ways androgynous. Highly androgynous people do not always follow traditional sex roles.

Whereas gender roles are an expression of cultural expectations for behavior, **gender identity** is a sense or awareness of being male or a female. A person's gender identity does not always match his or her biological sex; this is called being **transgendered**. There is a broad spectrum of expression among transgendered persons that reflects degree of dissatisfaction with sexual anatomy. Some transgendered persons are comfortable with their bodies and content simply to dress and live as the other gender. At the other end of the spectrum are **transsexuals,** who feel extremely trapped in their bodies and may opt for interventions such as sex reassignment surgery.

Sexual Orientation

Sexual orientation refers to a person's enduring emotional, romantic, sexual, or affectionate attraction to others. You may be primarily attracted to members of the opposite sex **(heterosexual)**, the same sex

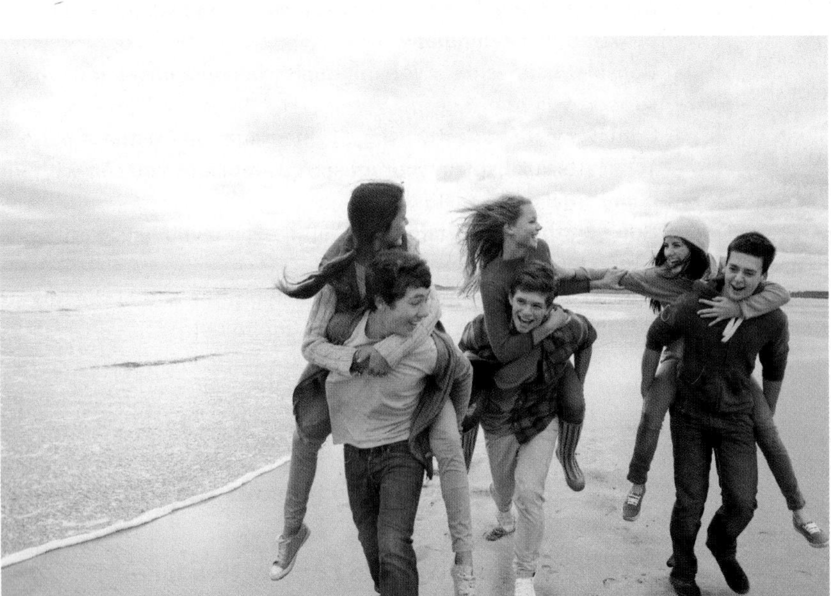

What influences sexual identity besides biology?

How you perceive yourself as a sexual being is influenced by socialization and personal experience. Your understanding of gender roles, your contact with people of various gender identities or sexual orientations, and your own degree of emotional maturity can all affect your sense of sexual identity.

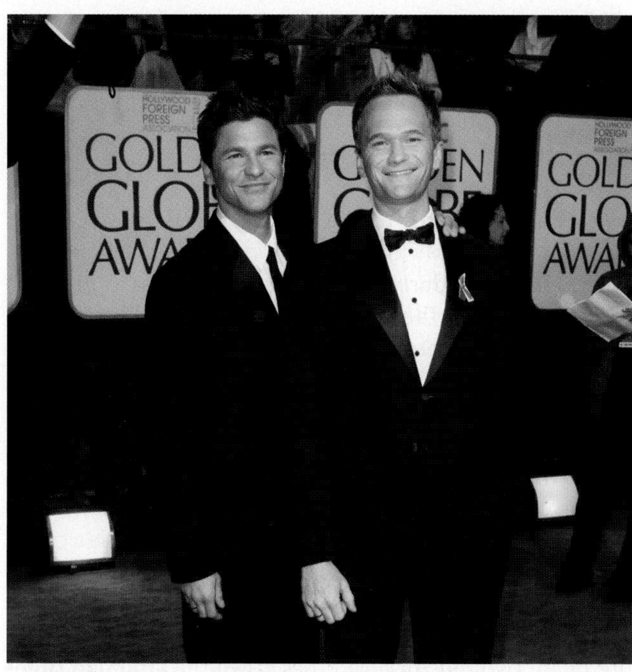

The presence of gay and lesbian celebrities in the media—such as actor Neil Patrick Harris and his partner David Burtka—contributes to the increasing acceptance of gay relationships in everyday life.

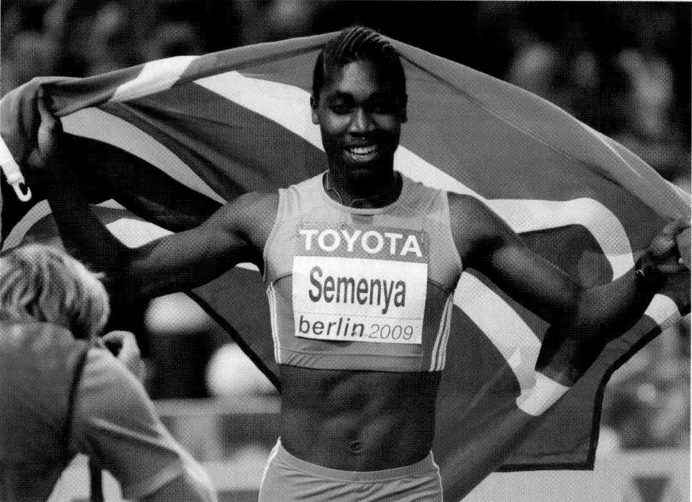

After South African middle-distance runner Caster Semenya won the gold medal in the 800-meter race at the 2009 World Championships, she was required to undergo gender testing and was subsequently barred from competition. Officials wanted to determine whether Semenya has a DSD resulting in testosterone levels that give her an unfair athletic advantage over other women competitors. After 11 months, a panel of medical experts announced that Semenya was again eligible to compete against other women. Her case highlights the challenges facing athletes and other people with both male and female characteristics.

(homosexual), or both sexes **(bisexual)**. Many homosexuals prefer the terms **gay,** queer, or **lesbian** to describe their sexual orientation. *Gay* and *queer* can apply to both men and women, but *lesbian* refers specifically to women.

Researchers today agree that sexual orientation is best understood using a model that incorporates biological, psychological, and socioenvironmental factors. Biological explanations focus on research into genetics, hormones, and differences in brain anatomy, whereas psychological and socioenvironmental explanations examine parent–child interactions, sex roles, and early sexual and interpersonal interactions. Collectively, this growing body of research suggests that the origins of homosexuality, like heterosexuality, are complex. To diminish the complexity of sexual orientation to "a choice" is a clear misrepresentation of current research. Homosexuals do not "choose" their sexual orientation any more than heterosexuals do.

Gay, lesbian, and bisexual persons are often the targets of **sexual prejudice** (or *sexual bias*). Prejudice refers to negative attitudes and hostile actions directed at a social group. Hate crimes, discrimination, and hostility toward sexual minorities are evidence of ongoing sexual prejudice. Bias regarding sexual orientation is the motivation for approximately 21 percent of all hate crimes reported in the United States.[40]

Sexual orientation is often viewed as based entirely on whom one has sex with, but this is inaccurate and overly simplistic. It depends not only on who you are sexually attracted to, fantasize about, and have sex with, but also factors such as who you feel close to emotionally and socialize with and in which "community" you feel comfortable. From this viewpoint, there are not just three (homosexual, heterosexual, bisexual) orientations, but a range of complex, interacting, and fluid factors influencing sexuality over time.

Disorders of Sexual Development

Sometimes chromosomes are added, lost, or rearranged at conception, and the sex of the offspring is unclear, a condition known as **intersex.** *Disorders of sexual development* (*DSDs*) is a less confusing term that has been recommended to refer to intersex conditions, which may occur as often as 1 in 4,500 live births.[41]

People with DSDs are born with various levels of male and female biological characteristics, ranging from different chromosomal arrangements to altered hormone production to variation in primary and secondary sex characteristics. Whereas most people are born with either XX or XY chromosomes, some are born with XXY or XO chromosomes (where O signifies a missing or damaged chromosome). In some people, gonads do not develop fully into ovaries or testicles, although there may be no external signs to indicate this; in others, external genitalia may be ambiguous.

Many, but not all, DSDs require some degree of hormonal or surgical intervention to ensure physical health. It is also necessary to "assign" a gender to children as early as possible to ensure psychological health. If this assignment is later found to be inconsistent with the child's own sense of gender, he or she may adopt a different gender identity. Most people born with DSDs today are allowed to grow up, establish their own gender identity, and choose as adults whether to have additional surgeries to alter any sexual tissues they feel are incongruent with their gender.[42]

check yourself

- **What is sexual identity?**
- **What are the major components of sexual identity?**

4.12 Female Sexual Anatomy and Physiology

learning outcome

4.12 Identify the major features and functions of female sexual anatomy and physiology.

The female reproductive system includes two major groups of structures, the external genitals and the internal organs (Figure 4.5).

The external female genitals are collectively known as the **vulva.** The **mons pubis** is a pad of fatty tissue covering and protecting the pubic bone; after the onset of puberty, it becomes covered with coarse hair. The **labia majora** are folds of skin and erectile tissue that enclose the urethral and vaginal openings; the **labia minora**, or inner lips, are folds of mucous membrane found just inside the labia majora.

The **clitoris** is located at the upper end of the labia minora and beneath the mons pubis; its only known function is to provide sexual pleasure, and it is the most sensitive part of the genital area. Directly below the clitoris is the **urethral opening**, through which urine is expelled from the body; below it is the vaginal opening. In some women, the vaginal opening is covered by a thin membrane called the **hymen.** The hymen can be stretched or torn by physical activity, and is not present in all women to begin with. The **perineum** is the area of smooth tissue between the vulva and the anus. The tissue in this area has many nerve endings and is sensitive to touch; it can play a part in sexual excitement.

The internal female genitals include the vagina, uterus, fallopian tubes, and ovaries. The **vagina** is a tubular organ that serves as a passageway from the uterus to the outside of the body. It allows menstrual flow to exit from the uterus during a woman's monthly cycle, receives the penis during intercourse, and serves as the birth canal during childbirth. The **uterus (womb)** is a hollow, muscular, pear-shaped organ. Hormones acting on the inner lining of the uterus (the **endometrium**) either prepare the uterus for implantation and development of a fertilized egg or signal that no fertilization has taken place, in which case the endometrium deteriorates and becomes menstrual flow.

The lower end of the uterus, the **cervix**, extends down into the vagina. The **ovaries**, almond-sized organs on either side of the uterus, produce the hormones estrogen and progesterone and are the reservoir for immature eggs. (All the eggs a woman will ever have are present in her ovaries at birth.) Extending from the upper end of the uterus are two thin, flexible tubes called the **fallopian tubes** (or **oviducts**). The fallopian tubes capture eggs as they are released from the ovaries during ovulation and are the site where sperm and egg meet and fertilization takes place. They then serve as the passageway to the uterus, where the fertilized egg becomes implanted.

The Onset of Puberty and the Menstrual Cycle

With the onset of puberty, the female reproductive system matures, and secondary sex characteristics, including breasts, widened hips,

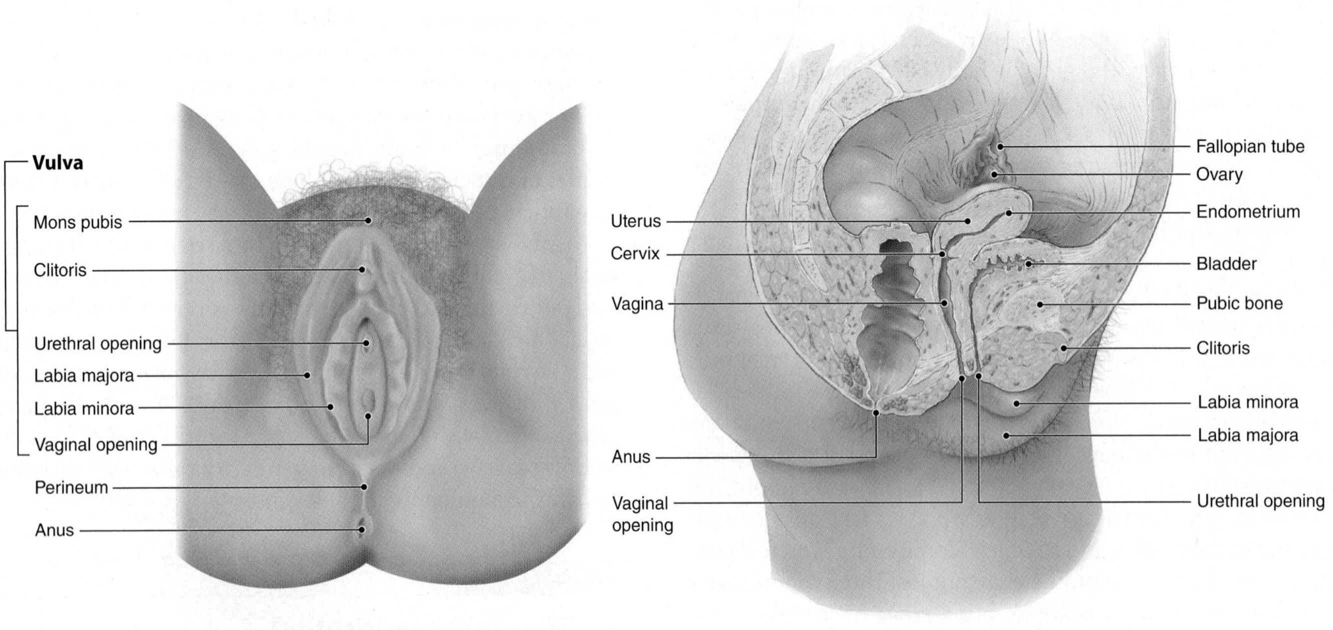

Figure 4.5 Female Reproductive System

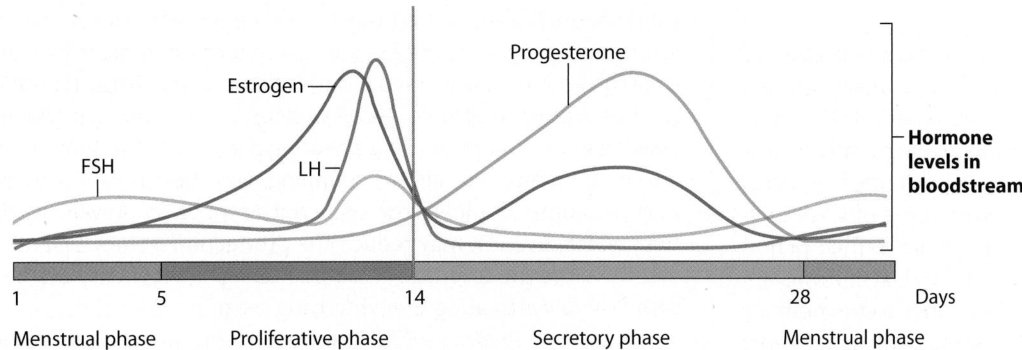

Figure 4.6 Hormonal Control and Phases of the Menstrual Cycle

and underarm and pubic hair, develop. The first sign of puberty is the beginning of breast development, around age 11. The pituitary gland, **hypothalamus,** and ovaries all secrete hormones that act as chemical messengers among them.

Around the same time, the hypothalamus receives a message to begin secreting *gonadotropin-releasing hormone* (*GnRH*). This, in turn, signals the pituitary gland to release hormones called *gonadotropins.* Two specific gonadotropins, *follicle-stimulating hormone* (*FSH*) and *luteinizing hormone* (*LH*), signal the ovaries to start producing **estrogens** and **progesterone.** The age range for the onset of the first menstrual period, or **menarche,** is 9 to 17 years, with the average 11 to 13 years. Body fat heavily influences the onset of puberty, and increasing rates of obesity in children may account for the fact that girls seem to be reaching puberty much earlier than they used to.[43]

The average menstrual cycle lasts 28 days and consists of the proliferative, secretory, and menstrual phases (Figure 4.6). The *proliferative phase* begins with the end of menstruation. During this time, the endometrium develops, or proliferates. The hypothalamus, sensing low levels of estrogen and progesterone in the blood, increases its secretions of GnRH, which, in turn, triggers the pituitary gland to release FSH. When FSH reaches the ovaries, it signals several **ovarian follicles** to begin maturing. Normally, only one of the follicles, the **graafian follicle**, reaches full maturity in the days preceding ovulation. While the follicles mature, they begin producing estrogen, which, in turn, signals the endometrial lining of the uterus to proliferate. High estrogen levels signal the pituitary to slow down FSH production and increase release of LH. Under the influence of LH, the graafian follicle ruptures and releases a mature **ovum** (plural: *ova*), a single egg cell, near a fallopian tube. This event, which usually occurs around day 14 of the cycle, is referred to as **ovulation.** The other ripening follicles degenerate and are reabsorbed by the body. Occasionally, two ova mature and are released during ovulation. If both are fertilized, fraternal (nonidentical) twins develop. Identical twins develop when one fertilized ovum (called a *zygote*) divides into two separate zygotes.

The phase following ovulation is called the *secretory phase.* The ruptured graafian follicle, which has remained in the ovary, is transformed into the **corpus luteum** and begins secreting large amounts of estrogen and progesterone. These secretions peak around the twentieth day of the cycle and cause the endometrium to thicken. If fertilization and implantation take place, cells surrounding the developing embryo release *human chorionic gonadotropin* (*HCG*), increasing estrogen and progesterone secretions that maintain the endometrium and signal the pituitary not to start a new menstrual cycle. If no implantation occurs, the hypothalamus signals the pituitary to stop producing FSH and LH, thus causing the levels of progesterone in the blood to peak. The corpus luteum begins to decompose, leading to rapid declines in estrogen and progesterone, the hormones needed to sustain the uterine lining. Without them, the endometrium is sloughed off in the menstrual flow, beginning the *menstrual phase.* Low estrogen levels signal the hypothalamus to release GnRH, which acts on the pituitary to secrete FSH—and the cycle begins again.

check yourself

- **What are the major features and functions of female sexual anatomy and physiology?**
- **Describe a 28-day menstrual cycle, starting with the proliferative phase.**

4.13 Menstrual Problems and Menopause

learning **outcome**

4.13 **Discuss possible menstrual problems.**

Premenstrual Syndrome

Premenstrual syndrome (PMS) is a term used for a collection of physical, emotional, and behavioral symptoms that many women experience 7 to 14 days prior to their menstrual period. The most common symptoms are tender breasts, food cravings, fatigue, irritability, and depression. It is estimated that 75 percent of menstruating women experience some signs and symptoms of PMS each month. For the majority of women, these disappear as their period begins, but for a small subset of women (3%–5%), symptoms are severe enough to affect daily routines and activities to the point of being disabling. This severe form of PMS has its own designation, **premenstrual dysphoric disorder (PMDD)**, with symptoms that include severe depression, hopelessness, anger, anxiety, low self-esteem, difficulty concentrating, irritability, and tension.

Several natural approaches to managing PMS can also help PMDD. These include eating more carbohydrates (grains, fruits, and vegetables), reducing caffeine and salt intake, exercising regularly, and taking measures to reduce stress. Recent investigation into methods of controlling severe emotional swings has led to the use of antidepressants for treating PMDD, primarily selective serotonin reuptake inhibitors (e.g., Prozac, Paxil, and Zoloft).

Dysmenorrhea

Dysmenorrhea is a medical term for menstrual cramps, the pain or discomfort in the lower abdomen that many women experience just before or after menstruation. Along with cramps, some women can experience nausea and vomiting, loose stools, sweating, and dizziness. Primary dysmenorrhea doesn't involve any physical abnormality and usually begins 6 months to a year after a woman's first period, whereas secondary dysmenorrhea has an underlying physical cause such as endometriosis or uterine fibroids.[44] If you experience primary dysmenorrhea, you can reduce discomfort by using over-the-counter nonsteroidal anti-inflammatory drugs (NSAIDs) such as aspirin, ibuprofen (Advil or Motrin), or naproxen (Aleve). Soaking in a hot bath or using a heating pad on your abdomen may also ease cramps. For severe cramping, your health care provider may recommend a low-dose oral contraceptive to prevent ovulation, which, in turn, may reduce the production of prostaglandins and therefore the severity of cramps. Managing secondary dysmenorrhea involves treating the underlying cause.

Toxic shock syndrome (*TSS*), although rare today, is still something women should be aware of. It is caused by a bacterial infection facilitated by tampon or diaphragm use. Symptoms, which occur during one's period or a few days afterward, can be hard to recognize because they mimic the flu and include sudden high fever, vomiting, diarrhea, dizziness, fainting, or a rash that looks like sunburn. Proper treatment usually assures recovery in 2 to 3 weeks.

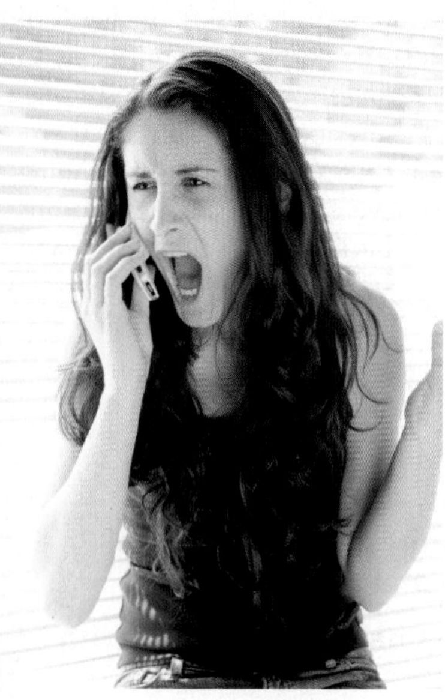

Do all women get PMS?

About 75 percent of menstruating women experience some PMS symptoms every month, but for most women these symptoms are mild and short-lived. Stress reduction, regular exercise, and a healthy diet are all good strategies for coping with PMS symptoms, which can include irritability and moodiness, fatigue, breast tenderness, and food cravings.

Changes in the Menstrual Cycle: Menopause

Just as menarche signals the beginning of a woman's potential reproductive years, **menopause**—the permanent cessation of menstruation—signals the end. Generally occurring between the ages of 45 and 55, menopause results in decreased estrogen levels, which may produce symptoms such as decreased vaginal lubrication, hot flashes, headaches, dizziness, and joint pain.

Synthetic forms of estrogen and progesterone have long been prescribed as **hormone replacement therapy** to relieve menopausal symptoms and reduce the risk of heart disease and osteoporosis. (The National Institutes of Health prefers the term **menopausal hormone therapy**, because hormone therapy is not a replacement and does not restore the physiology of youth.) However, recent studies suggest that hormone therapy may actually do more harm than good.[45] All women need to discuss the risks and benefits of menopausal hormone therapy with their health care provider to make an informed decision. A healthy lifestyle including regular exercise, a balanced diet, and adequate calcium intake can also help protect postmenopausal women from heart disease and osteoporosis.

check yourself

- **What are some common problems associated with menstruation?**

Male Sexual Anatomy and Physiology

learning outcome

4.14 Identify major features and functions of male sexual anatomy and physiology.

The structures of the male reproductive system are divided into external and internal genitals (Figure 4.7).

The external genitals are the penis and the scrotum. The **penis** is the organ that deposits sperm in the vagina during intercourse. The urethra, which passes through the center of the penis, acts as the passageway for both semen and urine to exit the body. During sexual arousal, the spongy tissue in the penis becomes filled with blood, making the organ stiff (erect). Further sexual excitement leads to **ejaculation**, a series of rapid, spasmodic contractions that propels semen out of the penis.

Situated behind the penis and also outside the body is a sac called the **scrotum**. The scrotum encases the testes, protecting them and helping control their internal temperature, which is vital to proper sperm production. The **testes** (singular: *testis*) manufacture sperm and **testosterone**, the hormone responsible for development of male secondary sex characteristics, including deepening of the voice and growth of facial, body, and pubic hair.

The development of sperm is referred to as **spermatogenesis**. Like the maturation of eggs in the female, this process is governed by the pituitary gland. Follicle-stimulating hormone (FSH) is secreted into the bloodstream to stimulate the testes to manufacture sperm. Immature sperm are released into a comma-shaped structure on the back of each testis called the **epididymis** (plural: *epididymides*), where they ripen and reach full maturity.

Each epididymis contains coiled tubules that gradually "unwind" to become the **vas deferens**. The two vasa deferentia make up the tubes whose sole function is to store and move sperm. Along the way, the **seminal vesicles** provide sperm with nutrients and other fluids that compose **semen**.

The vasa deferentia eventually connect each epididymis to the **ejaculatory ducts**, which pass through the prostate gland and empty into the urethra. The **prostate gland** contributes more fluids to the semen, including chemicals that help the sperm fertilize an ovum and neutralize the acidic environment of the vagina to make it more conducive to sperm motility and potency. Just below the prostate gland are two pea-shaped nodules called the **Cowper's glands**. The Cowper's glands secrete a fluid that lubricates the urethra and neutralizes any acid that may remain in the urethra after urination. During ejaculation of semen, a small valve closes off the tube to the urinary bladder.

Circumcision

Debate continues over the practice of *circumcision*, the surgical removal of a fold of skin covering the end of the penis known as the *foreskin*. Approximately 55 percent of all newborn boys are circumcised in the United States each year. Circumcision can be a controversial issue for parents, who must balance personal, cultural, and health issues in deciding whether to circumcise a son.[46]

Arguments for circumcision include religious or cultural reasons (Jewish and Muslim cultures have historically circumcised) and easier genital hygiene. There is also a lower risk of penile cancer, urinary tract infections during infancy, and foreskin infections.

Arguments against circumcision include the possibility of pain during the surgery and potential complications such as infection or improper healing. Families may feel the foreskin is needed for reasons of identity, culture, or sexual pleasure.

Andropause

Men do not experience a rapid hormone decline in middle age as women do during menopause. Instead, men typically experience a gradual decline in testosterone levels throughout adulthood, averaging 1 percent a year after age 30.[47] Many doctors use the term *andropause* to describe age-related hormone changes in some men, with symptoms including reduced sexual desire, infertility, changes in sleep patterns or insomnia, increased body fat, reduced muscle bulk, decreased bone density, and hair loss. Men may also experience emotional changes such as decreased motivation, depression, or memory problems.[48] For some men, testosterone therapy relieves bothersome symptoms. For others, especially older men, the benefits aren't clear.

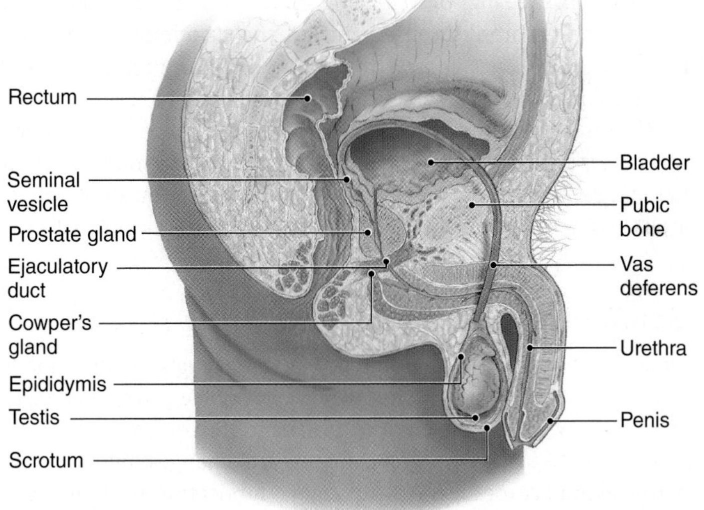

Figure 4.7 Male Reproductive System

check yourself

- **Identify major features and functions of male sexual anatomy and physiology.**

4.15 Human Sexual Response and Expression

learning outcome

4.15 Discuss the human sexual response, and give examples of human sexual expression.

For both men and women, sexual response is a physiological process of four stages: excitement/arousal, plateau, orgasm, and resolution; of course, individuals can vary in their experiences of this pattern.

During *excitement/arousal,* **vasocongestion** (increased blood flow causing swelling in the genitals) stimulates genital responses. The vagina begins to lubricate, and the penis becomes partially erect.

During the *plateau phase,* initial responses intensify. Voluntary and involuntary muscle tensions increase. The woman's nipples and the man's penis become erect. The penis secretes a few drops of pre-ejaculatory fluid, which may contain sperm.

During the *orgasmic phase,* vasocongestion and muscle tension reach their peak, and rhythmic contractions occur through the genital regions. In women, these contractions are centered in the uterus, outer vagina, and anal sphincter. In men, the contractions occur in two stages. First, contractions within the prostate gland begin propelling semen through the urethra. In the second stage, the muscles of the pelvic floor, urethra, and anal sphincter contract. Semen usually, but not always, is ejaculated from the penis.

Muscle tension and congested blood subside in the *resolution phase* as the genital organs return to prearousal states. Both sexes usually experience feelings of well-being and profound relaxation. Many women can become rearoused and experience additional orgasms; most men experience a refractory period of a few minutes to a few hours, during which they are incapable of subsequent arousal.

Although men and women experience the same stages in the sexual response cycle, time spent in any one stage varies; one partner may be in the plateau phase while the other is in the excitement/arousal or orgasmic phase. Such variations are entirely normal.

Sexual Responses among Older Adults

Older adults are commonly stereotyped as incapable of or uninterested in sex. In truth, although we do experience physical changes as we age, they generally do not cause us to stop enjoying sex.

In women, the most significant physical changes follow menopause. Skin becomes less elastic; vaginal lubrication may decrease. (Use of artificial lubricants usually resolves this problem.) Men's bodies also change; they require more direct and prolonged stimulation to achieve erection and are slower to reach orgasm, with less intense ejaculation.

Sexual Behavior: What Is "Normal"?

Which sexual behaviors are considered normal? Whose criteria should we use? Every society sets standards and attempts to regulate sexual behavior. Some common sociocultural standards for sexual behavior in Western culture today include the following:[49]

- **The coital standard.** Penile–vaginal intercourse (coitus) is viewed as the ultimate sex act.
- **The orgasmic standard.** Sexual interaction should lead to orgasm.
- **The two-person standard.** Sex is an activity to be experienced by two people.
- **The romantic standard.** Sex should be related to love.
- **The safer-sex standard.** If we choose to be sexually active, we should act to prevent unintended pregnancy or disease transmission.

These are not rules, but social scripts. Sexual standards often shift over time, and many people choose not to follow them. Rather than making blanket judgments about normal versus abnormal, we might ask: Is a sexual behavior healthy and fulfilling for a particular person? Is it safe? Does it involve exploitation of others? Does it take place between responsible, consenting adults?[50]

In this way, we can view behavior along a continuum that takes into account many individual factors.

Options for Sexual Expression

The range of human sexual expression is virtually infinite. What you find enjoyable may not be an option for someone else. How you meet your sexual needs may change over time. Accepting yourself as a sexual person with individual desires and preferences is the first step in achieving sexual satisfaction.

Celibacy **Celibacy** is avoidance of or abstention from sexual activities with others. Some people choose celibacy for religious or moral reasons. Others may be celibate for a period of time due to illness, the breakup of a long-term relationship, or lack of an acceptable partner. For some, celibacy is lonely, but others find it an opportunity for introspection and personal growth.

Autoerotic Behaviors **Autoerotic behaviors** involve sexual self-stimulation. **Sexual fantasies** are sexually arousing thoughts and dreams. Fantasies may reflect real-life experiences, forbidden desires, or the opportunity to practice new or anticipated sexual experiences. The fact that you fantasize about a particular experience does not mean that you want to, or have to, act it out. **Masturbation**, or self-stimulation of the genitals, is one of the most common ways humans seek sexual pleasure. In one survey of college students, 48 percent of women and 92 percent of men reported masturbating.[51]

Kissing and Erotic Touching Kissing and erotic touching are two common forms of nonverbal sexual communication. Both men and women have **erogenous zones,** areas of the body that lead to sexual arousal when touched. These may include genitals as well as areas such as the earlobes, mouth, breasts, and inner thighs. Spending

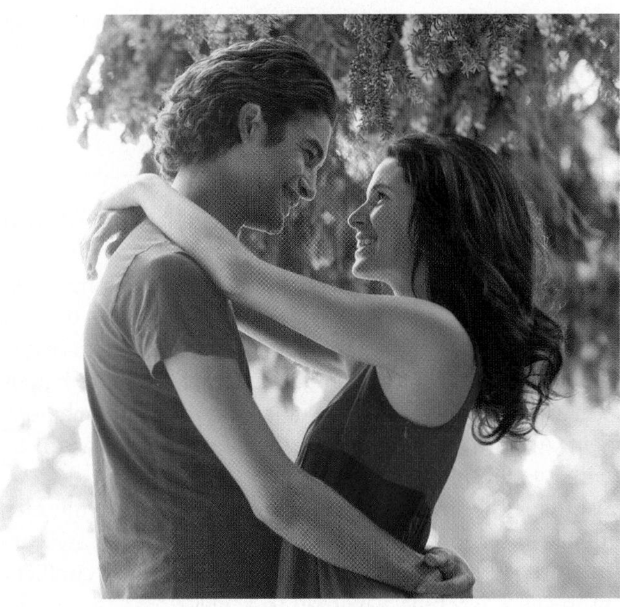

You may think everyone else on campus is having more sex with more partners than you are, but generally speaking, the actual numbers don't measure up to college students' perceptions.

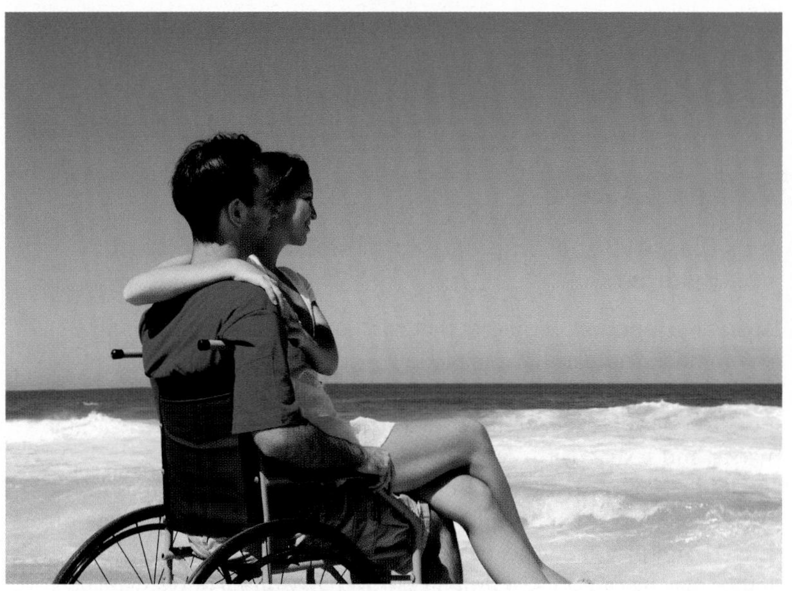

Whether able-bodied or disabled, we are all sexual beings deserving of intimacy and fulfilling sexual relationships.

time with your partner to explore and learn about his or her erogenous areas is a pleasurable and safe means of sexual expression.

Manual Stimulation Both men and women can be sexually aroused and achieve orgasm through manual stimulation of the genitals. For many women, orgasm is more likely through manual stimulation than through intercourse. *Sex toys* (such as vibrators and dildos) can be used alone or with a partner. Toys must be cleaned after each use.

Oral–Genital Stimulation **Cunnilingus** refers to oral stimulation of a woman's genitals and **fellatio** to oral stimulation of a man's genitals. Many partners find oral stimulation intensely pleasurable. Forty-two percent of college students reported having oral sex in the past month.[52] Note that HIV and other sexually transmitted infections (STIs) can be transmitted via unprotected oral–genital sex just as through intercourse. Use of an appropriate barrier device is strongly recommended if either partner's disease status is unknown.

Vaginal Intercourse The term *intercourse* generally refers to **vaginal intercourse** (*coitus*, or insertion of the penis into the vagina), the most frequently practiced form of sexual expression. Almost 50 percent of college students reported having vaginal intercourse in the past month.[53] Whatever your circumstances, you should practice safer sex to avoid disease and unintended pregnancy.

Anal Intercourse The anal area is highly sensitive to touch, and some couples find pleasure in stimulation there. **Anal intercourse** is insertion of the penis into the anus. Research indicates that 5 percent of college-aged men and women had anal sex in the past month.[54] Stimulation of the anus by the mouth, fingers, or sex toys is also practiced. If you enjoy this form of sexual expression, use condoms and/or dental dams to avoid transmitting disease. Also, anything inserted into the anus should not then be directly inserted into the vagina without cleaning, as bacteria commonly found in the anus can cause vaginal infections.

Variant Sexual Behavior

Although attitudes toward sexuality have changed substantially over time, some people still believe that any sexual behavior other than heterosexual intercourse is abnormal. People who study sexuality prefer to use the neutral term **variant sexual behavior** to describe sexual behaviors that most people do not engage in. Examples include group sex (sexual activity involving more than two people), swinging (partner swapping), and fetishism (sexual arousal achieved by looking at or touching inanimate objects, such as underclothing or shoes).

Some variant sexual behaviors can be harmful to the individual, to others, or to both. Examples include exhibitionism (exposing one's genitals to strangers in public places); voyeurism (observing other people for sexual gratification); sadomasochism (getting gratification from inflicting pain, verbal or physical, on a partner, or by being the object of such infliction); and pedophilia (sexual activity or attraction between an adult and a child). Autoerotic asphyxiation is the practice of reducing oxygen to the brain, usually by tying a cord around one's neck while masturbating to orgasm. Tragically, some individuals accidentally strangle themselves.

check yourself

- **What are the steps of the typical human sexual response?**
- **What are three examples of sexual expression?**

4.16 Sexual Dysfunction

learning outcome

4.16 Classify types and causes of sexual dysfunction disorders.

Sexual dysfunction, problems that can hinder sexual functioning, is common. You can have breakdowns involving sexual function just as in any other body system. Sexual dysfunction can be divided into disorders of sexual desire, sexual arousal, orgasm, sexual performance, and sexual pain. All can be treated successfully.

Libido is a person's sexual drive or desire. A common reason people seek out a sex therapist is **inhibited sexual desire**, a lack of interest and pleasure in sexual activity. A low sex drive (decreased libido) may be caused by a drop in estrogen in women or testosterone in men and women or by fatigue, stress, depression, or anxiety. Antidepressant medications (e.g., Prozac, Zoloft, Paxil) can often reduce sexual desire.[55] **Sexual aversion disorder** is characterized by sexual phobias (unreasonable fears) and anxiety about sexual contact. Causes may include the psychological stress of a punitive upbringing, a rigid religious background, or a history of physical or sexual abuse.

The most common sexual arousal disorder is **erectile dysfunction (ED)**—difficulty achieving or maintaining a penile erection sufficient for intercourse. At some time, every man experiences ED. Risk factors include many medical conditions, medications, and treatments; being overweight; injuries; psychological conditions, drug, alcohol, or tobacco use; and prolonged bicycling.[56] Some 30 million men in the United States, half under age 65, suffer from ED. The condition generally becomes more common with age, affecting 1 in 5 men in their sixties.[57] Drugs treat ED by relaxing the smooth muscle cells in the penis, allowing increased blood flow to erectile tissues.

Premature ejaculation—ejaculation that occurs before or very soon after insertion of the penis into the vagina—affects up to 70 percent of men at some time.[58] Treatment first involves physical examination to rule out organic causes. If the cause is not physiological, therapy can help a man learn how to control timing of his ejaculation. Fatigue, stress, performance pressure, and alcohol use can all contribute to this problem.

In a woman, the inability to achieve orgasm is called **female orgasmic disorder**. A woman with this disorder often blames herself and learns to fake orgasm to avoid embarrassment or preserve her partner's ego. The first step is a physical exam to rule out organic causes. However, the problem is often solved by self-exploration to learn more about self-stimulation. Once a woman has become orgasmic through masturbation, she learns to communicate her needs to her partner.

Both men and women can experience **sexual performance anxiety**. A man may become anxious and unable to maintain an erection or experience premature ejaculation. A woman may be unable to achieve orgasm or to allow penetration because of involuntary contraction of vaginal muscles. Both can overcome performance anxiety by learning to focus on immediate sensations rather than orgasm.

Dyspareunia is pain experienced by a woman during intercourse, which may be caused by endometriosis, uterine tumors, chlamydia, gonorrhea, or urinary tract infections. Damage to tissues during childbirth and insufficient lubrication during intercourse may also cause discomfort. Dyspareunia can also be psychological in origin. As with other sexual problems, dyspareunia can be treated, with good results.

Vaginismus is the involuntary contraction of vaginal muscles, making penile insertion painful or impossible. Most cases are related to fear of intercourse or to unresolved sexual conflicts. Treatment involves teaching a woman to achieve orgasm through nonvaginal stimulation.

While sexual dysfunction can happen at any age, the incidence of dysfunction increases during the menopause years in women and after age 50 in men.[59] Don't be afraid to talk to a counselor or medical professional; most colleges and universities have services available. The American Association of Sex Educators, Counselors, and Therapists (AASECT) also lists highly trained and certified counselors, sex therapists, and clinics that treat sexual dysfunctions at www.aasect.org.

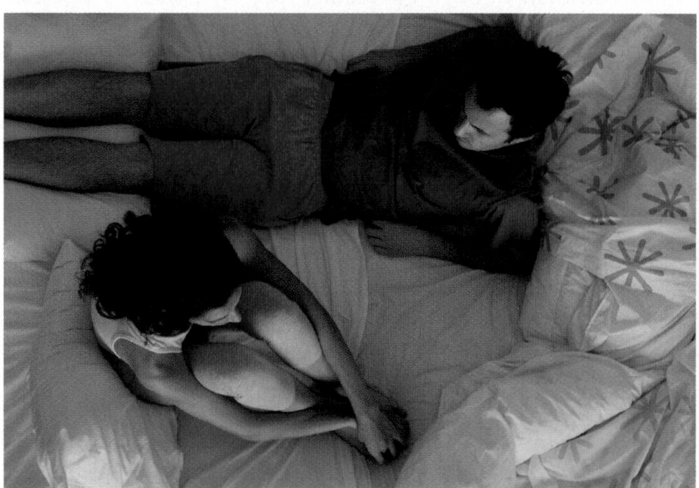

Sexual disorders can have both physical and psychological roots. Interpersonal problems can contribute to dysfunction as well.

check yourself

- **What are some types and causes of sexual dysfunction?**
- **Would you consider physical or psychological causes of sexual dysfunction easer to treat? Why?**

Alcohol, Drugs, and Sex

learning outcome

4.17 Examine the negative outcomes associated with combining sex with drugs or alcohol.

Because psychoactive drugs and alcohol affect the body's entire physiological functioning, it is only logical that they affect sexual behavior. Promises of increased pleasure make drugs very tempting to people seeking greater sexual satisfaction. Too often, however, drugs and alcohol become central to sexual activities and damage the relationship.

Drug and alcohol use can also lead to undesired sexual activity, as well as a tendency to blame the drug for negative behavior or unsafe sexual activities. "I can't help what I did last night because I was drunk" is a statement that demonstrates sexual immaturity. A sexually mature person carefully examines risks and benefits and makes decisions accordingly. If drugs are necessary to increase erotic feelings, it is likely that the partners are being dishonest about their feelings for each other. Good sex should not depend on chemical substances.

Alcohol is notorious for reducing inhibitions and promoting feelings of well-being and desirability. At the same time, alcohol inhibits sexual response—the mind may be willing, but not the body.

In addition to alcohol use, an increasing number of young men have begun experimenting with recreational use of drugs intended to treat erectile dysfunction, including Viagra, Cialis, and Levitra. Young men who take this type of medication are hoping to increase their sexual stamina or counteract sexual performance anxiety or the effects of alcohol or other drugs. However, these drugs probably have only a placebo effect in men with normal erections, and combining them with other drugs, such as cocaine, MDMA (Ecstasy), amyl nitrate ("poppers"), or methamphetamine, can lead to potentially fatal drug interactions. In particular, when combined with amyl nitrate, these drugs can lead to a sudden drop in blood pressure and possible cardiac arrest.[60]

"Date rape" drugs have been a growing concern in recent decades. They have become prevalent on college campuses, where they are often used in combination with alcohol. Rohypnol ("roofies," "rope," "forget pill"), GHB (gamma hydroxybutyrate, or "liquid X," "Grievous Bodily Harm," "easy lay," "Mickey Finn"), and ketamine ("K," "Special K," "cat valium") have all been used to facilitate rape. Rohypnol and GHB are difficult-to-detect drugs that depress the central nervous system. Ketamine can cause dreamlike states, hallucinations, delirium, amnesia, and impaired motor function. These drugs are often introduced to unsuspecting women through alcoholic drinks to render them unconscious and vulnerable to rape. This problem is so serious that the U.S. Congress passed the Drug-Induced Rape Prevention and Punishment Act of 1996 to increase federal penalties for using drugs to facilitate sexual assault.

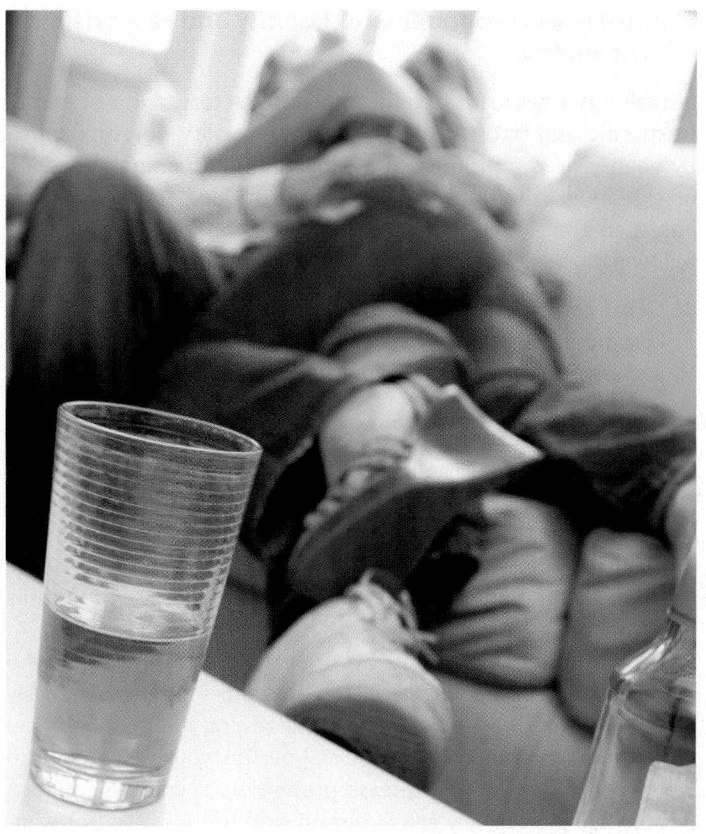

Drugs and alcohol can lead to decisions that you later regret.

18% of college men and 17% of college women who drank alcohol in the past year reported having **unprotected sex as a consequence of their drinking.**

check yourself

- **Give three potential negative outcomes from combining sex with drugs or alcohol.**

4.18 Responsible and Satisfying Sexual Behavior

learning outcome

4.18 Discuss components of healthy and responsible sexuality.

Sexuality is a fascinating, complex, contradictory, and sometimes frustrating aspect of our lives. Healthy sexuality doesn't happen by chance. It is a product of assimilating information and skills, of exploring values and beliefs, and of making responsible and informed choices. Healthy and responsible sexuality includes the following:

- **Good communication as the foundation.** Open and honest communication with your partner is the basis for establishing respect, trust, and intimacy. Do you communicate with your partner in caring and respectful ways? Can you share your thoughts and emotions freely with your partner? Do you talk about being sexually active and what that means? Can you share your sexual history with your partner? Do you discuss contraception and disease prevention? Are you able to communicate what you like and don't like? All of these are components of the open communication that accompanies healthy, responsible sexuality.
- **Acknowledging that you are a sexual person.** People who can see and accept themselves as sexual beings are more likely to make informed decisions and take responsible actions. If you see yourself as a potentially sexual person, you will plan ahead for contraception and disease prevention. If you are comfortable being a sexually active person, you will not need or want your sexual experiences clouded by alcohol or other drug use. If you choose not to be sexually active, you do so consciously, as a personal decision based on your convictions. Even if you are not sexually active, it is important to acknowledge that sex is a natural aspect of life and to recognize that you are in charge of your own decisions about your sexuality.
- **Understanding sexual structures and their functions.** If you understand how your body works, sexual pleasure and response will not be mysterious events. You will be able to pleasure yourself as well as communicate to your partner how best to please you. You will understand how pregnancy and sexually transmitted infections can be prevented. You will be able to recognize sexual dysfunction and take responsible actions to address the problem.
- **Accepting and embracing your gender identity and your sexual orientation.** "Being comfortable in your own skin" is an old saying that is particularly relevant when it comes to sexuality. It is difficult to feel sexually satisfied if you are conflicted about your gender identity or sexual orientation. You should explore and address questions and feelings you may have about your gender identity and/or your sexual orientation. Having good communication skills, acknowledging that you are a sexual person, and understanding your sexual structures and their functions will allow you to do so.

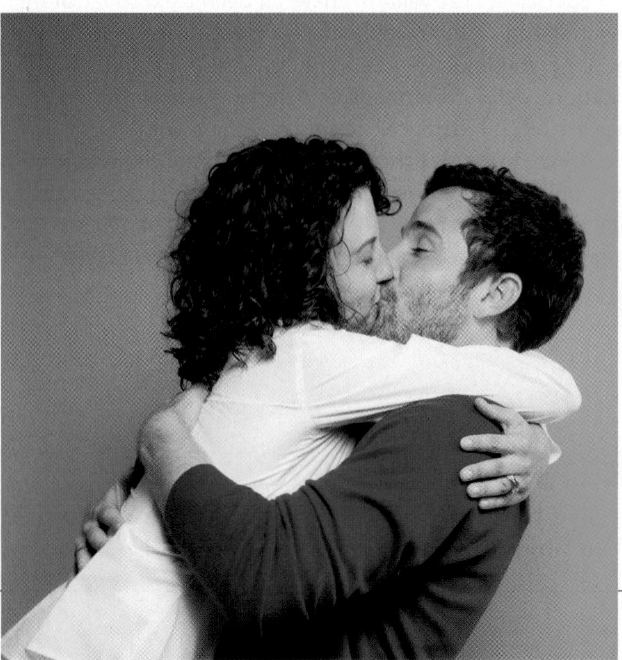

Skills for Behavior Change

TAKING STEPS TOWARD HEALTHY SEXUALITY

Healthy and responsible sexuality means having information and skills, exploring values and beliefs, and making responsible and informed choices. The following tips can help you:

- **Give some thought to your own sexuality. Do you choose to be sexually active now, or are you more comfortable waiting? If you are sexually active, which sexual practices are you comfortable with, and with whom?**
- **Get to know sexual structures and their functions in order to make communicating easier and sex better. If you understand the workings of your body and your partner's, it can improve your sexual satisfaction and your relationship as a whole.**
- **If you have a partner now, sit down and talk about your sexual relationship. Are you both comfortable and satisfied with all aspects of the relationship? Discuss what you like and don't like, and what you might like to change.**
- **Explore and address any questions and feelings you may have about your gender identity and/or your sexual orientation.**

check yourself

- **What are three components of healthy and responsible sexuality?**

How Well Do You Communicate?

An interactive version of this assessment is available online in MasteringHealth.

How do you think you rate as a communicator? How do you think others might rate you? Are you generally someone who expresses his or her thoughts easily, or are you more apt to say nothing for fear of saying the wrong thing? Read the following scenarios and indicate how each describes you, based on the following rating scale.

5 = Would describe me *all* or *nearly all* of the time
3 = Would describe me *sometimes*, but it would be a struggle for me
1 = Would describe me *never* or *almost never*

_____ 1. In a roomful of mostly strangers, you would find it easy to mingle and strike up conversations with just about anyone in the room.

_____ 2. Someone you respect is very critical/hateful about someone that you like a lot. You would be comfortable speaking up and saying you disagree and why you feel this way.

_____ 3. Someone in your class is not doing her part on a group project and her work is substandard. You would be direct and tell her the work isn't acceptable.

_____ 4. One of your friends asks you to let him look at your class assignment because he hasn't had time to do his. You know that he skips class regularly and seems to never do his own work, so you politely tell him no.

_____ 5. You realize that the person you are dating is not right for you and you are probably not right for him or her. When he or she blurts out, "I love you," you say, "I'm sorry, but I don't have those same feelings for you."

_____ 6. Your instructor asks you to give a speech at a state conference, discussing health problems faced by students on campus. You tell the instructor that you'd love to do it and begin planning what you will say.

_____ 7. You don't want to go out drinking at a party on Friday night, even though all of your good friends are going to go. When asked what time they should pick you up, you tell them you appreciate the offer, but you really don't want to go.

_____ 8. Your best friend, Bill, is in an abusive relationship with his girlfriend, Molly. You tell him that you think he might benefit by visiting the campus counseling center.

_____ 9. Students in your class have done poorly on a recent exam and believe that the test was unfair. You volunteer to be the spokesperson and talk with the instructor, telling her what the class thinks of the exam.

_____ 10. You see someone you are really attracted to. You walk up to him or her at a party and strike up a conversation, with the intention of asking him or her out on a date.

How Did You Do?

The higher your score on the above scenarios (the more 5s you have), the more likely it is that you are a direct and clear communicator. Are there areas that you rated as 3s or as 1s? Why do you think you have difficulties in these situations? How might you best communicate in these situations to achieve the results you want? Anytime you have to communicate with others about difficult topics, it is best to speak and listen carefully, keep the other person's feelings in mind, and show respect for the individual. Try to think about what you might say ahead of time so that you are prepared to speak.

Your Plan for Change

The Assess Yourself activity gave you the chance to look at how you communicate. Now that you have considered your responses, you can take steps toward becoming a better communicator and improving your relationships.

Today, you can:

◯ Call a friend you haven't talked to in a while or arrange a coffee date with a new acquaintance you'd like to get to know better.

◯ Start a journal in which you keep track of communication and relationship issues that arise. Look for trends and think about ways you can change your behavior to address them.

Within the next 2 weeks, you can:

◯ Consider if you want to have children now or in the future. If now is not the right time for children and you are sexually active, make sure you are using an effective birth control method.

◯ If there is someone with whom you have a conflict, arrange a time to sit down with that person in a neutral setting away from distractions to talk about the issues.

By the end of the semester, you can:

◯ Practice being an active listener and notice when your mind wanders while you are listening to someone.

◯ Consider your sexual activity. Are you happy with your choices? Consider removing yourself from an unhappy relationship or exploring new options with a partner in a satisfying relationship.

Summary

To hear an MP3 Tutor session, scan here or visit the Study Area in **MasteringHealth.**

LO 4.1–4.2 Characteristics of intimate relationships include behavioral interdependence, need fulfillment, emotional attachment, and emotional availability. Issues that can cause problems in relationships include jealousy, differences over gender roles, and unmet expectations.

LO 4.3 It's important to use social media appropriately when dating.

LO 4.4 To improve our ability to communicate, we need to listen effectively, convey and interpret nonverbal communication, practice self-disclosure, and establish a proper climate for communicating.

LO 4.5 Be cautious when sharing personal information on social networking sites.

LO 4.6–4.8 Being a good listener and communicator enhances relationships and allows us to manage and resolve conflicts.

LO 4.9 For most people, commitment is an important ingredient in successful relationships.

LO 4.10 Relationships end for many reasons, and the uncoupling process can be very painful.

LO 4.11 Biological sex, gender identity, gender roles, and sexual orientation are all blended into our *sexual identity.*

LO 4.12–4.13 The major structures of the female sexual anatomy include the mons pubis, labia minora and majora, clitoris, vagina, uterus, cervix, fallopian tubes, and ovaries.

LO 4.14 The major structures of the male sexual anatomy are the penis, scrotum, testes, epididymides, vasa deferentia, ejaculatory ducts, urethra, and the accessory glands.

LO 4.15 Physiologically, both males and females experience four stages of sexual response: excitement/arousal, plateau, orgasm, and resolution.

LO 4.16 Problems with sexual dysfunction are common and can be treated successfully.

LO 4.17 Alcohol and drug use can lead to undesired and/or unsafe sexual activity.

LO 4.18 Responsible and satisfying sexuality involves good communication, understanding of sexual functions, and acceptance of your gender identity and sexual orientation.

Pop Quiz

Visit MasteringHealth to personalize your study plan with Chapter Review Quizzes and Dynamic Study Modules.

LO 4.1 1. Intimate relationships fulfill our psychological need for someone to listen to our worries and concerns. This is known as our need for
a. dependence.
b. social integration.
c. enjoyment.
d. spontaneity.

LO 4.1 2. Lovers tend to pay attention to the other person even when they should be involved in other activities. This is called
a. inclusion.
b. exclusivity.
c. fascination.
d. authentic intimacy.

LO 4.1 3. Terms such as *behavioral interdependence, need fulfillment,* and *emotional availability* describe which type of relationship?
a. Dysfunctional
b. Sexual
c. Intimate
d. Behavioral

LO 4.2 4. All of the following are typical causes of jealousy *except*
a. overdependence on the relationship.
b. low self-esteem.
c. a past relationship that involved deception.
d. belief that relationships can easily be replaced.

LO 4.10 5. Jamie has just broken up with her boyfriend. Which is a recommended way to cope with the breakup?
a. Initiate a new relationship as soon as possible to recover.
b. Cut off contact with friends, who will be painful reminders of the relationship.
c. Avoid dwelling on sad feelings.
d. Find ways to express emotions through exercise or listening to music.

LO 4.11 6. Your personal inner sense of maleness or femaleness is known as your
a. sexual identity.
b. sexual orientation.
c. gender identity.
d. gender.

LO 4.12 7. The most sensitive or erotic spot in the female genital region is the
a. mons pubis.
b. vagina.
c. clitoris.
d. labia.

LO 4.12 8. When a woman is ovulating,
a. she has released an egg cell.
b. she has menstrual bleeding.
c. an egg has been fertilized.
d. the lining of her uterus thins.

LO 4.13 9. A condition in which a woman experiences pain when menstruating is known as
a. premenstrual syndrome.
b. dysmenorrhea.
c. premenstrual dysphoric disorder.
d. amenorrhea.

LO 4.14 10. What is the role of testosterone in the male reproductive system?
a. It is used to produce sperm for reproduction.
b. It is the hormone that stimulates development of secondary male sex characteristics.
c. It allows the penis to harden during sexual arousal.
d. It secretes the seminal fluid preceding ejaculation.

Answers to these questions can be found on page A-1. If you answered a question incorrectly, review the module identified by the Learning Outcome. For even more study tools, visit MasteringHealth.

Reproductive Choices

5

Today, we understand the intimate details of reproduction and possess technologies to control **fertility**. Along with information comes choice and responsibility, and one measure of maturity is the ability to discuss birth control with one's sexual partner. Too often, no one brings up the topic, and unprotected sex is the result. In fact, only 54 percent of college women and 49 percent of college men report having used contraception the last time they had vaginal intercourse.[1] The sad outcome is too many unwanted pregnancies and **sexually transmitted infections (STIs)**. If you're thinking about becoming sexually active, or you are but haven't used birth control, visit your health clinic to discuss contraceptives.

Birth control (or **contraception**) refers to methods of preventing **conception**, which occurs when a sperm fertilizes an egg. To evaluate a contraceptive method's effectiveness, look at its **perfect use failure rate**, or percentage of pregnancies likely in the first year of use if the method is used entirely without error. Even more important, and more useful, is its **typical use failure rate**, the percentage of pregnancies likely in the first year with *typical* use—that is, with the normal number of errors, memory lapses, and so on.

5.1 Barrier Methods: Male and Female Condoms

learning outcome

5.1 List the advantages, disadvantages, and effectiveness of the male and female condoms in preventing pregnancy and STIs.

Barrier methods of contraception work on the principle of preventing sperm from reaching the egg by use of a physical or chemical barrier during intercourse. Some barrier methods prevent semen from having contact with the woman's body, whereas others prevent sperm from going past the cervix. In addition, many barrier methods contain, or are used in combination with, a substance that kills sperm.

The Male Condom

The **male condom** is a thin sheath designed to cover the erect penis and catch semen before it enters the vagina. Most male condoms are made of latex, though polyurethane or lambskin condoms are also available. Condoms in a wide variety of styles may be purchased in pharmacies, supermarkets, public bathrooms, and many health clinics. A new condom must be used for each act of vaginal, oral, or anal intercourse.

A condom must be rolled onto the penis before the penis touches the vagina and must be held in place when removing the penis from the vagina after ejaculation (see Figure 5.1). Condoms come with or without **spermicide** and with or without lubrication. If desired, users can lubricate their own condoms with contraceptive foams, creams, jellies, or other water-based lubricants. Never use products such as baby oil, cold cream, petroleum jelly, vaginal yeast infection medications, or body lotion with a condom. These products contain substances that will cause the latex to disintegrate.

Condoms are less effective, and more likely to break during intercourse, if they are old or improperly stored. To maintain their effectiveness, store them in a cool place (not in a wallet or pocket) and inspect them for small tears before use. Lightly squeeze the package before opening to feel that air is trapped inside and the package has not been punctured. Discard all condoms that have passed their expiration date.

Advantages When used consistently and correctly, condoms can be up to 98 percent effective.[2] The condom is the only temporary means of birth control available for men, and latex and polyurethane condoms are the only barriers that effectively prevent the spread of some STIs and HIV. (Skin condoms, made from lamb intestines, are not effective against STIs.) Many people choose condoms for birth control because they are inexpensive and readily available without a prescription, and their use is limited to times of sexual activity, with no negative health effects. Some men find that condoms help them stay erect longer or help prevent premature ejaculation.

Disadvantages The easy availability of condoms is accompanied by considerable potential for user error; the typical use effectiveness of condoms in preventing pregnancy is around 82 percent.[3] Improper use of a condom can lead to breakage, leakage, or slipping, potentially exposing users to STIs or an unintended pregnancy. Even when used perfectly, a condom doesn't protect against STIs that may have external areas of infection (e.g., herpes). Some people feel that condoms ruin the spontaneity of sex because stopping to put one on may break the mood. Others report that condoms decrease sensation. These inconveniences and perceptions contribute to improper use or avoidance of condoms altogether. Partners who apply a condom as part of foreplay are generally

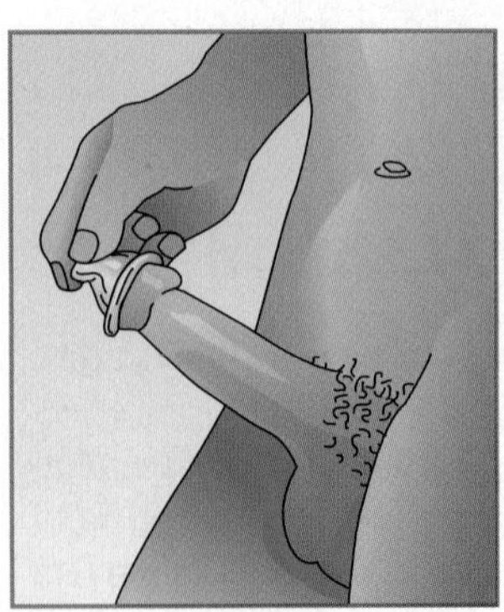

1 Pinch the air out of the top half-inch of the condom to allow room for semen.

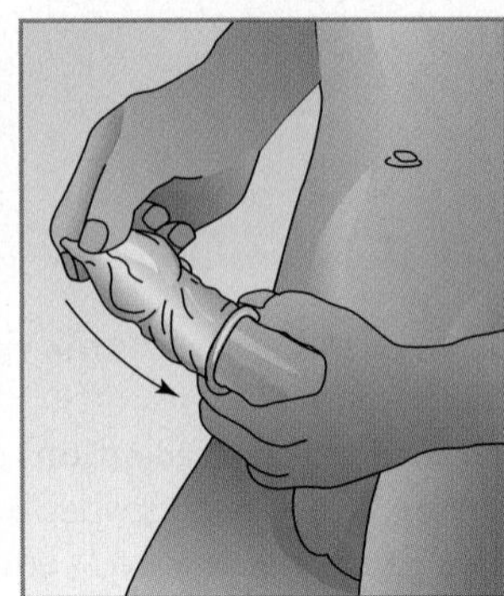

2 Holding the tip of the condom with one hand, use the other hand to unroll it onto the penis.

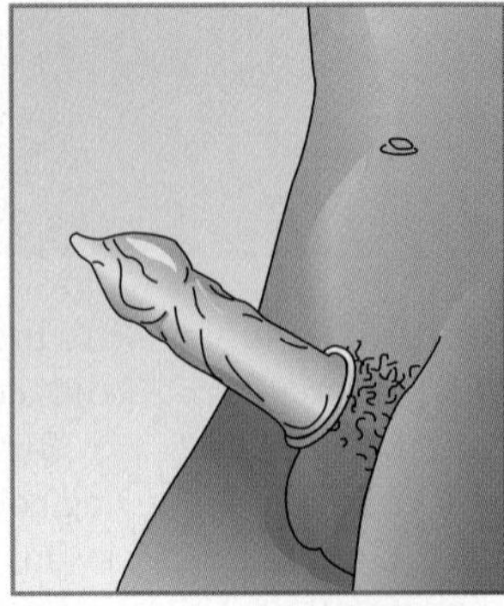

3 Unroll the condom all the way to the base of the penis, smoothing out any air bubbles.

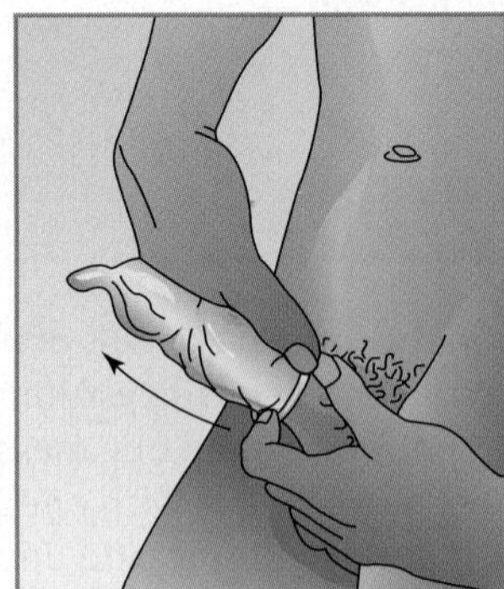

4 After ejaculation, hold the condom around the base until the penis is totally withdrawn to avoid spilling any semen.

Figure 5.1 How to Use a Male Condom

Inner ring is used for insertion and to help hold the sheath in place during intercourse.
Outer ring covers the area around the opening of the vagina.

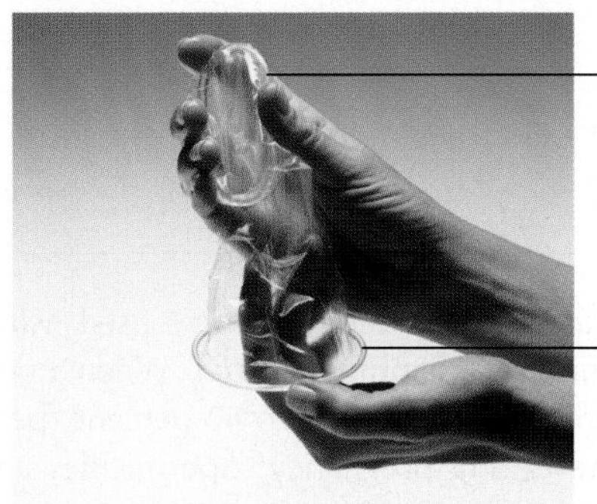

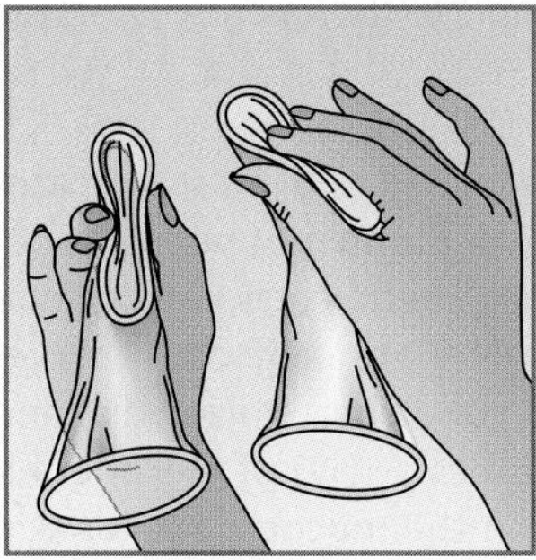

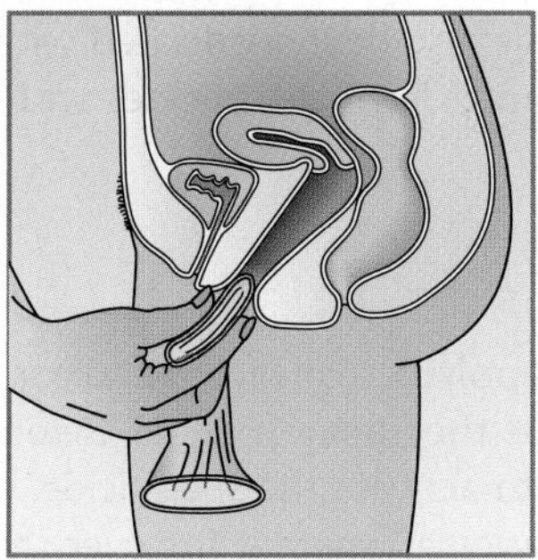

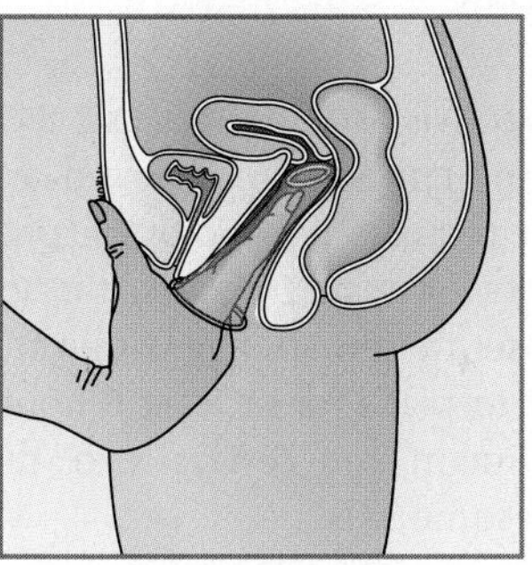

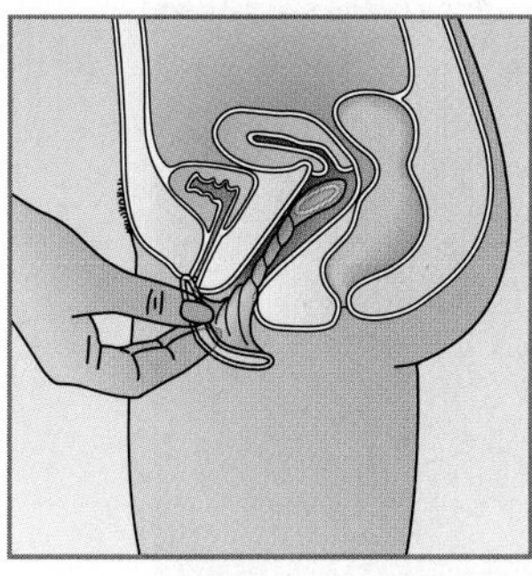

Figure 5.2 How to Use a Female Condom

more successful with this form of birth control. As a new condom is required for each act of intercourse, some users find it difficult to be sure to have a condom available when needed.

The Female Condom

The **female condom (FC2)** is a single-use, soft, loose-fitting sheath for internal vaginal use. The newest, improved versions are made from nitrile rather than polyurethane. The sheath has a flexible ring at each end. One ring lies inside the sheath and serves as an insertion mechanism and internal anchor. The other remains outside the vagina once the device is inserted and protects the labia and the base of the penis from infection. Figure 5.2 shows proper use of the female condom.

Advantages Used consistently and correctly, female condoms are 95 percent effective at preventing pregnancy.[4] They also can prevent the spread of HIV and other STIs, including those that can be transmitted by external genital contact. The female condom can be inserted in advance, so its use doesn't have to interrupt lovemaking. Some women choose the female condom because it gives them more personal control over prevention of pregnancy and STIs or because they cannot rely on their partners to use the male condom. Because the nitrile is thin and pliable, there is less loss of sensation with the female condom than with the latex male condom. The female condom can be used with or without lubrication. The female condom is relatively inexpensive, readily available without a prescription, and causes no negative health effects.

Disadvantages As with the male condom, there is potential for user error with the female condom, including possible breaking, slipping, or leaking, all of which could lead to STI transmission or an unintended pregnancy. Because of the potential problems, the typical use effectiveness of the female condom is 79 percent.[5] Some people dislike using the female condom because they find it disruptive, noisy, odd looking, or difficult to use. Some women have reported external or vaginal irritation from using the female condom. As with the male condom, a new condom is required for each act of intercourse, so users may not always have one available when needed. Remember that male and female condoms should never be used simultaneously.

check yourself

- **What are the advantages and disadvantages of the male and female condoms?**
- **How effective are the male and female condoms in preventing pregnancy and STIs?**
- **What are some reasons you might give to persuade a partner to use a condom?**

5.2 Other Barrier Methods

learning outcome

5.2 List the advantages, disadvantages, and effectiveness of different types of barrier methods in preventing pregnancy and STIs.

There are options beyond the male and female condoms for those who wish to use other barrier methods, including spermicides, the sponge, the diaphragm, and the cervical cap.

Spermicides

Some barrier methods—jellies, creams, foams, suppositories, and film—require no prescription. These are spermicides, substances designed to kill sperm. The active ingredient in most is nonoxynol-9 (N-9).

Jellies and creams come in tubes and **foams** in aerosol cans with applicators for vaginal insertion. They must be inserted far enough to cover the cervix, providing both a chemical barrier that kills sperm and a physical barrier that stops sperm from continuing toward an egg.

Suppositories are capsules inserted into the vagina, where they melt. They must be inserted 10 to 20 minutes before intercourse, but no more than 1 hour before or they lose their effectiveness. Additional contraceptive chemicals must be applied for each subsequent act of intercourse.

With **vaginal contraceptive film**, a thin film infused with spermicidal gel is inserted into the vagina so that it covers the cervix. The film dissolves into a spermicidal gel effective for up to 3 hours. As with other spermicides, a new film must be inserted for each act of intercourse.

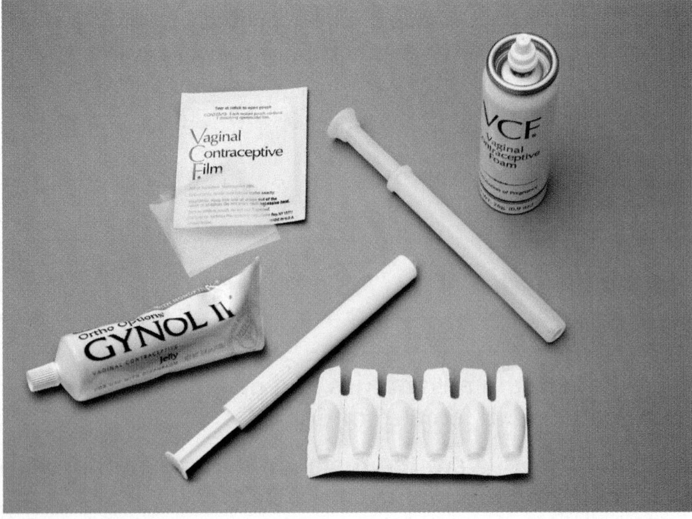

Spermicides come in many forms, including jellies, creams, films, foam, and suppositories.

Advantages Spermicides are most effective when used with another barrier method (condom, diaphragm, etc.). When used alone, they offer only 72 percent (typical use) to 82 percent (perfect use) effectiveness at preventing pregnancy.[6] Spermicides are inexpensive, require no prescription or pelvic examination, and are available over the counter. They are simple to use, and use is limited to the time of sexual activity.

Disadvantages Spermicides can be messy and must be reapplied for each act of intercourse. A small number of people experience irritation or allergic reactions to spermicides, and studies indicate that spermicides containing N-9 are ineffective in preventing transmission of STIs such as gonorrhea, chlamydia, and HIV. In fact, frequent use (multiple times a day) of N-9 spermicides can cause irritation and breaks in the mucous layer or skin of the genital tract, creating a point of entry for viruses and bacteria. Spermicides containing N-9 have also been associated with increased risk of urinary tract infection.[7] New spermicides without N-9 are under development.

Contraceptive Sponge

The **contraceptive sponge** is made of polyurethane foam and contains N-9 (sold in the United States as the Today Sponge). Before insertion, it is moistened with water to activate the spermicide. It is then folded and inserted into the vagina, where it fits over the cervix and creates a barrier against sperm.

Advantages The sponge is fairly effective (91% perfect use; 84% typical use) when used consistently and correctly.[8] A main advantage of the sponge is convenience; it requires no doctor's fitting. Protection begins on insertion and lasts for up to 24 hours. It is not necessary to reapply spermicide or insert a new sponge within the same 24-hour period; it must be left in place for at least 6 hours after last intercourse. Like the diaphragm and cervical cap, the sponge offers limited protection from some STIs.

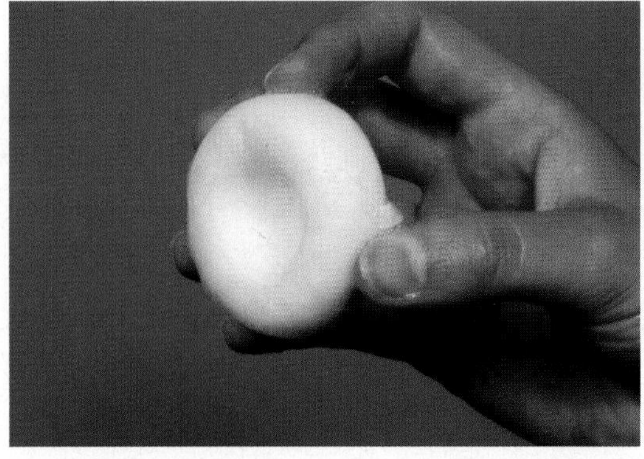

The Today Sponge is a combination barrier method and spermicide that is most effective when used in conjunction with male condoms.

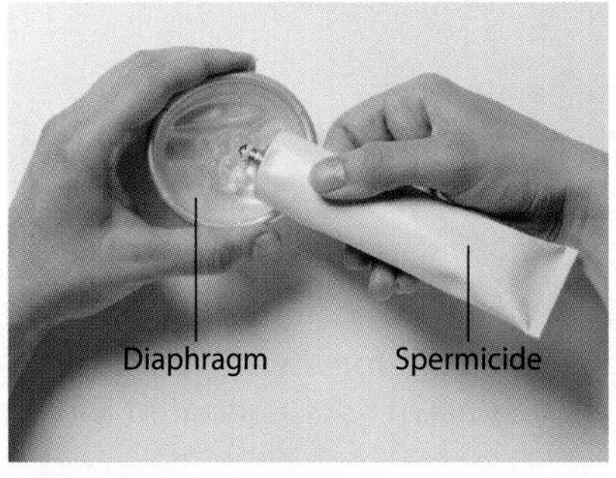

1 Place spermicidal jelly or cream inside the diaphragm and all around the rim.

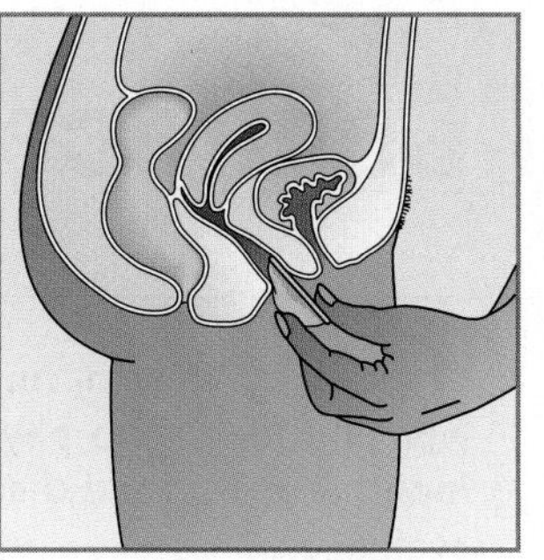

2 Fold the diaphragm in half and insert dome-side down (spermicide-side up) into the vagina, pushing it along the back wall as far as it will go.

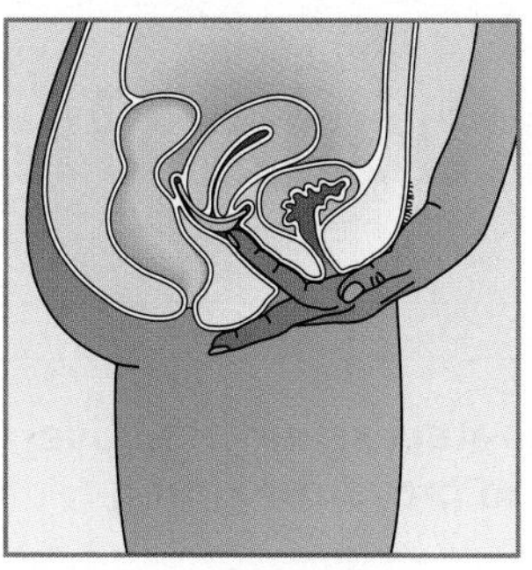

3 Position the diaphragm with the cervix completely covered and the front rim tucked up against your pubic bone; you should be able to feel your cervix through the rubber dome.

Figure 5.3 The Proper Use and Placement of a Diaphragm

Disadvantages The sponge is less effective for women who have given birth (80% perfect use; 68% typical use).[9] Allergic reactions, such as irritation of the vagina, are more common than with other barrier methods. Should the vaginal lining become irritated, the risk of yeast infections and other STIs may increase. Some cases of **toxic shock syndrome (TSS)** have been reported in women using the sponge; precautions should be taken as with the diaphragm and cervical cap. Some women find the sponge difficult or messy to remove.

The Diaphragm

Invented in the mid-nineteenth century, the **diaphragm** was the first widely used birth control method for women. The device is a soft, shallow cup made of thin latex rubber. Its flexible, rubber-coated ring is designed to fit behind the pubic bone in front of the cervix and over the back of the cervix on the other side. Diaphragms must be used with spermicidal cream or jelly that is applied to the inside of the diaphragm before inserting. A diaphragm may be inserted up to 6 hours before intercourse. The diaphragm holds the spermicide in place, creating a physical and chemical barrier against sperm (Figure 5.3). Diaphragms come in different sizes and must be fitted by a trained practitioner, who should ensure that the user knows how to insert her diaphragm correctly before leaving the practitioner's office.

Advantages If used consistently and correctly, diaphragms can be 94 percent effective in preventing pregnancy.[10] When used with spermicidal jelly or cream, the diaphragm also offers protection against gonorrhea and possibly chlamydia and human papillomavirus (HPV). After the initial prescription and fitting, the only ongoing expense is spermicide. Because the diaphragm can be inserted up to 6 hours in advance and used for multiple acts of intercourse, some users find it less disruptive than other barrier methods.

Disadvantages Although the diaphragm can be left in place for multiple acts of intercourse, additional spermicide must be applied each time, and the diaphragm must then stay in place for 6 to 8 hours afterward to allow the chemical to kill any sperm remaining in the vagina. Some women find insertion awkward. When inserted incorrectly, diaphragms are much less effective. A diaphragm may also slip out of place, be difficult to remove, or require refitting (e.g., following pregnancy or significant weight gain or loss).

The Cervical Cap

One of the oldest methods used to prevent pregnancy, early **cervical caps** were made from beeswax, silver, or copper. The currently available FemCap is a clear silicone cup that fits over the cervix. It comes in three sizes and must be fitted by a practitioner. The FemCap is designed for use with spermicidal jelly or cream. It is held in place by suction created during application and works by blocking sperm from the uterus.

Advantages Cervical caps can be reasonably effective (up to 86%) with typical use.[11] They may also offer some protection against transmission of gonorrhea, HPV, and possibly chlamydia. They are relatively inexpensive—the only ongoing cost is for spermicide.

The FemCap can be inserted up to 6 hours before intercourse, making it potentially less disruptive than other barrier methods. The device must be left in place for 6 to 8 hours afterward; after that, if removed and cleaned, it can be reinserted immediately. Because the FemCap is made of surgical-grade silicone, it is a suitable alternative for people allergic to latex.

Disadvantages The FemCap is somewhat more difficult to insert than a diaphragm because of its size. Like a diaphragm, it requires a fitting and may require subsequent refitting if a woman's cervix size changes, as after giving birth. Because the FemCap can become dislodged during intercourse, placement must be checked frequently. It cannot be used during the menstrual period or for longer than 48 hours because of the risk of TSS. Some women report unpleasant vaginal odors after use.

check yourself

- **What are the advantages and disadvantages of different types of barrier methods?**
- **What factors influence effectiveness and proper use of different types of barrier methods?**

5.3 Hormonal Methods: Oral Contraceptives

learning outcome

5.3 List the advantages, disadvantages, and effectiveness of oral contraceptives in preventing pregnancy and STIs.

The term *hormonal contraception* refers to birth control containing synthetic estrogen, progestin, or both. These ingredients are similar to the hormones estrogen and progesterone, which a woman's ovaries produce naturally for the process of ovulation and the menstrual cycle. In recent years, hormonal contraception has become available in a variety of forms (transdermal, injection, and oral). All forms require a prescription from a health care provider.

Hormonal contraception alters a woman's biochemistry, preventing ovulation (release of the egg) from taking place and producing changes that make it more difficult for the sperm to reach the egg if ovulation does occur. Synthetic estrogen works to prevent the ovaries from releasing an egg. If no egg is released, there is nothing to be fertilized by sperm and pregnancy cannot occur. Progestin, too, can prevent ovulation. It also thickens cervical mucus, which hinders sperm movement, inhibits the egg's ability to travel through the fallopian tubes, and suppresses sperm's ability to unite with the egg. Progestin also thins the uterine lining, rendering the egg unlikely to implant in the uterine wall.

Oral Contraceptives

Oral contraceptive pills were first marketed in the United States in 1960. Their convenience quickly made them the most widely used reversible method of fertility control. Most modern pills are more than 99 percent effective at preventing pregnancy with perfect use.[12] Today, oral contraceptives are the most commonly used birth control method among college women (Table 5.1).[13]

Most oral contraceptives work through the combined effects of synthetic estrogen and progesterone (*combination pills*). Combination pills are taken in a cycle. At the end of each 3-week cycle, the user discontinues the drug or takes placebo pills for 1 week. The resultant drop in hormones causes the uterine lining to disintegrate; the user then has a menstrual period, usually within 1 to 3 days. Menstrual flow is generally lighter than for women who don't use the pill, because the hormones in the pill prevent thick endometrial buildup.

Several newer brands of pills have extended cycles, such as the 91-day Seasonale and Seasonique. A woman using this type of regimen takes active pills for 12 weeks, followed by 1 week of placebos. On this cycle, women can expect to have a menstrual period every 3 months. Women often have increased occurrence of spotting or bleeding in the first few months of an extended cycle pill.[14] Lybrel, another extended-cycle pill, is taken continuously for 1 year, eliminating menstruation completely. While the idea of never having a period may be unsettling to some women, there is no physiological need for a woman to have a monthly period, and there are no known risks associated with its avoidance.

Advantages Combination pills are highly effective at preventing pregnancy: more than 99 percent with perfect use and 91 percent with typical use.[15] It is easier to achieve perfect use with pills than with barrier contraceptives, because there is less room for user error. Aside from its effectiveness, much of the pill's popularity is due to convenience and discreetness. Users like the fact that it does not interfere with lovemaking.

In addition to preventing pregnancy, the pill may lessen menstrual difficulties such as cramps and premenstrual syndrome (PMS). Oral contraceptives also lower the risk of conditions including endometrial and ovarian cancers, noncancerous breast disease, osteoporosis, ovarian cysts, pelvic inflammatory disease (PID), and iron-deficiency anemia.[16] Many different brands of combination pills are on the market, some of which contain progestin, which offer benefits such as reducing acne or minimizing fluid retention. Less-expensive generic versions are also available for many brands. With the extended-cycle pills, the major additional benefit is reduction in or absence of menstruation and associated cramps or PMS symptoms. Users of these pills also like that they don't need to remember when to stop or start a cycle of pills, or when to use placebos.

TABLE 5.1 Top Reported Means of Contraception Sexually Active Students or Their Partner Used the Last Time They Had Intercourse

Method	Male	Female	Total
Male condom	67%	60%	62%
Birth control pills (monthly or extended cycle)	60%	58%	59%
Withdrawal	26%	30%	29%
Fertility awareness (calendar, mucus, basal body temperature)	5%	7%	6%
Intrauterine device	6%	8%	7%
Cervical ring	4%	4%	4%
Birth control shots	4%	4%	4%
Spermicide (foam, jelly, cream)	5%	3%	4%

Note: Survey respondents could select more than one method.

Source: Data from American College Health Association, *American College Health Association—National College Health Assessment II: Reference Group Data, Fall 2013* (Baltimore, MD: American College Health Association, 2014).

Disadvantages Estrogen in combination pills is associated with increased risk of several serious health problems among older women, but the risk is low for most healthy women under 35 who do not smoke. Potential problems include increased risk for blood clots (which can lead to strokes or heart attacks) and higher risk for increased blood pressure, thrombotic stroke, and myocardial infarction. These risks increase with age and cigarette smoking. Early warning signs of complications associated with oral contraceptives include severe abdominal, chest, or leg pain, severe headache, and/or eye problems.[17]

Different brands of pills can cause varying minor side effects. Some of the most common are spotting between periods (particularly with extended-cycle regimens), breast tenderness, and nausea. With most pills, these clear up within a few months. Other potential side effects include change in sexual desire, acne, weight gain, and hair loss or growth. Because so many brands are available, most women who wish to use the pill are able to find one that works for them with few side effects.

The pill's other major disadvantage is that it must be taken every day. If a woman misses one pill, she should use an alternative form of contraception for the remainder of that cycle. A backup method of birth control is also necessary during the first week of use. After a woman discontinues the pill, return of fertility may be delayed, though the pill is not known to cause infertility. Another drawback is that the pill does not protect against STIs.

The costs associated with the pill (and all other hormonal contraceptives) have long been reported as a barrier to use, but in the United States the Affordable Care Act (ACA) is changing that. The ACA requires new private health insurance plans to cover "preventive services," including birth control and yearly physical exams, with no co-payments or deductibles.

Progestin-Only Pills

Progestin-only pills (or minipills) contain small doses of progesterone and no estrogen. These pills are available in 28-day packs of active pills (menstruation usually occurs during the fourth week even though the active dose continues through the entire month).

Advantages Progestin-only pills are a good choice for women who are at high risk for estrogen-related side effects or who cannot take estrogen-containing pills because of diabetes, high blood pressure, or other cardiovascular conditions. They can also be used safely by women over 35 and breast-feeding mothers. The effectiveness rate of these pills is more than 99 percent with perfect use and 91 percent with typical use.[18] Progestin-only pills share some health benefits associated with combination pills and carry no estrogen-related cardiovascular risks. Also, some typical side effects of combination pills, including nausea and breast tenderness, seldom occur with progestin-only pills. With progestin-only pills, menstrual periods generally become lighter or stop altogether.

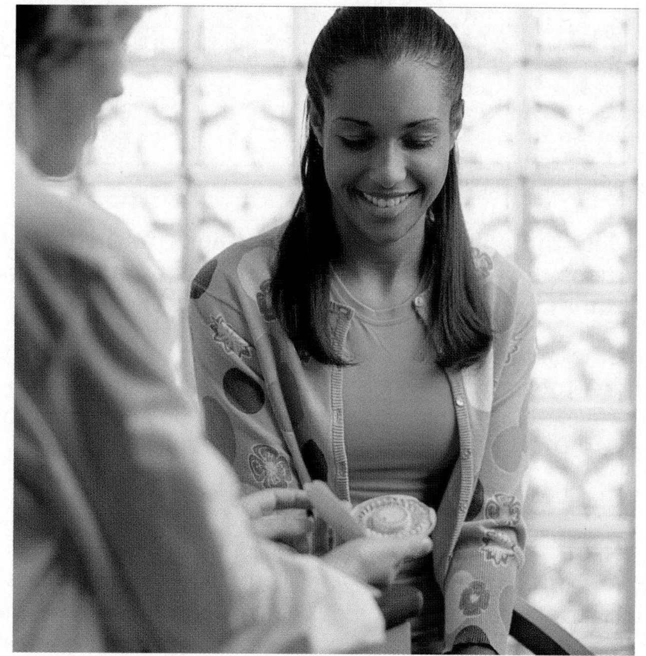

Does the birth control pill have any side effects?

There are many different brands and regimens of oral contraceptives available to women today, some of which are associated with various health benefits such as acne reduction or lessening of PMS symptoms. Some women experience minor side effects from pill use—the most common being headaches, breast tenderness, nausea, and breakthrough bleeding—but these usually clear up within 2 to 3 months.

Disadvantages Because of the lower dose of hormones in progestin-only pills, it is especially important that they be taken at the same time each day. If a woman takes a pill 3 or more hours later than usual, she will need to use a backup method of contraception for the next 48 hours. The most common side effect of progestin-only pills is irregular menstrual bleeding or spotting. Less common side effects include mood changes, changes in sex drive, and headaches. As with all oral contraceptives, progestin-only pills do not protect against STI transmission.

check yourself

- **What are the advantages and disadvantages of oral contraceptives?**
- **How effective are oral contraceptives in preventing pregnancy and STIs?**
- **What are the differences between combination pills and progestin-only pills (minipills)? Who should take progestin-only pills?**

5.4 Hormonal Methods: The Patch, Ring, Injections, and Implants

learning outcome

5.4 List the advantages, disadvantages, and effectiveness of various hormonal methods of contraception in preventing pregnancy and STIs.

Some hormonal methods, such as oral contraceptives, require the user to remember to take the pill every day. Others, such as the skin patch, ring, injections, and implants, do not require daily action.

Contraceptive Skin Patch

Ortho Evra is a square transdermal (through the skin) adhesive patch. It is as thin as a plastic strip bandage, is worn for 1 week, and is replaced on the same day of the week for 3 consecutive weeks; the fourth week is patch-free. Ortho Evra works by delivering continuous levels of estrogen and progestin through the skin and into the bloodstream. The patch can be worn on one of four areas of the body: buttocks, abdomen, upper torso (front and back, excluding the breasts), or upper outer arm. It should not be used by women over age 35 who smoke cigarettes and is less effective in women who weigh more than 198 pounds.[19]

Advantages Ortho Evra is 99.7 percent effective with perfect use and 91 percent with typical use.[20] As with other hormonal methods, there is less room for user error than with barrier methods. Women who choose to use the patch often do so because they find it easier to remember than taking a daily pill, and they like the fact that they need to change the patch only once a week. Ortho Evra probably offers similar potential health benefits as combination pills (reduction in risk of certain cancers and diseases, lessening of PMS symptoms, etc.). Like other hormonal methods, the patch regulates a woman's menstrual cycle.

Disadvantages Using the patch requires an initial exam and prescription, weekly patch changes, and the ongoing monthly expense of patch purchase. A backup method is required during the first week of use. Similar to other hormonal methods of birth control, the patch offers no protection against HIV or other STIs. Some women experience minor side effects, such as those associated with combination pills. The estrogen in the patch is associated with cardiovascular risks, particularly in women who smoke and women over the age of 35. Amid evidence that the patch may increase a woman's risk for life-threatening blood clots, the U.S. Food and Drug Administration (FDA) mandated an additional warning label explaining that patch use exposes women to about 60 percent more total estrogen than if they were taking a typical combination pill.[21]

Vaginal Contraceptive Ring

NuvaRing is a soft, flexible plastic hormonal contraceptive ring about 2 inches in diameter. The user inserts the ring into her vagina, leaves it in place for 3 weeks, and removes it for 1 week for her menstrual period. Once the ring is inserted, it releases a steady flow of estrogen and progestin.

Advantages When used properly, the ring is 99.7 percent effective and 91 percent with typical use.[22] Advantages of NuvaRing include less likelihood of user error, protection against pregnancy for 1 month, no pill to take daily or patch to change weekly, no need to be fitted by a clinician, no requirement to use spermicide, and rapid return of fertility when use is stopped. It also exposes the user to a lower dosage of estrogen than do the patch and some combination pills, so it may have fewer estrogen-related side effects. It probably offers some of the same potential health benefits as combination pills and, like other hormonal contraceptives, it regulates the menstrual cycle.

Disadvantages NuvaRing requires an initial exam and prescription, monthly ring changes, and the ongoing monthly expense of purchasing the ring (a generic version is not currently available). A backup method must be used during the first week, and the ring provides no protection against STIs. Like combination pills, the ring poses possible minor side effects and potentially more serious health risks for some women. Possible side effects unique to the ring include increased vaginal discharge and vaginal irritation or infection. Oil-based vaginal medicines to treat yeast infections cannot be used when the ring is in place, and a diaphragm or cervical cap cannot be used as a backup method for contraception.

Ortho Evra is an adhesive patch that delivers estrogen and progestin through the skin for 3 weeks.

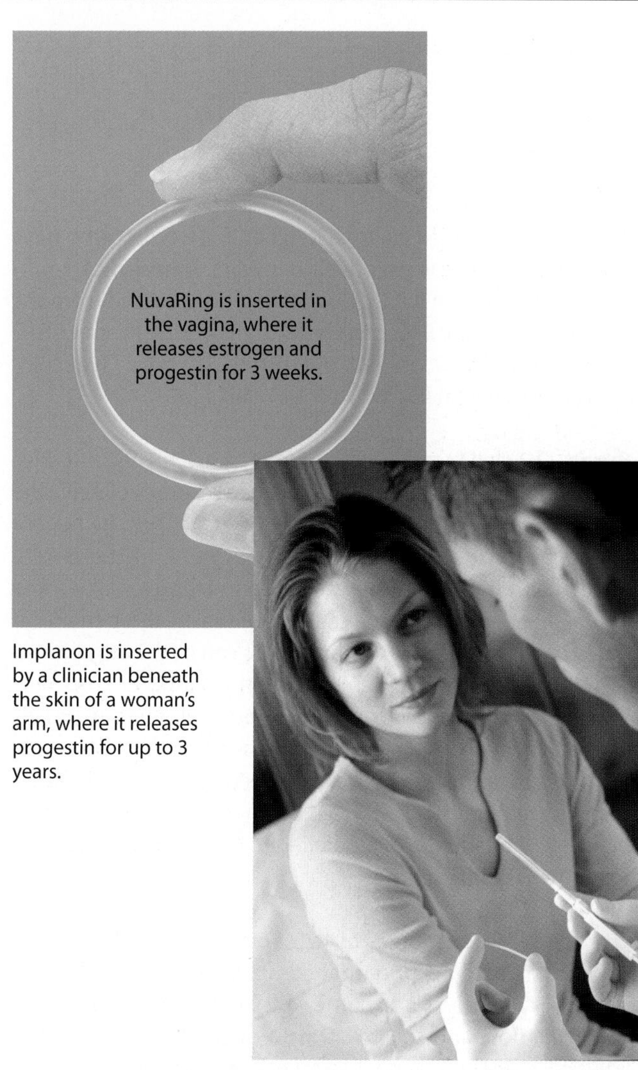

NuvaRing is inserted in the vagina, where it releases estrogen and progestin for 3 weeks.

Implanon is inserted by a clinician beneath the skin of a woman's arm, where it releases progestin for up to 3 years.

Contraceptive Injections

Depo-Provera (injected intra-muscularly) and the newer **Depo-SubQ Provera** (injected just below the skin in a lower dose) are long-acting synthetic progesterones that are injected every 3 months by a health care provider. Both prevent ovulation, thicken cervical mucus, and thin the uterine lining, all of which prevent pregnancy.

Advantages Depo-Provera takes effect within 24 hours of the first shot, so there is usually no need to use a backup method. There is little room for user error with the shot (because it is administered by a clinician every 3 months): With perfect use, the shot is 99.8 percent effective, and with typical use it is 94 percent effective.[23] Some women feel Depo-Provera encourages sexual spontaneity because they do not have to remember to take a pill or insert a device. With continued use of this method, a woman's menstrual periods become lighter and may eventually stop altogether. No estrogen-related health risks are associated with Depo-Provera, and it offers the same potential health benefits as progestin-only pills. Unlike estrogen-containing hormonal methods, Depo-Provera can be used by women who are breast-feeding.

Disadvantages Using Depo-Provera requires an initial exam and prescription, as well as follow-up visits every 3 months to have the shot administered. It offers no protection against STIs. The main disadvantage of Depo-Provera use is irregular bleeding, which can be troublesome at first, but within a year most women are amenorrheic (have no menstrual periods). Weight gain is commonly reported. Prolonged use of Depo-Provera has been linked to loss of bone density.[24] Other possible side effects include dizziness, nervousness, and headache. Unlike other methods of contraception, this method cannot be stopped immediately if problems arise, and the drug and its side effects may linger for up to 6 months after the last shot. A disadvantage for women who want to get pregnant is that fertility may not return for up to 1 year after the final injection.

Contraceptive Implants

A single-rod implantable contraceptive, **Nexplanon** (formerly called **Implanon**) is a small (about the size of a matchstick), soft plastic capsule that is inserted just beneath the skin on the inner side of a woman's upper underarm by a health care provider. Implanon continually releases a low, steady dose of progestin for up to 3 years, suppressing ovulation during that time.

Advantages After insertion, Nexplanon is generally not visible, making it a discreet method of birth control. The main advantages of Nexplanon are that it is highly effective (99.95%), it is not subject to user error, and it only needs to be replaced every 3 years.[25] It has similar benefits to those of other progestin-only forms of contraception, including the lightening or cessation of menstrual periods, the lack of estrogen-related side effects, and safety for use by breast-feeding women. Fertility usually returns quickly after removal of the implant.

Disadvantages Insertion and removal of Nexplanon must be performed by a clinician. The initial cost is higher for this method, and it may not be covered by all health plans. Potential minor side effects include irritation, allergic reaction, swelling, or scarring around the area of insertion; there is also a possibility of infection or complications with removal. Nexplanon may be less effective in women who are overweight.[26] As with other progestin-only contraceptives, users can experience irregular bleeding. Nexplanon offers no protection against transmission of STIs, and it may require a backup method during the first week of use.

check yourself

- **What are the advantages and disadvantages of the various hormonal methods of contraception?**
- **How effective are various hormonal methods of contraception in preventing pregnancy and STIs?**
- **The methods of contraception discussed in this module remain in place for days or weeks. What are the benefits and drawbacks of this characteristic?**

5.5 Intrauterine Contraceptives

learning outcome

5.5 List the advantages, disadvantages, and effectiveness of intrauterine contraceptives in preventing pregnancy and STIs.

The **intrauterine device (IUD)** is a small, plastic, flexible device with a nylon string attached that is placed in the uterus through the cervix and left there for 3 to 10 years at a time. The exact mechanism by which it works is not clearly understood, but researchers believe IUDs affect the way sperm and egg move, thereby preventing fertilization and/or affecting the lining of the uterus to prevent a fertilized ovum from implanting.

The IUD was once extremely popular in the United States, and used by about 10 percent of those using contraceptives. However, as evidence of pelvic infections, heavy bleeding, cramping, infertility, and even death grew, most brands were removed from the market and the stigma of IUDs grew. New, safe, and more effective IUDs are now on the market and the IUD is experiencing a resurgence in the U.S. and internationally. Today IUDs are the most commonly used method of reversible contraception in the world, with use ranging from 2 to 40 percent among countries. Misinformation about these highly effective methods of contraception persists and distribution and access is often difficult due to costs, international policies, and inadequate health care systems.[27]

ParaGard, Mirena, and Skyla IUDs

Three IUDs are currently available in the United States. *ParaGard* is a T-shaped plastic device with copper wrapped around the shaft. It does not contain any hormones and can be left in place for 10 years before replacement. *Mirena* is effective for 5 years and releases small amounts of progestin. The newest IUD, Skyla, is a lower dose and smaller-sized version of Mirena. It is designed for women who have not yet had a baby, and it is effective for 3 years. A health care provider must fit and insert an IUD. One or two strings extend from the IUD into the vagina so the user can check to make sure that her IUD is in place. The American Congress of Obstetricians and Gynecologists supports the use of IUDs for women of all ages.[28]

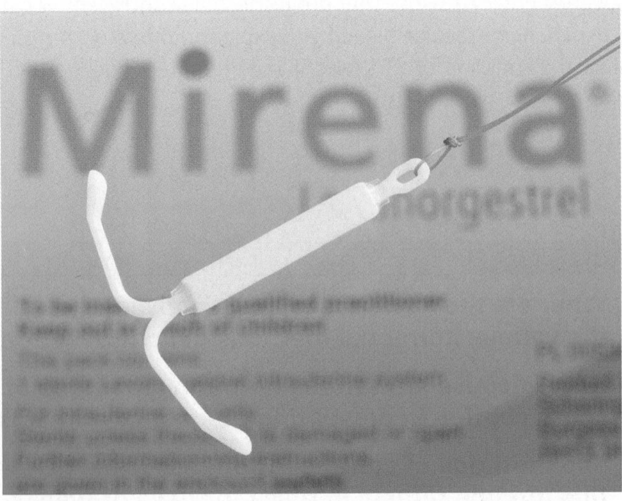

Mirena IUD is a flexible plastic device inserted by a clinician into a woman's uterus, where it releases progestin for up to 5 years.

Advantages The IUD is a safe, discreet, and highly effective method of birth control (99%).[29] It is effective immediately and needs to be replaced only every 3-10 years. ParaGard has the benefit of containing no hormones at all, and so has none of the potential negative health impacts of hormonal contraceptives. Skyla and Mirena probably offer some of the same potential health benefits as other progestin-only methods. All three IUDs can be used by breastfeeding women. With Mirena, periods become lighter or stop altogether. The IUDs are fully reversible; after removal, there is usually no delay in return of fertility. All three of these methods offer sexual spontaneity, because there is no need to keep supplies on hand or to interrupt lovemaking. The devices begin working immediately, and there is a low incidence of side effects. A health care provider can remove the IUD at any time.

Disadvantages Disadvantages of IUDs include possible discomfort, cost of insertion, and potential complications. Also, the IUD does not protect against STIs. In some women, the device can cause heavy menstrual flow and severe cramps for the first few months. Other side effects include acne, headaches, nausea, breast tenderness, mood changes, uterine cramps, and backache, which seem to occur most often in women who have never been pregnant. Women using IUDs have a higher risk of benign ovarian cysts.

See It! Videos

Why are IUDs gaining popularity? Watch **New Support for IUDs** in the Study Area of MasteringHealth.

check yourself

- **What are the advantages and disadvantages of intrauterine contraceptives?**
- **How effective are intrauterine contraceptives in preventing pregnancy and STIs?**
- **Why do you think the IUD is gaining popularity in the U.S. and worldwide?**

Emergency Contraception

learning outcome

5.6 Describe how emergency contraception prevents pregnancy.

Emergency contraception is the use of a contraceptive to prevent pregnancy after unprotected intercourse, a sexual assault, or the failure of another birth control method. Combination estrogen-progestin pills and progestin-only pills are two common types of **emergency contraceptive pills (ECPs)**, sometimes referred to as "morning-after pills." They are not the same as the "abortion pill," although the two are often confused. ECPs contain the same type of hormones as regular birth control pills and are used after unprotected intercourse but before a woman misses her period. A woman taking ECPs does so to prevent pregnancy; the method will not work if she is already pregnant, nor will it harm an existing pregnancy. In contrast, Mifeprex or mifepristone (formerly known as RU-486), the *early abortion pill*, is used to terminate a pregnancy that is already established—after a woman is sure she is pregnant. It and other methods of abortion are discussed later in the chapter.

ECPs prevent pregnancy by delaying or inhibiting ovulation, inhibiting fertilization, or blocking implantation of a fertilized egg, depending on the phase of the menstrual cycle. Although ECPs use the same hormones as birth control pills, not all brands of pills can be used for emergency contraception. When taken within 24 hours, ECPs reduce the risk of pregnancy by up to 95 percent; when taken 2 to 5 days later, ECPs reduce the risk of pregnancy by 88 percent.[30]

Multiple name-brand and generic ECPs are available in the United States including Plan B One Dose, Take Action, Next Choice One Dose, and My Way, all of which are available without a prescription and must be taken within 72 hours (3 days) of intercourse. The FDA has more recently approved ella. Unlike other ECPs, ella is only available by prescription. A progesterone receptor modulator, ella works by inhibiting or preventing ovulation. It can prevent pregnancy when taken up to 120 hours (5 days) after unprotected intercourse.

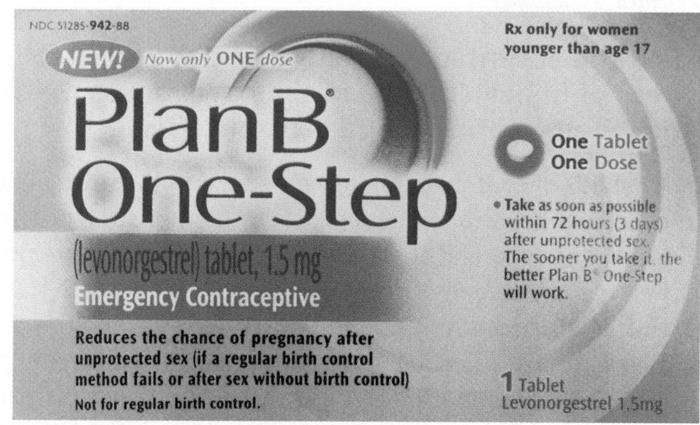

What is emergency contraception?

Emergency contraception is hormone-containing pills used after an act of unprotected intercourse. When taken within 24 hours of unprotected intercourse, ECPs reduce the risk of pregnancy by up to 95 percent. In the United States, Plan B One Dose, Take Action, Next Choice One Dose, and My Way are all available without a prescription; ella, which can prevent pregnancy up to 5 days after unprotected intercourse, requires a prescription.

Although ECPs are no substitute for taking proper precautions before having sex (such as using a condom), widespread availability of emergency contraception has the potential to significantly reduce the rates of unintended pregnancies and abortions, particularly among young women. The 2013 federal court decision requiring the FDA to make emergency contraception available over the counter to all ages was a major win for reproductive health advocates because it removed two barriers for users: the potential embarrassment of asking the pharmacist for ECP and the need to have proper identification to prove age.[31]

99% of U.S. women who have ever been sexually active report having used at least one form of birth control.

check yourself

- **How does emergency contraception prevent pregnancy?**
- **What restrictions, if any, do you think there should be on providing emergency contraception?**

5.7

Behavioral Methods and Fertility Awareness Methods

learning outcome

5.7 List the advantages, disadvantages, and effectiveness of behavioral and fertility awareness methods in preventing pregnancy and STIs.

Some methods of contraception rely on one or both partners altering their sexual behavior. In general, these methods require more self-control, diligence, and commitment, making them more prone to user error than other methods.

Withdrawal, or *coitus interruptus*, involves removing the penis from the vagina just prior to ejaculation. In a recent survey, 29 percent of respondents reported using withdrawal the last time they had intercourse.[32] This statistic is startlingly high, considering the very high risk of pregnancy (78% with typical use) and STI transmission associated with this method of birth control.[33] Withdrawal is highly unreliable, even with "perfect" use; there can be up to half a million sperm in the drop of fluid at the tip of the penis *before* ejaculation. Timing withdrawal is also difficult. Withdrawal offers no protection against transmission of STIs.

Strictly defined, **abstinence** means "deliberately avoiding intercourse," which would allow one to engage in such forms of intimacy as massage, kissing, and masturbation. Couples who go beyond fondling and kissing to activities such as oral sex and mutual masturbation, but not vaginal or anal sex, are sometimes said to be engaging in "outercourse."

Abstinence is the only method of avoiding pregnancy that is 100 percent effective. It is also the only one that is 100 percent effective against transmitting disease. Outercourse can be 100 percent effective for birth control as long as the male does not ejaculate near the vaginal opening, though it is not 100 percent effective against STIs. Oral–genital contact can transmit disease, although the practice can be made safer by using a condom on the penis or a latex barrier, such as a dental dam, on the vaginal opening. Both abstinence and outercourse require discipline and commitment for couples to sustain over long periods of time.

Fertility awareness methods (FAMs) of birth control rely on altering sexual behavior during certain times of the month (Figure 5.4) based on the facts that an ovum can survive for up to 48 hours after ovulation and sperm can live for up to 5 days in the vagina. Strategies include the *cervical mucus method*, which requires tracking changes in vaginal secretions; the *body temperature method*, which requires tracking subtle changes in a woman's basal body temperature; and the *calendar method*, which involves recording the menstrual cycle for 12 months and assuming that ovulation occurs during the midpoint of the cycle. All these methods require abstaining from penis–vagina contact during fertile times.

Fertility awareness methods are the only birth control complying with certain religious teachings, including those of the Roman Catholic Church. They require no medical visit or prescription and have no negative health effects. Their effectiveness depends on diligence and self-discipline; they are only 76 percent effective with typical use.[34] They offer no STI protection and may not work for women with irregular menstrual cycles.

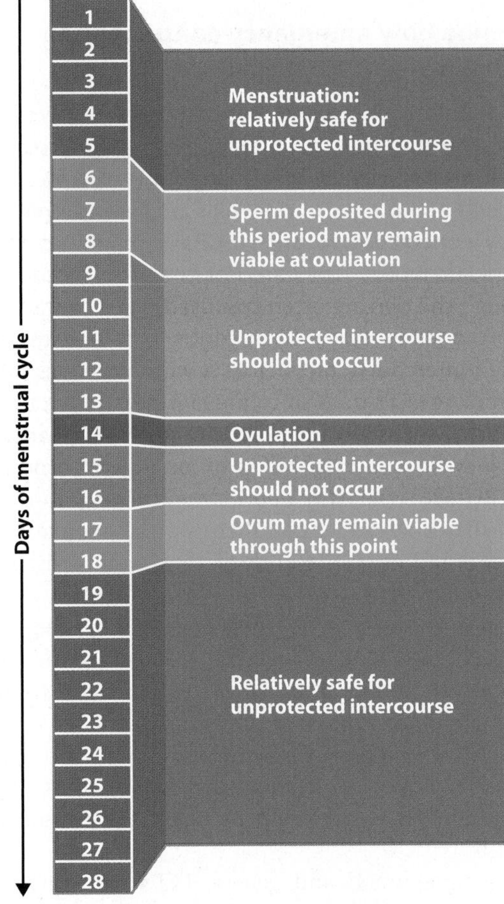

Figure 5.4 The Fertility Cycle
It is important to remember that most women do not have a consistent 28-day cycle.

check yourself

- **What are the advantages and disadvantages of behavioral and fertility awareness methods?**
- **How effective are these methods in preventing pregnancy and STIs?**
- **Why do many people use highly ineffective methods of birth control, such as withdrawal? What do you think it will take to change these behaviors?**

5.8 Surgical Methods

learning outcome

5.8 List the advantages, disadvantages, and effectiveness of surgical methods in preventing pregnancy and STIs.

In the United States, **sterilization** has become the second leading method of contraception for women of all ages and the leading method among married women and women over 30.[35] Because sterilization is permanent, anyone considering it should think through possibilities such as divorce and remarriage or improvement in financial status that might make a pregnancy desirable.

Female Sterilization

In **tubal ligation**, the woman's fallopian tubes are sealed to block sperm's access to released eggs (Figure 5.5). The operation is usually done laparoscopically on an outpatient basis and takes less than an hour. Tubal ligation does not affect ovarian and uterine function. The menstrual cycle continues; released eggs disintegrate and are absorbed by the lymphatic system. As soon as her incision heals, the woman may resume intercourse with no fear of pregnancy.

A newer procedure, Essure, involves placement of microcoils into the fallopian tubes via the vagina. The microcoils expand, promoting growth of scar tissue that blocks the tubes. Essure is recommended for women who cannot have a tubal ligation because of health conditions such as obesity or heart disease. With Adiana, another new method, a small flexible instrument is used to place a tiny insert into each fallopian tube. Scar tissue grows around the insert and eventually blocks the tubes.

A **hysterectomy**, or removal of the uterus, is a method of sterilization requiring major surgery. It is usually done only when a woman's uterus is diseased or damaged.

The main advantage to female sterilization is that it is highly effective (99.5%) and permanent.[36] Afterward, no other cost or action is required. Sterilization has no negative effect on sex drive.

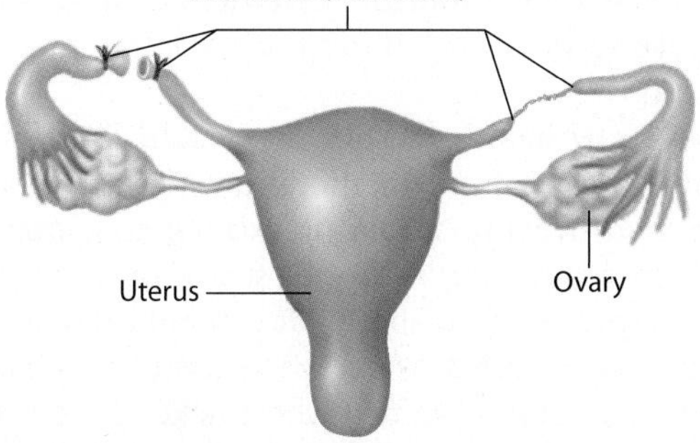

Figure 5.5 Female Sterilization: Tubal Ligation

The Essure and Adiana methods require no incision. As with any surgery, there are risks involved. Sterilization offers no protection against STIs and is initially expensive.

Male Sterilization

Sterilization in men is less complicated. A **vasectomy** is frequently done on an outpatient basis, using a local anesthetic (see Figure 5.6). It involves making a small incision in each side of the scrotum to expose the vasa deferentia, cutting and either tying or cauterizing the ends. Because sperm constitute only a small percentage of semen, the amount of ejaculate is not changed significantly. The testes continue to produce sperm, which disintegrate and are absorbed into the lymphatic system.

A vasectomy is highly effective and permanent: After 1 year, the pregnancy rate in women whose partners have had vasectomies is 0.15 percent.[37] The procedure requires minimal recovery time, and afterward no cost or action is required. Vasectomy has no effect on sex drive or sexual performance.

Male sterilization offers no protection against STI transmission. Also, a vasectomy is not immediately effective; because sperm are stored in other areas besides the vasa deferentia, couples must use alternative birth control for at least 1 month afterward. A physician's semen analysis determines when unprotected intercourse can take place. As with any surgery, there are some risks. Very infrequently the vas deferens may create a new path, negating the procedure.

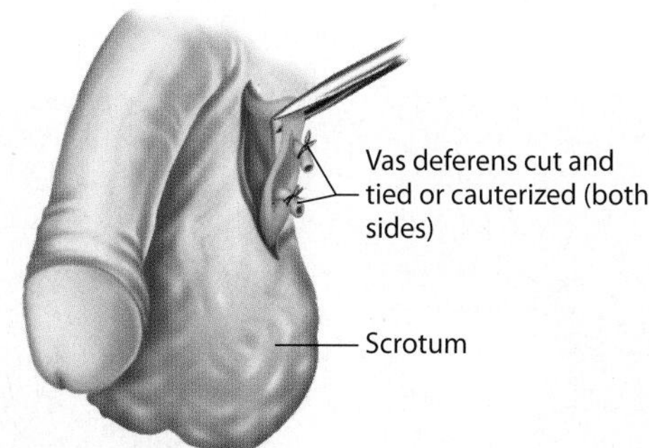

Figure 5.6 Male Sterilization: Vasectomy

check yourself

- **What are the advantages, disadvantages, and effectiveness of surgical methods in preventing pregnancy and STIs?**

5.9 Choosing a Method of Contraception

learning outcome

5.9 Explore questions to consider when choosing a method of contraception and strategies for discussing contraception with a partner.

With all the options available, how does a person or a couple decide what method of contraception is best? Take some time to research the various methods, ask questions of your health care provider, and be honest with yourself and your partner about your own preferences. Questions to ask yourself include the following:

- **How comfortable would I be using a particular method?** If you aren't at ease with a method, you may not use it consistently, and it probably will not be a reliable choice for you. Think about whether the method may cause discomfort for you or your partner, and consider your own comfort level with touching your body. For women, methods such as the diaphragm, sponge, and NuvaRing require inserting an apparatus into the vagina and taking it out. For men, using a condom requires rolling it onto the penis.
- **Will this method be convenient for me and my partner?** Some methods require more effort than do others. Be honest with yourself about how likely you are to use the method consistently. Are you willing to interrupt lovemaking, to abstain from sex during certain times of the month, or to take a pill every day? You may feel condoms are easy and convenient to use, or you may prefer something that requires little ongoing thought, such as Nexplanon or an IUD.
- **Am I at risk for the transmission of STIs?** If you have multiple sex partners or are uncertain about the sexual history or disease status of your current sex partner, then you are at risk for transmission of STIs and HIV (the virus that causes AIDS). Condoms (both male and female) are the *only* birth control methods that protect against STIs and HIV (although some other barrier methods offer limited protection).
- **Do I want to have a biological child in the future?** If you are unsure about your plans for future childbearing, you should use a temporary birth control method rather than a permanent one such as sterilization. Keep in mind that you may regret choosing a permanent method if you are young, if you have few or no children, if you are choosing this method because your partner wants you to, or if you believe this option will fix relationship problems. If you know you want to have children in the future, consider how soon that will be, because some methods, such as Depo-Provera, cause a delay in return to fertility.
- **How would an unplanned pregnancy affect my life?** If an unplanned pregnancy would be a potentially devastating event for you or would have a serious impact on your plans for the future, then you should choose a highly effective birth control method, for example, the pill, patch, ring, implant, or IUD. If, however, you are in a stable relationship, have a reliable source of income, are planning to have children in the future, and would embrace a pregnancy should it occur now, then you may be comfortable with a less reliable method such as condoms, fertility awareness, the diaphragm, cervical cap, or spermicides.
- **What are my religious and moral values in relation to contraception?** If your beliefs prevent you from considering other birth control methods, fertility awareness methods are a good option. When both partners are motivated to use these methods, they can be successful at preventing unintended pregnancy. If you are considering this option, sign up for a class to get specific training on using the method effectively.
- **How much will the birth control method cost?** Some contraceptive methods involve an initial outlay of money and few continuing costs (e.g., sterilization, IUD), whereas others are fairly inexpensive but must be purchased repeatedly (e.g., condoms, spermicides, monthly pill prescriptions). Remember that any prescription method requires routine checkups, which may involve some cost to you. Be sure to check your health insurance to determine if the Affordable Care Act's requirement to cover "preventive services" makes hormonal contraceptives available to you at no cost.
- **Do I have any health factors that could limit my choice?** Hormonal birth control methods can pose potential health risks to women with certain preexisting conditions, such as high blood pressure, a history of stroke or blood clots, liver disease, migraines, or diabetes. You should discuss this issue with your health care provider when considering birth control methods. In addition, women who smoke or are over the age of 35 are at risk from complications of combination hormonal

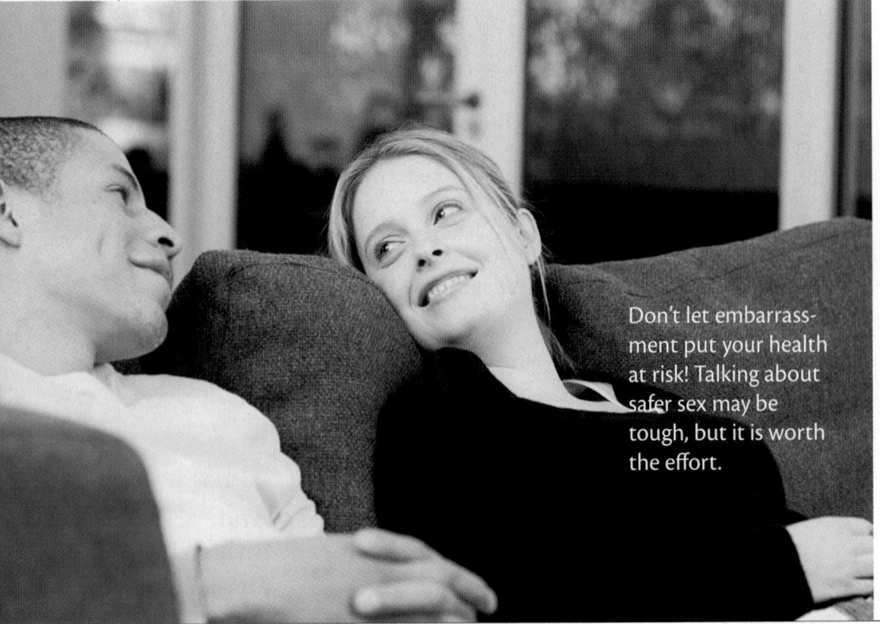

Don't let embarrassment put your health at risk! Talking about safer sex may be tough, but it is worth the effort.

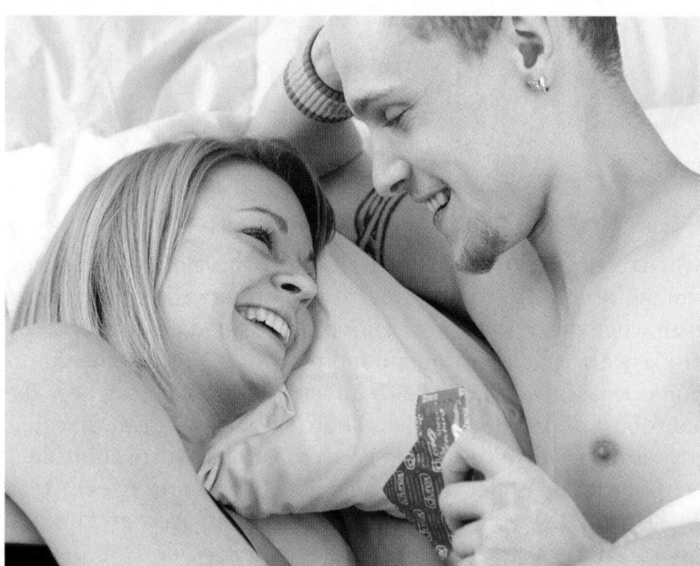

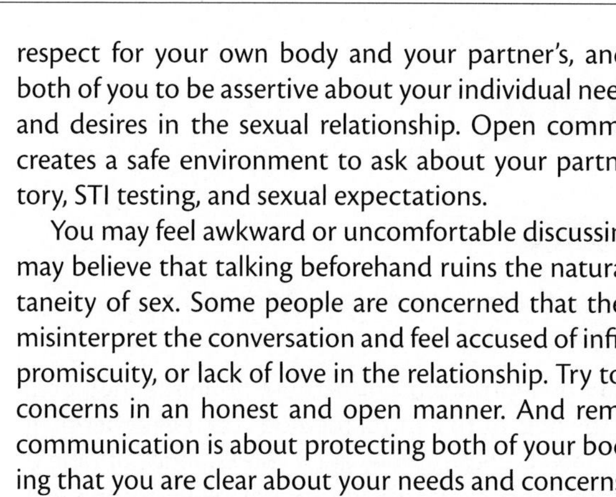

How do I choose a method of birth control?

VIDEO TUTOR
Choosing Contraception

Many different methods of birth control are on the market: barrier methods, hormonal methods, surgical methods, and other options. When you choose a method, you'll need to consider several factors, including cost, comfort level, convenience, and health risks. All of these factors together will influence your ability to consistently and correctly use the contraceptive and prevent unwanted pregnancy.

contraceptives. Breast-feeding women can use progestin-only methods, but should avoid methods containing estrogen. Men and women with latex allergies can use barrier methods made of polyurethane, silicone, or other materials, rather than latex condoms.

- **Are there any additional benefits I'd like to get from my contraceptive?** Hormonal birth control methods may have desirable secondary effects, such as the reduction of acne or the lessening of premenstrual symptoms. Certain pills are marketed as having specific effects, so it is possible to choose one that is known to clear skin or reduce mood changes caused by menstruation. Hormonal birth control methods are also associated with reduced risks of certain cancers. Extended-cycle pills and some progestin-only methods cause menstrual periods to be less frequent or to stop altogether, which some women find desirable. Condoms carry the added health benefit of protecting against STIs.

Communicating about Contraception

Communication is key to a healthy relationship, and it is especially so between those who are sexually intimate. It is a sign of care and respect for your own body and your partner's, and it empowers both of you to be assertive about your individual needs, likes, limits, and desires in the sexual relationship. Open communication also creates a safe environment to ask about your partner's sexual history, STI testing, and sexual expectations.

You may feel awkward or uncomfortable discussing sex, and you may believe that talking beforehand ruins the naturalness or spontaneity of sex. Some people are concerned that their partner will misinterpret the conversation and feel accused of infidelity, distrust, promiscuity, or lack of love in the relationship. Try to address these concerns in an honest and open manner. And remember: Sexual communication is about protecting both of your bodies and ensuring that you are clear about your needs and concerns.

If you are afraid that talking about sex beforehand is going to make your partner think you don't trust him or her, take some time to examine the strength of your relationship. Trust is about being open and honest. If you're afraid to talk with your partner, the chances are you actually don't trust your partner and you might be better off with a partner you do trust.

Before you talk with your partner, it's a good idea to talk with your health care provider about your options for practicing safer sex. Remember, you need to think about getting pregnant and avoiding STIs.

With your partner, try to find a time and place where you are both comfortable and free of distractions, and you have time to have a full conversation. It's generally better to have this conversation outside of the bedroom, so that you're not pressured by the heat of the moment to do things you don't want to do.

Some tips to boost your confidence in negotiating safer sex include the following:

- It can be helpful to have condoms and/or dental dams around, so when things start to really heat up you will be ready.
- Talk to your partner about using protection before getting intimate. This will help both of you be more comfortable and prepared to use a condom or dental dam when the time comes.
- Practice makes perfect. The best way to learn how to use condoms correctly and guarantee their effectiveness is to practice putting them on yourself or your partner.
- If you are concerned about the interruption of using either condoms or dental dams, try to incorporate them into your foreplay. By helping your partner put on protection together, you both will stay aroused and in the moment.
- If your partner complains that sex "doesn't feel as good with a condom/dental dam," remind him or her that it will make you feel more relaxed to worry less about the risk of STIs and pregnancy. You can also use lubricants to increase sensation.

check yourself

- **What are some questions to consider when choosing a method of contraception?**
- **What are some potential obstacles to communicating about contraception, and how can you overcome them?**

5.10 Abortion

learning outcome

5.10 Summarize the various types of abortion procedures.

The vast majority of abortions occur because of unintended pregnancies.[38] Even the best birth control methods can fail; other pregnancies are terminated because they are a consequence of rape or incest. Other commonly cited reasons are not being ready financially or emotionally to care for a child at the time.[39]

In 1973, the landmark U.S. Supreme Court decision in *Roe v. Wade* stated that the "right to privacy . . . founded on the Fourteenth Amendment's concept of personal liberty . . . is broad enough to encompass a woman's decision whether or not to terminate her pregnancy."[40] The decision maintained that during the first trimester of pregnancy a woman and her practitioner have the right to terminate the pregnancy through **abortion** without legal restrictions. It allowed individual states to set conditions for second-trimester abortions. Third-trimester abortions were ruled illegal unless the mother's life or health was in danger. Prior to this, women wishing to terminate a pregnancy had to travel to a country where the procedure was legal, consult an illegal abortionist, or perform their own abortions. These procedures sometimes led to death from hemorrhage or infection or infertility from internal scarring.

The Debate over Abortion

Abortion is a highly charged issue in America. In a recent national poll, 53 percent of people reported that *Roe v. Wade* should be kept in place, 29 percent felt it should be overturned, and 18 percent had no opinion.[41] Pro-choice individuals feel it is a woman's right to make decisions about her own body and health, including the decision to continue or terminate a pregnancy. On the other side of the issue, pro-life, or anti-abortion, individuals believe that the embryo or fetus is a human being with rights that must be protected. Pro-life groups lobby for laws prohibiting the use of public funds for abortion and abortion counseling at the same time that pro-choice groups lobby for laws that make abortions more widely available. At times, violence has arisen as a result of this controversy in the form of attacks on clinics or on individual physicians who perform abortions.

In the 40 years since *Roe v. Wade* legalized abortion nationwide, hundreds of laws have been passed at the state and federal level to narrow or expand its limits. In 2013, 70 new abortion related laws were passed in the United States, most of which focused on regulation of abortion providers or facilities, limitations on provision of medication abortions, or bans on private insurance coverage of abortion. These types of laws make abortions more difficult and costly to provide, consequently reducing the number of clinics and providers willing and able to provide abortion services. Thus, while abortion remains legal in all 50 states, for many women, due to difficulty accessing abortion services, abortion availability is severely limited.[42]

Abortion in the Developing World

When contraceptives are unavailable in developing countries, women often turn to abortion to end an unwanted pregnancy, even when death is a potential risk. Unintended pregnancy is the primary driver of abortion around the world, but whether abortion is legal or not has little to do with its overall incidence. The abortion rate in Africa, where abortion is illegal in most countries, is higher than the rate in Western Europe, where abortion is generally legal (29 per 1,000 women of childbearing age in Africa vs. 12 per 1,000 women of childbearing age in Western Europe). Abortions are also less safe in the developing world: 56 percent of all abortions in developing countries are defined as "unsafe," compared with just 6 percent in the developed world. An estimated 47,000 women died from unsafe abortions last year, nearly all in developing nations where abortion is illegal.[43] When abortion is legalized, it becomes safer. After the legalization of abortion in 1997, South Africa experienced a 91 percent reduction in abortion-related deaths.[44]

Emotional Aspects of Abortion

The best scientific evidence published indicates that among adult women who have an unplanned pregnancy, the risk of mental health problems is no greater if they have an abortion than if they deliver a baby. Although feelings such as regret, guilt, sadness, relief, and happiness are normal, no evidence has shown that an abortion causes long-term negative mental health outcomes.[45] Researchers found that the best predictor of a woman's emotional well-being following an abortion was her emotional well-being prior to the procedure.[46] Factors that place a woman at higher risk for negative psychological responses following an abortion include perception of stigma, need for secrecy, low levels of social support for the abortion decision, prior mental health issues, low self-esteem, and avoidance and denial coping strategies.[47] Certainly a support network is helpful to any woman struggling with the emotional aspects of her abortion decision.

Methods of Abortion

The choice of abortion procedure is determined by how many weeks the woman has been pregnant. Length of pregnancy is calculated from the first day of her last menstrual period.

Surgical Abortions The majority of abortions performed in the United States today are surgical. If performed during the first trimester of pregnancy, abortion presents a relatively low health risk to the mother. About 89 percent of abortions occur during the first 12 weeks of pregnancy (see Figure 5.7).[48] The most commonly used method of first-trimester abortion is **suction curettage,** also called vacuum aspiration or dilation and curettage (D&C) (Figure 5.8).

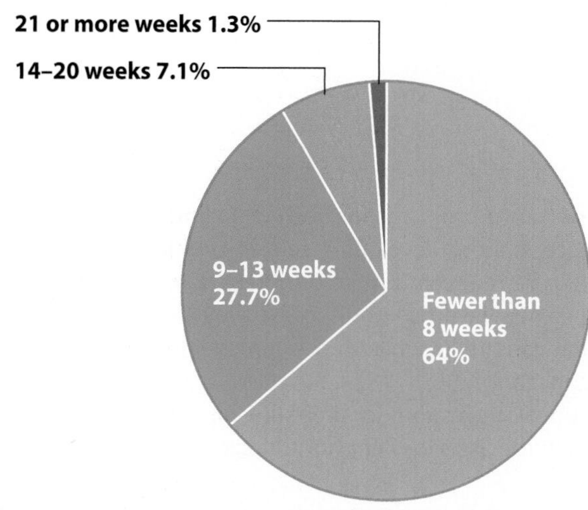

Figure 5.7 When Women Have Abortions (in weeks from the last menstrual period)

Source: K. Pazol et al., "Abortion Surveillance—United States 2009," *Surveillance Summaries* 61, no. SS08 (2012): 1–44, Available at www.cdc.gov.

The vast majority of abortions in the United States are done using this procedure, usually under local anesthetic. The cervix is dilated with instruments or by placing laminaria, a sterile seaweed product, into the cervical canal, where it slowly dilates the cervix. After the laminaria is removed, a long tube is inserted through the cervix and into the uterus, and gentle suction removes fetal tissue from the uterine walls.

Pregnancies in the second trimester (after week 12) can be terminated through **dilation and evacuation (D&E)**. For this procedure, the cervix is dilated for 1 to 2 days and a combination of instruments and vacuum aspiration is used to empty the uterus. Second-trimester abortions may be done under general anesthetic. The D&E can be performed on an outpatient basis, with or without pain medication. Generally, however, the woman is given a mild tranquilizer to help her relax. This procedure may cause moderate to severe uterine cramping and blood loss. After a D&E, a return visit to the clinic is an important follow-up.

Abortions during the third trimester are very rare (less than 2% of abortions in the United States).[49] When they are performed, a D&E or saline **induction abortion** can be performed. The much debated, **intact dilation and extraction (D&X)**, often referred to as "partial birth abortion," is no longer legal in the United States.

The risks associated with surgical abortion include infection, incomplete abortion (when parts of the placenta remain in the uterus), missed abortion, excessive bleeding, and cervical and uterine trauma. Follow-up and attention to danger signs decrease the chances of long-term problems.

The mortality rate for women undergoing first-trimester abortions in the United States averages 1 death per every 1 million procedures at 8 or fewer weeks. At 16 to 20 weeks, the mortality rate is 1 per 29,000; at 21 weeks or more, it increases to 1 per 11,000.[50] This higher rate later in the pregnancy is due to the increased risk of uterine perforation, bleeding, infection, and incomplete abortion; these complications occur because the uterine wall becomes thinner as the pregnancy progresses.

Medical Abortions Unlike surgical abortions, **medical abortions** are performed without entering the uterus. Mifepristone, formerly called RU-486 and currently sold in the United States under the name Mifeprex, is a steroid hormone that induces abortion by blocking the action of progesterone, which maintains the lining of the uterus. As a result, the uterine lining and embryo are expelled from the uterus, terminating the pregnancy.

Mifepristone's nickname, "the abortion pill," may imply an easy process; however, this treatment actually involves more steps than a suction curettage abortion. With mifepristone, a first visit involves a physical exam and a dose of three tablets, which may cause minor side effects, such as nausea, headaches, weakness, and fatigue. The patient returns 2–3 days later for a dose of prostaglandins (misoprostol), which causes uterine contractions that expel the fertilized egg. The patient is required to stay under observation for 4 hours and to make a follow-up visit within 2 weeks.[51]

More than 99 percent of women who use mifepristone early in pregnancy will experience a complete abortion.[52] The side effects are similar to those reported during heavy menstruation and include cramping, minor pain, and nausea. Less than 1 percent have more serious outcomes requiring a blood transfusion because of severe bleeding or intravenous antibiotics.[53]

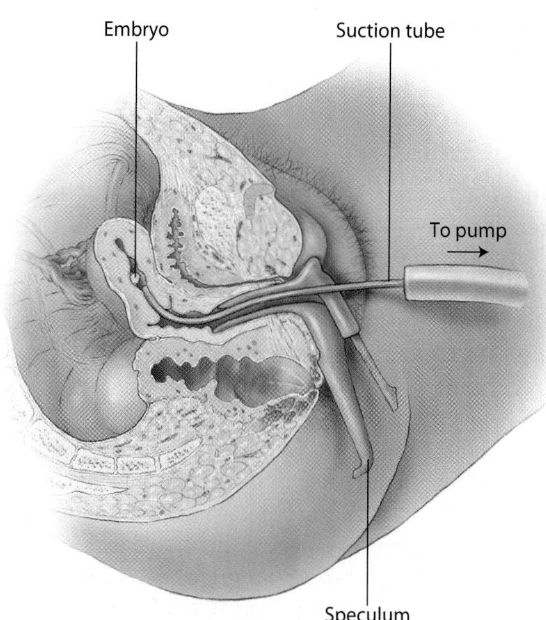

Figure 5.8 Suction Curettage Abortion

This procedure, in which a long tube with gentle suction is used to remove fetal tissue from the uterine walls, can be performed up to the twelfth week of pregnancy.

check yourself

- **What is the current legal status of abortion?**
- **What are the various types of abortion procedures?**

5.11 Planning a Pregnancy

learning outcome

5.11 Discuss key issues to consider when planning a pregnancy.

The many methods available to control fertility give you choices that did not exist when your parents—and even you—were born. If you are in the process of deciding whether, or when, to have children, take the time to evaluate your emotions, finances, and physical health.

Emotional Health

First and foremost, consider why you may want to have a child. To fulfill an inner need to carry on the family? To share love? To give your parents grandchildren? Because it's expected? Then, consider the responsibilities involved with becoming a parent. Are you ready to make all the sacrifices necessary to bear and raise a child? Can you care for this new human being in a loving and nurturing manner? Do you have a strong social support system? This emotional preparation for parenthood can be as important as the physical preparation.

Maternal Health

The birth of a healthy baby depends in part on the mother's **preconception care**. Maternal factors that can affect a fetus or infant include drug use (illicit or otherwise), alcohol consumption, and whether the mother smokes or is obese. To promote preconception health, get the best medical care you can, practice healthy behaviors, build a strong support network, and encourage safe environments at home and at work.[54]

During a preconception care visit, a health care provider performs a thorough medical evaluation and talks with the woman about any conditions she might have, such as diabetes or high blood pressure. The health care provider will also determine if the woman has had any problems with prior pregnancies, if any genetic disorders run in the family, and if the woman's immunizations are up-to-date. If, for example, she has never had rubella (German measles), a woman needs to be immunized prior to becoming pregnant. A rubella infection can kill the fetus or cause blindness or hearing disorders in the infant. The health care provider will encourage the woman to eliminate alcohol consumption and tobacco use and may adjust some medications, such as antidepressants, to safer levels.

Nutrition counseling is another important part of preconception care. Among the many important nutrition issues is folic acid (folate) intake. When consumed the month before conception and during early pregnancy, folate reduces the risk of spina bifida, a congenital birth defect resulting from failure of the spinal column to close.

Why is preconception care so important? Beginning prenatal care at week 11 or 12 of a pregnancy is often late to prevent a variety of health problems for both child and mother. The fetus is most susceptible to developing certain problems in the first 4 to 10 weeks after conception, before prenatal care is normally initiated. Since many women don't realize they are pregnant until later, they often can't reduce health risks unless intervention had begun before conception.[55]

Additional suggestions for preparing for a healthy pregnancy can be found in the Skills for Behavior Change feature.

Maternal Age The average age at which a woman has her first child has been rising. Although births to women in their twenties are declining, the rate of first births to women between the ages of 30 and 39 is the highest in four decades, and births to women over 39 have increased slightly.[56] The chances of having a baby with age-related risks, including miscarriage and Down syndrome, rises after the age of 35.[57] However, many doctors note that older mothers tend to be more conscientious about self-care during pregnancy and are more psychologically mature and ready to include an infant in their family than are some younger women.

Paternal Health

It is common wisdom that mothers-to-be should steer clear of toxic chemicals that can cause birth defects, should eat a healthy diet, and should stop smoking and drinking alcohol. Today, similar precautions are recommended for fathers-to-be. New research suggests that a man's exposure to chemicals influences not only his ability to father a child, but also the future health of that child.

By one route or another, dozens of chemicals studied so far (from occupational exposures to by-products of cigarette smoke) appear to harm sperm.[58] Chemical exposure can reduce the number of sperm, reduce the sperms' ability to fertilize an egg, cause miscarriage, or cause health

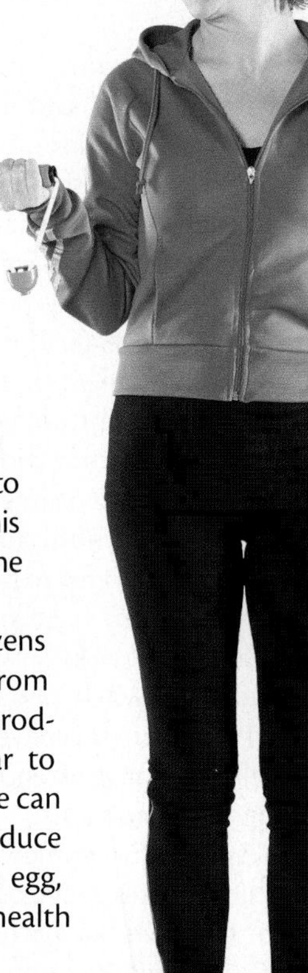

Being in good physical shape will help prepare you for the demands of pregnancy.

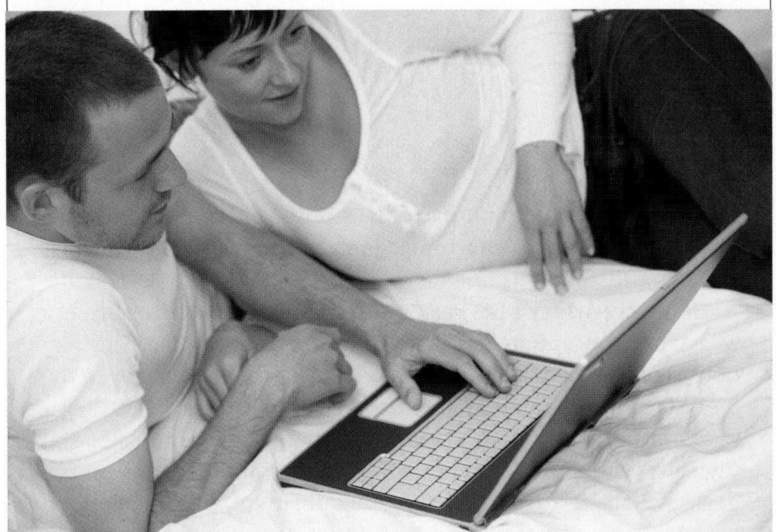

How can I prepare to be a parent?

Following a doctor-approved exercise program during pregnancy is just one aspect of healthy preparation for parenthood. Even before they conceive, prospective mothers and fathers should evaluate their emotional, physical, social, and financial well-being and implement healthy change where needed to better ready themselves for bringing a child into the world.

problems in the baby. Fathers' age also plays a role; men age 40 and over are more likely to father a child with autism, schizophrenia, or Down syndrome.

Financial Evaluation

Finances are another important consideration. Are you prepared to go out to dinner less often, forgo a new pair of shoes, or drive an older car? What about health insurance, disability insurance, life insurance, child care, and preschool? Clothes and shoes that are outgrown every 3 to 12 months? Maybe even orthodontia, glasses, summer camp, college savings accounts? These are important questions to ask yourself when considering the financial aspects of being a parent. Can you afford to give your child the life you would like him or her to enjoy?

First, check your medical insurance: Does it provide pregnancy and delivery benefits? If not, you can expect to pay, on average, $18,000 for a normal delivery and up to $38,000 for a cesarean section birth. Complications during delivery can increase the cost substantially.[59] Both partners should investigate their employers' policies concerning parental leave, including length of leave available and conditions for returning to work.

The U.S. Department of Agriculture estimates that it can cost an average of $241,080 to raise a child born in 2010 to age 18, not including college tuition.[60] While housing costs and food are the two largest expenditures, quality child care is also expensive. According to the National Association of Child Care Resource and Referral Agencies (NACCRRA), full-time child care costs for an infant range from $4,863 in Mississippi to $16,430 a year in Massachusetts.[61]

Contingency Planning

A final consideration is how to provide for your child should something happen to you and your partner. If both of you were to die, do you have relatives or close friends who could raise your child? If you have more than one child, would they have to be split up or could they be kept together? Although unpleasant to think about, this sort of contingency planning is crucial. Children who lose their parents are heartbroken and confused. A prearranged plan of action can smooth their transition into new families; without one, a judge will usually decide who will raise them.

Skills for Behavior Change

PREPARING FOR PREGNANCY

Before becoming pregnant, parents-to-be should take stock of, and possibly improve, their own health to help ensure the health of their child. Among the most important factors to consider are the following.

FOR WOMEN:

- **If you smoke, drink alcohol, or use drugs, stop.**
- **Reduce or eliminate your caffeine intake.**
- **Maintain a healthy weight; lose or gain weight, if necessary.**
- **Avoid X-rays and environmental chemicals, such as lawn and garden herbicides and pesticides.**
- **Take prenatal vitamins, which are especially important in providing adequate folic acid.**

FOR MEN:

- **If you smoke, quit.**
- **Drink alcohol only in moderation, and avoid drug use.**
- **Get checked for sexually transmitted infections and seek treatment if you have one.**
- **Avoid exposure to toxic chemicals in your work or home environment.**
- **Maintain a healthy weight; lose or gain weight, if necessary.**

check yourself

- **What are key issues to consider when planning a pregnancy?**
- **Of the issues discussed, which do you think are the most important?**
- **When considering the lifestyle changes needed for a successful pregnancy, which do you think would be the most challenging to implement?**

5.12

The Process of Pregnancy

learning outcome

5.12 Describe the process of pregnancy, from ovulation to implantation.

Pregnancy is an important event in a woman's life. Actions taken before, as well as behaviors engaged in during, pregnancy can significantly affect the health of both infant and mother.

The process of pregnancy begins the moment a sperm fertilizes an ovum in the fallopian tubes (Figure 5.9). From there, the single fertilized cell, now called a *zygote*, multiplies and becomes a sphere-shaped cluster of cells called a *blastocyst* that travels toward the uterus, a journey that may take 3 to 4 days. Upon arrival, the embryo burrows into the thick, spongy endometrium—in a process called implantation—and is nourished from this carefully prepared lining.

Pregnancy Testing A pregnancy test scheduled in a medical office or birth control clinic will confirm a pregnancy. Women who wish to know immediately can purchase home pregnancy test kits, sold over the counter in drugstores. A positive test is based on the secretion of **human chorionic gonadotropin (HCG)**, which is found in the woman's urine.

Home pregnancy tests vary, but some can be used as early as a week after conception and many are 99 percent reliable.[62] Instructions must be followed carefully. If the test is done too early in the pregnancy, it may show a false negative. Other causes of false negatives are unclean testing devices, ingestion of certain drugs, and vaginal or urinary tract infections. Accuracy also depends on the quality of the test itself and the user's ability to follow directions. Blood tests administered and analyzed by a medical laboratory are more accurate than home tests.

Early Signs of Pregnancy A woman's body undergoes substantial changes during the course of a pregnancy (Figure 5.10). The first sign of pregnancy is usually a missed menstrual period (although some women "spot" in early pregnancy, which may be mistaken for a period). Other signs include breast tenderness,

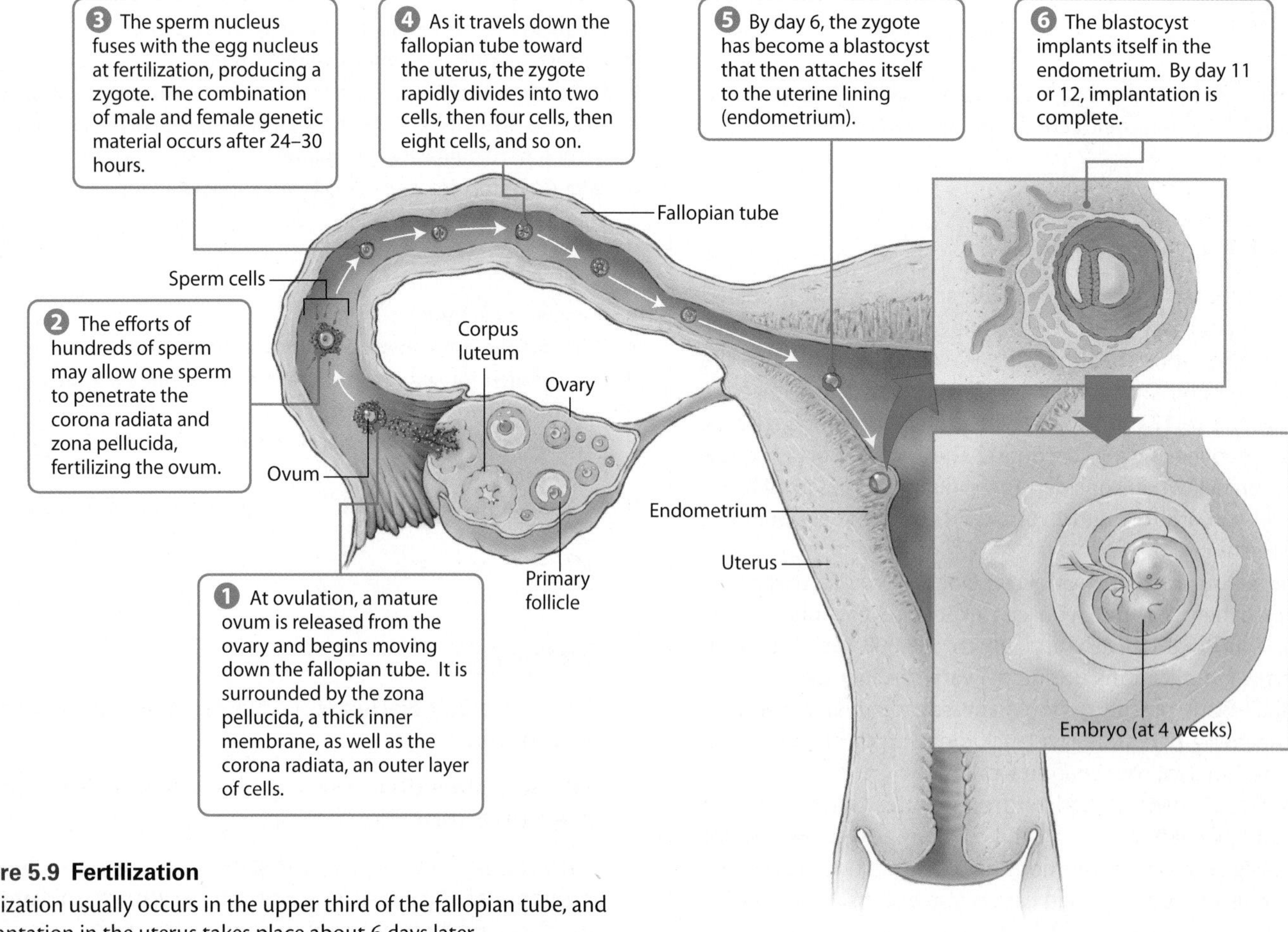

Figure 5.9 Fertilization

Fertilization usually occurs in the upper third of the fallopian tube, and implantation in the uterus takes place about 6 days later.

emotional upset, extreme fatigue, and sleeplessness, as well as nausea and vomiting, especially in the morning.

Pregnancy typically lasts 40 weeks and is divided into three phases, or **trimesters**, of approximately 3 months each. The due date is calculated from the expectant mother's last menstrual period.

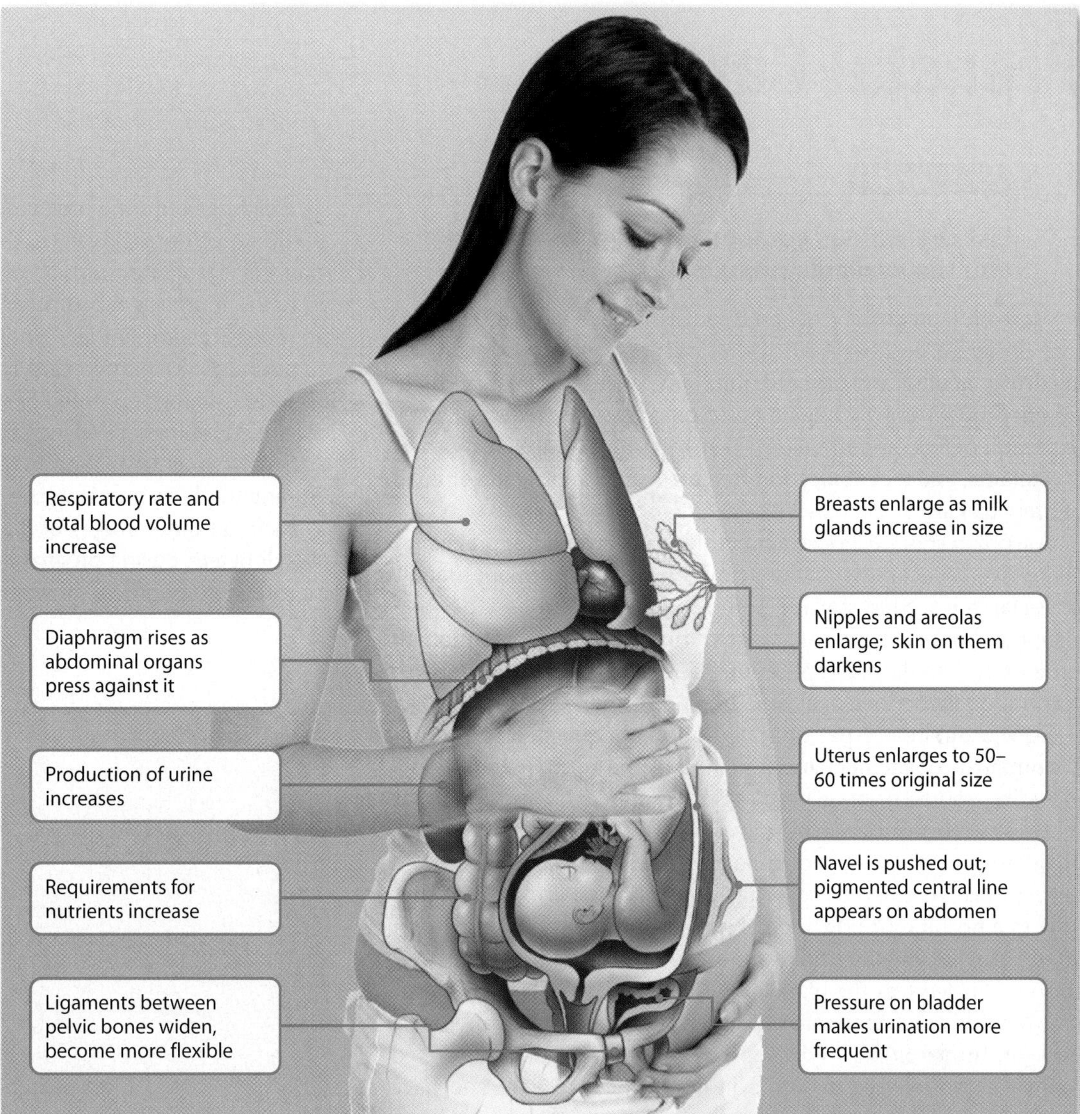

Figure 5.10 Changes in a Woman's Body during Pregnancy

The First Trimester During the first trimester, few visually noticeable changes occur in the mother's body. She may urinate more frequently and experience morning sickness, swollen breasts, or undue fatigue. These symptoms may or may not be frequent or severe, so she may not even realize she is pregnant unless she takes a pregnancy test.

During the first 2 months after conception, the **embryo** differentiates and develops its various organ systems, beginning with the nervous and circulatory systems. At the start of the third month, the embryo is called a **fetus**, a term indicating that all organ systems are in place. For the rest of the pregnancy, growth and refinement occur in each major body system so that each can function independently, yet in coordination with all the others.

The Second Trimester At the beginning of the second trimester, physical changes in the mother become more visible. Her breasts swell and her waistline thickens. During this time, the fetus makes greater demands on the mother's body. In particular, the **placenta**, the network of blood vessels that carries nutrients and oxygen to the fetus and fetal waste products to the mother, becomes well established.

The Third Trimester From the end of the sixth month through the ninth month is the third trimester. This is the period of greatest fetal growth, when the fetus gains most of its weight. The growing fetus depends entirely on its mother for nutrition and must receive large amounts of calcium, iron, and protein from the mother's diet.

Although the fetus may survive if it is born during the seventh month, it needs the layer of fat it acquires during the eighth month and time for the organs (especially respiratory and digestive organs) to develop fully. Infants born prematurely usually require intensive medical care.

Emotional Changes Of course, the process of pregnancy involves much more than the changes in a woman's body and the developing fetus. Many important emotional changes occur from the time a woman learns she is pregnant through the *postpartum period* (the first 6 weeks after her baby is born). Throughout pregnancy, women may experience fear of complications, anxiety about becoming a parent, and wonder and excitement over the developing baby.

check yourself

- **What is the process of pregnancy, from ovulation to implantation?**
- **What are some physical changes experienced by a mother during the three trimesters of pregnancy?**

5.13 Prenatal Care

learning outcome

5.13 List the various components of prenatal care and the available prenatal tests.

A successful pregnancy depends on a mother who takes good care of herself and her fetus. Good nutrition and exercise; avoiding drugs, alcohol, and other harmful substances; and regular medical checkups from the beginning of pregnancy are essential. Early detection of fetal abnormalities, identification of high-risk mothers and infants, and a complication-free pregnancy are the major goals of prenatal care.

A woman should choose a practitioner to attend her pregnancy and delivery. Recommendations from friends and from one's family physician are a good starting point; she should also consider philosophy about pain management during labor, the practitioner's experience handling complications, and his or her willingness to accommodate her personal beliefs on these and other issues.

Several different types of practitioners are qualified to care for a woman through pregnancy, birth, and the postpartum period, including obstetrician-gynecologists, family practitioners, and midwives. Obstetrician-gynecologists are medical doctors (MDs). They are specialists trained to handle all types of pregnancy- and delivery-related emergencies. They generally can perform deliveries only in a hospital setting and cannot serve as the baby's physician after birth. Family practitioners provide care for people of all ages, so they can serve as the baby's physician after birth. However, they may provide pregnancy care only to low-risk pregnancies and rarely perform home births. Midwives may be lay or certified. Certified midwives can oversee deliveries in nonhospital settings and have access to traditional medical facilities. They cannot provide any medication and may need to refer high-risk pregnancies to a clinician. Lay midwives are educated through informal routes such as apprenticeship and may not have training to handle an emergency.

Ideally, a woman should begin prenatal appointments within the first 3 months of becoming pregnant. This early care reduces infant mortality and the likelihood of low birth weight. On the first visit, the practitioner should obtain a complete medical history of the mother and her family and note any hereditary conditions that could put a woman or her fetus at risk. Regular checkups to measure weight gain and blood pressure and to monitor the fetus's size and position should continue throughout the pregnancy. The American Congress of Obstetricians and Gynecologists recommends seven or eight prenatal visits for women with low-risk pregnancies.

Nutrition and Exercise Despite "eating for two," pregnant woman only need about 300 additional calories a day. Special attention should be paid to getting enough folic acid (found in dark leafy greens), iron (dried fruits, meats, legumes, liver, egg yolks), calcium (nonfat or low-fat dairy products and some canned fish), and fluids. Babies born to poorly nourished mothers run high risks of substandard mental and physical development.

Weight gain during pregnancy helps nourish a growing baby. For a woman of normal weight, the recommended gain during pregnancy is 25 to 35 pounds.[63] For overweight women, weight gain of 15 to 25 pounds is recommended, and for obese women, 11 to 20 pounds is recommended. Underweight women should gain 28 to 40 pounds, and women carrying twins should gain about 35 to 45 pounds. Gaining too much or too little weight can lead to complications. With higher weight gains, women may develop gestational diabetes, hypertension, or increased risk of delivery complications. Gaining too little increases the chance of a low birthweight baby.

As in all other stages of life, exercise is an important factor in overall health during pregnancy. Regular exercise is recommended for pregnant women; however, they should consult with their

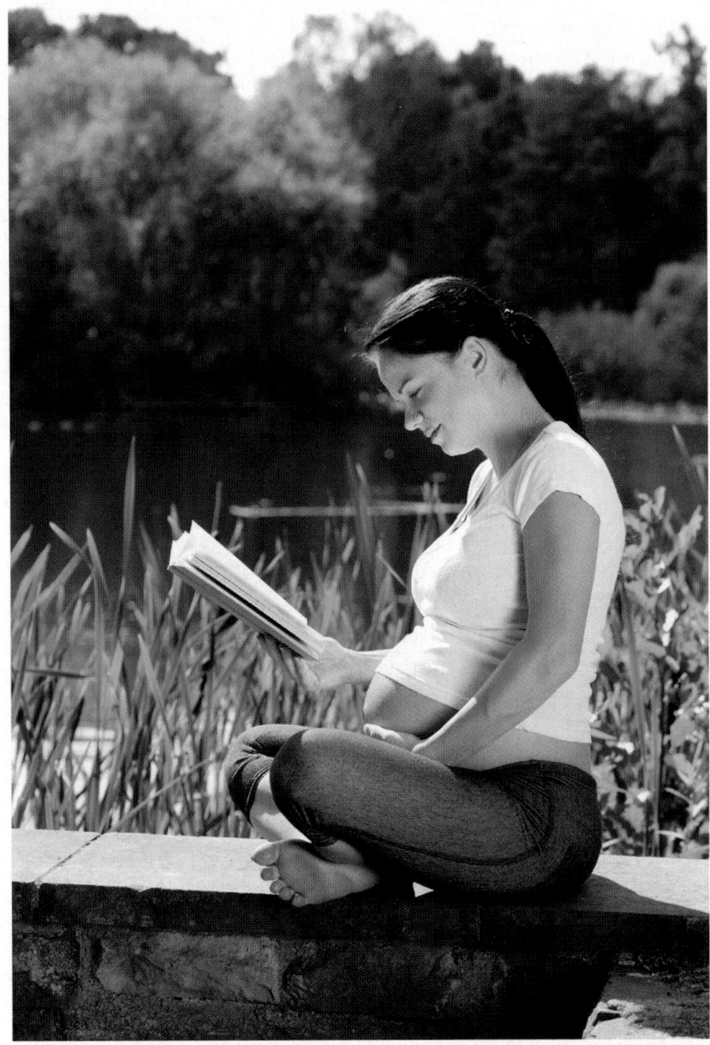

A pregnant woman who exercises, eats well, avoids harmful substances, and has regular medical checkups is more likely to have a successful pregnancy.

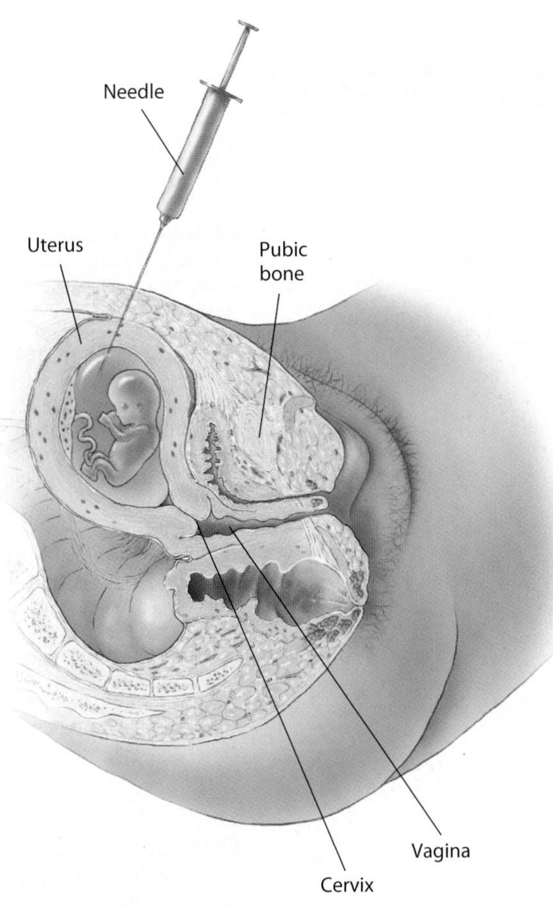

Figure 5.11 Amniocentesis
The process of amniocentesis, in which a long needle is used to withdraw a small amount of amniotic fluid for genetic analysis, can detect certain congenital problems as well as the fetus's sex.

health care provider before starting any exercise program. Exercise can help control weight, make labor easier, and help with a faster recovery because of increased strength and endurance. Women can usually maintain their customary level of activity during most of the pregnancy, although there are some cautions: Pregnant women should avoid exercise that puts them at risk of falling or having an abdominal injury, such as horseback riding, soccer, or skiing, and in the third trimester, exercises that involve lying on the back should be avoided as they can restrict blood flow to the uterus.

Drugs and Alcohol A woman should consult with a health care provider regarding the safety of any drugs she might use during pregnancy. Even too much of common over-the-counter medications such as aspirin can damage a developing fetus. During the first 3 months of pregnancy, the fetus is especially subject to the **teratogenic** (birth defect–causing) effects of drugs, environmental chemicals, X-rays, and diseases. The fetus can also develop an addiction to or tolerance for drugs that the mother uses.

Maternal consumption of alcohol is detrimental to a growing fetus. Symptoms of **fetal alcohol syndrome (FAS)** include mental retardation, slowed nerve reflexes, and small head size. The exact amount of alcohol that causes FAS is not known; therefore, researchers recommend abstinence during pregnancy.[64]

Smoking Tobacco use, and smoking in particular, harms every phase of reproduction. Smokers have more difficulty becoming pregnant and a higher risk of infertility. Women who smoke during pregnancy have a greater chance of complications, premature births, low birth weight infants, stillbirth, and infant mortality.[65] Smoking restricts blood supply to the developing fetus, limiting oxygen and nutrition delivery and waste removal. Tobacco use appears to be a significant factor in the development of cleft lip and palate.

Other Teratogens A pregnant woman should avoid exposure to X-rays, toxic chemicals, heavy metals, pesticides, gases, and other hazardous compounds. She shouldn't clean cat litter boxes; cat feces can contain organisms that cause **toxoplasmosis**—a disease that can cause a baby to be stillborn or suffer mental disabilities or other birth defects.

Prenatal Testing and Screening Modern technology enables detection of fetal health defects as early as the fourteenth week of pregnancy. One common test is **ultrasonography**, or **ultrasound**, which uses high-frequency sound waves to create a *sonogram* of the fetus in the uterus—a visual image used to determine the fetus's size and position; sonograms can also detect birth defects in the central nervous and digestive systems.

Chorionic villus sampling (CVS) involves snipping tissue from the developing fetal sac. It can be used at 10 to 12 weeks of pregnancy and is an attractive option for couples at high risk for having a baby with Down syndrome or a debilitating hereditary disease.

The **triple marker screen (TMS)** is a maternal blood test done at 16 to 18 weeks. TMS can detect susceptibility to a birth defect or genetic abnormality, but is not meant to diagnose any condition. A *quad screen test* screens for an additional protein in maternal blood; it is more accurate than the triple marker screen. Even more precise is the *integrated screen*, which uses the quad screen, results from an earlier blood test, and ultrasound to screen for abnormalities.

Amniocentesis, a common test recommended for women over 35, involves inserting a needle through the abdominal and uterine walls into the **amniotic sac** surrounding the fetus (Figure 5.11). The needle draws out 3 to 4 teaspoons of fluid, which is analyzed for genetic information. Amniocentesis can be performed between weeks 14 and 18.

If a test reveals a serious birth defect, parents are advised to undergo genetic counseling. In the case of a chromosomal abnormality such as Down syndrome, the parents are usually offered the option of a therapeutic abortion. Some parents choose this option; others research the disability and decide to go ahead with the pregnancy.

check yourself

- **What are the key components of prenatal care?**
- **Which, if any, prenatal tests would you choose if you or your partner were pregnant? Why?**

Childbirth and the Postpartum Period

learning outcome

5.14 Describe the stages of labor and the postpartum period.

Childbirth

During the few weeks preceding delivery, the baby normally shifts to a head-down position, and the cervix begins to dilate (widen). The pubic bones loosen to permit expansion during birth. Strong uterine contractions signal the beginning of labor. Another common signal is the breaking of the amniotic sac (commonly referred to as "water breaking"). The birth process (Figure 5.12) can last from several hours to more than a day.

If the baby is in physiological distress, a **cesarean section (C-section)**—a surgical procedure that involves making an incision across the mother's abdomen and through the uterus to remove the baby—may be used. A C-section may also be performed if labor is extremely difficult, maternal blood pressure falls rapidly, the placenta separates from the uterus too soon, or other problems occur. A C-section can be traumatic if the mother is not prepared for it. Risks are the same as for any major abdominal surgery, and recovery takes considerably longer afterward.

The rate of C-section delivery in the United States increased from 5 percent in the mid-1960s to 33 percent in 2012.[66] Although C-sections are sometimes necessary, some feel they are performed too frequently. Natural birth advocates suggest that hospitals driven by profits and worried about malpractice are too quick to intervene in the birth process. Some doctors attribute the increase to demand from mothers.

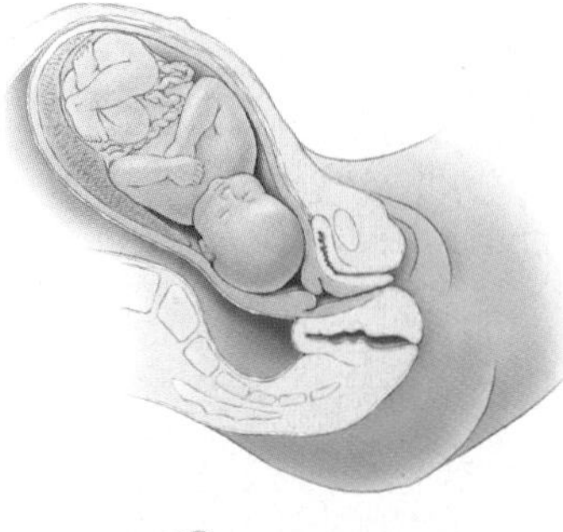

1 Stage I: Dilation of the cervix Contractions in the abdomen and lower back push the baby downward, putting pressure on the cervix and dilating it. The first stage of labor may last from a couple of hours to more than a day for a first birth, but it is usually much shorter during subsequent births.

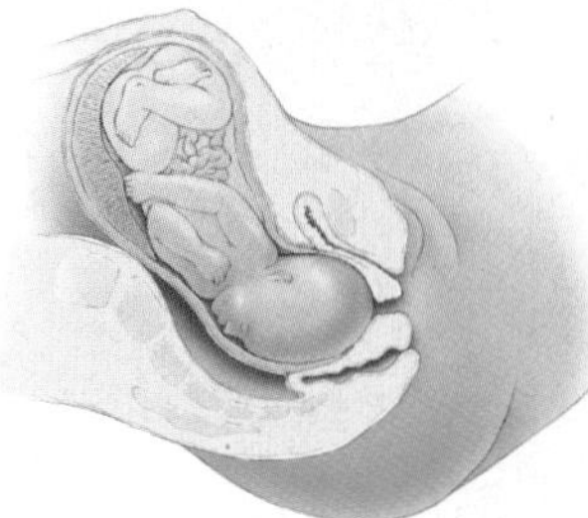

2 End of Stage I: Transition The cervix becomes fully dilated, and the baby's head begins to move into the vagina (birth canal). Contractions usually come quickly during transition, which generally lasts 30 minutes or less.

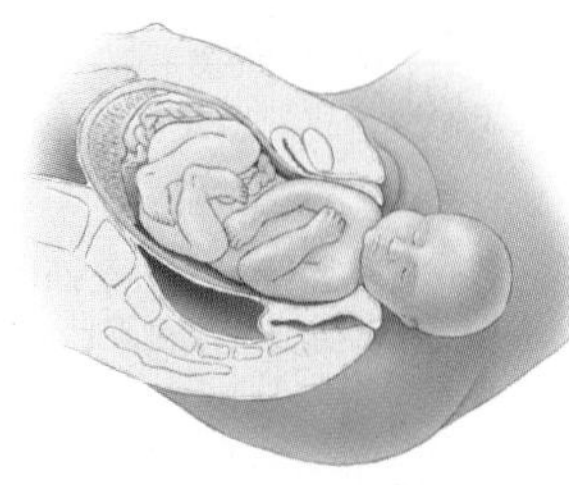

3 Stage II: Expulsion Once the cervix has become fully dilated, contractions become rhythmic, strong, and more intense as the uterus pushes the baby headfirst through the birth canal. The expulsion stage lasts 1 to 4 hours and concludes when the infant is finally pushed out of the mother's body.

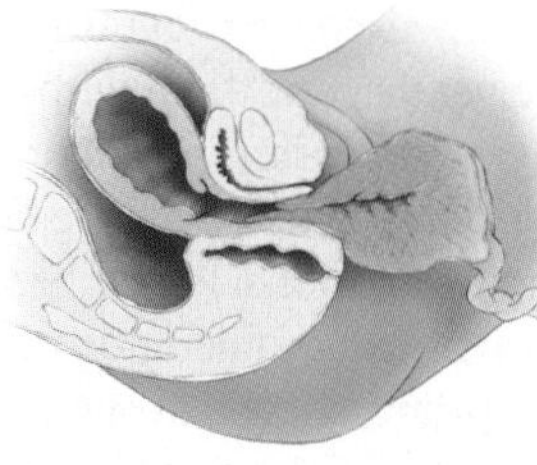

4 Stage III: Delivery of the placenta In the third stage, the placenta detaches from the uterus and is expelled through the birth canal. This stage is usually completed within 30 minutes after delivery.

Figure 5.12 The Birth Process

The entire process of labor and delivery usually takes from 2 to 36 hours. Labor is generally longer for a woman's first delivery and shorter for subsequent births.

Complications of Pregnancy and Childbirth

Pregnancy carries the risk of complications that can interfere with fetal development or threaten the health of mother and child.

Preeclampsia and Eclampsia **Preeclampsia** is characterized by high blood pressure, protein in the urine, edema, and swelling in the hands and face. Symptoms may include sudden weight gain, headache, nausea or vomiting, changes in vision, racing pulse, mental confusion, and stomach or right shoulder pain. If untreated, preeclampsia can cause *eclampsia*, with outcomes including seizures, liver and kidney damage, internal bleeding, stroke, poor fetal growth, and fetal and maternal death. Preeclampsia tends to occur in the late second or third trimester. The cause is unknown. The incidence is higher in first-time mothers; women over 40 or under 18; women carrying multiple fetuses; and women with a history of chronic hypertension, diabetes, kidney disorder, or previous preeclampsia.

Ectopic Pregnancy Implantation of a fertilized egg in the fallopian tube or pelvic cavity is called an **ectopic pregnancy**. If an ectopic pregnancy goes undiagnosed and untreated, the fallopian tube can rupture, putting the woman at risk of hemorrhage, peritonitis (abdominal infection), and even death. Ectopic pregnancy occurs in about 2 percent of pregnancies in North America and is a leading cause of maternal mortality in the first trimester.[67]

Miscarriage Unfortunately, not every pregnancy ends in delivery. In the United States, 15 to 20 percent of pregnancies end in

miscarriage (also referred to as *spontaneous abortion*).[68] Most miscarriages occur during the first trimester.

Reasons for miscarriage vary. In some cases, the fertilized egg has failed to divide correctly. In others, genetic abnormalities, maternal illness, or infections are responsible. In most cases, the cause is not known.

Stillbirth One of the most traumatic events a couple can face is a **stillbirth**, the death of a fetus *after* the twentieth week of pregnancy but before delivery. Each year in the United States, there is about 1 stillbirth in every 160 births.[69] Birth defects, placental problems, poor fetal growth, infections, and umbilical cord accidents all may contribute to stillbirth.

The Postpartum Period

The postpartum period typically lasts 6 weeks after delivery. During this period, many women experience fluctuating emotions and physical challenges.

For many new mothers, the physical stress of labor, dehydration and blood loss, and other stresses challenge their stamina. Many experience the "baby blues," characterized by sadness, anxiety, headache, sleep disturbances, and irritability. For most women, these symptoms disappear after a short while. About 1 in 7 new mothers experience **postpartum depression**, a more disabling syndrome characterized by mood swings, lack of energy, crying, guilt, and depression, that can happen anytime within the first year after childbirth. Mothers who experience postpartum depression should seek professional treatment.[70]

Breast-feeding Although the new mother's milk will not begin to flow for 2 or more days after delivery, her breasts secrete a yellow fluid called *colostrum*. Because colostrum contains vital antibodies to help fight infection, the newborn should be allowed to suckle.

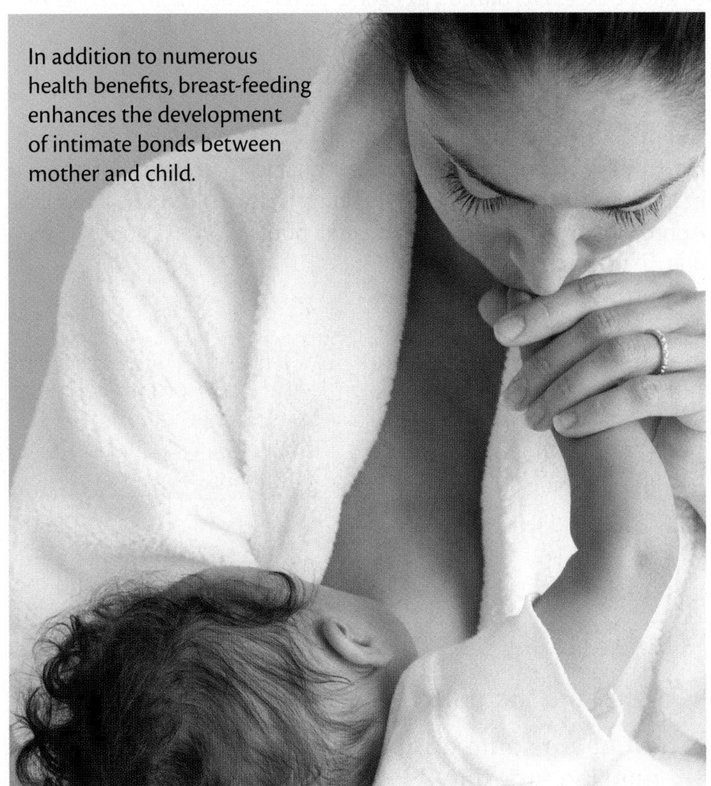

In addition to numerous health benefits, breast-feeding enhances the development of intimate bonds between mother and child.

The American Academy of Pediatrics strongly recommends that infants be breast-fed for at least 6 months, and as a supplement for 12 months or more. Breast-fed babies have fewer illnesses and a much lower hospitalization rate; breast milk contains maternal antibodies and immunological cells that stimulate the infant's immune system. When breast-fed babies do get sick, they recover more quickly. They are less likely to be obese than babies fed on formula and have fewer allergies. Researchers also theorize that breast milk contains substances that enhance brain development.[71] Breast-feeding has the added benefit of helping mothers lose weight after birth because the production of milk burns hundreds of calories a day. Breast-feeding also causes the hormone oxytocin to be released, which makes the uterus return to its normal size faster.

Some women are unable or unwilling to breast-feed; women with certain medical conditions or receiving certain medications are advised not to breast-feed. Prepared formulas can provide nourishment that allows a baby to grow and thrive. When deciding whether to breast- or bottle-feed, mothers must consider their own desires and preferences, too. Both feeding methods can supply the physical and emotional closeness so essential to the parent–child relationship.

Infant Mortality After birth, infant death can be caused by birth defects, low birth weight, injuries, or unknown causes. In the United States, the unexpected death of a child under 1 year of age, for no apparent reason, is called **sudden infant death syndrome (SIDS)**. SIDS is responsible for about 2,500 deaths a year. It is the leading cause of death for children age 1 month to 1 year and most commonly occurs in babies less than 6 months old.[72] It is not a specific disease; rather, it is ruled a cause of death after all other possibilities are ruled out. A SIDS death is sudden and silent; death occurs quickly, often during sleep, with no signs of suffering.

The exact cause of SIDS is unknown, but a few risk factors are known. For example, babies placed to sleep on their stomachs are more likely to die from SIDS than those placed on their backs, as are babies who are placed on or covered by soft bedding; however, breast-feeding and avoiding exposure to tobacco smoke are known protective factors.[73]

check yourself

- **What are the stages of labor, from Stage I to Stage III?**
- **What are the advantages and drawbacks of breast-feeding?**
- **What steps can be taken to reduce the risk of SIDS?**

5.15 Infertility

learning outcome

5.15 Discuss the primary causes of and treatments for infertility.

An estimated 1 in 10 American couples experiences **infertility**, the inability to conceive after trying for a year or more. Both partners should be evaluated; in about 20 percent of cases, infertility is due to a cause involving only the male partner, and in about 30 to 40 percent of cases, both partners.[74]

Reasons for high levels of infertility in the United States include the trend toward delaying childbirth (older women are less likely to conceive), endometriosis, pelvic inflammatory disease, and low sperm count. Environmental contaminants known as *endocrine disrupters*, such as some pesticides and emissions from burning plastics, appear to affect fertility in both men and women. Stress, anxiety, obesity, and diabetes also have reproductive implications.

Most infertility in women results from problems with ovulation. The most common is polycystic ovary syndrome (PCOS). When an egg is mature, its follicle breaks open, releasing it to travel to the uterus for fertilization. In women with PCOS, follicles bunch together to form cysts. Eggs mature, but their follicles don't open to release them. Approximately 5 to 10 percent of women of childbearing age have PCOS.[75]

In *premature ovarian failure*, the ovaries stop functioning before natural menopause. In **endometriosis**, parts of the endometrial lining of the uterus block the fallopian tubes. In **pelvic inflammatory disease (PID)**, chlamydia, or gonorrhea, bacteria invade the fallopian tubes, forming scar tissue that blocks the movement of eggs into the uterus. About 1 in 10 women with PID becomes infertile.[76]

Among men, the largest fertility problem is **low sperm count**.[77] Although only one viable sperm is needed, other sperm in the ejaculate aid in fertilization. There are normally 60 to 80 million sperm per milliliter of semen; below 20 million, fertility declines. Low sperm count may be attributable to environmental factors (such as exposure of the scrotum to intense heat or cold, radiation, or altitude) or even to wearing excessively tight pants. Other factors, such as the mumps virus, can also damage the cells that make sperm.

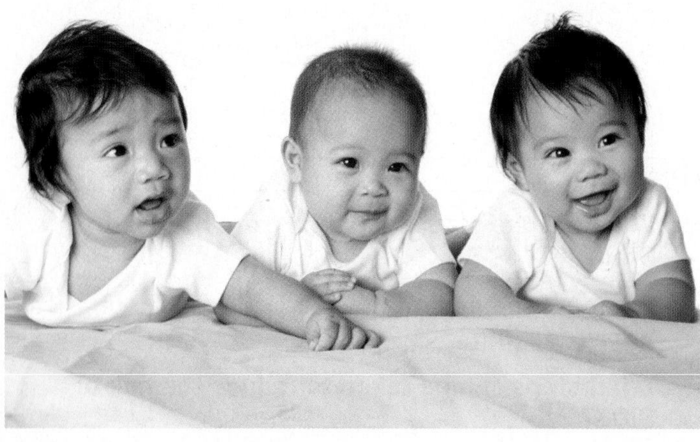

Infertility Treatments

Medical treatment can identify the cause of infertility in about 90 percent of cases.[78] The chances of becoming pregnant after a cause is determined range from 30 to 70 percent, depending on the cause.[79] The expense, countless tests, and invasion of privacy that characterize some couples' efforts to conceive can put stress on an otherwise healthy relationship.

Fertility drugs stimulate ovulation in women who are not ovulating. Following administration of fertility drugs, 60 to 80 percent of women begin to ovulate; of those, about half conceive.[80] The drugs sometimes trigger the release of more than one egg; as many as 1 in 3 women will become pregnant with more than one child.[81]

Other treatment options include **alternative insemination** (or *artificial insemination*) of a woman with her partner's sperm or that of a donor. In **in vitro fertilization (IVF)**, the most common type of *assisted reproductive technology (ART)*, eggs and sperm are combined in a laboratory dish to fertilize; fertilized eggs (zygotes) are then transferred to the uterus. Other ART techniques may combine an egg and sperm at different points, inside or outside the body.

In *nonsurgical embryo transfer*, a donor egg is fertilized by the man's sperm and implanted in the woman's uterus. In *embryo transfer*, an egg donor is artificially inseminated by the man's sperm, and the resulting embryo is transplanted into the birth mother's uterus. Another alternative—embryo adoption—allows infertile couples to adopt excess fertilized eggs generated by treatments such as IVF.

Adoption

Adoption benefits children whose birth parents are unable or unwilling to raise them, and gives adults unable to conceive or carry a pregnancy to term a means to bring children into their families. Approximately 2 percent of the adult population has adopted children.[82] In *confidential adoption*, the birth parents and adoptive parents never know each other. In *open adoption*, birth parents and adoptive parents know some things about each other and may have a defined ongoing relationship.

See It! Videos

Infertility can be troubling issue. Watch **What Are the Reasons for Infertility?** in the Study Area of MasteringHealth.

check yourself

- **What are the primary causes of infertility?**
- **What are some options available for people experiencing infertility?**

Are You Comfortable with Your Contraception?

An interactive version of this assessment is available online in MasteringHealth.

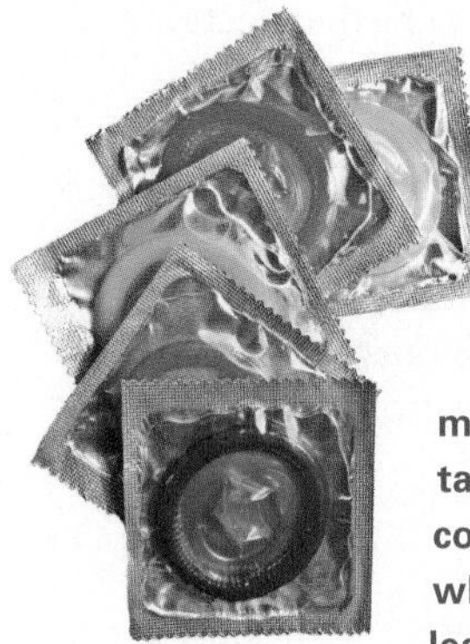

These questions will help you assess whether your current method of contraception or one you may consider using in the future will be effective for you. Answering yes to any of these questions predicts potential problems. If you have more than a few yes responses, consider talking to a health care provider, counselor, partner, or friend to decide whether to use a given method or to learn how to use it so that it will really be effective.

Method of contraception you use now or are considering: ____________

1. Have I or my partner ever become pregnant while using this method? Ⓨ Ⓝ
2. Am I afraid of using this method? Ⓨ Ⓝ
3. Would I really rather not use this method? Ⓨ Ⓝ
4. Will I have trouble remembering to use this method? Ⓨ Ⓝ
5. Will I have trouble using this method correctly? Ⓨ Ⓝ
6. Does this method make menstrual periods longer or more painful for me or my partner? Ⓨ Ⓝ Ⓨ Ⓝ
7. Does this method cost more than I can afford? Ⓨ Ⓝ
8. Could this method cause serious complications? Ⓨ Ⓝ
9. Am I, or is my partner, opposed to this method because of any religious or moral beliefs? Ⓨ Ⓝ
10. Will using this method embarrass me or my partner? Ⓨ Ⓝ
11. Will I enjoy intercourse less because of this method? Ⓨ Ⓝ
12. Am I at risk of being exposed to HIV or other sexually transmitted infections if I use this method? Ⓨ Ⓝ

Total number of yes answers: ____________

Source: Adapted from R. A. Hatcher et al., *Contraceptive Technology,* 19th rev. ed. Copyright © 2007 by R. A. Hatcher. Reprinted with permission of Ardent Media, Inc.

Your Plan for Change

The Assess Yourself activity gave you the chance to assess your comfort and confidence with a contraceptive method you are using now or may use in the future. Depending on the results of the assessment, you may consider changing your birth control method.

Today, you can:

◯ Visit your local drugstore and study the forms of contraception that are available without a prescription. Think about which of them you would consider using and why.

◯ If you are not currently using any contraception or are not in a sexual relationship but might become sexually active, purchase a package of condoms (or pick up a few free samples from your campus health center) to keep on hand just in case.

Within the next 2 weeks, you can:

◯ Make an appointment for a checkup with your health care provider. Be sure to ask him or her any questions you have about contraception.

◯ Sit down with your partner and discuss contraception. Decide who will be responsible and which form will work best for you.

By the end of the semester, you can:

◯ Periodically reevaluate whether your new or continued contraception is still effective for you. Review your experiences, and take note of any consistent problems you may have encountered.

◯ Always keep a backup form of contraception on hand. Check this supply periodically and throw out and replace any supplies that have expired.

Summary

To hear an MP3 Tutor session, scan here or visit the Study Area in **MasteringHealth**.

LO 5.1–5.9 Latex or polyurethane male condoms and female condoms, when used correctly for oral sex or intercourse, provide the most effective protection against sexually transmitted infections (STIs). Other contraceptive methods include spermicides, the diaphragm, cervical cap, Today Sponge, oral contraceptives, Ortho Evra, NuvaRing, Depo-Provera, Nexplanon, and intrauterine devices. Emergency contraception may be used within 72 hours of unprotected intercourse or failure of another contraceptive method. Fertility awareness methods rely on altering sexual practices to avoid pregnancy, as do abstinence, outercourse, and withdrawal. All these methods of contraception are reversible; sterilization is permanent.

LO 5.10 Abortion is legal in the United States, but strongly opposed by many Americans. Abortion methods include suction curettage, dilation and evacuation (D&E), and medical abortions. Intact dilation and extraction (D&X) is no longer legal in the United States.

LO 5.11 Parenting is a demanding job. Prospective parents must consider emotional and physical health and financial plans.

LO 5.12–5.13 Full-term pregnancy covers three trimesters. Prenatal care includes a complete physical exam within the first trimester, follow-up checkups throughout the pregnancy, nutrition and exercise, and avoidance of substances that could have teratogenic effects on the fetus. Prenatal tests can be used to detect birth defects during pregnancy.

LO 5.14 Childbirth occurs in three stages. Partners should choose a labor method early in the pregnancy to be better prepared when labor occurs. Possible complications include preeclampsia/eclampsia, ectopic pregnancy, miscarriage, and stillbirth.

LO 5.15 Infertility in women may be caused by pelvic inflammatory disease (PID) or endometriosis. In men, it may be caused by low sperm count. Treatments may include fertility drugs, alternative insemination, in vitro fertilization (IVF), and assisted reproductive technology (ART).

Pop Quiz

Visit MasteringHealth to personalize your study plan with Chapter Review Quizzes and Dynamic Study Modules.

LO 5.1 1. What lubricant could you safely use with a latex condom?
a. Mineral oil
b. Water-based lubricant
c. Body lotion
d. Petroleum jelly

LO 5.1 2. Why is it recommended not to use lambskin condoms?
a. They are less elastic than latex condoms.
b. They cannot be stored for as long as latex condoms.
c. They don't protect against transmission of STIs.
d. They're likely to cause allergic reactions.

LO 5.1 3. What is meant by the *failure rate* of contraceptive use?
a. The number of times a woman fails to get pregnant when she wants to
b. The number of times a woman gets pregnant when she doesn't want to
c. The number of pregnancies that occur for women using a particular method of birth control
d. The reliability of alternative methods of birth control that do not use condoms

LO 5.2 4. Which of the following is a barrier contraceptive?
a. Seasonale
b. FemCap
c. Ortho Evra
d. Contraceptive patch

LO 5.9 5. Twenty-year-old Lani is in a monogamous relationship with her boyfriend. She has a hard time remembering to take the pill or to carry her diaphragm with her. Which form of contraception would you recommend that she try?
a. Female condom
b. Tubal ligation
c. Nexplanon
d. The FemCap

LO 5.10 6. What is the most commonly used method of first-trimester abortion?
a. Suction curettage
b. Dilation and evacuation (D&E)
c. Medical abortion
d. Induction abortion

LO 5.13 7. Toxic chemicals, pesticides, X-rays, and other hazardous compounds causing birth defects are called
a. carcinogens.
b. teratogens.
c. mutants.
d. environmental assaults.

LO 5.13 8. What prenatal test involves snipping tissue from the developing fetal sac?
a. Fetoscopy
b. Ultrasound
c. Amniocentesis
d. Chorionic villus sampling

LO 5.14 9. In an ectopic pregnancy, the fertilized egg implants itself in the
a. fallopian tube.
b. uterus.
c. vagina.
d. ovaries.

LO 5.15 10. The number of American couples who experience infertility is
a. 1 in 10.
b. 1 in 24.
c. 1 in 60.
d. 1 in 100.

Answers to these questions can be found on page A-1. If you answered a question incorrectly, review the module identified by the Learning Outcome. For even more study tools, visit MasteringHealth.

Addiction and Drug Abuse

6

It's easy to find high-profile cases of compulsive and destructive behavior. Stories of celebrities, athletes, and politicians struggling with addictions to drugs, sex, and alcohol are often splashed in the headlines. But millions of people of all ages and from a wide range of socioeconomic conditions throughout the world are waging their own battles with addiction.

Drug misuse and abuse are enormous problems, and drug addiction wreaks havoc on individuals, families, businesses, and society. Approximately 9 percent of Americans report using illicit drugs during the past month.[1] By late adolescence, 42 percent of Americans report having used illicit drugs in their lifetime,[2] and over 21 percent of high school students have taken prescription drugs without a doctor's permission.[3] Drug misuse and abuse can cause problems ranging from deterioration of relationships to loss of employment to death. It's impossible to put a dollar amount on the pain, suffering, and dysfunction that drugs cause in our every-day lives.

Why do people use drugs? Human beings appear to have a need to alter their consciousness, or mental state, and they do so in many ways: Children spin until they become dizzy; adults enjoy the thrill of extreme sports. Some listen to music, skydive, meditate, pray, or have sex. Others turn to drugs.

6.1 What Is Addiction?

learning outcome

6.1 List the characteristics of addiction.

Addiction is a persistent, compulsive dependence on a behavior or substance, despite ongoing negative consequences. Some researchers speak of two types of addictions: *substance addictions* (e.g., alcoholism, drug abuse, and smoking) and *process addictions* (e.g., gambling, shopping, eating, and sex). Regardless of the addictive behavior, the person experiencing it usually feels a sense of pleasure or control that is beyond the addict's power to achieve in other ways. Eventually, the addicted person needs to do the behavior in order to feel normal.

Physiological dependence, the adaptive state that occurs with regular addictive behavior and results in withdrawal syndrome, is one indicator of addiction. Chemicals are responsible for the most profound addictions because they cause cellular changes to which the body adapts so well that it eventually requires the chemical to function normally.

Psychological dynamics also play an important role, which explains why behaviors not related to chemicals may also be addictive. Addictive behaviors have the potential to produce a positive mood change; some behaviors, such as gambling, working, and sex, also create changes at the cellular level.[4] A person with an intense, uncontrollable urge to continue engaging in a particular activity is said to have developed a *psychological dependence*. Psychological and physiological dependence are intertwined and nearly impossible to separate; all forms of addiction probably reflect dysfunction of certain biochemical systems in the brain.[5]

Five symptoms are present in addictions: (1) **compulsion** characterized by **obsession**, or excessive preoccupation, with the behavior and an overwhelming need to perform it; (2) **loss of control**, or inability to reliably predict whether any occurrence of the behavior will be healthy or damaging; (3) **negative consequences**, such as physical damage, financial problems, academic failure, and family dissolution, that don't occur with healthy involvement in the behavior; (4) **denial**, the inability to perceive the behavior as self-destructive; and (5) an **inability to abstain**.[6]

Addiction evolves over time, beginning when a person repeatedly seeks the illusion of relief to avoid unpleasant feelings or situations. This pattern, known as *nurturing through avoidance*, is a maladaptive way of taking care of emotional needs. As a person becomes increasingly dependent on the addictive behavior, relationships with family, friends, and coworkers, performance at work or school, and personal life deteriorate. Eventually, addicts do not find the addictive behavior pleasurable but consider it preferable to the unhappy realities they are seeking to escape. Figure 6.1 illustrates the cycle of psychological addiction.

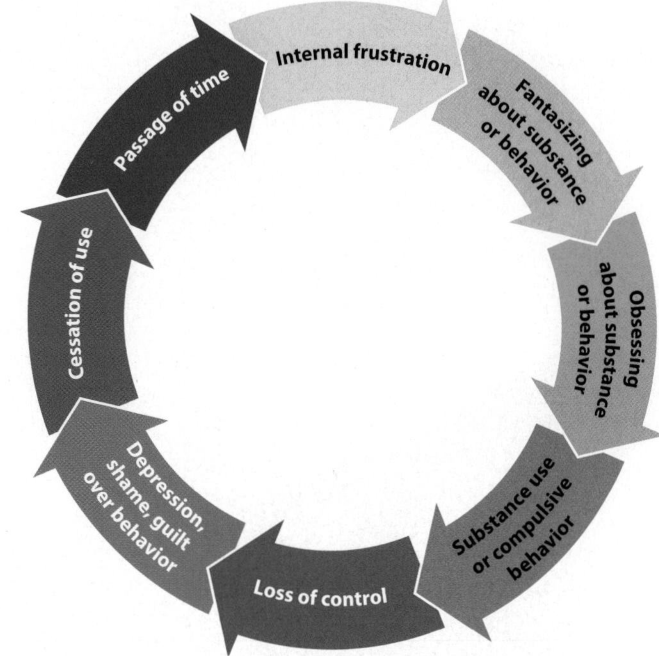

Figure 6.1 Cycle of Psychological Addiction
Source: Adapted from Recovery Connection, Cycle of Addiction, 2012, www.recoveryconnection.org

VIDEO TUTOR
Addiction Cycle

The Physiology of Addiction

Virtually all intellectual, emotional, and behavioral functions occur as a result of biochemical interactions in the body. Biochemical messengers called **neurotransmitters** exert their influence at specific receptor sites on nerve cells. Drug use and chronic stress can alter these receptor sites, leading to either production or breakdown of neurotransmitters. Some people's bodies naturally produce insufficient quantities of these neurotransmitters, predisposing them to seek out chemicals, such as alcohol, as substitutes and making them more susceptible to addiction.

Mood-altering substances and experiences produce **tolerance**—when progressively larger doses or more intense involvement are needed to obtain the desired effects. Addicts tend to seek more intense mood-altering experiences and eventually increase the amount and intensity to the point of negative effects.

An addictive substance or activity replaces an effect that the body normally provides on its own. If the experience is repeated often enough, the body adjusts by requiring the drug or experience to obtain the effect. Stopping causes a **withdrawal** syndrome. Mood-altering chemicals, for example, fill receptor sites for the body's "feel-good" neurotransmitters (endorphins), and nerve cells shut down production of these substances temporarily. When drug use stops, those receptor sites sit empty, resulting in uncomfortable feelings that remain until the body resumes normal neurotransmitter production or the person consumes more of the drug.

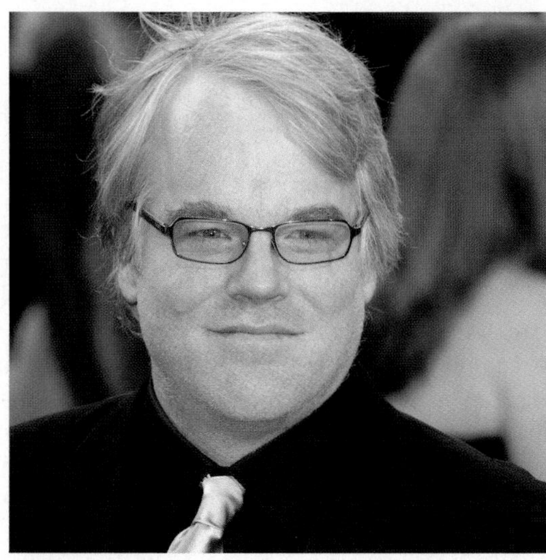

Addiction affects all kinds of people. In 2014, widely respected actor Philip Seymour Hoffman was found dead in his apartment with a needle in his arm. A mix of cocaine, heroin, and other drugs ultimately proved fatal.

Withdrawal symptoms of chemical dependencies are generally the opposite of the effects of the drugs. An addict who feels a high from cocaine will experience a "crash" (depression and lethargy) when he stops taking it. Withdrawal symptoms for addictive behaviors usually involve psychological discomfort and preoccupation with or craving for the behavior.

The Biopsychosocial Model of Addiction

The most effective treatment today is based on the **biopsychosocial model of addiction**, which proposes that addiction is caused not by a single influence but by multiple biological, psychological, social, and environmental factors operating in complex interaction.

Psychological Factors People with low self-esteem, tendencies for risk-taking behavior, or poor coping skills are more likely to develop addictive behavior. Individuals who consistently look outside themselves for solutions and explanations for life events (who have an external locus of control) are more likely to experience addiction.

Biological or Disease Influences Brain processes controlling memory, motivation, and emotional state are subjects for genetic research into risk for addiction, particularly to mood-altering substances. Studies show that drug addicts metabolize these substances differently than do others; for example, genes affecting activity of the neurotransmitters serotonin and GABA (gamma-aminobutyric acid) are likely involved in the risk for alcoholism.[7]

Research also supports a genetic influence on addiction. Identical twins, who share the same genes, are about twice as likely as fraternal twins, who share an average of 50 percent of genes, to resemble each other in terms of the presence of alcoholism. Approximately half of the risk for alcoholism is genetically determined.[8]

Environmental Influences Cultural expectations and mores help determine whether people engage in certain behaviors. Low rates of alcoholism typically exist in countries, like Italy, where children are gradually introduced to alcohol in diluted amounts, on special occasions, and within a strong family group; intoxication is not viewed as socially acceptable, stylish, or funny.[9] Such traditions and values are less widespread in the United States, where the incidence of alcohol addiction is very high.

Societal attitudes and messages also influence addictive behavior. Media emphasis on appearance and the ideal body plays a significant role in exercise addiction. Societal changes, in turn, influence individual norms. People living in cities characterized by rapid social change or social disorganization often feel disenfranchised and disconnected, leading to increased addiction rates.[10]

Social learning theory proposes that people learn behaviors by watching role models—parents, caregivers, and significant others. Many studies show that modeling by parents and by idolized celebrities exerts a profound influence on young people.[11]

On an individual level, major life events such as marriage, divorce, change in work status, or death of a loved one may trigger addictive behaviors. One thing that makes addictive behaviors so attractive is that they reliably alleviate personal pain, at least for a while—though in the long term they cause more pain than they relieve.

Family members whose needs for love, security, and affirmation are not consistently met; who are refused permission to express feelings or needs; and who frequently submerge their personalities to "keep the peace" are prone to addiction. Children whose parents are not consistently available (physically or emotionally); who are subjected to abuse; or who receive inconsistent or disparaging messages about their self-worth may experience addiction in adulthood.

Effect on Family and Friends

Family and friends of an addicted person often struggle with **codependence**. Codependents find it hard to set healthy boundaries and often live in the chaotic, crisis-oriented mode occurring around addicts. They assume responsibility for meeting others' needs to the point that they subordinate or even cease being aware of their own. Family and friends can also become **enablers**, knowingly or unknowingly protecting addicts from the consequences of their behavior. Both addicts and those around them must learn to see how addicts' behavior affects others and work to establish healthier relationships and boundaries.

check yourself

- **What are the characteristics of addiction?**
- **How does addiction affect the family and friends of the addict?**
- **According to the biopsychosocial model of addiction, what types of factors combine to cause addiction?**

6.2 Addictive Behaviors

learning outcome

6.2 Give examples of process addictions.

Process addictions are behaviors known to be addictive because they are mood altering. Traditionally, the word *addiction* was used mainly with regard to psychoactive substances. However, new knowledge suggests that, as far as the brain is concerned, a reward is a reward, whether brought on by a chemical or a behavior.[12]

Gambling Disorder

More than 2 million Americans suffer from **gambling disorder**, and 4 to 6 million more are considered to be at risk for gambling addiction.[13] Characteristic behaviors include preoccupation with gambling, unsuccessful efforts to quit, and lying to conceal the extent of one's involvement.[14]

There is strong evidence that gambling disorder has a biological component. A study of individuals with gambling disorder found the participants to have decreased blood flow to a key section of the brain's reward system. Individuals with gambling disorder, like people who abuse drugs, compensate for this deficiency in their brain's reward system by overdoing it and getting hooked.[15] Most compulsive gamblers seek excitement even more than money. Their cravings can be as intense as those of drug abusers; they show tolerance in their need to increase the amount of bets; and they experience intense highs. Up to half show withdrawal symptoms, including sleep disturbance, sweating, irritability, and craving.

Men, lower-income individuals, those who are divorced, African Americans, older adults, and individuals who begin gambling at a younger age are more likely to have gambling problems.

Obsession with a substance or behavior, even a generally positive activity such as exercise, can eventually develop into an addiction. If there are negative consequences from exercising, such as overuse injuries or withdrawal from friends and other activities, then addiction is a possibility.

Is my roommate's constant exercising an addiction?

Compulsive Buying Disorder

Compulsive buying is estimated to affect up to 5 percent of the U.S. population, mostly women.[16] Individuals with **compulsive buying disorder** are preoccupied with shopping and spending and exercise little control over impulses to buy. Signs that a person has crossed the line into compulsive buying include buying more than one of the same item, repeatedly buying much more than one needs or can afford, and buying to the point that it interferes with social activities or work and creates financial problems. Compulsive buying frequently results in depression and feelings of guilt, as well as conflict with friends and between couples.[17]

Compulsive buying disorders most often begin in the late teens and early twenties, coinciding with establishment of credit and independence from parents. It can be seasonal (shopping during the winter to alleviate seasonal anxiety and depression) and can occur when people feel depressed, lonely, or angry. Both compulsive gambling and compulsive buying frequently lead to repeated borrowing to help support the addiction.

Technology Addictions

Do you have friends who seem more concerned with texting or Web surfing than with eating, going out, or studying? These attitudes and behaviors are not unusual. An estimated 1 in 8 Internet users will likely experience **Internet addiction**.[18] Approximately 11 percent of college students report that Internet use and computer games have interfered with their academic performance.[19]

What you do online may be as important as how long you spend; some activities, such as gaming and cybersex, seem to be more potentially addictive than others. Technology addicts typically exhibit symptoms such as general disregard for their health, sleep deprivation, depression, neglecting family and friends, lack of physical activity, euphoria when online, uncomfortable feelings when not online, and poor grades or job performance. Addicts may be compensating for loneliness, marital or work problems, a poor social life, or financial problems.

$25,000 is the average amount of debt that a compulsive shopper owes.

Work Addiction

To understand work addiction, we must understand the concept of healthy work. Healthy work provides a sense of identity, helps develop our strengths, and is a means of satisfaction and mastery. Although work may occasionally keep them from family, friends, and personal interests, healthy workers generally maintain balance in their lives.

Conversely, **work addiction** is the compulsive use of work and the work persona to fulfill needs of intimacy, power, and success. Work addicts usually fail to set boundaries regarding work and feel driven to work even when away from the workplace.[20]

Work addiction, found among all age, racial, and socioeconomic groups, typically develops in people in their forties and fifties. Males outnumber females, but this is changing as women gain more equality in the workforce.[21] Most work addicts come from alcoholic, rigid, violent, or otherwise dysfunctional homes. While work addiction can bring admiration from society at large, as addicts often excel in their professions, the negative effects on individuals and those around them may be far-reaching.[22]

Exercise Addiction

Exercise addicts use exercise compulsively to try to meet needs—for nurturance, intimacy, self-esteem, and self-competency—that an object or activity cannot truly meet. Consequently, addictive or compulsive exercise results in negative consequences similar to those of other addictions: alienation of family and friends, injuries from overdoing it, and craving for more.

Warning signs of exercise addiction include only exercising by yourself; adhering to a rigid workout plan; working out longer than 2 hours daily, repeatedly; exercising through illness or injury; becoming fixated on burning calories or losing weight; missing work or class to exercise; or working out beyond the point of pain.[23]

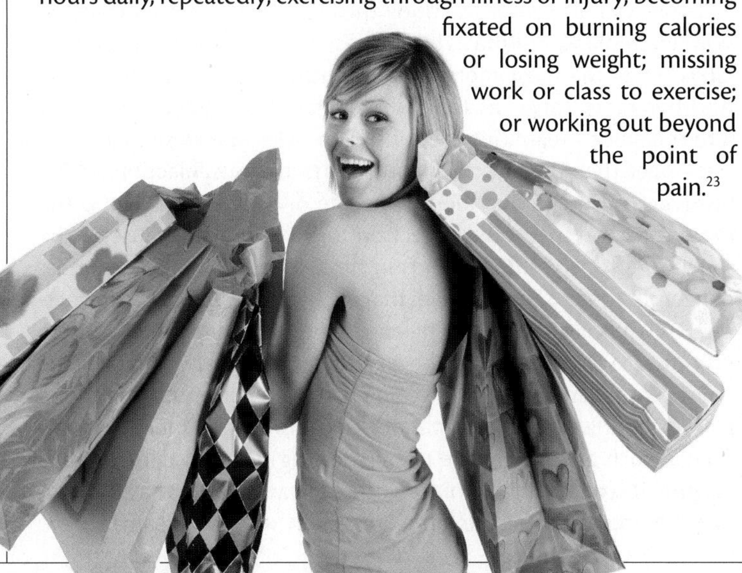

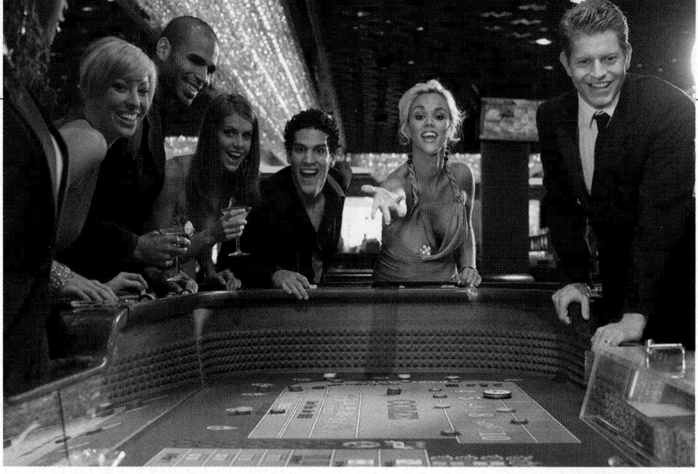

Call, fold, or raise? For increasing numbers of college students, gambling and the debts it can incur are becoming serious problems.

Sexual Addiction

See It! Videos

How do you battle compulsive shopping? Watch **Woman's Shopping Addiction Revealed** in the Study Area of **MasteringHealth**.

Sexual addiction is compulsive involvement in sexual activity. Compulsive sexual behavior may involve a normally enjoyable sexual experience that becomes an obsession, or it may involve fantasies or activities outside the bounds of culturally, legally, or morally acceptable sexual behavior.[24] In fact, people with sexual addictions may be satisfied by masturbation, whether alone or during phone sex or while reading or watching erotica. They may participate in affairs, sex with strangers, prostitution, voyeurism, exhibitionism, rape, incest, and pedophilia. People addicted to sex frequently experience depression and anxiety fueled by fear of discovery. The toll that sexual addiction exacts is seen in loss of intimacy with loved ones, which frequently leads to family disintegration.

Sexual addictions affect men and women of all ages, married and single people, and people of any sexual preference. Most had dysfunctional childhood families, often characterized by addiction. Many were physically, emotionally, and/or sexually abused.

Multiple Addictions

Although addicts tend to have a "favorite" drug or behavior, 55 percent of people in treatment have problems with more than one addiction.[25] For example, alcohol addiction and eating disorders are commonly paired in women, whereas individuals trying to break a chemical dependency frequently resort to compulsive eating. Multiple addictions complicate recovery, but don't make it impossible.

check yourself

- **What is an example of a process addiction?**
- **How can a positive behavior such as exercise become addictive?**

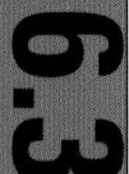

Drug Dynamics

learning **outcome**

6.3 Describe the six major categories of drugs and the interactions that can result from polydrug use.

Most bodily processes result from chemical reactions or changes in electrical charge. Drugs possess an electrical charge and chemical structure similar to those of chemicals occurring naturally in the body and thus can affect physical functions in many ways.

How Drugs Affect the Brain

Pleasure, which scientists call *reward*, is a powerful biological force for survival. If you do something that you experience as pleasurable, the brain is wired so you tend to do it again. Life-sustaining activities, such as eating, activate a circuit of specialized nerve cells devoted to producing and regulating pleasure. One important set of these cells, which uses a chemical neurotransmitter called *dopamine*, sits at the top of the brain stem in the *ventral tegmental area* (*VTA*). Here, dopamine-containing neurons relay messages about pleasure to nerve cells in the limbic system—brain structures that regulate emotions. Still other fibers connect to a related part of the frontal region of the cerebral cortex, the area of the brain that plays a key role in memory, perception, thought, and consciousness. So this "pleasure circuit," the *mesolimbic dopamine* system, spans the survival-oriented brain stem, the emotional limbic system, and the thinking frontal cerebral cortex.

All drugs that are addicting can activate the brain's pleasure circuit. Drug addiction is a biological, pathological process that alters how the pleasure center and other parts of the brain function. Almost all **psychoactive drugs** (those that change the way the brain works) do so by affecting chemical neurotransmission—enhancing, suppressing, or interfering with it. Some drugs, such as heroin and lysergic acid diethylamide (LSD), mimic the effects of natural neurotransmitters. Others, such as phencyclidine (PCP), block receptors, preventing neuronal messages from getting through. Still others, such as cocaine, block neurons' reuptake of neurotransmitters, increasing neurotransmitter concentration in the synaptic gap between individual neurons. Finally, some drugs, such as methamphetamine, act by causing neurotransmitters to be released in greater than normal amounts.

Categories of Drugs

Scientists divide drugs into six categories. Each includes some drugs that stimulate the body, some that depress body functions, and others that produce hallucinations (sensory perceptions that are not real). Each category also includes psychoactive drugs.

- *Prescription drugs* can be obtained only with a prescription from a licensed health care practitioner. Approximately 47 percent of Americans have reported using at least one prescription medication in the past month.[26]
- *Over-the-counter drugs (OTCs)* can be purchased without a prescription. They treat everything from headaches to pain, cold, stomach upsets, and athlete's foot, and provide an important access to medicine. They create substantial savings for the health care system through decreased visits to health care providers and decreased use of prescription medications.[27] However, there is a risk of OTC drugs being used improperly or misused.[28]
- *Recreational drugs* belong to a category whose boundaries depend upon how the term *recreation* is defined. Generally, recreational drugs contain chemicals used to help people relax or socialize. Most, like alcohol, tobacco, and caffeine, are legal even though they are psychoactive.
- *Herbal preparations* encompass approximately 750 substances, including herbal teas and other products of botanical (plant) origin believed to have medicinal properties.
- *Illicit (illegal) drugs* are the most notorious type of drug. Although laws governing their use, possession, cultivation, manufacture, and sale differ from state to state, illicit drugs are generally recognized as harmful. All are psychoactive.
- *Commercial preparations* are the most universally used, yet least commonly recognized, chemical substances. More than 1,000 exist, including seemingly benign items such as perfumes, cosmetics, household cleansers, paints, glues, inks, dyes, and pesticides.

Routes of Drug Administration

Route of administration refers to how a drug is taken into the body. The route of administration largely determines the rapidity of a drug's effect (**Figure 6.2**). The most common is **oral ingestion**—swallowing a tablet, capsule, or liquid. A drug taken orally may not reach the bloodstream for 30 minutes.

Drugs can also enter the body through the respiratory tract via sniffing, smoking, or **inhalation**. Drugs inhaled and absorbed by the lungs travel the most rapidly of all routes of drug administration. Another rapid form of drug administration is **injection** directly into the bloodstream (intravenously), muscles (intramuscularly), or just under the skin (subcutaneously). Intravenous injection, which involves inserting a hypodermic needle directly into a vein, is the most common method of injection for drug users because of the speed of effect (within seconds in most cases). It is also the most dangerous, due to the risk of damaging blood vessels and contracting HIV (human immunodeficiency virus) and hepatitis (a severe liver disease). Drugs can also be absorbed through the skin or tissue lining (**transdermal**)—the nicotine patch is a common example of a drug administered in this manner—or through the mucous membranes, such as those in the nose (snorting) or the vagina or anus (**suppositories**, typically mixed with a waxy medium that melts at body temperature, releasing the drug into the bloodstream).

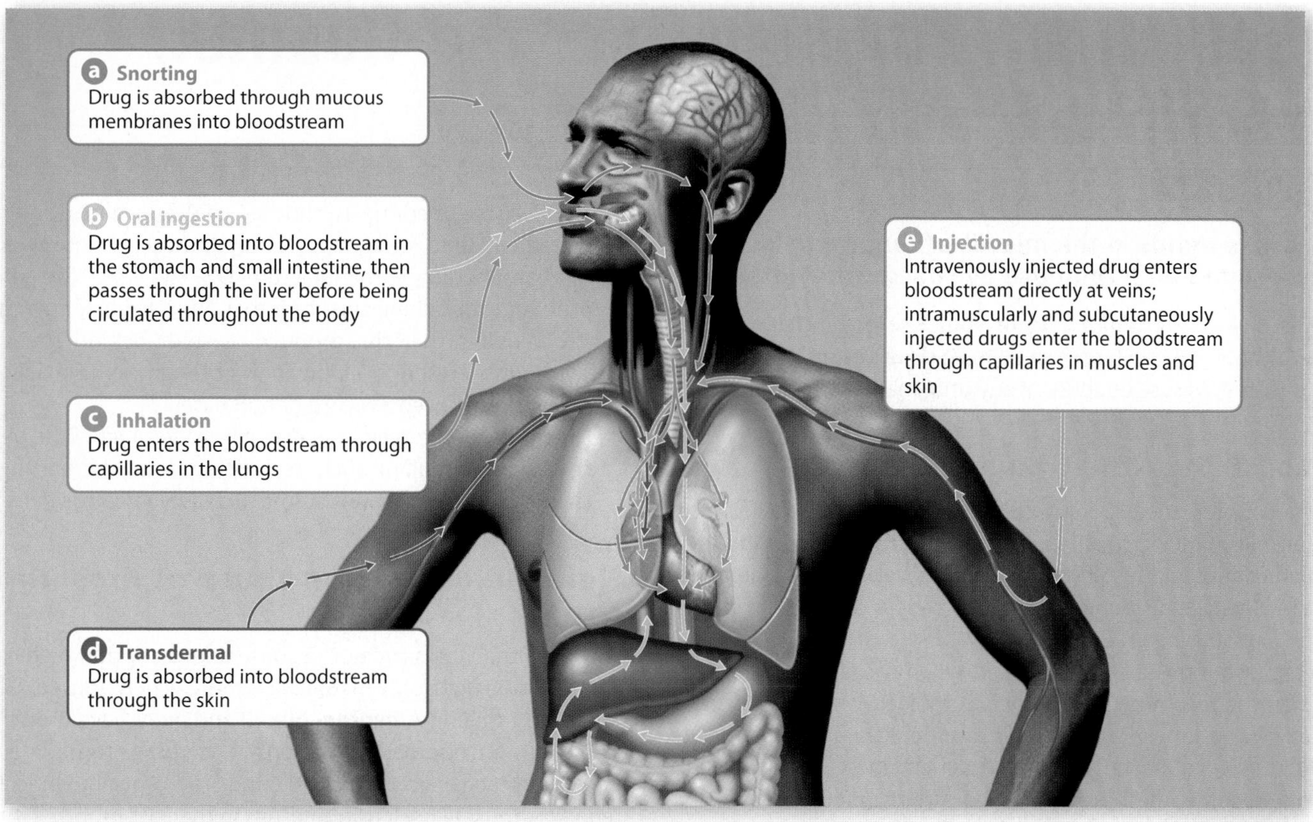

Figure 6.2 Routes of Drug Administration
Drugs are most commonly swallowed, inhaled, or injected. They can also be absorbed through the skin or mucous membranes (as in snorting and suppository use, not shown here).

VIDEO TUTOR
Psychoactive Drugs Acting on the Brain

However a drug enters the system, it eventually finds its way to the bloodstream and is circulated throughout the body to **receptor sites** where chemicals, enzymes, and other substances interact. Psychoactive drugs can cross the blood–brain barrier to reach receptor sites in the brain, where they can affect cognition, emotion, and physiological functioning. Once a drug reaches receptor sites in the brain and other organs, it may remain active for several hours before it dissipates and is carried by the blood to the liver, where it is metabolized (broken down by enzymes). The products of enzymatic breakdown, called *metabolites,* are then excreted, primarily through the kidneys (in urine) or bowels (in feces), but also through the skin (in sweat) or lungs (in expired air).

Drug Interactions

Polydrug use—taking several drugs simultaneously—can lead to dangerous health problems. Alcohol in particular frequently has dangerous interactions with other drugs.

Synergism, also called *potentiation,* is an interaction of two or more drugs in which the effects of the individual drugs are multiplied beyond what would normally be expected if they were taken alone. You might think of synergism as 2 + 2 = 10. A synergistic reaction can be very dangerous and even deadly.

Antagonism, though usually less serious than synergism, can also produce unwanted and unpleasant effects. In an antagonistic reaction, drugs work at the same receptor site; one blocks the action of the other. The blocking drug occupies the receptor site and prevents the other drug from attaching, altering its absorption and action.

With **inhibition**, the effects of one drug are eliminated or reduced by the presence of another drug at the receptor site. **Intolerance** occurs when drugs combine in the body to produce extremely uncomfortable reactions. The drug Antabuse (disulfiram), used to help alcoholics give up alcohol, works by producing this type of interaction. A final type of interaction, **cross-tolerance**, occurs when a person develops a physiological tolerance to one drug and shows a similar tolerance to certain other drugs as a result.

check yourself

- **What are the six major categories of drugs?**
- **What is polydrug use, and what are its risks?**

6.4 Misusing and Abusing Over-the-Counter, Prescription, and Illicit Drugs

learning outcome

6.4 Discuss trends in the misuse of drugs and factors associated with drug use by college students.

Drug misuse involves using a drug for a purpose for which it was not intended. This is not too far removed from **drug abuse**, or excessive use of any drug. Misuse or abuse of any drug may lead to addiction.

Abuse of Over-the-Counter Drugs

Over-the-counter medications come in many different forms, including pills, liquids, nasal sprays, and topical creams. Abusing OTC medications can result in health complications and potential addiction. Teenagers, young adults, and people over 65 are most vulnerable to abusing OTC drugs.

Over-the-counter drugs are abused when the drug is taken in more than the recommended dosage, combined with other drugs, or taken over a longer time than recommended. Tolerance from continued use can create unintended dependence. Teenagers and young adults sometimes abuse OTC medications in search of a cheap high—by drinking large amounts of cough medicine, for instance. Several types of OTC drugs are subject to misuse and abuse:

- **Sleep aids.** In excess, these drugs can cause sleep problems, weaken areas of the body, or induce narcolepsy (excessive, intrusive sleepiness). Continued use can lead to tolerance and dependence.
- **Cold medicines (cough syrups and tablets).** Dextromethorphan (DXM) is present in about 125 OTC medications; as many as 4 percent of high school seniors report taking drugs containing DXM to get high.[29] Large doses can cause hallucinations, loss of motor control, and "out-of-body" sensations. Other effects include impaired judgment, blurred vision, dizziness, paranoia, excessive sweating, slurred speech, irregular heartbeat, and numbness of fingers and toes. Abuse can lead to seizures, brain damage, and death. Some states have passed laws limiting the amount of products containing DXM a person can purchase or prohibiting sale to individuals under 18.[30]

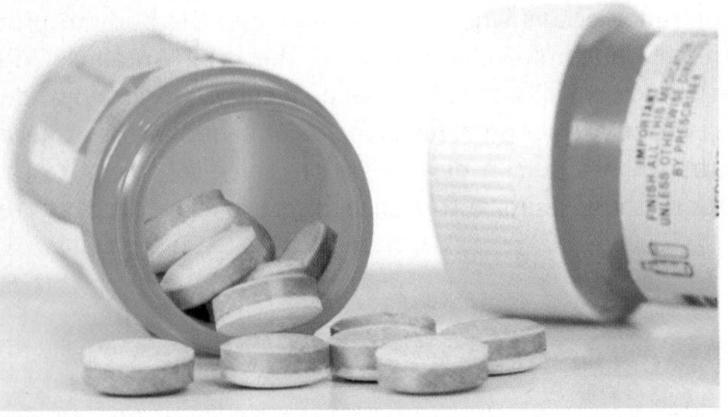

Painkillers such as Percocet, Percodan, Vicodin, and OxyContin are highly addictive.

Pseudoephedrine is another cold and allergy medication ingredient that is frequently abused, most commonly in illegal methamphetamine manufacture. U.S. law limits the amount of products containing this drug that an individual may purchase and requires that the product be sold "behind the counter" (without a prescription, but only through a pharmacist). Pharmacists must keep a record of purchasers.[31]

- **Diet pills.** Some teens use diet pills to get high. Diet pills often contain a stimulant such as caffeine or an herbal ingredient claimed to promote weight loss such as *Hoodia gordonii*.

Nonmedical Use or Abuse of Prescription Drugs

In the United States today, the abuse of prescription medications is at an all-time high; only marijuana is more widely abused.[32] Approximately 6.1 million Americans age 12 and older have used prescription drugs for nonmedical reasons in the past month.[33] In 2012, 3 percent of teenagers age 12 to 17 and 5 percent of people 18 to 25 reported abusing prescription drugs in the past month.[34] The problem may be getting worse, with nearly 15 percent of twelfth-graders reporting abuse of prescription drugs by the time they graduate from high school.[35]

Abusing opioids, narcotics, and pain relievers can result in life-threatening respiratory depression (reduced breathing). Overdoses involving prescription painkillers now kill more Americans than heroine and cocaine combined.[36] Individuals who abuse depressants place themselves at risk of seizures, respiratory depression, and decreased heart rate. Stimulant abuse can cause elevated body temperature, irregular heart rate, cardiovascular system failure, and fatal seizures. Individuals who abuse prescription drugs by injecting them expose themselves to additional risks, including contracting HIV, hepatitis B and C, and other bloodborne viruses.

Prescription drugs are often easier to obtain than illegal ones. In some cases, unscrupulous pharmacists or other medical professionals steal the drugs or sell fraudulent prescriptions. Abusers visit several doctors to obtain multiple prescriptions, fake or exaggerate symptoms to get prescriptions, or call pharmacies with fraudulent prescriptions. Some teenagers and college students who have legitimate prescriptions sell or give away their medications to other students or trade them for others.

College Students and Prescription Drug Abuse College students' prescription drug abuse has increased dramatically over the past decade; 11.8 percent of students surveyed in 2013 reported illegally using one or more prescription drugs in the last year.[37] Many students see prescription drugs as safer than illicit drugs. However, when these drugs are misused, they can be even more unsafe than illegal drugs. Students who illegally use prescription drugs are also more likely to use other illegal drugs and binge drink.[38]

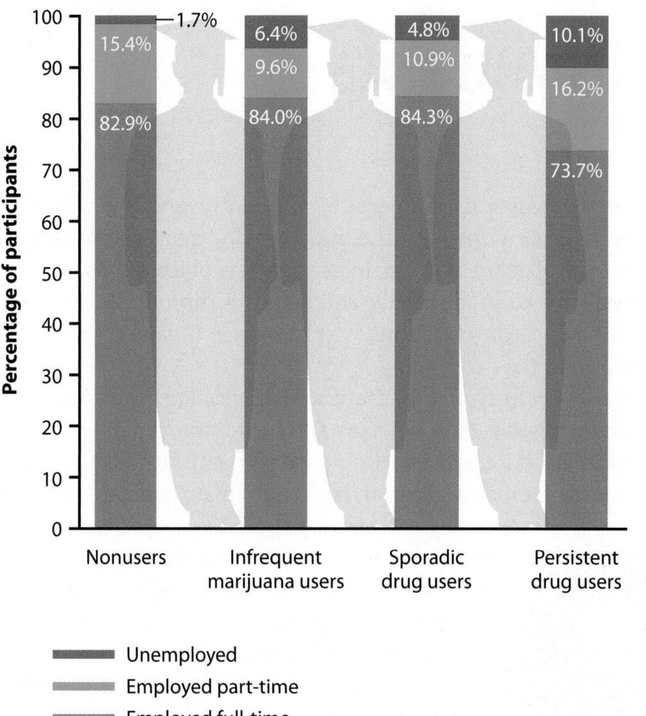

Figure 6.3 Employment After College Based on College Drug Use
Even periodically using drugs increases the chances of unemployment after college.

Source: A. M. Arria, "Drug Use Patterns in Young Adulthood and Post-College Employment," *Drug and Alcohol Dependence* 1, no. 127 (2013): 23–30, DOI: 10.1016/j.drugalcdep.2012.06.001.

One of the most commonly abused prescription drugs on college campuses are painkillers (e.g., OxyContin and Vicodin). Approximately 5.8 percent of students (6.2% of men and 5.5% of women) report using painkillers that were not prescribed to them in the past 12 months.[39] Taking prescription painkillers daily for several weeks is enough time to develop an addiction.

Also of concern is increased abuse of stimulants, such as Adderall and Ritalin, intended to treat attention-deficit/hyperactivity disorder (ADHD). Students primarily report using ADHD drugs for academic gain. Approximately six percent of students (7.1 percent of men and 5.4 percent of women) report using stimulants that were not prescribed to them in the past 12 months.[40] Friends with prescriptions were the most common sources of prescription stimulants.[41]

Illicit Drugs

The problem of illicit drug use touches us all. We may use illicit substances ourselves, watch someone we love struggle with drug abuse, or become the victim of a drug-related crime. At the very least, we are forced to pay increasing taxes for law enforcement and drug rehabilitation. Illicit drug use spans ages, genders, ethnicities, occupations, and socioeconomic groups.

Use of illicit drugs in the United States peaked between 1979 and 1986 and then declined until 1992, and it has since remained stable at around 24 million users per year. Among youth, however, illicit drug use, notably of marijuana, has been rising in recent years.[42]

See It! Videos

Is illegal painkiller use spiraling out of control? Watch **Government Crackdown on Painkillers** in the Study Area of MasteringHealth.

Illicit Drug Use on Campus Illicit drug use has seen a resurgence on college campuses. Close to 50 percent of college-aged students nationwide have tried an illicit drug at some point; the vast majority of them reported using marijuana.[43] Daily use of marijuana is at its highest point since 1989.[44] Cocaine use is down sharply, but LSD use has more than doubled.[45]

College staff are concerned about the link between substance abuse and poor academic performance, depression, anxiety, suicide, vandalism, fights, serious medical problems, and death.[46] A longer-term consequence of illicit drug use among college students is a significantly increased chance of unemployment after college (**Figure 6.3**).

Research has identified factors in a student's life that increase the risk of substance abuse. The more factors, the greater the risk:

- **Positive expectations.** Some students take drugs such as Adderall and Ritalin believing that the drugs will help their ability to study. Many students say they take drugs to relax or reduce stress.
- **Genetics and family history.** These play a significant role in risk for addiction.
- **Substance use in high school.** Two-thirds of college students who use illicit drugs began doing so in high school.[47]
- **Mental health problems.** Students who report being diagnosed with depression are more likely to have abused prescription drugs or to have used marijuana or other illicit drugs.
- **Sorority and fraternity membership.** Being a member of a sorority or fraternity increases the likelihood of using alcohol, marijuana, cocaine, or abusing prescription drugs.
- **Stress.** For some students under academic and social stress, seemingly easy relief comes in the form of drugs or alcohol.

Many factors influence students to avoid drugs; the most commonly reported include these:[48]

- **Parental attitudes and behavior.** Students who are more influenced by their parents' concerns or expectations drink, use marijuana, and smoke significantly less than those less influenced.
- **Religion and spirituality.** The greater students' level of religiosity, the less likely they are to drink, smoke, or use other drugs.
- **Student engagement.** The more a student is involved in learning and extracurricular activities, the less likely he or she is to binge drink, use marijuana, or abuse prescription drugs.
- **College athletics.** College athletes drink at higher rates than nonathletes but are less likely to use illicit drugs.

check yourself

- **What are recent trends in how college students misuse and abuse drugs?**
- **What factors increase or decrease a college student's risk of substance abuse?**
- **Just because a drug is legal, does that mean it's safe? Explain your answer.**

6.5 Common Drugs of Abuse: Stimulants

learning outcome

6.5 Discuss the effects and health risks of stimulants that are commonly misused or abused.

Hundreds of drugs are subject to abuse—some are legal, such as recreational drugs and prescription medications, whereas many others are illegal and classified as "controlled substances." Some of the drugs of most concern are stimulants, marijuana, depressants, hallucinogens, inhalants, and anabolic steroids.

Stimulants

A **stimulant** is a drug that increases activity of the central nervous system. Its effects usually involve increased activity, anxiety, and agitation; users often seem jittery or nervous while high. Commonly used illegal stimulants include cocaine, amphetamines, and methamphetamine. Legal stimulants include caffeine and nicotine.

Caffeine is a legal stimulant.

Cocaine A white crystalline powder derived from the leaves of the South American coca shrub (not related to cocoa plants), *cocaine* ("coke") has been described as one of the most powerful naturally occurring stimulants.

Cocaine can be taken in several ways, including snorting, smoking, and injecting. The powdered form is snorted through the nose, which can damage mucous membranes and cause sinusitis. It can destroy the user's sense of smell, and occasionally it even eats a hole through the septum. When snorted, the drug enters the bloodstream through the lungs in less than 1 minute and reaches the brain in less than 3 minutes. It binds at receptor sites in the central nervous system, producing an intense high that usually disappears quickly, leaving a powerful craving for more.

Cocaine alkaloid, or *freebase*, is obtained by removing the hydrochloride salt from cocaine powder. *Freebasing* refers to smoking freebase by placing it at the end of a pipe and holding a flame near it to produce a vapor, which is then inhaled. *Crack* is identical pharmacologically to freebase, but the hydrochloride salt is still present and is processed with baking soda and water. It is a cheap, widely available drug that is smokable and very potent. Crack is commonly smoked in the same manner as freebase. Because crack is such a pure drug, it takes little time to achieve the desired high, and a crack user can become addicted quickly.

Some cocaine users inject the drug intravenously, which introduces large amounts into the body rapidly, creating a brief, intense high and subsequent crash. Injecting users place themselves at risk not only for contracting HIV and hepatitis through shared needles, but also for skin infections, vein damage, inflamed arteries, and infection of the heart lining.

Cocaine is both an anesthetic and a central nervous system stimulant. In tiny doses, it can slow the heart rate. In larger doses, the physical effects are dramatic: increased heart rate and blood pressure, loss of appetite that can lead to dramatic weight loss, convulsions, muscle twitching, irregular heartbeat, and even death resulting from an overdose. Other effects of cocaine include temporary relief of depression, decreased fatigue, talkativeness, increased alertness, and heightened self-confidence. However, as the dose increases, users become irritable and apprehensive, and their behavior may turn paranoid or violent.

Amphetamines The **amphetamines** include a large and varied group of synthetic agents that stimulate the central nervous system. Small doses of amphetamines improve alertness, lessen fatigue, and generally elevate mood. With repeated use, however, physical and psychological dependencies develop. Sleep patterns are affected (insomnia); heart rate, breathing rate, and blood pressure increase; and restlessness, anxiety, appetite suppression, and vision problems are common. High doses over long periods of time can produce hallucinations, delusions, and disorganized behavior.

Certain types of amphetamines or amphetamine-like drugs are used for medicinal purposes. As discussed earlier, drugs prescribed to treat ADHD are stimulants and are increasingly abused on campus.

Methamphetamine An increasingly common form of amphetamine, *methamphetamine* (commonly called "meth") is a potent, long-acting, addictive drug that strongly activates the brain's reward center by producing a sense of euphoria. Over 439,000 Americans are regular users of methamphetamine, and it is believed that more than 12 million Americans have tried it.[49] In 2012, about 2 percent of high school seniors reported using

Methamphetamine users often damage their teeth beyond repair because of the toxic chemicals in the substance. This condition is commonly referred to as "meth mouth."

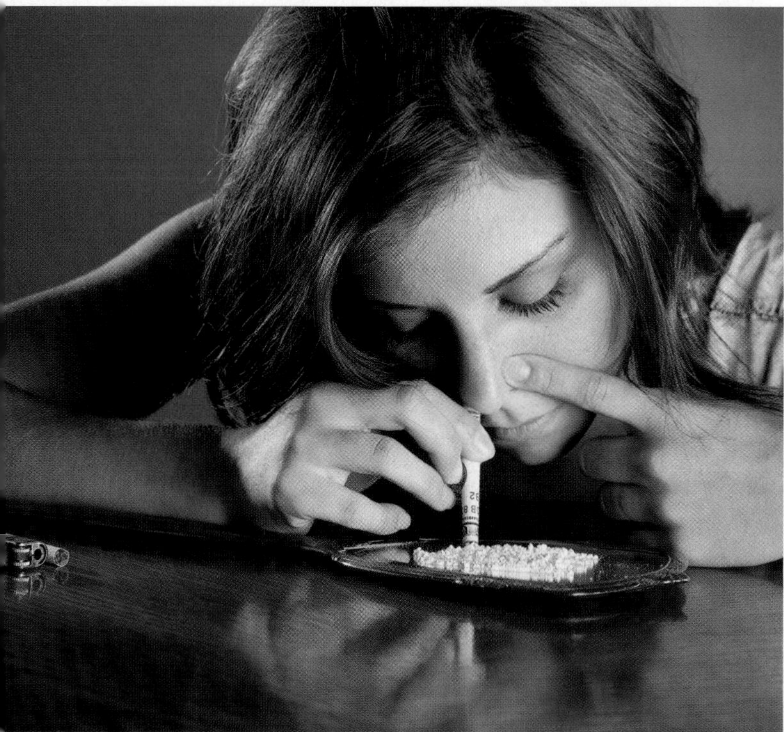

Although cocaine use has declined from its peak in the 1980s, it continues to be a commonly abused illicit drug.

methamphetamine in their lifetime.[50] The rate of methamphetamine use may be increasing because it is relatively easy to make. Recipes often include common OTC ingredients such as ephedrine and pseudoephedrine.

In the short term, methamphetamine produces increased physical activity, alertness, euphoria, rapid breathing, increased body temperature, insomnia, tremors, anxiety, confusion, and decreased appetite; the drug's effects quickly wear off, leaving the user seeking more.

Methamphetamine can be snorted, smoked, injected, or orally ingested. When snorted, the effects can be felt in 3 to 5 minutes; if orally ingested, effects occur within 15 to 20 minutes. The pleasurable effects of methamphetamine are typically an intense rush lasting only a few minutes when snorted; in contrast, smoking the drug can produce a high lasting more than 8 hours. Users often experience tolerance after the first use, making methamphetamine a highly addictive drug.

Methamphetamine increases the release and blocks the reuptake of the neurotransmitter dopamine, leading to high levels of the chemical in the brain. This action occurs rapidly and produces the intense euphoria, or "rush," that many users feel. Over time, methamphetamine destroys dopamine receptors, making it impossible to feel pleasure. Due to the destruction of dopamine receptors, people who abuse methamphetamine (or cocaine) are at increased risk for developing Parkinson's disease later in life.[51]

Other long-term effects of methamphetamine can include severe weight loss, cardiovascular damage, increased risk of heart attack and stroke, hallucinations, extensive tooth decay and tooth loss, violence, paranoia, psychotic behavior, and even death. Recent studies of chronic methamphetamine abusers have revealed severe structural and functional changes in areas of the brain associated with emotion and memory, which may account for the emotional and cognitive problems observed in chronic methamphetamine abusers. Some of these changes persist after the methamphetamine abuse has stopped. Other changes reverse after sustained periods of abstinence from methamphetamine, typically longer than a year, but problems often remain.

Caffeine Unlike cocaine and methamphetamine, **caffeine** is a legal stimulant. More than half of all Americans drink coffee every day, and many others consume caffeine in some other form, making it the most popular and widely consumed drug in the United States.[52] Coffee, tea, soft drinks, chocolate, and other caffeine-containing products are loved for their wake-up effects. Caffeine may be commonplace, but excessive consumption is associated with addiction and certain health problems.

Caffeine is derived from the chemical family called *xanthines*, which are found in plant products from which coffee, tea, and chocolate are made. The xanthines are mild central nervous system stimulants that enhance mental alertness and reduce feelings of fatigue. Other stimulant effects include increased heart muscle contractions, oxygen consumption, metabolism, and urinary output. Side effects of the xanthines include wakefulness, insomnia, irregular heartbeat, dizziness, nausea, indigestion, and sometimes mild delirium. Some people also experience heartburn. A person feels these effects within 15 to 45 minutes of ingesting a caffeinated product. It takes 4 to 6 hours for the body to metabolize half of the caffeine ingested, so, depending on the amount of caffeine taken in, it may continue to exert effects for a day or longer.

As the effects of caffeine wear off, frequent users may feel let down—mentally or physically depressed, exhausted, and weak. To counteract this, they commonly choose to drink another cup of coffee. Habitually engaging in this practice leads to tolerance and psychological dependence. Symptoms of excessive caffeine consumption include chronic insomnia, jitters, irritability, nervousness, anxiety, and involuntary muscle twitches. Withdrawing from caffeine may compound the effects and produce headaches, fatigue, and nausea. Because caffeine meets the requirements for addiction—tolerance, psychological dependence, and withdrawal symptoms—it can be classified as addictive.

Long-term caffeine use has been suspected of being linked to several serious health problems. However, no strong evidence exists to suggest that moderate caffeine use (less than 300 mg, or approximately 3 cups or less of regular coffee, a day) produces harmful effects in healthy, nonpregnant people. For most people, caffeine poses few health risks and may actually have some benefits. Drinking coffee has been associated with lower prostate cancer rates in men, lower depression rates among women, and lower risk of stroke for both men and women. Caffeine may also protect against Alzheimer's disease, Parkinson's disease, liver disease, and some additional types of cancer.[53]

check yourself

- **What is a stimulant?**
- **What are the effects and health risks of commonly abused stimulants?**
- **Compare caffeine to illicit stimulants.**

6.6 Common Drugs of Abuse: Marijuana

learning outcome

6.6 Discuss the effects and health risks of marijuana.

Although archaeological evidence indicates that **marijuana** ("grass," "weed," "pot") was used as long as 6,000 years ago, the drug did not become popular in the United States until the 1960s. Today, marijuana is the most commonly used illicit drug in the country. Approximately 43 percent of Americans over the age of 12 have tried marijuana at least once,[54] some 32 million have used marijuana in the past year, and more than 19 million have done so in the past month. Marijuana use is on the rise on college campuses, following the trend of increased use in the general population.[55]

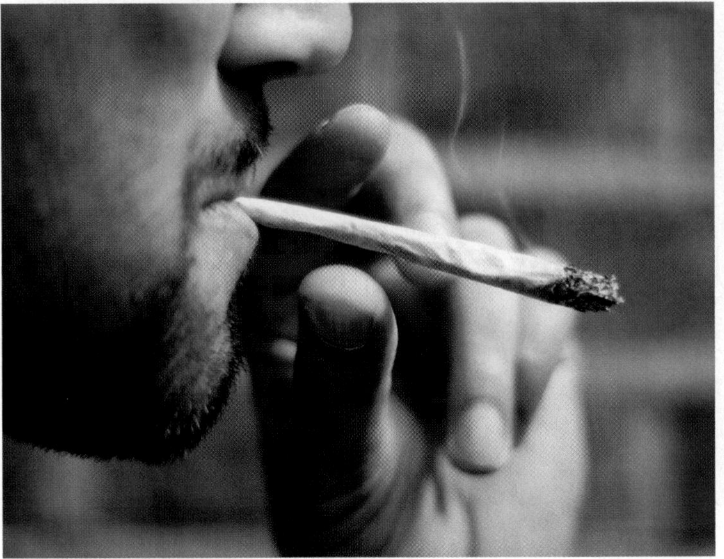

Methods of Use and Physical Effects

Marijuana is derived from either the *Cannabis sativa* or *Cannabis indica* (hemp) plant. Most of the time, marijuana is smoked, although it can also be ingested, as in brownies baked with marijuana in them. When marijuana is smoked, it is usually rolled into cigarettes (joints) or placed in a pipe or water pipe (bong).

Tetrahydrocannabinol (THC) is the psychoactive substance in marijuana and the key to determining how powerful a high it will produce. More potent forms of the drug can contain up to 27 percent THC, but most average 15 percent.[56] *Hashish*, a potent cannabis preparation derived mainly from the plant's thick, sticky resin, contains high THC concentrations. Hash oil, a substance produced by percolating a solvent such as ether through dried marijuana to extract the THC, is a tar-like liquid that may contain up to 300 mg of THC in a dose.

The effects of smoking marijuana are generally felt within 10 to 30 minutes and usually wear off within 3 hours. The most noticeable visible effect of THC is dilation of the eyes' blood vessels, which gives the smoker bloodshot eyes. Marijuana smokers also exhibit coughing; dry mouth and throat ("cotton mouth"); increased thirst and appetite; lowered blood pressure; and mild muscular weakness, primarily exhibited in drooping eyelids. Users can also experience severe anxiety, panic, paranoia, and psychosis and may have intensified reactions to various stimuli—colors, sounds, and the speed at which things move may seem altered. High doses of hashish may produce vivid visual hallucinations.

Marijuana and Driving

Marijuana use presents clear hazards for drivers of motor vehicles and others on the road with them. The drug substantially reduces a driver's ability to react and make quick decisions. Perceptual and other performance deficits may persist for some time after the high subsides. Users who attempt to drive, fly, or operate heavy machinery often fail to recognize their impairment. Overall, marijuana is the most prevalent illegal drug detected in impaired drivers, fatally injured drivers, and motor vehicle crash victims.[57] Recent research indicates you are two and a half times more likely to be involved in a motor vehicle accident if you drive under the influence of marijuana.[58] Combining even a low dose of marijuana with alcohol enhances the impairing effects of both drugs.

Effects of Chronic Marijuana Use

Because marijuana has been widely used only since the 1960s, long-term studies of its effects have been difficult to conduct. Also, studies conducted in the 1960s involved marijuana with THC levels only a fraction of today's levels; their results may not apply to stronger forms available today.

Marijuana smoke contains 50 to 70 percent more carcinogenic hydrocarbons than does tobacco smoke. Because marijuana smokers typically inhale more deeply and hold their breath longer than tobacco smokers, the lungs are exposed to more carcinogens. Likewise, effects from irritation (e.g., cough, excessive phlegm, and increased lung infections) similar to those experienced by tobacco smokers can occur.[59] Lung conditions such as chronic bronchitis, emphysema, and other lung disorders are also associated with smoking marijuana.

Inhaling marijuana smoke introduces carbon monoxide into the bloodstream. Because the blood has a greater affinity for carbon monoxide than it does for oxygen, its oxygen-carrying capacity is diminished; the heart must work harder to pump oxygen to oxygen-starved tissues. Furthermore, the tar from cannabis contains higher levels of carcinogens than does tobacco smoke.

Study results show that frequent and/or long-term marijuana use may significantly increase a man's risk of developing testicular cancer. The risk is particularly elevated (about twice that of those who never smoked marijuana) for those who use marijuana at least weekly or who have long-term exposure to the substance beginning in adolescence. The results also suggested that the association with marijuana use might be limited to *nonseminoma*, an aggressive, fast-growing testicular malignancy that tends to strike early, between ages 20 and 35, and accounts for about 40 percent of all testicular cancer cases.[60]

The link between marijuana and common mental health disorders is somewhat conflicting, because marijuana is said to potentially cause as well as relieve symptoms of depression and anxiety. While marijuana may ease the symptoms of depression, depression may actually worsen once the positive effects wear off.[61] Marijuana users are more likely to suffer from depression and depressive symptoms than nonusers, with risk increasing for people using both marijuana and alcohol.[62]

Some research suggests that frequent or heavy use of marijuana during adolescence may be associated with developing anxiety disorders in young adulthood.[63] Certain personality disorders, interpersonal violence, and suicidal ideation are also correlated with marijuana use. In general, the younger marijuana use started, the greater the risk of eventually developing a mental health disorder.[64]

Other risks associated with marijuana use include suppression of the immune system, blood pressure changes, impaired memory function, and disrupted sleep. Pregnant women who smoke marijuana may have children who have subtle brain changes that can cause cognitive difficulties, and marijuana use can more than double the risk of giving birth prematurely.[65]

Legalization of Marijuana and Medicinal Uses

Although recognized as a dangerous drug by the U.S. government, marijuana has been legalized for medicinal uses in 23 states and the District of Columbia. While marijuana's legal status for medicinal purposes continues to be hotly debated, marijuana has several medical purposes. Marijuana also reduces the muscle pain and spasticity caused by diseases such as multiple sclerosis.

Medications that harness therapeutic benefits of cannabinoids (the active chemicals in marijuana) while reducing or eliminating side effects have been developed. FDA-approved drugs **dronabinol** (Marinol) and **nabilone** (Cesamet) both contain THC and are used to lessen the chemotherapy-induced nausea, as well as the effects of wasting disease (extreme weight loss) caused by AIDS. A drug called **Sativex** is currently moving through clinical trials in the United States as an option for treating cancer pain. Although not yet FDA tested or approved, another drug, **Epidiolex**, has been developed for the treatment of different types of childhood epilepsy.[66]

Voters in Washington and Colorado recently passed ballot initiatives to legalize marijuana for recreational use and it is on the ballot for possible legalization in other states such as Oregon. Many arguments have been made for legalization, including the revenue boost to state and local governments (Colorado will receive an estimated $99 million in tax revenues from marijuana); more effective law enforcement and criminal justice since police officers will have more time and money to pursue criminals for other crimes; a decrease in the violence associated with selling marijuana as a result of cutting off revenue streams to organized crime; and safety controls that help eliminate the risk of smoking marijuana potentially laced with toxic substances.[67]

On the other side of the coin, people have argued that marijuana is addictive—with research suggesting that as many as 10 percent of users will develop dependence over time. Additionally, others have suggested marijuana alters the way users perceive things while under the influence; can be a gateway drug with the potential to introduce users to more serious illegal substances; and has negative health impacts as a result of high levels of carcinogens, ability to raise heart rate, and links to mental health issues such as depression, anxiety, and suicidal ideation.[68]

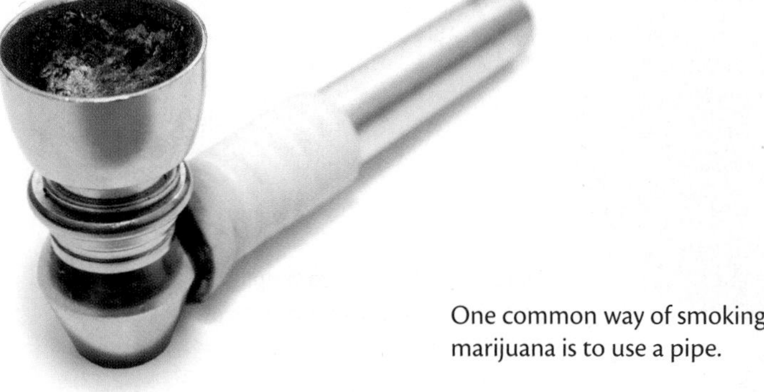

One common way of smoking marijuana is to use a pipe.

Synthetic Marijuana

Synthetic marijuana is used to describe a diverse family of herbal blends marketed under many names, including K2, spice, fake marijuana, Yucatan Fire, Skunk, Moon Rocks, and others. These products contain dried, shredded plant material and one or more synthetic cannabinoids, with results that mimic marijuana intoxication but with longer duration and poor detection on urine drug screens. K2 is sold legally as herbal blend incense; however, it is smoked by people to gain effects similar to marijuana, hashish, and other forms of cannabis.[69]

K2 is used by nearly 1 in 10 college students; students who reported using K2 were more likely to have smoked cigarettes, marijuana, and hookahs. It is also gaining more attention among high school seniors, with reports that 1 in every 9 high school seniors are using this drug.[70]

People smoking K2 may experience several adverse health effects such as hallucinations, severe agitation, extremely elevated heart rate and blood pressure, coma, suicide attempts, and drug dependence, which is not common among cannabis users. Emergency departments are also reporting a significant increase in the numbers of people being treated for K2 use.[71]

check yourself

- **What are the effects and health risks of marijuana?**
- **How is marijuana used for medicinal purposes?**
- **What are the differences between marijuana and synthetic marijuana?**

6.7

Common Drugs of Abuse: Depressants and Narcotics

learning outcome

6.7 Discuss the effects and health risks of depressants and narcotics that are commonly misused or abused.

Whereas central nervous system stimulants increase muscular and nervous system activity, **depressants** have the opposite effect. These drugs slow down neuromuscular activity and cause sleepiness or calmness. If the dose is high enough, brain function can stop, causing death. Alcohol is the most widely used central nervous system depressant; others include opioids, benzodiazepines, and barbiturates.

Benzodiazepines and Barbiturates

A *sedative* drug promotes mental calmness and reduces anxiety, whereas a *hypnotic* drug promotes sleep or drowsiness. The most common sedative-hypnotic drugs are **benzodiazepines**, more commonly known as *tranquilizers.* These include prescription drugs such as Valium, Ativan, and Xanax. Benzodiazepines are most commonly prescribed for tension, muscular strain, sleep problems, anxiety, panic attacks, and alcohol withdrawal. **Barbiturates** are sedative-hypnotic drugs that include Amytal and Seconal. Today, benzodiazepines have largely replaced barbiturates, which were used medically in the past for relieving tension and inducing relaxation and sleep.

Sedative-hypnotics have a synergistic effect when combined with alcohol, another central nervous system depressant. Taken together, these drugs can lead to respiratory failure and death. All sedative or hypnotic drugs can produce physical and psychological dependence in several weeks. A complication specific to sedatives is cross-tolerance, which occurs when users develop tolerance for one sedative or become dependent on it and develop tolerance for others as well. Withdrawal from sedative or hypnotic drugs may range from mild discomfort to severe symptoms, depending on the degree of dependence.

Rohypnol One benzodiazepine of concern is Rohypnol, a potent tranquilizer similar in nature to Valium but many times stronger. The drug produces a sedative effect, amnesia, muscle relaxation, and slowed psychomotor responses. The most publicized "date rape" drug, Rohypnol has gained notoriety as a growing problem on college campuses. The drug has been added to punch and other drinks at parties, where it is reportedly given to women in hopes of lowering their inhibitions and facilitating potential sexual conquests.

GHB

Gamma-hydroxybutyrate (GHB) is a central nervous system depressant known to have euphoric, sedative, and anabolic (bodybuilding) effects. It was originally sold over the counter to bodybuilders to help reduce body fat and build muscle. The FDA banned OTC sales of GHB in 1992, and it is now a Schedule I controlled substance.[72] GHB is an odorless, tasteless fluid that can be made easily at home or in a chemistry lab. Like Rohypnol, GHB has been slipped into drinks without being detected, resulting in loss of memory, unconsciousness, amnesia, and even death. Other dangerous side effects include nausea, vomiting, seizures, hallucinations, coma, and respiratory distress.

Opioids (Narcotics)

Opioids cause drowsiness, relieve pain, and produce euphoria. Also called *narcotics,* opioids are derived from the parent drug **opium**, a dark, resinous substance made from the milky juice of the opium poppy seedpod. All opioids are highly addictive. Opium and heroin are both illegal in the United States, but some opioids are available by prescription for medical purposes: Morphine is sometimes prescribed for severe pain, and codeine is found in prescription cough syrups and other painkillers.

Synthetic Opioids Several prescription drugs, including the painkillers Vicodin, Percodan, OxyContin, Demerol, and Dilaudid, contain synthetic opioids. College students are increasingly abusing these drugs; a 2012 study found that approximately 3.8 percent of college students had used Vicodin and 1.2 percent used OxyContin without a doctor's prescription in the past year.[73] These prescription painkillers are highly addictive. OxyContin, in particular, can be a highly addictive and dangerous narcotic when abused. The "rush" is similar to that of heroin. In fact, it's common for people who are addicted to OxyContin to turn to heroin when they can't afford to buy OxyContin. Chronic use can also result in increasing tolerance, as more of the drug is needed to achieve the desired effect.

Physical Effects of Opioids Opioids are powerful depressants of the central nervous system. In addition to relieving pain, these drugs lower heart rate, respiration, and blood pressure. Side effects include weakness, dizziness, nausea, vomiting, euphoria, decreased sex drive, visual disturbances, and lack of coordination.

Opium is extracted from opium poppy seedpods like this one.

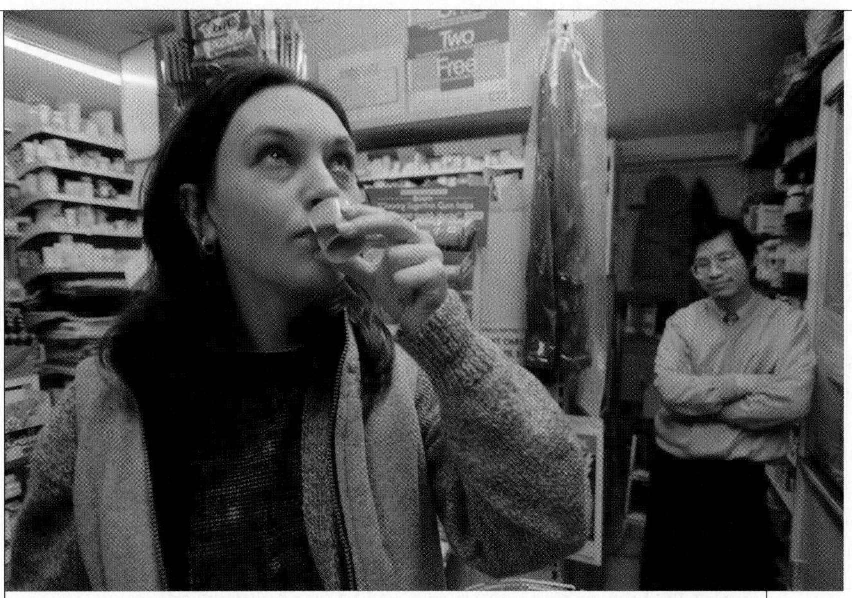

Why is it so hard to quit using heroin?

Heroin's effect on the body is similar to the painless well-being created by endorphins. Stopping heroin use causes withdrawal symptoms that are very difficult to withstand or tolerate, which keeps many addicts from attempting to quit. Methadone is a synthetic narcotic that blocks the effects of withdrawal. Although it is still a narcotic and must be administered under the supervision of clinic or pharmacy staff, methadone allows many heroin addicts to lead somewhat normal lives.

The human body's physiology could be said to make us particularly susceptible to opioid addiction. Opioid-like hormones called **endorphins** are manufactured in the body and have multiple receptor sites, particularly in the central nervous system. When endorphins attach themselves at these sites, they create feelings of painless well-being; medical researchers refer to them as "the body's own opioids." When endorphin levels are high, people feel euphoric. The same euphoria occurs when opioids or related chemicals are active at the endorphin receptor sites. Of all the opioids, heroin has the greatest notoriety as an addictive drug. The following section discusses the progression of heroin addiction; addiction to any opioid follows a similar path.

Heroin Use *Heroin* is a white powder derived from morphine. *Black tar heroin* is a sticky, dark brown, foul-smelling form of heroin that is relatively pure and inexpensive. Once considered a cure for morphine dependence, heroin was later discovered to be even more addictive and potent than morphine. Today, heroin has no medical use.

10.3 million people reported driving under the influence of illicit drugs in the past year.

Heroin is a depressant that produces drowsiness and a dreamy, mentally slow feeling. It can cause drastic mood swings, with euphoric highs followed by depressive lows. Heroin slows respiration and urinary output and constricts the pupils of the eyes. Symptoms of tolerance and withdrawal can appear within 3 weeks of first use.

In 2012, 669,000 Americans reported using heroin in the past year, a considerable increase since 2002.[74] This trend appears to be driven largely by 18- to 25-year-olds, among whom there have been the largest increases. This younger age group may be more likely to purchase heroin since it is both cheaper and generally easier to obtain than prescription opioids.

The most common route of administration for heroin addicts is "mainlining"—intravenous injection of powdered heroin mixed in a solution—though the contemporary version of heroin is so potent that users can get high by snorting or smoking the drug. This has attracted a more affluent group of users who may not want to inject, for reasons such as the increased risk of contracting diseases such as HIV. Still, it is estimated that within 2–3 weeks of beginning snorting or smoking, the majority of users experience an increase in tolerance and begin injecting their heroin.

Many users describe the "rush" they feel when injecting themselves as intensely pleasurable, whereas others report unpredictable and unpleasant side effects. The temporary nature of the rush contributes to the drug's high potential for addiction—many addicts shoot up four or five times a day. Mainlining can cause veins to scar and eventually collapse. Once a vein has collapsed, it can no longer be used to introduce heroin into the bloodstream. Addicts become expert at locating new veins to use: in the feet, the legs, the temples, under the tongue, or in the groin.

Heroin addicts experience a distinct pattern of withdrawal. Symptoms of withdrawal include intense desire for the drug, sleep disturbance, dilated pupils, loss of appetite, irritability, goose bumps, and muscle tremors. The most difficult time in the withdrawal process occurs 24 to 72 hours following last use. All of the preceding symptoms continue, along with nausea, abdominal cramps, restlessness, insomnia, vomiting, diarrhea, extreme anxiety, hot and cold flashes, elevated blood pressure, and rapid heartbeat and respiration. Once the peak of withdrawal has passed, all these symptoms begin to subside.

check yourself

- **What is a depressant?**
- **What are the effects and health risks of commonly abused depressants?**
- **Why has use of heroin increased so dramatically in recent years?**

Common Drugs of Abuse: Hallucinogens

learning outcome

6.8 Discuss the effects and health risks of hallucinogens that are commonly misused or abused.

Hallucinogens, or *psychedelics*, are substances capable of creating auditory or visual hallucinations and unusual changes in mood, thoughts, and feelings.

Major receptor sites for hallucinogens are in the reticular formation (located in the brain stem at the upper end of the spinal cord), which is responsible for interpreting outside stimuli before allowing these signals to travel to other parts of the brain. When a hallucinogen is present at a reticular formation site, messages become scrambled; the user may see wavy walls instead of straight ones or, in a mixing of sensory messages known as *synesthesia*, "smell" colors and "hear" tastes. Users may also become less inhibited or recall events long buried in the subconscious mind.

LSD

First synthesized in the late 1930s, *lysergic acid diethylamide* (*LSD*) received media attention in the 1960s when young people used it to "turn on and tune out." In 1970, federal authorities placed LSD on the list of controlled substances (Schedule I).

Today, LSD, or "acid," has been making a comeback. It is estimated that 6 percent of Americans aged 18 to 25 have used LSD at least once.[75] A national survey of college students showed that 3 percent had used the drug.[76]

The most popular form is blotter acid—small squares of paper impregnated with LSD that are swallowed or chewed. LSD also comes in gelatin squares called *windowpane* and tiny tablets called *microdots*.

One of the most powerful drugs known to science, LSD can produce strong effects in doses as low as 20 micrograms (μg). (A postage stamp weighs 60,000 μg.) The potency of a typical dose currently ranges from 20 to 80 μg, compared to 150 to 300 μg commonly used in the 1960s.

Depending on the quantity users have eaten, LSD usually takes 20 to 60 minutes to take effect and can last 6 to 8 hours. Psychological effects of LSD vary. Euphoria is common, but dysphoria (a sense of evil and foreboding) may also be experienced. LSD also causes distortions of perception and auditory or visual hallucinations. Thoughts may be interposed so the user experiences several thoughts simultaneously. Users become introspective, and suppressed memories may surface. Other possible effects include decreased aggressiveness and enhanced sensory experiences.

Physical effects include increased heart rate, elevated blood pressure, muscle twitches, perspiration, chills, headaches, and mild nausea. Because the drug also stimulates uterine muscle contractions, it can lead to premature labor and miscarriage in pregnant women. Research into long-term effects has been inconclusive.

Although there is no evidence that LSD creates physical dependency, it may well create psychological dependence. Many users become depressed for 1 or 2 days following a trip and turn to the drug to relieve this depression. The result is a cycle of LSD use to relieve post-LSD depression, which can lead to psychological addiction.

Ecstasy

Ecstasy is the most common name for the drug *methylene-dioxymethamphetamine* (*MDMA*), a synthetic compound with stimulant and mildly hallucinogenic effects. It is one of the most well-known **club drugs** or "designer drugs," synthetic analogs of illicit drugs popular at nightclubs and all-night parties. Ecstasy creates feelings of extreme euphoria, increased willingness to communicate, feelings of warmth and empathy, and heightened appreciation for music. Like other hallucinogenics, Ecstasy can enhance sensory experience and distort perceptions, but it does not create visual hallucinations. Effects begin within 20 to 90 minutes and can last for 3 to 5 hours.

Some of the risks associated with Ecstasy use are similar to those of other stimulants. Because of the nature of the drug, Ecstasy users are at greater risk of inappropriate or unintended emotional bonding. Physical consequences may include jaw clenching, short-term memory loss or confusion, increased body temperature as a result of dehydration and heat stroke, and increased heart rate and blood pressure. Combined with alcohol, Ecstasy can be extremely dangerous and sometimes fatal. As the effects begin to wear off, the user can experience mild depression, fatigue, and a hangover that can last from days to weeks. Chronic use appears to damage the brain's ability to think and to regulate emotion, memory, sleep, and pain. Some studies indicate that the drug may cause long-lasting neurotoxic effects by damaging brain cells that produce serotonin.[77]

MDMA in powder or crystal form—called "Molly"—has become a popular festival drug. Unlike Ecstasy, which tends to be laced with ingredients like caffeine or methamphetamine, Molly is considered pure MDMA. Still, many powders sold as Molly contain zero actual MDMA. Typical side effects include teeth grinding, dehydration, anxious feelings, sleep troubles, fever, appetite loss, uncontrollable seizures, elevated blood pressure, high body temperature, and depression.[78]

Psilocybe mushrooms produce hallucinogenic effects when ingested.

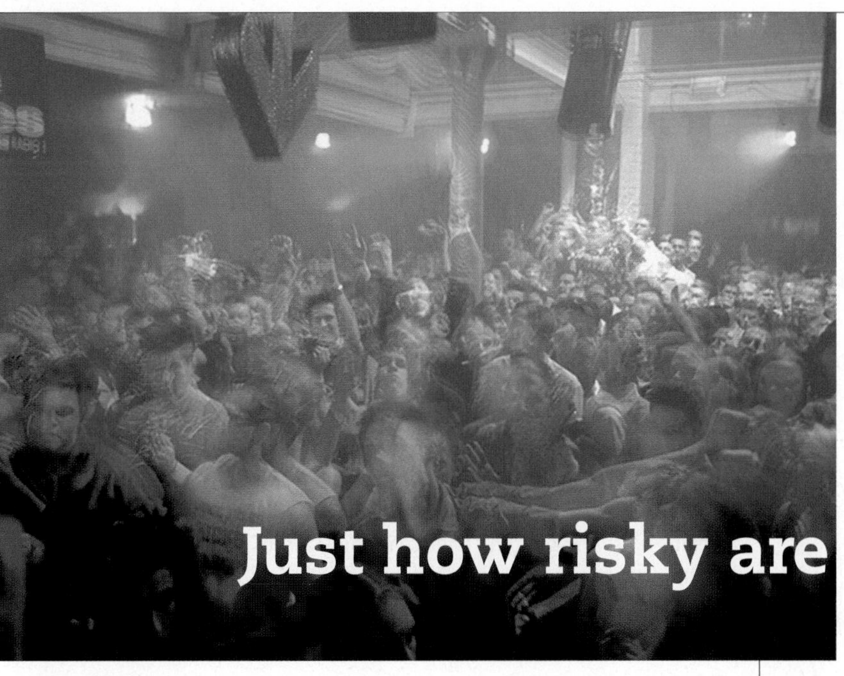

So-called "club drugs" are a varied group of synthetic drugs, including Ecstasy, GHB, ketamine, Rohypnol, and methamphetamine, that are often abused by teens and young adults at nightclubs, bars, or all-night dances. The sources and chemicals used to make these drugs vary, so dosages are unpredictable and the drugs may not be "pure." Although users may think them relatively harmless, research has shown that club drugs can produce hallucinations, paranoia, amnesia, dangerous increases in heart rate and blood pressure, coma, and in some cases, death. Some club drugs work on the same brain mechanisms as alcohol and can be particularly dangerous when used in combination with alcohol. In addition, some club drugs can be easily slipped into unsuspecting partygoers' drinks, facilitating sexual assault and other crimes.

Just how risky are "club drugs"?

Mescaline

Mescaline is both a powerful hallucinogen and a central nervous system stimulant. Products sold on the street as mescaline are likely to be synthetic relatives of the true drug.

Users typically swallow 10 to 12 buttons. They taste bitter and generally induce immediate nausea or vomiting. Those able to keep the drug down feel its effects within 30 to 90 minutes. Effects may persist for up to 9 or 10 hours.

Psilocybin

Psilocybin and *psilocin* are the active chemicals in a group of mushrooms sometimes called "magic mushrooms." Psilocybe mushrooms, which grow throughout the world, can be cultivated from spores or harvested wild. When consumed, they can cause hallucinations. Because many mushrooms resemble the psilocybe variety, people who harvest wild mushrooms for any purpose should be certain of what they are doing. Mushroom varieties can be easily misidentified, and mistakes can be fatal. Psilocybin is similar to LSD in its physical effects, which generally wear off in 4 to 6 hours.

Mescaline comes from the "buttons" of the peyote cactus, like this one.

PCP

Phencyclidine (*PCP*) was originally developed as a dissociative anesthetic—patients administered it could keep their eyes open, apparently remain conscious, and feel no pain during a medical procedure. Afterward, they would experience amnesia for the time that the drug was in their system. The unpredictability and drastic effects (postoperative delirium, confusion, and agitation) made doctors abandon it, and it was withdrawn from the legal market.

On the illegal market, PCP is a white, crystalline powder that users often sprinkle onto marijuana cigarettes. It is dangerous and unpredictable regardless of method of administration. Effects depend on dosage. A dose as small as 5 mg will produce effects similar to those of strong central nervous system depressants—slurred speech, impaired coordination, reduced sensitivity to pain, and reduced heart and respiratory rate. Doses between 5 and 10 mg cause fever, salivation, nausea, vomiting, and total loss of sensitivity to pain. Doses greater than 10 mg result in a drastic drop in blood pressure, coma, muscular rigidity, violent outbursts, and possible convulsions and death.

Psychologically, PCP may produce either euphoria or dysphoria. It is also known to produce hallucinations, delusions, and overall delirium. Long-term effects of PCP use are unknown.

Ketamine

The liquid form of *ketamine* ("Special K") is used as an anesthetic in hospital and veterinary clinics. After stealing it from hospitals or medical suppliers, dealers typically dry the liquid (usually by cooking it) and grind the residue into powder. Special K inhibits the relay of sensory input, triggering hallucinations as the brain fills the resulting void with visions, memories, and sensory distortions. Effects are similar to those of PCP—confusion, agitation, aggression, and lack of coordination—and less predictable. The aftereffects are less severe than those of Ecstasy, so it has grown in popularity as a club drug.

check yourself

- **What is a hallucinogen?**
- **What are the effects and health risks of commonly abused hallucinogens?**
- **Why do you think some users mistakenly consider hallucinogens to be less harmful than other types of drugs?**

6.9 Common Drugs of Abuse: Inhalants

learning outcome

6.9 Discuss the effects and health risks of inhalants that are commonly misused or abused.

Inhalants are chemicals whose vapors, when inhaled, can cause hallucinations and create intoxicating and euphoric effects. Not commonly recognized as drugs, inhalants are legal to purchase and universally available but dangerous. They generally appeal to young people who can't afford or obtain illicit substances. Some misused products include rubber cement, model glue, paint thinner, aerosol sprays, lighter fluid, varnish, wax, spot removers, and gasoline. Most of these substances are sniffed or "huffed" by users in search of a quick, cheap high.

Because they are inhaled, the volatile chemicals in these products reach the bloodstream and then the brain within seconds. This characteristic, along with the fact that dosages are extremely difficult to control because everyone has unique lung and breathing capacities, makes inhalants particularly dangerous. The effects of inhalants usually last for fewer than 15 minutes and resemble those of central nervous system depressants. Users may experience dizziness, disorientation, impaired coordination, reduced judgment, and slowed reaction times. Combining inhalants with alcohol produces a synergistic effect and can cause severe and sometimes fatal liver damage. An overdose of fumes from inhalants can cause unconsciousness. If the user's oxygen intake is reduced during the inhaling process, death can result within 5 minutes. Sudden sniffing death (SSD) syndrome can be a fatal consequence, whether it's the user's first time or not. This syndrome can occur if a user inhales deeply and then participates in physical activity or is startled.

Amyl Nitrite

Sometimes called "poppers" or "rush," *amyl nitrite* is packaged in small, cloth-covered glass capsules that can be crushed to release the active chemical for the user to inhale. The drug is often prescribed to alleviate chest pain in heart patients, because it dilates small blood vessels and reduces blood pressure. Dilation of blood vessels in the genital area is thought to enhance sensations or perceptions of orgasm. It also produces fainting, dizziness, warmth, and skin flushing.

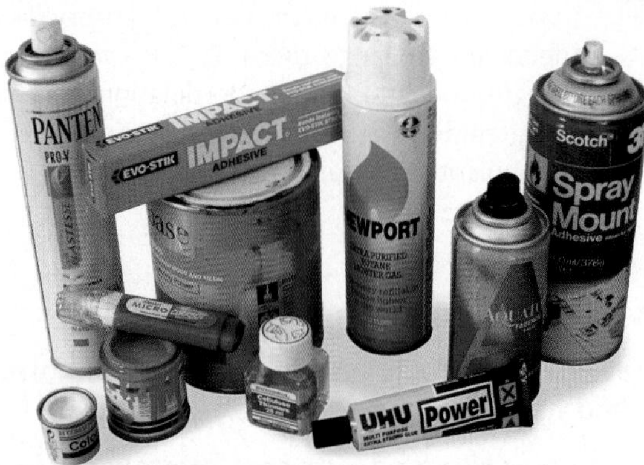

Common household products, such as aerosol sprays, solvents, or glues, can be inhaled for a quick high.

Nitrous Oxide

Nitrous oxide is sometimes used as an adjunct to dental anesthesia or minor surgical anesthesia. It is also a propellant chemical in aerosol products such as whipped toppings. Users who inhale nitrous oxide experience a state of euphoria, floating sensations, and illusions. Effects also include pain relief and a silly feeling, demonstrated by laughing and giggling (hence its nickname "laughing gas"). Regulating dosages of this drug can be difficult. Sustained inhalation can lead to unconsciousness, coma, and death.

Skills for Behavior Change

RESPONDING TO AN OFFER OF DRUGS

No matter what your experience until now, it is likely that you will be invited to use drugs at some point in your life. Here are some questions to consider *before* you find yourself in a situation in which you have the opportunity or feel pressure to use illicit drugs:

- **Why am I considering trying drugs? Am I trying to fit in or impress my friends? What does this say about my friends if I need to take drugs to impress them? Are my friends really looking out for what is best for me?**
- **Am I using this drug to cope or feel different? Am I depressed?**
- **What could taking drugs cost me? Will this cost me my career if I am caught using? Could using drugs prevent me from getting a job?**
- **What are the long-term consequences of using this drug?**
- **What will this cost me in terms of my friendships and family? How would my close family and friends respond if they knew I was using drugs?**

Even when you make the decision not to use drugs, it can be difficult to say no gracefully. Some good ways to turn down an offer include the following:

- **"Thanks, but I've got a big test (game, meeting) tomorrow morning."**
- **"I've already got a great buzz right now. I really don't need anything more."**
- **"I don't like how (insert drug name here) makes me feel."**
- **"I'm driving tonight. So I'm not using."**
- **"I want to go for a run in the morning."**
- **"No."**

check yourself

- **What is an inhalant?**
- **What are the effects and health risks of inhalants?**

Common Drugs of Abuse: Anabolic Steroids

learning outcome

6.10 Discuss the effects and health risks of anabolic steroids.

Anabolic steroids are artificial forms of the male hormone testosterone that promote muscle growth and strength. Steroids are available in two forms: injectable solutions and pills. These **ergogenic drugs** are used primarily by people who believe the drugs will increase their strength, power, bulk (weight), speed, and athletic performance.

It was once estimated that up to 20 percent of college athletes used steroids. Now that stricter drug-testing policies have been instituted by the National Collegiate Athletic Association (NCAA), reported use of anabolic steroids among intercollegiate athletes has decreased.[79] Few data exist on the extent of steroid abuse by adults; it has been estimated that approximately 1 million adults have used anabolic steroids.[80] Among both adolescents and adults, steroid abuse is higher among men than it is among women. However, steroid abuse is growing most rapidly among young women.[81]

Physical Effects of Steroids

In both sexes, anabolic steroids produce a state of euphoria, diminished fatigue, and increased bulk and power. These characteristics give steroids an addictive quality. When users stop, they can experience psychological withdrawal and sometimes severe depression, in some cases leading to suicide attempts. If untreated, depression associated with steroid withdrawal has been known to last for a year or more after steroid use stops.

Men and women who use steroids experience a variety of adverse effects, including mood swings (aggression and violence, sometimes known as "roid rage"); acne; liver tumors; elevated cholesterol levels; hypertension; kidney disease; and immune system disturbances. There is also a danger of transmitting HIV and hepatitis through shared needles. In women, large doses of anabolic steroids may trigger the development of masculine attributes such as lowered voice, increased facial and body hair, and male pattern baldness; they may also result in an enlarged clitoris, smaller breasts, and changes in or absence of menstruation. When taken by healthy males, anabolic steroids shut down the body's production of testosterone, causing men's breasts to grow and testicles to atrophy.

Steroid Use and Society

To combat the growing problem of steroid use, Congress passed the Anabolic Steroids Control Act (ASCA) of 1990. This law makes it a crime to possess, prescribe, or distribute anabolic steroids for any use other than the treatment of specific diseases. Penalties for illegal use include up to 5 years' imprisonment and a $250,000 fine for the first offense and up to 10 years' imprisonment and a $500,000 fine for subsequent offenses.

The use of steroids and related substances among professional athletes periodically makes the news. In recent years, high-profile athletes in sports such as cycling, track and field, swimming, and baseball have garnered media attention for suspected use of steroids or other banned performance-enhancing drugs. Six athletes were barred from the 2014 Winter Olympic Games for illegal drug use.

Cyclist Alberto Contador was suspended from the Tour de France for 2 years and stripped of his 2010 victory after testing positive for performance-enhancing drug use.

check yourself

- **What are anabolic steroids?**
- **What are the effects and health risks of anabolic steroids?**

6.11 Treatment and Recovery

learning outcome

6.11 Discuss treatment and recovery options for people with an addiction.

Recovery from addiction is a lifelong process, starting with treatment—and before that, recognition—of the addiction. This can be difficult because of the power of denial—the inability to see the truth. Denial can be so powerful that intervention is sometimes necessary to break down the addict's defenses against recognizing the problem.

Intervention

Intervention is a planned process of confrontation by people who are important to the addict, including spouses, parents, children, bosses, and friends. Its purpose is to break down denial compassionately so that the person can see the addiction's destructive nature. Getting addicts to admit that they have a problem is not enough; they must come to perceive that the behavior is destructive and requires treatment.

Individual confrontation is difficult and often futile. However, an addict's defenses generally crumble when significant others collectively share their observations and concerns about the addict's behavior. Effective interventions include (1) emphasizing care and concern for the addicted person; (2) describing the behavior that is the cause for concern; (3) expressing how the behavior affects the addict, each person taking part in the intervention, and others; and (4) outlining specifically what you would like to see happen.

Participants in the intervention must clarify how they plan to end their enabling. Persons contemplating interventions must also choose consequences they are ready to stick to if the addict refuses treatment—and be ready to give support if the addict is willing to begin a recovery program.

Treatment for Addiction

Treatment and recovery for any addiction generally begin with **abstinence**—refraining from the addictive behavior. For people addicted to behaviors such as work and sex, abstinence means restoring balance to their lives through noncompulsive engagement in the behaviors. An estimated 21.6 million Americans aged 12 or older needed treatment for an illicit drug or alcohol use problem in 2011. Of these, only 2.3 million—approximately 11 percent—received treatment.[82]

Detoxification refers to the early period during which an addict adjusts physically and cognitively to being free from the addiction's influence. It occurs in virtually every recovering addict. Detoxification is uncomfortable and can be dangerous. For some addicts, early abstinence may involve profound withdrawal that requires medical supervision.

Abstinence alone does little to change the psychological, biological, and environmental dynamics underlying addictive behavior. Without treatment, an addict is apt to relapse or to change addictions. Treatment involves learning new ways of looking at oneself, others, and the world. It may require exploring a traumatic past so psychological wounds can heal. It also involves learning interdependence with significant others and new ways of caring for oneself physically and emotionally.

Finding a Treatment Program

For many addicts, recovery begins with a period of formal treatment. A good treatment program includes the following:

- Staff familiar with the specific addictive disorder for which help is being sought
- Availability of both inpatient and outpatient services
- Medical personnel who can assess the addict's health and treat medical concerns, as needed

How can I approach someone who needs help and treatment?

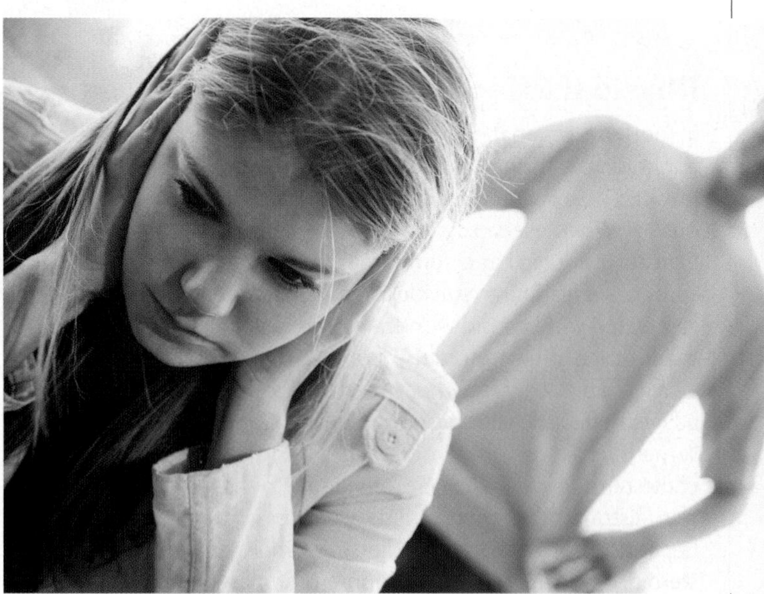

Confronting a person about addiction is a difficult task, and one that usually requires intervention by a group of family members and friends. It is more effective for an addict to be faced with the facts from a group of the people most important to him or her than by one person. Most addiction treatment centers have specialists who can help plan an intervention.

How do people recover from drug addiction?

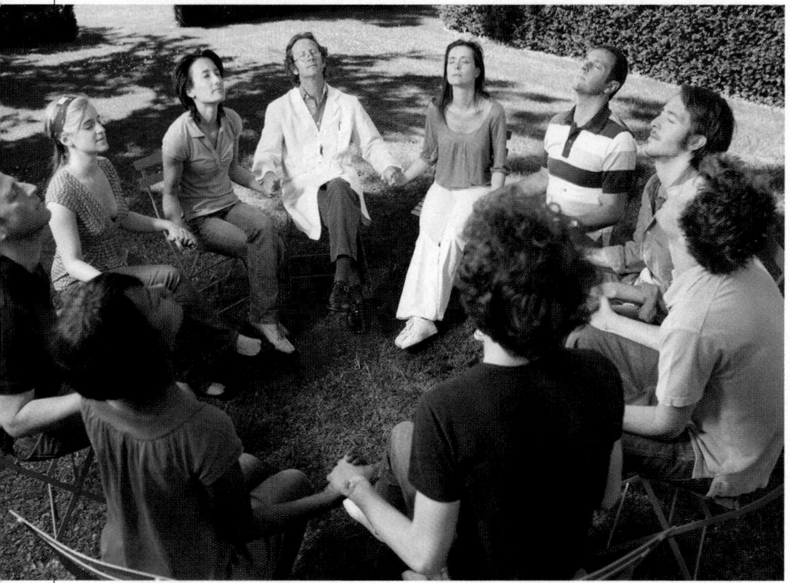

For most addicts, recovery is a long, difficult process—for some people it can be a lifelong journey. Treatment and recovery usually begin with detoxification. Once the person's body has adjusted, the addict usually enters therapy to learn how to cope without the drug and avoid relapse. Therapy often takes the form of group meetings, such as those held by 12-step programs.

- Medical supervision of addicts at risk for complicated detoxification
- Involvement of family members in the treatment process
- A coordinated team approach to treating addictive disorders (e.g., medical personnel, counselors, psychotherapists, clergy, and dietitians)
- Group and individual therapy options
- Peer-led support groups that encourage involvement after treatment ends
- Structured aftercare and relapse-prevention programs
- Accreditation by the Joint Commission (a national organization that accredits and certifies health care organizations and programs) and a license from the state in which it operates

Treatment Approaches

Outpatient behavioral treatment encompasses a variety of programs for addicts who visit a clinic at regular intervals. Most involve individual or group counseling. *Residential treatment programs* can be effective for those with more severe problems. For example, therapeutic communities are highly structured programs in which addicts remain at a residence, typically for 6 to 12 months. The focus is on resocialization to a drug-free lifestyle.

The first *12-step program*, Alcoholics Anonymous (AA), began in 1935. The 12-step program has since become the most widely used approach to dealing with addictive or dysfunctional behaviors. More than 200 recovery programs are based on the program, including Narcotics Anonymous and Gamblers Anonymous.

The 12-step program is nonjudgmental and based on the idea that its purpose is to work on personal recovery. Working the 12 steps involves admitting to having a problem, recognizing there is an outside power that could help, consciously relying on that power, admitting and listing character defects, seeking deliverance from defects, apologizing to those one has harmed, and helping others with the same problem. Free meetings, held at a variety of times and locations in almost every city, are open to anyone who wishes to attend.

Medicinal Treatments Methadone maintenance is one treatment available for people addicted to heroin or other opioids. Methadone is chemically similar enough to opioids to control the tremors, chills, vomiting, diarrhea, and severe abdominal pains of withdrawal. Critics of methadone maintenance contend that the program merely substitutes one addiction for another. Proponents argue that people on methadone maintenance are less likely to engage in criminal activities to support their habits than heroin addicts are.

A number of new drug therapies for opioid dependence are emerging as well, such as naltrexone (Trexan), an opioid antagonist. While on naltrexone, recovering addicts do not have the compulsion to use heroin, and if they do use it, they don't get high, so there is no point in using the drug.

Vaccines against Addictive Drugs A promising new cocaine vaccine, currently in development, keeps the user from getting high by stimulating the immune system to attack the drug when it's taken. Vaccines against nicotine and methamphetamine are also in development.

Relapse

Relapse, an isolated occurrence of or full return to addictive behavior, is a defining characteristic of addiction. Addicts are set up to relapse because of their tendency to meet change and other forms of stress with the same kind of denial once used to justify addictive behavior (e.g., "I don't have a problem; I can handle this").

Treatment programs recognize this tendency and teach clients and significant others how to recognize and respond to signs of imminent relapse. Without such a plan, recovering addicts are likely to relapse more frequently, and perhaps permanently.

Relapse should not be interpreted as failure to change or lack of desire to stay well. The appropriate response is to remind addicts that they are addicted and redirect them to strategies that have worked for them. Relapse prevention may involve connecting the recovering person with support groups or counselors.

check yourself

- **What are the steps in treatment and recovery from addiction?**

6.12 Addressing Drug Misuse and Abuse in the United States

learning outcome

6.12 Identify strategies to address drug misuse and abuse.

Illegal drug use in the United States costs about $193 billion per year.[83] This includes costs associated with health care, lost productivity, and criminal investigation and prosecution.

Preventing Drug Use and Abuse on Campus

College and university campuses should consider multiple strategies to reduce substance use among students:

- Changing student expectations that college is a time to experiment with drugs
- Engaging parents and encouraging them to continue open communication with their children
- Identifying high-risk students through early detection programs
- Providing programs specifically tailored for students needing treatment and recovery support

The pressure to take drugs is often tremendous, and reasons for use complex. People who develop drug problems generally believe they can control their use when they start out. Peer influence is also a strong motivator, especially among adolescents.

Solving the Drug Problem

Respondents in public opinion polls feel that the most important strategy for fighting drug abuse is educating young people, in addition to strategies such as:

- Stricter border surveillance to reduce drug trafficking
- Longer prison sentences for drug dealers
- Increased government spending on prevention
- Enforcing antidrug laws
- Greater cooperation between government agencies and private groups and individuals providing treatment assistance

Drug abuse has been a part of human behavior for thousands of years, and it is unlikely to disappear. We must educate ourselves and develop the self-discipline necessary to avoid dangerous drug dependence.

For many years, the most popular antidrug strategy has been total prohibition—an approach that has proved ineffective. Prohibition of alcohol during the 1920s created more problems than it solved, as did prohibition of opioids in 1914. A recent U.S. government campaign, commonly referred to as the "War on Drugs," includes laws and policies intended to reduce illegal drug trade and to diminish and discourage production, distribution, and consumption of illicit substances.

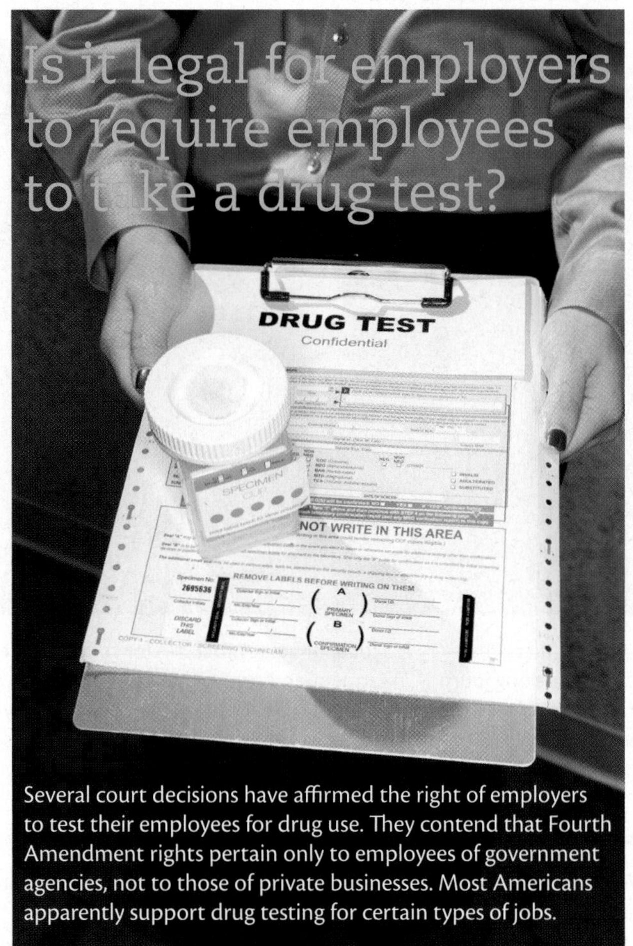

Several court decisions have affirmed the right of employers to test their employees for drug use. They contend that Fourth Amendment rights pertain only to employees of government agencies, not to those of private businesses. Most Americans apparently support drug testing for certain types of jobs.

In general, drug education researchers agree that students should be taught the difference between drug use, misuse, and abuse. Factual information that is free of scare tactics must be presented; lecturing and moralizing have proved not to work.

Harm reduction is a set of practical approaches to reducing negative consequences of drug use, incorporating a spectrum of strategies from safer use to abstinence. Harm reduction may involve changing the legal sanctions associated with drug use, increasing the availability of treatment services to drug abusers, making use safer through programs like needle exchange, and attempting to change drug users' behavior through education. Harm reduction strategies recognize that people always have and always will use drugs and, therefore, attempt to minimize the potential hazards associated with drug use rather than the use itself.

check yourself

- **What are some strategies to address substance abuse? Which, if any, of these are present on your campus?**

Do You Have a Problem with Drugs?

An interactive version of this assessment is available online in MasteringHealth.

Answering the following questions will help you determine whether you have developed a drug problem:

	Yes	No
1. In the past year, did you have a hard time paying attention in classes, work, or at home?	◯	◯
2. Have you ever felt you should cut down on your drug use?	◯	◯
3. Have you had blackouts or flashbacks as a result of your drug use?	◯	◯
4. Have people annoyed (irritated, angered, etc.) you by criticizing your drug use?	◯	◯
5. Have you ever been arrested or in trouble with the law because of your drug use?	◯	◯

	Yes	No
6. Have you lost friends because of your drug use?	◯	◯
7. Have you ever felt bad or guilty about your drug use?	◯	◯
8. Have you ever thought you might have a drug problem?	◯	◯

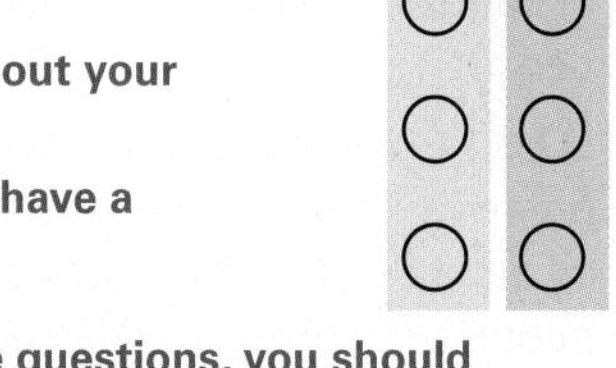

If you answered "yes" to any of the questions, you should consider talking to a counselor or health care provider either on campus or at your health or counseling center.

Source: Adapted from U.S. Department of Health and Human Services, Substance Abuse and Mental Health Services Administration, Center for Substance Abuse Treatment, "Should You Talk to Someone About a Drug, Alcohol or Mental Health Problem?," 2011, www.samhsa.gov.

Your Plan for Change

The Assess Yourself activity describes signs of being controlled by drugs or by a drug user. Depending on your results, you may need to change certain behaviors that may be detrimental to your health.

Today, you can:

◯ **Imagine a situation in which someone offers you a drug and think of several different ways of refusing. Rehearse these scenarios in your head.**

◯ **Think about the drug use patterns among your social group. Are you ever uncomfortable with these people because of their drug use? Is it difficult to avoid using drugs when you are with them? If the answers are yes, begin exploring ways to expand your social circle.**

Within the next 2 weeks, you can:

◯ **Stop by your campus health center to find out about any drug treatment programs or support groups they may have.**

◯ **If you are concerned about your own drug use or the drug use of a close friend, make an appointment with a counselor to talk about the issue.**

By the end of the semester, you can:

◯ **Participate in clubs, activities, and social groups that do not rely on substance abuse for their amusement.**

◯ **If you have a drug problem, make a commitment to enter a treatment program. Acknowledge that you have a problem and that you need the assistance of others to help you overcome it.**

Summary

To hear an MP3 Tutor session, scan here or visit the Study Area in **MasteringHealth.**

LO 6.1 Addiction is continued use of a substance or activity despite ongoing negative consequences. All addictions share four common symptoms: compulsion, loss of control, negative consequences, and denial.

LO 6.1 Codependents are typically friends or family members who are controlled by an addict's addictive behavior. Enablers are people who protect addicts from consequences of their behavior.

LO 6.1 The biopsychosocial model of addiction takes into account biological (genetic) factors as well as psychological and environmental influences in understanding the addiction process.

LO 6.2 Addictive behaviors include disordered gambling, compulsive buying, compulsive Internet or technology use, work addiction, compulsive exercise, and sexual addiction.

LO 6.3 The six categories of drugs are prescription drugs, over-the-counter (OTC) drugs, recreational drugs, herbal preparations, illicit drugs, and commercial preparations.

LO 6.4 Over-the-counter medications are drugs that do not require a prescription. Some OTC medications can be addictive.

LO 6.4 Prescription drug abuse is at an all-time high, particularly among college students. The most commonly abused prescription drugs are painkillers.

LO 6.4 People from all walks of life use illicit drugs. Drug use declined from the mid-1980s to the early 1990s but has remained steady since then. However, among young people, use of drugs has been rising in recent years.

LO 6.5–6.10 Controlled substances include cocaine and its derivatives, amphetamines, methamphetamine, marijuana, opioids, depressants, hallucinogens/psychedelics, inhalants, and steroids.

LO 6.11 Treatment begins with abstinence from the drug or addictive behavior, usually instituted through intervention by close family, friends, or other loved ones. Treatment programs may include individual, group, or family therapy, as well as 12-step programs.

Pop Quiz

Visit MasteringHealth to personalize your study plan with Chapter Review Quizzes and Dynamic Study Modules.

LO 6.1 1. Which of the following is *not* a characteristic of addiction?
a. Denial
b. Acknowledgment of self-destructive behavior
c. Loss of control
d. Obsession with a substance or behavior

LO 6.1 2. Aaliyah is addicted to the Internet. She is so preoccupied with it that she is failing her classes. What symptom of addiction does her preoccupation characterize?
a. Denial
b. Compulsion
c. Loss of control
d. Negative consequences

LO 6.1 3. An individual who knowingly tries to protect an addict from natural consequences of his or her destructive behaviors is
a. enabling.
b. helping the addict to recover.
c. practicing intervention.
d. controlling.

LO 6.3 4. Cross-tolerance occurs when
a. drugs work at the same receptor site so that one blocks the action of the other.
b. the effects of one drug are eliminated or reduced by the presence of another drug at the receptor site.
c. a person develops a physiological tolerance to one drug and shows a similar tolerance to selected other drugs as a result.
d. two or more drugs interact so their effects are multiplied.

LO 6.3 5. Jayden takes Prinivil (an antihypertensive drug), insulin (a diabetic medication), and Claritin (an antihistamine). This is an example of
a. synergism.
b. illegal drug use.
c. polydrug use.
d. antagonism.

LO 6.4 6. The most widely used illicit drug in the United States is
a. alcohol.
b. heroin.
c. marijuana.
d. methamphetamine.

LO 6.5 7. Which of the following is classified as a stimulant drug?
a. Amphetamines
b. Alcohol
c. Marijuana
d. LSD

LO 6.7 8. Drugs that depress the central nervous system are called
a. amphetamines.
b. hallucinogens.
c. depressants.
d. psychedelics.

LO 6.8 9. The psychoactive drug mescaline is found in what plant?
a. Mushrooms
b. Peyote cactus
c. Marijuana
d. Belladonna

LO 6.11 10. Chemical dependency *relapse* refers to
a. a person experiencing a blackout.
b. a gap in one's drinking or drug-taking patterns.
c. a full return to addictive behavior.
d. failure to change one's behavior.

Answers to these questions can be found on page A-1. If you answered a question incorrectly, review the module identified by the Learning Outcome. For even more study tools, visit MasteringHealth.

7 Alcohol and Tobacco

People throughout history have used alcohol. Alcohol consumption is part of many traditions, and moderate use can enhance special times. Although alcohol can play a positive role in some people's lives, it is a drug, and if used irresponsibly, can become dangerous.

Approximately half of all Americans consume alcohol regularly, while 21 percent abstain altogether.[1] Alcohol consumption levels among Americans declined steadily from the late 1970s until 2000, when consumption began to increase slightly; this has been linked to the downturn of the U.S. economy.[2] Since 2009, consumption levels have again been declining, a trend tied to a stronger economy and growing attention to personal health.[3]

Meanwhile, the prevalence of cigarette smoking among adults has declined significantly over the last 50 years.[4] However, tobacco use is still the single most preventable cause of death in the United States: Nearly 480,000 Americans die each year from tobacco-related diseases, and another 16 million people will suffer from health disorders caused by tobacco. Smoking cigarettes kills more Americans than alcohol, car accidents, suicide, AIDS, homicide, and illegal drugs combined.[5] Any contention by the tobacco industry that tobacco use is not dangerous completely ignores scientific evidence.

7.1 Alcohol and College Students

learning outcome

7.1 Discuss the alcohol use patterns of college students and the factors that make college students vulnerable to alcohol-related problems.

Alcohol is the most popular drug on college campuses, where large numbers of students report having consumed alcoholic beverages in the past 30 days (Figure 7.1).[6] In a new trend on college campuses, women's consumption of alcohol has come close to equaling that of men.

Approximately 40 percent of all college students engage in **binge drinking**,[7] consuming five or more drinks (men), or four or more drinks (women), in about 2 hours.[8] Students who drink only once a week are considered binge drinkers if they consume these amounts within 2 hours. Binge drinking can quickly lead to extreme intoxication, unconsciousness, alcohol poisoning, and even death.

For some students, independence is symbolized by alcohol use. Others drink to "have fun"—which often means drinking simply to get drunk. This may be a way of coping with stress, boredom, anxiety, or academic and social pressures.

In the past 12 months, a significant number of college students who drank experienced at least one negative consequence of alcohol consumption (Figure 7.2). About 32 percent of college students who drank reported doing something they later regretted; 27 percent forgot where they were or what they did due to intoxication; 17 percent had unprotected sex; and 12 percent accidentally injured themselves.[9]

Fortunately, many students report always or usually practicing protective behaviors when consuming alcohol. About 84 percent said they stayed with the same group of friends the entire time they drank; 83 percent reported using a designated driver; 78 percent reported eating before or during drinking; and 65 percent kept track of how many drinks they consumed.[10]

However, some students don't drink responsibly, and the stakes are high. According to one study, 1,825 college students die each year because of alcohol-related unintentional injuries, including car accidents.[11] Alcohol consumption is the top cause of preventable death among U.S. undergraduates.

Who Drinks?

It's likely that students who enter college will drink at some point, but some groups are more likely to drink more, and more often. For example, students who believe that their parents approve of their drinking are more likely to drink.[12] Students who drank heavily in high school are also at risk for heavy drinking in college.[13] A recent study also found students who played intramural sports, were in abusive relationships, had high stress levels, belonged to a fraternity or sorority, or were depressed reported higher levels of drinking and negative alcohol-related effects.[14]

Why Do College Students Drink So Much?

College students seem to be particularly vulnerable to alcohol-related problems. In addition to newfound freedom, several factors encourage drinking during college:

- Many student customs (Greek rush), norms (reputation as party schools), and traditional celebrations (St. Patrick's Day) encourage drinking.
- Alcohol advertising and promotions target students.
- College students are particularly vulnerable to peer influence.
- Drink specials enable students to consume large amounts of alcohol cheaply.
- College administrators often deny the extent of alcohol problems on their campuses.

Student Drinking Behavior

College students are more likely than their noncollegiate peers to drink recklessly and to engage in dangerous drinking practices. One such practice, **pre-gaming** (also preloading or front-loading), involves planned heavy drinking prior to going out to a bar, nightclub, or sporting event. In a recent study, 75 percent of students reported pre-gaming in the past month. College men are more likely than women to pre-game.[15] Pre-gamers have more negative consequences, such as blackouts, hangovers, passing out, and alcohol poisoning.

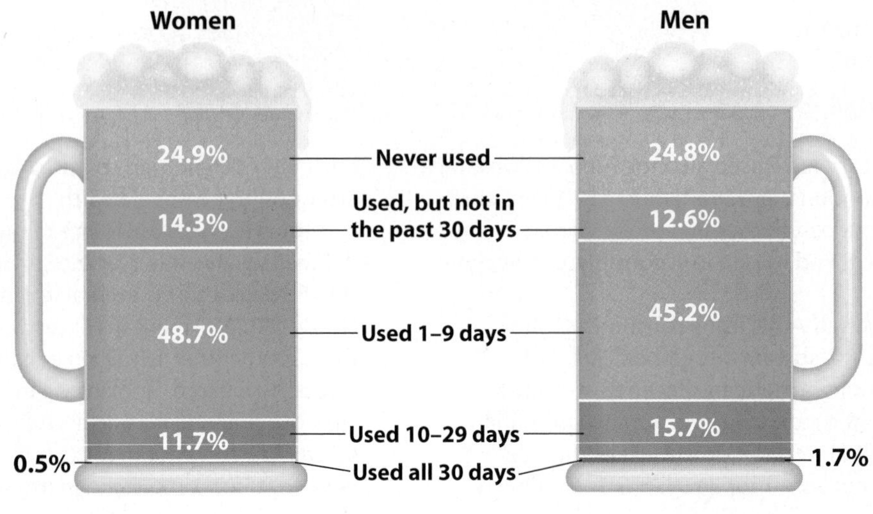

Figure 7.1 College Students' Patterns of Alcohol Use in the Past 30 Days
Source: Data from American College Health Association, *American College Health Association—National College Health Assessment II (ACHA-NCHA II) Reference Group Data Report, Fall 2013* (Baltimore, MD: American College Health Association, 2014).

More than 80 percent of college students drink alcohol to celebrate their twenty-first birthday.[16] Nearly half of students celebrating experienced at least one negative consequence of drinking (e.g., headache, feeling very sick to their stomach, etc.).[17]

Two-thirds of college students engage in drinking games that involve binge drinking.[18] Those who participate in drinking games are much less likely to monitor or regulate how much they are drinking and are at risk for extreme intoxication.

Some college students use extreme measures to control their eating and/or exercise excessively so that they can save calories, consume more alcohol, and become intoxicated faster.[19] *Drunkorexia* describes the combination of two dangerous behaviors: disordered eating and heavy drinking. Potential risks of drunkorexia include risk of blackouts, forced sexual activity, unintended sexual activity, and alcohol poisoning.

What Is the Impact of Student Drinking?

The more students drink, the more likely they are to miss class, do poorly on tests and papers, have lower grade point averages, and fall behind on assigned work. Some students even drop out of school as a result of their drinking.

One study indicated that over 696,000 students 18 to 24 were assaulted by another student who had been drinking.[20] There is significant evidence that campus rape is linked to binge drinking; an estimated 97,000 students between the ages of 18 and 24 experience alcohol-related sexual assault or date rape each year in the United States.[21] The laws regarding sexual consent are clear: A person who is drunk or passed out cannot consent to sex. If you have sex with someone who is drunk or unconscious, you are committing rape. Claiming you were also drunk does not absolve you of legal and moral responsibility for this crime.

Did something they later regretted	**31.7%** **1 in 3**
Forgot where they were or what they did	**27.3%** **1 in 4**
Had unprotected sex	**17.4%** **1 in 6**
Physically injured self	**12.4%** **1 in 8**

Figure 7.2 Prevalence of Negative Consequences of Drinking among College Students, Past Year

Source: Data from American College Health Association, *American College Health Association—National College Health Assessment II (ACHA-NCHA II) Reference Group Data Report, Fall 2013* (Hanover, MD: American College Health Association, 2014).

Colleges' Efforts to Reduce Student Drinking

Some colleges are instituting strong policies against drinking; at the same time, schools are making more help available to students with drinking problems. Programs that have proven effective include cognitive-behavioral skills training with *motivational interviewing*, a nonjudgmental approach to behavior change, and e-Interventions, alcohol education interventions via text message.

Schools are also trying a *social norms* approach to reducing alcohol consumption, sending a consistent message to students about actual drinking behavior on campus. Many students perceive that their peers drink more than they actually do, which may cause them to feel pressured to drink more themselves. In a national survey, for example, college students perceived that 40.5 percent of students used alcohol 10 to 29 days a month; the actual rate is 13 percent.[22] As a result of such campaigns, binge drinking has declined on campuses across the country.

See It! Videos

Heavy drinking during spring break can lead to bad decisions, or worse. Watch **Sloppy Spring Breaker** in the Study Area of MasteringHealth.

Skills for Behavior Change

TIPS FOR DRINKING RESPONSIBLY

- Eat before and while you drink.
- Don't drink before the party.
- Avoid drinking if you are angry, anxious, or depressed.
- Drink no more than one alcoholic drink an hour.
- Alternate alcoholic and nonalcoholic drinks.
- Determine ahead of time how many drinks you'll have.
- Avoid drinking games.
- Keep track of how much you drink.
- Don't drink and drive. Volunteer to be the sober driver.
- Avoid parties where you can expect heavy drinking.

check yourself

- **How does this module's description of college student drinking compare to drinking on your campus?**
- **What is binge drinking?**
- **What factors make college students vulnerable to alcohol-related problems? Which of these factors exist on your campus?**

7.2 Alcohol in the Body

learning outcome

7.2 Explain the processes by which alcohol is absorbed and metabolized in the human body and the factors that affect blood alcohol concentration.

Learning about the metabolism and absorption of alcohol can help you understand how it is possible to drink safely—and how to avoid life-threatening circumstances such as alcohol poisoning. This information can be critical for your safety and that of your friends.

The Chemistry and Potency of Alcohol

The intoxicating substance found in beer, wine, liquor, and liqueurs is **ethyl alcohol**, or **ethanol**. It is produced during **fermentation**, in which yeast organisms break down plant sugars, yielding ethanol and carbon dioxide. For beers, ales, and wines, the process ends with fermentation. Hard liquor is produced through further processing called **distillation**, in which alcohol vapors are condensed and mixed with water to make the final product.

The **proof** of an alcoholic drink is a measure of its percentage of alcohol, and therefore its strength. Alcohol percentage by volume is half of the given proof: 80 proof whiskey is 40 percent alcohol by volume. Lower-proof drinks produce fewer alcohol effects than do the same amount of higher-proof drinks. Most wines are 12 to 15 percent alcohol, and most beers are 2 to 8 percent.

As defined by the National Institute on Alcohol Abuse and Alcoholism (NIAAA), a **standard drink** contains about 14 grams (0.6 fluid ounce or 1.2 tablespoons) of pure alcohol (Figure 7.3). A 12-ounce can of beer, a 5-ounce glass of wine, and a 1.5-ounce shot of vodka are each considered one standard drink—each contains the same amount of alcohol. If estimating blood alcohol concentration using standard drinks as a measure, keep in mind both proof and drink size. You may have bought one beer at the ballpark, but if it came in a 22-ounce cup, you actually consumed two standard drinks.

Absorption and Metabolism

Unlike the molecules in most foods and drugs, alcohol molecules are sufficiently small and fat soluble to be absorbed throughout the entire gastrointestinal system. Approximately 20 percent of ingested alcohol diffuses through the stomach lining into the bloodstream and nearly 80 percent through the lining of the upper third of the small intestine.

Several factors influence how quickly your body will absorb alcohol: the alcohol concentration in your drink; the amount you consume; the amount of food in your stomach; and your metabolism, weight, body mass index, and mood. The higher the concentration of alcohol in your drink, the more rapidly it will be absorbed in your digestive tract. As a rule, wine and beer are absorbed more slowly than distilled beverages. "Fizzy" alcoholic beverages, carbonated beverages, and drinks served with mixers cause the pyloric valve to relax, emptying stomach contents more rapidly into the small intestine and increasing the rate of absorption.

Students often mix energy drinks with alcohol, and these drinks can be particularly dangerous. Students who consume alcohol mixed energy drinks often report not noticing signs of intoxication (e.g., dizziness, fatigue, headache, and trouble walking). Caffeine may delay the onset of normal sleepiness, increasing the amount of time a person would normally stay awake and drink. Caffeine also reduces the subjective feeling of drunkenness without actually reducing alcohol-related impairment. Students who reported drinking alcohol-mixed energy drinks were more likely to consume large amounts of alcohol; have unprotected sex or sex under the influence; be hurt or injured; and meet criteria for alcohol dependency.[23]

The more alcohol you consume, the longer absorption takes. High concentrations of alcohol can cause irritation of the digestive system or vomiting. Alcohol also takes longer to absorb if there is food in your stomach, because the surface area exposed to alcohol is smaller; a full stomach also retards emptying of alcoholic beverages into the small intestine.

Mood also affects how long it takes for the stomach's contents to empty into the intestine. Alcohol is absorbed much more rapidly when people are tense than when they are relaxed.

Once absorbed into the bloodstream, alcohol circulates throughout the body and is metabolized in the liver, where it is converted

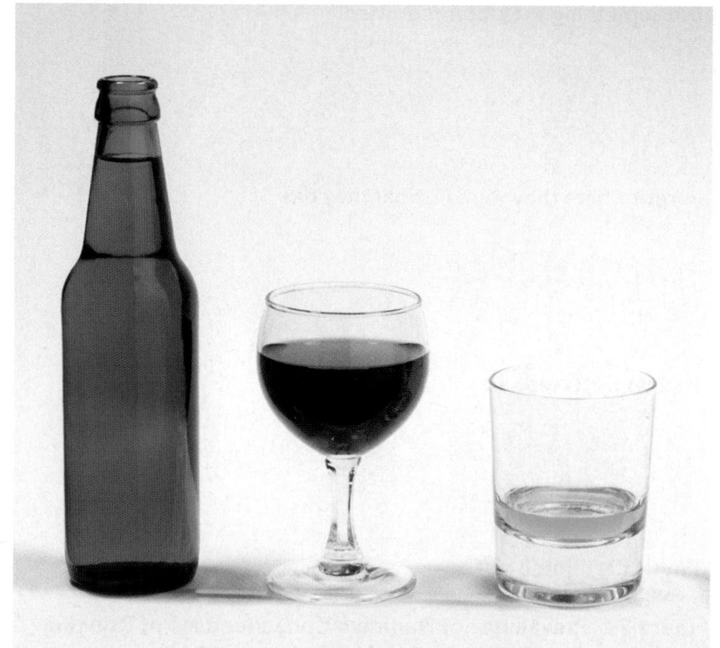

Figure 7.3 What Is a Standard Drink?
One standard drink of beer (12 ounces), wine (5 ounces), or liquor (1.5 ounces) contains the same amount of alcohol.

Blood Alcohol Concentration (BAC)	Psychological and Physical Effects
Not Impaired	
<0.01%	Negligible
Sometimes Impaired	
0.01–0.04%	Slight muscle relaxation, mild euphoria, slight body warmth, increased sociability and talkativeness
Usually Impaired	
0.05–0.07%	Lowered alertness, impaired judgment, lowered inhibitions, exaggerated behavior, loss of small muscle control
Always Impaired	
0.08–0.14%	Slowed reaction time, poor muscle coordination, short-term memory loss, judgment impaired, inability to focus
0.15–0.24%	Blurred vision, lack of motor skills, sedation, slowed reactions, difficulty standing and walking, passing out
0.25–0.34%	Impaired consciousness, disorientation, loss of motor function, severely impaired or no reflexes, impaired circulation and respiration, uncontrolled urination, slurred speech, possible death
0.35% and up	Unconsciousness, coma, extremely slow heartbeat and respiration, unresponsiveness, probable death

Figure 7.4 The Psychological and Physical Effects of Alcohol

to *acetaldehyde* by the enzyme *alcohol dehydrogenase.* It is then rapidly oxidized to *acetate*, converted to carbon dioxide and water, and eventually excreted from the body. Acetaldehyde is a toxic chemical that can cause immediate symptoms such as nausea and vomiting, as well as long-term effects such as liver damage. A very small portion of alcohol is excreted unchanged by the kidneys, lungs, and skin.

Alcohol contains 7 calories (kcal) per gram; the average regular beer contains about 150 calories. Mixed drinks may contain more. The body uses the calories in alcohol in the same manner it uses those in carbohydrates: for immediate energy or for storage as fat if not immediately needed.

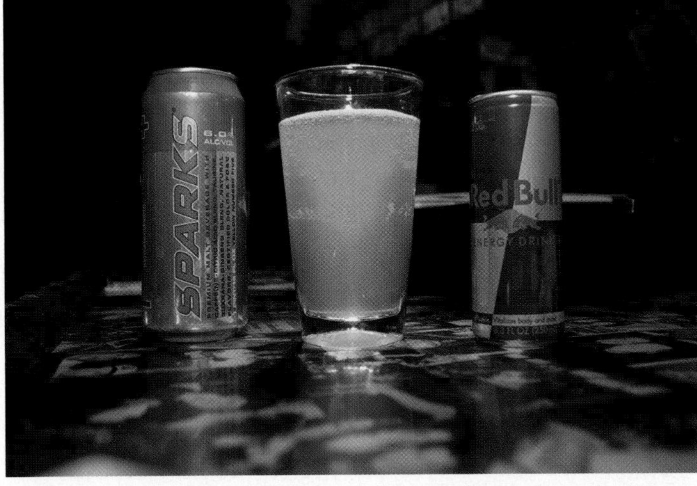

Combining alcohol with energy drinks can have dangerous results.

Breakdown of alcohol occurs at a fairly constant rate of 0.5 ounce (slightly less than one standard drink) per hour. Unmetabolized alcohol circulates in the bloodstream until enough time passes for the body to break it down.

Blood Alcohol Concentration

Blood alcohol concentration (BAC), the ratio of alcohol to total blood volume, is the primary method used to measure physiological and behavioral effects of alcohol. Despite individual differences, alcohol produces some general effects, depending on BAC (Figure 7.4).

At a BAC of 0.02 percent, a person feels relaxed and in a good mood. At 0.05 percent, relaxation increases, and there is some motor impairment and a willingness to talk. At 0.08 percent comes euphoria and further motor impairment. At 0.10 percent, the depressant effects of alcohol become apparent, drowsiness sets in, and motor skills are further impaired, followed by a loss of judgment. A driver may not be able to estimate distance or speed; some drinkers lose their ability to make value-related decisions and may do things they wouldn't do when sober. As BAC increases, the drinker suffers increased negative physiological and psychological effects.

BAC depends on weight and body fat, concentration of alcohol in a beverage, rate of consumption, and volume of alcohol consumed. Heavier people have more body surface through which to diffuse alcohol, so have lower concentrations of blood alcohol than do thin people after drinking the same amount.

Alcohol does not diffuse as rapidly into body fat as into body tissues; BAC is higher in those with more body fat. Because a woman is likely to have proportionately more body fat than a man of the same weight, she will be more intoxicated after drinking the same amount of alcohol.

Breath analysis (breathalyzer tests) and urinalysis are used to determine whether an individual is legally intoxicated, though blood tests are more accurate. An increasing number of states require blood tests for people suspected of driving under the influence of alcohol. In some states, refusal to take a breath, urine, or blood test results in immediate driver's license revocation.

People can develop physical and psychological tolerance of the effects of alcohol through regular use. The nervous system adapts over time, so greater amounts of alcohol are required to produce the same effects. Though BAC may be quite high, the individual has learned to modify his or her behavior to appear sober, an ability called **learned behavioral tolerance.**

check yourself

- **What is a standard drink of alcohol?**
- **How does alcohol enter the bloodstream?**
- **What are some of the factors that increase and decrease blood alcohol concentration?**

7.3 Alcohol and Your Health: Short-Term Effects

learning outcome

7.3 Discuss the short-term health effects of alcohol consumption.

Immediate and long-term effects of alcohol consumption can vary greatly (Figure 7.5). The effects you experience depend on you as an individual, how much alcohol you consume, and your circumstances.

The most dramatic effects produced by ethanol occur within the central nervous system (CNS). Alcohol depresses CNS function, which decreases respiratory rate, pulse rate, and blood pressure. As CNS depression deepens, vital functions become affected. In extreme cases, coma and death can result.

Alcohol is a diuretic that increases urinary output. Although this might be expected to lead to **dehydration** (loss of water), the body actually retains water, most of it in the muscles and cerebral tissues. Because water is pulled out of the *cerebrospinal fluid* (fluid within the brain and spinal cord), drinkers may suffer symptoms that include "morning-after" effects.

Alcohol irritates the gastrointestinal system and may cause indigestion and heartburn if consumed on an empty stomach. People who consume unusually high amounts of alcohol in a short time also put themselves at risk for irregular heartbeat or even total loss of heart rhythm, which can disrupt blood flow and damage the heart muscle.

Hangover

A **hangover** is often experienced the morning after a drinking spree. Its symptoms are familiar to most people who drink: headache, muscle aches, upset stomach, anxiety, depression, diarrhea, and thirst. Hangovers kick in for more than half of people after their blood alcohol content reaches 0.11.[24] **Congeners**, forms of alcohol that are metabolized more slowly than ethanol and are more toxic, are thought to play a role in the development of a hangover; the body metabolizes congeners after ethanol is gone from the system, and their toxic by-products may contribute to hangover. Alcohol upsets the body's water balance, resulting in hangover symptoms including excess urination, dehydration, and thirst. Increased production of hydrochloric acid can irritate the stomach lining and cause nausea. Recovery from a hangover usually takes 12 hours. Bed rest, solid food, plenty of water, and aspirin or ibuprofen may help relieve a hangover's discomforts. But the only way to avoid one is to abstain from excessive alcohol use in the first place.

Alcohol and Injuries

Alcohol use plays a significant role in the types of injuries people experience. Hospitalizations from alcohol overdoses among 18- to 24-year-olds rose by 25 percent over the past 10 years, and about 30 percent of young adults hospitalized for overdoses involve excessive consumption of alcohol.[25] Alcohol use is involved in approximately 70 percent of fatal injuries during activities such as swimming and boating[26] and 40 percent of fatal injuries due to house fires.[27]

Alcohol use also plays a role in approximately one-third of suicides in the United States. Alcohol may increase the risk for suicide by intensifying depressive thoughts, lowering inhibitions to hurt oneself, and interfering with the ability to assess future consequences of one's actions.[28]

Alcohol and Sexual Decision Making

Alcohol affects your ability to make good decisions about sex because it lowers inhibitions. Intoxicated people are less likely to use safer sex practices and more likely to engage in high-risk sexual activity. The chances of sexually transmitted infection and unplanned pregnancy also increase among people who drink more heavily, compared with those who drink moderately or not at all.

Alcohol and Rape and Sexual Assault

More than 30 percent of rape victims reported that their assailant was under the influence of alcohol.[29] Almost 20 percent of undergraduate women reported experiencing some type of sexual assault since entering college—with most incidents involving alcohol or unknowingly consuming a drug placed in their drinks.[30] Most college assault victims know their attacker, and assaults occur frequently at parties.

Alcohol and Weight Gain

Freshman college year weight gain may have more to do with alcohol consumption than the food served in the dining halls. By drinking an extra 150 calories a day (the amount in a typical serving of beer), you can gain 1 pound a month and up to 12 pounds a year.[31]

Alcohol Poisoning

Alcohol poisoning (*acute alcohol intoxication*) occurs much more frequently than people realize and can be fatal. Drinking large amounts of alcohol in a short period of time can cause one's BAC to quickly reach the lethal range. Alcohol, used either alone or in combination with other drugs, is responsible for more toxic overdose deaths than any other substance.

The amount of alcohol that causes loss of consciousness is dangerously close to the lethal dose. Death from alcohol poisoning can be caused by either CNS and respiratory depression or by inhalation of vomit or fluid into the lungs. Alcohol depresses the nerves that control involuntary actions such as breathing and the gag reflex (which prevents choking). At higher BAC levels, these functions can

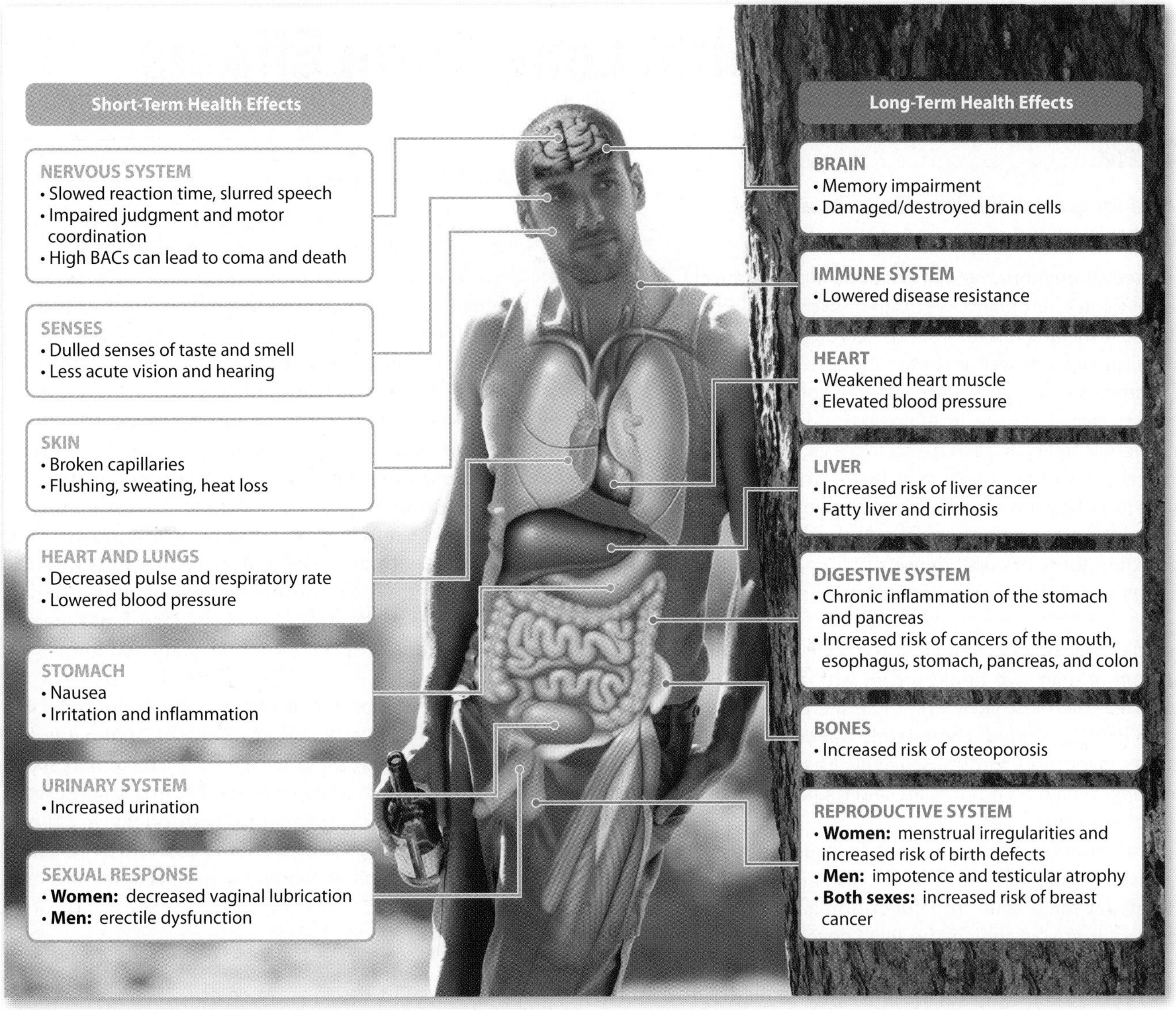

Short-Term Health Effects

NERVOUS SYSTEM
- Slowed reaction time, slurred speech
- Impaired judgment and motor coordination
- High BACs can lead to coma and death

SENSES
- Dulled senses of taste and smell
- Less acute vision and hearing

SKIN
- Broken capillaries
- Flushing, sweating, heat loss

HEART AND LUNGS
- Decreased pulse and respiratory rate
- Lowered blood pressure

STOMACH
- Nausea
- Irritation and inflammation

URINARY SYSTEM
- Increased urination

SEXUAL RESPONSE
- **Women:** decreased vaginal lubrication
- **Men:** erectile dysfunction

Long-Term Health Effects

BRAIN
- Memory impairment
- Damaged/destroyed brain cells

IMMUNE SYSTEM
- Lowered disease resistance

HEART
- Weakened heart muscle
- Elevated blood pressure

LIVER
- Increased risk of liver cancer
- Fatty liver and cirrhosis

DIGESTIVE SYSTEM
- Chronic inflammation of the stomach and pancreas
- Increased risk of cancers of the mouth, esophagus, stomach, pancreas, and colon

BONES
- Increased risk of osteoporosis

REPRODUCTIVE SYSTEM
- **Women:** menstrual irregularities and increased risk of birth defects
- **Men:** impotence and testicular atrophy
- **Both sexes:** increased risk of breast cancer

Figure 7.5 Effects of Alcohol on the Body and Health

VIDEO TUTOR
Long- and Short-Term Effects of Alcohol

be completely suppressed. If a drinker becomes unconscious and vomits, there is danger of deadly asphyxiation through choking on one's own vomit. BAC can rise even after a drinker becomes unconscious, because alcohol in the stomach and intestine continues to empty into the bloodstream.

Skills for Behavior Change

DEALING WITH AN ALCOHOL EMERGENCY

Heavy drinking can be life threatening. Anyone who has passed out from drinking should be watched very closely. Roll an unconscious drinker onto his or her side with knees bent to minimize the chance of vomit obstructing the airway. If the drinker vomits, you may need to reach into his or her mouth and clear the airway.

If you suspect that someone has alcohol poisoning, call 9-1-1 immediately to get help. For the safety of you and your friends, know the signs of acute alcohol intoxication:

- **Mental confusion, stupor, coma, or inability to be roused**
- **Vomiting and/or seizures**
- **Slow breathing (fewer than eight breaths per minute)**
- **Rapid or irregular pulse (100 beats or more per minute) or irregular breathing (10 seconds or more between breaths)**
- **Cool, clammy skin; bluish skin, fingernails, or lips.**

check yourself

- **What are the short-term health effects of alcohol consumption?**
- **What actions should you take if you're with someone who shows symptoms of alcohol poisoning?**

7.4 Alcohol and Your Health: Long-Term Effects

learning outcome

7.4 Discuss the long-term health effects of alcohol consumption.

Alcohol is distributed throughout most of the body and may affect many organs and tissues. Problems associated with long-term, habitual alcohol abuse include diseases of the nervous system, cardiovascular system, and liver, as well as some cancers.

The nervous system is especially sensitive to alcohol. Even moderate drinkers experience shrinkage in brain size and weight and some loss of intellectual ability. Research also suggests that alcohol damages the frontal areas of the adolescent brain, which are crucial for controlling impulses and thinking through consequences.[32] People who begin drinking at an early age are at much higher risk of experiencing alcohol abuse or dependence, drinking five or more drinks per occasion, and driving under the influence of alcohol at least weekly.[33]

Numerous studies have associated light-to-moderate alcohol consumption (no more than two drinks a day) with reduced risk of coronary artery disease, most likely due to an increase in high-density lipoprotein (HDL), or "good" cholesterol.[34] However, alcohol consumption causes many more cardiovascular health hazards than benefits, contributing to high blood pressure and slightly increased heart rate and cardiac output.

One of the most common diseases related to alcohol abuse is **cirrhosis** of the liver (Figure 7.6). With heavy drinking, the liver begins to store fat; fat-filled cells stop functioning. Continued drinking can cause *fibrosis*, in which the liver develops fibrous scar tissue. If the person continues to drink, cirrhosis results—the liver cells die and the damage becomes permanent. In **alcoholic hepatitis**, another serious condition, chronic inflammation of the liver develops, which may be fatal in itself or progress to cirrhosis.

Long-term alcohol use has been linked to cancers of the esophagus, stomach, mouth, tongue, and liver. One study discovered a possible link between acetaldehyde and DNA damage that could help explain this connection.[35]

Substantial evidence indicates that women who consume three to six drinks per week have a higher risk of breast cancer than do abstainers, and the risk is even higher for women who consume more than two drinks per day.[36] In a study, girls and young women who drank 6 or 7 days a week were 5.5 times more likely to have benign breast disease—which itself increases the risk for breast cancer—than those who had less than one drink per week.[37]

The pancreas produces digestive enzymes and insulin. Chronic alcohol abuse reduces enzyme production, inhibiting nutrient absorption. Alcohol may also impair the body's ability to recognize and fight bacteria and viruses. Drinking alcohol can block absorption of calcium—of particular concern to women because of their risk for osteoporosis. Drinking alcohol also significantly increases trouble with both falling asleep and staying asleep.

Alcohol and Pregnancy

Teratogenic substances cause birth defects. Of 30 known teratogens, alcohol is one of the most dangerous. More than 7.6 percent of children have been exposed to alcohol *in utero*, and 1.4 percent of pregnant women reported binge drinking.[38] Consuming four or more drinks a day during pregnancy may significantly increase risk of childhood mental health and learning problems. Alcohol consumed during the first trimester poses the greatest threat to organ development; exposure during the last trimester, when the brain develops rapidly, is most likely to affect the CNS.

Fetal alcohol syndrome (FAS), which is associated with alcohol consumption during pregnancy, is the third most common birth defect and the second leading cause of mental retardation in the United States, with an estimated incidence of 0.2 to 1.5 in every 1,000 live births.[39] Symptoms include mental retardation; small head; tremors; abnormalities of the face, limbs, heart, and brain; poor memory; reduced attention span; and impulsive behavior.

Children with some symptoms of FAS may be diagnosed with partial fetal alcohol syndrome (PFAS) or alcohol-related neurodevelopmental disorder (ARND); these, like FAS, are *fetal alcohol spectrum disorders* (FASD). Infants whose mothers habitually consumed more than 3 ounces of alcohol (approximately six drinks) in a short time when pregnant are at high risk for FASD.[40] To avoid any chance of harming her fetus, any woman who is or may become pregnant should not consume alcohol.

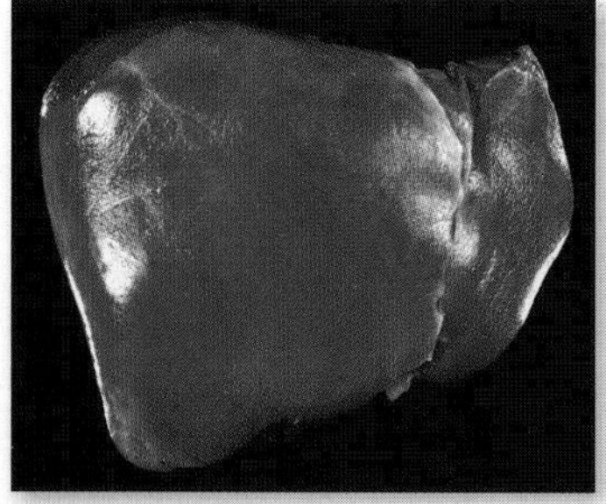

(a) A normal liver

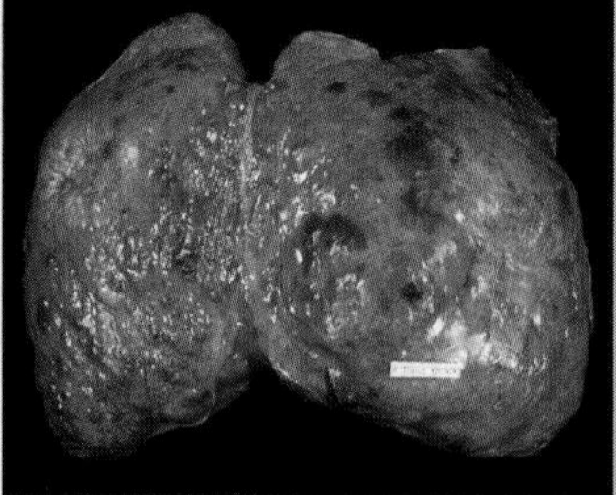

(b) A liver with cirrhosis

Figure 7.6 Comparison of a Healthy Liver with a Cirrhotic Liver

check yourself

- **What are some long-term health effects of alcohol consumption?**
- **How does awareness of these effects influence your decision whether to consume alcohol?**

7.5

Drinking and Driving

learning outcome

7.5 List effects of alcohol use on the ability to drive safely.

Traffic accidents are the leading cause of accidental death for all age groups from 1 to 44 years old.[41] In the United States, adults drank too much and got behind the wheel approximately 112 million times in a year.[42] Alcohol-impaired drivers are involved in about 1 in 3 crash deaths, resulting in nearly 11,000 deaths a year.[43] This number represents roughly one traffic fatality every 51 minutes.[44] Some groups are more likely to drink and drive than others. Men were responsible for 81 percent of the drinking and driving episodes, and 85 percent of people drinking and driving were reportedly binge drinking.[45] Unfortunately, college students are overrepresented in alcohol-related crashes. A recent survey reported that about 23 percent of college students reported having driven after drinking and about 2 percent said they had driven after drinking five or more drinks in the past 30 days.[46]

Over the past 20 years, the percentage of drivers involved in fatal crashes who were intoxicated (BAC of 0.08 percent or greater) has decreased for all age groups (Figure 7.7). Several factors have probably contributed to these reductions in fatalities: laws that increased the drinking age to 21; stricter law enforcement; laws prohibiting anyone under 21 from driving with any detectable BAC; increased automobile safety; and educational programs designed to discourage drinking and driving. The legal limit for BAC in all states is 0.08 percent. Furthermore, all states have zero-tolerance laws for driving while intoxicated, and the penalty is usually suspension of the driver's license.

Despite all these measures, the risk of being involved in an alcohol-related automobile crash remains substantial. Laboratory and test track research shows that the vast majority of drivers are impaired even at 0.08 BAC with regard to critical driving tasks. The likelihood of a driver being involved in a fatal crash rises significantly with a BAC of 0.05 percent and even more rapidly after 0.08 percent.[47]

Alcohol-related fatal car crashes occur more often at night than during the day, and the hours between 9:00 P.M. and 6:00 A.M. are the most dangerous. Sixty-seven percent of fatally injured drivers involved in nighttime single-vehicle crashes had BACs at or above 0.08 percent.[48] The risk of being involved in an alcohol-related crash increases not only with the time of day, but also with the day of the week; 24 percent of all fatal crashes during the week were alcohol related, compared with 46 percent on weekends.[49]

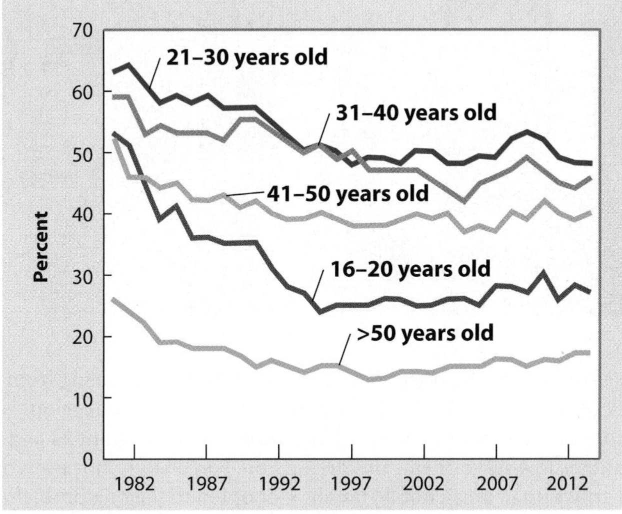

Figure 7.7 Percentage of Fatally Injured Drivers with BACs Greater Than 0.08 Percent, by Driver Age, 1982–2012

Source: Insurance Institute for Highway Safety, "Fatality Facts 2012: Alcohol," http://www.iihs.org. Copyright 2013. Reprinted with permission.

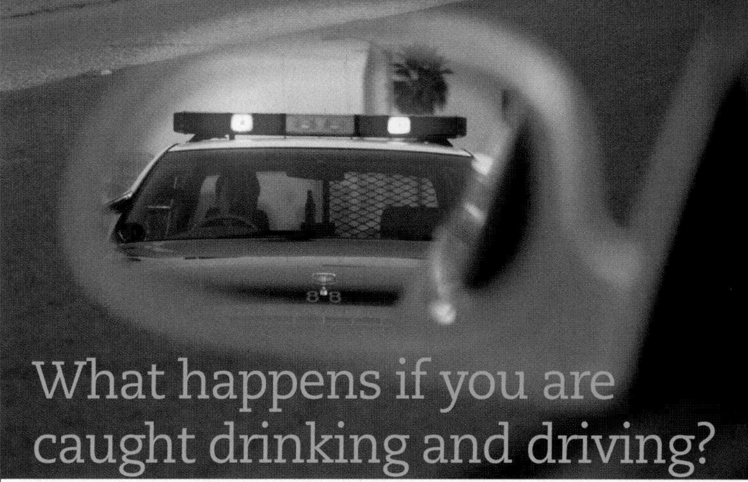

What happens if you are caught drinking and driving?

Getting behind the wheel if you have consumed alcohol is a dangerous choice, with serious legal consequences if you are caught and convicted of driving under the influence (DUI). If you are under age 21 and have any detectable alcohol in your bloodstream, your license can be revoked. Other common penalties for DUI include driver's license restrictions, fines, mandatory counseling, and jail time, even for a first offense. In many states, if you are convicted three times for DUI, you are considered a habitual violator and penalized as a felon, meaning that you lose your right to vote and to own a weapon, among other rights, as well as possibly losing your license permanently. If you are involved in an accident in which someone is injured or killed, the consequences are even more serious. Involvement in such an incident is considered a felony in many states. If a person dies as a result of the accident, the drunk driver may be charged with manslaughter or second-degree murder.

3 in 10

Americans will be involved in an alcohol-related accident at some time in their lives.

check yourself

- **How does alcohol impact the ability to drive?**

7.6 Alcohol Abuse and Alcoholism

learning outcome

7.6 Discuss biological and psychological causes of alcoholism.

Alcohol use becomes alcohol abuse when it interferes with work, school, or social and family relationships or when it entails any violation of the law, including driving under the influence (DUI). **Alcoholism**, or **alcohol dependency**, results when personal and health problems related to alcohol use are severe and stopping alcohol use causes withdrawal symptoms.

Identifying an Alcoholic

As with other drug addictions, tolerance, psychological dependence, and withdrawal symptoms must be present to qualify a drinker as an addict. Irresponsible and problem drinkers, such as people who get into fights or embarrass themselves or others when they drink, aren't necessarily alcoholics. About 15 percent of people in the United States are problem drinkers; about 5 to 10 percent of male and 3 to 5 percent of female drinkers would be diagnosed as alcohol dependent.[50]

Among full-time college students, 1 in 4 experienced alcohol abuse or dependence in the past year.[51] In a recent study, the progression to alcohol dependency based on college students' drinking patterns when they entered showed that 1.9 percent of nondrinkers, 4.3 percent of light drinkers, 12.8 percent of moderate drinkers, and 19 percent of heavy drinkers developed alcohol dependency.[52]

Causes of Alcohol Abuse and Alcoholism

Biological and Family Factors Children of alcoholics have higher rates of alcoholism than the general population. Development of alcoholism among individuals with a family history of alcoholism is four to eight times more common than it is among those with no such history.[53]

Despite such evidence, scientists do not yet understand the precise role of genes in increased risk for alcoholism, nor have they identified a specific "alcoholism" gene. Adoption studies demonstrate a strong link between individuals' substance use and their biological children's risk for addiction. Recently, scientists have found a gene that, by controlling the way that alcohol stimulates the brain to release dopamine, can trigger feelings of reward, giving individuals with the gene a stronger sense of reward from alcohol.[54] No single gene causes addiction, though, and multiple genes can affect the ability to develop addiction.

Social and Cultural Factors Some people begin drinking as a way to dull the pain of an acute loss or an emotional or social problem. Unfortunately, the discomfort that causes many people to turn to alcohol ultimately causes even more discomfort as the drug's depressant effect takes its toll. Eventually, the drinker becomes physically dependent.

Family attitudes also seem to be an influence; people raised in cultures in which alcohol is a part of religious or ceremonial activities or a traditional part of the family meal are less prone to alcohol dependence. In contrast, in societies in which alcohol purchase is carefully controlled and drinking regarded as a rite of passage, the tendency for abuse appears greater.

The amount of alcohol a person consumes seems to be directly related to the drinking habits of that individual's social group. Those whose friends and relatives drink heavily are 50 percent more likely

How does it affect you to grow up in a family with alcoholism?

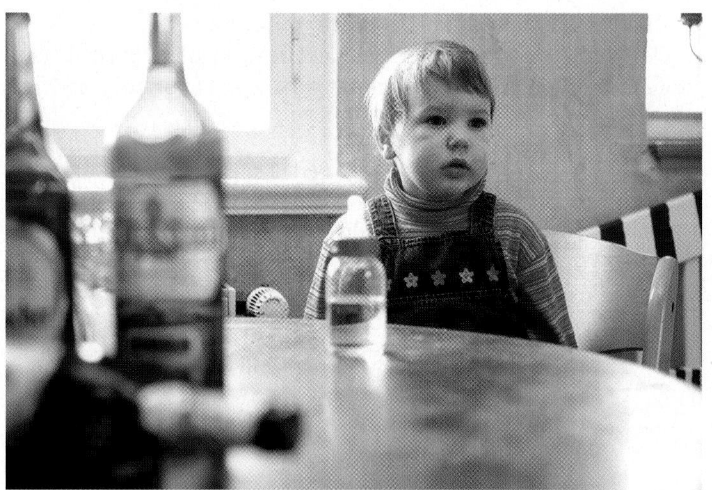

Adult children of alcoholics have unique problems stemming from a lack of parental nurturing during childhood: difficulty developing social attachments, a need to be in control of all emotions and situations, low self-esteem, and depression. Fortunately, not everyone who grows up in an alcoholic family is doomed to lifelong problems. As they mature, many develop resiliency in response to their families' problems and enter adulthood armed with positive strengths and valuable skills.

to drink heavily themselves[55]—a finding with importance for individuals who need to sever ties with heavy drinkers to maintain abstinence.

Women and Alcoholism

Women tend to become alcoholics at later ages and after fewer years of heavy drinking than do men. Women also get addicted faster with less alcohol use. With greater risks for cirrhosis; excessive memory loss and shrinkage of the brain; heart disease; and cancers of the mouth, throat, esophagus, liver, and colon than male alcoholics, women suffer the consequences of alcoholism more profoundly.[56]

The highest risks for alcoholism occur among women who are unmarried but living with a partner, are in their twenties or early thirties, or have a husband or partner who drinks heavily. Other risks for women include a family history of drinking problems, pressure to drink from a peer or spouse, depression, and stress.

Different Ethnicities and Alcoholism

Among Native American populations, alcohol is the most widely used drug; the rate of alcoholism is two to three times higher than the national average, and the death rate from alcohol-related causes is eight times higher than the national average.[57] Poor economic conditions and the cultural belief that alcoholism is a spiritual problem, not a physical disease, may partially account for high alcoholism rates.

On average, African Americans drink less than white Americans; however, those who do drink tend to be heavy drinkers, and twice as many African Americans die of cirrhosis of the liver.[58] Alcohol also contributes to high rates of hypertension, esophageal cancer, and homicide in African Americans.

Among Latino populations, men have a higher than average rate of alcohol abuse and alcohol-related health problems, though recent evidence shows drinking rates among Latina women are matching or surpassing those of young Latino men.[59] Many researchers agree that a major factor for alcohol problems in this ethnic group is the key role that drinking plays in Latino culture.[60]

Asian Americans have a very low rate of alcoholism[61] and alcohol-related injuries. Social and cultural influences, such as strong kinship ties, are thought to discourage heavy drinking in Asian American groups. Asians also have a genetic predisposition that might influence their low risk for alcohol abuse.[62]

Effects on Family and Friends

An estimated 7.5 million children in the United States live with a parent who has experienced an alcohol use disorder in the past year. These children are at increased risk for physical illness, emotional disturbances, behavioral problems, lower educational performance, and susceptibility to alcoholism or other addictions later in life.[63]

In dysfunctional families, children learn certain unspoken rules that allow the family to avoid dealing with real problems—don't talk, don't trust, and don't feel. Unfortunately, these behaviors enable the alcoholic to keep drinking. Children in such families generally assume at least one of the following roles:

- **Family hero.** Tries to divert attention from the problem by being too good to be true.
- **Scapegoat.** Draws attention from the family's primary problem through delinquency or misbehavior.
- **Lost child.** Becomes passive and withdraws from upsetting situations.
- **Mascot.** Disrupts tense situations with comic relief.

Children in alcoholic homes have to deal with constant stress, anxiety, and embarrassment. The alcoholic is the center of attention; children's needs are often ignored. It is not uncommon for these children to be victims of violence, abuse, neglect, or incest.

Living with a family member (or friend or roommate) who is an alcoholic can be extremely stressful. People in close proximity to alcoholics can find themselves in codependent relationships that are often emotionally destructive or abusive and that enable the alcoholic's addiction. Codependents try to cover up for the addicted person: They may make excuses for the drinker's behavior or lie to others to cover for him or her.

Costs to Society

Alcohol-related costs to society are estimated at well over 223.5 billion, including health insurance, criminal justice costs, treatment costs, and lost productivity.[64]Alcoholism is directly or indirectly responsible for over 25 percent of the nation's medical expenses and lost earnings.[65]

A study estimated that underage drinking costs society $68 billion annually.[66] The largest costs were related to violence ($35 billion) and drunk-driving accidents ($9.955 billion), followed by high-risk sex ($5 billion), property crime ($3 billion), and addiction treatment programs (nearly $2.5 billion). The study estimated that every underage drinker costs society an average of $2,070 a year.[67]

check yourself

- **What is the difference between alcohol abuse and alcoholism?**
- **What factors can make a person more likely to abuse alcohol or become an alcoholic?**
- **How does alcoholism affect the family and friends of the alcoholic?**

7.7 Reducing Alcohol Intake

learning outcome

7.7 List practical steps for reducing alcohol intake.

Alcoholism is characterized by symptoms including craving, loss of control, physical dependence, and tolerance. People who recognize one or more of these behaviors in themselves may wish to seek professional help to determine whether alcohol has become a controlling factor in their lives.

There are some steps that you can take on your own if you are concerned about the amount of alcohol that you consume. Being worried about your consumption is a strong signal that there may be cause for alarm. If a counselor or health care practitioner advises you to reduce or eliminate alcohol intake, you should follow their suggestions and guidance. There are also ways for you to cut down your drinking on your own, depending on their recommendations.

Skills for Behavior Change

HOW TO CUT DOWN ON YOUR DRINKING

If you suspect that you drink too much, talk with a counselor or clinician at your student health center. Either of these professionals can tell you whether you should cut down or abstain. If you have a severe drinking problem, alcoholism in your family, or other medical problems, you should stop drinking completely. Your counselor or clinician will advise you about what is right for you.

If you need to cut down on your drinking, these steps can help you:

- **Write your reasons for cutting down or stopping.** There are many reasons you may want to cut down or stop drinking. You may want to improve your health, sleep better, or get along better with your family or friends.
- **Set a drinking goal.** Determine a limit for how much you will drink. You may choose to cut down, or to not drink at all. If you aren't sure what goal is right for you, talk with your counselor. Once you determine your goal, write it down on a piece of paper. Put it someplace you can see it, such as on your refrigerator or bathroom mirror.
- **Keep a journal of your drinking.** Write down every time you have a drink. Try to keep your journal for 3 or 4 weeks. This will show you how much you drink and when. You may be surprised. How different is your goal from the amount you drink now?
- **Keep little or no alcohol at home.** You don't need the temptation.
- **Drink slowly.** When you drink, sip slowly. Take a break of 1 hour between drinks. Drink a nonalcoholic beverage, such as soda, water, or juice, after every alcoholic drink you consume. Do not drink on an empty stomach! Eat food when you are drinking.
- **Take a break from alcohol.** Pick a day or two each week when you will not drink at all. Then try to stop drinking for 1 week. Think about how you feel physically and emotionally on these days. When you succeed and feel better, you may find it easier to cut down for good.
- **Learn how to say no.** You do not have to drink when other people are or take a drink when offered one. Practice ways to say no politely. Stay away from people who give you a hard time about not drinking.
- **Stay active.** Use the time and money once spent on drinking to do something fun with your family or friends. Go out to eat, see a movie, or play sports or a game.
- **Get support.** Cutting down on your drinking may be difficult at times. Ask your family and friends for support to help you reach your goal. Talk to your counselor if you are having trouble cutting down. Get the help you need to reach your goal.

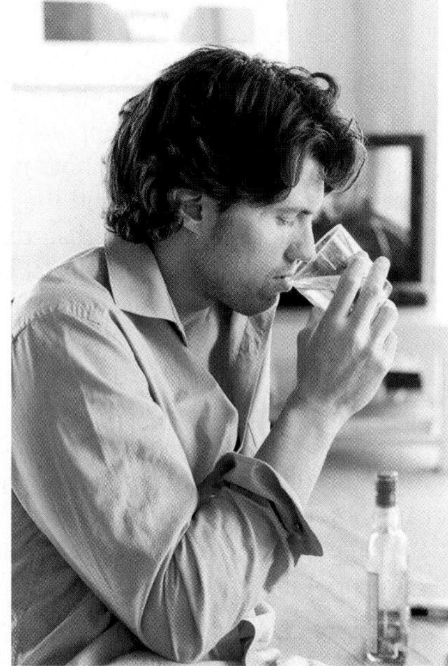

- **Avoid temptations.** Watch out for people, places, or times that lead you to drink, even if you did not want to. Plan ahead of time what you will do to avoid drinking when you are tempted. Do not drink when you are angry, upset, or having a bad day.
- **Remember, don't give up!** Most people don't cut down or give up drinking all at once. As with a diet, it is not easy to change. That's OK. If you don't reach your goal the first time, try again. Remember, get support from people who care about you and want to help.

check yourself

- What are some practical steps to cut down on your drinking?
- Have you ever decided to reduce the amount of alcohol you consume? If so, what were the steps that you took?

Treatment and Recovery

learning outcome

7.8 Explain treatment options available to alcoholics.

Despite growing recognition of our national alcohol problem, only a very small percentage of alcoholics ever receive care in special treatment facilities. Contributing factors include inability or unwillingness to admit to a problem, social stigma, inability to pay for treatment, breakdowns in referral and delivery systems, and failure of medical providers to recognize or diagnose symptoms among patients.[68] Most problem drinkers who seek help reach a turning point—finally recognizing that alcohol controls their lives.

An alcoholic's family sometimes takes action before the alcoholic does. An effective method of helping an alcoholic confront the disease is **intervention**, a planned confrontation involving family and friends plus professional counselors.

Alcoholics who quit drinking experience detoxification, the process by which addicts end their dependence on a drug. Withdrawal symptoms include hyperexcitability, confusion and agitation, sleep disorders, convulsions, tremors, depression, headaches, and seizures. A small percentage of people have **delirium tremens (DTs)**—confusion, delusions, agitation, and hallucinations.

Treatment Programs

Private Treatment Facilities Upon admission to a private treatment facility, the patient receives a complete physical exam to determine whether underlying medical problems will interfere with treatment. Shortly after detoxification, alcoholics begin treatment for psychological addiction. Most treatment facilities keep patients from 3 to 6 weeks and charge several thousand dollars; some insurance programs or employers assume most of the expense.

Therapy Several types of therapy are commonly used in alcoholism recovery. In family therapy, the person and family members examine psychological reasons underlying the addiction. In individual and group therapy with fellow addicts, alcoholics learn positive coping skills for situations that have caused them to turn to alcohol.

On some college campuses, the problems associated with alcohol abuse are so great that student health centers are opening their own treatment programs. At some schools, students in recovery live together in special housing. Programs such as these hope to provide the support and comfortable environment recovering students need.

Pharmacological Treatment Disulfiram (trade name Antabuse) is a drug commonly used for treating alcoholism. If users drink alcohol or consume foods with alcohol content, disulfiram causes acetaldehyde to build up in the liver, triggering nausea, vomiting, headache, bad breath, drowsiness, and impotence. Naltrexone is used to reduce alcohol cravings and decrease the pleasant effects of alcohol, without making the user ill. Acamprosate (Campral) is thought to restore normal brain balance, which has been disturbed in the alcohol dependent, and to reduce the physical and emotional discomfort often associated with staying alcohol free. All pharmacological treatments for alcoholism should be used in conjunction with psychotherapy or support groups.

Support Groups **Alcoholics Anonymous (AA)** is a nonprofit self-help organization with more than 1 million members; it offers group support to help people stop drinking. Related *Al-Anon* and *Alateen* groups help relatives, friends, and children of alcoholics understand the disease and how they can contribute to the recovery process. Other self-help groups include Women for Sobriety, which addresses the specific needs of female alcoholics, and Secular Organizations for Sobriety (SOS), founded to help those uncomfortable with AA's spiritual emphasis.

Relapse

Success with recovery varies. Over half of alcoholics relapse (resume drinking) within the first 3 months of treatment. Treating an addiction requires more than getting the addict to stop using a substance; it also requires getting the person to break a pattern of behavior that has dominated his or her life. Many alcoholics refer to themselves as "recovering" throughout their lifetime rather than "cured."

People in recovery must not only confront addictions but also guard against relapse. It is important to identify situations that could trigger a relapse, such as becoming angry or frustrated and being around others who drink. During the initial recovery period, it can help to join a support group, maintain stability (resisting the urge to relocate, travel, take a new job, or make other drastic life changes), set aside time each day for reflection, and maintain a pattern of assuming responsibility for one's own actions. To be effective, recovery programs must offer alcoholics ways to increase self-esteem and resume personal growth.

check yourself

- **Why do so few alcoholics receive treatment?**
- **What treatment options are available for alcoholics?**

7.9

Tobacco Use in the United States

learning outcome

7.9 Examine reasons that people start smoking and factors that contribute to tobacco use by college students.

Approximately 70 million Americans report using tobacco products (cigarettes, cigars, smokeless tobacco, and pipe tobacco) at least once in the past month.[69] In 2012, 20.5 percent of men and 15.8 percent of women were current cigarette smokers. Adults 25 to 44 years old had the highest percentage of current cigarette smoking (22 percent).[70]

Education is closely linked to cigarette use: Adults with a bachelor's degree or higher education are two times *less* likely to smoke than are those with less than a high school education. Cigarette smoking also varies by ethnicity and gender, with the highest rates of smoking found among American Indian and Alaska Native men.[71]

More than 20 percent of Americans are former smokers; about 60 percent have never smoked. The most commonly used tobacco product is cigarettes, more common among men (20.5%) than women (15.8%), followed by cigars (9.1% of men and 2.0% of women) and smokeless tobacco (3.5 percent of people 12 and older).[72]

Why Do People Use Tobacco?

Nicotine Addiction Beginning smokers usually feel the effects of nicotine with their first puff. These symptoms, called **nicotine poisoning**, can include dizziness, lightheadedness, rapid and erratic pulse, clammy skin, nausea, vomiting, and diarrhea. Symptoms cease as tolerance develops, which happens as quickly as the second or third cigarette. Many regular smokers experience no "buzz," but continue to smoke because stopping is too difficult.

Studies have found genetic factors to be significantly influential in smoking initiation and nicotine dependence. Specifically, one study found that teenagers carrying variants in two genes were three times more likely to become regular smokers in adolescence and twice as likely to be persistent smokers in adulthood, compared to noncarriers.[73] These two specific genes may influence smoking behavior by affecting the action of the brain chemical dopamine.[74] Understanding the influence of genetics on nicotine addiction could be crucial to developing more effective smoking-cessation treatments.[75]

Behavioral Dependence People who smoke are not just physically but also psychologically dependent. Nicotine "tricks" the brain into creating pleasurable associations with sensory stimuli or environmental cues that may trigger the urge for a cigarette.[76] Some former smokers remain vulnerable to sensory and environmental cues for many years after they quit.

Weight Control Nicotine is an appetite suppressant and slightly increases basal metabolic rate. After smoking a cigarette, one's metabolism quickly increases then returns to normal; heavy smokers have such surges throughout the day. When a smoker quits, the metabolic rate slows down and appetite returns. People tend to eat more, particularly sweets. Fear of gaining weight is one of the biggest reasons smokers are reluctant to quit. To avoid weight gain after quitting smoking, avoid crash diets, keep low-calorie treats handy, and drink plenty of water.

Advertising The tobacco industry spends an estimated $24 million per day on advertising and promotion.[77] With the number of smokers declining by about 1 million each year, the industry must actively recruit new smokers. Tobacco advertising encourages young people to begin smoking before they are old enough to understand the long-term health risks.[78] Of adult smokers, 90 percent started by age 21, and half became regular smokers by age 18. Tobacco companies have also targeted children and teens with products using candy, fruit, or alcohol flavorings, thus making them more palatable to young people.[79]

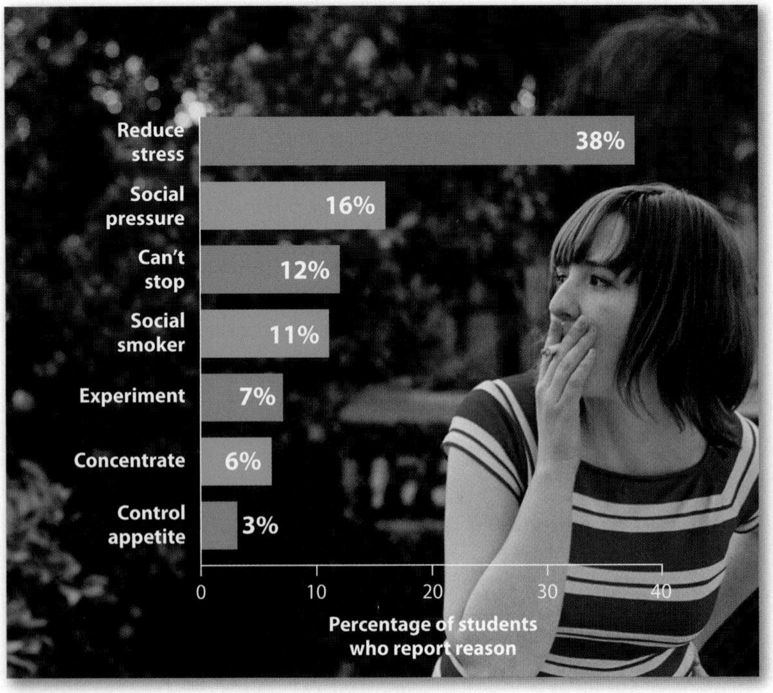

Reduce stress 38%
Social pressure 16%
Can't stop 12%
Social smoker 11%
Experiment 7%
Concentrate 6%
Control appetite 3%
0 10 20 30 40
Percentage of students who report reason

Figure 7.8 Reasons for Smoking among College Student Smokers

Source: National Center on Addiction and Substance Abuse at Columbia University, *Wasting the Best and the Brightest: Substance Abuse at America's Colleges and Universities* (New York, NY: National Center on Addiction and Substance Abuse at Columbia University, 2007), 48. Copyright © 2007. Used with permission.

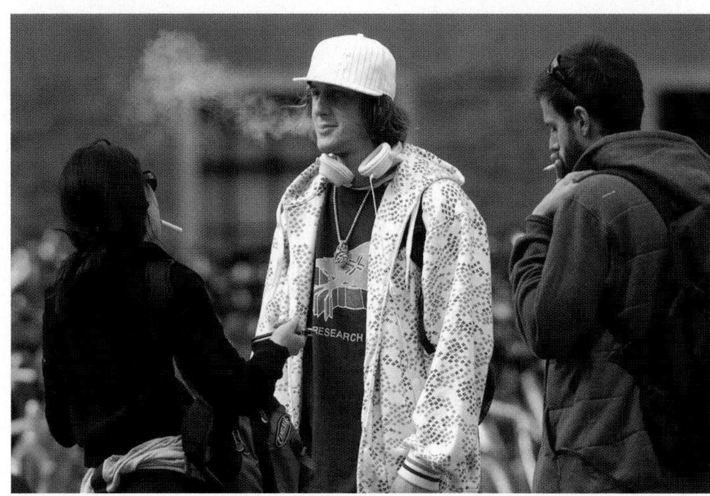

Is social smoking that bad for me?

An occasional puff once in a while when you are out with friends can't hurt, right? Wrong! There is no "safe" amount of tobacco use—any smoking or exposure to smoke increases your risks for negative health effects such as heart disease and lung cancer.

Advertisements in women's magazines imply that smoking is the key to financial success, thinness, independence, and social acceptance. These ads have apparently been working. From the mid-1970s through the early 2000s, cigarette sales to women increased dramatically. Not coincidentally, by 1987 cigarette-induced lung cancer had surpassed breast cancer as the leading cancer killer among women and has remained the leading cancer killer in every year since.[80]

Women are not the only targets of gender-based cigarette advertisements. Men are depicted in locker rooms, charging over rugged terrain in off-road vehicles, or riding stallions into the sunset in blatant appeals to a need to feel and appear masculine. Minorities are also often targeted. Tobacco advertising, particularly menthol cigarettes, is much more common in magazines aimed at African Americans. Billboards and posters spreading the cigarette message have dotted the landscape in Hispanic communities for many years, especially in low-income areas.

Financial Costs to Society

Estimates show annual costs attributed to smoking in the United States are between $289 and $333 billion. The economic burden of tobacco use totals more than $132 to $176 billion in direct medical expenditures and $156 billion in lost productivity.[81] These costs far exceed the tax revenues on the sale of tobacco products, even though the average cigarette tax in 2012 was $1.53 per pack and is rising in some states.[82]

College Students and Tobacco Use

Although college students are the targets of heavy tobacco advertising campaigns, cigarette smoking among U.S. college students has decreased in recent years. In a 2013 study, about 11.7 percent of college students reported having smoked cigarettes in the past 30 days.[83] College men have slightly higher rates of smoking (15 percent) compared to women (10 percent).[84] Men also use more cigars and smokeless tobacco.[85]

Why Do College Students Smoke?

Some of the reasons college students smoke are to relax or reduce stress (Figure 7.8). Other key reasons students smoke are to fit in or because they are addicted. For some students, weight control is an important motivator, and fear of weight gain is a common reason for smoking relapse. Students diagnosed or treated for depression are much more likely to use tobacco compared to students who are not.

Many college-age smokers identify themselves as "social smokers"—those who smoke when they are with people, rather than alone. Up to half of college smokers deny being smokers, even though they reported smoking in the past 30 days. Many of these students smoke in social situations where they also drink alcohol.[86] Like regular smokers, social smokers engage in more alcohol use, illicit drug use, and higher sexual risk taking behaviors than nonsmokers.[87] Even occasional smoking is not without risks of damaging health effects. Social smoking in college can lead to a complete dependence on nicotine and thus to all the same health risks as smoking regularly.

Smoking less than a pack of cigarettes a week has been shown to damage blood vessels and to increase the risk of heart disease and cancer.[88] Occasional or social smokers also experience an increased occurrence of colds, sore throats, shortness of breath, and fatigue.[89] In women taking birth control pills, even a few cigarettes a week can increase the likelihood of heart disease, blood clots, stroke, liver cancer, and gallbladder disease.[90] Pregnant women who smoke only occasionally still run a risk of giving birth to unhealthy babies.

Unlike social smokers, most students who smoke regularly and are nicotine dependent do want to stop smoking, but in spite of their efforts or desire to quit, they continue to smoke throughout college. To reduce the incidence of smoking among students, colleges and universities need to engage in antismoking efforts, control tobacco advertising, provide smoke-free residence halls, and offer greater access to smoking-cessation programs.

As policies designed to reduce cigarette smoking increase, the use of electronic cigarettes poses an additional challenge. E-cigarette use is banned on many campuses. Because e-cigarettes are not yet regulated by the FDA and health effects remain in question, many campuses are being proactive in reducing potential health threats.

check yourself

- **The tobacco industry has been accused of targeting college students in its marketing campaigns. Do you agree? If so, give examples of tobacco marketing that target young adults.**
- **What factors make college students more likely to use tobacco?**

7.10 Tobacco: Its Components and Effects

learning **outcome**

7.10 Compare and contrast tobacco products on the market.

Smoking, the most common form of tobacco use, delivers a strong dose of nicotine directly to the lungs, along with 7,000 other chemical substances, including 69 known or suspected carcinogens (cancer-causing agents).[91] Inhaling hot toxic gases exposes sensitive mucous membranes to irritating chemicals that weaken the tissues and contribute to cancers of the mouth, larynx, and throat. The heat from tobacco smoke is also harmful to tissues.

Nicotine

The highly addictive chemical stimulant **nicotine** is the major psychoactive substance in all tobacco products. When tobacco leaves are burned in a cigarette, pipe, or cigar, nicotine is inhaled into the lungs. Sucking or chewing tobacco releases nicotine into the saliva; it is then absorbed through the mucous membranes in the mouth.

Nicotine is a powerful central nervous system stimulant that produces a variety of physiological effects. In the cerebral cortex, it produces an aroused, alert mental state. It stimulates production of adrenaline, increases heart and respiratory rates, constricts blood vessels, and, in turn, increases blood pressure because the heart must work harder to pump blood through narrowed vessels.

Tar and Carbon Monoxide

Cigarette smoke is a complex mixture of chemicals and gases produced by the burning of tobacco and its additives. Particulate matter condenses in the lungs to form a sludge called **tar**, which contains carcinogenic agents, such as benzopyrene, and chemical irritants, such as phenol. Phenol has the potential to combine with other chemicals that contribute to developing lung cancer.

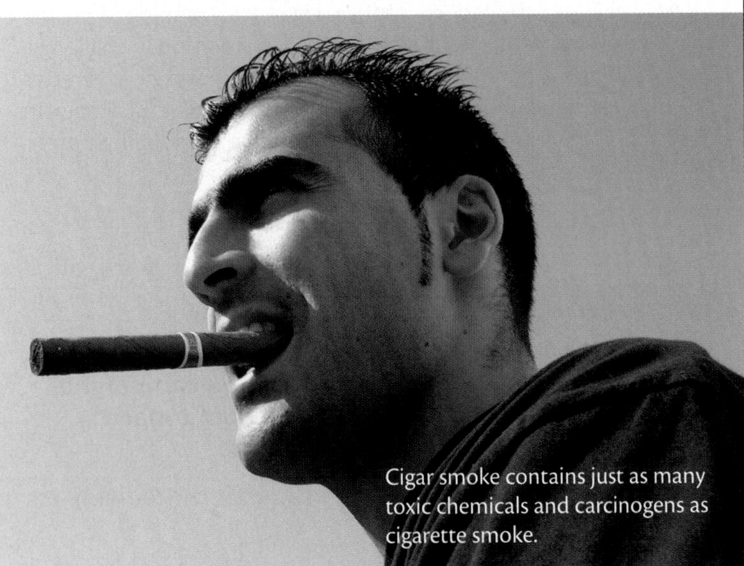

Cigar smoke contains just as many toxic chemicals and carcinogens as cigarette smoke.

In healthy lungs, millions of tiny hairlike projections (*cilia*) on the surfaces lining the upper respiratory passages sweep away foreign matter, which is then expelled from the lungs by coughing. However, in smokers, nicotine paralyzes the cilia for up to 1 hour following a single cigarette, impairing their cleansing function. This allows tars and other solids in tobacco smoke to accumulate and irritate sensitive lung tissue.

Cigarette smoke also contains poisonous gases, the most dangerous of which is **carbon monoxide**, the deadly gas emitted in car exhaust. In the human body, carbon monoxide reduces the oxygen-carrying capacity of red blood cells by binding with the receptor sites for oxygen; this causes oxygen deprivation in many body tissues. It is at least partly responsible for increased risk of heart attacks and strokes in smokers.

Tobacco Products

Cigarettes *Filtered cigarettes* are the most common form of tobacco available today. Almost all manufactured cigarettes have filters designed to reduce levels of gases such as hydrogen cyanide and carbon monoxide, but these products may actually deliver more hazardous gases to the user than nonfiltered brands. Some smokers use low-tar and low-nicotine products as an excuse to smoke more cigarettes, but they wind up exposing themselves to more harmful substances than they would with a smaller number of regular-strength cigarettes.

Clove cigarettes contain about 40 percent ground cloves and 60 percent tobacco. Many users mistakenly believe that these products are made entirely of ground cloves and that smoking them eliminates the risks associated with tobacco. In fact, clove cigarettes contain higher levels of tar, nicotine, and carbon monoxide than do regular cigarettes. In addition, the numbing effect of eugenol, an ingredient in cloves, allows smokers to inhale more deeply. The same effect is true of *menthol cigarettes:* The throat-numbing effect of the menthol allows for deeper inhalation. Menthol cigarettes also have higher carbon monoxide concentrations than do regular cigarettes.

Cigars Many people believe that cigars are safer than cigarettes, when in fact the opposite is true. Cigar smoke contains 23 poisons and 43 carcinogens. Most cigars contain as much nicotine as several cigarettes, and when cigar smokers inhale nicotine it is absorbed as rapidly as it is with cigarettes. For those who don't inhale, nicotine is still absorbed through the mucous membranes in the mouth.

While cigar use has declined in recent years, the sale of little cigars has increased approximately 240 percent.[92] Little cigars are roughly the same size and shape as cigarettes, come in packs of 20 as do cigarettes, can be flavored, and cost much less than cigarettes. In a recent study, users of little cigars were more likely to be younger, male, black, and current cigarette, cigar, hookah, or marijuana smokers. Users also tended to have a lower perception of harm, greater sensation-seeking behaviors, and higher perceived levels of stress.[93]

Pipes and Hookahs Pipes have had a long history of use throughout the world, including ritualistic and ceremonial usage for many cultures.

Often thought to be safer than cigarettes or cigars, pipes are not risk-free. According to cumulative research by the National Cancer Institute and the American Cancer Society, pipe smoking carries similar risks to cigar smoking. Of concern in recent years is the increasing prevalence, particularly among college students, of the use of "hookahs," or water pipes. Hookah smoking originated in the Middle East and involves burning flavored tobacco in a water pipe and inhaling the smoke through a long hose. Hookahs are marketed as reducing risks from hazardous chemicals by filtering the smoke through water before you inhale. Water pipes may cool the smoke, but they do not filter out harmful substances.[94] In addition to the health risks associated with all tobacco products, risks associated with hookah use include the possibility of infectious disease transmission by sharing a pipe.

Bidis Generally made in India or Southeast Asia, **bidis** are small, hand-rolled cigarettes in a variety of flavors, such as vanilla, chocolate, and cherry. They have become increasingly popular with college students. Though often viewed as safer than cigarettes, they are actually far more toxic. Smoke from a bidi contains three times more carbon monoxide and nicotine and five times more tar than cigarettes.[95] The leaf wrappers are nonporous, which means that smokers must suck harder to inhale and must inhale more to keep the bidi lit, resulting in much more exposure to the higher amounts of tar, nicotine, and carbon monoxide. Bidi smoking increases risks of oral cancer, lung cancer, stomach cancer, and esophageal cancer. It is also associated with emphysema and chronic bronchitis.[96]

Smokeless Tobacco Smokeless tobacco is just as addictive as cigarettes and actually contains more nicotine—holding an average-sized dip or chew in the mouth for 30 minutes delivers as much nicotine as smoking four cigarettes. A 2-can-a-week snuff user gets as much nicotine as a 10-pack-a-week smoker.

Chewing tobacco comes in three forms—loose leaf, plug, or pouch—and contains tobacco leaves treated with molasses and other flavorings. The user "dips" the tobacco by placing a small amount between the lower lip and teeth to stimulate the flow of saliva and release the nicotine. **Dipping** rapidly releases nicotine into the bloodstream. Use of chewing tobacco by teenagers, especially white males, has increased in recent years.[97]

Snuff is a finely ground form of tobacco that can be inhaled, chewed, or placed against the gums. It comes in dry or moist powdered form or sachets (tea bag–like pouches). In 2009, "snus" became the latest form of smokeless tobacco to hit the market in the United States. Popular for more than 100 years in Sweden, these small sachets of tobacco are placed inside the cheek and sucked.

Electronic cigarettes Electronic cigarettes, also called e-cigarettes, are increasingly used worldwide, even though there is limited information on their health effects. A recent report from the Centers for Disease Control and Prevention (CDC) showed that in 2012 10 percent of U.S. middle and high school students experimented with e-cigarettes.[98] With various colors, fruity flavors, clever designs, and other options, e-cigarettes may offer young people an easy gateway to nicotine addiction.[99]

Although manufacturers claim that electronic cigarettes are a safe alternative to conventional cigarettes, the U.S. Food and Drug Administration (FDA) analyzed samples of two popular brands and found variable amounts of nicotine and traces of toxic chemicals, including known carcinogens.[100]

Most e-cigarettes consist of a battery, a charger, an atomizer, and a cartridge containing nicotine and propylene glycol. When a smoker draws air through an e-cigarette, a sensor activates the battery and heats the atomizer to vaporize the propylene glycol and nicotine (users refer to this as "vaping"). Upon inhalation, the aerosol vapor delivers a dose of nicotine into the lungs; residual aerosol is exhaled into the environment.

E-cigarettes are often marketed as a method to quit smoking, but health professionals recommend using FDA-approved medications and aids that have been shown to be safe and effective for this purpose.

As e-cigarettes have increased in popularity, the CDC has also reported a dramatic increase in calls to poison control centers regarding e-cigarettes and liquid nicotine poisoning. Over 51 percent of these calls involved children under 5 years of age.[101]

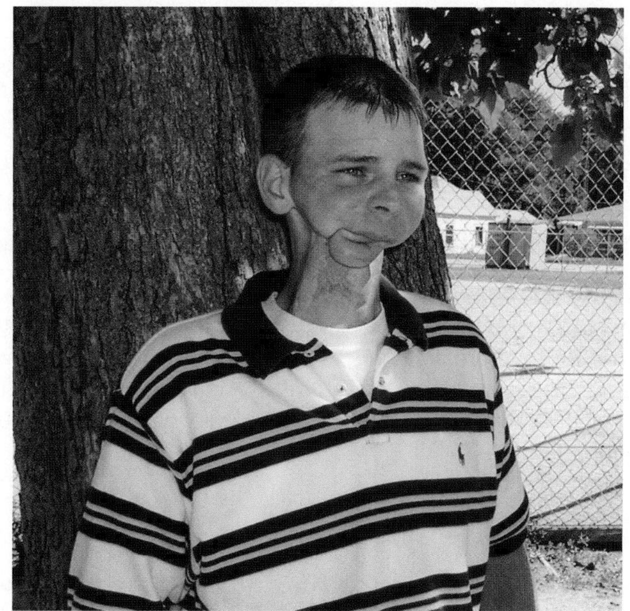

Is chewing tobacco as harmful as smoking cigarettes?

Dental problems are common among users of smokeless tobacco. Contact with tobacco juice causes receding gums, tooth decay, bad breath, and discolored teeth. Damage to both the teeth and jawbone can contribute to loss of teeth. This young cancer survivor began using smokeless tobacco at age 13; by age 17, he was diagnosed with squamous cell carcinoma. He has undergone surgery to remove neck muscles, lymph nodes, and his tongue, and he now educates others about the dangers of chewing tobacco.

check yourself

- **How does nicotine affect the body?**
- **Why do some people mistakenly believe that some tobacco products are less harmful than others?**

7.11 Health Hazards of Tobacco Products

learning outcome

7.11 Summarize the health risks of tobacco products.

Cigarette smoking adversely affects the health of every person who smokes, as well as the health of everyone nearby. Each day, cigarettes contribute to approximately 1,200 deaths from cancer, cardiovascular disease, and respiratory disorders.[102] In addition, tobacco use can negatively affect the health of almost every system in your body (Figure 7.9).

Cancer

Lung cancer is the leading cause of cancer deaths in the United States. Tobacco smoking causes 90 percent of all cases of lung cancer in men and 78 percent in women.[103] There were an estimated 242,550 *new* cases of lung cancer in the United States in 2013 alone, and an estimated 163,660 Americans died from the disease in 2013.[104]

Lung cancer can take 10 to 30 years to develop, and the outlook for its victims is poor; the 5-year survival rate is only 17 percent.[105] Smokers' risk of developing lung cancer depends on several factors. Someone who smokes two packs a day is 15 to 25 times more likely to develop lung cancer than a nonsmoker. A second factor is when you started smoking; an earlier start greatly increases risk. A third factor is whether you inhale deeply when you smoke.

A major risk of chewing tobacco is **leukoplakia**, leathery white patches inside the mouth produced by contact with irritants in tobacco juice (Figure 7.10). Approximately 1 out of 5 leukoplakias is either cancerous or precancerous, eventually progressing to cancer if not treated.[106]

There were over 42,440 cases of oral cancer diagnosed in 2014—the vast majority of which were caused by smokeless tobacco or cigarettes.[107] Smokeless tobacco users have significantly higher rates of oral cancer than do nonusers. Warning signs include lumps in the jaw, neck, or lips; white, smooth, or scaly patches in the mouth or on the neck, lips, or tongue; mouth sores or bleeding that don't heal in 2 weeks; and difficulty speaking or swallowing. The time between first use and contracting cancer is shorter for smokeless tobacco users than for smokers.

Tobacco is linked to other cancers as well. The rate of pancreatic cancer is more than twice as high for smokers as for nonsmokers. Smokers are at increased risk to develop cancers of the lip, tongue, salivary glands, and esophagus. Long-term use of smokeless tobacco increases the risk of cancers of the larynx, esophagus, nasal cavity, pancreas, colon, kidney, and bladder.

Cardiovascular Disease

Over a third of all tobacco-related deaths occur from heart disease.[108] Daily cigar smoking, especially for people who inhale, also increases the risk of heart disease (double the risk of heart attack and stroke compared to nonsmokers).[109] Smoking and exposure to environmental tobacco smoke (ETS) accelerates buildup of fatty deposits (plaque) in the heart and major blood vessels (atherosclerosis). People regularly exposed to ETS can have a 20 to 25 percent increase in plaque buildup.[110]

Smoking also contributes to **platelet adhesiveness**, the sticking together of red blood cells associated with blood clots. Smoking decreases oxygen supplied to the heart and contributes to irregular heart rhythms, which can trigger a heart attack. Smokers are also two to four times as likely to suffer strokes as nonsmokers.[111] A stroke occurs when a small blood vessel in the brain bursts or is blocked by a blood clot, denying the brain oxygen and nourishment. Depending on the brain area affected, stroke can result in paralysis, loss of mental functioning, or death. Smoking contributes to strokes by raising blood pressure, which increases stress on vessel walls. Platelet adhesiveness contributes to blood clot formation.

50% of regular smokers eventually die of smoking-related diseases.

The risk of dying from a heart attack falls by half after only 1 year without smoking, and declines steadily thereafter. After about 15 years, the ex-smoker's risk of cardiovascular disease and stroke is similar to that of people who have never smoked.[112]

Respiratory Disorders

Smokers are more prone to breathlessness, chronic cough, and excess phlegm production than are nonsmokers their age. Ultimately, smokers are up to 25 times more likely to die of lung disease than are nonsmokers.[113]

Chronic bronchitis may develop in smokers, because their inflamed lungs produce more mucus, which they constantly try to expel along with foreign particles. This results in the persistent cough known as "smoker's hack." Smokers are also more prone to respiratory ailments such as influenza, pneumonia, and colds, and smoking exacerbates asthma symptoms.

Emphysema is a chronic disease in which the alveoli (the tiny air sacs in the lungs) are destroyed, impairing the lungs' ability to obtain oxygen and remove carbon dioxide and making breathing very difficult. Because the heart has to work harder to do even the simplest tasks, it may become enlarged and death from heart damage may result. There is no known cure, and the damage is irreversible. Approximately 80 percent of all cases of emphysema are related to cigarette smoking.[114]

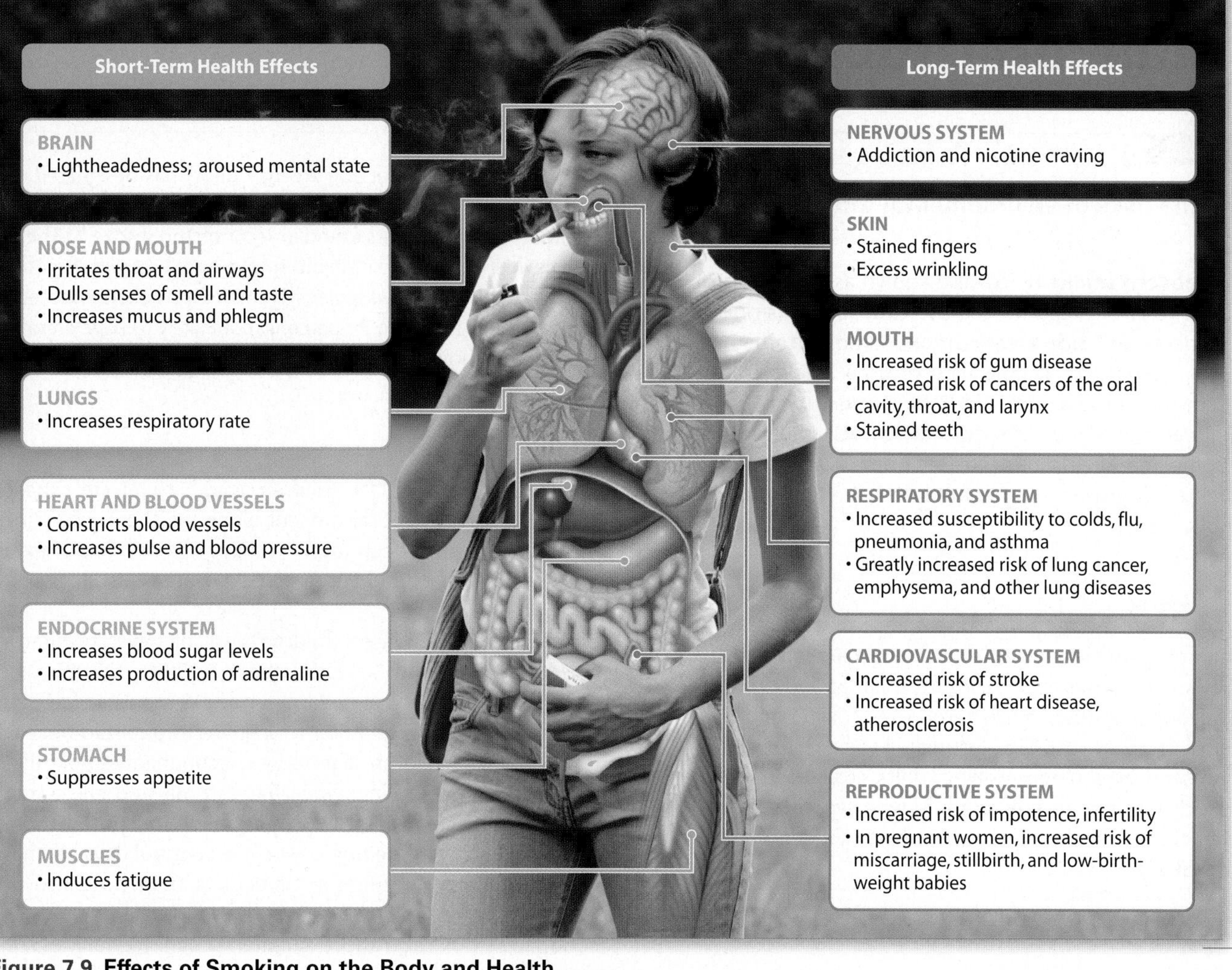

Figure 7.9 Effects of Smoking on the Body and Health

VIDEO TUTOR
Long- and Short-Term Effects of Tobacco

Sexual Dysfunction and Fertility Problems

Despite tobacco advertisers' attempts to make smoking appear sexy, male smokers are much more likely to experience erectile dysfunction than are nonsmokers.[115] Women who smoke increase their risk for infertility, ectopic pregnancy, spontaneous abortion, and stillbirth. They also increase their baby's risk of sudden infant death syndrome and chances of being born with a cleft lip or palate.[116] Smoking during pregnancy increases the chances of premature births and the risk of low birth weight, which, in turn, increases babies' likelihood of illness or death.[117]

Figure 7.10 Leukoplakia
Leukoplakia, which can appear on the tongue or in the mouth as shown here, can be a precursor to oral cancer.

Other Health Effects

Studies have shown tobacco use to be a serious risk factor in the development of gum disease.[118] In addition, smoking increases the risk of macular degeneration, one of the most common causes of blindness in older adults. It also causes premature skin wrinkling, staining of the teeth, yellowing of the fingernails, and bad breath. Nicotine speeds up the process by which the body uses and eliminates drugs, making medications less effective. In addition, research suggests that smoking significantly increases the risk of Alzheimer's disease.[119]

check yourself

- **What do lung cancer and emphysema have in common? How do they differ?**
- **Explain how the use of tobacco products affects the lungs and heart.**
- **Name at least four types of cancer that are linked to the use of tobacco.**

7.12 Environmental Tobacco Smoke

learning **outcome**

7.12 Describe the risks of environmental tobacco smoke.

Environmental tobacco smoke (ETS), also known as *secondhand smoke*, is divided into two categories: **mainstream smoke** (smoke exhaled by a smoker) and **sidestream smoke** (smoke from the burning end of a cigarette).[120] People who breathe smoke from someone else's smoking product are said to be *involuntary* or *passive* smokers. Between 1988 and 2008, detectable levels of nicotine exposure in nonsmoking Americans decreased from 87.9 percent to 40.1 percent due to the growing number of laws banning smoking in work and public places.[121]

Risks from ETS

Although involuntary smokers breathe less tobacco than active smokers do, they still face risks from exposure; it has about 2 times more tar and nicotine, 5 times more carbon monoxide, and 50 times more ammonia. Every year, ETS is estimated to be responsible for 3,400 lung cancer deaths in nonsmoking adults, 46,000 coronary and heart disease deaths in nonsmoking adults who live with smokers, and a higher risk of deaths in newborns from sudden infant death syndrome (SIDS).[122]

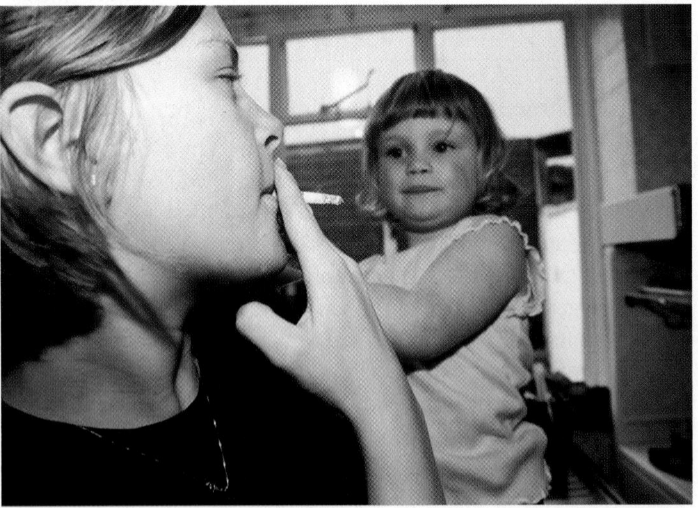

What are the health risks of secondhand smoke?

ETS is linked to deaths from cancer and heart disease in adults and SIDS in infants. Because their bodies and brains are still developing, babies and children are particularly vulnerable to the toxins in secondhand smoke.

The Environmental Protection Agency (EPA) has designated secondhand smoke as a known (group A) carcinogen. There are more than 69 cancer-causing agents found in secondhand smoke.[123] There is also strong evidence that secondhand smoke interferes with functioning of the heart, blood, and vascular systems. Nonsmokers exposed to secondhand smoke are 20 to 30 percent more likely to have coronary heart disease than nonsmokers not exposed to smoke.[124]

Children and ETS

More than 53 percent of U.S. children aged 3 to 11 are exposed to ETS.[125] Disparities in ETS also occur along racial and class lines. African Americans have been found to have higher levels of exposure to ETS than whites and Hispanics; exposure is also higher for low-income persons.[126]

Exposure to ETS increases children's risk of lower respiratory tract infections, leading to an estimated 150,000 to 300,000 lower respiratory tract infections in children under 18 months of age and lung infections resulting in 7,500 to 15,000 hospitalizations each year.[127] In addition, children exposed to secondhand smoke have a greater chance of coughing, wheezing, asthma, and chest colds, along with a decrease in lung function. Children exposed to secondhand smoke daily in the home miss more school days and have more colds and acute respiratory infections than do those not exposed.

Secondhand smoke also affects children's cognitive abilities. One study found that children exposed to high levels of secondhand smoke were twice as likely to develop learning disabilities, conduct disorders, and other behavioral disorders.[128] Boys were more likely to be at risk of developing learning disabilities than girls.[129]

ETS and Additional Health Problems

Environmental tobacco smoke can cause allergic reactions such as itchy eyes, difficulty breathing, headaches, nausea, and dizziness. It may also increase risk of breast cancer in women; cancers of the nasal sinus cavity and pharynx in adults; and leukemia, lymphoma, and brain tumors in children.[130] The level of carbon monoxide in cigarette smoke contained in enclosed places is 4,000 times higher than that allowed in the clean-air standard recommended by the EPA.

check yourself

- **What are the health risks of exposure to ETS?**
- **Considering the risks of ETS to children, do you think parents should be prohibited from using tobacco?**

Tobacco Use Prevention Policies

learning outcome

7.13 Describe policy efforts to discourage tobacco use.

It has been more than 40 years since the U.S. government began warning that tobacco use was hazardous to the nation's health. Despite all the education on the health hazards of tobacco use, health care spending and lost productivity associated with smoking costs between $289 and $333 billion each year.[131]

In 1998, the tobacco industry reached the Master Settlement Agreement with 46 states. The agreement requires tobacco companies to pay out more than $206 billion over 25 years. The agreement includes a variety of measures to support antismoking education and advertising and to fund research to determine effective smoking-cessation strategies. The agreement also curbs certain advertising and promotions directed at youth.

Unfortunately, most of the money designated for tobacco control and prevention at the state level has not been used for this purpose. Facing budget woes, many states have drastically cut spending on antismoking programs. In the few states that have spent the settlement money on smoking-cessation programs, there has been some reported success in decreasing cigarette use.[132]

The Family Smoking Prevention and Tobacco Control Act, signed into law in 2009, allows the U.S. Food and Drug Administration (FDA) to forbid advertising geared toward children, to lower the amount of nicotine in tobacco products, to ban sweetened cigarettes that appeal to young people, and to prohibit labels such as "light" and "low tar."[133] The FDA recently ordered four tobacco products (bidis) to be taken off the market when the company that created them was unwilling to provide ingredient information—the first time since being given the authority in 2009.

One of the most significant impacts of the law is that it requires more prominent health warnings on advertising of tobacco products. Smokeless tobacco ads must contain a warning that fills 20 percent of the advertising space. The FDA attempted to require cigarette packages and advertising to have larger, graphical warnings depicting the negative consequences of smoking (Figure 7.11), but a federal judge declared the requirement unconstitutional in 2012.

Recently, questions about the safety of e-cigarettes have prompted the FDA to issue a warning about potential health risks. There is no quality control in the manufacturing of the product, with many e-cigarettes manufactured in China under uncontrolled conditions.

As cities in the past took action to ban cigarette smoking in public places, some cities are following suit with e-cigarettes as well, including New York City, Chicago, and Los Angeles. Additionally, many employers are struggling with employees wanting to "vape" indoors on break, and some employers are charging employees who use e-cigarettes and tobacco a higher price for their insurance premiums.[134]

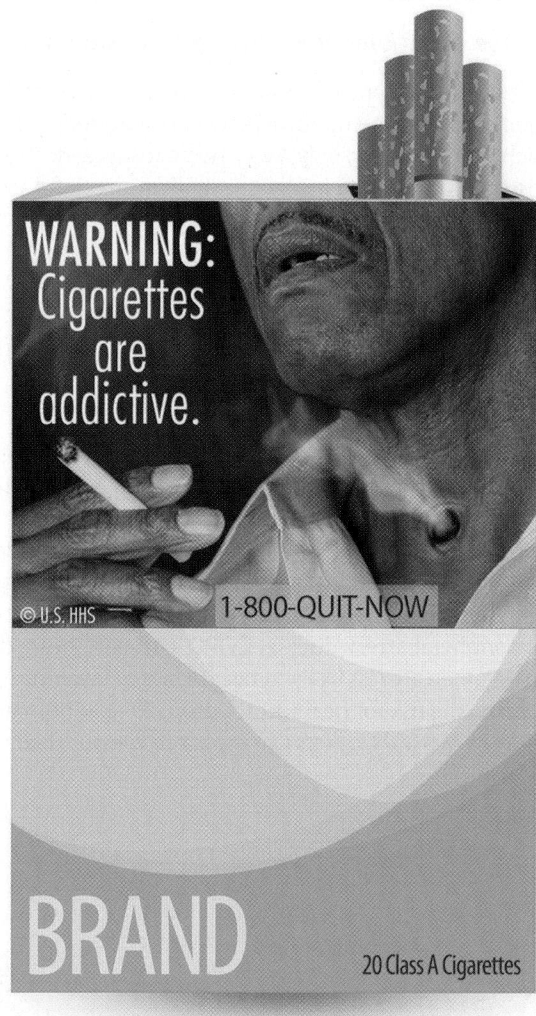

Figure 7.11 Proposed New Cigarette Warning Labels
The U.S. Food and Drug Administration proposed that graphic warning images such as this one be placed on all cigarette packages and advertisements. However, lawsuits prevented their implementation, and the FDA is now in the process of creating new warning labels.
Source: U.S. Food and Drug Administration, "Proposed Cigarette Product Warning Labels," www.fda.gov.

check yourself

- **Which policies do you think have been most successful in discouraging tobacco use?**
- **What would you recommend as further steps?**

7.14 Quitting the Tobacco Habit

learning outcome

7.14 Discuss strategies for quitting tobacco use.

Approximately 70 percent of adult smokers in the United States want to quit smoking, and up to 44 percent make a serious attempt to quit each year. However, only 4 to 7 percent succeed.[135] Quitting smoking isn't easy and often involves several unsuccessful attempts before success is finally achieved.

Benefits of Quitting

Many tissues damaged by smoking repair themselves (see Figure 7.12). Within 8 hours, carbon monoxide and oxygen levels return to normal, and "smoker's breath" disappears. Within weeks, the mucus that clogs airways is eliminated, and circulation and sense of taste and smell improve. Many ex-smokers have more energy, sleep better, and feel more alert.

After 1 year, risk for lung cancer and stroke decreases. Ex-smokers considerably reduce their chances of developing cancers of the mouth, throat, esophagus, larynx, pancreas, bladder, and cervix, as well as peripheral artery disease, COPD, coronary heart disease, and ulcers. Women are less likely to bear babies of low birth weight. Within 2 years, the risk for heart attack drops to near normal. After 10 smoke-free years, ex-smokers can expect to live out their normal life span.

Another benefit is money saved. A pack of cigarettes ranges from about $5.00 (including tax) to as much as $11.00 to $14.50 in the most expensive states; a pack-a-day smoker who lives in an area where cigarettes cost $8.00 per pack spends $56.00 per week, or $2,912 per year.[136] That is money that could have gone toward school expenses, a down payment on a car, a vacation, or family-related expenses.

How Can You Quit?

Many people quit "cold turkey"—they simply decide not to smoke again. Others choose programs based on behavior modification and self-reward, treatment centers, or work privately with a physician. Plans that combine several approaches have shown the most promise.

Nicotine addiction may be one of the toughest addictions to overcome. Symptoms of **nicotine withdrawal** include irritability, restlessness, nausea, vomiting, and intense cravings. Pharmacological treatments can help: 25 to 33 percent of people who have used nicotine replacement therapy or smoking-cessation medications continue to abstain from cigarettes for over 6 months.[137]

Nicotine Replacement Products Nontobacco products that replace depleted levels of nicotine in the bloodstream have helped some people stop using tobacco; the dose of nicotine is gradually

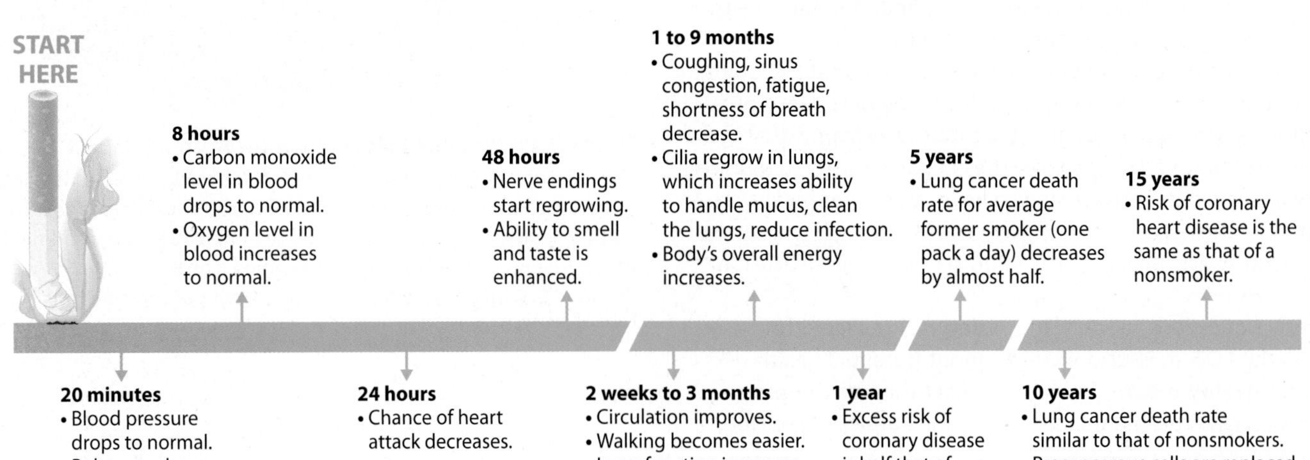

Figure 7.12 When Smokers Quit

Will quitting smoking reverse the damage that's already done?

When you quit using tobacco, your body immediately starts to repair the damage. Over time, the body's repair processes reduce the former smoker's risks of heart disease and cancer; after 10 years, heart disease and lung cancer risks are comparable to those of nonsmokers.

reduced until the smoker is fully weaned from the drug. Nicotine gum delivers about as much nicotine as a cigarette but doesn't produce the same rush. Users experience no withdrawal symptoms and fewer cravings. Nicotine lozenges, like the gum, are available over the counter. The nicotine patch is a small, thin patch that, when placed on the smoker's upper body, delivers a continuous flow of nicotine through the skin, helping relieve cravings. Some insurance plans will pay for the patch.

Nicotine nasal spray, which requires a prescription, is much more powerful. Patients must be careful not to overdose; as little as 40 mg of nicotine at once could be lethal. The spray should be used for no more than 3 months and never for more than 6 months, so smokers don't find themselves dependent on it; also, those with nasal or sinus problems, allergies, or asthma shouldn't use the spray. The nicotine inhaler also requires a prescription. The smoker inhales air saturated with nicotine, which is absorbed through the lining of the mouth, entering the body much more slowly than the nicotine in cigarettes does.

Smoking-Cessation Medications Some smoking-cessation aids are aimed at reducing withdrawal symptoms and decreasing cravings. Zyban (bupropion) is an antidepressant thought to work on dopamine and norepinephrine receptors in the brain. Chantix (varenicline) reduces cravings and the urge to smoke while blocking the effects of nicotine at receptor sites in the brain. Both drugs may cause changes in behavior such as hostility, agitation, depressed mood, and suicidal thoughts or actions. People taking one of these drugs who experience any unusual changes in mood are advised to stop taking the drug immediately and contact their health care professional.[138]

See It! Videos

What tools should you use to quit smoking? Watch **Do Nicotine Patches and Gum Work?** in the Study Area of MasteringHealth.

Antismoking Therapy For some smokers, the road to quitting includes antismoking therapy. Operant conditioning often pairs the act of smoking with an external stimulus; in one technique, smokers carry a timer that sounds a buzzer at intervals. When the buzzer sounds, the patient is required to smoke a cigarette. Once the smoker is conditioned to associate the sound with smoking, the buzzer is eliminated and, one hopes, so is the smoking. Self-control strategies are tied to viewing smoking as a learned habit associated with specific situations such as driving, studying, drinking, or watching TV. Therapy is aimed at identifying these situations and teaching smokers the skills necessary to resist smoking.

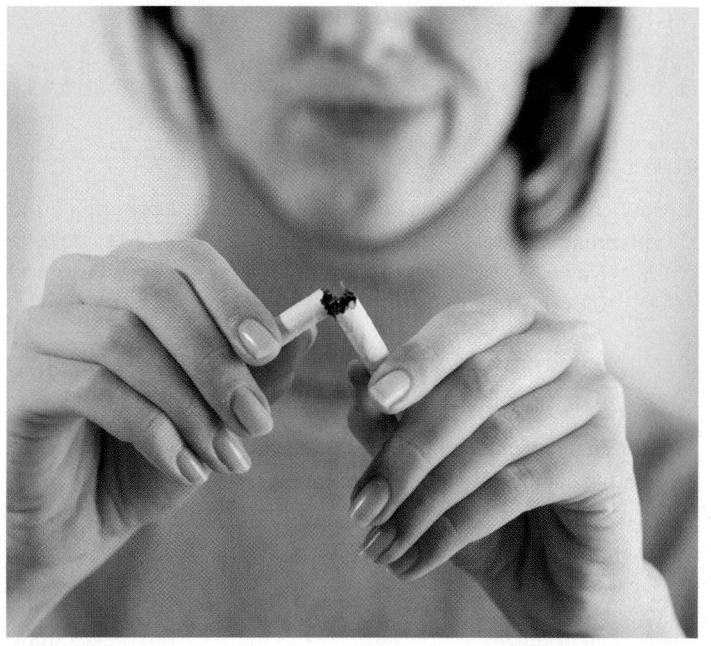

Skills for Behavior Change

TIPS FOR QUITTING SMOKING

If you're a smoker and you're ready to quit, try these tips:

- Use the four Ds: Delay (put off smoking for 10 minutes, then another 10 after that, etc.), Deep breathing, Drink water, Do something else.
- Keep "mouth toys" like hard candy, gum, toothpicks, and carrot sticks handy.
- If you've had trouble stopping before, ask your doctor about nicotine gum, patches, nasal sprays, inhalers, or lozenges.
- Have your teeth cleaned.
- Examine associations that trigger your urge to smoke.
- Tell family and friends that you've stopped so they won't offer you cigarettes.
- Spend time in places that prohibit smoking.
- To shake up your routine and distract you from smoking, take up a new sport, hobby, or organizational commitment.
- Throw out your cigarettes or keep them in a place that makes smoking inconvenient, such as in the freezer or at a friend's house.

check yourself

- **What are the benefits of stopping the use of tobacco products?**
- **Discuss products that can help people stop using tobacco.**
- **Discuss strategies that can help smokers break the habit of smoking.**

What's Your Risk of Alcohol Abuse?

An interactive version of this assessment is available online in MasteringHealth.

1. How often do you have a drink containing alcohol?
- 0 Never
- 1 Monthly or less
- 2 2 to 4 times a month
- 3 2 to 3 times a week
- 4 4 or more times a week

2. How many alcoholic drinks do you have on a typical day when you are drinking?
- 0 1 or 2
- 1 3 or 4
- 2 5 or 6
- 3 7 to 9
- 4 10 or more

3. How often do you have six drinks or more on one occasion?
- 0 Never
- 1 Less than monthly
- 2 Monthly
- 3 Weekly
- 4 Daily or almost daily

4. How often during the past year have you been unable to stop drinking once you had started?
- 0 Never
- 1 Less than monthly
- 2 Monthly
- 3 Weekly
- 4 Daily or almost daily

5. How often during the past year have you failed to do what was normally expected of you because of drinking?
- 0 Never
- 1 Less than monthly
- 2 Monthly
- 3 Weekly
- 4 Daily or almost daily

6. How often during the past year have you needed a first drink in the morning to get yourself going after a heavy drinking session?
- 0 Never
- 1 Less than monthly
- 2 Monthly
- 3 Weekly
- 4 Daily or almost daily

7. How often during the past year have you had a feeling of guilt or remorse after drinking?
- 0 Never
- 1 Less than monthly
- 2 Monthly
- 3 Weekly
- 4 Daily or almost daily

8. How often during the past year have you been unable to remember what happened the night before because you had been drinking?
- 0 Never
- 1 Less than monthly
- 2 Monthly
- 3 Weekly
- 4 Daily or almost daily

9. Have you or someone else been injured as a result of your drinking?
- 0 No
- 1 Yes, but not in the past year
- 2 Yes, during the past year

10. Has a relative, friend, or health care professional been concerned about your drinking or suggested you cut down?
- 0 No
- 1 Yes, but not in the past year
- 2 Yes, during the past year

Scoring

Scores above 8: Your drinking patterns are putting you at high risk for illness, unsafe sexual situations, or alcohol-related injuries, and may even affect your academic performance.

Source: Reproduced, with the permission of the publisher, from the AUDIT Manual, box 4, p. 17, World Health Organization, Division of Mental Health and Prevention of Substance Abuse. http://whqlibdoc.who.int/hq/2001/WHO_MSD_MSB_01.6a.pdf.

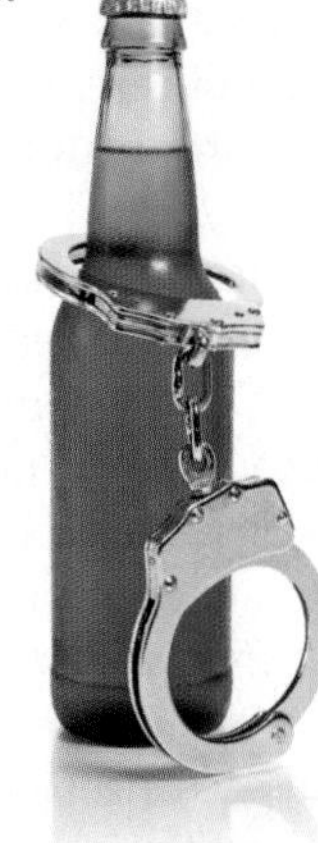

Your Plan for Change

The Assess Yourself activity gave you a chance to evaluate your alcohol use. If some of your answers concerned you, consider taking steps to change your behavior.

Today, you can:

◯ Start a journal of your drinking habits—how much you drink, how much money you spend on drinks, and how you feel when you are drinking.

◯ Spend some time thinking about the ways your family members use alcohol. Consider whether your current alcohol use is healthy, or whether it is likely to create problems for you in the future.

Within the next 2 weeks, you can:

◯ Make your first drink a nonalcoholic beverage the next time you go to a party.

◯ Intersperse alcoholic drinks with nonalcoholic beverages to help you pace yourself.

By the end of the semester, you can:

◯ Cultivate friendships and explore activities that do not center on alcohol. If your current group of friends drinks heavily, and it is becoming a problem for you, you may need to step back.

Why Do You Smoke?

An interactive version of this assessment is available online in MasteringHealth.

Identifying why you smoke can help you develop a plan to quit. Answer the following questions and evaluate your reasons for smoking.

1. **I smoke to keep from slowing down.** __Often __Sometimes __Never
2. **I feel more comfortable with a cigarette in my hand.** __Often __Sometimes __Never
3. **Smoking is pleasant and enjoyable.** __Often __Sometimes __Never
4. **I light up a cigarette when something makes me angry.** __Often __Sometimes __Never
5. **When I run out of cigarettes, it's almost unbearable until I get more.** __Often __Sometimes __Never
6. **I spoke cigarettes automatically without even being aware of it.** __Often __Sometimes __Never
7. **I reach for a cigarette when I need a lift.** __Often __Sometimes __Never
8. **Smoking relaxes me in a stressful situation.** __Often __Sometimes __Never

Interpreting Your Score

Use your answers to identify some of the key reasons why you smoke, then use the tips presented in this chapter to develop a plan for quitting.

Source: Abridged and adapted from National Institutes of Health, Why Do You Smoke? NIH Pub. No. 93-1822. (Washington, DC: U.S. Department of Health and Human Services, 1990).

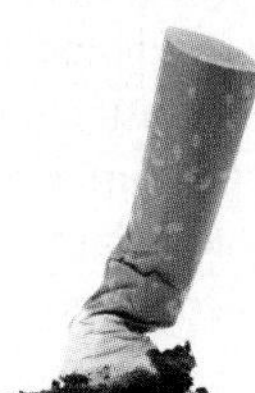

Your Plan for Change

The Assess Yourself activity gave you the chance to evaluate your current smoking habits. Regardless of your current level of nicotine addiction, now is the time to take steps toward kicking the habit.

Today, you can:

- ◯ Develop a plan to kick the tobacco habit. The first step in quitting smoking is to identify why you want to quit. Write your reasons down on a sheet of paper.
- ◯ Think about the times and places you usually smoke. What could you do instead of smoking at those times? Make a list of positive tobacco alternatives.

Within the next 2 weeks, you can:

- ◯ Pick a day to stop smoking, fill out a behavior change contract, and have a family member or friend sign it.
- ◯ Throw away all your cigarettes, lighters, and ashtrays.

By the end of the semester, you can:

- ◯ Focus on the positives. Now that you have stopped smoking, your mind and your body will begin to feel better. Make a list of the good things about not smoking. Carry a copy with you, and look at it whenever you have the urge to smoke.
- ◯ Reward yourself for stopping. Go to a movie, go out to dinner, or buy yourself a gift.

Summary

To hear an MP3 Tutor session, scan here or visit the Study Area in **MasteringHealth**.

LO 7.1 Although consumption trends are creeping downward, students are under extreme pressure to consume alcohol. Negative consequences associated with alcohol use among college students are academic problems, traffic accidents, dropping out of school, unplanned sex, alcohol poisoning, and injury.

LO 7.2 Alcohol's effect on the body is measured by blood alcohol concentration (BAC), the ratio of alcohol to total blood volume.

LO 7.3 Alcohol depresses the central nervous system (CNS); short-term effects include decreased respiratory rate, pulse rate, and blood pressure. Alcohol use is a contributing factor to injuries, poor sexual decision-making, rape, and weight gain. Drinking large amounts quickly can lead to alcohol poisoning.

LO 7.4 Long-term alcohol overuse can cause nervous system damage, cardiovascular damage, liver disease, and increased cancer risk. Drinking during pregnancy can cause fetal alcohol spectrum disorders (FASDs).

LO 7.5 Drinking impairs driving abilities. Alcohol-impaired drivers are involved in 1 out of 3 crash deaths in the United States.

LO 7.6 Alcohol use becomes alcoholism when it interferes with school, work, or relationships or entails legal violations. Causes are biological, social, and cultural.

LO 7.7 Being worried about one's alcohol consumption is a cause for concern. A counselor or clinician can advise steps to cut down on drinking.

LO 7.8 Most alcoholics deny having a problem until reaching a major crisis. Treatment options include detoxification at private facilities, therapy, and self-help programs such as Alcoholics Anonymous. Most alcoholics relapse; alcoholism is a behavioral and chemical addiction.

LO 7.9 Tobacco use is widespread in the United States and costs the nation $289 to $333 billion per year. Tobacco companies target college students in their marketing campaigns.

LO 7.10 Tobacco is available in smoking and smokeless forms, both of which contain nicotine, an addictive psychoactive substance. Little is known about the health risks of electronic cigarettes, which are growing in popularity.

LO 7.11 Hazards of smoking include increased rates of cancer, heart and circulatory disorders, and respiratory and gum diseases. Smoking during pregnancy presents risks for the fetus. Smokeless tobacco dramatically increases oral cancer risk.

LO 7.12 Environmental tobacco smoke (secondhand smoke) puts nonsmokers at risk for cancer and heart disease.

LO 7.13 The U.S. Food and Drug Administration (FDA) regulates the sale and advertising of tobacco products.

LO 7.14 To quit, smokers must kick a chemical addiction *and* a behavioral habit. Nicotine replacement products or drugs can help wean smokers off nicotine. Therapy methods can also help.

Pop Quiz

Visit MasteringHealth to personalize your study plan with Chapter Review Quizzes and Dynamic Study Modules.

LO 7.1 1. When Amanda goes out with her friends, she usually has four or five beers in a row. This type of high-risk drinking is called
a. tolerance.
b. alcoholic addiction.
c. alcohol overconsumption.
d. binge drinking.

LO 7.2 2. BAC is the
a. concentration of plant sugars in the bloodstream.
b. percentage of alcohol in a beverage.
c. ratio of alcohol to body weight.
d. ratio of alcohol to total blood volume.

LO 7.3 3. Drinking large amounts of alcohol in a short period of time that leads to passing out is known as
a. learned behavioral tolerance.
b. alcoholic unconsciousness.
c. alcohol poisoning.
d. acute metabolism syndrome.

LO 7.6 4. To adapt to his father's alcoholic behavior, Jake played the obedient son. What role did he assume?
a. Family hero
b. Mascot
c. Scapegoat
d. Lost child

LO 7.8. 5. The alcohol withdrawal syndrome that results in confusion, delusion, agitated behavior, and hallucination is known as
a. automatic detoxification.
b. delirium tremens.
c. acute withdrawal.
d. transient hyperirritability.

LO 7.10 6. What does carbon monoxide do to smokers?
a. Makes it difficult for a smoker to breathe
b. Causes dizzy spells and lightheadedness
c. Reduces the ability of blood hemoglobin to carry oxygen
d. Impairs the cleaning function of the lung's cilia

LO 7.10. 7. What is the major psychoactive ingredient in tobacco products?
a. Carbon monoxide
b. Tar
c. Formaldehyde
d. Nicotine

LO 7.10 8. What does nicotine do to cilia?
a. Instantly destroys them
b. Thickens them
c. Paralyzes them
d. Accumulates on them

LO 7.11 9. A major health risk of chewing tobacco is
a. lung cancer.
b. leukoplakia.
c. heart disease.
d. emphysema.

LO 7.14 10. Quitting smoking
a. usually results in minor withdrawal symptoms.
b. does little to reverse damage to the lungs.
c. can be aided by nicotine replacement.
d. is best done by transitioning to "light" cigarettes.

Answers to these questions can be found on page A-1. If you answered a question incorrectly, review the module identified by the Learning Outcome. For even more study tools, visit MasteringHealth.

8 Nutrition

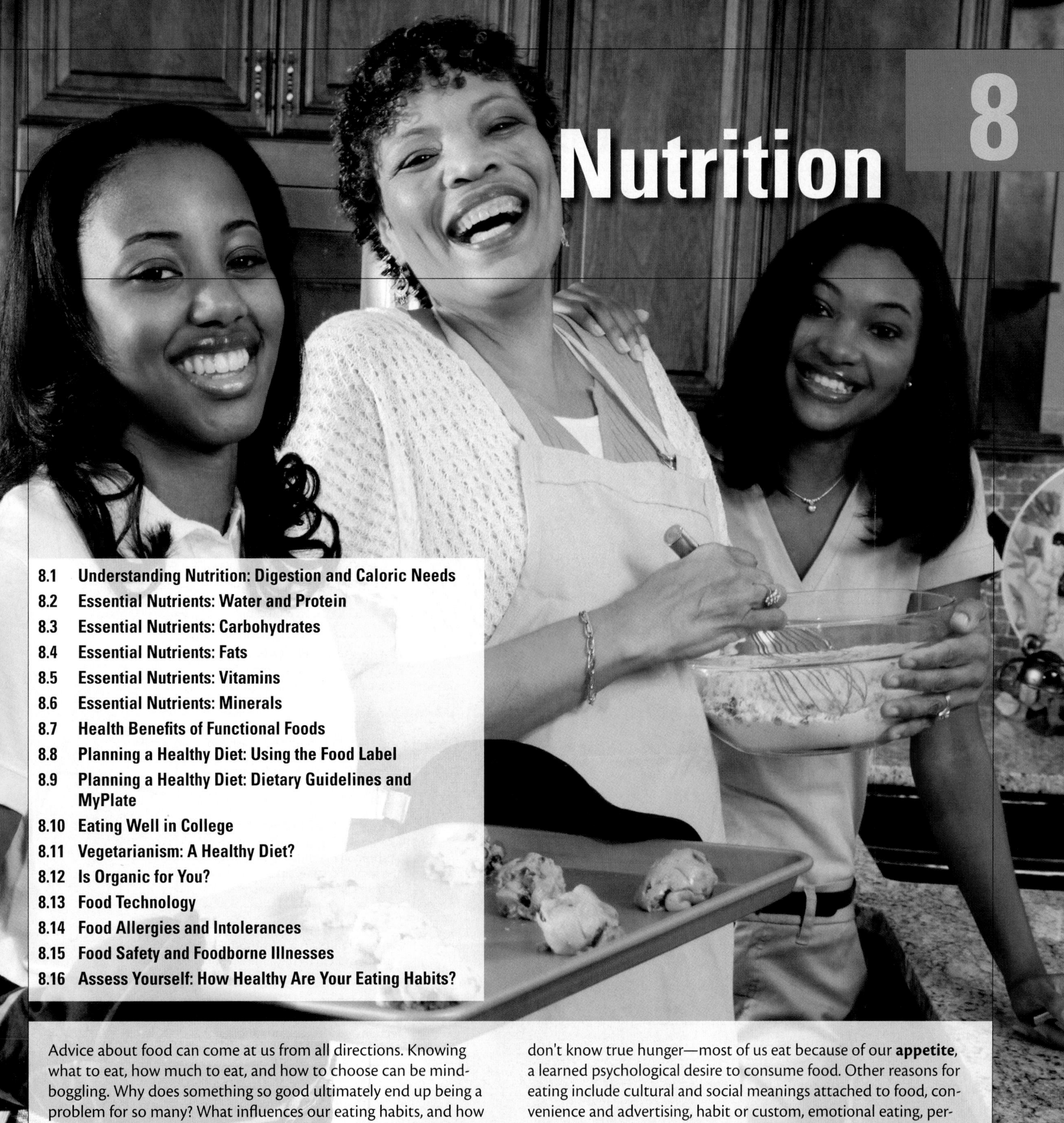

Advice about food can come at us from all directions. Knowing what to eat, how much to eat, and how to choose can be mind-boggling. Why does something so good ultimately end up being a problem for so many? What influences our eating habits, and how can we learn to eat more healthfully?

True **hunger** occurs when there is a lack of basic foods. When we're hungry, our brains initiate a physiological response that prompts us to seek food for the energy and **nutrients** our bodies need for proper functioning. Most people in the United States don't know true hunger—most of us eat because of our **appetite**, a learned psychological desire to consume food. Other reasons for eating include cultural and social meanings attached to food, convenience and advertising, habit or custom, emotional eating, perceived nutritional value, social interaction, and financial means.

Nutrition is the science that investigates the relationship between physiological function and the essential elements of the foods we eat. Your health largely depends on what and how much you eat.

8.1 Understanding Nutrition: Digestion and Caloric Needs

learning outcome

8.1 Describe the digestive process and identify daily calorie needs.

Food provides the chemicals we need for activity and body maintenance. Our bodies cannot synthesize certain *essential nutrients* (or cannot synthesize them in adequate amounts)—we must obtain them from the foods we eat. Of the six groups of essential nutrients, the four we need in the largest amounts—water, proteins, carbohydrates, and fats—are called *macronutrients*. The other two groups—vitamins and minerals—are needed in smaller amounts, so they are called *micronutrients*.

Before the body can use foods, the digestive system must break down larger food particles into smaller, more usable forms. The sequence of functions by which the body breaks down foods and either absorbs or excretes them is the digestive process (Figure 8.1).

Recommended Intakes for Nutrients

The recommended amounts of each nutrient group are known as the *Dietary Reference Intakes (DRIs)*. The DRIs are published by the Food and Nutrition Board of the Institute of Medicine, and they establish the amount of each nutrient needed to prevent deficiencies or reduce the risk of chronic disease, as well as identify maximum safe intake levels for healthy people. The DRIs are umbrella guidelines and include the following categories:

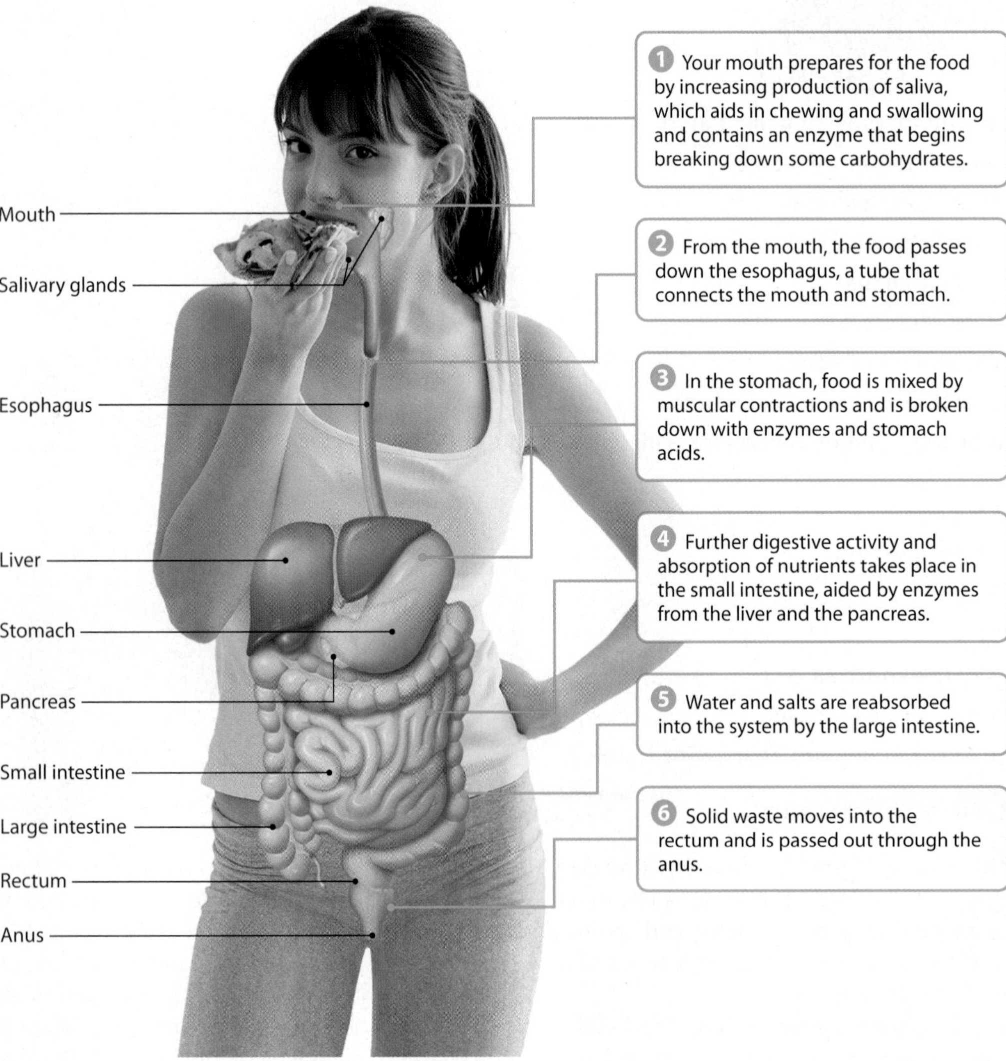

Figure 8.1 The Digestive Process
The entire digestive process takes approximately 24 hours.

- **Recommended Dietary Allowances (RDAs)** are daily nutrient intake levels meeting the nutritional needs of 97 to 98 percent of healthy individuals.
- **Adequate Intakes (AIs)** are daily intake levels assumed to be adequate for most healthy people. AIs are used when there isn't enough research to support establishing an RDA.
- **Tolerable Upper Intake Levels (ULs)** are the highest amounts of a nutrient that an individual can consume daily without risking adverse health effects.
- **Acceptable Macronutrient Distribution Ranges (AMDRs)** are ranges of protein, carbohydrate, and fat intake that provide adequate nutrition, and they are associated with a reduced risk for chronic disease.

Whereas the RDAs, AIs, and ULs are expressed as amounts—usually milligrams (mg) or micrograms (μg)—AMDRs are expressed as percentages. The AMDR for protein, for example, is 10 to 35 percent, meaning that no less than 10 percent and no more than 35 percent of the calories you consume should come from proteins. But that raises a new question: What are calories?

TABLE 8.1 **Estimated Daily Calorie Needs**

	Calorie Range	
	Sedentary[a]	Active[b]
CHILDREN		
2–3 years old	1,000	1,400
FEMALES		
4–8 years old	1,200	1,800
9–13	1,400	2,200
14–18	1,800	2,400
19–30	1,800	2,400
31–50	1,800	2,200
51+	1,600	2,200
MALES		
4–8 years old	1,200	2,000
9–13	1,600	2,600
14–18	2,000	3,200
19–30	2,400	3,000
31–50	2,200	3,000
51+	2,000	2,800

[a] A lifestyle that includes only the light physical activity associated with typical day-to-day life.
[b] A lifestyle that includes physical activity equivalent to walking more than 3 miles per day at 3 to 4 miles per hour, in addition to the light physical activity associated with typical day-to-day life.

Source: U.S. Department of Agriculture and U.S. Department of Health and Human Services, *Dietary Guidelines for Americans, 2010*, 7th ed. (Washington, DC: U.S. Government Printing Office).

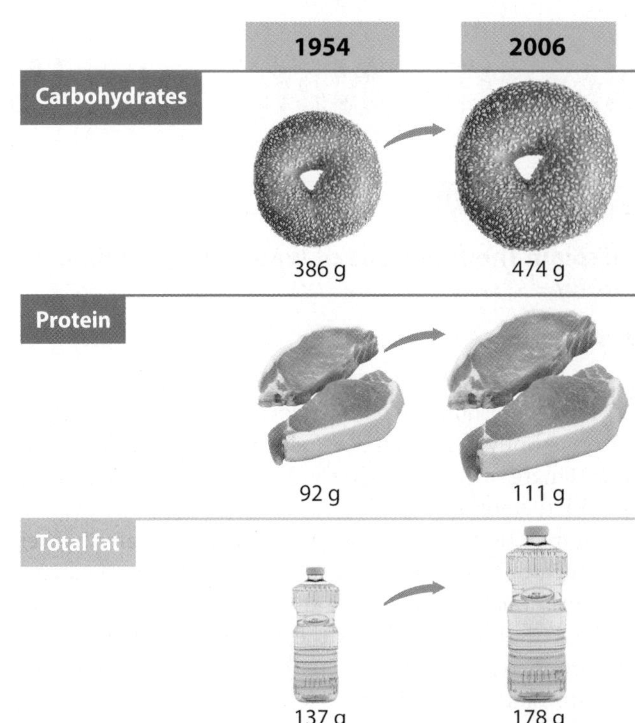

Figure 8.2 Trends in Per Capita Nutrient Consumption
Since 1954, Americans' daily caloric intake has increased by about 25 percent, as has daily consumption of carbohydrates and protein. Daily total fat intake has increased by 30 percent.
Source: Data from USDA Economic Research Service, "Nutrient Availability," Updated August 2012, www.ers.usda.gov.

Calories

A *kilocalorie* is a unit of measure used to quantify the amount of energy in food. On nutrition labels and in consumer publications, the term is shortened to **calorie**. *Energy* is defined as the capacity to do work. We derive energy from the energy-containing nutrients in the foods we eat. These nutrients—proteins, carbohydrates, and fats—provide calories. Vitamins, minerals, and water do not. It's important to know your approximate caloric needs, based on your age, gender, and activity level. Table 8.1 shows the caloric needs for various individuals.

Overall, Americans today eat more food than ever before. From 1970 to 2008, average calorie consumption increased from 2,157 to 2,614 calories per day (see Figure 8.2).[1] In general, it isn't the actual amount of food, but the number of calories in the foods we choose to eat that has increased. When these trends are combined with our increasingly sedentary lifestyle, it is not surprising that we have seen a dramatic rise in obesity.[2] With an understanding of nutrition, you will be able to make more informed choices about your diet and lifestyle.

check yourself

- **Describe the digestive process, from mouth to excretion.**
- **What are your estimated daily calorie needs?**

8.2 Essential Nutrients: Water and Protein

learning outcome

8.2 Explain the functions of water and protein in the body.

Water

Humans can survive for several weeks without food but only for about 1 week without water. **Dehydration**, a state of abnormal depletion of body fluids, can develop within a single day, especially in a hot climate. Too much water—*hyponatremia*—can also pose a serious risk to your health.

The human body consists of 50 to 70 percent water by weight. The water in our system bathes cells, aids in fluid and electrolyte balance, maintains pH balance, and transports molecules and cells throughout the body. Water is the major component of blood, which carries oxygen and nutrients to the tissues, removes metabolic wastes, and keeps cells in working order.

Individual needs for water vary according to dietary factors, age, size, overall health, environmental temperature and humidity, and exercise. The latest DRIs suggest that most people can meet their hydration needs simply by eating a healthy diet and drinking in response to thirst. The general recommendations for women are approximately 9 cups of total water from all beverages and foods each day, and for men, an average of 13 cups.[3]

About 20 percent of our daily water needs are met through the food we eat. Fruits and vegetables are 80 to 95 percent water, meats more than 50 percent water, and bread and cheese about 35 percent water! Contrary to popular opinion, caffeinated drinks, including coffee, tea, and soda, also count toward total fluid intake for those who regularly consume them. Caffeinated beverages have not been found to dehydrate people whose bodies are used to caffeine.[4]

Of course, there are situations in which a person needs additional fluids to stay properly hydrated. It is important to drink extra fluids when you have a fever or an illness in which there is vomiting or diarrhea. People with kidney problems, diabetes, or cystic fibrosis may need more water, as may the elderly and very young. When the weather heats up or when you sweat profusely, extra water is needed to keep your core temperature within a normal range; visit the American College of Sports Medicine's website (www.acsm.org) to download its brochure, "Selecting and Effectively Using Hydration for Fitness."[5]

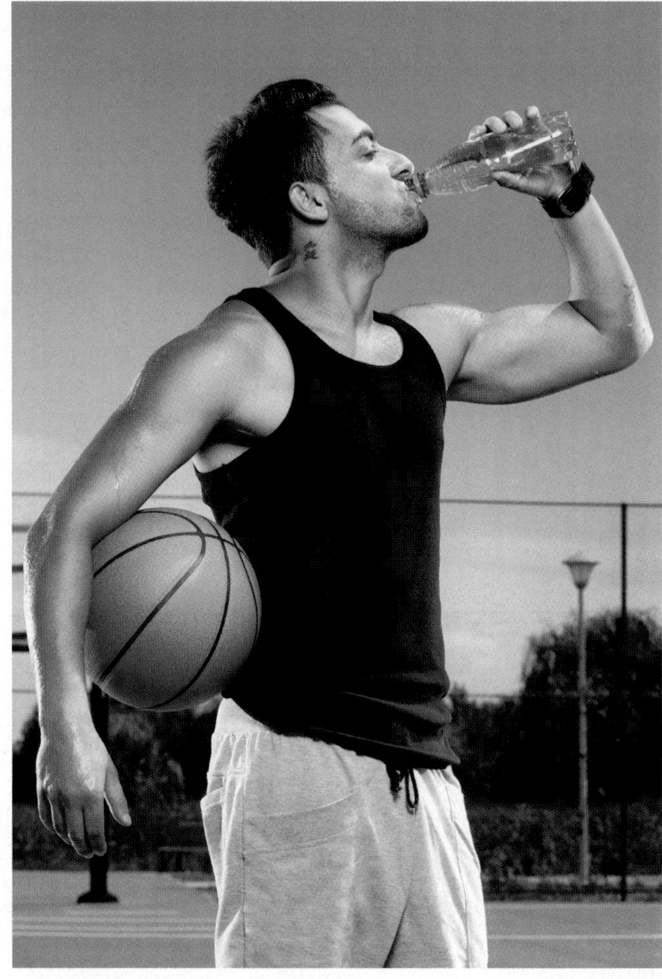

Drinking water is important to maintain normal body functioning. If you're exercising in hot weather or sweating profusely, it's crucial to stay adequately hydrated.

Protein

Next to water, **proteins** are the most abundant substances in the human body. Proteins are major components of nearly every cell; they've been called the "body builders" because of their role in developing and repairing bone, muscle, skin, and blood cells. They are the key elements of antibodies that protect us from disease, of enzymes that control chemical activities in the body, and of hormones that regulate body functions. Proteins help transport iron, oxygen, and nutrients to all body cells and supply another source of energy to cells when fats and carbohydrates are not available. Every gram of protein you eat provides 4 calories. Adequate amounts of protein in the diet are vital to many body functions and, ultimately, to survival.

Your body breaks down proteins into smaller nitrogen-containing **amino acids**. Nine of the 20 amino acids are **essential amino acids**, which the body must obtain from the diet; the other 11 can be produced by the body. Dietary protein that supplies all the essential amino acids is called **complete protein.** Typically, protein from animal products is complete.

Legumes and grains
Green leafy vegetables and grains and legumes
Legumes and nuts and seeds
Green leafy vegetables and nuts and seeds and legumes

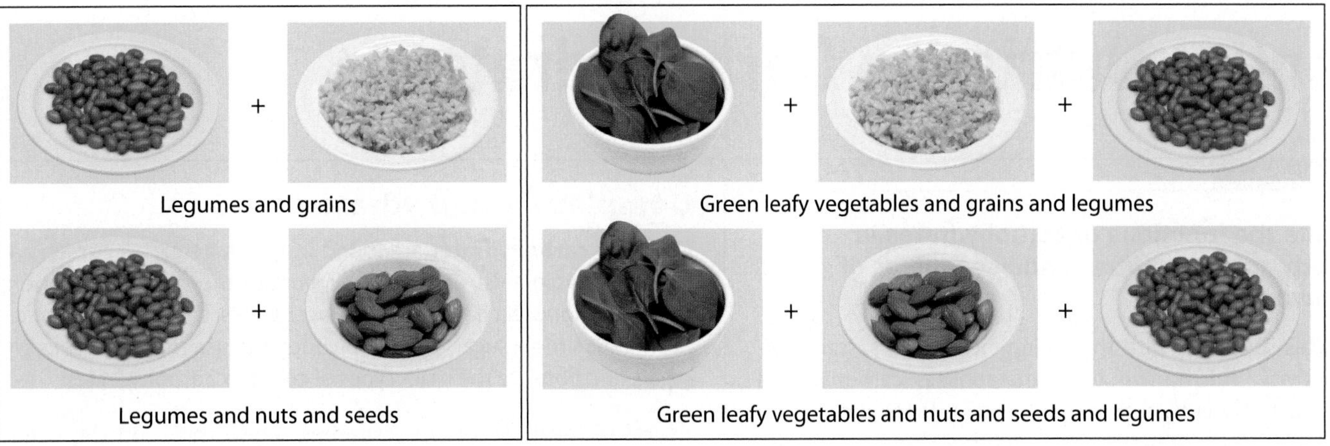

Figure 8.3 Complementary Proteins
Eaten in the right combinations, plant-based foods can provide complementary proteins and all essential amino acids.

Nearly all proteins from plant sources are **incomplete proteins** that lack one or more of the essential amino acids. However, it is easy to combine plant foods to produce a complete protein meal (Figure 8.3). Plant sources of protein fall into three general categories: *legumes* (e.g., beans, peas, peanuts, and soy products), *grains* (e.g., wheat, corn, rice, and oats), and *nuts and seeds.* Certain vegetables, such as leafy green vegetables and broccoli, also contribute valuable plant proteins. Consuming a variety of foods from these categories will provide all the essential amino acids.

Although protein deficiency poses a threat to the global population, few Americans suffer from protein deficiencies. In fact, the average American consumes more than 79 grams of protein daily, much of it from high-fat animal flesh and dairy products.[6] The AMDR for protein is 10 to 35 percent of calories. Adults should consume about 0.8 grams per kilogram of body weight.[7] To calculate your recommended protein intake per day, divide your body weight in pounds by 2.2 to get your weight in kilograms, then multiply by 0.8. For example, a woman who weighs 130 pounds should consume about 47 grams of protein each day. A 6-ounce steak provides 53 grams of protein—more than she needs!

A person might need extra protein if she is pregnant, fighting off a serious infection, recovering from surgery or blood loss, or recovering from burns. In these instances, proteins that are lost to cellular repair and development must be replaced. Athletes also require more protein to build and repair muscle fibers.[8] In addition, a sedentary person or one who gets little exercise may find it easier to stay in energy balance if more of his calories come from protein and fewer from carbohydrates. Why? Because proteins make a person feel full and satisfied for a longer period of time.

Toward Sustainable Seafood The U.S. Department of Agriculture (USDA) recommends consuming fish twice a week to reduce saturated fat and cholesterol levels and increase omega-3 fatty acid levels. However, the many environmental concerns surrounding the seafood industry today call into question the sustainability and safety of such consumption. More than 70 percent of the world's natural fishing grounds have been overfished, and whole stretches of the oceans are dead zones where fish and shellfish can no longer live.

To counteract the loss of wild fish populations, increasing numbers of fish are being farmed, which poses additional health risks and environmental concerns. Some farmed fish are laden with antibiotics, while highly concentrated levels of parasites and bacteria from fish farm runoff may enter the ocean and river fish populations through adjacent waterways. And some farmed fish are fed wild fish, resulting in a net loss of fish from the sea.

At the same time, high levels of chemicals, parasites, bacteria, and toxins are also found in many of the fish available on the market. Mercury, a waste product of many industries, binds to proteins and stays in an animal's body, accumulating as it moves up the food chain. In humans, mercury can damage the nervous system and kidneys and cause birth defects and developmental problems. Polychlorinated biphenyls (PCBs), chemicals that can build up in the fatty tissue of fish, are another cause of concern.

Purchasing seafood from regularly inspected, environmentally responsible sources will support fisheries and fish farms that are healthier for you and the environment. Several major environmental groups have developed guides to inform consumers of safe and sustainable seafood choices. The Monterey Bay Aquarium in California provides a national guide for seafood available for purchase in the United States; you can find the guide online at http://mobile.seafoodwatch.org or as a free smartphone application.

check yourself

- **Why is water considered an essential nutrient?**
- **What are the functions of protein in the body?**

8.3 Essential Nutrients: Carbohydrates

learning outcome

8.3 **Describe the functions of carbohydrates in the body, including fiber, and list sources of carbohydrates.**

Carbohydrates supply us with the energy needed to sustain normal daily activity. The human body metabolizes carbohydrates more quickly and efficiently than it does proteins for a quick source of energy for the body. Carbohydrates are easily converted to glucose, the fuel for the body's cells. Carbohydrates also play an important role in the functioning of internal organs, the nervous system, and muscles. They are the best fuel for moderate to intense exercise because they can be readily broken down to glucose even when we're breathing hard and our muscle cells are getting less oxygen.

Like proteins, carbohydrates provide 4 calories per gram. The RDA for adults is 130 grams of carbohydrate per day.[9] There are two major types of carbohydrates: simple and complex.

Simple Carbohydrates

Simple carbohydrates, or *simple sugars*, are found naturally in fruits, many vegetables, and dairy. The most common form of simple carbohydrates is *glucose*. Fruits and berries contain *fructose* (commonly called *fruit sugar*). Glucose and fructose are **monosaccharides**. Eventually, the human body converts all types of simple sugars to glucose to provide energy to cells.

Disaccharides are combinations of two monosaccharides. Perhaps the best-known example is *sucrose* (granulated table sugar). *Lactose* (milk sugar), found in milk and milk products, and *maltose* (malt sugar) are other common disaccharides. Disaccharides must be broken down into monosaccharides before the body can use them.

Americans typically consume far too many refined carbohydrates (i.e., carbohydrates containing only sugars and starches, discussed below), which have few health benefits and are a major factor in our growing epidemic of overweight and obesity. Many of the simple sugars in these foods come from *added sugars*, sweeteners put in during processing to flavor foods, make sodas taste good, and ease our craving for sweets. A classic example is the amount of added sugar in one can of soda: more than 10 teaspoons per can! All that refined sugar can cause tooth decay and put on pounds.

Sugar is found in high amounts in a wide range of food products. Such diverse items as ketchup, barbecue sauce, and flavored coffee creamers derive 30 to 65 percent of their calories from sugar. Knowing what foods contain these sugars, considering the amounts you consume each day that are hidden in foods, and then trying to reduce these levels can be a great way to reduce excess weight. Read food labels carefully before purchasing. If *sugar* or one of its aliases (including *high fructose corn syrup* and *cornstarch*) appears near the top of the ingredients list, then that product contains a lot of sugar and is probably not your best nutritional bet. Also, most labels list the amount of sugar as a percentage of total calories.

Complex Carbohydrates

Complex carbohydrates are found in grains, cereals, legumes, and other vegetables. Also called *polysaccharides*, they are formed by long chains of monosaccharides. Like disaccharides, they must be broken down into simple sugars before the body can use them. *Starches, glycogen*, and *fiber* are the main types of complex carbohydrates.

Starches and Glycogen **Starches**, which make up the majority of the complex carbohydrate group, come from flours, breads, pasta, rice, corn, oats, barley, potatoes, and related foods. The body breaks down these complex carbohydrates into the monosaccharide glucose, which can be easily absorbed by cells and used as energy. Polysaccharides can also be stored in body muscles and the liver as **glycogen**. When the body requires a sudden burst of energy, it breaks down glycogen into glucose.

Fiber **Fiber**, sometimes referred to as "bulk" or "roughage," is the indigestible portion of plant foods that helps move foods through the digestive system, delays absorption of cholesterol and other nutrients, and softens stools by absorbing water. Dietary fiber is found only in plant foods, such as fruits, vegetables, nuts, and grains.

Fiber is either *soluble* or *insoluble*. Soluble fibers, such as pectins, gums, and mucilages, dissolve in water, form gel-like substances, and can be digested easily by bacteria in the colon. Major food sources

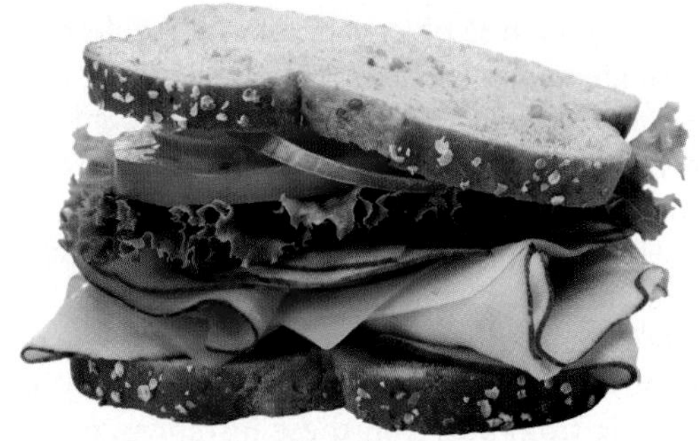

Why are whole grains better than refined grains?

Whole-grain foods contain fiber, a crucial form of carbohydrate that protects against some gastrointestinal disorders and reduces risk for certain cancers. Fiber is also associated with lowered blood cholesterol levels. Studies have shown that eating 2.5 servings of whole grains per day can reduce cardiovascular disease risk by as much as 21 percent. But are people getting the message? One nutrition survey showed that only 8 percent of U.S. adults consume three or more servings of whole grains each day, and 42 percent ate no whole grains at all on a given day.

Source: Dietary Guidelines Advisory Committee 2010, "What is the Relationship between Whole Grain Intake and Cardiovascular Disease?," *United States Department of Agriculture Nutrition Evidence Library*, 2010, www.nel.gov.

The average American consumes 15.9 grams of fiber daily—much less than the recommended

25 to 38

grams per day.

of soluble fiber include citrus fruits, berries, oat bran, dried beans (e.g., kidney, garbanzo, pinto, and navy beans), and some vegetables. Insoluble fibers, such as lignins and cellulose, are those that typically do not dissolve in water and that cannot be fermented by bacteria in the colon. They are found in most fruits and vegetables and in **whole grains**, such as brown rice, wheat, bran, and whole-grain breads and cereals (see Figure 8.4). The AMDR for carbohydrates is 45 to 60 percent of total calories, and heath experts recommend that the majority of this intake be fiber-rich carbohydrates.

Despite growing evidence supporting the benefits of whole grains and high-fiber diets, fiber intake among the general public remains low. Most experts believe that Americans should double their current consumption of dietary fiber. The AI for fiber is 25 grams per day for women and 38 grams per day for men.[10]

Research supports many benefits of fiber. Colorectal cancer, one of the leading causes of cancer deaths in the United States, is much less common in countries whose populations eat diets high in fiber and low in animal fat. A recent analysis found support for the hypothesis that high dietary fiber intake is associated with a reduced colorectal cancer risk.[11] Fiber also protects against constipation and *diverticulosis* (a condition in which tiny bulges form on the large intestinal wall and can become irritated under strain from constipation). Insoluble fiber helps reduce constipation and discomfort by absorbing moisture and producing softer stools. In addition, fiber helps delay or reduce the absorption of dietary cholesterol, a factor in heart disease.[12] Soluble fiber also improves control of blood sugar and can reduce the need for insulin or medication in people with type 2 diabetes.[13] And because most high-fiber foods are high in carbohydrates and low in fat, they help control caloric intake for those wishing to lose unhealthy weight. Fiber also stays in the digestive tract longer than other nutrients, making you feel full sooner.

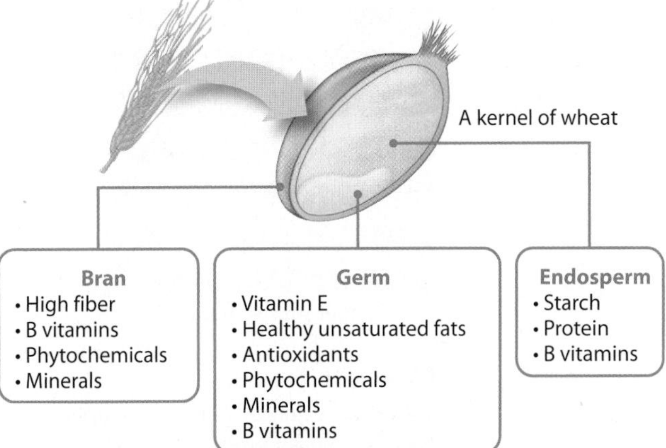

Figure 8.4 Anatomy of a Whole Grain

Whole grains are more nutritious than refined grains, because they contain the bran, germ, and endosperm of the seed—sources of fiber, vitamins, minerals, and beneficial phytochemicals (chemical compounds that occur naturally in plants).

Source: Adapted from Joan Salge Blake, Kathy D. Munoz, and Stella Volpe, *Nutrition: From Science to You*, 1st ed., © 2010. Reprinted by permission of Pearson Education, Inc., Upper Saddle River, New Jersey.

See It! Videos

Cut back on sugar while satisfying your sweet tooth! Watch **Ditching Sugar** in the Study Area of MasteringHealth.

To increase your fiber intake, eat fewer refined or processed carbohydrates in favor of more whole grains, fruits, vegetables, legumes, nuts, and seeds. If you haven't been eating enough fiber, however, make any such change gradually—in this case, too much of a good thing too quickly can pose problems. Sudden increases in dietary fiber may cause flatulence (intestinal gas), cramping, or bloating. Consume plenty of water or other (sugar-free!) liquids to reduce such side effects.

See It! Videos

Are whole grain product labels telling the truth? Watch **Grain Labels Do Not Reflect "Whole" Truth** in the Study Area of MasteringHealth.

Skills for **Behavior Change**

BULK UP YOUR FIBER INTAKE!

To increase your intake of dietary fiber:

- **Whenever possible, select whole-grain breads low in fat and sugars, with 3 or more grams of fiber per serving. Read labels—just because bread is brown doesn't mean it's better for you.**
- **Eat whole, unpeeled fruits and vegetables rather than drinking their juices. The fiber in whole fruit tends to slow blood sugar increases and helps you feel full longer.**
- **Substitute whole-grain pastas, bagels, and pizza crust for the refined, white flour versions.**
- **Add wheat crumbs or grains to meat loaf and burgers to increase fiber intake.**
- **Toast grains to bring out their nutty flavor and make foods more appealing.**
- **Sprinkle ground flaxseed on cereals, yogurt, and salads or add it to casseroles, burgers, and baked goods. Flaxseeds have a mild flavor and are also high in beneficial fatty acids.**

check yourself

- **What are the functions of carbohydrates in the body?**
- **What are the preferred sources of carbohydrates?**
- **Why is fiber important in the diet?**

8.4 Essential Nutrients: Fats

learning outcome

8.4 **Describe the functions of fats in the body.**

Fats, perhaps the most misunderstood nutrient, are the most energy dense, providing 9 calories per gram. Fats are a significant source of our body's fuel. The body can store only a limited amount of carbohydrate, so the longer you exercise, the more fat your body burns. Fats also play a vital role in maintaining healthy skin and hair, insulating body organs against shock, maintaining body temperature, and promoting healthy cell function. Fats make foods taste better and carry vitamins A, D, E, and K to cells. They also make you feel full after eating. So why are we constantly urged to cut back on fats? Because some fats are less healthy than others and because excessive consumption of fats can lead to weight gain.

Triglycerides, which make up about 95 percent of total body fat, are the most common form of fat circulating in the blood. When we consume too many calories from any source, the liver converts the excess into triglycerides, which are stored throughout our bodies.

Another oily substance in foods derived from animals is **cholesterol**. We don't need to consume any dietary cholesterol because our liver can make all that we need; the recommended intake for cholesterol is less than 300 milligrams a day (one egg contains about 215 milligrams).[14]

Neither triglycerides nor cholesterol can travel independently in the bloodstream. Instead, they are "packaged" inside protein coats to form compounds called lipoproteins. **High-density lipoproteins (HDLs)** are relatively high in protein and low in cholesterol and triglycerides. A high level of HDLs in the blood is healthful because HDLs remove cholesterol from dying cells and from plaques within blood vessels, eventually transporting cholesterol to the liver and eliminating it from the body. **Low-density lipoproteins (LDLs)** are much higher in both cholesterol and triglycerides than HDLs. They travel in the bloodstream delivering cholesterol to body cells; however, LDLs not taken up by cells degrade and release their cholesterol into the bloodstream. This cholesterol can then stick to the lining of blood vessels, contributing to the plaque that causes heart disease.

Types of Dietary Fats

Fat molecules include *fatty acid* chains of oxygen, carbon, and hydrogen atoms. Fatty acid chains that cannot hold any more hydrogen in their chemical structure are called **saturated fats**. These generally come from animal sources such as meat, dairy, and poultry and are solid at room temperature. **Unsaturated fats** have room for additional hydrogen atoms in their chemical structure and are liquid at room temperature. They come from plants and include most vegetable oils.

The terms *monounsaturated fatty acids (MUFAs)* and *polyunsaturated fatty acids (PUFAs)* refer to the relative number of hydrogen atoms missing in a fatty acid chain. Peanut and olive oils are high in monounsaturated fats. Corn, sunflower, and safflower oils are high in polyunsaturated fats.

There is controversy about which unsaturated fats are most beneficial. Monounsaturated fatty acids, such as olive oil, which seem to lower LDL levels and increase HDL levels, are currently preferred. Figure 8.5 shows fats in common vegetable oils.

Polyunsaturated fatty acids come in two forms: *omega-3 fatty acids* (in many fatty fish) and *omega-6 fatty acids* (in corn, soybean, and cottonseed oils). Both are classified as *essential fatty acids*—we must receive them from our diets. *Linoleic acid*, an omega-6 fatty acid, and alpha-linolenic acid, an omega-3 fatty acid, are needed to

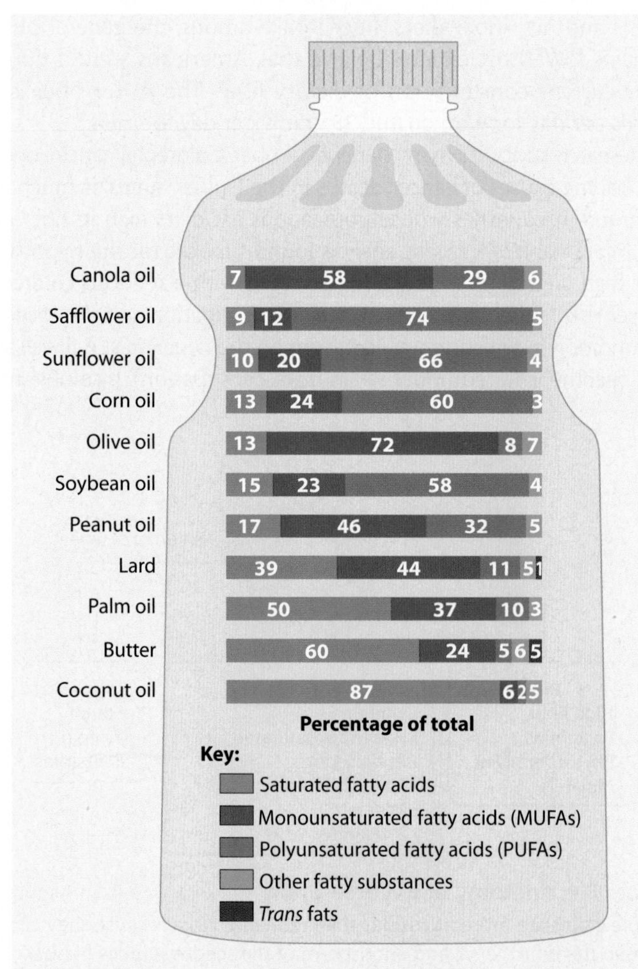

Figure 8.5 Percentages of Saturated, Polyunsaturated, Monounsaturated, and *Trans* Fats in Common Vegetable Oils

make hormone-like compounds that control immune function, pain perception, and inflammation and reduce cardiovascular disease (CVD) risks. EPA and DHEA, derivatives of alpha-linolenic acid that are found abundantly in oily fish such as salmon and tuna, are also associated with a reduced risk for heart disease.[15]

The AMDR for fats is 20 to 35 percent of calories, with 5 to 10 percent coming from essential fatty acids. Within this range, we should minimize our intake of saturated fats.

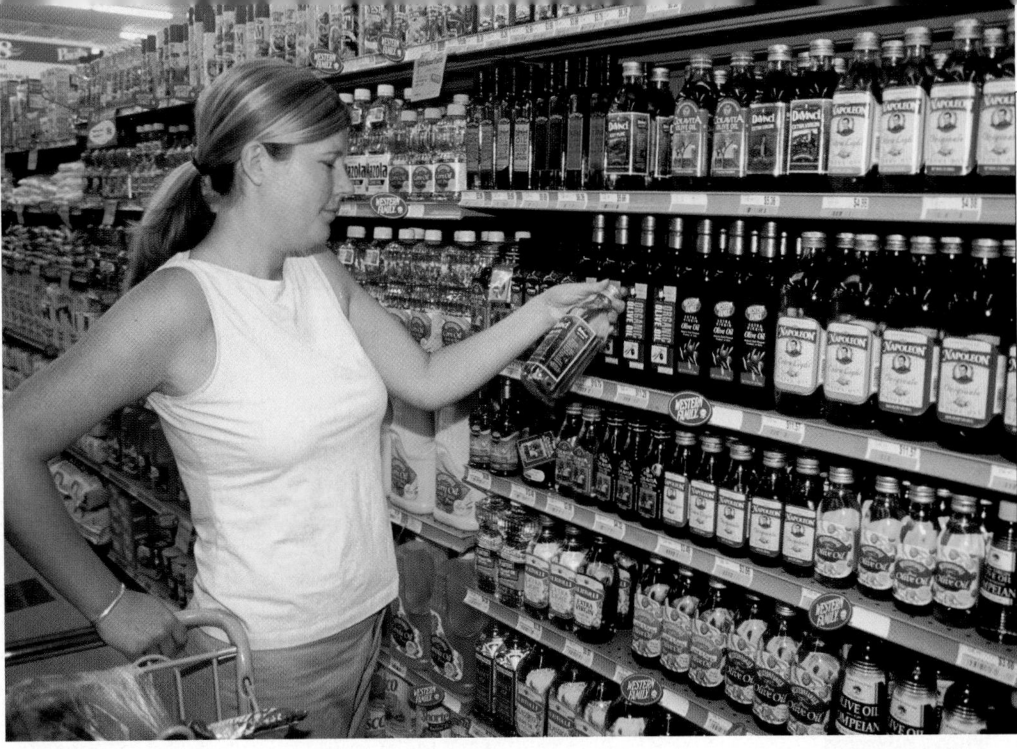

Are all fats bad for me?

All fats are not the same, and your body needs some fat to function healthily. Try to reduce saturated fats, those that come in meat, dairy, and poultry products; avoid *trans* fats, those that can come in stick margarine, commercially baked goods, and deep-fried foods; and replace these with monounsaturated fats, such as those in peanut and olive oils.

Avoiding *Trans* Fatty Acids

For decades, Americans shunned butter, red meat, and other foods because of their saturated fats. What they didn't know is that foods low in saturated fat, such as margarine, could be just as harmful because they contain ***trans* fatty acids**. Research shows that just a 2 percent caloric intake of these fats is associated with a 23 percent increased risk for heart disease and a 47 percent increased chance of sudden cardiac death.[16]

The great majority of *trans* fatty acids are found in processed foods made with partially hydrogenated oils (PHOs).[17] PHOs are produced when food manufacturers add hydrogen to a plant oil, solidifying it, helping it resist rancidity, and giving the food in which it is used a longer shelf life. This process straightens out the fatty acid chain so that it is more like a saturated fatty acid, and it has similar harmful effects, lowering HDLs and raising LDLs. *Trans* fats have been used in margarines, many commercial baked goods, and restaurant deep-fried foods.

In 2013, the U.S. Food and Drug Administration (FDA) issued a preliminary determination that PHOs are no longer recognized as safe for consumption. If it is finalized, foods containing PHOs will no longer be sold legally in the United States.[18] In the meantime, *trans* fats are being removed from most foods, and if they are present, they must be clearly indicated on food packaging. If you see the words *partially hydrogenated oils, fractionated oils, shortening, lard*, or *hydrogenation* on a food label, then *trans* fats are present.

Is More Fat Ever Better?

Despite all this, some studies have shown that balanced high-fat diets produce significant improvements in weight loss, blood fat, and blood glucose measures.[19]

Balance is the key. No more than 7 to 10 percent of your total calories should come from saturated fat, and no more than 35 percent should come from all forms of fat.[20] Follow these dietary guidelines to add more healthy fats to your diet:

- Eat sustainable fatty seafood (bluefish, herring, mackerel, salmon, sardines, or tuna) at least twice weekly.
- Use olive, peanut, soy, and canola oils instead of butter or lard.
- Add green leafy vegetables, walnuts, walnut oil, and ground flaxseed to your diet.
- Read the Nutrition Facts panel on food labels to find out how much fat is in your food.
- Chill meat-based soups and stews, scrape off any fat that hardens on top, then reheat to serve.
- Fill up on fruits and vegetables.
- Avoid all products with *trans* fatty acids. For healthy toppings on your bread, try vegetable spreads, bean spreads, nut butters, sugar-free jams, fat-free cheese, etc.
- Choose lean meats, fish, or skinless poultry. Broil, steam, poach, or bake whenever possible. Drain off fat after cooking.
- Choose fewer cold cuts, bacon, sausages, hot dogs, and organ meats.
- Select nonfat and low-fat dairy products, but remember that many nonfat and low-fat foods have higher amounts of carbohydrates and sugars. Choose wisely.

check yourself

- **What are the functions of fats in the body?**
- **What are more and less healthful sources of fats?**

8.5 Essential Nutrients: Vitamins

learning outcome

8.5 Describe the functions of vitamins in the body.

Vitamins are organic compounds that promote growth and help maintain life and health. They help maintain nerves and skin, produce blood cells, build bones and teeth, heal wounds, and convert food energy to body energy.

Vitamins can be *fat soluble* (absorbed through the intestinal tract with the help of fats) or *water soluble* (dissolvable in water). See Table 8.2 for the fat-soluble vitamins and Table 8.3 for the water-soluble vitamins. Vitamins A, D, E, and K are fat soluble; C- and B-complex vitamins are water soluble. Fat-soluble vitamins tend to be stored in the body; over-accumulation in the liver may cause cirrhosis-like symptoms. Water-soluble vitamins generally are excreted and cause few toxicity problems.

Vitamin D and folate are vitamins of special concern. Vitamin D is formed from a compound in the skin when exposed to the sun's ultraviolet rays. It's essential for the body's regulation of calcium, the primary mineral component of bone. An adequate amount of vitamin D can be synthesized with 5 to 30 minutes of sun on the body twice a week, without sunscreen,[21] or by consuming vitamin D–fortified milk, yogurt, soy milk, cereals, and fatty fish.

Folate is particularly important for proper cell division during embryonic development. Deficiencies during early pregnancy can

TABLE 8.2 **Fat-Soluble Vitamins**

Vitamin Name	Primary Functions	Recommended Intake[a]	Reliable Food Sources	Toxicity/Deficiency Symptoms
A (retinol, retinal, retinoic acid)	Required for ability of eyes to adjust to changes in light Protects color vision Assists cell differentiation Required for sperm production in men and fertilization in women Contributes to healthy bone Contributes to healthy immune system	RDA: Men: 900 μg Women: 700 μg UL: 3,000 μg/day	Preformed retinol: beef and chicken liver, egg yolks, milk Carotenoid precursors: spinach, carrots, mango, apricots, cantaloupe, pumpkin, yams	*Toxicity:* fatigue; bone and joint pain; spontaneous abortion and birth defects of fetuses in pregnant women; nausea and diarrhea; liver damage; nervous system damage; blurred vision; hair loss; skin disorders *Deficiency:* night blindness and xerophthalmia; impaired growth, immunity, and reproductive function
D (cholecalciferol)	Regulates blood calcium levels Maintains bone health Assists cell differentiation	RDA: Adult aged 19–70: 600 IU/day Adult aged >70: 800 IU/day UL: 4,000 IU/day	Canned salmon and mackerel, fortified milk and milk alternatives, fortified cereals	*Toxicity:* hypercalcemia *Deficiency:* rickets in children; osteomalacia and/or osteoporosis in adults
E (tocopherol)	As a powerful antioxidant, protects cell membranes, polyunsaturated fatty acids, and vitamin A from oxidation Protects white blood cells Enhances immune function Improves absorption of vitamin A	RDA: Men: 15 mg/day Women: 15 mg/day UL: 1,000 mg/day	Sunflower seeds, almonds, vegetable oils, fortified cereals	*Toxicity:* rare *Deficiency:* hemolytic anemia; impairment of nerve, muscle, and immune function
K (phylloquinone, menaquinone, menadione)	Serves as a coenzyme during production of specific proteins that assist in blood coagulation and bone metabolism	AI: Men: 120 μg/day Women: 90 μg/day	Kale, spinach, turnip greens, brussels sprouts	*Toxicity:* none known *Deficiency:* impaired blood clotting; possible effect on bone health

[a]Note: RDA, Recommended Dietary Allowance; UL, upper limit; AI, Adequate Intake.

TABLE

8.3 Water-Soluble Vitamins

Vitamin Name	Primary Functions	Recommended Intake[a]	Reliable Food Sources	Toxicity/Deficiency Symptoms
Thiamin (vitamin B1)	Required as enzyme cofactor for carbohydrate and amino acid metabolism	RDA: Men: 1.2 mg/day Women: 1.1 mg/day	Pork, fortified cereals, enriched rice and pasta, peas, tuna, legumes	*Toxicity:* none known *Deficiency:* beriberi; fatigue, apathy, decreased memory, confusion, irritability, muscle weakness
Riboflavin (vitamin B2)	Required as enzyme cofactor for carbohydrate and fat metabolism	RDA: Men: 1.3 mg/day Women: 1.1 mg/day	Beef liver, shrimp, milk and other dairy foods, fortified cereals, enriched breads and grains	*Toxicity:* none known *Deficiency:* ariboflavinosis; swollen mouth and throat; seborrheic dermatitis; anemia
Niacin, nicotinamide, nicotinic acid	Required for carbohydrate and fat metabolism Plays role in DNA replication and repair and cell differentiation	RDA: Men: 16 mg/day Women: 14 mg/day UL: 35 mg/day	Beef liver, most cuts of meat/fish/poultry, fortified cereals, enriched breads and grains, canned tomato products	*Toxicity:* flushing, liver damage, glucose intolerance, blurred vision differentiation *Deficiency:* pellagra; vomiting, constipation, or diarrhea; apathy
Pyridoxine, pyridoxal, pyridoxamine (vitamin B6)	Required as enzyme cofactor for carbohydrate and amino acid metabolism Assists synthesis of blood cells	RDA: Men and women aged 19–50: 1.3 mg/day Men aged >50: 1.7 mg/day Women aged >50: 1.5 mg/day UL: 100 mg/day	Chickpeas (garbanzo beans), most cuts of meat/fish/poultry, fortified cereals, white potatoes	*Toxicity:* nerve damage, skin lesions *Deficiency:* anemia; seborrheic dermatitis; depression, confusion, and convulsions
Folate (folic acid)	Required as enzyme cofactor for amino acid metabolism Required for DNA synthesis Involved in metabolism of homocysteine	RDA: Men: 400 μg/day Women: 400 μg/day UL: 1,000 μg/day	Fortified cereals, enriched breads and grains, spinach, legumes (lentils, chickpeas, pinto beans), greens (spinach, romaine lettuce), liver	*Toxicity:* masks symptoms of vitamin B12 deficiency, specifically signs of nerve damage *Deficiency:* macrocytic anemia; neural tube defects in a developing fetus; elevated homocysteine levels
Cobalamin (vitamin B12)	Assists with formation of blood Required for healthy nervous system function Involved as enzyme cofactor in metabolism of homocysteine	RDA: Men: 2.4 μg/day Women: 2.4 μg/day	Shellfish, all cuts of meat/fish/poultry, milk and other dairy foods, fortified cereals and other fortified foods	*Toxicity:* none known *Deficiency:* pernicious anemia; tingling and numbness of extremities; nerve damage; memory loss, disorientation, and dementia
Pantothenic acid	Assists with fat metabolism	AI: Men: 5 mg/day Women: 5 mg/day	Meat/fish/poultry, shiitake mushrooms, fortified cereals, egg yolk	*Toxicity:* none known *Deficiency:* rare
Biotin	Involved as enzyme cofactor in carbohydrate, fat, and protein metabolism	RDA: Men: 30 μg/day Women: 30 μg/day	Nuts, egg yolk	*Toxicity:* none known *Deficiency:* rare
Ascorbic acid (vitamin C)	Antioxidant in extracellular fluid and lungs Regenerates oxidized vitamin E Assists with collagen synthesis Enhances immune function Assists in synthesis of hormones, neurotransmitters, and DNA Enhances iron absorption	RDA: Men: 90 mg/day Women: 75 mg/day Smokers: 35 mg more per day than RDA UL: 2,000 mg	Sweet peppers, citrus fruits and juices, broccoli, strawberries, kiwi	*Toxicity:* nausea and diarrhea, nosebleeds, increased oxidative damage, increased formation of kidney stones in people with kidney disease *Deficiency:* scurvy; bone pain and fractures, depression, and anemia

[a]Note: RDA, Recommended Dietary Allowance; UL, upper limit; AI, Adequate Intake

prompt a neural tube defect, in which the primitive tube that eventually forms the brain and spinal cord fails to close properly. All bread, cereal, rice, and pasta products sold in the United States must be fortified with folic acid, the synthetic form of folate.

check yourself

- **What are some functions of vitamins in the body?**
- **What are key vitamins and some recommended food sources for them? Are there any that are difficult for you to eat in the recommended quantity?**

8.6 Essential Nutrients: Minerals

learning outcome

8.6 Describe the functions of minerals in the body.

Minerals are the inorganic, indestructible elements that aid physiological processes within the body. Without minerals, vitamins could not be absorbed.

Minerals are readily excreted and, with a few exceptions, are usually not toxic. **Major minerals** are the minerals that the body needs in fairly large amounts: sodium, calcium, phosphorus, magnesium, potassium, sulfur, and chloride. **Trace minerals** include iron, zinc, manganese, copper, fluoride, selenium, chromium, and iodine. Only very small amounts of trace minerals are needed, and serious problems may result if excesses or deficiencies occur (see Tables 8.4 and 8.5).

Sodium and calcium are two minerals of particular concern. Sodium enhances flavors and acts as a preservative, so it's often present in high quantities in the foods we eat—particularly processed foods. The average American consumes 3,463 milligrams of sodium per day,[22] much

TABLE 8.4 **Major Minerals**

Mineral Name	Primary Functions	Recommended Intake[a]	Reliable Food Sources	Toxicity/Deficiency Symptoms
Sodium	Fluid balance Acid–base balance Transmission of nerve impulses Muscle contraction	AI: Adults: 1.5 g/day (1,500 mg/day)	Table salt, pickles, most canned soups, snack foods, cured luncheon meats, canned tomato products	*Toxicity:* water retention, high blood pressure, loss of calcium *Deficiency:* muscle cramps, dizziness, fatigue, nausea, vomiting, mental confusion
Potassium	Fluid balance Transmission of nerve impulses Muscle contraction	AI: Adults: 4.7 g/day (4,700 mg/day)	Most fresh fruits and vegetables: potatoes, bananas, tomato juice, orange juice, melons	*Toxicity:* muscle weakness,vomiting, irregular heartbeat *Deficiency:* muscle weakness,paralysis, mental confusion,irregular heartbeat
Phosphorus	Fluid balance Bone formation Component of ATP, which provides energy for our bodies	RDA: UL: 1,100 µg/day	Milk/cheese/yogurt, soy milk and tofu, legumes (lentils, black beans), nuts (almonds, peanuts and peanut butter), poultry	*Toxicity:* muscle spasms, convulsions, low blood calcium *Deficiency:* muscle weakness, muscle damage, bone pain, dizziness
Calcium	Primary component of bone Acid–base balance Transmission of nerve impulses Muscle contraction	RDA: Adults aged 19 to 50 and men aged 51–70: 1,000 mg/day Women aged 51–70 and adults aged >70: 1,200 mg/day UL for adults 19–50: 2,500 mg/day UL for adults aged 51 and above: 2,000 mg/day	Milk/yogurt/cheese (best-absorbed form of calcium), sardines, collard greens and spinach, calcium fortified juices and milk alternatives	*Toxicity:* mineral imbalances, shock, kidney failure, fatigue, mental confusionw *Deficiency:* osteoporosis, convulsions, heart failure
Magnesium	Component of bone Muscle contraction Assists more than 300 enzyme systems	RDA: Men aged 19–30: 400 mg/day Men aged >30: 420 mg/day Women aged 19–30: 310 mg/day Women aged >30: 320 mg/day UL: 350 mg/day	Greens (spinach, kale, collard greens), whole grains, seeds, nuts, legumes (navy and black beans)	*Toxicity:* none known *Deficiency:* low blood calcium, muscle spasms or seizures, nausea, weakness, increased risk for chronic diseases, such as heart disease, hypertension, osteoporosis, and type 2 diabetes

[a]Note: RDA, Recommended Dietary Allowance; UL, upper limit; AI, Adequate Intake.

TABLE 8.5 Trace Minerals

Mineral Name	Primary Functions	Recommended Intake[a]	Reliable Food Sources	Toxicity/Deficiency Symptoms
Selenium	Required for carbohydrate and fat metabolism	RDA: Adults: 55 μg/day UL: 400 μg/day	Nuts, shellfish, meat/fish/poultry, whole grains	*Toxicity:* brittle hair and nails, skin rashes, nausea and vomiting, weakness, liver disease *Deficiency:* specific forms of heart disease and arthritis, impaired immune function, muscle pain and wasting, depression, hostility
Fluoride	Development and maintenance of healthy teeth and bones	RDA: Men: 4 mg/day Women: 3 mg/day UL: 2.2 mg/day for children aged 4–8; 10 mg/day for children aged >8	Fish, seafood, legumes, whole grains, drinking water (variable)	*Toxicity:* fluorosis of teeth and bones *Deficiency:* dental caries, low bone density
Iodine	Synthesis of thyroid hormones Temperature regulation Reproduction and growth	RDA: Adults: 150 μg/day UL: 1,100 μg/day	Iodized salt, saltwater seafood	*Toxicity:* goiter *Deficiency:* goiter, hypothyroidism, cretinism in infant of mother who is iodine deficient
Chromium	Glucose transport Metabolism of DNA and RNA Immune function and growth	AI: Men aged 19–50: 35 μg/day Men aged >50: 30 μg/day Women aged 19–50: 25 μg/day Women aged >50: 20 μg/day	Whole grains, brewer's yeast	*Toxicity:* none known *Deficiency:* elevated blood glucose and blood lipids, damage to brain and nervous system
Iron	Component of hemoglobin in blood cells Component of myoglobin in muscle cells Assists many enzyme systems	RDA: Adult men: 8 mg/day Women aged 19–50: 18 mg/day Women aged >50: 8 mg/day	Meat/fish/poultry (best-absorbed form of iron), fortified cereals, legumes, spinach	*Toxicity:* nausea, vomiting, and diarrhea; dizziness, confusion; rapid heartbeat, organ damage, death *Deficiency:* iron-deficiency microcytic (small red blood cells), hypochromic anemia
Zinc	Assists more than 100 enzyme systems Immune system function Growth and sexual maturation Gene regulation	RDA: Men: 11 mg/day Women: 8 mg/day UL: 40 mg/day	Meat/fish/poultry (best-absorbed form of zinc), fortified cereals, legumes	*Toxicity:* nausea, vomiting, and diarrhea; headaches, depressed immune function, reduced absorption of copper *Deficiency:* growth retardation, delayed sexual maturation, eye and skin lesions, hair loss, increased incidence of illness and infection

[a]Note: RDA, Recommended Dietary Allowance; UL, upper limit; AI, Adequate Intake.

more than the recommend AI, 500 milligrams.[23] High sodium intake is a major concern because a high-sodium diet increases blood pressure (hypertension), which contributes to heart disease and strokes.

The issue of calcium consumption has gained attention with the rising incidence of osteoporosis. Most Americans do not consume the recommended 1,000 to 1,200 milligrams of calcium per day.[24] For optimal absorption, consume calcium-rich foods (broccoli, collard greens, kale) and beverages (dairy products, calcium-fortified juices) throughout the day.

check yourself

- **What are some functions of minerals in the body?**
- **What are key minerals and some recommended food sources for them?**
- **Are there any key minerals that are difficult for you to eat in the recommended quantity? How could you incorporate more of these into your diet?**

8.7 Health Benefits of Functional Foods

learning outcome

8.7 Describe how functional foods impact health.

Increasingly, nutrition research is focusing on components of foods that interact with nutrients to promote human health, rather than solely as sources of macro- and micronutrients.[25] Foods that may confer health benefits beyond the nutrients they contribute to the diet—whole foods, fortified foods, enriched foods, or enhanced foods—are called **functional foods**. When functional foods are included as part of a varied diet, they have the potential to positively impact health.[26]

Some of the most popular functional foods today are those containing **antioxidants.** These substances appear to protect against oxidative stress, a complex process in which *free radicals* (atoms with unpaired electrons) destabilize other atoms and molecules, prompting a chain reaction that can damage cells, cell proteins, or genetic material in the cells. Free radical formation is a natural process that cannot be avoided, but antioxidants combat it by donating their electrons to stabilize free radicals, activating enzymes that convert free radicals to less damaging substances, or reducing or repairing the damage they cause.

Among the more commonly cited antioxidants are vitamins C and E, as well as the minerals copper, iron, manganese, selenium, and zinc. Other potent antioxidants are **phytochemicals**, compounds that occur naturally in plants and are thought to protect them against ultraviolet radiation, pests, and other threats. Common examples include the *carotenoids*, pigments found in red, orange, and dark green fruits and vegetables. Beta-carotene, the most researched carotenoid, is a precursor of vitamin A, meaning that vitamin A can be produced in the body from beta-carotene. Both vitamin A and beta-carotene have antioxidant properties. Phenolic phytochemicals, which include a group known as *flavonoids*, are found in an array of fruits and vegetables as well as soy products, tea, and chocolate. Like carotenoids, they are thought to have antioxidant properties that may prevent cardiovascular disease.[27]

To date, many such claims about the health benefits of antioxidant nutrients and phytochemicals have not been fully investigated. However, studies do show that individuals deficient in antioxidant vitamins and minerals have an increased risk for age-related diseases and that antioxidants consumed in whole foods, mostly fruits and vegetables, may reduce these individuals' risks. In contrast, antioxidants consumed as supplements do not confer such a benefit and may be harmful.[28]

Health Claims of Superfoods

In food advertisements, fitness and food magazines, and even among health care organizations, functional foods are increasingly being referred to as "superfoods." Do superfoods live up to their new name? Let's look at a few.

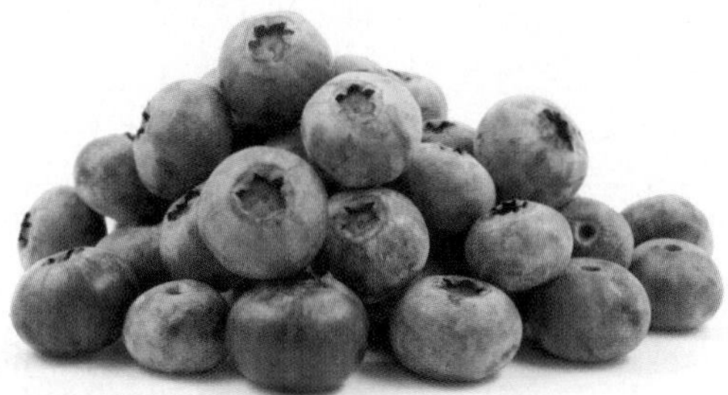

Blueberries are a great source of antioxidants.

Salmon is a rich source of the omega-3 fatty acids EPA and DHA, which combat inflammation, improve HDL/LDL blood profiles, and reduce the risk for cardiovascular disease. DHA may also promote a healthy nervous system, reducing the risk for age-related dementia.[29]

Yogurt makes it onto most superfood lists because, like other fermented milk products, it contains living, beneficial bacteria called probiotics. Probiotics colonize the large intestine, where they help complete digestion, produce certain vitamins, and are thought to reduce the risk of diarrhea and other bowel disorders, boost immunity, and help regulate body weight.[30]

Cocoa is particularly rich in a class of chemicals called flavonols that have been shown in many studies to reduce the risk for cardiovascular disease, diabetes, and even arthritis.[31] Dark chocolate is believed to have a higher level of flavonols than milk chocolate. However, while it is widely believed that dark chocolate contains the highest levels of flavonols, newer research indicates that processing can drastically reduce flavonal levels. Buying higher quality dark chocolate with a higher percentage of cocoa may be a good idea, but it isn't foolproof. When in doubt, your best bet is still dark over milk chocolate, but remember that moderation is key!

Given such claims, it's easy to get carried away by the idea that superfoods have superpowers. But eating a square of dark chocolate won't rescue you from the ill effects of a fast-food burger and fries. What matters is your whole diet. Focus on including superfoods as components of a varied diet rich in fresh fruits, legumes and other vegetables, whole grains, lean sources of protein, and nuts and seeds.

check yourself

- **How do functional foods benefit health?**
- **How can you incorporate more functional foods into your diet?**

Planning a Healthy Diet: Using the Food Label

learning outcome

8.8 Understand each component of the food label.

To help consumers evaluate the nutritional values of packaged foods, the FDA and the USDA developed the Nutrition Facts panel that is typically displayed on the side or back of packaged foods. One of the most helpful items on the panel is the **% daily values (%DVs)** list, which tells you how much of an average adult's allowance for a particular substance (fat, fiber, calcium, etc.) is provided by a serving of the food. The %DV is calculated based on a 2,000 calorie per day diet, so your values may be different from those listed on a label. The panel also includes information on the serving size and calories. In 2014, the FDA announced plans to make the data on the panel more helpful for consumers by identifying the calories per serving in much larger type, and adjusting the serving size so that it better reflects the amount of the food that people typically eat.[32] Figure 8.6 walks you through a typical Nutrition Facts panel.

Start here. The size of the serving on the food package influences the number of calories and all the nutrient amounts listed on the top part of the label. Pay attention to the serving size, especially how many servings there are in the food package. Then ask yourself, "How many servings am I consuming?"

Limit these nutrients. The nutrients listed first are the ones Americans generally eat in adequate amounts, or even too much of. Eating too much fat, saturated fat, *trans* fat, cholesterol, or sodium may increase your risk of certain chronic diseases, such as heart disease, some cancers, or high blood pressure.

Get enough of these nutrients. Most Americans don't get enough dietary fiber, vitamin A, vitamin C, calcium, and iron in their diets. Eating enough of these nutrients can improve your health and help reduce the risk of some diseases and conditions.

The footnote is not specific to the product. It shows recommended dietary advice for all Americans. The Percent Daily Values are based on a 2,000-calorie diet, but the footnote lists daily values for both a 2,000- and 2,500-calorie diet.

Sample Label for Macaroni and Cheese

Nutrition Facts
Serving size 1 cup (228g)
Servings Per Container 2

Amount Per Serving

Calories 250	Calories from Fat 110
	% Daily Value*
Total Fat 12g	**18%**
Saturated Fat 3g	**15%**
Trans Fat 1.5g	
Cholesterol 30mg	**10%**
Sodium 470mg	**20%**
Total Carbohydrate 31g	**10%**
Dietary Fiber 0g	**0%**
Sugars 5g	
Protein 5g	
Vitamin A	4%
Vitamin C	2%
Calcium	20%
Iron	4%

* Percent Daily Values are based on a 2,000 calorie diet. Your Daily Values may be higher or lower depending on your calorie needs:

	Calories:	2,000	2,500
Total Fat	Less than	65g	80g
Sat Fat	Less than	20g	25g
Cholesterol	Less than	300mg	300mg
Sodium	Less than	2,400mg	2,400mg
Total Carbohydrate		300g	375g
Dietary Fiber		25g	30g

Pay attention to calories (and calories from fat). Many Americans consume more calories than they need. Remember: The number of servings you consume determines the number of calories you actually eat (your portion amount). Dietary guidelines recommend that no more than 30% of your daily calories consumed come from fat.

5% DV or less is low and 20% DV or more is high. The %DV helps you determine if a serving of food is high or low in a nutrient, whether or not you consume the 2,000-calorie diet it is based on. It also helps you make easy comparisons between products (just make sure the serving sizes are similar).

Note that a few nutrients—*trans* fats, sugars, and protein—do not have a %DV. Experts could not provide a reference value for *trans* fat, but it is recommended that you keep your intake as low as possible. There are no recommendations for the total amount of sugar to eat in one day, but check the ingredient list to see information on added sugars, such as high fructose corn syrup. A %DV for protein is required to be listed if a claim is made (such as "high in protein") or if the food is meant for infants and children under 4 years old. Otherwise, none is needed.

Figure 8.6 Reading a Food Label

Source: Center for Food Safety and Applied Nutrition, "A Key to Choosing Healthful Foods: Using the Nutrition Facts on the Food Label," Updated May 2009, www.fda.gov.

VIDEO TUTOR
Understanding Food Labels

check yourself

- **What are the key components of a food label? How can they help you make better food choices?**

8.9 Planning a Healthy Diet: Dietary Guidelines and MyPlate

learning outcome

8.9 Explain the principles for a healthy diet contained in the MyPlate food guidance system.

Now that you have some idea of your nutritional needs, let's discuss what a healthy diet looks like, how you can begin to meet your needs, and how you can meet the challenge of getting the foods you need on campus.

Dietary Guidelines for Americans

The *Dietary Guidelines for Americans* are a set of recommendations for healthy eating; they are revised every 5 years. The 2010 *Dietary Guidelines for Americans* are designed to help bridge the gap between the standard American diet and the key recommendations that aim to combat the growing obesity epidemic by balancing calories with adequate physical activity.[33] They provide advice about consuming fewer calories, making informed food choices, and being physically active to attain and maintain a healthy weight, reduce your risk for chronic disease, and improve your overall health. The 2010 *Dietary Guidelines for Americans* are presented as an easy-to-follow graphic and guidance system called MyPlate, found at www.choosemyplate.gov and illustrated in Figure 8.7.

The MyPlate Food Guidance System

The MyPlate food guidance system takes into consideration the dietary and caloric needs for a wide variety of individuals, such as pregnant or breast-feeding women, those trying to lose weight, and adults with different activity levels. When you visit the interactive website, you can create personalized dietary and exercise recommendations based on the information you enter.

MyPlate also encourages consumers to eat for health through three general areas of recommendation:

1. **Balance calories.** Find out how many calories you need for a day is a first step in managing your weight. Go to www.choosemyplate.gov to find your calorie level. Being physically active also helps you balance calories.
   - Enjoy your food, but eat less. Take time to fully enjoy your food as you eat it. Eating too fast or when your attention is elsewhere may lead to eating too many calories. Pay attention to hunger cues before, during, and after meals. Use them to recognize when to eat and when you've had enough.
   - Avoid oversized portions. Use a smaller plate, bowl, and glass. Portion out food before you eat. When eating out, choose a smaller size option, share a dish, or take home part of your meal.
2. **Increase some foods.** Eat more vegetables, fruits, whole grains, and fat-free or 1 percent milk and dairy products, These foods have the nutrients you need for health—including potassium, calcium, vitamin D, and fiber. Make them the basis for meals and snacks.
   - Make half your plate fruits and vegetables. Choose red, orange, and dark-green vegetables like tomatoes, sweet pota-

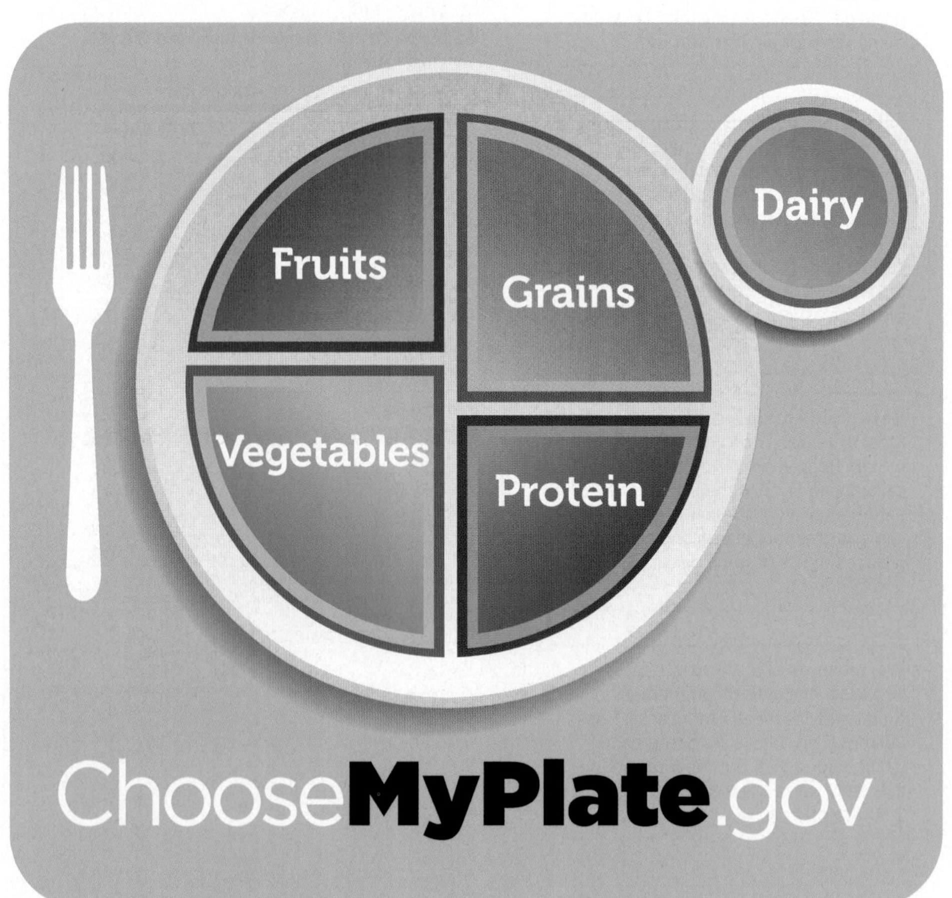

Figure 8.7 The MyPlate Food Guidance System
The USDA MyPlate food guidance system takes a new approach to dietary and exercise recommendations. Each colored section of the plate represents a food group. An interactive tool on www.choosemyplate.gov can provide individualized recommendations for users.
Source: U.S. Department of Agriculture, 2011, www.choosemyplate.gov.

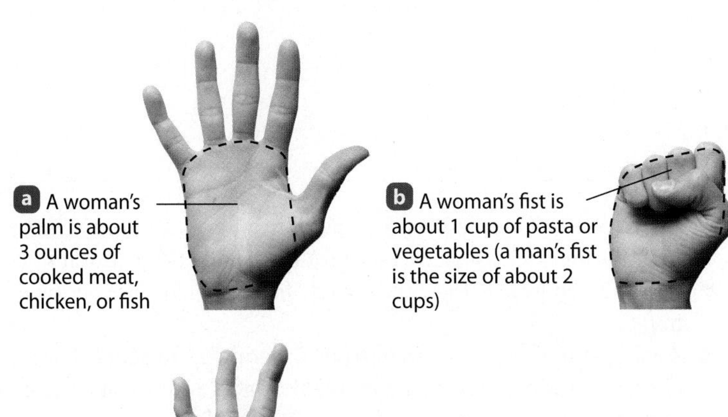

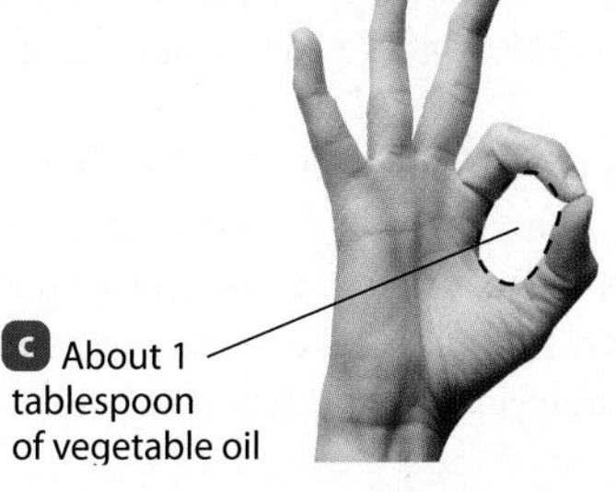

Figure 8.8 What's a Serving?
Your hands can guide you in estimating portion sizes.

toes, and broccoli. Add fruit to meals as part of main or side dishes or as dessert.
- Make at least half your grains whole grains. Substitute whole-wheat bread for white bread or brown rice for white rice.
- Switch to fat-free or 1 percent milk. They have the same amount of calcium and other essential nutrients as whole milk, but fewer calories and less saturated fat.
- Experiment with some spices and herbs. They have interesting flavors that can "spice up" food without the extra hit of sodium. Remember to replace them when they get old or lose flavor.

3. **Reduce some foods.** Cut back on foods high in solid fats, added sugars, and salt. Enjoy these foods as occasional treats, not everyday foods.
   - Compare sodium in foods like soup, bread, and frozen meals—and choose the foods with lower numbers. Look for "low sodium," "reduced sodium," or "no salt added" on the food label.
   - Drink water instead of sugary drinks. Cut calories by drinking water or unsweetened beverages. Soda, energy drinks, and sports drinks are a major source of added sugar and calories in American diets.

Understand Serving Sizes MyPlate presents personalized dietary recommendations in terms of numbers of servings of particular nutrients. But how much is one serving? Is it different from a portion? Although these two terms are often used interchangeably, they actually mean very different things. A *serving* is the recommended amount you should consume, whereas a *portion* is the amount you choose to eat at any one time. Many people select portions that are much bigger than recommended servings. See Figure 8.8 for an easy way to recognize serving sizes.

Unfortunately, we don't always get a clear picture from food producers and advertisers about what a serving really is. Consider a bottle of chocolate milk: The food label may list one serving size as 8 fluid ounces and 150 calories. However, note the size of the entire bottle. If it holds 16 ounces, drinking the whole thing serves up 300 calories.

Eat Nutrient-Dense Foods Although eating the proper number of servings from MyPlate is important, it is also important to recognize that there are large caloric, fat, and energy differences among foods within a given food group. For example, salmon and hot dogs provide vastly different nutrient levels per ounce. Salmon is rich in essential fatty acids and is considered nutrient dense. Hot dogs are loaded with saturated fats, cholesterol, and sodium—all substances we should limit. It is important to eat foods that have a high nutritional value for their caloric content.

Reduce Empty Calorie Foods Avoid *empty calories*, that is, calories that have little or no nutritional value. Sugar is sugar, but when you eat it in a piece of fruit, you're getting dietary fiber, lots of vitamins and minerals, and phytochemicals. In contrast, when you drink a 12-ounce soft drink, you're getting nearly 200 empty calories. Don't be fooled by fruit drinks, either. Unless the label states that they're 100 percent juice, they may also be loaded with added sugar. Even 100 percent fresh-squeezed orange juice has 20 grams (5 teaspoons!) of naturally occurring sugar in an 8-ounce serving. Bottled coffees, teas, and energy drinks usually are even higher in sugar and empty calories.

MyPlate recommends we limit our intake of sugary drinks as well as the following sugar- and fat-laden items:[34]

- **Cakes, cookies, pastries, and donuts:** One slice of chocolate cake contains 77 percent empty calories.
- **Cheese:** Switching from whole milk mozzarella cheese to nonfat mozzarella cheese saves you 76 empty calories per ounce.
- **Pizza:** One slice of pepperoni pizza adds 139 empty calories to your meal.
- **Ice cream:** More than 75 percent of the 275 calories in ice cream are empty calories.
- **Sausages, hot dogs, bacon, and ribs:** Adding a sausage link to your breakfast adds 96 empty calories.
- **Wine, beer, and all alcoholic beverages:** A whopping 155 empty calories are consumed with each 12 fluid ounces of beer.
- **Refined grains, including crackers, cookies, and white rice:** Switching to whole wheat versions can save you 25 fat-laden empty calories per serving.

Physical Activity Strive to be physically active for at least 30 minutes per day, preferably with moderate to vigorous activity levels on most days. Physical activity does not mean you have to go to the gym, jog 3 miles a day, or hire a personal trainer. Any activity that gets your heart pumping (e.g., gardening, playing basketball, heavy yard work, or dancing) is a good way to get moving. In addition to personalized recommendations on diet, MyPlate personalized plans will also offer recommendations for weekly physical activity.

check yourself

- **What are the main guidelines of the MyPlate food guidance system?**
- **Which parts of MyPlate can you most easily adopt in your diet? Which are the most challenging? Why?**

8.10 Eating Well in College

learning outcome

8.10 Provide examples of what college students can do to eat more healthfully.

Many college students may find it hard to fit a well-balanced meal into the day, but eating breakfast and lunch are important if you are to keep energy levels up and get the most out of your classes. Eating a complete breakfast that includes fiber-rich carbohydrates, protein, and healthy unsaturated fat (such as a banana, peanut butter, and whole-grain bread sandwich, or a bowl of oatmeal topped with dried fruit and nuts) is key. If you are short on time, bring a container of yogurt and some trail mix to your morning class.

If your campus is like many others, you've probably noticed a distinct move toward fast-food restaurants in your student unions. Generally speaking, you can eat more healthfully and for less money if you bring food from home or your campus dining hall. If you must eat fast food, follow the tips below to get more nutritional bang for your buck:

- Ask for nutritional analyses of items. Most fast-food chains now have them.
- Order salads, but be careful about what you add to them. Taco salads and Cobb salads are often high in fat, calories, and sodium. Ask for dressing on the side, and use it sparingly. Try the vinaigrette or low-fat dressings. Stay away from eggs and other high-fat add-ons, such as bacon bits, croutons, and crispy noodles.
- If you crave french fries, try baked "fries," which may be lower in fat.
- Avoid giant sizes, and refrain from ordering extra sauce, bacon, cheese, dressings, and other extras that add additional calories, sodium, carbohydrates, and fat.
- Limit sodas and other beverages that are high in added sugars.
- At least once per week, substitute a vegetable-based meat substitute into your fast-food choices. Most places now offer veggie burgers or similar products, which provide excellent sources of protein and often have considerably less fat and fewer calories.

In the dining hall, try these ideas:

- Choose lean meats, grilled chicken, fish, or vegetable dishes. Avoid fried chicken, fatty cuts of red meat, or meat dishes smothered in creamy or oily sauce.
- Hit the salad bar and load up on leafy greens, beans, tuna, or tofu. Choose items such as avocado or nuts for a little "good" fat, and go easy on the dressing.
- When choosing items from a made-to-order food station, ask the preparer to hold the butter, oil, mayonnaise, sour cream, or cheese- or cream-based sauces.
- Avoid going back for seconds and consuming large portions.
- Pass on high-calorie, low-nutrient foods such as sugary cereals, ice cream, and other sweet treats. Choose fruit or low-fat yogurt to satisfy your sweet tooth.
- If there is something you'd like but don't see in your dining hall, speak to your food services manager and provide suggestions.

Between classes, avoid vending machines. Reach into your backpack for an apple, banana, some dried fruit and nuts, a single serving of unsweetened applesauce, or whole-grain crackers spread with peanut butter. Energy bars can be a nutritious option if you choose right. Check the Nutrition Facts panel for bars that are below 200 calories and provide at least 3 grams of dietary fiber. Cereal bars usually provide less protein than energy bars; however, they also tend to be much lower in calories and sugar, and high in fiber.

Many college students tend to think that fruits and vegetables are beyond their budget. Contrary to popular opinion, people on a tight budget can eat healthfully and spend less on food. Throughout the United States, five of the least expensive, perennially available fresh vegetables are carrots, eggplant, lettuce, potatoes, and summer squash. Five fresh fruit options are apples, bananas, pears, pineapple, and watermelon.[35] Additionally, choose fruits and veggies in season—they'll cost less. If you can freeze them, stock up. If not, enjoy them fresh while you can. Canned and frozen produce, especially when it's on sale, may also be less expensive than some fresh produce.

Maintaining a nutritious diet within the confines of student life can be challenging. However, if you take the time to plan healthy

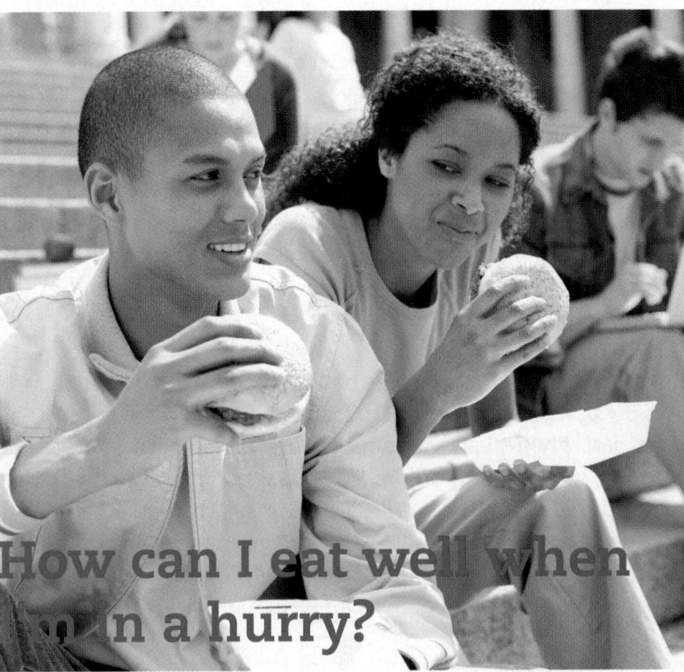

Meals like this one may be convenient, but they are high in fat, calories, sodium, and refined carbohydrates. Even when you are short on time and money, it is possible—and worthwhile—to make healthier choices. If you are ordering fast food, opt for foods prepared by baking, roasting, or steaming; ask for the leanest meat option; and request that sauces, dressings, and gravies be served on the side.

College males spend an average of

$99.17

and college females spend an average of

$52.11

on fast food in a month.

meals, you will find that you are eating better, enjoying it more, and actually saving money.

What's Healthy on the Menu?

No matter what type of cuisine you enjoy, there will always be healthier and less healthy options on the menu. To help you order wisely, here are lighter options and high-fat pitfalls. "Best" choices contain fewer than 30 grams of fat, a generous meal's worth for an active, medium-sized woman. "Worst" choices have up to 100 grams of fat.

Breakfast

- Best: Hot or cold cereal with low fat milk; pancakes or French toast with syrup; scrambled eggs with hash browns and plain toast
- Worst: Belgian waffle with sausage; sausage and eggs with biscuits and gravy; ham-and-cheese omelet with hash browns and toast
- Tips: Ask for whole-grain cereal or shredded wheat with low-fat milk or whole wheat toast without butter or margarine. Order omelets without cheese, and order fried eggs without bacon or sausage.

Sandwiches

- Best: Ham and Swiss cheese; roast beef; turkey; hummus and red pepper
- Worst: Tuna salad; Reuben; submarine
- Tips: Ask for mustard; hold the mayonnaise and high-fat cheese. Load up sandwiches with veggies such as tomatoes, lettuce, cucumbers, sprouts, and bell peppers.

Seafood

- Best: Broiled bass, halibut, or snapper; grilled scallops; steamed crab or lobster
- Worst: Fried seafood platter; blackened catfish
- Tips: Order fish broiled, baked, grilled, or steamed—not panfried or sautéed. Ask for lemon instead of tartar sauce. Avoid creamy and buttery sauces.

Italian

- Best: Pasta with red or white clam sauce; spaghetti with marinara or tomato-and-meat sauce
- Worst: Eggplant parmigiana; fettuccine Alfredo; fried calamari; lasagna
- Tips: Stick with plain bread instead of garlic bread made with butter or oil. Avoid cream- or egg-based sauces. Try vegetarian pizza, and don't ask for extra cheese.

Mexican

- Best: Bean burrito (no cheese); chicken fajitas
- Worst: Beef chimichanga; quesadilla; chile relleno; refried beans
- Tips: Choose soft tortillas (not fried) with fresh salsa, not guacamole. Ask for beans made without lard or fat, and have cheeses and sour cream provided on the side or left out altogether.

See It! Videos

How accurate are restaurant calorie counts? Watch **Menu Calorie Counts** in the Study Area of MasteringHealth.

Skills for **Behavior Change**

HEALTHY EATING SIMPLIFIED

Messages from nutrition experts, marketing campaigns, and media blitzes may leave you scratching your head about how to eat healthfully. When it all starts to feel too complicated to be worthwhile, here are some simple tips to follow for health-conscious eating:

- **You don't need foods from fancy packages to improve your health. Fruits, vegetables, and whole grains should make up the bulk of your diet. Shop the perimeter of the store and the bulk foods aisle.**
- **Let the MyPlate method guide you. Your plate should be half vegetables, a quarter lean protein, and a quarter whole grains/bread. Have a serving of fruit for dessert.**
- **Limit processed and packaged foods. This will assist you in limiting added sodium, sugar, and fat. If you can't make sense of the ingredients, don't eat it.**
- **Eat natural snacks such as dried fruit, nuts, fresh fruits, string cheese, yogurt without added sugar, hard-boiled eggs, and vegetables.**
- **Be mindful of your eating. Eat until you are satisfied but not overfull.**
- **Bring healthful foods with you when you head out the door. Whether going to class, to work, or on a road trip, you *can* control the foods that are available. Don't put yourself in a position where you're forced to buy from a vending machine or convenience store.**

Source: M. Pollan, *Food Rules: An Eater's Manual* (New York, NY: Penguin Books, 2010).

check yourself

- **What challenges do you face when trying to eat more healthfully?**
- **What are some steps that you can take to eat more healthfully?**

8.11 Vegetarianism: A Healthy Diet?

learning outcome

8.11 Describe the benefits and drawbacks of a vegetarian diet.

More than 3 percent of U.S. adults, approximately 4 to 9 million people, are vegetarians.[36] Countless other Americans are heeding the advice of health, environmental, and animal ethics groups to reduce their meat consumption in favor of other "faceless" forms of protein. The word **vegetarian** can mean different things to different people—*vegans* eat no animal products at all, while many vegetarians eat dairy or other animal products but not animal flesh, and some eat seafood but not beef, pork, or poultry.

Common reasons for such eating choices include concern for animal welfare, improving health, environmental concerns, natural approaches to wellness, food safety, and weight loss or maintenance. Generally, people who follow a balanced vegetarian diet weigh less and have better cholesterol levels, less constipation and diarrhea, and a lower risk of heart disease than do nonvegetarians. Some studies suggest that vegetarianism may also reduce the risk of some cancers, particularly colon cancer.[37]

With proper meal planning, vegetarianism provides a healthful alternative to a high-fat, high-calorie, meat-based diet. Eating a variety of healthful foods throughout the day helps to ensure proper nutrient intake. Purely vegan diets may be deficient in some important vitamins and minerals, though many foods are fortified with these nutrients, or vegans can obtain them from supplements. Pregnant women, older adults, sick people, and children who are vegans or vegetarians need to take special care to ensure that their diets are adequate. In all cases, seek advice from a health care professional if you have questions.

Do Vegetarians Need to Take Supplements?

Dietary supplements are products intended to supplement existing diets. Ingredients range from vitamins, minerals, and herbs to enzymes, amino acids, fatty acids, and organ tissues. Supplement sales have skyrocketed in the last few decades. The FDA does not evaluate the safety and efficacy of supplements prior to their marketing; it can take action to remove a supplement from the market only after it has been proved harmful.

But do you really need any dietary supplements? That's a matter of some debate. The Office of Dietary Supplements, part of the National Institutes of Health, states that some supplements may help ensure that you get adequate amounts of essential nutrients if you don't consume a variety of foods, as recommended in the *Dietary Guidelines for Americans*. However, dietary supplements are not intended to prevent or treat disease, and recently the U.S. Preventive Services Task Force concluded that there is insufficient evidence to recommend that healthy people take multivitamin/mineral supplements to prevent cardiovascular disease or cancer.[38]

Taking high-dose supplements of the fat-soluble vitamins A, D, and E can be harmful or even fatal. Too much vitamin A, for example, can damage the liver, and excessive vitamin E increases the risk for a stroke.[39] Though some people—including vegans—benefit from taking supplements, The Academy of Nutrition and Dietetics recommends that a healthy diet is the best way to give your body what it needs.[40]

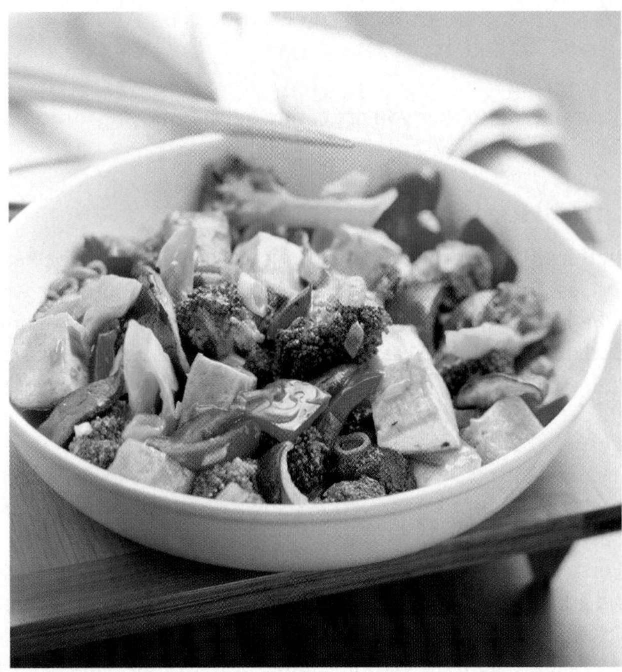

Are vegetarian diets healthy?

Adopting a vegan or vegetarian diet can be a very healthy way to eat. Take care to prepare your food healthfully by limiting the use of oils and avoiding added sugars and sodium. Make sure you get all the essential amino acids by eating meals like this tofu and vegetable stir fry. To further enhance it, add a whole grain such as brown rice.

check yourself

- **What are some of the benefits and drawbacks of a vegetarian diet?**
- **Should vegetarians supplement their diet in any way?**

Is Organic for You?

learning outcome

8.12 Explain the nature of organic foods.

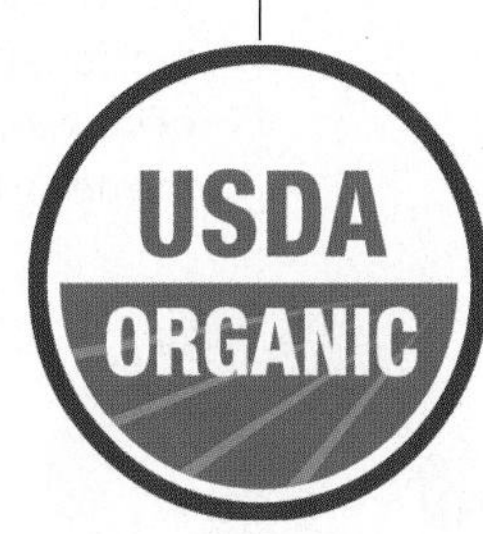

USDA label for certified organic foods.

Concerns about food safety, genetically modified foods, and the health impacts of chemicals used in the growth and production of food have led many people to turn to foods that are **organic**—foods and beverages developed, grown, or raised without the use of synthetic pesticides, chemicals, or hormones. Any food sold in the United States as organic has to meet criteria set by the USDA under the National Organic Rule and can carry a USDA seal verifying products as "certified organic."

Under the National Organic Rule, a product that is certified may carry one of the following terms: "100 percent Organic" (100% compliance with organic criteria), "Organic" (must contain at least 95% organic materials), "Made with Organic Ingredients" (must contain at least 70% organic ingredients), or "Some Organic Ingredients" (contains less than 70% organic ingredients—usually listed individually). Products that are labeled "all natural," "free-range," or "hormone free" are not necessarily organic. To be labeled with any of the above "organic" terms, the foods must be produced without hormones, antibiotics, herbicides, insecticides, chemical fertilizers, genetic modification, or germ-killing radiation. However, reliable monitoring systems to ensure credibility are still under development.

The market for organic foods has been increasing faster than food sales in general for many years. Whereas only a small subset of the population once bought organic, 81 percent of all U.S. families are now buying organic foods at least occasionally.[41] In 2010, annual organic food sales were estimated to be $31 billion.[42] Common reasons why people chose to buy organic include preferring the taste and wanting to limit exposure to pesticides and food additives. Some people purchase organics because of environmental concerns, since organic farming limits pesticide use and takes other measures to reduce pollution. One drawback is that organic foods are often more expensive than conventional foods, due in part to the higher costs associated with these organic farming practices.[43]

Is buying organic better for you? That all depends on what aspect of the food is being studied, and how the research is conducted. Two recent review studies, both of which examined decades of research into the nutrient quality of organic versus traditionally grown foods, reached opposite conclusions: One found organic foods more nutritious, and the other did not.[44] However, we do know that pesticide residues remain on conventionally grown produce. The U.S. Environmental Protection Agency warns that food pesticides can lead to health problems like cancer, nerve damage, and birth defects.[45] In 2013, the USDA reported that 3.7 percent of food samples harvested in 2011 had pesticide residues that exceeded the established tolerance level or for which no tolerance level has been established.[46] Both agencies advise consumers to wash fruits and vegetables before cooking or consuming them.

The word **locavore** has been coined to describe people who eat only food grown or produced locally, usually within close proximity to their homes. Farmers' markets or homegrown foods or those grown by independent farmers are thought to be fresher and to require far fewer resources to get them to market and keep them fresh for longer periods of time. Locavores believe that locally grown organic food is preferable to foods produced by large corporations or supermarket-based organic foods because they have a smaller impact on the environment and are believed to retain more of their nutritive value. Although there are many reasons organic farming is better for the environment, the fact that pesticides, herbicides, and other products are not used is perhaps the greatest benefit.

See It! Videos

Is organic produce better for you? Watch **Organic Produce** in the Study Area of MasteringHealth.

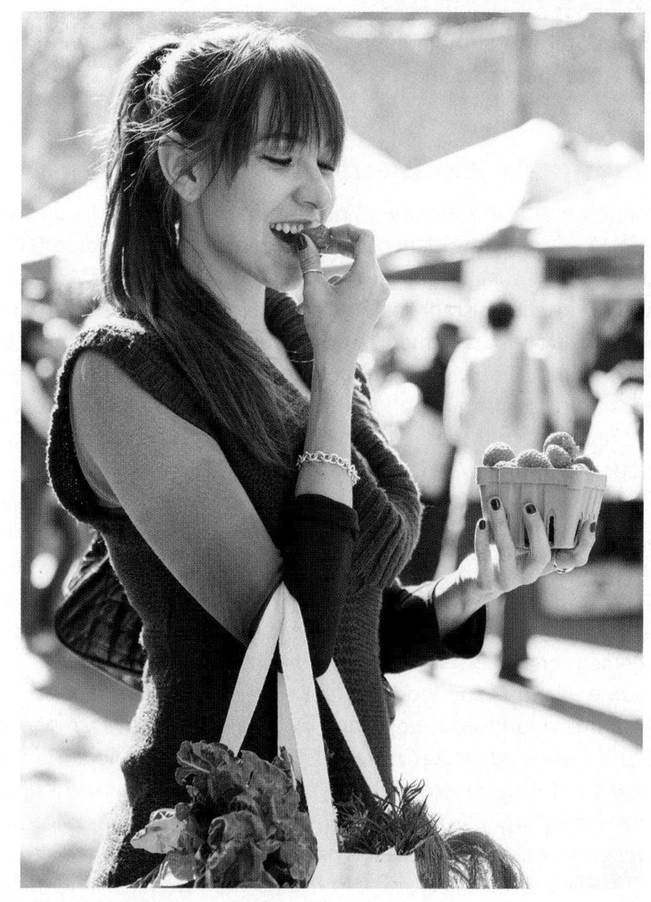

check yourself

- **What are organic foods?**
- **What are your reasons for buying or for not buying organic foods?**

8.13

Food Technology

learning outcome

8.13 **Identify technologies being used in food production today.**

Food Irradiation

Food irradiation involves exposing foods to low doses of radiation, or ionizing energy, which breaks chemical bonds in the DNA of harmful bacteria, destroying them or keeping them from reproducing. Essentially, the rays pass through the food without leaving any radioactive residue.[47]

Irradiation lengthens food products' shelf life and prevents spread of deadly microorganisms, particularly in high-risk foods such as ground beef and pork. Use of food irradiation is limited because of consumer concerns about safety and because irradiation facilities are expensive to build. Still, food irradiation is now common in over 40 countries. Irradiated foods are marked with the "radura" logo.

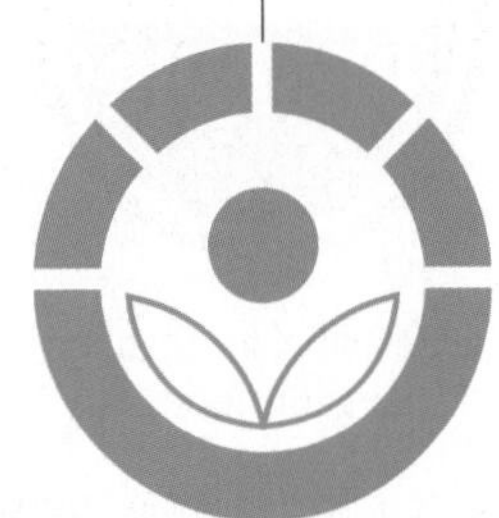

U.S. FDA label for irradiated foods.

Genetically Modified Food Crops

Genetic modification involves insertion or deletion of genes into the DNA of an organism. In the case of **genetically modified (GM) foods**, this is usually done to enhance production by making disease- or insect-resistant plants, improving yield, or controlling weeds. GM foods are sometimes created to improve foods' appearance or enhance nutrients; GM technology has been used to create rice containing vitamin A and iron, designed to help reduce disease in developing countries. Another use under development is the production and delivery of vaccines through GM foods.

The first genetically modified food crop was the FlavrSavr tomato, developed in 1996 to ripen without getting soft, increasing shipping capacity and shelf life. Since then, U.S. farmers have widely accepted GM crops.[48] Soybeans and cotton are the most common GM crops, followed by corn. On supermarket shelves, an estimated 75 percent of processed foods are genetically modified.[49]

Some scientists and food producers believe that GM crops could help address worldwide hunger and malnutrition, but many researchers and health advocates believe GM foods carry serious risks to humans and the ecosystem. Others are concerned about seeds being controlled by large corporations, while organic farmers are concerned about genetically modified seeds drifting into their fields.

The long-term safety of GM foods—for humans and other species—is still in question. Although the genetic engineering of insect-resistant crops has reduced the use of insecticides, it has simultaneously increased the use of herbicides (which kill weeds). This has not only led to the evolution of so-called "superweeds," but has also killed off beneficial weeds such as milkweed.[50] As a result, butterfly populations that depend on these weeds, particularly the monarch butterfly, have been decimated.[51] In addition, unintentional transfer of potentially allergy-provoking proteins has occurred, and although rigorous, validated tests of crops are performed to screen for known allergens, there is a potential for the transfer of new, unknown allergens.[52] However, the American Association for the Advancement of Science reports that foods containing genetically modified (GM) ingredients are no more a risk than are the same foods composed of crops modified over time with conventional plant breeding techniques, and the World Health Organization states that no adverse effects on human health have been shown from consumption of GM foods in countries that have approved their use.[53] Thus, the debate surrounding the risks and benefits of GM foods is not likely to end soon.

Arguments for the Development of GM Foods

- People have been manipulating food crops through selective breeding since the beginning of agriculture.
- Genetically modified seeds and products are tested for safety, and there has never been a substantiated claim for human illness resulting from their consumption.
- Insect- and weed-resistant GM crops allow farmers to use fewer chemical insecticides and herbicides.
- GM crops can be created to grow more quickly than conventional crops, increasing food yield. Nutrient-enhanced crops can address malnutrition.

Arguments against the Development of GM Foods

- Genetic modification is fundamentally different from and more problematic than selective breeding.
- There haven't been enough independent studies of GM products to confirm their safety. There are potential health risks if GM products approved for other uses are mistakenly or inadvertently used in production of food for human consumption.
- Inadvertent cross-pollination leads to "superweeds." Insect-resistant crops harm insect species that are not pests, and insect- and disease-resistant crops prompt evolution of even more virulent species, which then require aggressive control measures.
- Because corporations create and patent GM seeds, they control the market, forcing farmers worldwide to become reliant on these corporations.

check yourself

- **What are two technologies being used in our food?**
- **Are you more or less likely to buy foods that have been modified or irradiated? Why?**

Food Allergies and Intolerances

learning outcome

8.14 Define food allergies and intolerances.

About 33 percent of people today *think* they have a food allergy; however, it is estimated that only 5 percent of children and 4 percent of adults actually do.[54] Still, the prevalence of reported food allergies is on the rise. Data suggest the prevalence of peanut allergies among children tripled between 1997 and 2008.[55]

Food Allergies

A **food allergy**, or hypersensitivity, is an abnormal response to a food that is triggered by the immune system. Symptoms of an allergic reaction vary in severity and may include a tingling sensation in the mouth; swelling of the lips, tongue, and throat; difficulty breathing; hives; vomiting; abdominal cramps; diarrhea; drop in blood pressure; loss of consciousness; and death. Approximately 100 to 200 deaths per year occur from the *anaphylaxis* (the acute systemic immune and inflammatory response) that occurs with allergic reactions. These symptoms may appear within seconds to hours after eating the foods to which one is allergic.[56]

The Food Allergen Labeling and Consumer Protection Act (FALCPA) requires food manufacturers to label foods clearly to indicate the presence of (or possible contamination by) any of the eight major food allergens: milk, eggs, peanuts, wheat, soy, tree nuts (walnuts, pecans, etc.), fish, and shellfish. Although over 160 foods have been identified as allergy triggers, these 8 foods account for 90 percent of all food allergies in the United States.[57]

If you suspect that you have an actual allergic reaction to food, see an allergist to be tested to determine the source of the problem. Because there are several diseases that share symptoms with food allergies (ulcers and cancers of the gastrointestinal tract can cause vomiting, bloating, diarrhea, nausea, and pain), you should have persistent symptoms checked out as soon as possible. If particular foods seem to bother you consistently, look for alternatives or modify your diet. In true allergic instances, you may not be able to consume even the smallest amount of a substance safely.

Food Intolerance

In contrast to allergies, **food intolerance** can cause symptoms of gastric upset, but the upset is not the result of an immune system response. Probably the best example of a food intolerance is *lactose intolerance,* a problem that affects about 1 in every 10 adults. Lactase is an enzyme in the lining of the gut that degrades lactose, which is in dairy products. If you don't have enough lactase, you cannot digest lactose, and it remains in the gut to be used by bacteria. Gas is formed, causing bloating, abdominal pain, and sometimes diarrhea. Americans of European descent typically have rates of lactose intolerance as low as 2 to 3 percent, whereas 24 percent or more of minority populations are lactose intolerant.[58] Food intolerance also occurs in response to some food additives, such as the flavor enhancer MSG, certain dyes, sulfites, gluten, and other substances. In some cases, the food intolerance may have psychological triggers.

Celiac Disease

Celiac disease is an immune disorder that causes malabsorption of nutrients from the small intestine in genetically susceptible people. It is thought to affect over 2 million Americans, most of whom are undiagnosed.[59] When a person with celiac disease consumes gluten, a protein found in wheat, rye, and barley, the person's immune system attacks the small intestine and stops nutrient absorption. Pain, cramping, and other symptoms often follow in the short term. Untreated, celiac disease can lead to other health problems, such as osteoporosis, nutritional deficiencies, and cancer. Individuals diagnosed with celiac disease are encouraged to consult a dietitian for help designing a gluten-free diet. If you suspect you have celiac disease, see a doctor. Blood tests looking for specific antibodies or a small intestine biopsy can help determine whether you have celiac disease or other GI issues.

For those who need to achieve a gluten-free diet, there are increasing numbers of products available. Specially formulated gluten-free breads, pasta, and cereal products can allow people with celiac disease to enjoy meals similar to those without the disease. Reading food labels is particularly important, because many foods that seem safe may have hidden sources of gluten. Bouillon cubes, cold cuts, and soups are three examples of processed foods that may contain wheat, barley, or rye.

Peanuts are among the eight most common food allergens.

check yourself

- **What causes food allergies and intolerances?**
- **What is the difference between a food allergy and an intolerance?**

8.15

Food Safety and Foodborne Illnesses

learning outcome

8.15 Provide examples of food safety concerns and tips for reducing exposure to unsafe food.

Eating unhealthy food is one thing. Eating food that has been contaminated with a pathogen, toxin, or other harmful substance is quite another. As outbreaks of foodborne illness (commonly called food poisoning) make the news, the food industry has come under fire. The Food Safety Modernization Act, passed into law in 2011, included new requirements for food processors to take actions to prevent contamination of foods. The act gave the FDA greater authority to inspect food-manufacturing facilities and to recall contaminated foods.[60]

Are you concerned that the chicken you are buying doesn't look pleasingly pink or that your "fresh" fish smells a little *too* fishy? You may have good reason to be worried. In increasing numbers, Americans are becoming sick from what they eat, and many of these illnesses are life threatening. Scientists estimate that foodborne illnesses sicken 1 in 6 Americans (over 48 million people) and cause some 128,000 hospitalizations and 3,000 deaths in the United States annually.[61] Although the incidence of infection with certain microbes has declined, current data from the U.S. Centers for Disease Control and Prevention (CDC) shows a lack of recent progress in reducing foodborne infections and highlights the need for improved prevention.[62]

Most foodborne infections and illnesses are caused by several common types of bacteria and viruses; the following are some of the most common:[63]

- **Norovirus.** Transmitted through contact with the vomit or stool of infected people, norovirus is the most common cause of foodborne illness in the United States annually. Washing hands and all kitchen surfaces can help prevent transmission.
- ***Salmonella.*** Commonly found in the intestines of birds, reptiles, and mammals, the species *Salmonella* can spread to humans through foods of animal origin. Infection is more likely in people with poor underlying health or weakened immune systems.
- ***Clostridium perfringens.*** This is a bacterial species found in the intestinal tracts of humans and animals.
- ***Campylobacter.*** Most raw poultry has *Campylobacter* in it; bacterial infection most frequently results from eating undercooked chicken, raw eggs, or foods contaminated with juices from raw chicken. Shellfish and unpasteurized milk are also sources.
- ***Staphylococcus aureus.*** *Staph* lives on human skin, in infected cuts, and in the nose and throat.

Foodborne illnesses can also be caused by a toxin in food originally produced by a bacterium or other microbe in the food. These toxins can produce illness even if the microbes that produced them are no longer there. For example, botulism is caused by a deadly neurotoxin produced by the bacterium *Clostridium botulinum*. This bacterium is widespread in soil, water, plants, and intestinal tracts, but it can grow only in environments with limited or no oxygen. Potential food sources include improperly canned food and vacuum-packed or tightly wrapped foods. Though rare, botulism is fatal if untreated.

Signs of foodborne illnesses vary tremendously and usually include one or several symptoms: diarrhea, nausea, cramping, and vomiting. Depending on the amount and virulence of the pathogen, symptoms may appear as early as 30 minutes after eating contaminated food or as long as several days or weeks later. Most of the time, symptoms occur 5 to 8 hours after eating and last only a day or two. For certain populations, such as the very

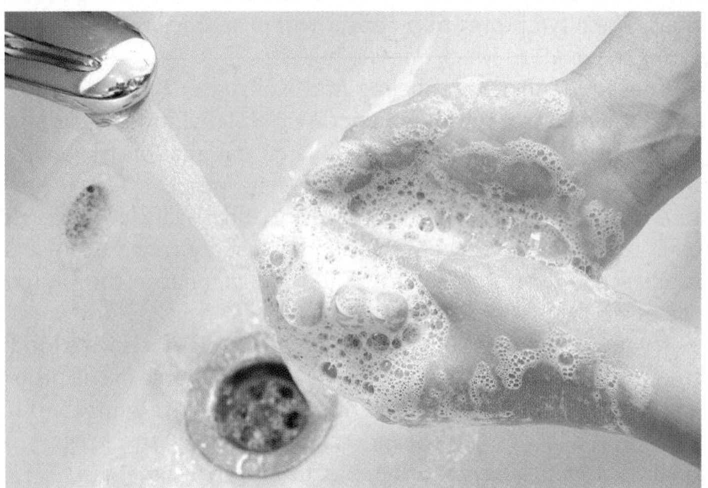

88% percent of college students said they understood the importance of hand washing in preventing foodborne illness. Yet only 49 percent of those surveyed actually washed their hands always or most of the time before meals.

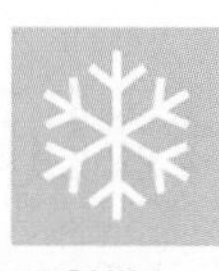

Figure 8.9 Education's Fight BAC!
This logo reminds consumers how to prevent foodborne illness.
Source: Partnership for Food Safety and Education, www.fightbac.org.

young; older adults; or people with severe illnesses such as cancer, diabetes, kidney disease, or AIDS, foodborne diseases can be fatal.

Several factors contribute to foodborne illnesses. Since fresh foods are not in season much of the year, the United States imports $18 billion in fresh fruits and vegetables from other countries, often from great distances. These countries include Mexico (36% of imports), several Central and South American countries (about 25%), and China (8%).[64] Although we are told when we travel to developing countries to "boil it, peel it, or don't eat it," we bring these foods into our kitchens at home and eat them, often without even washing them.

Food can become contaminated by being watered with tainted water, fertilized with animal manure, or harvested by people who have not washed their hands properly after using the toilet. Food-processing equipment, facilities, or workers may contaminate food, or it can become contaminated if not kept clean and cool during transport or on store shelves. To give you an idea of the implications, studies have shown that the bacterium *Escherichia coli* can survive in cow manure for up to 70 days and can multiply in foods grown with manure unless heat or additives such as salt or preservatives are used to kill the microbes.[65] No regulations prohibit farmers from using animal manure to fertilize crops. In addition, *E. coli* actually increases in summer months as factory-farmed cows await slaughter in crowded, overheated pens. This increases the chances of meat coming to market already contaminated.

Other key factors associated with the increasing spread of foodborne diseases include the inadvertent introduction of pathogens into new geographic regions and insufficient education about food safety. Globalization of the food supply, climate change, and global warming are also factors that may influence increasing spread.

Avoiding Risks in the Home

Part of the responsibility for preventing foodborne illness lies with consumers—more than 30 percent of all such illnesses result from unsafe handling of food at home. Fortunately, consumers can take several steps to reduce the likelihood of contaminating their food (see Figure 8.9). Among the most basic precautions is to wash your hands and wash all produce before eating it. Also, avoid cross-contamination in the kitchen by using separate cutting boards and utensils for meats and produce.

Temperature control is also important—refrigerators must be set at 40 degrees or less. Be sure to cook meats to the recommended temperature to kill contaminants before eating. Hot foods must be kept hot and cold foods kept cold in order to avoid unchecked bacterial growth. Eat leftovers within 3 days; if you're unsure how long something has been sitting in the fridge, don't take chances. When in doubt, throw it out. See Skills for Behavior Change for more tips about reducing risk of foodborne illness when shopping for and preparing food.

Skills for Behavior Change

REDUCE YOUR RISK FOR FOODBORNE ILLNESS

- **When shopping, put perishable foods in your cart last. Check for cleanliness throughout the store, especially at the salad bar and at the meat and fish counters. Never buy dented cans of food. Check the "sell by" or "use by" date on foods.**
- **Once you get home, put dairy products, eggs, meat, fish, and poultry in the refrigerator immediately. If you don't plan to eat meats within 2 days, freeze them. You can keep an unopened package of hot dogs or luncheon meats for about 2 weeks.**
- **When refrigerating or freezing raw meats, make sure their juices can't spill onto other foods.**
- **Never thaw frozen foods at room temperature. Put them in the refrigerator to thaw or thaw in the microwave, following manufacturer's instructions.**
- **Wash your hands with soap and warm water before preparing food. Wash fruits and vegetables before peeling, slicing, cooking, or eating them—but not meat, poultry, or eggs! Wash cutting boards, countertops, and other utensils and surfaces with detergent and hot water after food preparation.**
- **Use a meat thermometer to ensure that meats are completely cooked. To find out proper cooking temperatures for different types of meat, visit http://foodsafety.gov.**
- **Refrigeration slows the secretion of bacterial toxins into foods. Never leave leftovers out for more than 2 hours. On hot days, don't leave foods out for longer than 1 hour.**

check yourself

- **What are some current food safety concerns?**
- **Have you ever experienced a foodborne illness? If so, what were possible causes and how could you have avoided it?**

8.16

How Healthy Are Your Eating Habits?

An interactive version of this assessment is available online in MasteringHealth.

1 Keep Track of Your Food Intake

Keep a food diary for 5 days, writing down everything you eat or drink. Be sure to include the approximate amount or portion size. Add up the number of servings from each of the major food groups on each day and enter them into the chart below.

Number of Servings of:						
	Day 1	Day 2	Day 3	Day 4	Day 5	Average
Fruits						
Vegetables						
Grains						
Protein foods						
Dairy						
Fats and oils						
Sweets						

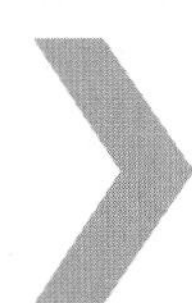

2A Does Your Diet Have Proportionality?

	Yes	No
1. Are grains the main food choice at all your meals?	○	○
2. Do you often forget to eat vegetables?	○	○
3. Do you typically eat fewer than three pieces of fruit daily?	○	○
4. Do you often have fewer than 3 cups of milk daily?	○	○
5. Is the portion of meat, chicken, or fish the largest item on your dinner plate?	○	○

Scoring 2A

If you answered yes to three or more of these questions, your diet probably lacks proportionality. Review the recommendations in this chapter, particularly the MyPlate guidelines, to learn how to balance your diet.

2 Evaluate Your Food Intake

Now compare your consumption patterns to the MyPlate recommendations. Visit www.choosemyplate.gov to evaluate your daily caloric needs and the recommended consumption rates for the different food groups. How does your diet match up?

	Less than the recommended amount	About equal to the recommended amount	More than the recommended amount
1. How does your daily fruit consumption compare to the recommendation for your age and activity level?	○	○	○
2. How does your daily vegetable consumption compare to the recommendation for your age and activity level?	○	○	○
3. How does your daily grain consumption compare to the recommendation for your age and activity level?	○	○	○
4. How does your daily protein food consumption compare to the recommendation for your age and activity level?	○	○	○
5. How does your daily fats and oils consumption compare to the recommendation for your age and activity level?	○	○	○

Scoring

If you found that your food intake is consistent with the MyPlate recommendations, congratulations! If, however, you are falling short in a major food group or overdoing it in certain categories, consider taking steps described in this chapter to adopt healthier eating habits.

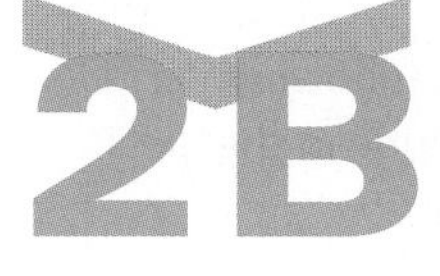

Are You Getting Enough Fat-Soluble Vitamins in Your Diet?

	Yes	No
1. Do you eat at least 1 cup of deep yellow or orange vegetables, such as carrots and sweet potatoes, or dark green vegetables, such as spinach, every day?	◯	◯
2. Do you consume at least two glasses (8 ounces each) of milk daily?	◯	◯
3. Do you eat a tablespoon of vegetable oil, such as corn or olive oil, daily? (Tip: Salad dressings, unless they are fat free, count.)	◯	◯
4. Do you eat at least 1 cup of leafy green vegetables in your salad and/or put lettuce in your sandwich every day?	◯	◯

Scoring 2B

If you answered yes to all four questions, you are on your way to acing your fat-soluble vitamin needs! If you answered no to any of the questions, your diet needs some fine-tuning. Deep orange and dark green vegetables are excellent sources of vitamin A, and milk is an excellent choice for vitamin D. Vegetable oils provide vitamin E; if you put them on top of your vitamin K–rich leafy green salad, you'll hit the vitamin jackpot.

2C Are You Getting Enough Water-Soluble Vitamins in Your Diet?

	Yes	No
1. Do you consume at least 1/2 cup of rice or pasta daily?	◯	◯
2. Do you eat at least 1 cup of a ready-to-eat cereal or hot cereal every day?	◯	◯
3. Do you have at least one slice of bread, a bagel, or a muffin daily?	◯	◯
4. Do you enjoy a citrus fruit or fruit juice, such as an orange, a grapefruit, or orange juice, every day?	◯	◯
5. Do you have at least 1 cup of vegetables throughout your day?	◯	◯

Scoring 2C

If you answered yes to all of these questions, you are a vitamin B and C superstar! If you answered no to any of the questions, your diet could use some refinement. Rice, pasta, cereals, bread, and bread products are all excellent sources of B vitamins. Citrus fruits are a ringer for vitamin C. In fact, all vegetables can contribute to meeting your vitamin C needs daily.

Source: Adapted from J. Blake, *Nutrition and You*, 2nd ed. (San Francisco, CA: Benjamin Cummings, 2011).

Your Plan for Change

The Assess Yourself activity gave you the chance to evaluate your current nutritional habits. Now that you have considered these results, you can decide whether you need to make changes in your daily eating for long-term health.

Today, you can:

◯ Start keeping a more detailed food log. The easy-to-use SuperTracker at www.supertracker.usda.gov can help you keep track of your food intake and analyze what you eat. Take note of the nutritional information of the various foods you eat and write down particulars about the number of calories, grams of fat, grams of sugar, milligrams of sodium, and so on of each food. Try to find specific weak spots: Are you consuming too many calories or too much salt or sugar? Do you eat too little calcium or iron? Use the SuperTracker to plan a healthier food intake to overcome these weak spots.

◯ Take a field trip to the grocery store. Forgo your fast-food dinner and instead spend some time in the produce section of the supermarket. Purchase your favorite fruits and vegetables, and try something new to expand your tastes.

Within the next 2 weeks, you can:

◯ Plan at least three meals that you can make at home or in your dorm room, and purchase the ingredients you'll need ahead of time. Something as simple as a chicken sandwich on whole-grain bread will be more nutritious, and probably cheaper, than heading out for a fast-food meal.

◯ Start reading labels. Be aware of the amount of calories, sodium, sugars, and fats in prepared foods; aim to buy and consume those that are lower in all of these and are higher in calcium and fiber.

By the end of the semester, you can:

◯ Get in the habit of eating a healthy breakfast every morning. Combine whole grains, proteins, and fruit in your breakfast—for example, eat a bowl of cereal with milk and bananas or a cup of yogurt combined with granola and berries. Eating a healthy breakfast will jump-start your metabolism, prevent drops in blood glucose levels, and keep your brain and body performing at their best through those morning classes.

◯ Commit to one or two healthful changes to your eating patterns for the rest of the semester. You might resolve to eat five servings of fruits and vegetables every day, to switch to low-fat or nonfat dairy products, to stop drinking soft drinks, or to use only olive oil in your cooking. Use your food diary to help you spot places where you can make healthier choices on a daily basis.

Summary

To hear an MP3 Tutor session, scan here or visit the Study Area in **MasteringHealth**.

LO 8.1 Recognizing that we eat for more reasons than just survival is the first step toward improving our nutritional habits.

LO 8.1–8.7 The essential nutrients include water, proteins, carbohydrates, fats, vitamins, and minerals. Water makes up 50 to 60 percent of our body weight and is necessary for nearly all life processes. Proteins are major components of our cells and are key elements of antibodies, enzymes, and hormones. Carbohydrates are our primary sources of energy. Fats play important roles in maintaining body temperature and cushioning and protecting organs. Vitamins are organic compounds, and minerals are inorganic compounds. We need both in relatively small amounts to maintain healthy body function. Functional foods may provide health benefits in addition to the nutrients they contribute to the diet.

LO 8.8 Food labels provide information on serving size and number of calories in a food, as well as the amounts of various nutrients and the percentage of recommended daily values those amounts represent.

LO 8.9 A healthful diet is adequate, moderate, balanced, varied, and nutrient dense. The *Dietary Guidelines for Americans* and the MyPlate food guidance system provide guidelines for healthy eating. These recommendations, developed by the USDA, place emphasis on balancing calories and making appropriate food choices.

LO 8.10 College students face unique challenges in eating healthfully. Learning to make better choices at restaurants, to eat healthfully on a budget, and to eat nutritionally in the dorm are all possible when you use the information in this chapter.

LO 8.11 Vegetarianism can provide a healthy alternative for people wishing to eat less or no meat.

LO 8.12 Organic foods are grown and produced without the use of synthetic pesticides, chemicals, or hormones. The USDA offers certification of organics. These foods have become increasingly available and popular, as people take a greater interest in eating healthfully and sustainably.

LO 8.11–8.15 Foodborne illnesses, food irradiation, allergies, food intolerances, GM foods, and other food safety and health concerns are becoming increasingly important to health-wise consumers. Recognizing potential risks and taking steps to prevent problems are part of a sound nutritional plan.

Pop Quiz

Visit MasteringHealth to personalize your study plan with Chapter Review Quizzes and Dynamic Study Modules.

LO 8.2 **1.** What is the most crucial nutrient for life?
- a. Water
- b. Fiber
- c. Minerals
- d. Protein

LO 8.2 **2.** Which of the following nutrients is required for the repair and growth of body tissue?
- a. Carbohydrates
- b. Proteins
- c. Vitamins
- d. Fats

LO 8.3 **3.** Which of the following nutrients moves food through the digestive tract?
- a. Water
- b. Fiber
- c. Minerals
- d. Starch

LO 8.4 **4.** What substance plays a vital role in maintaining healthy skin and hair, insulating body organs against shock, maintaining body temperature, and promoting healthy cell function?
- a. Fats
- b. Fibers
- c. Proteins
- d. Carbohydrates

LO 8.4 **5.** Triglycerides make up about ________ percent of total body fat.
- a. 5
- b. 35
- c. 55
- d. 95

LO 8.4 **6.** Which of the following is a healthier fat to include in the diet?
- a. *Trans* fat
- b. Saturated fat
- c. Unsaturated fat
- d. Hydrogenated fat

LO 8.5 **7.** Which vitamin maintains bone health?
- a. B_{12}
- b. D
- c. B_6
- d. Niacin

LO 8.6 **8.** Which of the following is a trace mineral?
- a. Calcium
- b. Sodium
- c. Potassium
- d. Iron

LO 8.9 **9.** Which of the following foods would be considered a healthy, *nutrient-dense* food?
- a. Nonfat milk
- b. Celery
- c. Soft drink
- d. Potato chips

LO 8.14 **10.** Lucas's doctor diagnoses him with celiac disease. Which of the following foods should Lucas cut out of his diet to eat gluten-free?
- a. Shellfish
- b. Eggs
- c. Peanuts
- d. Wheat

Answers to these questions can be found on page A-1. If you answered a question incorrectly, review the module identified by the Learning Outcome. For even more study tools, visit MasteringHealth.

Weight Management and Body Image

9

The keys to weight management sound simple enough: Eat too many calories without exercising and you will gain weight; reduce calories and increase exercise, and the pounds will slide right off. But if all it took were eating less and exercising more, Americans would merely reevaluate their diets, cut calories, and exercise. Unfortunately, it's not that easy. And the problem goes beyond body weight to increasingly common issues of self-perception and disordered eating, among both men and women.

What factors predispose us to problems with weight? Although diet and exercise are clearly major contributors, genetics and physiology are also important. Learned behaviors in the home and influences at school, in social environments, in the media, and in the environments where we live, work, and play are all important to our weight profiles.[1] Experts realize that a complex web of interactive factors influences what we eat, how much we eat, and when we eat, as well as how we expend energy. Figuring out what these factors are and developing key strategies to reduce risk are key.[2]

9.1 Obesity in the United States and Worldwide

learning outcome

9.1 Examine obesity trends in the United States.

The United States currently has the dubious distinction of being among the fattest nations on Earth. Young and old, rich and poor, rural and urban, educated and uneducated Americans share one thing in common—they are fatter than virtually all previous generations.[3]

The word **obesogenic**, meaning characterized by environments that promote increased food intake, nonhealthful foods, and physical inactivity, has increasingly become an apt descriptor of our society. The maps in Figure 9.1 illustrate the rapidly increasing levels of obesity in the United States over the last two decades. Indeed, the prevalence of obesity has tripled among children and doubled among adults in recent decades.[4] While previous research has shown some stabilization in overweight and obesity rates between 2003–2004 and 2011–2012, current rates are still extremely high. More than 68 percent of U.S. adults overall (over 170 million people) are *overweight* (have a body mass index [BMI] of 25.0–29.9) or obese (have a BMI of 30.0 or higher).[5] Rates of obesity are 34.4 percent among men and 36.1 among women, with rates of extreme obesity on the rise.[6] This has staggering implications for increased risks from heart disease, diabetes, and other health complications associated with obesity.

A bright spot in the obesity profile appears to be among the very youngest populations. Rates for 2- to 5-year-olds have dropped significantly, from a high of nearly 14 percent in 2003–2004 to just over 8 percent in 2011–2012.[7] Possible reasons for this include greater public awareness; more options for healthy foods in child care centers, restaurants, and grocery stores; improved labeling; improvements in physical activity programs; and decreases in sugar consumption.

Research points to higher obesity rates and risks among some ethnic groups. Mexican American men (81 percent) and non-Hispanic whites (73 percent) are more likely to be overweight/obese than non-Hispanic blacks (69 percent). Non-Hispanic black women (80 percent) and Mexican-American women (78 percent) are more likely to be overweight or obese than are non-Hispanic white women (60 percent). In sharp contrast, nearly 58 percent of Asian populations are at a healthy weight.[8] Of youth aged 2 to 19, over 39 percent of Hispanics, Mexican Americans, and non-Hispanic blacks, as well as nearly 28 percent of non-Hispanic whites, are overweight/obese. Low parental education, low-income, and higher unemployment are related to increased risk of overweight/obesity in youth.[9]

The United States is not alone in the obesity epidemic. In fact, overweight and obesity have become the fifth leading risks for global death, and nearly 1.5 billion adults aged 20 and over and 40 million children under the age of 5 are overweight/obese.[10] While obesity was once predominantly a problem in high-income countries, today, increasing numbers of low- and middle-income countries have overweight/obesity problems.[11] The global epidemic of high rates of overweight and obesity in multiple regions of the world has come to be known as **globesity**.

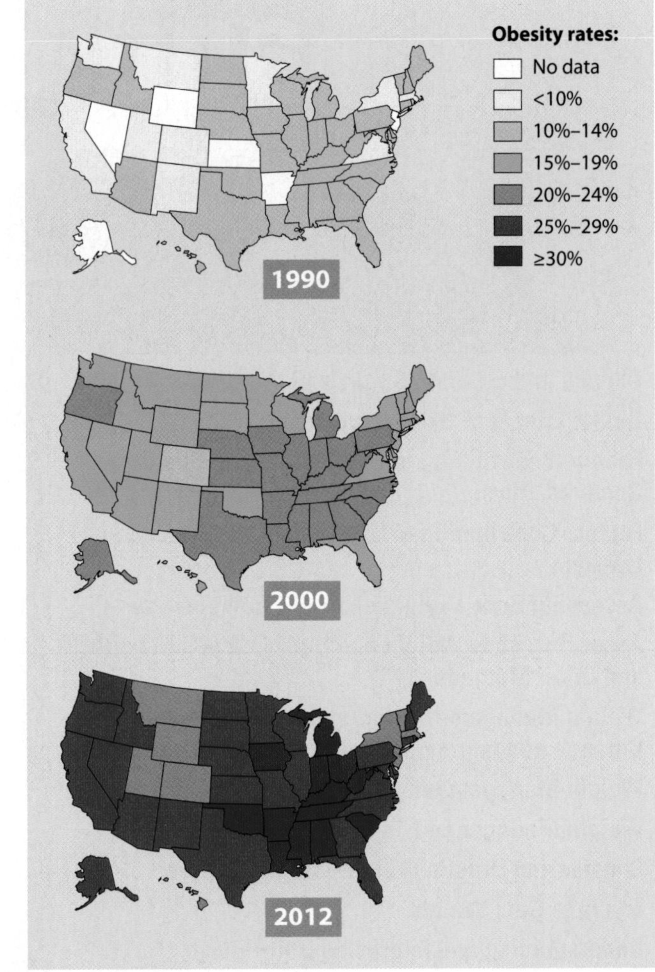

Figure 9.1 Obesity Trends among U.S. Adults, 1990, 2000, and 2012

Sources: Centers for Disease Control and Prevention (CDC), "U.S. Obesity Trends: 1999–2010," 2012, www.cdc.gov; CDC, "Prevalence of Self-Reported Obesity among U.S. Adults," 2013, www.cdc.gov.

Note: Historical maps are provided for reference only, as differences in the analysis of prevalence rates for 2012 make direct comparisons to previous years incompatible.

check yourself

- **How have levels of obesity changed in the United States over the last two decades?**
- **Why do you think disparities in obesity levels exist among certain populations in the United States?**

9.2 Health Effects of Overweight and Obesity

learning outcome

9.2 List health effects associated with overweight and obesity.

Although smoking is still the leading cause of preventable death in the United States, obesity is rapidly gaining ground on this killer as associated health problems soar. Cardiovascular disease (CVD), stroke, cancer, hypertension, diabetes, depression, digestive problems, gallstones, sleep apnea, osteoarthritis, and other ailments lead the list of life-threatening, weight-related problems. Diabetes, strongly associated with overweight and obesity, is another major concern. Nearly 26 million Americans have diabetes and another 79 million adults have prediabetes.[12] Figure 9.2 summarizes these and other potential health consequences of obesity.

Short- and long-term health consequences of obesity are not our only concern: According to new estimates, obesity accounts for nearly 21 percent of U.S. health care costs, more than double previous estimates. Morbidly obese individuals may cost between $6,500 and $15,000 more per year in additional health care costs when factors such as longer hospital stays, recovery, and increased medications are included.[13] Of course, it is impossible to place a dollar value on a life lost prematurely due to diabetes, stroke, or heart attack or to assess the cost of the social isolation of and discrimination against overweight individuals. Of growing importance is the recognition that obese individuals suffer significant disability during their lives, in terms of both mobility and activities of daily living.[14]

Other effects of overweight and obesity can be more subtle. Consequences can include depression, anxiety, low self-esteem, poor body image, and suicidal acts and thoughts; binge eating and unhealthy weight-control practices; lack of adequate health care due to doctors spending less time with and doing fewer interventions on overweight patients and doctor reluctance to perform preventive health screenings; and reluctance to visit the doctor and get necessary preventive health care services.

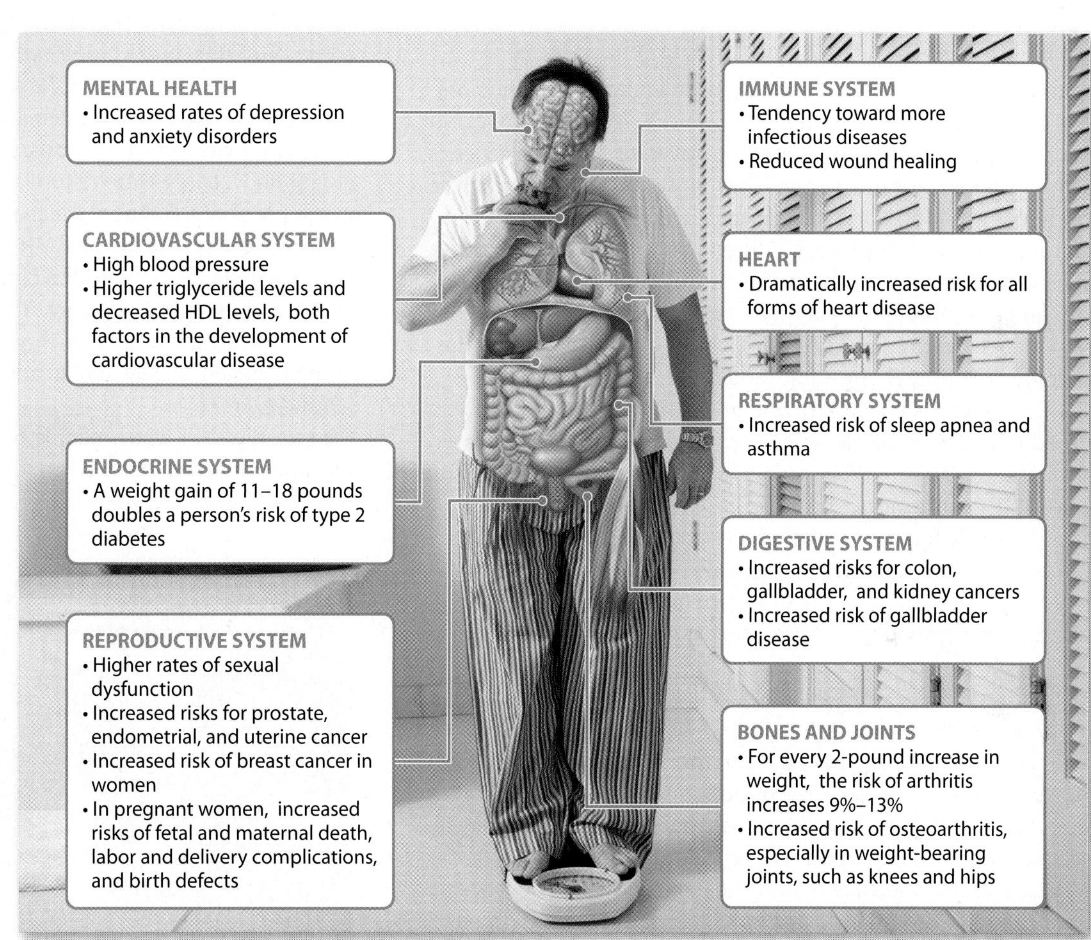

Figure 9.2 Potential Negative Health Effects of Overweight and Obesity

VIDEO TUTOR
Obesity Health Effects

check yourself

- **What are some potential effects on the body of overweight and obesity?**
- **Do you consider the most significant consequences of overweight and obesity to be physical, financial, emotional, or other?**

9.3 Factors Contributing to Overweight and Obesity: Genetics, Physiology, and the Environment

learning outcome

9.3 Explain the impact of genetics, physiology, and environment on body weight.

Several factors appear to influence why one person becomes obese and another remains thin.

Body Type and Genes

In spite of decades of research, the exact role of genes in one's predisposition toward obesity remains in question. We know that children whose parents are obese tend to be overweight. Both genetics and the gene–environment interaction are thought to play a role in body composition. One gene in particular, the *FTO gene*, may be among the most important.[15] Specifically, people with certain genetic variations may tend to graze for food more often, eat more meals, and consume more calories every day. Also, different genes may influence weight gain at certain periods of life, particularly during adolescence and young adulthood.[16]

So, if your genes play a key role in obesity tendencies, are you doomed to a lifelong battle with your weight? Probably not, based on exciting new research that points to the fact that even if obesity does run in your family, a healthy lifestyle can override "obesity" genes. The study found that the effects of the *FTO* gene on obesity are over 30 percent less among physically active adults. Those who seemed to be beating their obesity tendencies exercised at least 90 minutes a day compared to those who exercised 30 minutes.[17]

Thrifty Gene Theory Researchers have noted higher body fat and obesity levels in certain Indian and African tribes than in the general population.[18] The theory: Their ancestors struggled through centuries of famine and survived by adapting with slowed metabolism. If this "thrifty gene" hypothesis is true, certain people may be genetically programmed to burn fewer calories. Today, critics of this theory believe that there are many other factors, such as obesogenic behaviors and environments, that influence obesity development.

Physiological Factors

Metabolic Rates Although number of calories consumed is important, metabolism also helps determine weight. The **basal metabolic rate (BMR)** is the minimum rate at which the body uses energy when working to maintain basic vital functions. BMR for the average healthy adult is 1,200 to 1,800 calories per day.

The **resting metabolic rate (RMR)** includes the BMR plus any energy expended through daily sedentary activities such as food digestion, sitting, studying, or standing. The **exercise metabolic rate (EMR)** accounts for all remaining daily calorie expenditures. For most of us, these calories come from activities such as walking, climbing stairs, and mowing the lawn.

In general, the younger you are, the higher your BMR. Growth consumes a good deal of energy, and BMR is highest during infancy, puberty, and pregnancy. After age 30, a person's BMR slows down by 1 to 2 percent a year. Less activity, shifting priorities from fitness to family and career, and loss in muscle mass also contribute to weight gain in many middle-aged people.

Theories abound concerning mechanisms regulating metabolism and food intake. Some sources indicate that the hypothalamus (the part of the brain that regulates appetite) closely monitors levels of certain nutrients in the blood; when they fall, the brain signals us to eat. According to one theory, the monitoring system in obese people makes cues to eat more frequent and intense than in others. Another theory, **adaptive thermogenesis**, suggests the brain slows metabolic activity and energy expenditure as a form of defensive protection against possible starvation, which makes weight loss difficult.[19]

On the other side of the BMR equation is the **set point theory**, which suggests that our bodies fight to maintain our weight around a narrow range or at a set point. If we go on a drastic diet, our bodies slow our BMR to conserve energy. The good news is that set points can be changed, slowly and steadily, via healthy diet, steady weight loss, and exercise.

Yo-yo diets, in which people repeatedly gain weight then lose it quickly, are doomed to fail. When such dieters resume eating, their BMR

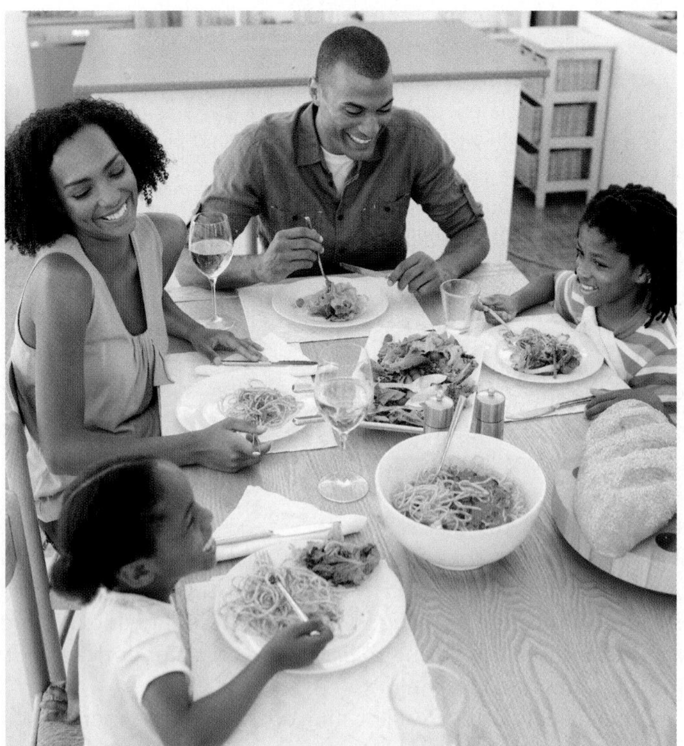

Do my genes affect my weight?
Many factors help determine weight and body type, including heredity and genetic makeup, environment, and learned eating patterns, which are often connected to family habits.

is set lower, making them almost certain to regain lost pounds. After repeated gains and losses, such people find it increasingly hard to lose weight and easy to regain it.

Hormonal Influences: Ghrelin and Leptin Obese people may be more likely than thin people to eat for reasons other than nutrition.[20] Many people have attributed obesity to problems with the thyroid gland and resultant hormone imbalances that impede the ability to burn calories. Although less than 2 percent of the obese population have a thyroid problem and can trace their weight problems to a metabolic or hormone imbalance,[21] hormones may still affect one's weight.

Problems with overconsumption may be related to **satiety**—the feeling of fullness when nutritional needs are satisfied and the stomach signals "no more." Researchers suspect that *ghrelin*, sometimes referred to as "the hunger hormone," influences satiety.[22] Ghrelin helps regulate appetite, food intake control, gastrointestinal motility, gastric acid secretion, endocrine and exocrine pancreatic secretions, glucose and lipid metabolism, and cardiovascular and immunological processes.[23] Another hormone, *leptin*, is produced by fat cells; its levels in the blood increase as fat tissue increases. Scientists believe leptin signals when you are getting full, slows food intake, and promotes energy expenditure.[24] When levels of leptin in the blood rise, appetite levels drop. Although obese people have adequate leptin and leptin receptors, the receptors do not seem to work properly—though why remains a mystery. It may be simply that environmental cues are stronger than our hunger pangs.

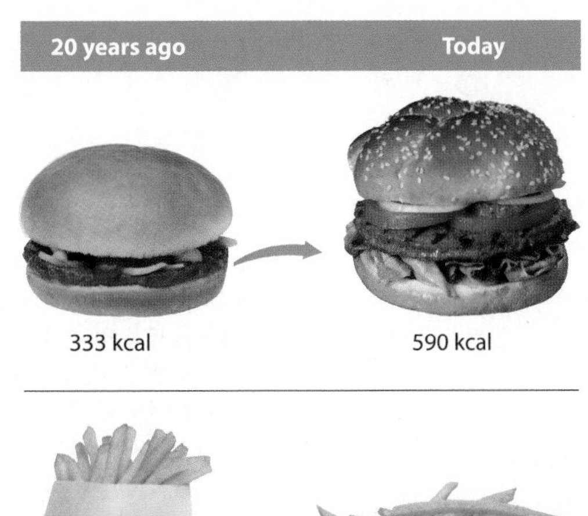

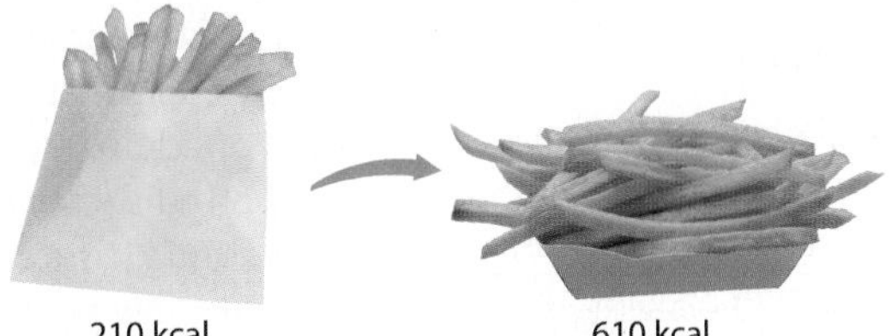

Figure 9.3 Today's Bloated Portions
The increase in average portion sizes has made it tougher than ever to manage your weight.
Source: Data are from the National Institutes of Health/National Heart, Lung, and Blood Institute (NHLBI), "Portion Distortion!," Updated February 2013, www.nhlbi.nih.gov.

Fat Cells and Predisposition to Fatness Some obese people may have excessive numbers of fat cells. An average-weight adult has approximately 25 to 35 billion fat cells, a moderately obese adult 60 to 100 billion, and an extremely obese adult as many as 200 billion.[25] This type of obesity, **hyperplasia**, usually appears in early childhood and perhaps, due to the mother's dietary habits, even prior to birth. Critical periods for development of hyperplasia are the last 2 to 3 months of fetal development, the first year of life, and from ages 9 to 13. Central to this theory is the belief that the number of fat cells in a body does not increase appreciably during adulthood. However, the ability of each cell to swell (**hypertrophy**) and shrink does carry over into adulthood. Weight gain may be tied to both the number of fat cells and the capacity of individual cells to enlarge.

Environmental Factors

Automobiles, remote controls, desk jobs, and computer use all lead us to sit more and move less; our culture also urges us to eat more. Combined, these environmental influences are a clear recipe for weight gain.

- We are bombarded with advertising for high-calorie foods at a low price and marketing of super-sized portions. Standard portions have increased dramatically in the past 20 years (Figure 9.3).
- Access to prepackaged, high-fat meals; fast food; and sugar-laden soft drinks are increasingly widespread, as are high-calorie coffee drinks and energy drinks.
- As society eats out more, higher-calorie, high-fat foods become the norm.
- Bottle-feeding infants may increase energy intake relative to breast-feeding.
- Misleading food labels confuse consumers about portion and serving sizes.

A Youthful Start on Obesity Children have always loved junk food. However, today's youth have easy access to a vast array of high-fat, high-calorie foods, have fewer physical education requirements in schools, and are more obese than ever before. Maternal nutrition, diabetes, and obesity may predispose children to overweight or obesity prior to puberty and early onset puberty.[26] Race and ethnicity also seem to be intricately interwoven with environmental factors in increasing risks to young people.[27]

Skills for Behavior Change

BEWARE OF PORTION DISTORTION

To make sure you're not overeating when you dine out, follow these strategies:

- **Order the smallest size available. Focus on taste, not quantity.**
- **Take your time, and let your fullness indicator have a chance to kick in while there is still time to quit.**
- **Dip your food in dressings, gravies, and sauces on the side rather than pour extra calories over the top.**
- **Order a healthy appetizer as your main meal along with a small side salad or veggie side.**
- **Split an entrée with a friend. Alternately, put half of your meal in a take-out box immediately, and finish the rest at the restaurant.**
- **Avoid buffets and all-you-can-eat establishments. If you go to them, use small plates and fill them with salads, veggies, and other high-protein, low-calorie, low-fat options.**

check yourself

- **What are the influences of genetics, physiology, and environment on body weight? Which do you consider most important?**
- **How does the importance of genetics and physiology affect strategies for weight management?**

9.4 Factors Contributing to Overweight and Obesity: Lifestyle

learning outcome

9.4 Explain the impact of psychosocial, economic, and lifestyle factors on body weight.

Psychosocial and Economic Factors

The relationship of weight problems to emotional needs and wants remains uncertain. Food often is used as a reward for good behavior in childhood. For adults facing economic and interpersonal stress, the bright spot in the day is often "what's for dinner." Again, the research here is controversial. What is certain is that eating is a social ritual associated with companionship, celebration, and enjoyment.

Socioeconomic factors can also affect weight control. When economic times are tough, people tend to eat more inexpensive, high-calorie processed foods. People living in poverty may have less access to fresh, nutrient-dense foods and have less time to cook nutritious meals due to shiftwork, longer commutes, or multiple jobs.[28] Unsafe neighborhoods and lack of recreational areas may make it difficult for less affluent people to exercise.[29]

Lifestyle Factors

Of all the factors affecting obesity, perhaps the most critical is the relationship between activity level and calorie intake. Determining activity levels using surveys, however, is difficult. One big problem in that people surveyed overestimate their daily exercise level and intensity. It is also difficult to determine which measures of fitness were actually used and how indicative of overall health these may ultimately be. Defining yourself as "active" can mean very different things for different people. According to data from the 2012 Health Interview Survey, 30 percent of adults reported being inactive, 20 percent of adults reported being insufficiently active, and 50 percent reported sufficient levels of activity—mostly through physical activity during leisure time.[30]

Do you know people who seemingly can eat whatever they want without gaining weight? With few exceptions, if you were to monitor the level and intensity of their activity, you would discover why. Even if their schedule does not include intense exercise, it probably includes a high level of activity.

Rather than focusing only on how much formal exercise we get in each day, health and fitness experts have begun to focus on how much time we spend sitting. If the body isn't moving, it's not burning many calories. Research indicates a dose-response association between sitting time and mortality from all causes and from cardiovascular disease, independent of leisure-time activity; that is, the more time you spend sitting, the worse your health is likely to be, regardless of whether you exercise or not. Because muscle activity burns energy, passive sitting is one of the worst things you can do if you are trying to burn calories. If you stood up while reading this chapter, the large and small muscle groups in your legs would be constantly working to keep you from falling over—and burning more calories. These little extra bouts of movement may make a big difference in daily calories burned, weight management, and overall health.

U.S. adults get

11.3 percent

of total daily calories from fast foods.

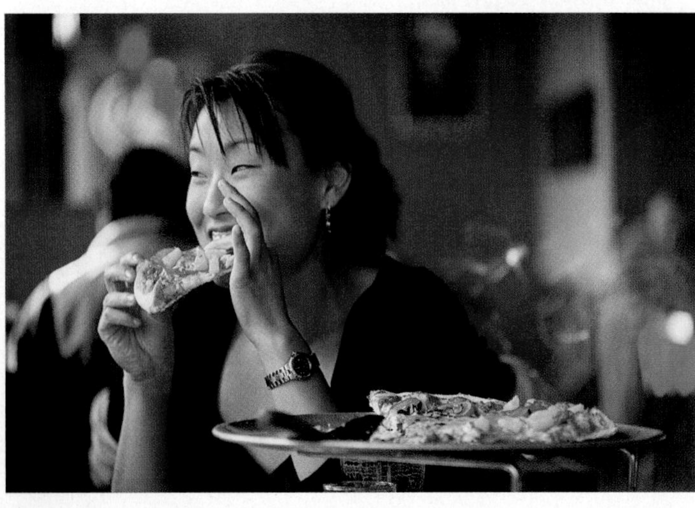

Skills for Behavior Change

FINDING THE FUN IN HEALTHY EATING AND EXERCISE

With a little creativity, you can make weight management a fun, positive part of your life. Try these tips:

- **Cook and eat with friends. Share the responsibility for making the meal while you spend time with people you like.**
- **Experiment with new foods to add variety to your meals.**
- **Vary your exercise routine. Change the exercise or your location, join a team for the social aspects in addition to exercise, decide to run a race for the challenge, or learn how to skateboard for fun.**

check yourself

- **What are some lifestyles changes that can contribute to weight management?**

Assessing Body Weight and Body Composition

learning outcome

9.5 Distinguish among overweight, obesity, and underweight.

Everyone has his or her own ideal weight, based on individual variables such as body structure, height, and fat distribution. Traditionally, experts used measurement techniques such as height-weight charts to determine whether an individual fell into the ideal weight, overweight, or obese category. However, these charts can be misleading because they don't take body composition (a person's ratio of fat to lean muscle) or fat distribution into account.

In fact, weight can be a deceptive indicator. Many a muscular athlete or a middle-aged adult who brags about weighing the same as in high school may be shocked to find out that he or she has relatively high fat levels based on BMI. More accurate measures of evaluating healthy weight and disease risk focus on a person's percentage of body fat and how that fat is distributed in his or her body.

Many people worry about becoming fat, but some fat is essential for healthy body functioning. Fat regulates body temperature, cushions and insulates organs and tissues, and is the body's main source of stored energy. Body fat is composed of two types of fat: essential and storage. *Essential fat* is the fat necessary for maintenance of life and reproductive functions. *Storage fat*, the nonessential fat that many of us try to shed, makes up the remainder of our fat reserves.

Overweight and Obesity

In general, **overweight** is increased body weight due to excess fat that exceeds healthy recommendations, whereas **obesity** refers to body weight that greatly exceeds health recommendations. Traditionally, *overweight* was defined as being 1 to 19 percent above one's ideal weight, based on a standard height-weight chart, and *obesity* was defined as being 20 percent or more above one's ideal weight. **Morbidly obese** people are 100 percent or more above their ideal weight. Experts now usually define *overweight* and *obesity* in terms of BMI, a measure discussed later, or percentage of body fat, as determined by some of the methods we'll discuss shortly. Although opinion varies somewhat, most experts agree that men's bodies should contain between 8 and 20 percent total body fat, and women should be within the range of 20 to 30 percent. At various ages and stages of life, these ranges also vary, but generally, men who exceed 22 percent body fat and women who exceed 35 percent are considered overweight (see Table 9.1).

Underweight

Men with only 3 to 7 percent body fat and women with approximately 8 to 15 percent are considered **underweight**, which can seriously compromise health. Extremely low body fat can cause hair loss, visual disturbances, skin problems, a tendency to fracture bones easily, digestive system disturbances, heart irregularities, gastrointestinal problems, difficulties in maintaining body temperature, and amenorrhea (in women). Rates of underweight individuals have declined in recent decades as overweight and obesity percentages have increased. Today, fewer than 4 percent of children and adolescents aged 2–19 and 2 percent of adults aged 20–74 are underweight.[31]

TABLE 9.1 **Body Fat Percentage Norms for Men and Women***

Men Age	Very Lean	Excellent	Good	Fair	Poor	Very Poor
20–29	<7%	7%–10%	11%–15%	16%–19%	20%–23%	>23%
30–39	<11%	11%–14%	15%–18%	19%–21%	22%–25%	>25%
40–49	<14%	14%–17%	18%–20%	21%–23%	24%–27%	>27%
50–59	<15%	15%–19%	20%–22%	23%–24%	25%–28%	>28%
60–69	<16%	16%–20%	21%–22%	23%–25%	26%–28%	>28%
70–79	<16%	16%–20%	21%–23%	24%–25%	26%–28%	>28%
Women Age	**Very Lean**	**Excellent**	**Good**	**Fair**	**Poor**	**Very Poor**
20–29	<14%	14%–16%	17%–19%	20%–23%	24%–27%	>27%
30–39	<15%	15%–17%	18%–21%	22%–25%	26%–29%	>29%
40–49	<17%	17%–20%	21%–24%	25%–28%	29%–32%	>32%
50–59	<18%	18%–22%	23%–27%	28%–30%	31%–34%	>34%
60–69	<18%	18%–23%	24%–28%	29%–31%	32%–35%	>35%
70–79	<18%	18%–24%	25%–29%	30%–32%	33%–36%	>36%

*Assumes nonathletes. For athletes, recommended body fat is 5 to 15 percent for men and 12 to 22 percent for women. Please note that there are no agreed-upon national standards for recommended body fat percentage.

Source: Based on data from The Cooper Institute, Dallas Texas, www.cooperinstitute.org.

check yourself

- **What are the differences between overweight and obesity?**

9.6 Assessing Body Weight and Body Composition: BMI and Other Methods

learning outcome

9.6 Compare and contrast different methods of body composition assessment.

Although people have a general sense that BMI is an indicator of how "fat" a person is, most do not really know what it assesses. **Body mass index (BMI)** is a description of body weight relative to height, numbers highly correlated with total body fat. Find your BMI in inches and pounds in Figure 9.4, or you can calculate your BMI by dividing your weight in kilograms by height in meters squared:

$$\text{BMI} = \text{weight(kg)/height squared (m}^2)$$

A BMI calculator is also available at www.nhlbi.nih.gov.

Desirable BMI levels may vary with age and by sex; however, most BMI tables for adults do not account for such variables. **Healthy weight** is defined as having a BMI of 18.5 to 24.9, the range of lowest statistical health risk.[32] A BMI of 25 to 29.9 indicates overweight and potentially significant health risks. A BMI of 30 or above is classified as obese. A BMI of 40 to 49.9 is morbidly obese, and a new category of BMI of 50 or higher has been labeled as super obese.[33] Nearly 3 percent of obese men and almost 7 percent of obese women are morbidly obese.[34]

Although useful, BMI levels don't include water, muscle, and bone mass or account for the fact that muscle weighs more than fat. BMI levels can be inaccurate for people who are under 5 feet tall, are highly muscled, or who are older and have little muscle mass. More precise methods of determining body fat, described below, should be used for these individuals.

Youth and BMI The labels *obese* and *morbidly obese* have been used for years for adults, though there is growing concern about the consequences of pinning these potentially stigmatizing labels on children.[35] BMI ranges above normal weight for children and teens are often labeled as "at risk of overweight" and "overweight." BMI ranges for children and teens take into account normal differences in body fat between boys and girls and the differences in body fat that occur at various ages. Specific guidelines for calculating youth BMI are available at the Centers for Disease Control and Prevention website, www.cdc.gov.

Key:
- Underweight
- Normal weight
- Overweight
- Obese

Height (feet and inches)	100		120		140		160		180		200		220		240		260
4′6″	24	27	29	31	34	36	39	41	43	46	48	51	53	55	58	60	63
4′8″	22	25	27	29	31	34	36	38	40	43	45	47	49	52	54	56	58
4′10″	21	23	25	27	29	31	33	36	38	40	42	44	46	48	50	52	54
5′0″	20	22	23	25	27	29	31	33	35	37	39	41	43	45	47	49	51
5′2″	18	20	22	24	26	27	29	31	33	35	37	38	40	42	44	46	48
5′4″	17	19	21	22	24	26	28	29	31	33	34	36	38	40	41	43	45
5′6″	16	18	19	21	23	24	26	27	29	31	32	34	36	37	39	40	42
5′8″	15	17	18	20	21	23	24	26	27	29	30	32	33	35	37	38	40
5′10″	14	16	17	19	20	22	23	24	26	27	29	30	32	33	34	36	37
6′0″	14	15	16	18	19	20	22	23	24	26	27	29	30	31	33	34	35
6′2″	13	14	15	17	18	19	21	22	23	24	26	27	28	30	31	32	33
6′4″	12	13	15	16	17	18	20	21	22	23	24	26	27	28	29	30	32
6′6″	12	13	14	15	16	17	19	20	21	22	23	24	25	27	28	29	30
6′8″	11	12	13	14	15	17	18	19	20	21	22	23	24	25	26	28	29
6′10″	11	12	13	14	15	16	17	18	19	20	21	22	23	24	25	26	27
7′0″	10	11	12	13	14	15	16	17	18	19	20	21	22	23	24	25	26

Weight (pounds)

Figure 9.4 Body Mass Index

Locate the intersection of your weight and height to determine BMI. Note that BMI values have been rounded off to the nearest whole number.

Waist Circumference and Ratio Measurements

Knowing where you carry your fat may be more important than knowing how much you carry. Men and postmenopausal women tend to store fat in the abdominal area. Premenopausal women usually store fat in the hips, buttocks, and thighs. Waist circumference measurement is increasingly recognized as

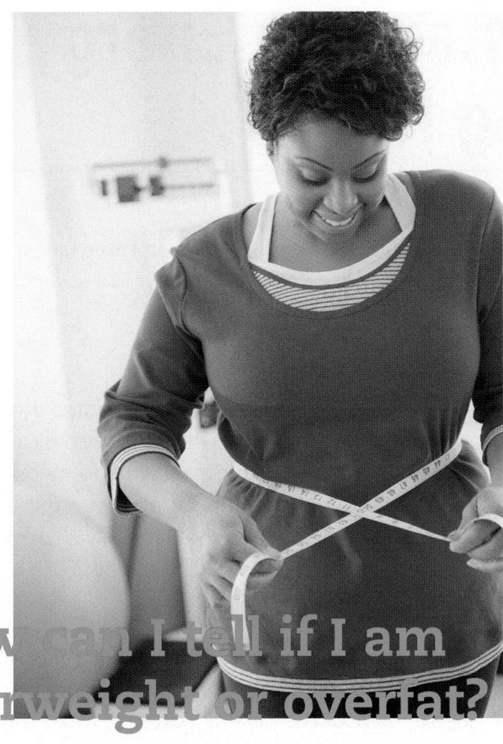

How can I tell if I am overweight or overfat?

Observing the way you look and how your clothes fit can give you a general idea of whether you weigh more or less than in the past. But for evaluating your weight and body fat levels in terms of potential health risks, it's best to use more scientific measures, such as BMI, waist circumference, waist-to-hip ratio, or a technician-administered body composition test.

a useful tool in assessing abdominal fat, which is considered more threatening to health than fat in other regions. In particular, as waist circumference increases, the risk for diabetes, cardiovascular disease, and stroke increases.[36] A waistline greater than 40 inches (102 centimeters) in men and 35 inches (88 centimeters) in women may be particularly indicative of greater health risk.[37] If a person is less than 5 feet tall or has a BMI of 35 or above, waist circumference standards used for the general population might not apply.

The **waist-to-hip ratio** measures regional fat distribution. A waist-to-hip ratio greater than 1 in men and 0.8 in women indicates increased health risks.[38] Measuring the waist-to-hip ratio is relatively inexpensive and accurate; however, it is less practical to use in clinical settings, and many believe that for most people, waist circumference and BMI are sufficient.[39]

Measures of Body Fat

There are many other ways to assess body fat levels. One low-tech way is simply to look in the mirror or consider how your clothes fit now compared with how they fit in the past. For those who wish to take a more precise measurement of their percentage of body fat, more accurate techniques are available, including caliper measurement, underwater weighing, and various body scans (Figure 9.5). These methods usually involve the help of a skilled professional and typically must be done in a lab or clinical setting. Before undergoing any procedure, make sure you understand the expense, potential for accuracy, risks, and training of the tester. Also, consider why you are seeking this assessment and what you plan to do with the results.

Underwater (hydrostatic) weighing:
Measures the amount of water a person displaces when completely submerged. Fat tissue is less dense than muscle or bone, so body fat can be computed within a 2%–3% margin of error by comparing weight underwater and out of water.

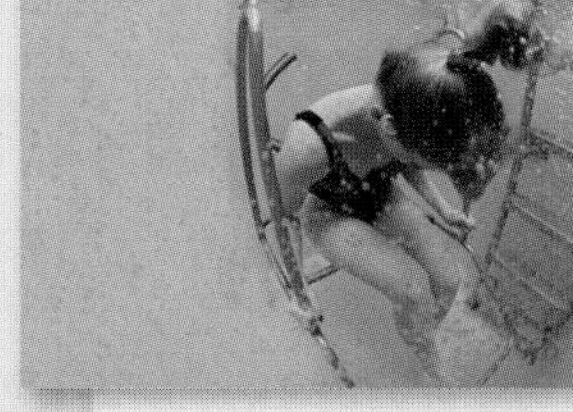

Skinfolds:
Involves "pinching" a person's fold of skin (with its underlying layer of fat) at various locations of the body. The fold is measured using a specially designed caliper. When performed by a skilled technician, it can estimate body fat with an error of 3%–4%.

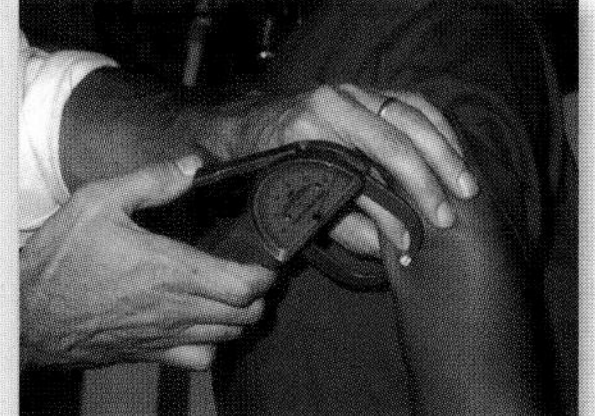

Bioelectrical impedance analysis (BIA):
Involves sending a very low level of electrical current through a person's body. As lean body mass is made up of mostly water, the rate at which the electricity is conducted gives an indication of a person's lean body mass and body fat. Under the best circumstances, BIA can estimate body fat with an error of 3%–4%.

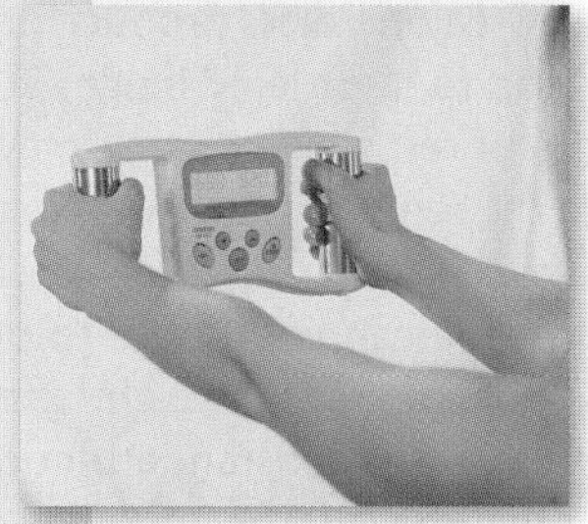

Dual-energy X-ray absorptiometry (DXA):
The technology is based on using very-low-level X-ray to differentiate between bone tissue, soft (or lean) tissue, and fat (or adipose) tissue. The margin of error for predicting body fat is 2%–4%.

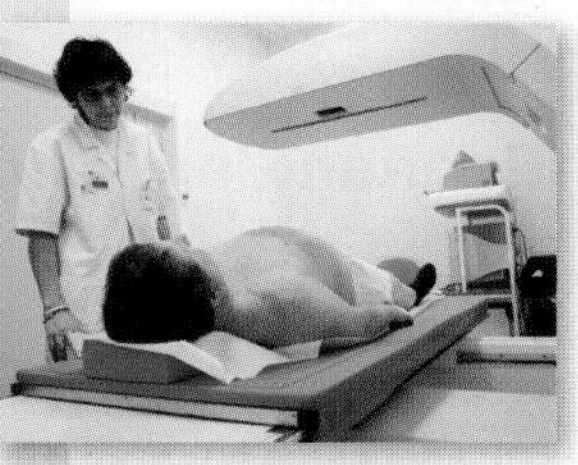

Bod Pod:
Uses air displacement to measure body composition. This machine is a large, egg-shaped chamber made from fiberglass. The person being measured sits in the machine wearing a swimsuit. The door is closed and the machine measures how much air is displaced. That value is used to calculate body fat, with a 2%–3% margin of error.

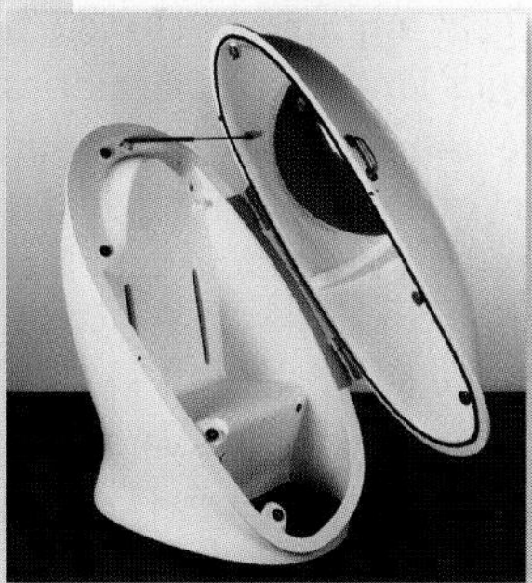

Figure 9.5 Overview of Various Body Composition Methods

Source: Adapted from J. Thompson and M. Manore, *Nutrition: An Applied Approach My Plate Edition*, 3rd ed., © 2012. Printed and electronically reproduced by permission of Pearson Education, Inc., Upper Saddle River, New Jersey.

check yourself

- **Which of the various assessment methods do you consider the most accurate? Which is the most accessible to the average person?**

9.7

Weight Management: Understanding Energy Balance and Improving Eating Habits

learning outcome

9.7 Explain how energy expenditure and energy intake affect weight management and ways to successfully manage your weight.

At some point in our lives, almost all of us will decide to lose weight or modify our diet. Many will have mixed success. Failure is often related to thinking about losing weight in terms of short-term "dieting" rather than adjusting long-term eating behaviors (such as developing the habit of healthy snacking).

Low-calorie diets produce only temporary losses and may actually lead to disordered binge eating or related problems.[40] Repeated bouts of restrictive dieting may be physiologically harmful; moreover, the sense of failure we experience each time we don't meet our goal can exact far-reaching psychological costs. Drugs and intensive counseling can contribute to positive weight loss, but, even then, many people regain weight after treatment. Maintaining a healthful body takes constant attention and nurturing over the course of your lifetime.

Understanding Calories and Energy Balance

A *calorie* is a unit of measure that indicates the amount of energy gained from food or expended through activity. Each time you consume 3,500 calories more than your body needs to maintain weight, you gain a pound of storage fat. Conversely, each time your body expends an extra 3,500 calories, you lose a pound of fat. If you consume 140 calories (the amount in one can of regular soda) more than you need every single day and make no other changes in diet or activity, you would gain 1 pound in 25 days (3,500 calories ÷140 calories ÷ 1 day = 25 days). Conversely, if you walk for 30 minutes each day at a pace of 15 minutes per mile (172 calories burned) in addition to your regular activities, you would lose 1 pound in 20 days (3,500 calories ÷ 172 calories ÷ 1 day = 20.3 days) due to the negative caloric balance. This is an example of the concept of energy balance described in Figure 9.6.

The Importance of Exercise

Any increase in the intensity, frequency, and duration of daily exercise can have a significant impact on total calorie expenditure because lean (muscle) tissue is more metabolically active than fat tissue. Exact estimates vary, but experts currently think that 2–50 more calories per day are burned per pound of muscle than for each pound of fat tissue. Thus, the base level of calories needed to maintain a healthy weight varies greatly from person to person.

The number of calories spent depends on three factors:

1. The number and proportion of muscles used
2. The amount of weight moved
3. The length of time the activity takes

An activity involving both the arms and legs burns more calories than one involving only the legs. An activity performed by a heavy person burns more calories than the same activity performed by a lighter person. And an activity performed for 40 minutes requires twice as much energy as the same activity performed for only 20 minutes.

Improving Your Eating Habits

Before you can change a behavior, such as unhealthy eating habits, you must first determine what causes or triggers it. Many people find it helpful to keep a chart of their eating patterns: when they feel like eating, where they are when they decide to eat, the amount of time they spend eating, other activities they engage in during the meal (watching television or reading), whether they eat alone or with others, what and how much they consume, and how they felt before they took their first bite. If you keep a detailed daily log of eating triggers for at least a week, you will discover useful clues about what in your environment or your emotional makeup causes you to want food. Typically, these

See It! Videos

A new strategy to keep off the weight? Watch **Keeping It Off** in the Study Area of MasteringHealth.

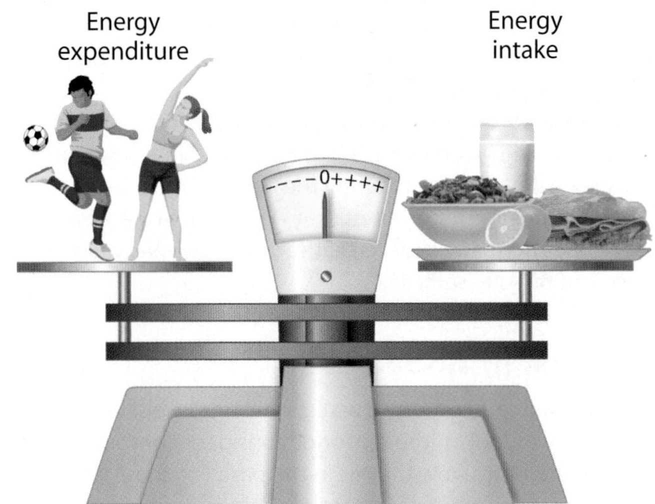

Figure 9.6 The Concept of Energy Balance
If you consume more calories than you burn, you will gain weight. If you burn more than you consume, you will lose weight. If both are equal, your weight will not change, according to this concept.

dietary triggers center on patterns and problems in everyday living rather than on real hunger pangs. Many people eat compulsively when stressed; however, for other people, the same circumstances diminish their appetite, causing them to lose weight.

Once you've evaluated your behaviors and determined your triggers, you can begin to devise a plan for improved eating. If you are unsure of where to start, seek assistance from reputable sources such as MyPlate (www.choosemyplate.gov). Registered dietitians, some physicians (not all doctors have a strong background in nutrition), health educators and exercise physiologists with nutritional training, and other health professionals can provide reliable information. Be wary of people who call themselves nutritionists; there is no such official designation. Avoid weight-loss programs that promise quick "miracle" results or those run by "trainees," often people with short courses on nutrition and exercise that are designed to sell products or services.

Before engaging in any weight-loss program, ask about the credentials of the adviser; assess the nutrient value of the prescribed diet; verify that dietary guidelines are consistent with reliable nutrition research; and analyze the suitability of the diet to your tastes, budget, and lifestyle. Any diet that requires radical behavior changes or sets up artificial dietary programs through prepackaged products that don't teach you how to eat healthfully is likely to fail. Supplements and fad diets that claim fast weight loss will invariably mean fast weight regain. The most successful plans allow you to make food choices in real-world settings and do not ask you to sacrifice everything you enjoy.

You will also need to address some of the triggers that you may have for eating that are unrelated to hunger. For example, if you tend to eat in stressful situations, try to acknowledge the feelings of stress and anxiety and develop stress management techniques to practice daily. If you find yourself eating when you are bored or tired, identify the times when you feel low energy, and fill them with activities other than eating, such as exercise breaks, or cultivate a new interest or hobby that keeps your mind and hands busy. If your trigger is feeling angry or upset, analyze your emotions and look for a noneating activity to deal with them, such as taking a quick walk or calling a friend. If it is the sight and smell of food, stop buying high-calorie foods that tempt you, or store them in an inconvenient place, out of sight. Avoid walking past or sitting or standing near the table of tempting treats at a meeting, party, or other gathering.

Some people drink diet soda to help maintain or control their weight. In fact, 11 percent of healthy weight, 19 percent of overweight, and 22 percent of obese adults drink diet sodas for weight control. They may not realize it, but in drinking diet sodas they could actually be sabotaging their weight loss plans. According to new research, overweight/obese individuals who opt for diet beverages actually consume more calories from food at meals and from snacks than people who choose sugared beverages.[41] Why is this the case? While the exact mechanism remains in question, researchers speculate that artificial sweeteners may change the way we perceive fullness and may increase appetite. Others suggest a form of "cognitive distortion" whereby we justify a few more snacks or dessert since our drinks have fewer calories.

Skills for Behavior Change

TIPS FOR SENSIBLE SNACKING

- **Keep healthy munchies around.** Buy 100 percent whole-wheat breads. If you need to spice up your snack, use low-fat or soy cheese, low-fat cream cheese, peanut butter, hummus, or other healthy favorites. Some baked or popped crackers are low in fat and calories and high in fiber. Look for these on your grocery shelves.
- **Keep "crunchies" on hand.** Apples, pears, red or green pepper sticks, carrots, and celery all are good choices. Wash the fruits and vegetables and cut them up to carry with you; eat them when a snack attack comes on.
- **Quench your thirst with hot drinks.** Hot tea, heated milk, plain or decaffeinated coffee, hot chocolate made with nonfat milk or water, or soup broths will help keep you satisfied.
- **Choose natural beverages.** Drink plain water, 100 percent juice in small quantities, or other low-sugar choices to satisfy your thirst. Avoid certain juices, energy drinks, and soft drinks that have added sugars, low fiber, and no protein. Usually, they are high in calories and low in longer-term satisfaction.
- **Eat nuts instead of candy.** Although nuts are relatively high in calories, they are also loaded with healthy fats and make a healthy snack when consumed in moderation.
- **If you must have a piece of chocolate, keep it small.** Note that dark chocolate is better than milk chocolate or white chocolate because of its antioxidant content.
- **Avoid high-calorie energy bars.** Eat these only if you are exercising hard and don't have an opportunity to eat a regular meal. If you buy energy bars, look for ones with a good mixture of fiber and protein and that are low in fat and calories.

check yourself

- **What are three potential triggers for overeating, and how can they be overcome?**
- **What steps should you take before engaging in any weight-loss program?**

9.8 Weight Management: Assessing Diet Programs

learning **outcome**

9.8 Identify strengths and weaknesses of popular diet programs.

People looking to lose weight and improve eating habits often turn to diet programs for advice and guidance. Table 9.2 analyzes several popular diets marketed today. For information on other plans, check out the regularly updated list of reviews on the website of the Academy of Nutrition and Dietetics at www.eatright.org.

See It! Videos

What makes one diet plan work better than another? Watch **Best Diet Plan Apparently Works** in the Study Area of MasteringHealth.

TABLE **9.2** **Analyzing Popular Diet Programs**

Diet Name	Basic Principles	Good for Diabetes and Heart Health?	Weight Loss Effectiveness	Pros, Cons, and Other Things to Consider
DASH (Dietary Approaches to Stop Hypertension)	A plan developed to fight high blood pressure. Eat fruits, veggies, whole grains, lean protein, and low-fat dairy. Avoid sweets, fats, red meat, and sodium.	Yes	Not specifically designed for weight loss.	A safe and healthy diet that can be complicated to learn. Although not designed for weight reduction, it is regarded as effective in improving cholesterol levels long term.
Mediterranean	A plan that emphasizes fruits, vegetables, fish, whole grains, beans, nuts, legumes, olive oil, and herbs and spices. Poultry, eggs, cheese, yogurt, and red wine are enjoyed in moderation; sweets and red meat are for special occasions.	Yes	Effective	Widely considered to be one of the more healthy, safe, and balanced diets. Weight loss may not be as dramatic, but long-term health benefits have been demonstrated.
Weight Watchers	The program assigns every food a point value based on its nutritional values and how hard your body has to work to burn it off. Total points allowed depend on activity level and personal weight goals.	Yes (depending on individual choices)	Effective	Experts consider Weight Watchers effective and easy to follow for both short- and long-term weight loss. Other pluses include an emphasis on group support and room for occasional indulgences. But while not as expensive as some plans, there are membership fees.
Jenny Craig	Prepackaged meals do the work of restricting calorie intake. Members get personalized meal and exercise plans, plus weekly counseling sessions.	Yes	Effective short term, long-term results dependent on adopting healthful eating later	Support and premade meals make weight loss easier; however, it may be difficult to maintain for the long run. Cons include cost—hundreds of dollars per month for food alone plus membership fees. No lactose- and gluten-free foods are available.
Atkins	Carbs (sugars and simple starches) are avoided in this plan, and protein and fat from chicken, meat, and eggs are embraced.	Not likely with so much fat eaten	Effective in short term, mixed long-term results	Atkins is extremely effective at short-term weight loss, but many experts worry that fat intake is up to three times higher than standard daily recommendations.
Paleo	Based on the theory that digestive systems have not evolved to deal with many modern foods such as diary, legumes, grains and sugar, this plan emphasizes meats, fish, poultry, fruits, and vegetables.	Unknown (too few studies)	Unknown (too few studies)	Gets low marks by health and nutrition experts due to avoidance of grains, legumes, and dairy and higher fat than the government recommends. Other cons include that it is missing essential nutrients, costly to maintain, hard to follow long term, and has had only a few very small studies done to document effectiveness.
Fast Diet (also known as the 5:2 diet or intermittent fasting diet)	Based on the theory that by drastically reducing calories on two days (500 cal/day) each week and eating normally the other five, you will lose weight	Not likely as it doesn't follow guidelines for carbohydrates	Effective but weight loss is slow unless calorie intake is monitored on non-fast days and exercise is part of regimen	Exceeds dietary guidelines for fat and protein and falls short on carbohydrate recommendation. Does encourage fruits and veggies, but feast and famine regimen is hard to sustain.

Sources: Opinions on diet pros and cons are based on *U.S. News & World Report*, "Best Diet Rankings," 2012, http://health.usnews.com; Dietary reviews available online from registered dieticians at the Academy of Nutrition and Dietetics, 2013, www.eatright.org.

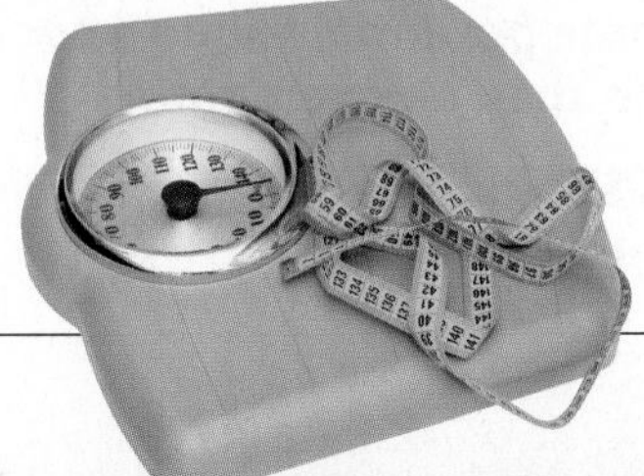

check yourself

- **What are important factors to consider when evaluating current diet programs?**

9.9 Weight Management: In Perspective

learning **outcome**

9.9 List steps to successful weight management.

Supportive friends, relatives, community resources, and policies that support healthy food choices and exercise options all increase the likelihood of successful weight loss. People of the same age, sex, height, and weight can have resting metabolic rates that differ by as much as 1,000 calories a day. This may explain why one person's extra food intake and weight gain may lead to weight loss and hunger in another person. Depression, stress, cultural influences, and the availability of high-fat, high-calorie foods can also make weight loss harder.

To reach and maintain the weight at which you will be healthy and feel your best, develop a program of exercise and healthy eating that you can maintain. It is unrealistic and potentially dangerous to try to lose weight in a short period of time. Instead, try to lose a healthy 1 to 2 pounds during the first week, and stay with this slow-and-easy regimen. Adding exercise and cutting back on calories to expend about 500 calories more than you consume each day will help you lose weight at a rate of 1 pound per week.

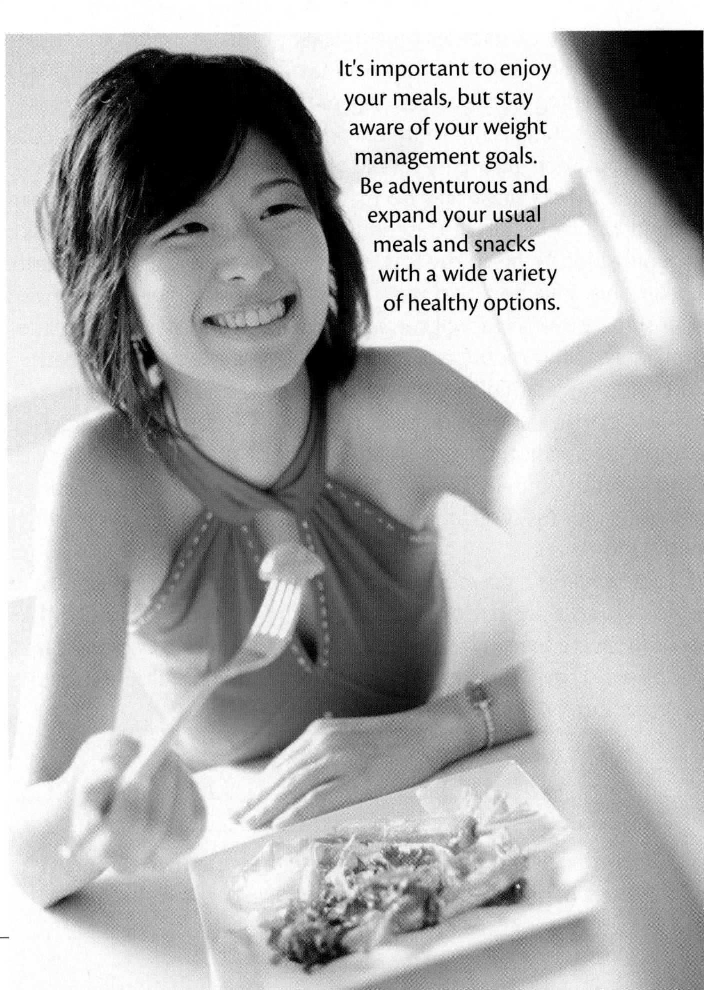

It's important to enjoy your meals, but stay aware of your weight management goals. Be adventurous and expand your usual meals and snacks with a wide variety of healthy options.

Skills for **Behavior Change**

KEYS TO SUCCESSFUL WEIGHT MANAGEMENT

The key to successful weight management is finding a sustainable way to control what you eat and to make exercise a priority.

- To get started, ask yourself some key questions. Why do you want to make this change right now? What are your ultimate goals?
- Write down the things you find positive about your diet and exercise behaviors. Then write down things that need to be changed. For each change you need to make, list three or four small things you could change right now.
- What resources on campus or in your community could help? Out of your friends and family members, who will help you?
- Keep a food and exercise log for 2 or 3 days. Note the good things you are doing, the things that need improvement, and the triggers you need to address.

Make a Plan

- Set realistic short- and long-term goals.
- Establish a plan. What diet and exercise changes can you make this week? Once you do 1 week, plot a course for 2 weeks, and so on.
- Look for balance. Remember that it is calories taken in and burned over time that make the difference.

Change Your Habits

- Notice whether you're hungry before starting a meal. Eat slowly, noting when you start to feel full. Stop before you are full.
- Eat breakfast. This will prevent you from being too hungry and overeating at lunch.
- Keep healthful snacks on hand for when you get hungry.
- Don't constantly deprive yourself or set unrealistic guidelines.

Incorporate Exercise

- Be active; slowly increase your time, speed, distance, or resistance levels.
- Vary your physical activity. Find activities you love; try things you haven't tried before.
- Find an exercise partner to help you stay motivated.
- Make exercise a fun break. Go for a walk in a place that interests you.

check yourself

- **What are the key components of a successful weight management plan?**

9.10 Considering Drastic Weight-Loss Measures

learning **outcome**

9.10 Explain measures that may be taken when body weight poses an extreme threat to health.

In certain limited instances, extreme measures may be considered to reduce weight.

In severe cases of obesity, patients may be given powdered formulas with daily values of 400 to 700 calories plus vitamin and mineral supplements. Such **very-low-calorie diets (VLCDs)** should never be undertaken without strict medical supervision.

One dangerous potential complication of VLCDs or starvation diets is *ketoacidosis,* in which a patient's blood becomes more acidic, causing severe damage to body tissues. Risk is greatest for those with untreated type 1 diabetes, anorexia nervosa, or bulimia nervosa. If fasting continues, the body turns to its last resort—protein—for energy, breaking down essential muscle and organ tissue to stay alive. Within about 10 days after the typical adult begins a complete fast, the body will have depleted its energy stores, and death may occur.

Dieters often turn to commercially marketed weight-loss supplements. U.S. Food and Drug Administration (FDA) approval is not required for over-the-counter "diet aids" or supplements, whose effectiveness is largely untested and unproven. Virtually all persons who use diet pills eventually regain their weight.[42]

In 2007, the FDA approved the first over-the-counter weight loss pill—a half-strength version of the drug orlistat (Xenical), marketed as Alli. This drug inhibits the action of lipase, an enzyme that helps the body digest fats, causing about 30 percent of fats consumed to pass through the digestive system. Side effects include gas with watery fecal discharge; frequent, often unexpected, bowel movements; and possible deficiencies of fat-soluble vitamins.

The FDA approved the drugs Belvig and Qsymia in 2012. Belvig affects serotonin levels, helping patients feel full, and Qsymia is an appetite suppressant and anti-seizure drug that reduces the desire for food.

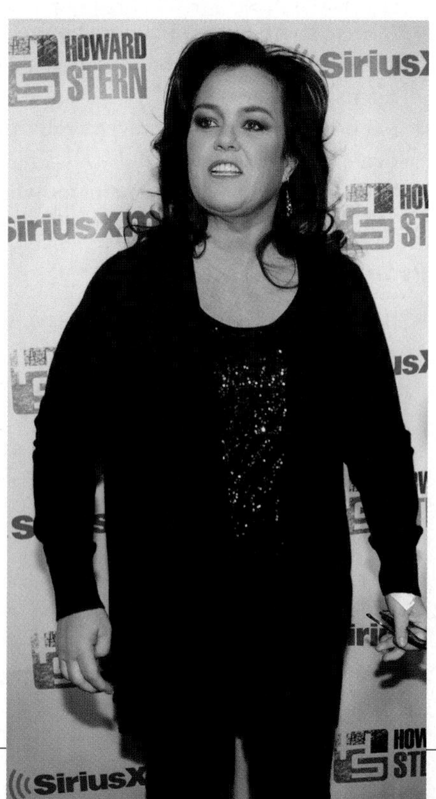

Comedian and talk show host Rosie O'Donnell underwent weight loss surgery in 2013, following a heart attack the previous year.

Several once-approved diet drugs have since been recalled due to a variety of problems like heart attacks, heart valve problems, stroke, and liver damage. View all diet drugs and supplements with caution, including these:

- **Human chorionic gonadotropin (HCG).** In prescription form, this is an approved treatment for some female fertility problems; it has recently become known as a crash-diet miracle drug. Results consistently show that hCG is no more effective for weight loss than cutting calories.[43]
- **Sibutramine (Meridia).** This prescription medication suppresses appetite by inhibiting serotonin uptake in the brain. Side effects include dry mouth, headache, and high blood pressure. The FDA has issued warnings about Meridia for people with hypertension or heart disease.[44]
- ***Hoodia gordonii.*** This plant native to Africa is a purported appetite suppressant. To date, it is not FDA approved and has not been tested in clinical trials.[45]
- **Herbal weight-loss aids.** Products containing *Ephedra* can cause rapid heart rate, seizures, insomnia, and raised blood pressure, all without significant effects on weight. *St. John's wort* and other herbs reported to suppress appetite have not been shown effective.

People who are severely overweight and have diabetes or hypertension may be candidates for surgical options. In *adjustable gastric banding,* an inflatable band partitions off the stomach, leaving only a small opening between its two parts so the stomach is smaller and the person feels full more quickly. Although weight loss isn't as dramatic as with gastric bypass surgery, the risks are fewer.

Gastric bypass drastically decreases how much food a person can eat and absorb. Results are fast and dramatic, but there are many risks, including blood clots in the legs, a leak in a staple line in the stomach, pneumonia, infection, and death. The stomach pouch that remains after surgery is small (about the size of a lime), so the person can eat or drink only a tiny amount at a time. Possible side effects include nausea and vomiting, vitamin and mineral deficiencies, and dehydration.

Research has shown unexpected results from gastric surgeries: complete remission of type 2 diabetes in the majority of cases, with drastic reductions in blood glucose levels in others.[46] Researchers are exploring surgical options for diabetes prevention in other populations.[47]

Liposuction is a cosmetic (not weight loss) surgical procedure in which fat cells are removed from specific areas of the body. Risks include severe scarring, and even death has resulted. In many cases, people who have liposuction regain fat or require multiple surgeries to repair lumpy, irregular surfaces.

check yourself

- **What measures can be taken when body weight poses a risk to health? What are their risks?**

Trying to Gain Weight

learning outcome

9.11 Describe healthy strategies for trying to gain weight.

For some people, trying to gain weight is a challenge for a variety of metabolic, hereditary, psychological, and other reasons. If you are one of these individuals, the first priority is to determine why you cannot gain weight.

Perhaps you're an athlete and you burn more calories than you manage to eat. Perhaps you're stressed out and skipping meals to increase study time. Or stress, depression, or other emotional issues may make it difficult to focus on food and take good care of your body. Among older adults, the senses of taste and smell may decline, which makes food taste different and therefore less pleasurable to eat. Visual problems and other disabilities may make meals more difficult to prepare, and dental problems may make eating more difficult.

People who engage in extreme energy-burning sports and exercise routines may be at risk for caloric and nutritional deficiencies, which can lead not only to weight loss, but to immune system problems and organ dysfunction; weakness, which leads to falls and fractures; slower recovery from diseases; and a host of other problems as well.

People who are too thin need to take the same kind of steps as those who are overweight or obese to find out what their healthy weight is and attain that weight.

The Skills for Behavior Change feature gives ideas and tips for gaining weight. Depending on your situation, you may aim to gain as much as a pound per week, which would mean adding up to 500 calories a day to your diet. It is important that these calories be added in the form of energy-dense, nutritious choices from a variety of foods. For example, you could choose to eat a thick slice of whole grain toast topped with peanut butter and a banana for breakfast or garnish a salad with olive oil, avocado, nuts, and sunflower seeds for lunch. One cup of whole-wheat flakes provides 128 calories, while a cup of granola is 464 calories. Similarly, plain low-fat yogurt is 154 calories per cup, while strawberry low-fat yogurt offers 238 calories per cup. Just be sure that the calories you add are coming from high-quality sources, not high-fat junk food.[48]

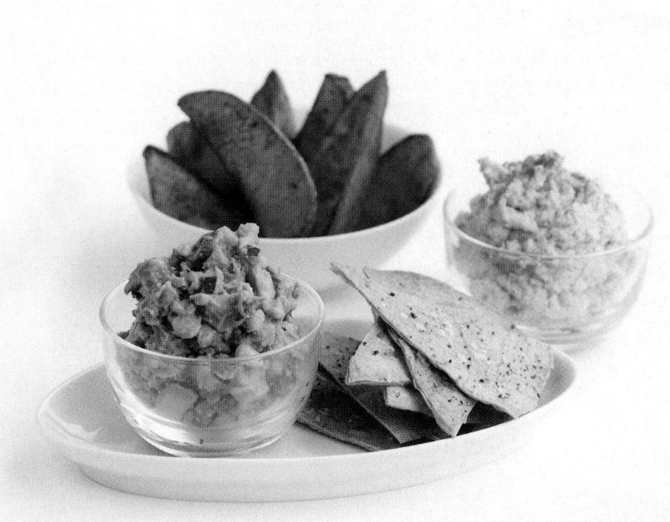

A snack of guacamole and whole-grain tortilla chips or hummus and baked potatoes is a healthy, nutrient-dense way to increase calorie intake.

Skills for Behavior Change

TIPS FOR GAINING WEIGHT

- **Eat at regularly scheduled times.**
- **Eat more frequently, spend more time eating, eat high-calorie foods first if you fill up fast, and always start with the main course.**
- **Take time to shop, to cook, and to eat slowly.**
- **Put extra spreads such as peanut butter, cream cheese, or cheese on your foods. Make your sandwiches with extra-thick slices of bread and add more filling. Take seconds whenever possible, and eat high-calorie, nutrient-dense snacks such as nuts and cheese during the day.**
- **Supplement your diet. Add high-calorie drinks that have a healthy balance of nutrients, such as whole milk.**
- **Try to eat with people you are comfortable with. Avoid people who you feel are analyzing what you eat or make you feel as if you should eat less.**
- **If you are sedentary, be aware that moderate exercise can increase appetite. If you are exercising, or exercising to extremes, moderate your activities until you've gained some weight.**
- **Avoid diuretics, laxatives, and other medications that cause you to lose body fluids and nutrients.**
- **Relax. Many people who are underweight operate in high gear most of the time. Slow down, get more rest, and take steps to control stress and anxiety.**

check yourself

- **What are some steps to be taken when weight needs to be gained? Do you think this is as difficult a task as trying to lose weight?**

9.12 Understanding and Improving Body Image

learning outcome

9.12 Identify the elements of the body image continuum, and list steps that can be taken to build a more positive body image.

When you look in the mirror, do you like what you see? If you feel disappointed, frustrated, or even angry, you're not alone. In a study, 93 percent of the women reported having negative thoughts about their appearance during the past week.[49] Negative feelings about one's body can contribute to behaviors that can threaten your health—and your life. In contrast, a healthy body image can contribute to reduced stress, an increased sense of personal empowerment, and more joyful living.

Body image includes several components:

- How you see yourself in your mind
- What you believe about your appearance
- How you feel about your body
- How you sense and control your body as you move

A *negative body image* is either a distorted perception of your shape or feelings of discomfort, shame, or anxiety about your body. A *positive body image* is a true perception of your appearance. You understand that everyone is different, and you celebrate your uniqueness. Figure 9.7 will help you identify whether your body image is positive, negative, or somewhere in between.

Factors Influencing Body Image

Images of celebrities in the media set the standard for what we find attractive, leading some people to go to dangerous extremes to have the biggest biceps or fit into size zero jeans. Though most of us think of this obsession with appearance as a recent phenomenon, it has long been part of American culture.

Social media has also increased concerns regarding negative body images.[50] Many sites actively warn against posts promoting self-harm, but images of unrealistically thin bodies—coupled with catch phrases telling young people to get "thin"—can still be hard to avoid.[51]

Body hate/ disassociation	Distorted body image	Body preoccupied/ obsessed	Body acceptance	Body is not an issue
I often feel separated and distant from my body—as if it belonged to someone else. I hate my body, and I often isolate myself from others. I don't see anything positive or even neutral about my body shape and size. I don't believe others when they tell me I look okay. I hate the way I look in the mirror.	I spend a significant amount of time exercising and dieting to change my body. My body shape and size keeps me from dating or finding someone who will treat me the way I want to be treated. I have considered changing (or have changed) my body shape and size through surgical means. I wish I could change the way I look in the mirror.	I weigh and measure myself a lot. I spend a significant amount of time viewing myself in the mirror. I compare my body to others. I have days when I feel fat. I accept society's ideal body shape and size as the best body shape and size. I'd be more attractive if I were thinner, more muscular, etc.	I pay attention to my body and my appearance because it is important to me, but it only occupies a small part of my day. I would like to change some things about my body, but I spend most of my time highlighting my positive features. My self-esteem is based on my personality traits, achievements, and relationships—not just my body image.	I feel fine about my body. I don't worry about changing my body shape or weight. I never weigh or measure myself. My feelings about my body are not influenced by society's concept of an ideal body shape. I know that the significant others in my life will always love me for who I am, not for how I look.

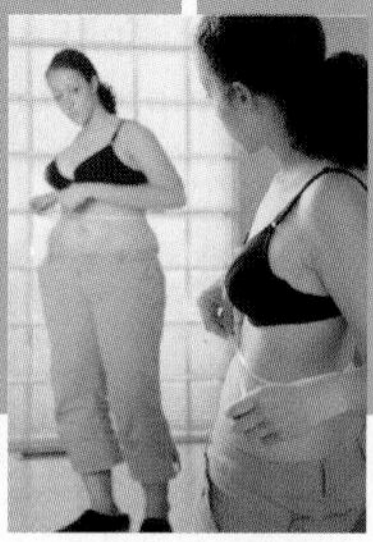

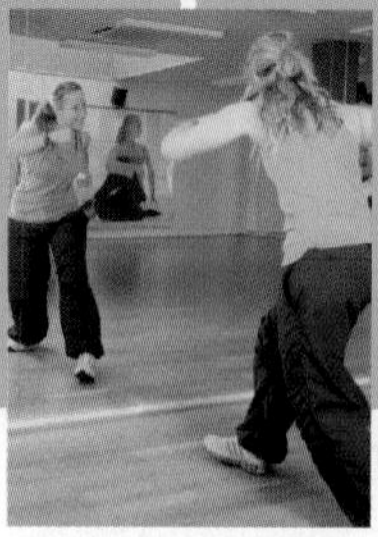

VIDEO TUTOR
Body Image Continuum

Figure 9.7 Body Image Continuum

This continuum shows a range of attitudes and behaviors toward body image. Functioning at either extreme—not caring at all or being obsessed—leads to problems. When you are functioning in the "body acceptance" area, you are taking care of your body and emotions.

Source: Adapted from Smiley/King/Avery, "Eating Issues and Body Image Continuum," Campus Health Service 1996.

Today, as more than 69 percent of Americans are overweight or obese, a significant disconnect exists between idealized images of male and female bodies and the typical American body.[52] At the same time, the media bombards us with messages telling us that we just don't measure up.

Others strongly influence how we see ourselves. Parents are especially influential in body image development. For instance, fathers who validate the acceptability of their daughters' appearance throughout puberty and mothers who model body acceptance can help their daughters maintain a positive body image.

Interactions with others outside the family—for instance, teasing and bullying from peers—can contribute to negative body image. Moreover, associations within one's cultural group appear to influence body image. For example, European American females experience the highest rates of body dissatisfaction; as a minority group becomes more acculturated into the mainstream, the body dissatisfaction levels of women in that group increase.[53]

People diagnosed with a body image disorder show differences in the brain's ability to regulate *neurotransmitters* linked to mood,[54] in a way similar to that of depression and anxiety disorders, including obsessive-compulsive disorder. One magnetic resonance imaging (MRI) study linked distortions in body image to malfunctions in the brain's visual processing region.[55]

See It! Videos

What does a "real" woman look like? Watch **A Real Look at Real Women** in the Study Area of MasteringHealth.

Building a Positive Body Image

If you want to develop a more positive body image, your first step might be to bust some toxic myths and challenge some commonly held attitudes in contemporary society:[56]

- **Myth 1: How you look is more important than who you are.** Is your weight important in defining who you are? How much does it matter to you to have friends who are thin? How important do you think being thin is in attracting a partner?
- **Myth 2: Anyone can be slender and attractive if they work at it.** When you see someone who is thin, or obese, what assumptions do you make? Have you ever berated yourself for not having the "willpower" to change some aspect of your body?
- **Myth 3: Extreme dieting is an effective weight-loss strategy.** Do you believe in fad diets or "quick-weight-loss" products? How far would you go to attain the "perfect" body?
- **Myth 4: Appearance is more important than health.** How do you evaluate whether a person is healthy? Is your desire to change your body motivated by health or appearance?

Body Image Disorders

Although most Americans are dissatisfied with some aspect of their appearance, only a few have a true body image disorder. Approximately 1 percent of people in the United States suffer from **body dysmorphic disorder (BDD)**.[57] Persons with BDD are obsessively concerned with their appearance and have a distorted view of their own body shape, body size, and so on. Although the precise cause of BDD isn't known, an anxiety disorder such as obsessive-compulsive disorder is often present. Contributing factors may include genetic susceptibility, childhood teasing, physical or sexual abuse, low self-esteem, and rigid sociocultural expectations of beauty.[58]

People with BDD may try to fix their perceived flaws through excessive bodybuilding, repeated cosmetic surgeries, or other appearance-altering behaviors. It is estimated that 10 percent of people seeking dermatology or cosmetic treatments have BDD.[59] Psychotherapy and/or antidepressant medications are often successful in treating BBD.

In **social physique anxiety (SPA)**, the desire to "look good" is so strong that it has a destructive effect on one's ability to function effectively in interactions with others. People suffering from SPA may spend a disproportionate amount of time fixating on their bodies, working out, and performing tasks that are ego centered and self-directed.[60] Experts speculate that this anxiety may contribute to disordered eating behaviors.

Skills for Behavior Change

STEPS TO A POSITIVE BODY IMAGE

One list cannot create a positive body image, but it can help you think about new ways of looking more healthfully and happily at yourself and your body.

- **Step 1. Celebrate all of the amazing things your body does for you—running, dancing, breathing, laughing, dreaming.**
- **Step 2. Keep a list of things you like about yourself—things unrelated to how much you weigh or how you look. Read your list often, and add to it regularly.**
- **Step 3. Remind yourself that true beauty is not simply skin deep. When you feel good about who you are, you carry yourself with confidence, self-acceptance, and openness that makes you beautiful.**
- **Step 4. Surround yourself with people who are supportive and who recognize the importance of liking yourself as you are.**
- **Step 5. Shut down voices in your head that tell you your body is not "right" or that you are a "bad" person. You can overpower those negative thoughts with positive ones.**
- **Step 6. Become a critical viewer of social and media messages. Identify and resist images, slogans, or attitudes that make you feel bad about yourself or your body.**
- **Step 7. Do something that lets your body know you appreciate it. Take a bubble bath, make time for a nap, or find a peaceful place outside to relax.**
- **Step 8. Use the time and energy you might have spent worrying about your appearance to do something to help others.**

Source: Adapted with permission from the National Eating Disorders Association, www.nationaleatingdisorders.org.

check yourself

- **Where do you place yourself on the body image continuum?**
- **Are there steps that you may take to improve your body image?**

9.13 What Is Disordered Eating?

learning outcome

9.13 Identify the elements of the eating issues continuum.

The eating issues continuum in Figure 9.8 identifies thoughts and behaviors associated with disordered eating.

Some people who exhibit disordered eating patterns progress to a clinical **eating disorder**—a diagnosis that can be applied only by a physician to a patient who exhibits severe disturbances in thoughts, behavior, and body functioning.

The American Psychiatric Association (APA) has defined several eating disorders: *anorexia nervosa, bulimia nervosa, binge-eating disorder,* and a cluster of conditions referred to as **Other Specified Feeding or Eating Disorder (OSFED).**[61]

In the United States, 10 percent or more of late adolescent and adult women report symptoms of eating disorders.[62] In 2013, 2.1 percent of college students reported dealing with either anorexia or bulimia.[63] Disordered eating and eating disorders are also common in college athletes in sports such as gymnastics, wrestling, swimming, and figure skating.[64] Eating disorders are on the rise among men, who represent up to 25 percent of anorexia and bulimia patients.[65]

Many people with these disorders feel disenfranchised in other aspects of their lives and try to gain a sense of control through food. Many are clinically depressed, suffer from obsessive-compulsive disorder, or have other psychiatric problems. Individuals with low self-esteem, negative body image, and a high tendency for perfectionism are most at risk.[66]

Eating disordered	Disruptive eating patterns	Food preoccupied/ obsessed	Concerned in a healthy way	Food is not an issue
I worry about what I will eat or when I will exercise all the time. I follow a very rigid eating plan and know precisely how many calories, fat grams, or carbohydrates I eat every day. I feel incredible guilt, shame, and anxiety when I break my diet. I regularly stuff myself and then exercise, vomit, or use laxatives to get rid of the food. My friends and family tell me I am too thin, but I feel fat. I am out of control when I eat. I am afraid to eat in front of others. I prefer to eat alone.	My food and exercise concerns are starting to interfere with my school and social life. I use food to comfort myself. I have tried diet pills, laxatives, vomiting, or extra time exercising in order to lose or maintain my weight. I have fasted or avoided eating for long periods of time in order to lose or maintain my weight. If I cannot exercise to burn off calories, I panic. I feel strong when I can restrict how much I eat. I feel out of control when I eat more than I wanted to.	I think about food a lot. I'm obsessed with reading books and magazines about dieting, fitness, and weight control. I sometimes miss school, work, and social events because of my diet or exercise schedule. I divide food into "good" and "bad" categories. I feel guilty when I eat "bad" foods or when I eat more than I feel I should be eating. I am afraid of getting fat. I wish I could change how much I want to eat and what I am hungry for.	I pay attention to what I eat in order to maintain a healthy body. Food and exercise are important parts of my life, but they only occupy a small part of my time. I enjoy eating, and I balance my pleasure with my concern for a healthy body. I usually eat three balanced meals daily, plus snacks, to fuel my body with adequate energy. I am moderate and flexible in my goals for eating well and being physically active. Sometimes I eat more (or less) than I really need, but most of the time I listen to my body.	I am not concerned about what or how much I eat. I feel no guilt or shame no matter what I eat or how much I eat. Exercise is not really important to me. I choose foods based on cost, taste, and convenience, with little regard to health. My eating is very sporadic and irregular. I don't worry about meals; I just eat whatever I can, whenever I can. I enjoy stuffing myself with lots of tasty food at restaurants, holiday meals, and social events.

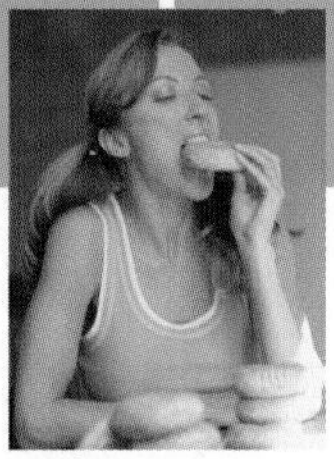

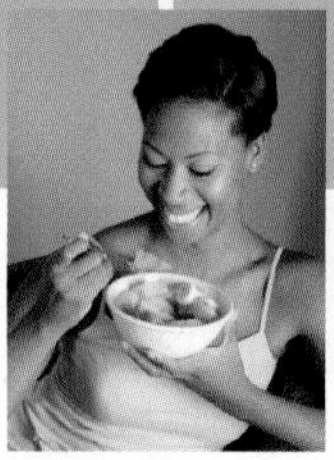

Figure 9.8 Eating Issues Continuum

This continuum shows progression from eating disorders to normal eating. The goal is to be concerned in a healthy way.

Source: Adapted from Smiley/King/Avery, "Eating Issues and Body Image Continuum," Campus Health Service 1996. Copyright © 1997 Arizona Board of Regents for University of Arizona.

check yourself

- **Where do you place yourself on the eating issues continuum?**

Eating Disorders: Anorexia Nervosa

learning outcome

9.14 List the criteria, effects, and treatment of anorexia nervosa.

Anorexia nervosa is a persistent, chronic eating disorder characterized by deliberate food restriction and severe, life-threatening weight loss. It involves self-starvation motivated by an intense fear of gaining weight along with an extremely distorted body image. Initially, most people with anorexia nervosa lose weight by reducing total food intake, particularly of high-calorie foods. Eventually, they progress to restricting their intake of almost all foods. The little they do eat, they may purge through vomiting or use of laxatives. Although they lose weight, people with anorexia nervosa never seem to feel thin enough.

An estimated 0.3 percent of females suffer from anorexia nervosa in their lifetime.[67] The American Psychiatric Association (APA) criteria for anorexia nervosa are:[68]

- Refusal to maintain body weight at or above a minimally normal weight for age and height
- Intense fear of gaining weight or becoming fat, even though considered underweight by all medical criteria
- Disturbance in the way in which one's body weight or shape is experienced, undue influence of body weight or shape on self-evaluation, or denial of the seriousness of the current low body weight

Physical symptoms and negative health consequences associated with anorexia nervosa are illustrated in Figure 9.9. Because it involves starvation and can lead to heart attacks and seizures, anorexia nervosa has the highest death rate (20%) of any psychological illness.[69]

The causes of anorexia nervosa are complex and variable. Many people with anorexia have other coexisting psychiatric problems, including low self-esteem, depression, an anxiety disorder such as obsessive-compulsive disorder, and substance abuse. Some people with anorexia nervosa have a history of being physically or sexually abused, and others have troubled interpersonal relationships with family members. Cultural norms that value people on the basis of their appearance and glorify thinness are of course a factor, as is weight-based teasing and weight bias.[70] Physical factors are thought to include an imbalance of neurotransmitters and genetic susceptibility.[71]

Once the patient is stabilized, treatment involves long-term therapy that focuses on the psychological, social, environmental, and physiological factors that have led to the problem. Through therapy, the patient works on adopting new eating behaviors, building self-confidence, and finding other ways to deal with life's problems. Support groups can also help.

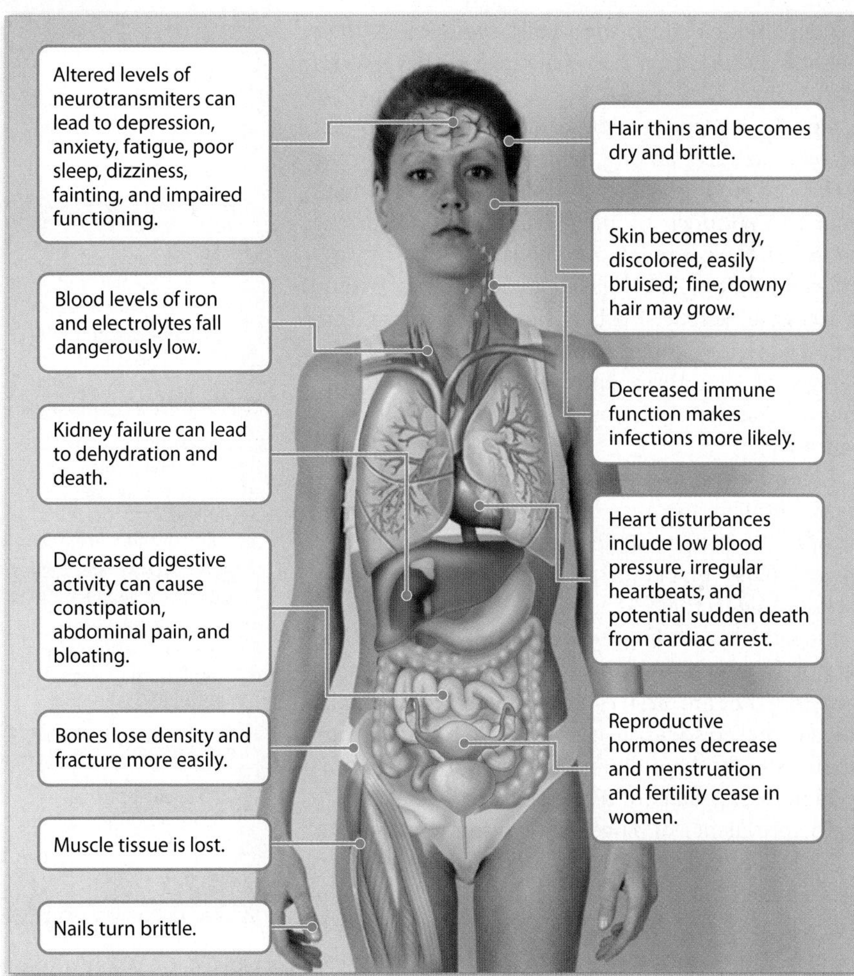

Figure 9.9 What Anorexia Nervosa Can Do to the Body

check yourself

- **What factors might put a person at risk for anorexia nervosa?**
- **How is anorexia nervosa treated?**

9.15 Eating Disorders: Bulimia Nervosa and Binge Eating

learning outcome

9.15 List the criteria, effects, and treatments for bulimia nervosa and binge eating.

Individuals with **bulimia nervosa** often binge on huge amounts of food and then engage in some kind of purging or "compensatory behavior," such as vomiting, taking laxatives, or exercising excessively, to lose the calories they have just consumed. People with bulimia are obsessed with their bodies, weight gain, and appearance, although their problem is often "hidden" from the public eye because their weight may fall within a normal range or they may be overweight.

Up to 3 percent of adolescents and young women are bulimic; rates among men are about 10 percent of the rate among women.[72] The APA criteria include recurrent episodes of binge eating and recurrent inappropriate compensatory behavior such as self-induced vomiting, use of laxatives or diuretics, fasting, or excessive exercise. The behavior must occur at least once a week for 3 months.[73]

Physical symptoms and negative health consequences associated with bulimia nervosa are shown in Figure 9.10.

A combination of genetic and environmental factors is thought to cause bulimia nervosa.[74] A family history of obesity, an underlying anxiety disorder, and an imbalance in neurotransmitters are all possible contributing factors.[75]

Individuals with **binge-eating disorder** gorge, but do not take excessive measures to lose the weight they gain; they are often clinically obese. As in bulimia, binge-eating episodes are characterized by eating large amounts of food rapidly, even when not feeling hungry, and feeling guilty or depressed after overeating.[76]

The prevalence of binge-eating disorder is thought to be 1.4 percent.[77] The APA criteria for binge-eating disorder are similar to those for bulimia nervosa, without compensatory behavior.[78] Those diagnosed with the condition also show three or more of the following behaviors: (1) eating much more rapidly than normal; (2) eating until uncomfortably full; (3) eating large amounts when not physically hungry; (4) eating alone because of embarrassment over how much one is eating; (5) feeling disgusted, depressed, or very guilty after overeating.

Without treatment, approximately 20 percent of people with a serious eating disorder will die from it; with treatment, long-term full recovery rates range from 44 to 76 percent.[79] Treatment for bulimia and binge eating is similar to treatment for anorexia. Support groups can help the family and the individual learn positive actions and interactions. Treatment of an underlying anxiety disorder or depression may also be a focus.

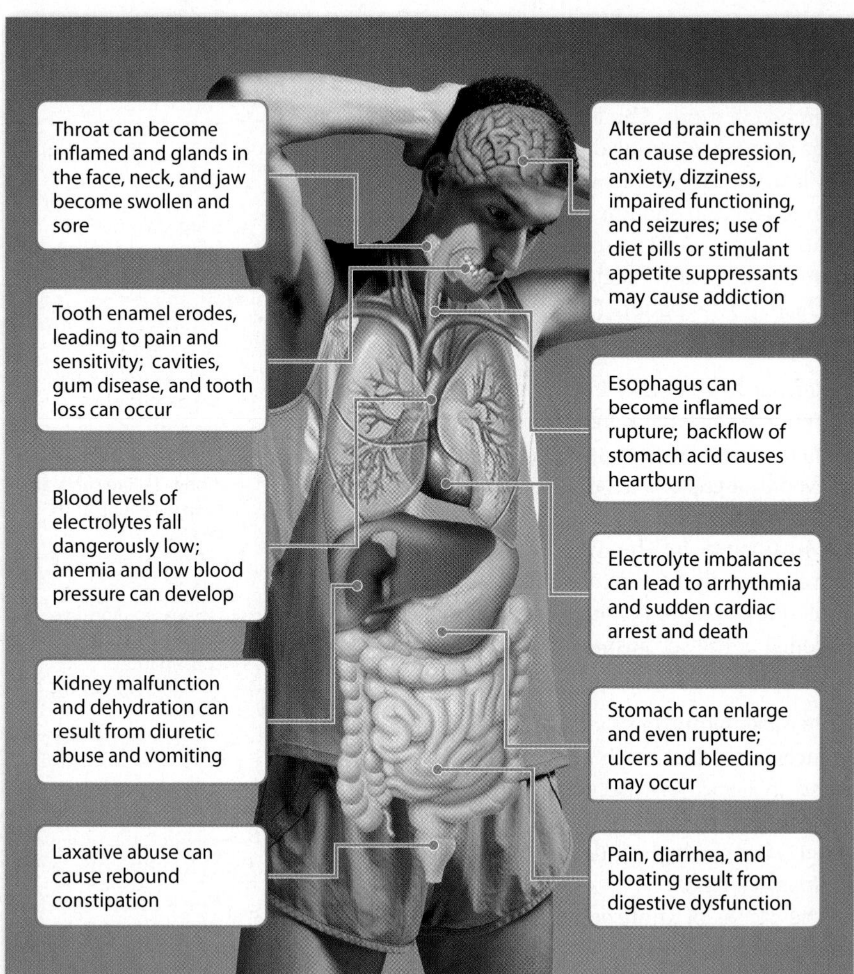

Figure 9.10 What Bulimia Nervosa Can Do to the Body

check yourself

- **What factors might put a person at risk for bulimia nervosa and binge-eating disorder?**
- **How are bulimia nervosa and binge-eating disorder treated?**

9.16

Exercise Disorders

learning outcome

9.16 List the criteria, effects, and treatment for exercise disorders.

Although exercise is generally beneficial to health, in excess it can be a problem. In addition to being a common compensatory behavior used by people with anorexia or bulimia, exercise can become a compulsion or contribute to muscle dysmorphia and the female athlete triad.

A recent study showed that participants used excessive exercise or compulsive exercise as a way to regulate their emotions.[80] **Compulsive exercise**, or *anorexia athletica*, is characterized not by a *desire* to exercise but a *compulsion* to do so, with guilt and anxiety if the person doesn't work out.

Compulsive exercise can contribute to injuries to joints and bones. It can also put significant stress on the heart, especially if combined with disordered eating. Psychologically, people who engage in compulsive exercise are often plagued by anxiety and/or depression.

Muscle Dysmorphia

Muscle dysmorphia appears to be a relatively new form of body image disturbance and exercise disorder in which a man believes that his body is insufficiently lean or muscular.[81] Men with muscle dysmorphia believe that they look "puny," when in reality they look normal or may even be unusually muscular. Behaviors characteristic of muscle dysmorphia include comparing oneself unfavorably to others, checking one's appearance in the mirror, and camouflaging one's appearance. Men with muscle dysmorphia also are likely to abuse anabolic steroids and dietary supplements.[82]

The Female Athlete Triad

Female athletes in competitive sports often strive for perfection. In an effort to be the best, they may put themselves at risk for a syndrome called the **female athlete triad**, with three interrelated problems (Figure 9.11): low energy intake, typically prompted by disordered eating; menstrual dysfunction such as amenorrhea; and poor bone density.[83]

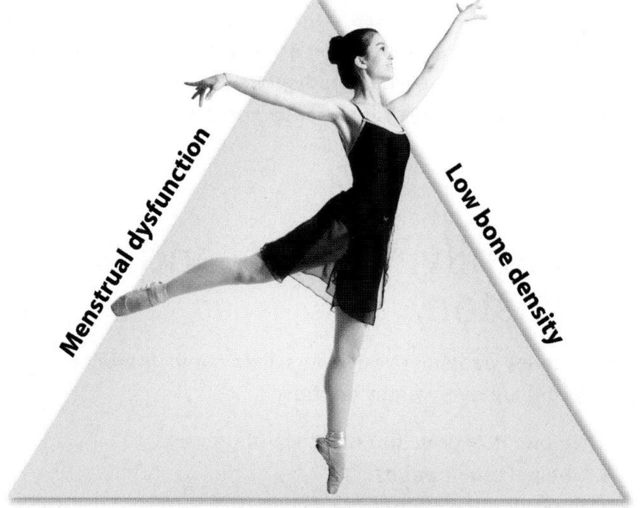

Figure 9.11 The Female Athlete Triad
The female athlete triad is a cluster of three interrelated health problems.

How does the female athlete triad develop? First, a chronic pattern of low food intake and intensive exercise depletes nutrients essential to health. The body begins to burn stores of fat tissue for energy, reducing levels of the female reproductive hormone *estrogen*, and so stopping menstruation. Depletion of fat-soluble vitamins, calcium, and estrogen weakens the athlete's bones, leaving her at high risk for fracture.

See It! Videos

Can you go too far with extreme exercise? Watch **Young Boys Exercising to Extremes** in the Study Area of MasteringHealth.

The triad is particularly prevalent in athletes in highly competitive individual sports that emphasize leanness—gymnasts, figure skaters, cross-country runners, and ballet dancers.

Warning signs include dry skin; light-headedness/fainting; fine, downy hair covering the body; multiple injuries; and changes in endurance, strength, or speed. Associated behaviors include preoccupation with food and weight, compulsive exercising, use of weight-loss products or laxatives, self-criticism, anxiety, and depression. Treatment requires a multidisciplinary approach involving the athlete's coach or trainer, a psychologist, and family members and friends.

Men with muscle dysmorphia may have unusually muscular bodies but suffer from very low self-esteem.

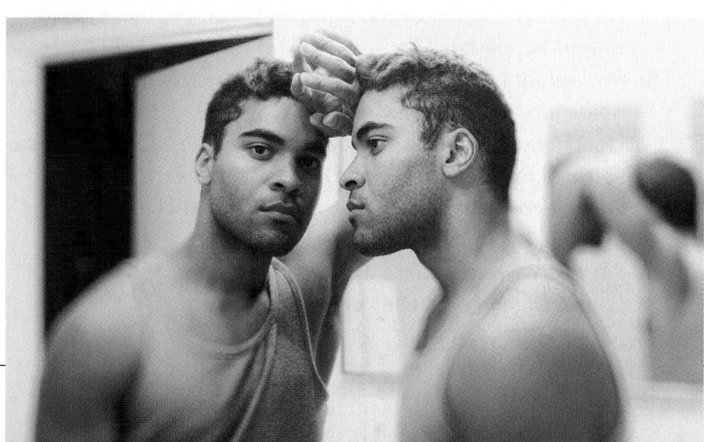

check yourself

- **What are the criteria, effects, and treatment for exercise disorders? How might these differ for men and women?**

Assessyourself

9.17

Are You Ready to Jump Start Your Weight Loss?

An interactive version of this assessment is available online in MasteringHealth.

If you are overweight or obese, complete each of the following questions by circling the response(s) that best represents your situation or attitudes, then total your points for each section. Section 1 indicates the factors that may predispose you to excess weight and make weight loss more challenging. Section 2 assesses how ready you are to begin losing weight right now.

1 Family, Weight, and Diet History

1. How many people in your immediate family (parents or siblings) are overweight or obese?

   a. No one is overweight or obese (0 points)
   b. One person (1 point)
   c. Two people (2 points)
   d. Three or more people (3 points)

2. During which periods of your life were you overweight or obese? (Circle all that apply.)

   a. Birth through age 5 (1 point)
   b. Ages 6 to 11 (1 point)
   c. Ages 12 to 13 (1 point))
   d. Ages 14 to 18 (2 points)
   e. Ages 19 to present (2 points)

3. How many times in the last year have you made an effort to lose weight but have had little or no success?

   a. None. I've never thought about it. (0 points)
   b. I've thought about it, but I've never tried hard to lose weight. (1 point)
   c. I have tried 2 to 3 times. (1 point)
   d. I have tried at least once a month. (2 points)
   e. I have tried so many times, I can't remember the number. (3 points)

4. How would you describe your weight right now?

   a. Normal and consistent (1 point)
   b. Normal but difficult to maintain (2 points)
   c. Overweight (3 points)
   d. Obese (4 points)

Total points: __________

Scoring

A score of 5 or higher suggests that you may have several challenges ahead as you begin a weight loss program. The higher your score, the greater the likelihood of challenges.

Your own weight problems may be related, at least in part, to the eating habits and preferences you learned at home, and it may take a conscious effort to change them. If in the past you tried repeatedly to lose weight but returned to your old behaviors, you may have to reframe your thinking.

2 Readiness to Change

Attitudes and Beliefs About Weight Loss

1. What is/are your main reason(s) for wanting to lose weight? (Circle all that apply.)

   a. I want to please someone I know or attract a new person. (0 points)
   b. I want to look great and/or fit into smaller size clothes for an upcoming event (wedding, vacation, date, etc.). (1 point)
   c. Someone I know has had major health problems because of being overweight/obese. (1 point)
   d. I want to improve my health and/or have more energy. (2 points)
   e. I was diagnosed with a health problem (pre-diabetes, diabetes, high blood pressure, etc.) because of being overweight/obese. (2 points)

2. What do you think about your weight and body shape? (Circle all that apply.)

   a. I'm fine with being overweight, and if others don't like it, tough! (0 points)
   b. My weight hurts my energy levels and my performance and holds me back. (1 point)
   c. I feel good about myself, but think I will be happier if I lose some of my weight. (1 point)
   d. I'm self-conscious about my weight and uncomfortable in my skin. (1 point)
   e. I'm really worried that I will have a major health problem if I don't change my behaviors now. (2 points)

Daily Eating Patterns

3. Which of the following statements describes you? (Circle all that apply.)

   a. I think about food several times a day, even when I'm not hungry. (0 point)

   b. There are some foods or snacks that I can't stay away from, and I eat them even when I'm not hungry. (0 point)

   c. I tend to eat more meat and fatty foods and never get enough fruits and veggies. (0 points)

   d. I've thought about the weaknesses in my diet and have some ideas about what I need to do. (1 point)

   e. I haven't really tried to eat a "balanced" diet, but I know that I need to start now. (1 point)

4. When you binge or eat things you shouldn't or too much at one sitting, what are you likely to do? (Circle all that apply.)

   a. Not care and go off of my diet. (0 points)

   b. Feel guilty for a while, but then do it again the next time I am out. (0 points)

   c. Fast for the next day or two to help balance the high consumption day. (0 points)

   d. Plan ahead for next time and have options in mind so that I do not continue to overeat. (1 point)

   e. Acknowledge that I have made a slip and get back on my program the next day. (1 point)

5. On a typical day, what are your eating patterns? (Circle all that apply.)

   a. I skip breakfast and save my calories for lunch and dinner. (0 point)

   b. I never really sit down for a meal. I am a "grazer" and eat whatever I find that is readily available. (0 point)

   c. I try to eat at least five servings of fruits and veggies and restrict saturated fats in my diet. (1 point)

   d. I eat several small meals, trying to be balanced in my portions and getting foods from different food groups. (1 point)

Commitment to Weight Loss and Exercise

6. How would you describe your current support system for helping you lose weight? (Circle all that apply.)

   a. I believe I can do this best by doing it on my own. (0 points)

   b. I am not aware of any sources that can help me. (0 points)

   c. I have two to three friends or family members I can count on to help me. (1 point)

   d. There are counselors on campus with whom I can meet to plan a successful approach to weight loss. (1 point)

   e. I have the resources to join Weight Watchers or other community or online weight loss programs. (1 point)

7. How committed are you to exercising? (Circle all that apply.)

   a. Exercise is uncomfortable, embarrassing, and/or I don't enjoy it. (0 points)

   b. I don't have time to exercise. (0 points)

   c. I'd like to exercise, but I'm not sure how to get started. (1 point)

   d. I've visited my campus recreation center or local gym to explore my options for exercise. (2 points)

   e. There are specific sports or physical activities I do already, and I can plan to do more of them. (2 points)

8. What statement best describes your motivation to start a weight loss/lifestyle change program?

   a. I don't want to start losing weight. (0 points)

   b. I am thinking about it sometime in the distant future. (0 points)

   c. I am considering starting within the next few weeks; I just need to make a plan. (1 point)

   d. I'd like to start in the next few weeks, and I'm working on a plan. (2 points)

   e. I already have a plan in place, and I'm ready to begin tomorrow. (3 points)

Total points: __________

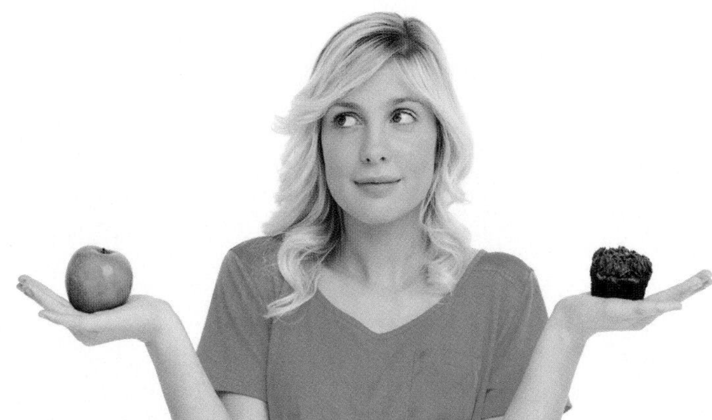

Scoring

A score higher than 8 indicates that you may be ready to change; the higher your score above 8, the more successful you may be. If you scored lower than 8, consider the following:

One of the first steps in making a plan to lose weight is to recognize your strengths and weaknesses and be ready to anticipate challenges. Think about the stages of change model (discussed in Chapter 1) to determine if your current thoughts and attitudes about weight loss reflect a good foundation for beginning a successful weight loss program. Which long-term motivations will you need to successfully lose weight? Which benefits of losing weight motivate you most strongly? Which behavioral changes are you ready to make to address your weight issues?

In order to lose weight, you will need to change your daily eating habits. Overeating (or eating poorly) may be a response to your food attitudes rather than to physical hunger. Poor eating may also reflect your emotional responses toward food, and/or unhealthy dietary choices. To increase your commitment to weight loss and exercise, think of friends or family who can support your efforts to stick to your plan. Also consider the wealth of available resources and where you can go for help. Having a plan and sticking to it will be crucial as you begin your weight loss journey!

Your Plan for Change

The Assess Yourself activity identifies areas of importance in determining your readiness for weight loss. If you wish to lose weight to improve your health, understanding your attitudes about food and exercise will help you succeed in your plan.

Today, you can:

◯ Set "SMART" goals for weight loss and give them a reality check: Are they specific, measurable, achievable, relevant, and time-oriented? For example, rather than aiming to lose 15 pounds this month (which probably wouldn't be healthy or achievable), set a comfortable goal to lose 5 pounds. Realistic goals will encourage weight-loss success by boosting your confidence in your ability to make lifelong healthy changes.

◯ Begin keeping a food log and identifying the triggers that influence your eating habits. Think about what you can do to eliminate or reduce the influence of your two most common food triggers.

Within the next 2 weeks, you can:

◯ Get in the habit of incorporating more fruits, vegetables, and whole grains in your diet and eating less fat. The next time you make dinner, look at the proportions on your plate. If vegetables and whole grains do not take up most of the space, substitute 1 cup of the meat, pasta, or cheese in your meal with 1 cup of legumes, salad greens, or a favorite vegetable. You'll reduce the number of calories while eating the same amount of food!

◯ Aim to incorporate more exercise into your daily routine. Visit your campus rec center or a local gym and familiarize yourself with the equipment and facilities that are available. Try a new machine or sports activity, and experiment until you find a form of exercise you really enjoy.

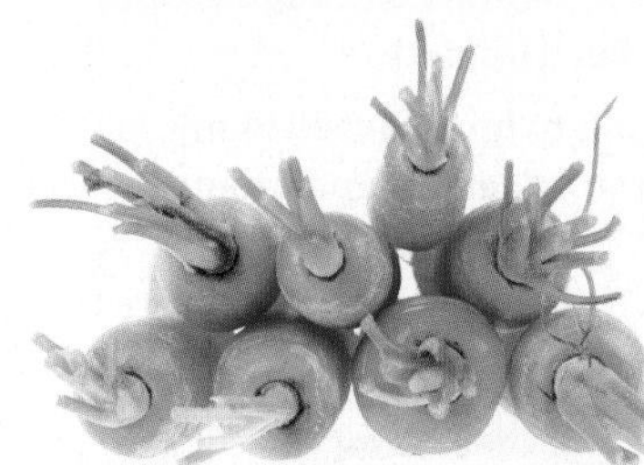

By the end of the semester, you can:

◯ Get in the habit of grocery shopping every week and buying healthy, nutritious foods while avoiding high-fat, high-sugar, or overly processed foods. As you make healthy foods more available and unhealthy foods less available, you'll find it easier to eat better.

◯ Chart your progress and reward yourself as you meet your goals. If your goal is to lose weight and you successfully take off 10 pounds, reward yourself with a new pair of jeans or other article of clothing (which will likely fit better than before!).

How Sensible Are Your Efforts to Be Thin?

An interactive version of this assessment is available online in MasteringHealth.

On one hand, just because you weigh yourself, count calories, or work out every day, don't jump to the conclusion that you have any of the health concerns discussed in this chapter. On the other hand, efforts to lose a few pounds can spiral out of control. To find out whether your efforts to be thin are harmful to you, take the following quiz from the National Eating Disorders Association (NEDA).

1. I constantly calculate numbers of fat grams and calories.	T	F
2. I weigh myself often and find myself obsessed with the number on the scale.	T	F
3. I exercise to burn calories and not for health or enjoyment.	T	F
4. I sometimes feel out of control while eating.	T	F
5. I often go on extreme diets.	T	F
6. I engage in rituals to get me through mealtimes and/or secretly binge.	T	F
7. Weight loss, dieting, and controlling my food intake have become my major concerns.	T	F
8. I feel ashamed, disgusted, or guilty after eating.	T	F
9. I constantly worry about the weight, shape, and/or size of my body.	T	F
10. I feel my identity and value are based on how I look or how much I weigh.	T	F

If any of these statements is true for you, you could be dealing with disordered eating. If so, talk about it! Tell a friend, parent, teacher, coach, youth group leader, doctor, counselor, or nutritionist what you're going through. Check out the NEDA's Sharing with EEEase handout at www.nationaleatingdisorders.org for help planning what to say the first time you talk to someone about your eating and exercise habits.

Source: Reprinted with permission from the National Eating Disorders Association, www.nationaleatingdisorders.org.

Your Plan for Change

The Assess Yourself activity gave you the chance to evaluate your feelings about your body, and to determine whether or not you might be engaging in eating or exercise behaviors that could undermine your health and happiness. Here are some steps you can take to improve your body image, starting today.

Today, you can:

◯ Talk back to the media. Write letters to advertisers and magazines that depict unhealthy and unrealistic body types. Boycott their products or start a blog commenting on harmful body image messages in the media.

◯ Visit www.choosemyplate.gov and create a personalized food plan. Just for today, eat the recommended number of servings from every food group at every meal, and don't count calories!

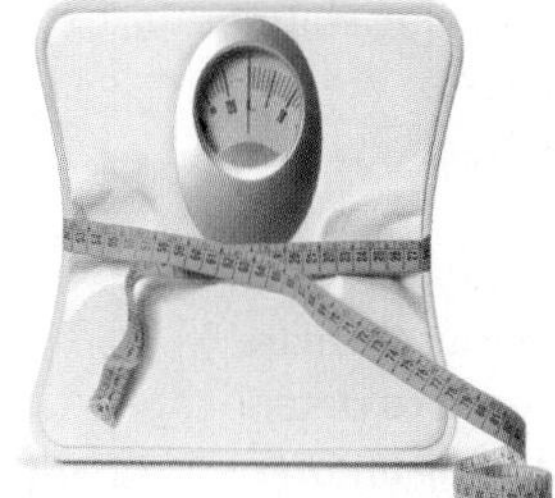

Within the next 2 weeks, you can:

◯ Find a photograph of a person you admire not for his or her appearance, but for his or her contribution to humanity. Paste it up next to your mirror to remind yourself that true beauty comes from within and benefits others.

◯ Start a journal. Each day, record one thing you are grateful for that has nothing to do with your appearance. At the end of each day, record one small thing you did to make someone's world a little brighter.

By the end of the semester, you can:

◯ Establish a group of friends who support you for who you are, not what you look like, and who get the same support from you. Form a group on a favorite social-networking site and keep in touch, especially when you start to feel troubled by self-defeating thoughts or have the urge to engage in unhealthy eating or exercise behaviors.

◯ Borrow from the library or purchase one of the many books on body image now available, and read it!

Summary

To hear an MP3 Tutor session, scan here or visit the Study Area in **MasteringHealth.**

LO 9.1 Overweight, obesity, and weight-related health problems have reached epidemic levels in the United States, largely due to obesogenic behaviors in an obesogenic environment.

LO 9.2 Societal costs from obesity include increased health care costs, lowered worker productivity, low self-esteem, and obesity-related stigma. Individual health risks from overweight and obesity include a variety of chronic diseases.

LO 9.3–9.4 Many factors contribute to risk for obesity, including environmental factors, poverty, education level, genetics, developmental factors, endocrine influences, psychosocial factors, eating cues, metabolic changes, and lifestyle.

LO 9.5–9.6 Percentage of body fat is a reliable indicator for levels of overweight and obesity. *Overweight* is most commonly defined as a BMI of 25 to 29 and *obesity* as a BMI of 30 or greater. Waist circumference is believed to be related to risk for several chronic diseases, particularly type 2 diabetes. Body mass index is one of the most commonly accepted measures of assessing body fat.

LO 9.7–9.9 Sensible eating and exercise offer the best options for weight loss and maintenance. The best diet programs allow you to make healthy choices in real-world settings without sacrificing everything enjoyable. Successful weight management includes making a plan and changing habits.

LO 9.10 Diet pills, surgery, and very-low-calorie diets are drastic measures for weight loss and may carry significant risks.

LO 9.11 To gain weight, increase intake of energy-dense, nutritious foods.

LO 9.12 Negative feelings about one's body can contribute to behaviors that can threaten health. In contrast, a healthy body image can contribute to reduced stress and personal empowerment. Body image disorders affect men and women of all ages. Body image can be affected by culture, media, and individual physiological and psychological factors.

LO 9.13–9.15 Disordered eating and eating disorders such as anorexia nervosa, bulimia nervosa, and binge-eating disorder can lead to serious health problems and even death.

LO 9.16 Although exercise is healthy in moderation, if it becomes a compulsion it can lead to disorders such as muscle dysmorphia and the female athlete triad.

Pop Quiz

Visit MasteringHealth to personalize your study plan with Chapter Review Quizzes and Dynamic Study Modules.

LO 9.3 1. The rate at which your body consumes food energy to sustain basic functions is your
- a. basal metabolic rate.
- b. resting metabolic rate.
- c. body mass index.
- d. set point.

LO 9.5 2. Which of the following statements is *false*?
- a. A slowing basal metabolic rate may contribute to weight gain after age 30.
- b. Hormones are implicated in hunger impulses and eating behavior.
- c. The more muscles you have, the fewer calories you'll burn.
- d. Overweight and obesity can have serious health consequences, even before middle age.

LO 9.6 3. Which of the following statements about BMI is *false*?
- a. BMI is based on height and weight measurements.
- b. BMI is accurate for everyone, including people with high muscle mass.
- c. Children's BMIs are used to determine a percentile ranking among their age peers.
- d. BMI stands for "body mass index."

LO 9.6 4. Which of the following BMI ratings is considered overweight?
- a. 20
- b. 25
- c. 30
- d. 35

LO 9.6 5. Which of the following body circumferences is most strongly associated with risk of heart disease and diabetes?
- a. Hip circumference
- b. Chest circumference
- c. Waist circumference
- d. Thigh circumference

LO 9.7 6. One pound of additional body fat is created through consuming how many extra calories?
- a. 1,500 calories
- b. 3,500 calories
- c. 5,000 calories
- d. 7,000 calories

LO 9.7 7. To lose weight, you must establish a(n)
- a. negative caloric balance.
- b. energy balance.
- c. positive caloric balance.
- d. set point.

LO 9.9 8. Successful, healthy weight loss is characterized by
- a. a lifelong pattern of healthful eating and exercise.
- b. cutting out fats and carbohydrates.
- c. never eating foods considered bad for you.
- d. a pattern of repeatedly losing and regaining weight.

LO 9.12 9. Which of the following is not a contributor to negative body image?
- a. Idealized media images of celebrities
- b. Increases in portion sizes
- c. Cultural attitudes about body ideals
- d. Neurotransmitter regulation in the brain

LO 9.15 10. Which of the following eating disorders includes compensatory behavior in its definition?
- a. Anorexia nervosa
- b. Bulimia nervosa
- c. Binge-eating disorder
- d. Muscle dysmorphia

Answers to these questions can be found on page A-1. If you answered a question incorrectly, review the module identified by the Learning Outcome. For even more study tools, visit MasteringHealth.

Fitness 10

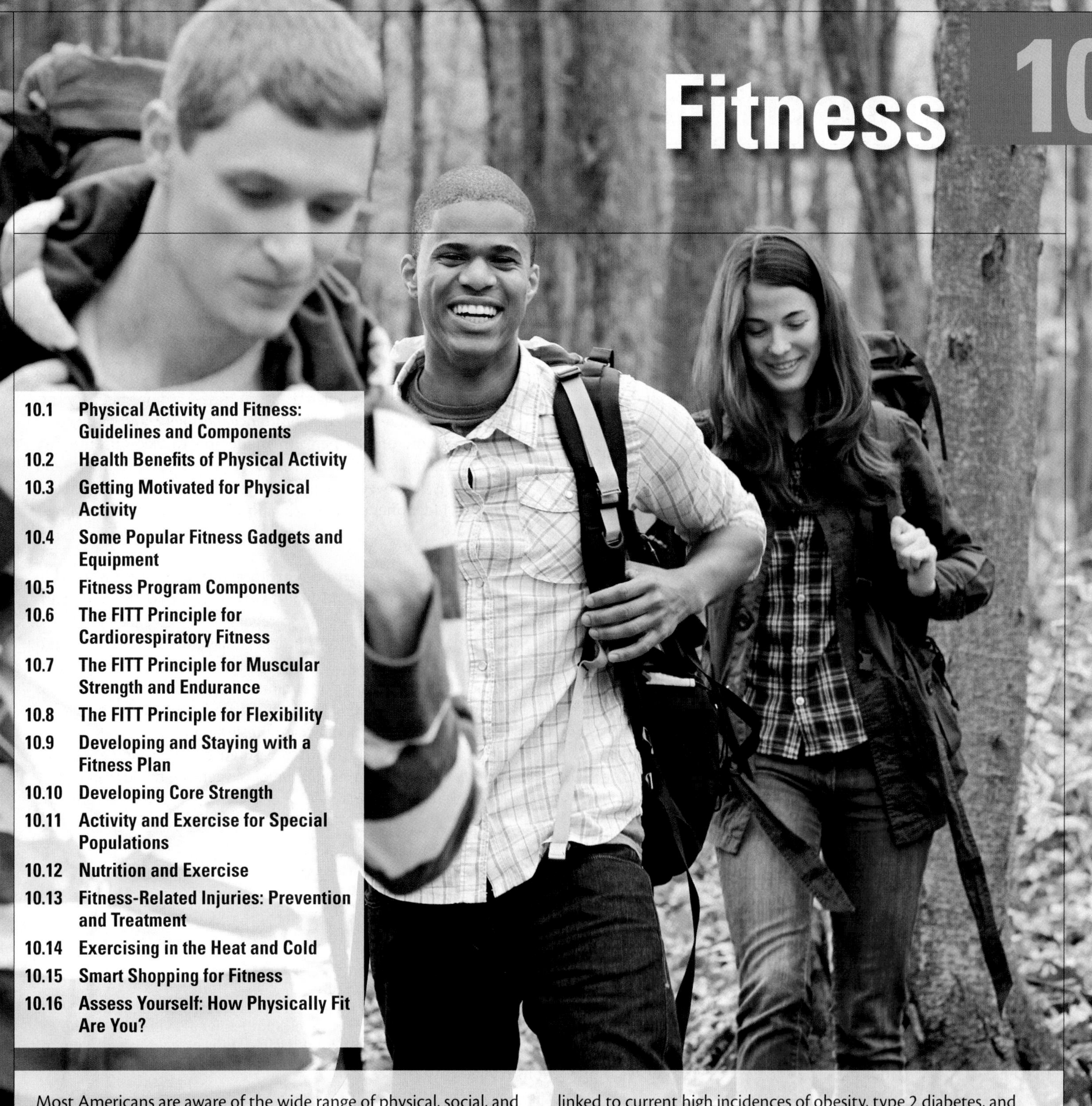

Most Americans are aware of the wide range of physical, social, and mental health benefits of physical activity—and that they should be more physically active. Physiological changes resulting from regular physical activity reduce the likelihood of coronary artery disease, high blood pressure, type 2 diabetes, obesity, and other chronic diseases. Engaging in physical activity regularly also helps to control stress and increase self-esteem.

Despite these benefits, however, 23.1 percent of American adults engage in no leisure-time physical activity[1]—a situation linked to current high incidences of obesity, type 2 diabetes, and other chronic and mental health diseases.[2]

In general, college students are more physically active than are older adults, but a recent survey indicated that 56 percent of college women and 49.3 percent of college men do not meet recommended guidelines for engaging in moderate or vigorous physical activities.[3]

College is a great time to develop attitudes and behaviors that can increase the quality and quantity of your life. This chapter offers knowledge and strategies to help you get moving.

10.1 Physical Activity and Fitness: Guidelines and Components

learning outcome

10.1 Distinguish among physical activity for health, for fitness, and for performance.

Physical activity is any body movement that works your muscles, uses more energy than when resting, and enhances health.[4] Physical activities can vary by intensity. For example, walking to class on flat ground typically requires little effort, while walking to class uphill is more intense and harder to do. The three general categories of physical activity are defined by their purpose: physical activity for health, physical activity for physical fitness, and physical activity for performance.

Exercise is defined as planned, structured, and repetitive bodily movement done to improve or maintain one or more components of physical fitness, such as cardiorespiratory endurance, muscular strength or endurance, or flexibility. Although all exercise is physical activity, not all physical activity would be considered exercise. For example, walking from your car to class is physical activity, whereas going for a brisk 30-minute walk is considered exercise.

Physical Activity for Health

Researchers have found that "there is irrefutable evidence of the effectiveness of regular physical activity in the primary and secondary prevention of several chronic diseases (e.g., cardiovascular disease, diabetes, cancer, hypertension, obesity, depression, and osteoporosis)."[5] Adding more physical activity to your day can benefit your health. In fact, if the number of adults meeting the 2008 Physical Activity Guidelines (Table 10.1) increased by 25 percent, there would be 1.3 million fewer deaths per year and the life expectancy would increase. In the United States, physical inactivity is responsible for 6.7 percent of the cases of coronary heart disease, 8.3 percent cases of type 2 diabetes, 12.4 percent cases of breast cancer, and 12.0 percent cases of colon cancer, and it accounts for approximately 10.8 percent of deaths.[6]

Physical Activity for Fitness

Physical fitness refers to a set of health- and performance-related attributes. The health-related attributes—cardiorespiratory fitness, muscular strength and endurance, flexibility, and body composition—allow one to perform moderate- to vigorous-intensity physical activities on a regular basis without getting too tired and with energy left over to handle physical or mental emergencies. Figure 10.1 identifies the major health-related components of physical fitness.

Cardiorespiratory Fitness **Cardiorespiratory fitness** is the ability of the heart, lungs, and blood vessels to supply the body with oxygen efficiently. The primary category of physical activity known to improve cardiorespiratory fitness is **aerobic exercise**. The word *aerobic* means "with oxygen" and describes any exercise that requires oxygen to make energy for prolonged activity. Aerobic activities such as swimming, cycling, and jogging are among the best exercises for improving or maintaining cardiorespiratory fitness.

Cardiorespiratory fitness is measured by determining **aerobic capacity** (or **power**), the volume of oxygen the muscles consume during exercise. Maximal aerobic power (VO_{2max}) is defined as the

TABLE 10.1 **Physical Activity Guidelines for Americans**

Key Guidelines for Health*	For Additional Fitness or Weight Loss Benefits*	PLUS
150 min/week moderate intensity OR 75 min/week of vigorous intensity OR Equivalent combination of moderate and vigorous intensity (i.e., 100 min moderate intensity + 25 min vigorous intensity)	300 min/week moderate intensity OR 150 min/week of vigorous intensity OR Equivalent combination of moderate and vigorous intensity (i.e., 200 min moderate intensity + 50 min vigorous intensity) OR More than the previously described amounts	Muscle strengthening activities for *all* the major muscle groups at least 2 days/week

*Accumulate this physical activity in sessions of 10 minutes or more at one time.
Source: Office of Disease Prevention and Health Promotion, U.S. Department of Health and Human Services, *2008 Physical Activity Guidelines for Americans: Be Active, Healthy, and Happy!* ODPHP Publication no. U0036 (Washington, DC: U.S. Department of Health and Human Services, 2008), available at www.health.gov.

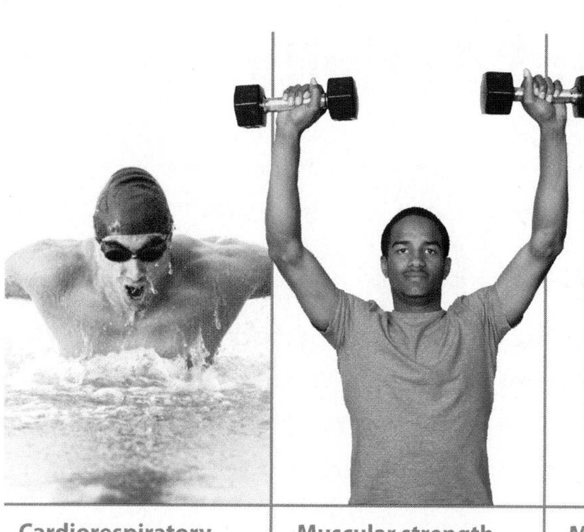

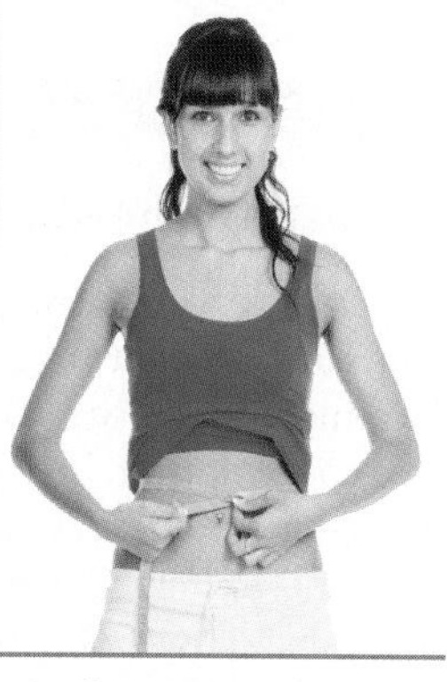

Cardiorespiratory fitness	**Muscular strength**	**Muscular endurance**	**Flexibility**	**Body composition**
Ability to sustain aerobic whole-body activity for a prolonged period of time	Maximum force able to be exerted by single contraction of a muscle or muscle group	Ability to perform high-intensity muscle contractions repeatedly without fatiguing	Ability to move joints freely through their full range of motion	The amount and relative proportions and distribution of fat mass and fat-free mass in the body

Figure 10.1 Components of Physical Fitness

maximal volume of oxygen that the muscles consume during exercise. The most common measure of maximal aerobic capacity is a walk or run test on a treadmill. For greatest accuracy, this is done in a lab and requires special equipment and technicians to measure the precise amount of oxygen entering and exiting the body during the exercise session. Submaximal tests can be used to get a more general sense of cardiorespiratory fitness; one such test, the 1-mile walk test, is described in the Assess Yourself module at the end of this chapter.

Muscular Strength **Muscular strength** refers to the amount of force a muscle or group of muscles is capable of exerting in one contraction. A common way to assess the strength of a particular muscle group is to measure the maximum amount of weight you can move one time (and no more), or your one repetition maximum (1 RM).

Muscular Endurance **Muscular endurance** is the ability of a muscle or group of muscles to exert force repeatedly without fatigue or the ability to sustain a muscular contraction. The more repetitions of an endurance activity (e.g., push-ups) you can perform successfully, or the longer you can hold a certain position (e.g., wall sit), the greater your muscular endurance. General muscular endurance is often measured using the number of curl-ups an individual can do; this test is described in the Assess Yourself module at the end of this chapter.

Flexibility **Flexibility** refers to the range of motion, or the amount of movement possible, at a particular joint or series of joints: the greater the range of motion, the greater the flexibility. One of the most common measures of general flexibility is the sit-and-reach test, described in the Assess Yourself module at the end of this chapter.

Body Composition **Body composition**, the fifth and final component of a comprehensive fitness program, describes the relative proportions and distribution of fat and lean (muscle, bone, water, organs) tissues in the body.

Physical Activity for Performance

Physical fitness for athletes involves attributes that improve their ability to perform athletic tasks. These attributes can also help general exercisers increase fitness levels and their ability to perform daily tasks. These skill-related components of physical fitness (also called sports skills) are the following: *agility*, *balance*, *coordination*, *power*, *speed*, and *reaction time*. Participating regularly in any sport or activity can improve your sport skills, as can performing drills that mimic a sport-specific skill.

check yourself

- **What are the differences between physical activity for health, for fitness, and for performance?**
- **What is the difference between exercise and physical activity?**
- **What are the core components of physical fitness?**

10.2 Health Benefits of Physical Activity

learning outcome

10.2 List the health benefits of physical activity.

The first step in starting a physical fitness program is identifying your goals for that program. You should next consider the things that might get in the way of your achieving those goals. Once you have contemplated these factors, you are ready to create an individual exercise program to meet your physical fitness goals. Before we start, and to help you get motivated, let's take a look at the many physical and psychological benefits of physical activity.

What Are the Health Benefits of Regular Physical Activity?

Regular participation in physical activity improves more than 50 different physiological, metabolic, and psychological aspects of human life. Figure 10.2 summarizes some of these major health-related benefits.

Reduced Risk of Cardiovascular Diseases Aerobic exercise is good for the heart and lungs and reduces risk for heart-related diseases. It improves blood flow and eases performance of everyday tasks. Regular exercise makes the cardiovascular and respiratory systems more efficient by strengthening the heart muscle, enabling more blood to be pumped with each stroke, and increasing the number of *capillaries* (small blood vessels that allow gas exchange between blood and surrounding tissues) in trained skeletal muscles, which supply more blood to working muscles. Exercise also improves the respiratory system by increasing the amount of oxygen inhaled and distributed to body tissues.[7]

Regular physical activity can reduce hypertension, or chronic high blood pressure—a form of cardiovascular disease and a significant risk factor for coronary heart disease and stroke.[8] Regular aerobic exercise also reduces low-density lipoproteins (LDLs, or "bad" cholesterol), total cholesterol, and triglycerides (a blood fat), thus reducing plaque buildup in the arteries while increasing high-density lipoproteins (HDLs, or "good" cholesterol), which are associated with lower risk for coronary artery disease.[9]

Reduced Risk of Metabolic Syndrome and Type 2 Diabetes Regular physical activity reduces the risk of metabolic syndrome, a combination of heart disease and diabetes risk factors that produces a synergistic increase in risk.[10] Specifically, metabolic syndrome includes high blood pressure, abdominal obesity, low levels of HDLs, high levels of triglycerides, and impaired glucose tolerance.[11] Regular participation in moderate-intensity physical activities reduces risk for these factors both individually and collectively.[12]

Research indicates that a healthy dietary intake combined with sufficient physical activity could prevent many current cases of type 2 diabetes.[13] In a major national clinical trial, researchers found that exercising 150 minutes per week and eating fewer calories and less fat could prevent or delay the onset of type 2 diabetes.[14]

30 minutes of physical activity a day—all at once or in three 10-minute sessions—provides health benefits.

Reduced Cancer Risk After decades of research, most cancer epidemiologists believe that the majority of cancers are preventable and can be avoided by healthier lifestyle and environmental choices.[15] In fact, a report recently released by the World Cancer Research Fund in conjunction with the American Institute for Cancer Research stated that one-third of cancers could be prevented by being physically active and eating well.[16]

Regular physical activity appears to lower the risk for some specific types of cancer, particularly colon and rectal cancer.[17] Regular exercise is also associated with lower risk for breast cancer. Research on exercise and breast cancer risk has found that the earlier in life a woman starts to exercise, the lower her breast cancer risk.[18]

Improved Bone Mass and Reduced Risk of Osteoporosis A common affliction for older people is *osteoporosis*, a disease characterized by low bone mass and deterioration of bone tissue, which increases fracture risk. Regular weight-bearing and strength-building physical activities are recommended to maintain bone health and prevent osteoporotic fractures. Although both men and women can be affected by osteoporosis, it is more common in women. Women (like men) have much to gain by remaining physically active as they age—bone mass levels are significantly higher among active individuals than among sedentary persons.[19] However, it appears that the full bone-related benefits of physical activity can be achieved only with sufficient hormone levels (estrogen in women; testosterone in men) and adequate calcium, vitamin D, and total caloric intakes.[20]

Improved Weight Control For many people, the desire to lose weight or maintain a healthy weight is the main reason for physical activity. Physical activity requires your body to generate energy through calorie expenditure; if calories expended exceed calories consumed over a span of time, the net result will be weight loss.

Physical activity also increases metabolic rate, keeping it elevated for several hours following vigorous physical activities. This increase in metabolic rate can lead to body composition changes that favor weight management. Increased physical activity also improves your chances of maintaining weight loss. If you are currently at a healthy body weight, regular physical activity can prevent significant weight gain.[21]

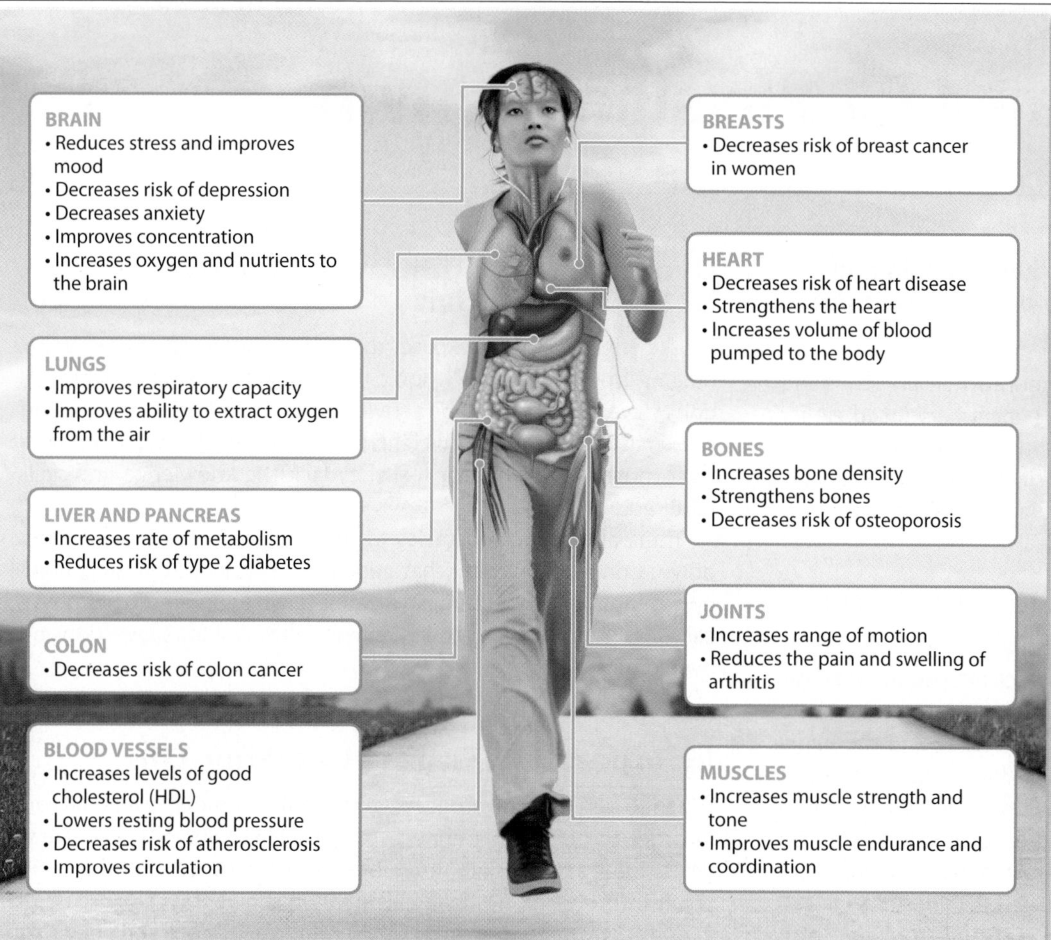

Figure 10.2 Some Health Benefits of Regular Exercise

VIDEO TUTOR
Health Benefits of Regular Exercise

Improved Immunity Research shows that regular moderate-intensity physical activity reduces individual susceptibility to disease.[22] Just how physical activity alters immunity is not well understood. We do know that moderate-intensity physical activity temporarily increases the number of white blood cells (WBCs), which are responsible for fighting infection.[23] Often the relationship of physical activity to immunity, or more specifically to disease susceptibility, is described as a J-shaped curve. In other words, susceptibility to disease decreases with moderate activity, but then increases as you move to more extreme levels of physical activity or exercise or if you continue to exercise without adequate recovery time.[24] Athletes engaging in marathon-type events or very intense physical training programs have been shown to be at greater risk for upper respiratory tract infections (colds and flu).[25]

Improved Back Strength Regular whole-body exercise, as well as exercises targeting the specific muscles of the back (and the rest of the core), create a strong platform for the entire body. A strong and healthy back helps you maintain proper posture and avoid posture-related stress in the neck, shoulders, hips, knees, and ankles. It also gives you a good foundation for a range of exercise and reduces the likelihood of injury.

Improved Mental Health and Stress Management Most people who engage in regular physical activity are likely to notice the psychological benefits, such as feeling better about oneself and an overall sense of well-being. Although these mental health benefits are difficult to quantify, they are frequently mentioned as reasons for continuing to be physically active.

Physical activity contributes to mental health in several ways. Learning new skills, developing increased ability and capacity in recreational activities, and sticking with a physical activity plan all improve self-esteem. In addition, regular physical activity can improve a person's physical appearance, further increasing self-esteem.

Regular aerobic activity can improve the way the body handles stress through its effect on neurotransmitters associated with mood enhancement. Physical activity might also help the body recover from the stress response more quickly as fitness increases.[26]

Increasing evidence suggests that regular physical activity improves cognitive function across the life span. Research has associated regular activity with improved academic and standardized test performance in school.[27] Regular aerobic activity has also been associated with improved function in adults and with the prevention and improvement of dementia in adults.[28]

Longer Life Span Experts have long debated the relationship between physical activity and longevity. Several studies indicate significant decreases in long-term health risk and increases in years lived, particularly among those who have several risk factors and who use physical activity as a means of risk reduction. Results from a study of nearly a million participants showed that the greatest benefits from physical activity occurred in sedentary individuals who added a little physical activity to their lives, with additional benefits added as physical activity levels were increased.[29]

check yourself

- **What are five health benefits of physical activity?**

10.3 Getting Motivated for Physical Activity

learning **outcome**

10.3 Explain factors to consider when choosing an exercise activity and ways to overcome common obstacles to physical activity.

There are many reasons for wanting to be more physically active and physically fit, including the many health benefits discussed earlier in this text. Taking some time to reflect on your personal circumstances, goals, and desires regarding physical fitness will probably make it easier for you to come up with a plan you can stick to.

What If I Have Been Inactive for a While?

If you have been physically inactive for the past few months or longer, first make sure that your physician clears you for exercise. Consider consulting a personal trainer or fitness instructor to help you get started. In this phase of your fitness program, the *initial conditioning stage*, you may begin at levels lower than those recommended for physical fitness. Starting slowly will ease you into a workout regime with a minimum of soreness. For example, you might start your cardiorespiratory program by simply moving more and reducing your sedentary time each day. Take the stairs instead of the elevator, walk farther from your car to the store, and plan for organized movement each day, such as a 10- to 15-minute walk. In addition, you can start your muscle fitness program with simple body weight exercises, emphasizing proper technique and body alignment before adding any resistance.

Overcoming Common Obstacles to Physical Activity

People offer a variety of excuses to explain why they do not exercise, ranging from personal ("I don't have time") to environmental ("I don't have a safe place to be active"). Some people may be reluctant to exercise if they are overweight, are embarrassed to work out with their more "fit" friends, or feel they lack the knowledge and skills required.

Think about your obstacles to physical activity and write them down. Consider anything that gets in your way of exercising, however minor. Once you honestly evaluate why you are not as physically active as you want to be, review Table 10.2 for suggestions on overcoming your hurdles.

Incorporating Fitness into Your Life

When designing your program, you should consider several factors in order to boost your chances of achieving your physical fitness goals. Some activities are more intense or vigorous than others and result in more calories used; Figure 10.3 shows the caloric cost of various activities when done for 30 minutes. Choose activities that are appropriate for you, that you genuinely like doing, and that are convenient. For example, you might choose jogging because you like to run and there are beautiful trails nearby, rather than swimming, since you do not really like the water and the pool is difficult to get to. Likewise, choose activities suitable for your current fitness level. If you are overweight or obese and have not exercised in months, do not sign up for the advanced aerobics classes. Start slow, plan fun activities, and progress to more challenging activities as your physical fitness improves. You may choose to simply walk more in an attempt to achieve the recommended goal of 10,000 steps per day; keep track with

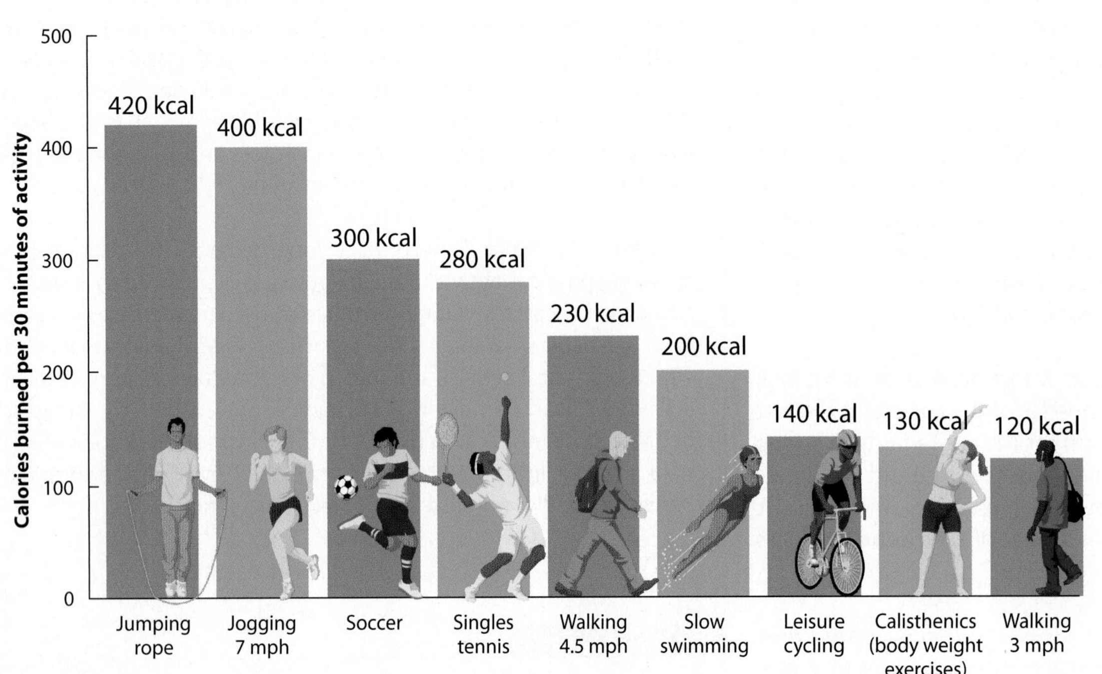

Figure 10.3 Calories Burned by Different Activities
The harder you exercise, the more energy you expend. Estimated calories burned for various moderate and vigorous activities are listed for a 30-minute bout of activity.

TABLE 10.2 Overcoming Obstacles to Physical Activity

Obstacle	Possible Solution
Lack of time	• Look at your schedule. Where can you find 30-minute time slots? Perhaps you need to focus on shorter times (10 minutes or more) throughout the day. • Multitask. Read while riding an exercise bike or listen to lectures or podcasts while walking. • Be physically active during your lunch and study breaks as well as between classes. Skip rope or throw a Frisbee with a friend. • Select activities that require less time, such as brisk walking or jogging. • Ride your bike to class, or park (or get off the bus) farther from your destination.
Social influence	• Invite family and friends to be active with you. • Join a class to meet new people. • Explain the importance of exercise and your commitment to physical activity to people who may not support your efforts. • Find a role model to support your efforts. • Plan for physically active dates—go dancing or bowling.
Lack of motivation, willpower, or energy	• Schedule your workout time just as you would any other important commitment. • Enlist the help of an exercise partner to make you accountable for working out. • Give yourself an incentive. • Schedule your workouts when you feel most energetic. • Remind yourself that exercise gives you more energy. • Get things ready for your workout; for example, if you choose to walk in the morning, set out your walking clothes the night before, or pack your gym bag before going to bed.
Lack of resources	• Select an activity that requires minimal equipment, such as walking, jogging, jumping rope, or calisthenics. • Identify inexpensive resources on campus or in the community. • Use active forms of transportation. • Take advantage of no-cost opportunities, such as playing catch in the park/green space on campus.

Source: Adapted from National Center for Chronic Disease Prevention and Health Promotion, "How Can I Overcome Barriers to Physical Activity?," Updated February 2011, www.cdc.gov.

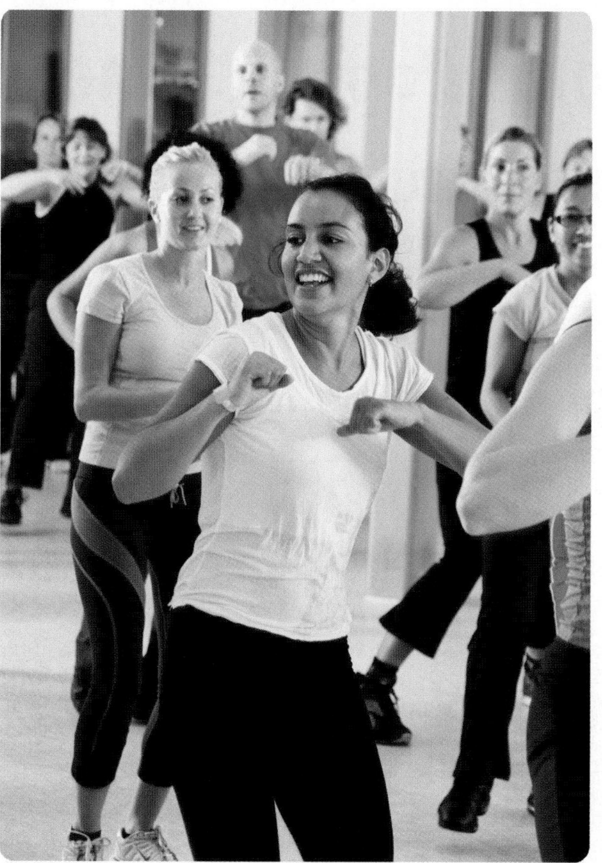

How can I motivate myself to be more physically active?

One great way to motivate yourself is to sign up for an exercise class. Find something that interests you—dance, yoga, aerobics, martial arts, acrobatics—and get yourself involved. The structure, schedule, social interaction, and challenge of learning a new skill can be terrific motivators that make exercising and being physically active exciting and fun.

a pedometer (or step counter; see Table 10.3 for more on this handy gadget and other fitness equipment you may consider purchasing or using at a health club). Try to make exercise a part of your routine by incorporating it into something you already have to do—such as getting to class or work.

check yourself

- **What are some common obstacles people face when deciding to be more physically active?**
- **How can these obstacles be overcome?**
- **What factors should you consider when choosing an exercise activity?**

10.4 Some Popular Fitness Gadgets and Equipment

learning outcome

10.4 **Identify common types of fitness equipment and their uses.**

TABLE 10.3 Some Popular Fitness Gadgets and Equipment

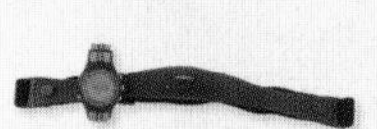 Heart rate monitor	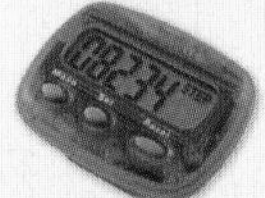 Pedometer	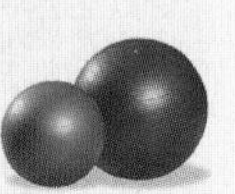 Stability ball	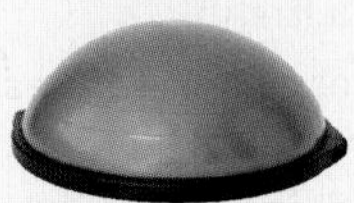 Balance Board	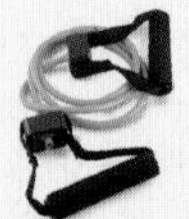 Resistance band	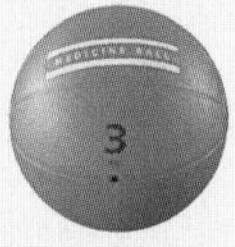 Medicine ball
Chest strap with watch device that measures heart rate during training. • Instant feedback about intensity of your workout. • Strap can be uncomfortable. Cost: $50–$200	Battery-operated device, usually worn on belt, that measures steps taken. Some models also monitor calories, distance, and speed. • Great motivation and feedback. • Must be calibrated for height, weight, and stride length. Cost: $25–$50	Ball made of burst-resistant vinyl used for strengthening core muscles or improving flexibility. • Balls must be inflated correctly to be most effective. Cost: $25–$50	Board with rounded bottom used to improve balance, core muscle strength, and flexibility. • Great for improving agility, coordination, reaction skills, and ankle strength. • Can be difficult for new users. Cost: $40–$80	Rubber or elastic material, sometimes with handles, used to build muscular strength and endurance or for flexibility. • Lightweight, durable, and portable. Cost: $5–$15	Heavy ball, about 14 inces in diameter, used in rehabilitation and strength training. Weight varies from 2–25 lb. • Can be used in plyometric training and to develop core strength. • If used incorrectly, risk of lower back injuries. Cost: $10–$150

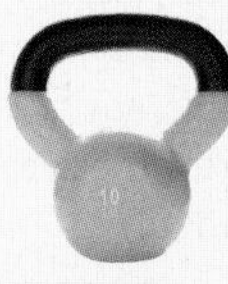 Kettlebell	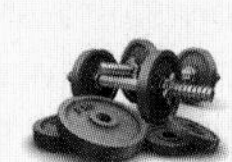 Free Weights	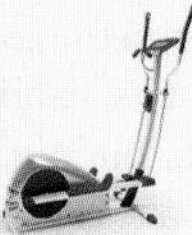 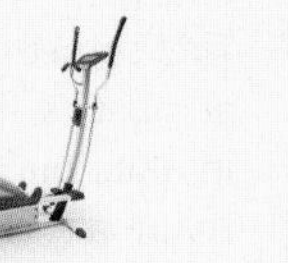 Elliptical Trainer	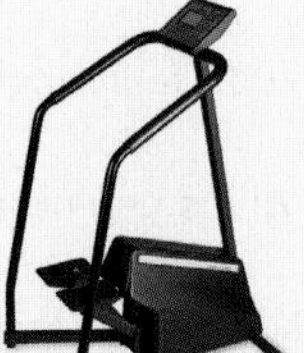 Stair Climber	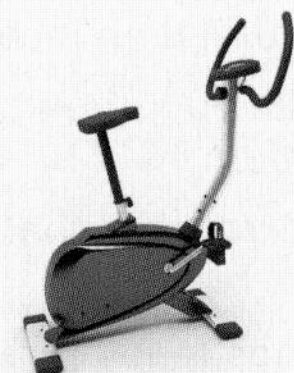 Stationary Bike	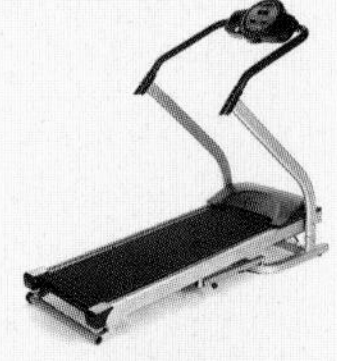 Treadmill
Heavy ball with a handle used for full body muscular strength and endurance exercises. Weight varies from 5 to 100 lb. • Movements can be complex; if used incorrectly, potential for lower back and/or wrist injuries. Cost: $10–$150	Dumbbells or barbells, often with adjustable weight. • Build muscular strength and endurance. • Potential for injury with incorrect form; concentrate on alignment and core strength. Cost: $10–$300	Stationary exercise machine that simulates walking or running without impact on bones and joints. Some include arm movements. • Nonimpact; less wear and tear on the joints and risk of shin splints. Cost: $300–$4,000	Stationary exercise machine that provides low-impact lower body workout by stair climbing. • Nonimpact; less wear and tear on the joints and risk of shin splints. • Various programs are available. Cost: $200–$3,000	Lower body exercise machine designed to simulate bike riding. • Generally easy to use; does not require balance. • Comes with varied resistance programs. • Recumbent styles offer less strain on back and knees. Cost: $200–$2,000	Exercise machine for walking or running on a moving platform. • Generally easy to use; comes with emergency shutoff. • Lower impact on joints than running on most pavements. Cost: $500–$4,000

check yourself

- **What are five types of fitness equipment? Which would you be likely to use and why?**

10.5 Fitness Program Components

learning **outcome**

10.5 Describe how to set SMART goals and list the parts of the FITT principle.

Set SMART Goals

Your physical fitness goals and objectives should be both achievable and in line with what you truly want. To set successful goals, try using the *SMART* system. SMART goals are **s**pecific, **m**easurable, **a**ction-oriented, **r**ealistic, and **t**ime-oriented. A vague goal would be "Improve fitness by exercising more." A SMART goal would be:

- *Specific*—"I'll participate in a resistance training program that targets all of the major muscle groups 3–5 days per week."
- *Measurable*—"I'll improve my fitness classification to average."
- *Action-oriented*—"I'll meet with a personal trainer to learn how to safely do resistance exercises and to plan a workout."
- *Realistic*—"I'll increase the weight I can lift by 20 percent."
- *Time-oriented*—"I'll try my new weight program for 8 weeks, then reassess."

Use the FITT Principle

The **FITT (frequency, intensity, time, and type)** principle shown in Figure 10.4 can be used to devise a workout plan. To achieve the desired level of fitness, consider the following elements:

- **Frequency** refers to how often you must exercise.
- **Intensity** refers to how hard your workout must be.
- **Time**, or *duration*, refers to how many minutes or repetitions of an exercise are required per session.
- **Type** refers to the kind of exercises performed.

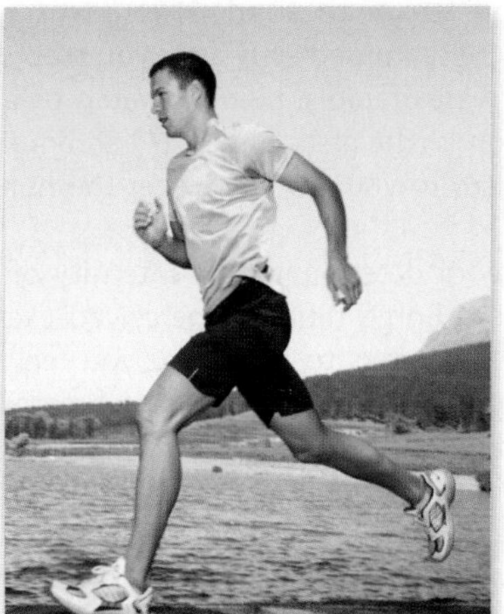
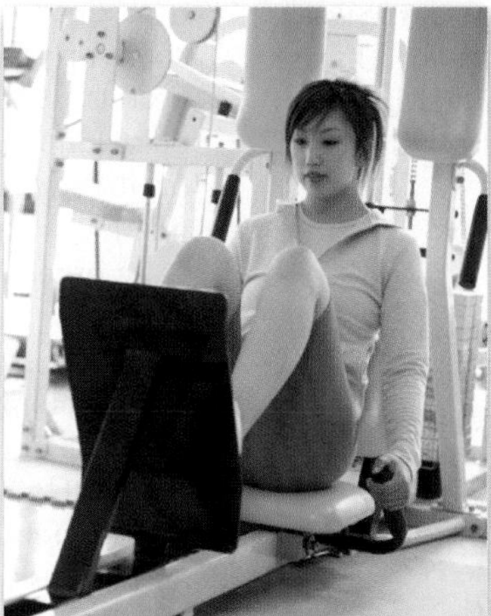
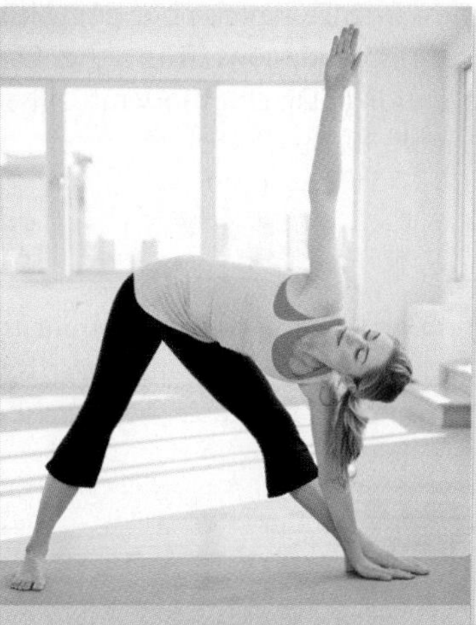

	Cardiorespiratory Endurance	Muscular Fitness	Flexibility
Frequency	3–5 days per week	2–3 days per week	Minimally 2–3 days per week
Intensity	64%–96% of maximum heart rate	60%–80% of 1 RM	To the point of mild tension
Time	20–60 minutes	8–10 exercises, 2–4 sets, 8–12 reps	10–30 seconds per stretch, 2–4 reps
Type	Any rhythmic, continuous, large muscle group activity	Resistance training (with body weight and/or external resistance) for all major muscle groups	Stretching, dance, or yoga exercises for all major muscle groups

Figure 10.4 The FITT Principle Applied to Cardiorespiratory Fitness, Muscular Strength and Endurance, and Flexibility

check yourself

- **What is an example of a SMART goal for fitness?**
- **What are the four parts of the FITT principle?**

10.6 The FITT Principle for Cardiorespiratory Fitness

learning outcome

10.6 List the FITT requirements for cardiorespiratory fitness.

The most effective aerobic exercises for building cardiorespiratory fitness are total-body activities involving the large muscle groups of your body. The FITT prescription for cardiorespiratory fitness includes 3 to 5 days per week of vigorous, rhythmic, continuous activity, at 64 to 95 percent of your estimated maximal heart rate, for 20 to 60 minutes.[30]

Frequency

To improve your cardiorespiratory fitness, you must exercise vigorously at least three times a week or moderately at least five times a week. If you are a newcomer to exercise, you can still make improvements by doing less intense exercise but doing it more days a week, following the recommendations from the Centers for Disease Control and Prevention (CDC) for moderate physical activity 5 days a week (refer to Table 10.1).

Intensity

The most common methods used to determine the intensity of cardiorespiratory endurance exercises are target heart rate, rating of perceived exertion, and the talk test. The exercise intensity required to improve cardiorespiratory endurance is a heart rate between 64 and 96 percent of your maximum heart rate. To calculate this target **heart rate**, first estimate your maximal heart rate with the formula 206.9 − (0.67 × age). Following is an example based on a 20-year-old. Substitute your age to determine your target heart rate training range, then multiply by 0.64 and 0.94 to determine the lower and upper limits of your target range. Figure 10.5 shows a range of target heart rates.

1. 206.9 − (0.67 × 20) = 193.5 (target heart rate for a 20-year-old)
2. 193.5 × 0.64 = 123.8 (lower target limit)
3. 193.5 × 0.94 = 181.89 (upper target limit)

Target range = 124–182 beats per minute

Take your pulse during your workout to determine how close you are to your target heart rate. Lightly place your index and middle fingers (not your thumb) over one of the major arteries in your neck, or on the artery on the inside of your wrist (Figure 10.6). Start counting your pulse immediately after you stop exercising, as your heart rate decreases rapidly. Using a watch or a clock, take your pulse for 6 seconds (the first pulse is "0") and multiply this number by 10 (add a zero to your count) to get the number of beats per minute.

Another way of determining the intensity of cardiorespiratory exercise is to use Borg's rating of perceived exertion (RPE) scale. Perceived exertion refers to how hard you feel you are working, which you might base on your heart rate, breathing rate, sweating, and level of fatigue. This scale uses a rating from 6 (no exertion at all) to 20 (maximal exertion). An RPE of 12 to 16 is generally recommended for training the cardiorespiratory system.

The easiest method of measuring cardiorespiratory exercise intensity is the "talk test." A "moderate" level of exercise (heart rate at 64 to 76 percent of maximum) is a conversational level of exercise. At this level you are able to talk with a partner while exercising.

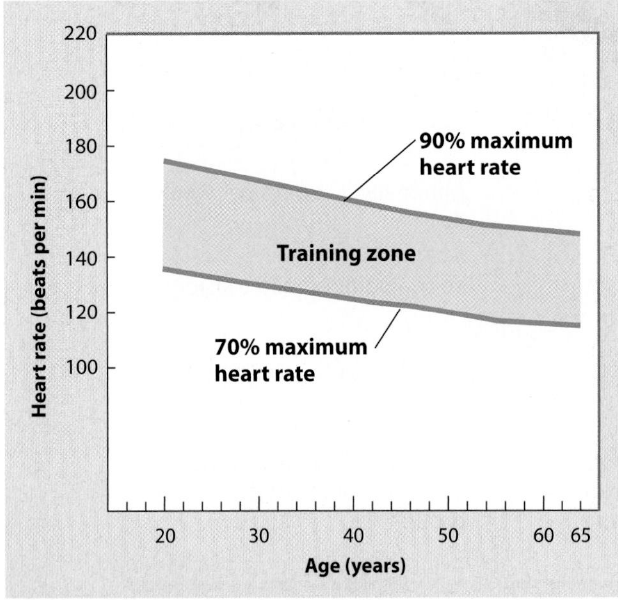

Figure 10.5 Target Heart Rate Ranges
These ranges are based on calculating the maximum heart rate as 206.9 − (0.67 × age), and the training zone as 64 percent to 96 percent of maximum heart rate. Individuals with low fitness levels should start below or at the low end of these ranges.

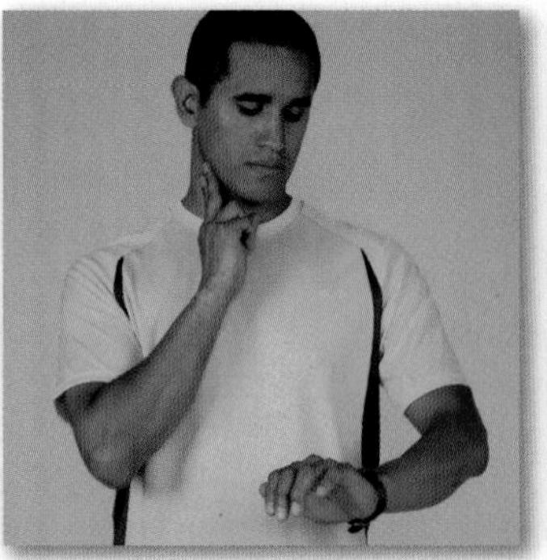

(a) Carotid pulse

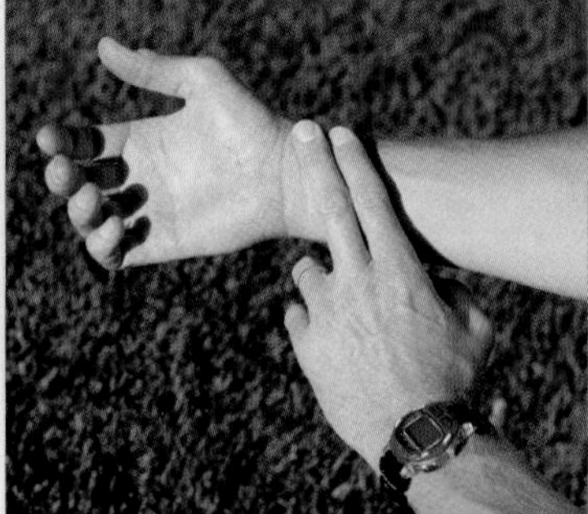

(b) Radial pulse

Figure 10.6 Taking a Pulse
Palpation of the carotid (neck) or radial (wrist) artery is a simple way of determining heart rate.

If you can talk but only in short fragments and not sentences, you may be at a "vigorous" level of exercise (heart rate at 76 to 96 percent of maximum). If you are breathing so hard that talking is difficult, the intensity of your exercise may be too high. Conversely, if you are able to sing or laugh heartily while exercising, the intensity of your exercise is insufficient for maintaining and/or improving cardiorespiratory fitness.

Time

For cardiorespiratory fitness benefits, the American College of Sports Medicine (ACSM) recommends that vigorous activities be performed for at least 20 minutes at a time, and moderate activities for at least 30 minutes.[31] You can also set a time goal for the entire week, as long as you keep your sessions to at least 10 minutes (150 minutes per week for moderate intensity, and 75 minutes per week for vigorous intensity).

Type

Any sort of rhythmic, continuous, and vigorous physical activity that can be done for 20 or more minutes will improve cardiorespiratory fitness. Examples include walking briskly, cycling, jogging, fitness classes, and swimming.

Incorporating Cardiorespiratory Fitness into Daily Life

Before we became a car culture, much of our transportation was human powered. Bicycling and walking historically were important means of transportation and recreation in the United States. These modes not only helped keep people in good physical shape, but they also had little or no impact on the environment. Even in the first few decades after the automobile started to be popularized, people continued to get around under their own power. Since World War II, however, the development of automobile-oriented communities has led to a steady decline of bicycling and walking. Currently, only about 10 percent of trips are made by foot or bike.[32]

The more we use our cars to get around, the more congested our roads, the more polluted our air, and the more sedentary our lives become. That is why many people are now embracing a movement toward more active transportation. *Active transportation* means getting out of your car and using your own power to get from place to place—whether walking, riding a bike, skateboarding, or roller skating. Each of these activities can also be incorporated into your life as a form of exercise that contributes to cardiorespiratory fitness.

The following are just a few of the many reasons to make active transportation a bigger part of your life:[33]

- **You will be adding more exercise into your daily routine.** People who walk, bike, or use other active forms of transportation to complete errands are physically active.
- **Walking or biking can save you money.** With rising gas prices and parking fees, in addition to increasing car maintenance and insurance costs, fewer automobile trips could add up to considerable savings. During the course of a year, regular bicycle commuters who ride 5 miles to work can save about $500 on fuel and more than $1,000 on other expenses related to driving.
- **Walking or biking may save you time!** Cycling is usually the fastest mode of travel door to door for distances up to 6 miles in city centers. Walking is simpler and faster for distances of about a mile.
- **You will enjoy being outdoors.** Research is emerging on the physical and mental health benefits of nature and being outdoors. So much of what we do is inside, with recirculated air and artificial lighting, that our bodies are deficient in fresh air and sunlight.
- **You will be making a significant contribution to the reduction of air pollution.** Driving less means fewer pollutants being emitted into the air. Annually, personal transportation accounts for the consumption of approximately 136 billion gallons of gasoline, or the production of 1.2 billion tons of carbon dioxide. Leaving your car at home just 2 days a week will reduce greenhouse gas emissions by an average of 1,600 pounds per year.

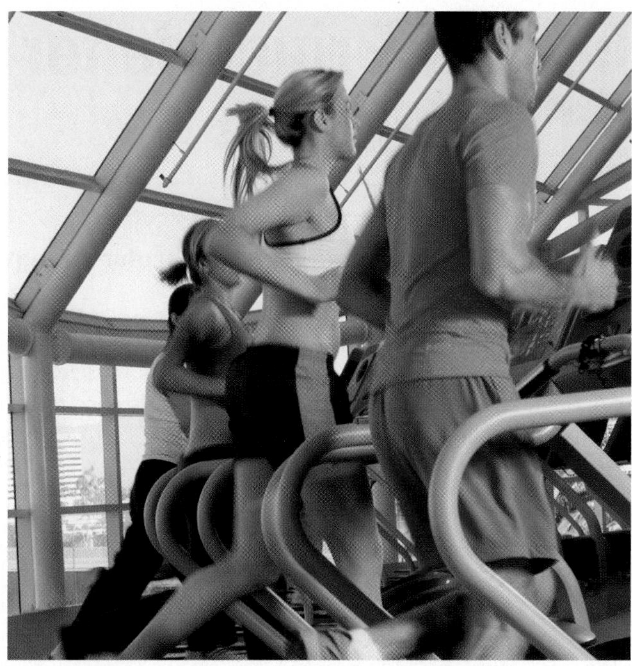

A typical 30-minute workout on a cardiorespiratory training device generates 50 watt hours of electricity—enough to operate a laptop for an hour. At least 20 colleges as well as several independent fitness clubs throughout the United States have retrofitted aerobic machines with equipment that converts the kinetic energy produced by the exercisers into renewable electric energy to help power the club.

check yourself

- **What are the FITT requirements for cardiorespiratory fitness?**
- **How can you incorporate cardiorespiratory fitness into your daily life?**

10.7 The FITT Principle for Muscular Strength and Endurance

learning outcome

10.7 List the FITT requirements for muscular strength and endurance.

The FITT prescription for muscular strength and endurance includes 2 to 3 days per week of exercises that train the major muscle groups, using enough sets and repetitions and enough resistance to maintain or improve muscular strength and endurance.[34]

Frequency

For frequency, the FITT principle recommends performing 8 to 10 exercises that train the major muscle groups 2 to 3 days a week. It is believed that overloading the muscles, a normal part of resistance training (described below), causes microscopic tears in muscle fibers. The rebuilding process that increases the muscle's size and capacity takes about 24 to 48 hours. Thus, resistance-training exercise programs should include at least 1 day of rest between workouts before the same muscles are overloaded again. But don't wait too long between workouts—one of the important principles of strength training is the idea of *reversibility*. Reversibility means that if you stop exercising, the body responds by deconditioning. Within 2 weeks, muscles begin to revert to their untrained state.[35] The saying "use it or lose it" applies here!

Intensity

To determine the intensity of exercise needed to improve muscular strength and endurance, you need to know the maximum amount of weight you can lift (or move) in one contraction. This value is called your **one repetition maximum (1 RM)** and can be individually determined or predicted from a 10 RM test. Once your 1 RM is determined, it is used as the basis for intensity recommendations for improving muscular strength and endurance. Muscular strength is improved when resistance loads are greater than 60 percent of your 1 RM, whereas muscular endurance is improved using loads of less than 60 percent of your 1 RM.

Everyone begins a resistance-training program at an initial level of strength. To become stronger, you must *overload* your muscles, that is, regularly create a degree of tension in your muscles greater than that to which you are accustomed. Overloading your muscles forces them to adapt by getting larger, stronger, and capable of producing more tension. If you "underload" your muscles, you will not increase strength. If you create too great an overload, you may experience muscle injury, muscle fatigue, and potentially a loss in strength. Once your strength goal is reached, no further overload is necessary; your challenge at that point is to maintain your level of strength by engaging in a regular (once or twice per week) total-body resistance exercise program.

Time

The time recommended for muscular strength and endurance exercises is measured not in minutes of exercise, but rather in repetitions and sets. The types of demands that you put on your body will result in the kind of adaptation that will follow.

Repetitions and Sets. To increase muscular strength, you need higher intensity and fewer repetitions and sets. Use a resistance of at least 60 percent of your 1 RM, performing 8 to 12 repetitions per set, with two to four sets performed overall. If improving muscular endurance is your goal, use less resistance and more repetitions and sets. The recommendations for improving muscular endurance are to perform one to two sets of 15 to 25 repetitions using a resistance that is less than 50 percent of your 1 RM.

Rest Periods. The amount of rest between exercises is key to an effective strength-training workout. Resting between exercises can

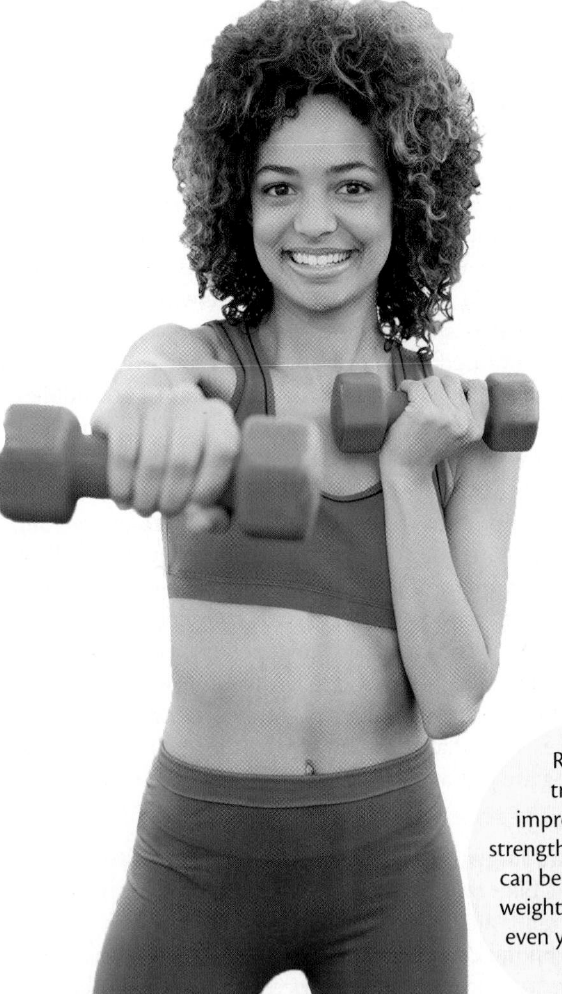

Resistance training to improve muscular strength and endurance can be done with free weights, machines, or even your own body weight.

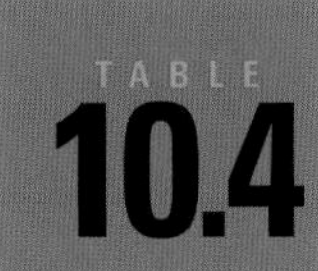

TABLE 10.4 Methods of Providing Exercise Resistance

Calisthenics (Body Weight Resistance)	Free Weights (Fixed Resistance)	Weight Machines (Variable Resistance)
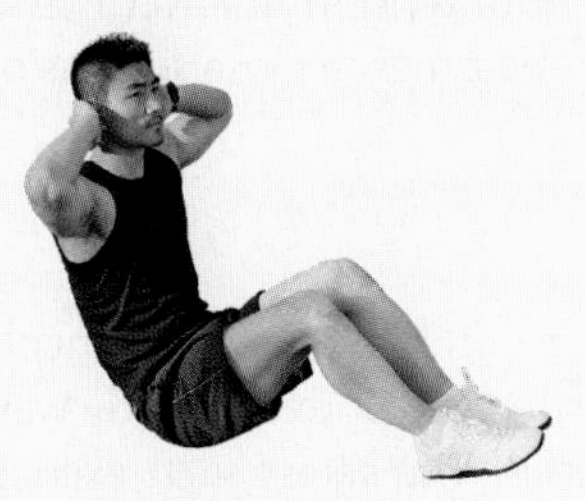	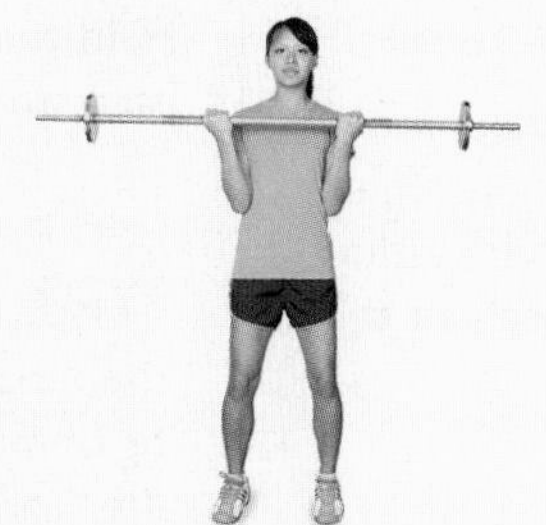	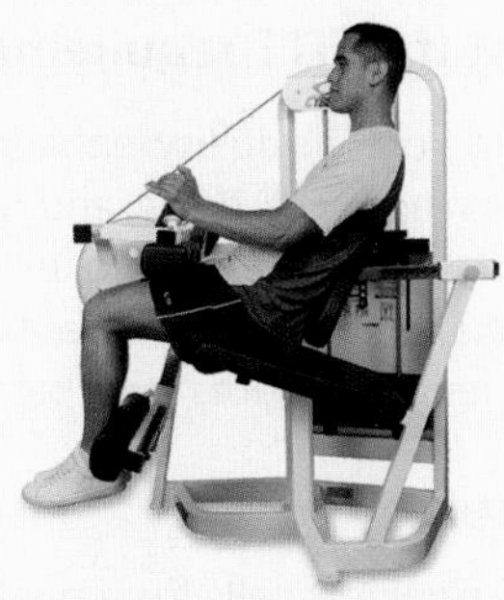
• Using your own body weight to develop muscular strength, endurance. • Improves overall muscular fitness—in particular core strength and overall muscle tone.	• Provides constant resistance throughout full range of movement. • Requires balance and coordination; promotes development of core strength.	• Resistance is altered so the muscle's effort is consistent throughout full range of motion. • Provides more controlled motion and isolates certain muscle groups.
Examples: Push-ups, pull-ups, curl-ups, dips, leg raises, chair sits. For an extra challenge, you can do these exercises on a stability ball or balance board.	**Examples:** Barbells, dumbbells, medicine balls, and kettlebells. Resistance bands can be used for resistance instead of weights.	**Examples:** Weight machines in gyms, homes (Nautilus or Bowflex), and rehabilitation centers.

reduce fatigue and help with performance and safety in subsequent sets. A rest period of 2 to 3 minutes is recommended when using the guidelines for general health benefits. However, the rest period when working to develop strength or endurance will vary. Note that the rest period refers specifically to the muscle group being exercised, and it is possible to alternate muscle groups. For example, you can alternate a set of push-ups with a set of curl-ups; the muscle groups worked in one set can rest while you are working the other muscle groups.

Type

To improve muscular strength or endurance, resistance training is most often recommended using either your own body weight or devices that provide a fixed or variable resistance (see Table 10.4). Some cardiorespiratory training activities also enhance muscular endurance: Thousands of repetitions are performed during a 20-minute (or longer) workout using relatively low resistance when jogging or when training on an exercise device such as a stationary bicycle, rowing machine, or stair-climbing machine.

When selecting the type of strength-training exercises to do, keep several important principles in mind. The first of these is *specificity.* According to the specificity principle, the effects of resistance-exercise training are specific to the muscles exercised; only the muscle or muscle group that is overloaded responds to the demands placed upon it. For example, if you regularly do curls, the muscles involved—your biceps—will become larger and stronger, but the other muscles in your body will not change. This sort of training may put opposing muscle groups—in this case the triceps—at increased risk for injury. To improve total body strength, you must include exercises for all the major muscle groups. You must also ensure that your overload is sufficient to increase strength and not only endurance.

Another important concept to consider is *exercise selection.* Exercises that work a single joint (e.g., chest presses) are effective for building specific muscle strength, whereas multiple-joint exercises (e.g., a squat coupled with an overhead press) are more effective for increasing overall muscle strength. Selecting 8 to 10 exercises targeting all major muscle groups is generally recommend and will ensure that exercises are balanced for opposing muscle groups.

Finally, for optimal training effects, it is important to pay attention to *exercise order.* When training all major muscle groups in a single workout, complete large-muscle group exercises (e.g., the bench press or leg press) before small-muscle group exercises, multiple-joint exercises before single-joint exercises (e.g., biceps curls, triceps extension), and high-intensity exercises before lower-intensity exercises.

check yourself

- **What are the FITT requirements for muscular strength and endurance?**

The FITT Principle for Flexibility

learning outcome

10.8 List the FITT requirements for flexibility.

Improving your flexibility enhances the efficiency of your movements, increases well-being, and reduces stress. Furthermore, inflexible muscles are susceptible to injury; flexibility training helps reduce incidence and severity of lower back problems and muscle or tendon injuries and reduces joint pain and deterioration.[36]

Frequency

The FITT principle calls for a minimum of 2 to 3 days per week for flexibility training; daily training is even better.

Intensity

Hold static (still) stretching positions at an individually determined "point of tension." You should feel tension or mild discomfort in the muscle(s) stretched, but not pain.[37]

Time

Hold each stretch at the "point of tension" for 10 to 30 seconds for each stretch; repeat two or three times in close succession.[38]

Type

The most effective exercises for building flexibility involve stretching of major muscle groups when the body is already warm, such as after cardiorespiratory activities. The safest such exercises involve **static stretching**, which slowly and gradually lengthens a muscle or group of muscles and their attached tendons.[39] With each repetition, your range of motion improves temporarily due to the slightly lessened sensitivity of tension receptors in the stretched muscles; when done regularly, range of motion increases.[40] Figure 10.7 shows some basic stretching exercises.

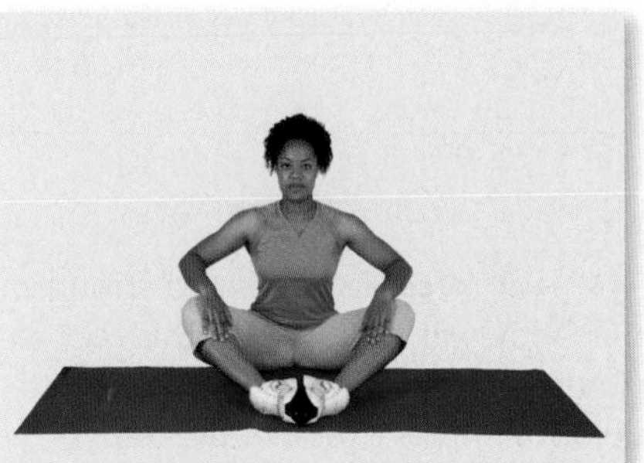

a Stretching the inside of the thighs

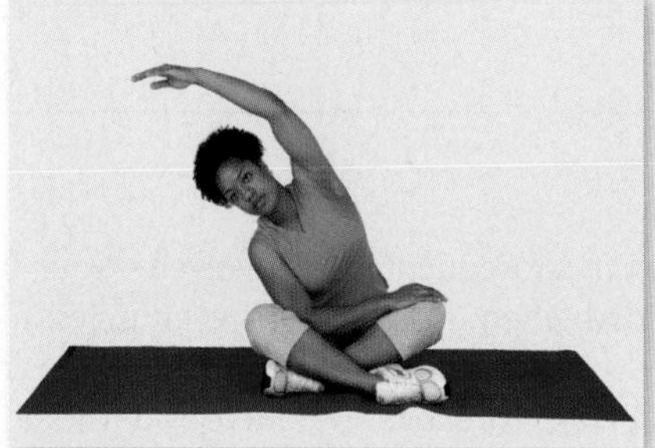

b Stretching the upper arm and the side of the trunk

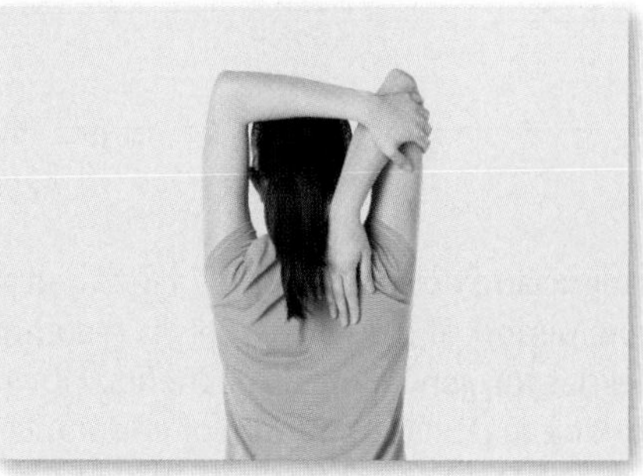

c Stretching the triceps

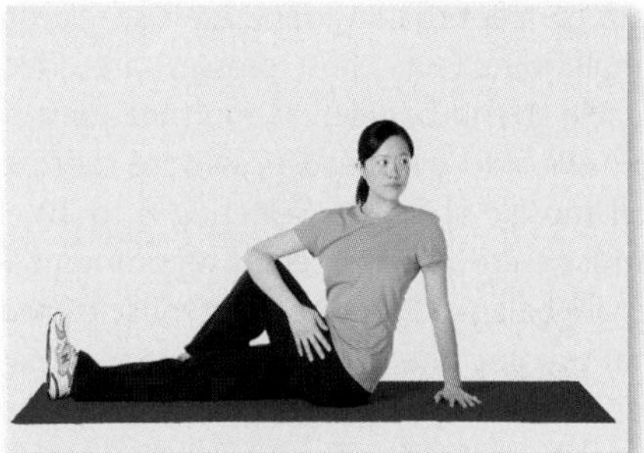

d Stretching the trunk and the hip

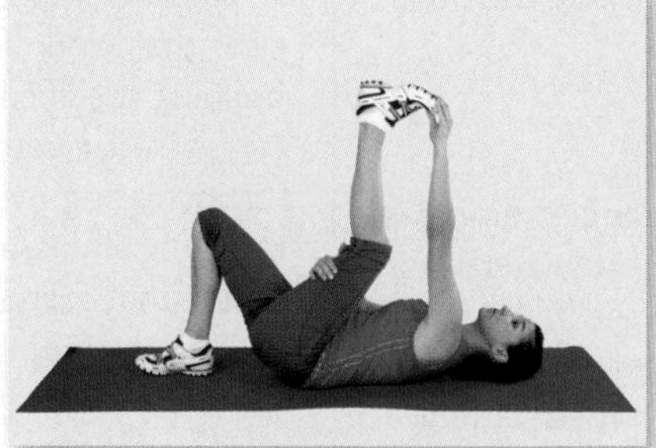

e Stretching the hip, back of the thigh, and the calf

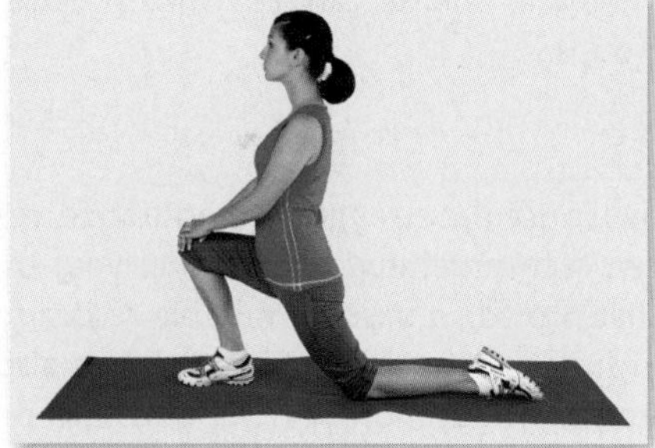

f Stretching the front of the thigh and the hip flexor

Figure 10.7 Stretching Exercises to Improve Flexibility and Prevent Injury
Use these stretches as part of your warm-up and cool-down. Hold each stretch for 10 to 30 seconds, and repeat two to three times for each limb.

check yourself

- **What are the FITT requirements for flexibility?**

10.9 Developing and Staying with a Fitness Plan

learning outcome

10.9 Describe how to stay with and adjust your fitness program over time.

As your physical fitness improves, in order to continue to improve and/or maintain your level of fitness you will need to adjust your frequency, intensity, time, and type of exercise.

Develop a Progressive Plan

Begin an exercise regimen by picking an exercise and gradually increasing workout frequency. For example, in week 1, you might exercise 3 days for 20 minutes per day, and then move to 4 days in week 3 or 4. Then, consider increasing your duration to 30 minutes per session over the next couple of weeks. In general, an increase of 5 to 10 minutes a session every 1 to 2 weeks is tolerated by most during the first month.

Be sure to vary your type of exercise—variety is a fundamental strength training principle also relevant to cardiorespiratory fitness and flexibility training. Changes in one or more parts of your workout not only produce a higher level of physical fitness and reduce the risk of overuse injuries (because different muscle groups are used), but also keep you motivated and interested.

It's also important to reevaluate your overall goals and plans every month or so. Too often, people deciding to become more physically active (or make any other behavior change) work hard on getting started, then lose steam as they go on. To keep yourself motivated, review your progress, make changes when necessary, and continue to reevaluate regularly.

Design Your Exercise Session

A comprehensive workout includes a warm-up, cardiorespiratory and/or resistance training, and then a cool-down to finish the session.

Warm-ups involve large body movements, generally using light cardiorespiratory activities, followed by range-of-motion exercises of the muscle groups to be used during the exercise session. Usually 5 to 15 minutes long, a warm-up is shorter when you are geared up and ready to go and longer when you are struggling to get moving or your muscles are cold or tight. Warm-ups slowly increase heart rate, blood pressure, breathing rate, and body temperature; improve joint lubrication; and increase muscles' and tendons' elasticity and flexibility.

The next stage of your workout, immediately following the warm-up, may involve cardiorespiratory training, resistance training, or a little of both. If you are in a fitness center, you may choose to use one or more of the aerobic training devices for the recommended time frame. If completing aerobic and resistance exercise in the same session, it is often recommended to perform your aerobic exercise first. This order will provide additional warm-up for the resistance session, and your muscles will not be fatigued for the aerobic workout.

Cool-down includes 5 to 10 minutes of low-intensity activity and 5 to 10 minutes of stretching. Because of the body's increased temperature, the cool-down is an excellent time to stretch to improve flexibility. The cool-down gradually reduces heart rate, blood pressure, and body temperature; reduces the risk of blood pooling in the extremities; and helps speed recovery between exercise sessions.

Skills for Behavior Change

PLAN IT, START IT, STICK WITH IT!

The most successful physical activity program is one that is realistic and appropriate for your skill level and needs.

- **Make it enjoyable.** Pick activities you like to do so you will make the effort and find the time to do it.
- **Start slowly.** If you have been physically inactive for a while or are a first-time exerciser, any type and amount of physical activity is a step in the right direction. Keep in mind that it is an achievement to get to the fitness center or to put your sneakers on for a walk! Make sure you start slowly and let your body adapt so that your new physical activity or exercise does not cause excess pain the next day (a real reaction to using muscles you have not used much or as intensely before). Do not be discouraged; you will be able to increase your activity each week, and soon you will be on your way to meeting the physical activity recommendations and your personal goals.
- **Make only one lifestyle change at a time.** It is not realistic to change everything at once. Plus, success with one behavioral change will increase your belief in yourself and encourage you to make other positive changes.
- **Set reasonable expectations for yourself and your physical fitness program.** You will not become "fit" overnight. It takes several months to really feel the benefits of your physical activity. Be patient.
- **Choose a time to exercise and stick with it.** Set priorities and keep to a schedule. Try exercising at different times of the day to learn what works best for you. Yet be flexible, so if something comes up that you cannot work around, you will find time later that day or evening to do some physical activity. Be careful of an all-or-none attitude.
- **Keep a record of your progress.** Include the intensity, time, type of physical activities, and your emotions and personal achievements.
- **Take lapses in stride.** Sometimes life gets in the way. Start again and do not despair; your commitment to physical fitness has ebbs and flows like everything else in life.

check yourself

- **What are strategies for staying with and adjusting your fitness program over time?**

10.10 Developing Core Strength

learning outcome

10.10 Explain the benefits of a strong core.

Yoga, tai chi, and Pilates have become increasingly popular in the United States. All three forms of exercise have the potential to improve **core strength**, flexibility, balance, coordination, and agility. They also develop the mind–body connection through concentration on breathing and body position.

Core Strength Training

The body's core muscles, including deep back and abdominal muscles that attach to the spine and pelvis, are the foundation for all movement.[41] Contraction of these muscles provides the basis of support for movements of the upper and lower body and powerful movements of the extremities. A weak core generally results in poor posture, low back pain, and muscle injuries. A strong core provides a stable center of gravity and so a more stable platform for movements, thus reducing the chance of injury.

You can develop core strength using exercises such as calisthenics, yoga, and Pilates. Core strength does not happen from one single exercise, but rather from a structured regime of postures and exercises.[42] Holding yourself in a front or reverse plank ("up" and reverse of a push-up position) and holding or doing abdominal curl-ups are examples of exercises that increase core strength. The use of instability devices (stability ball, wobble boards, etc.) and exercises to train the core have also become popular.[43]

Yoga

Yoga, based on ancient Indian practices, blends the mental and physical aspects of exercise—a union of mind and body that participants often find relaxing and satisfying. If done regularly, yoga improves flexibility, vitality, posture, agility, balance, coordination, and muscular strength and endurance. Many people report an improved sense of general well-being, too.

The practice of yoga focuses attention on controlled breathing as well as physical exercise and incorporates a complex array of static stretching exercises expressed as postures (*asanas*). During a session, participants move to different asanas and hold them for 30 seconds or longer.

Some forms of yoga are more meditative in their practice, whereas others are more athletic. *Ashtanga yoga,* also called "power yoga," focuses on a series of poses done in a continuous, repeated flow, with controlled breathing. *Bikram yoga,* also known as *hot yoga,* is unique in that classes are held in rooms heated to 105°F, which practitioners claim helps the potential for increasing flexibility.

See It! Videos

Yoga is a great way to exercise your body and your mind. Watch **Beginner's Guide to Yoga** in the Study Area of MasteringHealth.

Tai Chi

Tai chi is an ancient Chinese form of exercise that combines stretching, balance, muscular endurance, coordination, and meditation. It increases range of motion and flexibility while reducing muscular tension. Tai chi involves a series of positions called *forms* that are performed continuously. Tai chi is often described as "meditation in motion" because it promotes serenity through gentle movements, connecting the mind and body.

Pilates

Pilates was developed by Joseph Pilates in 1926 as an exercise style that combines stretching with movement against resistance, frequently aided by devices such as tension springs or heavy rubber bands. It teaches body awareness, good posture, and easy, graceful body movements while improving flexibility, coordination, core strength, muscle tone, and economy of motion.

Pilates differs from yoga and tai chi in that it includes sequences of movements specifically designed to increase strength. Some Pilates exercises are carried out on specially designed equipment, whereas others can be performed on mats.

Strengthening core body muscles can also enhance flexibility and help lower stress levels.

check yourself

- **What are some benefits of having a strong core?**
- **What types of exercise increase core strength?**

Activity and Exercise for Special Populations

learning outcome

10.11 Explain challenges and considerations related to physical activity for older people and those with common health conditions.

All individuals can benefit from a physically active lifestyle. People with the considerations mentioned here should consult a physician before beginning an exercise program.

Asthma

For individuals with asthma, regular physical activity strengthens respiratory muscles, improves immune system functioning, and helps in weight maintenance.

Before engaging in exercise, ensure that your asthma is under control. Ask about adjusting medications (for example, your doctor may recommend you use your inhaler 15 minutes prior to exercise). When exercising, keep your inhaler nearby. Warm up and cool down properly; it is particularly important that you allow your lungs and breathing rate to adjust slowly. Protect yourself from asthma triggers when exercising. Finally, if you have symptoms while exercising, stop and use your inhaler; if an asthma attack persists, call 9-1-1.[44]

Obesity

Limitations such as heat intolerance, shortness of breath during physical activity, lack of flexibility, frequent musculoskeletal injuries, and difficulty with balance in weight-bearing activities need to be addressed. Programs for individuals who are obese should emphasize physical activities that can be sustained for 30 minutes or more, such as walking, swimming, or bicycling, with caution recommended in heat or humidity. Start slow (5 to 10 minutes of activity at 55% to 65% of maximal heart rate), then work up to at least 30 to 60 minutes of exercise per day—150 to 300 minutes per week. Obese individuals can improve health with cardiorespiratory and resistance-training activities.[45]

Athletes like Jay Cutler, an NFL quarterback and a type 1 diabetic, are living proof that chronic conditions needn't prevent you from achieving your physical activity goals.

Coronary Heart Disease and Hypertension

Although regular physical activity reduces risk of coronary heart disease, vigorous activity acutely increases risk of sudden cardiac death and heart attack. Individuals with coronary heart disease must consult their physicians and might need to participate in a supervised exercise program for individuals with heart disease.[46]

Physical activity is an integral component for the prevention and treatment of hypertension. Using the FITT prescription, individuals who are hypertensive should engage in physical activity on most, if not all, days at moderate intensity for 30 minutes or more.[47]

Diabetes

Physical activity benefits individuals with diabetes by controlling blood glucose (for type 2 diabetics) by improving insulin transport into cells, controlling body weight, and reducing risk of heart disease.

Before individuals with type 1 diabetes engage in physical activity, they must learn how to manage their resting blood glucose levels. Individuals with type 1 diabetes should have an exercise partner; eat 1 to 3 hours before exercise; eat complex carbohydrates after exercise; avoid late-evening physical activities; and monitor blood glucose before, during, and after exercise.

One of the most important factors for individuals with type 2 diabetes is the time or length of their physical activity. Because a critical objective of the management of type 2 diabetes is to reduce body fat (obesity), the longer exercise periods are recommended—at least 30 minutes, working up to 60 minutes per session or 300 minutes per week. Multiple 10-minute sessions can be used to accumulate these totals. It is prudent to reduce the intensity of the activity to a target heart rate range of 40 to 60 percent of maximal heart rate.

Older Adults

A physically active lifestyle increases life expectancy by limiting development and progression of chronic diseases and disabling conditions; the general recommendation for older adults is to engage in regular physical activity. For individuals with arthritis, osteoarthritis, and other musculoskeletal problems, non-weight-bearing activities, such as cycling and swimming or other water exercises, are recommended.[48]

check yourself

- **What should older people and those with health conditions be aware of when choosing a program of physical exercise?**
- **Have you had to make any accommodations in your fitness program due to an existing health condition?**

10.12

Nutrition and Exercise

learning **outcome**

10.12 Explain nutritional habits that support healthy exercise.

To make the most of your workouts, follow the recommendations from the MyPlate plan and make sure that you eat sufficient carbohydrates, the body's main source of fuel. Your body stores carbohydrates as glycogen primarily in the muscles and liver and then uses this stored glycogen for energy when you are physically active. Fats are also an important source of energy, packing more than double the energy per gram of carbohydrates. Protein plays a role in muscle repair and growth, but is not normally a source of energy. Another important nutrient to consider is water (or fluids containing water).

How much do I need to drink before, during, and after physical activity?

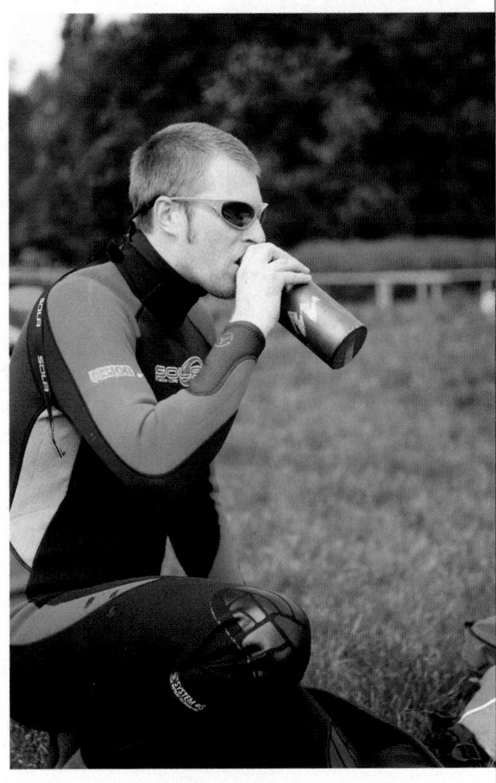

The American College of Sports Medicine and the National Athletic Trainers' Association recommend consuming 14 to 22 ounces of fluid several hours prior to exercise and about 6 to 12 ounces per 15 to 20 minutes during—assuming you are sweating.

Timing Your Food Intake

When you eat is almost as important as what you eat. Eating a large meal before exercising can cause upset stomach, cramping, and diarrhea, because your muscles have to compete with your digestive system for energy. After a large meal, wait 3 to 4 hours before you begin exercising. Smaller meals (snacks) can be eaten about an hour before activity. Not eating at all before a workout can cause low blood sugar levels that, in turn, cause weakness and slower reaction times.

It is also important to refuel after your workout. Help your muscles recover and prepare for the next bout of activity by eating a snack or meal that contains plenty of carbohydrates plus a bit of protein.

Staying Hydrated

In addition to eating well, staying hydrated is crucial for active individuals wanting to maintain a healthy, fully functional body. How much fluid do you need to stay well hydrated? Keep in mind that the goal of fluid replacement is to prevent excessive dehydration (greater than 2% loss of body weight). The ACSM and the National Athletic Trainers Association recommend consuming 5 to 7 mL per kg of body weight (approximately 0.7 to 1.07 oz per 10 pounds of body weight), 4 hours prior to exercise.[49] Drinking fluids during exercise is also important, though it is difficult to provide guidelines for how much or when because intake should be based on time, intensity, and type of activity performed. A good way to monitor how much fluid you need to replace is to weigh yourself before and after your workout. The difference in weight is how much you should drink. So, for example, if you lost 2 pounds during a training session, you should drink 32 ounces of fluid.[50]

For hydration, electrolytes, carbohydrates, and protein, low-fat chocolate milk may be the ideal post-workout drink.

What are the best fluids to drink? For exercise sessions lasting less than 1 hour, plain water is sufficient for rehydration. If your exercise session exceeds 1 hour—and you sweat profusely—consider a sports drink containing electrolytes. The electrolytes in these products are minerals and ions such as sodium and potassium needed for proper functioning of your nervous and muscular systems. Replacing electrolytes is particularly important for endurance athletes engaging in long bouts of exercise or competition. In endurance events lasting more than 4 hours, an athlete's overconsumption of plain water can dilute the sodium concentration in the blood with potentially fatal results, an effect called **hyponatremia** or **water intoxication**.

What about mixing alcohol and exercise? Drinking alcohol can contribute to weight gain, derailing efforts to stay fit. Additionally, a hangover from drinking the night before leads to dehydration and other negative symptoms that can inhibit exercise performance. Consuming

See It! Videos

Will that fancy sports drink help you exercise better? Watch **Sports Drinks Science: Is It Hype?** in the Study Area of MasteringHealth.

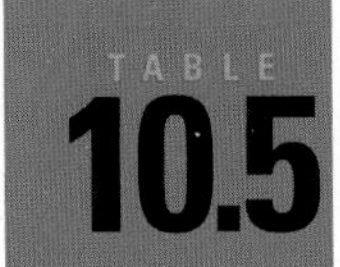

TABLE 10.5 Performance-Enhancing Dietary Supplements and Drugs—Their Uses and Effects

Substance	Primary Uses	Side Effects
Creatine Naturally occurring compound that helps supply energy to muscle	• Improve post-workout recovery • Increase muscle mass • Increase strength • Increase power	• Weight gain, nausea, muscle cramps • Large doses have a negative effect on the kidneys
Ephedra and ephedrine Stimulant that constricts blood vessels and increases blood pressure and heart rate Illegal; banned by FDA in 2006; banned by sports organizations	• Lose weight • Increase performance	• Nausea, vomiting • Anxiety and mood changes • Hyperactivity • In rare cases, seizures, heart attack, stroke, psychotic episodes
Anabolic steroids Synthetic versions of the hormone testosterone Nonmedical use is illegal; banned by major sports organizations	• Improve strength, power, and speed • Increase muscle mass	• In adolescents, stops bone growth; therefore reduces adult height • Masculinization of females; feminization of males • Mood swings • Severe acne, particularly on the back • Sexual dysfunction • Aggressive behavior • Potential heart and liver damage
Steroid precursors Substances that the body converts into anabolic steroids, e.g., androstenedione (andro), dehydroepiandrosterone (DHEA) Nonmedical use is illegal; banned by major sports organizations	• Converted in the body to anabolic steroids to increase muscle mass	• In addition to side effects noted with anabolic steroids: body hair growth, increased risk of pancreatic cancer
Human growth hormone Naturally occurring hormone secreted by the pituitary gland that is essential for body growth Nonmedical use is illegal; banned by major sports organizations	• Antiaging agent • Improve performance • Increase muscle mass	• Structural changes to the face • Increased risk of high blood pressure • Potential for congestive heart failure

Sources: Mayo Clinic Staff, "Performance-Enhancing Drugs and Your Teen Athlete," MayoClinic.com, August 2013, www.mayoclinic.com; Office of Diversion Control, Drug and Chemical Evaluation Section, "Drugs and Chemicals of Concern: Human Growth Hormone," August 2013, www.deadiversion.usdoj.gov; Office of Dietary Supplements, National Institutes of Health, "Ephedra and Ephedrine Alkaloids for Weight Loss and Athletic Performance," Reviewed July 2004, http://ods.od.nih.gov.

alcohol immediately before or during exercise also impairs judgment and motor coordination. After the workout, it's important to rehydrate with water (or other recovery fluids) and refuel first before drinking any alcohol. (See Chapter 7 for more on the effects of alcohol.)

Dietary Supplements

Today there is a burgeoning market for dietary supplements that claim to deliver the nutrients needed for muscle recovery, as well as some that include additional "performance-enhancing" ingredients. Supplements do not require FDA approval, and ingredients may cause side effects and interact with prescription medicines. See Table 10.5 for a list of some of the most popular performance-enhancing drugs and supplements, their purported benefits, and associated risks.

check yourself

- **What are some of the most important nutritional aspects of fitness?**
- **How does hydration affect exercise?**

10.13 Fitness-Related Injuries: Prevention and Treatment

learning outcome

10.13 Distinguish between traumatic injuries and overuse injuries, and discuss how to prevent common fitness-related injuries.

The two basic types of fitness-related injuries are traumatic and overuse injuries. **Traumatic injuries** occur suddenly and violently, typically by accident. Typical traumatic injuries are broken bones, torn ligaments and muscles, contusions, and lacerations.

Many traumatic injuries are unavoidable—for example, spraining your ankle by landing on another person's foot after jumping up for a rebound in basketball. Others are preventable through proper training, appropriate equipment and clothing, and common sense. If your traumatic injury causes a noticeable loss of function and immediate pain or pain that does not go away after 30 minutes, consult a physician.

Overtraining is the most frequent cause of injuries related to physical fitness training. Doing too much intense exercise, too much exercise without variation, or not allowing for sufficient rest and recovery time can increase the likelihood of **overuse injuries**. Overuse injuries occur because of the cumulative, day-after-day stresses placed on tendons, muscles, and joints.

Common Overuse Injuries

Common sites of overuse injuries are the hip, knee, shoulder, and elbow joints. Three of the most common overuse injuries are plantar fasciitis, shin splints, and runner's knee.

Plantar Fasciitis *Plantar fasciitis* is an inflammation of the plantar fascia, a broad band of dense, inelastic tissue (fascia) that runs from the heel to the toes on the bottom of your foot. The main function of the plantar fascia is to protect the nerves, blood vessels, and muscles of the foot from injury. In repetitive weight-bearing physical activities such as walking and running, the plantar fascia may become inflamed. Common symptoms are pain and tenderness under the ball of the foot, at the heel, or at both locations.[51] The pain of plantar fasciitis is particularly noticeable during your first steps in the morning. If not treated properly, this injury may progress to the point that weight-bearing activities are too painful to endure.

Shin Splints *Shin splints*, a general term for any pain that occurs on the front part of the lower legs, is used to describe more than 20 different medical conditions. The most common type of shin splints occurs along the inner side of the tibia and is usually a combination of muscle irritation and irritation of the tissues attaching the muscles to the bone. Specific pain on the tibia or on the fibula (the adjacent smaller bone) should be examined for a possible stress fracture.

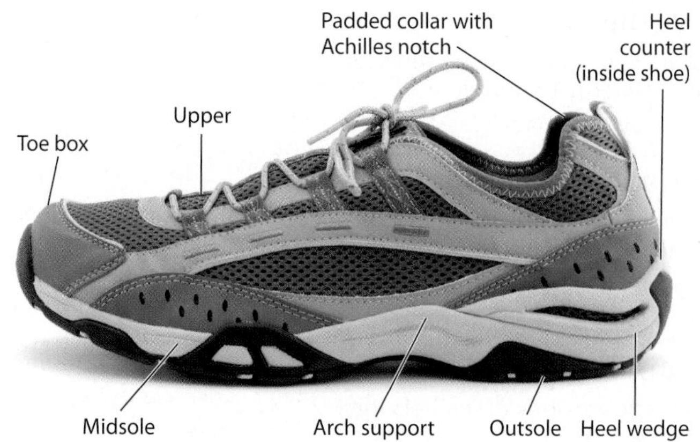

Figure 10.8 Anatomy of a Running Shoe
A good running shoe should fit comfortably; allow room for your toes to move; have a firm, but flexible, midsole; and have a firm grip on your heel to prevent slipping.

Sedentary people who start a new weight-bearing physical activity program are at the greatest risk for shin splints, although well-conditioned aerobic exercisers who rapidly increase their distance or pace may also be at risk.[52] Running and exercise classes are the most frequent cause of shin splints, but those who do a great deal of walking (such as postal carriers and restaurant workers) may also develop them.

Runner's Knee *Runner's knee* describes a series of problems involving the muscles, tendons, and ligaments of the knee. The most common cause is abnormal movements of the patella (kneecap). Women are more commonly affected because their wider pelvis results in a lateral pull on the patella by the muscles that act on the knee. In women (and some men), this causes irritation to cartilage on the back of the patella and to nearby tendons and ligaments. The main symptom is pain experienced when downward pressure is applied to the kneecap after the knee is straightened fully. Additional symptoms include pain, swelling, redness, and tenderness around the patella, and a dull aching pain in the center of the knee.[53]

Treatment of Fitness-Training Related Injuries

First-aid treatment for virtually all fitness-training related injuries involves **RICE**: rest, ice, compression, and elevation. *Rest* is required to avoid further irritation of the injured body part. *Ice* is applied to relieve pain and constrict the blood vessels to reduce internal or external bleeding. To prevent frostbite, wrap the ice or cold pack in a layer of wet toweling or

Applying ice to an injury such as a sprain can help relieve pain and reduce swelling, but never apply the ice directly to the skin, as that could lead to frostbite.

elastic bandage before applying to your skin. A new injury should be iced for approximately 20 minutes every hour for the first 24 to 72 hours. *Compression* of the injured body part can be accomplished with a 4- or 6-inch-wide elastic bandage; this applies indirect pressure to damaged blood vessels to help stop bleeding. Be careful, though, that the compression wrap does not interfere with normal blood flow. Throbbing or pain indicates that a compression wrap should be loosened. *Elevation* of an injured extremity above heart level also helps control internal or external bleeding by forcing the blood to flow upward to reach the injured area.

Preventing Injuries

Using common sense and identifying and using proper gear and equipment can help you avoid an injury. Varying your physical activities and setting appropriate and realistic short- and long-term goals will also help. It is important to listen to your body when working out. Warning signs include muscle stiffness and soreness, bone and joint pains, and whole-body fatigue that simply does not go away.

Appropriate Footwear Proper footwear decreases the likelihood of foot, knee, and back injuries. Biomechanics research has revealed that running is a collision sport—with each stride, a runner's foot collides with the ground with a force three to five times the runner's body weight.[54] Force not absorbed by a shoe is transmitted upward into the foot, leg, thigh, and back. Although our bodies can absorb forces such as these, they may be injured by the cumulative effect of repetitive impact. A shoe's ability to absorb shock is therefore critical—not just for runners, but for anyone engaged in weight-bearing activities.

In addition to providing shock absorption, an athletic shoe should provide a good fit for maximum comfort and performance (see Figure 10.8). To get the best fit, shop at a sports or fitness specialty store where there is a large selection to choose from and there are salespeople available who are trained in properly fitting athletic shoes. Because different activities place different stresses on your feet and joints, you should choose shoes specifically designed for your sport or activity. Shoes of any type should be replaced once they lose their cushioning.

Protective Equipment It is essential to use well-fitted, appropriate protective equipment for your physical activities. For some activities, that means choosing what is best for you and your body. For example, using the correct racquet with the proper tension helps prevent the general inflammatory condition known as tennis elbow. Likewise, eye injuries can occur in virtually all physical activities, although some activities (such as baseball, basketball, and racquet sports) are more risky than others.[55] As many as 90 percent of eye injuries could be prevented by wearing appropriate eye protection, such as goggles with polycarbonate lenses.[56]

Wearing a helmet while bicycle riding is an important safety precaution. An estimated 66 to 88 percent of head injuries among cyclists can be prevented by wearing a helmet.[57] Of the college students who rode a bike in the past 12 months, 39.2 percent reported never wearing a helmet, and 24 percent said they wore one only sometimes or rarely.[58] The direct medical costs from cyclists' failure to wear helmets is an estimated $81 million a year.[59] Cyclists aren't the only ones who should be wearing helmets—so should people who skateboard, use kick-scooters, ski, in-line skate, play contact sports, and snowboard. Look for helmets that meet standards established by the American National Standards Institute or the Snell Memorial Foundation.

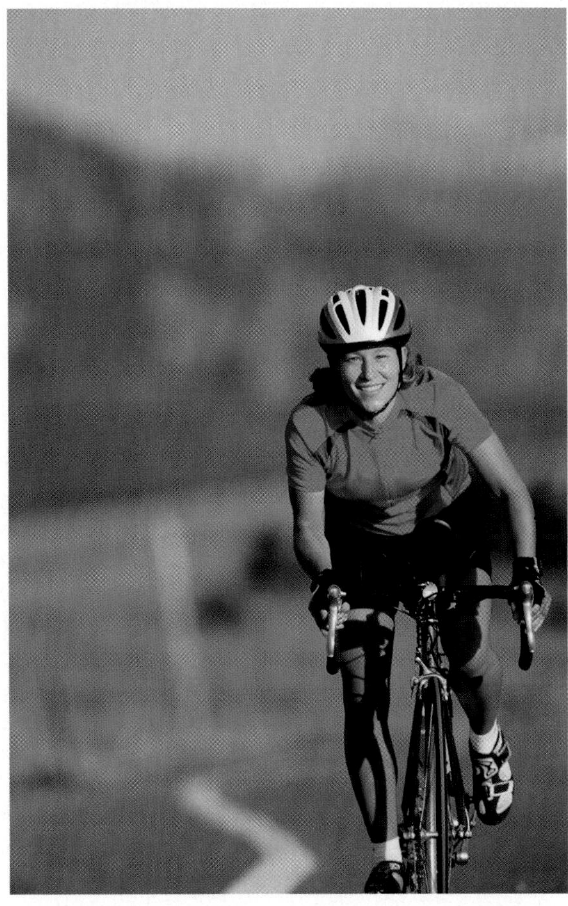

What can I do to avoid injury when I am physically active?

Reducing risk for exercise-related injuries requires common sense and some preventative measures. Wear protective gear, such as helmets, knee pads, elbow pads, eyewear, and supportive footwear, that is appropriate for your activity. Vary your activities to avoid overuse injuries. Dress for the weather, try to avoid exercising in extreme conditions, and always stay properly hydrated. Finally, respect your personal physical limitations, listen to your body, and respond effectively to it.

check yourself

- **What is the difference between traumatic injuries and overuse injuries?**
- **How can you prevent and treat fitness-related injuries?**

10.14 Exercising in the Heat and Cold

learning outcome

10.14 Describe signs and prevention of heat-related injuries and hypothermia.

Exercising in the Heat

Exercising in hot or humid weather increases the risk of a heat-related injury, in which the body's rate of heat production can exceed its ability to cool. The three heat stress illnesses, by increasing severity, are heat cramps, heat exhaustion, and heatstroke.

Heat cramps, heat-related involuntary and forcible muscle contractions that cannot be relaxed, can usually be prevented by intake of fluid and electrolytes lost during sweating. **Heat exhaustion** is a mild form of shock, in which blood pools in the arms and legs away from the brain and major organs, caused by excessive water loss because of intense or prolonged exercise or work in a hot and/or humid environment. Symptoms include nausea, headache, fatigue, dizziness and faintness, and, paradoxically, "goose bumps" and chills. In sufferers from heat exhaustion, the skin is cool and moist. **Heatstroke**, or *sunstroke*, is a life-threatening emergency condition with a high morbidity and mortality rate.[60] Heatstroke occurs when the body's heat production significantly exceeds its cooling capacities. Core body temperature can rise from normal (98.6°F) to 105°F to 110°F; this rapid increase can cause brain damage, permanent disability, or death. Common signs of heatstroke are dry, hot, and usually red skin; very high body temperature; and rapid heart rate. If you experience any of these symptoms, stop exercising immediately.

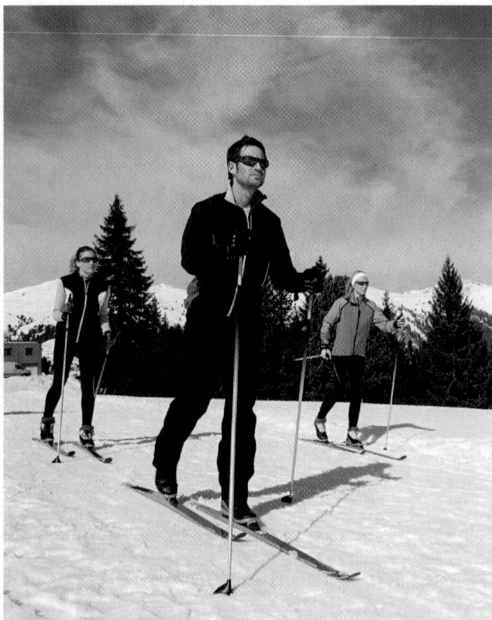

Staying with a friend and dressing in layers are two key tips for making cold weather exercise both safe and fun.

Move to the shade or a cool spot to rest, and drink plenty of cool fluids. If heatstroke is suspected, seek medical attention immediately.

Heat stress illnesses may also occur when the danger is not so obvious. Serious or fatal heat stroke may result from prolonged immersion in a sauna, hot tub, or steam bath or from exercising in a "sauna suit." Similarly, exercising in the heat with heavy clothing and equipment, such as a football uniform, puts one at risk.[61]

To prevent heat stress, follow certain precautions. If possible, acclimatize yourself to hot or humid climates through 10 to 14 days of gradually increased activity in the hot environment. Replace fluids before, during, and after exercise. Wear light, breathable clothing appropriate for the activity and environment. Use common sense—for example, when the temperature is 85°F and the humidity 80 percent, postpone a lunchtime run until evening when it is cooler.

Pay particular attention to your pets if you take them running or walking with you. Pets can quickly succumb to heatstroke and rely on you for hydration. They can also quickly burn their pads on hot pavement. Be responsible and take care of yourself and your pets.

Exercising in the Cold

When you exercise in cool weather, especially in windy conditions, your body's rate of heat loss is frequently greater than its rate of heat production. This may lead to **hypothermia**—a condition in which the body's core temperature drops below 95°F.[62] Hypothermia doesn't require frigid temperatures; it can result from prolonged, vigorous exercise in 40°F to 50°F temperatures, particularly if there is rain, snow, or strong wind.

As body core temperature drops from the normal 98.6°F to about 93.2°F, shivering begins, which increases body temperature using the heat given off by muscle activity. You may also experience cold hands and feet, poor judgment, apathy, and amnesia. Shivering ceases as core temperatures drop to between 87°F and 90°F, a sign the body has lost its ability to generate heat. Death usually occurs at body core temperatures between 75°F and 80°F.[63]

To prevent hypothermia, analyze weather conditions, including wind and humidity, before engaging in outdoor activity. Have a friend join you for cold-weather outdoor activities and wear layers of appropriate clothing to prevent excessive heat loss and frostbite. Keep your head, hands, and feet warm. Do not allow yourself to become dehydrated.

check yourself

- **What are the signs and treatment of heat cramps, heat exhaustion, and heatstroke?**
- **How can you prevent hypothermia?**

Smart Shopping for Fitness

learning outcome

10.15 List important factors to keep in mind when choosing fitness equipment, facilities, and clothing.

You can achieve your personal physical fitness goals without becoming a member of a fitness or wellness center, without buying equipment, and without spending lots of money on the latest fitness fashions. All you need is a good pair of shoes, comfortable clothing to suit the environment you will be physically active in, your own body to use as resistance, and a safe place for activity. However, you may enjoy the outing or experience created by going to a fitness or wellness center or prefer to have some exercise equipment in your home. The following will help guide your selections.

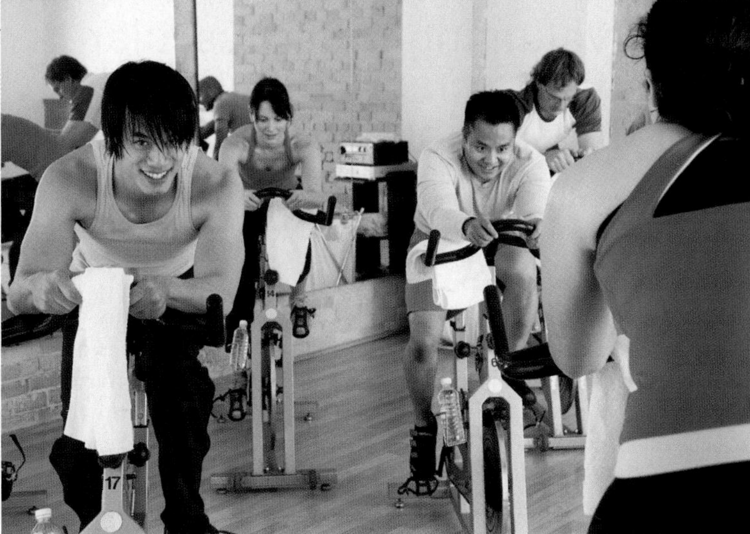

Before you sign on the dotted line, check out the classes, equipment, and personnel a fitness center offers.

Choosing Facilities

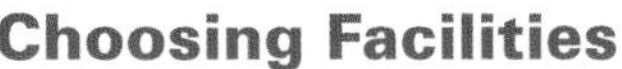

- Visit several facilities before making a decision—and if possible during the time when you intend to use them (so you can see how busy or crowded they are at that time).
- Determine the hours of operation. Are they convenient for you?
- Consider the exercise classes offered. What is the schedule? Can you try one for free? Are classes included in the price of membership or do they cost extra?
- Consider the equipment. Is it sufficient to cover your training needs (e.g., aerobic exercise machines; resistance-training equipment, including both free weights and machines; mats; and other items to assist with stretching)? Is it kept clean and in good condition? Do they offer instruction in how to use the equipment?
- Consider the locker room. Is it kept clean? Are there lockers free for your use if you need them?
- Consider the location. How convenient is it (e.g., on your way to or from work or school, close to your home)?
- Consider the personnel (including their training in first aid and CPR), options for working with a personal trainer, and how friendly and approachable staff members are.
- Consider the financial implications. What membership benefits, student rates, or other discounts are available? Will they hold your membership for the summer, so you do not have to continue paying if you are not attending school in the area? Steer clear of clubs that pressure you for a long-term commitment and do not offer trial memberships or grace periods that allow you to get a refund.

Buying Equipment

- Ignore claims that an exercise device provides lasting "no-sweat" results in a short time.
- Question claims that an exercise device can target or burn fat or lead to miracle cures for "cellulite."
- Be skeptical of testimonials and before-and-after pictures of satisfied customers.
- Calculate the cost including shipping and handling fees, sales tax, delivery and setup charges, or long-term commitments.
- Obtain details on warranties, guarantees, and return policies.
- Consider how this piece of equipment will fit in your home. Where will you store it? Will you be able to get to it easily?
- Check out consumer reports or online resources for the best product ratings and reviews.

Buying Exercise Clothing

- Choose your exercise clothing based on comfort, not looks. It should be neither too loose nor too tight.
- Invest in a good pair of sneakers.
- Consider the environment (temperature, humidity, ventilation) when making your selection.
- Choose clothing that helps you to feel good about yourself and the activity you are undertaking.

check yourself

- **What should you keep in mind when choosing fitness equipment, facilities, and clothing?**
- **Which of these factors are most important to you?**

How Physically Fit Are You?

An interactive version of this assessment is available online in MasteringHealth.

1 Evaluating Your Muscular Strength and Endurance (the 1-Minute Curl-Up Test)

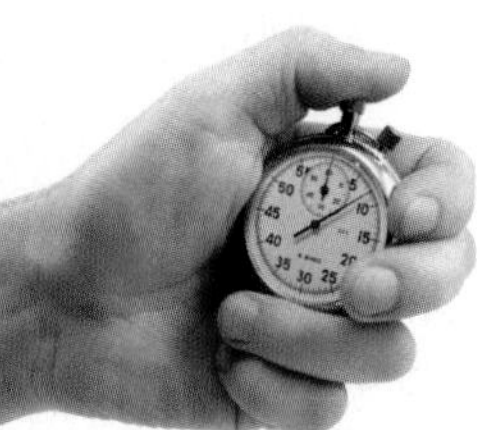

Your abdominal muscles are important for core stability and back support; this test will assess their muscular endurance.

Description/Procedure:

Lie on a mat with your arms by your sides, palms flat on the mat, elbows straight, and fingers extended. Bend your knees at a 90-degree angle. Your instructor or partner will mark your starting finger position with a piece of masking tape aligned with the tip of each middle finger. He or she will also mark with tape your ending position, 10 cm or 3 inches away from the first piece of tape, with one ending position tape for each hand.

Set a metronome to 50 beats per minute and curl up at this slow, controlled pace: one curl-up every two beats (25 curl-ups per minute). Curl your head and upper back upward, lifting your shoulder blades off the mat (your trunk should make a 30-degree angle with the mat) and reaching your arms forward along the mat to touch the ending tape. Then curl back down so that your upper back and shoulders touch the floor. During the entire curl-up, your fingers, feet, and buttocks should stay on the mat. Your partner will count the number of correct repetitions you complete. Perform as many curl-ups as you can in 1 minute without pausing, to a maximum of 25.

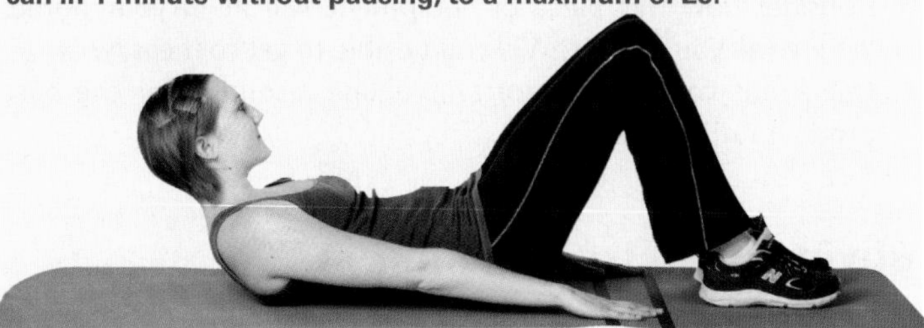

Healthy Musculoskeletal Fitness: Norms and Health Benefit Zones: Curl-Ups

Men	Excellent	Very Good	Good	Fair	Needs Improvement
Ages 20–29	25	21–24	16–20	11–15	≤ 10
Ages 30–39	25	18–24	15–17	11–14	≤ 10
Ages 40–49	25	18–24	13–17	6–12	≤ 5
Ages 50–59	25	17–24	11–16	8–10	≤ 7
Ages 60–69	25	16–24	11–15	6–10	≤ 5
Women	**Excellent**	**Very Good**	**Good**	**Fair**	**Needs Improvement**
Ages 20–29	25	18–24	14–17	5–13	≤ 4
Ages 30–39	25	19–24	10–18	6–9	≤ 5
Ages 40–49	25	19–24	11–18	4–10	≤ 3
Ages 50–59	25	19–24	10–18	6–9	≤ 5
Ages 60–69	25	17–24	8–16	3–7	≤ 2

Source: Adapted from *Canadian Physical Activity, Fitness & Lifestyle Approach: CSEP-Health & Fitness Program's Appraisal and Counselling Strategy*, 3rd edition, © 2003. Reprinted with permission from the Canadian Society for Exercise Physiology.

2 Evaluating Your Flexibility (the Sit-and-Reach Test)

This test measures the general flexibility of your lower back, hips, and hamstring muscles.

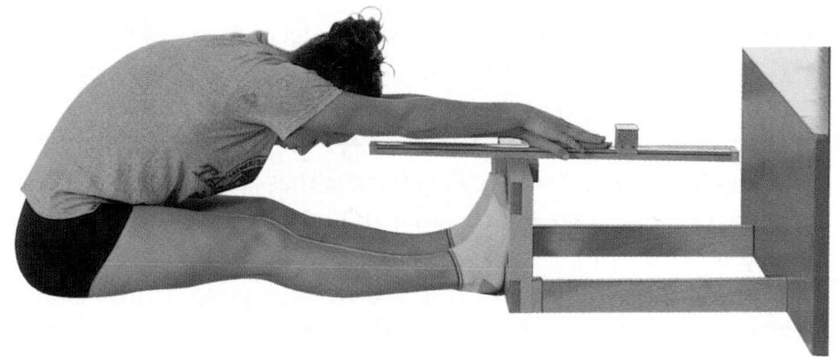

Description/Procedure:

Warm up with some light activity that involves the total body and range-of-motion exercises and stretches for the lower back and hamstrings. For the test, start by sitting upright, straight-legged on a mat with your shoes removed and soles of the feet flat against the flexometer (sit-and-reach box) at the 26-cm mark. Inner edges of the soles are placed within 2 cm of the measuring scale.

Have a partner on hand to record your measurements. Stretch your arms out in front of you and, keeping the hands parallel to each other, slowly reach forward with both hands as far as possible, holding the position for approximately 2 seconds. Your fingertips should be in contact with the measuring portion (meter stick) of the sit-and-reach box. To facilitate a longer reach, exhale and drop your head between your arms while reaching forward. Keep your knees extended the whole time and breathe normally.

Your score is the most distant point (in centimeters) reached with the fingertips; have your partner make note of this number for you. Perform the test twice, record your best score, and compare it with the norms presented in the tables.

Healthy Musculoskeletal Fitness: Norms and Health Benefit Zones: Sit-and-Reach Test

Men	Excellent	Very Good	Good	Fair	Needs Improvement	Women	Excellent	Very Good	Good	Fair	Needs Improvement
Ages 20–29	≥ 40 cm	34–39 cm	30–33 cm	25–29 cm	≤ 24 cm	Ages 20–29	≥ 41 cm	37–40 cm	33–36 cm	28–32 cm	≤ 27 cm
Ages 30–39	≥ 38 cm	33–37 cm	28–32 cm	23–27 cm	≤ 22 cm	Ages 30–39	≥ 41 cm	36–40 cm	32–35 cm	27–31 cm	≤ 26 cm
Ages 40–49	≥ 35 cm	29–34 cm	24–28 cm	18–23 cm	≤ 17 cm	Ages 40–49	≥ 38 cm	34–37 cm	30–33 cm	25–29 cm	≤ 24 cm
Ages 50–59	≥ 35 cm	28–34 cm	24–27 cm	16–23 cm	≤ 15 cm	Ages 50–59	≥ 39 cm	33–38 cm	30–32 cm	25–29 cm	≤ 24 cm
Ages 60–69	≥ 33 cm	25–32 cm	20–24 cm	15–19 cm	≤ 14 cm	Ages 60–69	≥ 35 cm	31–34 cm	27–30 cm	23–26 cm	≤ 22 cm

Note: These norms are based on a sit-and-reach box in which the zero point is set at 26 cm. When using a box in which the zero point is set at 23 cm, subtract 3 cm from each value in this table.

Source: Adapted from *Canadian Physical Activity, Fitness & Lifestyle Approach: CSEP-Health & Fitness Program's Appraisal and Counselling Strategy*, 3rd edition, © 2003. Reprinted with permission from the Canadian Society for Exercise Physiology.

3 Evaluating Your Cardiorespiratory Fitness (the 1-Mile Walk Test)

The 1-mile walk test assesses your cardiorespiratory fitness level.

Description/Procedure:

The objective of this test is to walk 1 mile as quickly as possible. This walk can be completed on an oval track or any properly measured course using a stopwatch to measure the time used. Do not eat a heavy meal for at least 2 to 3 hours prior to the test. Be sure to warm-up for 5 to 10 minutes before the test. It is best to pace yourself on this test and choose a pace/speed you think you can continue for the entire test. If you become extremely fatigued during the test, slow your pace—do not overstress yourself! If you feel faint or nauseated or experience any unusual pains in your upper body, stop and notify your instructor. Upon completion of the test, cool down and record your time and fitness category from the table below.

Cardiorespiratory Fitness Categories: 1-Mile Walk Test (min)

	Fitness Category						Fitness Category				
Men	Very Poor	Poor	Average	Good	Excellent	Women	Very Poor	Poor	Average	Good	Excellent
Ages 13–19	>17:30	16:01–17:30	14:01–16:00	12:30–14:00	<12:30	Ages 13–19	>18:01	16:31–18:00	14:31–16:30	13:31–14:30	< 13:30
Ages 20–29	>18:01	16:31–18:00	14:31–16:30	13:00–14:30	< 13:00	Ages 20–29	>18:31	17:01–18:30	15:01–17:00	13:31–15:00	< 13:30
Ages 30–39	>19:00	17:31–19:00	15:31–17:30	13:30–15:30	< 13:30	Ages 30–39	>19:31	18:01–19:30	16:01–18:00	14:01–16:00	< 14:00
Ages 40+	>21:30	18:31–21:30	16:01–18:30	14:00–16:00	< 14:00	Ages 40+	>20:01	19:31–20:00	18:01–19:30	14:31–18:00	< 14:30

Source: Adapted from *Rockport Walking Fitness Test*. Copyright © 1993 by The Rockport Company, LLC. Reprinted with permission.

Your Plan for Change

The Assess Yourself activity helped you determine your current level of physical fitness. Based on your results, you may decide to improve one or more components of your physical fitness.

Today, you can:

- ◯ **Visit your campus fitness facility and familiarize yourself with the equipment and resources.**
- ◯ **Walk between your classes; make an extra effort to take the long way to get from building to building. Use the stairs instead of the elevator.**
- ◯ **Take a stretch break. Spend 5 to 10 minutes between homework projects doing some stretches to release tension.**

Within the next 2 weeks, you can:

- ◯ **Shop for comfortable workout clothes and appropriate athletic footwear.**
- ◯ **Ask a friend to join you in your workout once a week. Agree on a date and time in advance so you'll both be committed to following through.**
- ◯ **Plan for a physically active outing with a friend or date; go dancing or bowling. Use active transportation (e.g., walk or cycle) to get to a movie.**

By the end of the semester, you can:

- ◯ **Establish a regular routine of engaging in physical activity or exercise at least three times a week. Mark your exercise times on your calendar and keep a log to track your progress.**
- ◯ **Take your workouts to the next level. If you are walking, perhaps try intermittent jogging or sign up for a fitness event such as a charity 5K.**

Summary

To hear an MP3 Tutor session, scan here or visit the Study Area in **MasteringHealth**.

LO 10.1 Physical fitness involves achieving minimal levels in the health-related components of fitness: cardiorespiratory, muscular strength, muscular endurance, flexibility, and body composition. Skill-related components of fitness, such as agility, balance, reaction time, speed, coordination, and power, are essential for elite and recreational athletes to increase performance and enjoyment in sport.

LO 10.2 Benefits of regular physical activity include reduced risk of heart attack, some cancers, hypertension, and type 2 diabetes and improved blood profile, bone mass, weight control, immunity, mental health and stress management, and physical fitness. Regular physical activity can also increase life span.

LO 10.3 Commit to your lifestyle of physical activity and increased fitness levels by incorporating fitness activities into your life. If you are new to exercise, start slowly, keep your fitness program simple, and consider consulting your physician and/or a fitness instructor for recommendations. Overcome your barriers or obstacles to exercise by identifying them and then planning specific strategies to address them.

LO 10.4 Fitness gadgets and equipment can encourage you to stay motivated and provide opportunities to try different types of exercises and movements.

LO 10.5 Planning to improve fitness involves setting SMART goals and designing a program to achieve them. The FITT principle can be used to develop a progressive program of physical fitness.

LO 10.6 For general health benefits, every adult should participate in moderate-intensity activities for 30 minutes at least 5 days a week. To improve cardiorespiratory fitness, engage in vigorous, continuous, and rhythmic activities 3 to 5 days per week.

LO 10.7 Three key principles for developing muscular strength and endurance are overload, specificity of training, and variation. Muscular strength and muscular endurance are improved via resistance-training exercises multiple times per week.

LO 10.8 Flexibility is improved by engaging in two to three repetitions of static stretching exercises at least 2 to 3 days a week.

LO 10.9 A regular comprehensive workout should include a warm-up with light stretching, strength-development exercises, aerobic activities, and a cool-down period with a heavier emphasis on stretching. A fitness program should be appropriate and realistic to the individual's skill level.

LO 10.10 Core strength training is important for maintaining full mobility and stability and for preventing back injury.

LO 10.11 Individuals with special conditions, such as asthma, heart disease, and diabetes, should consult with a physician before beginning an exercise program. Obese individuals need to take precautions to avoid excessive heat and musculoskeletal injuries. Non-weight-bearing activities are recommended for older adults.

LO 10.12 Fueling properly for exercise involves eating a balance of healthy foods 3 to 4 hours before exercise. Hydrating properly for exercise is important for performance and injury prevention.

LO 10.13–10.15 Fitness training injuries are generally caused by overuse or trauma. Proper footwear and equipment can help prevent injuries. Exercise in the heat or cold requires special precautions.

Pop Quiz

Visit MasteringHealth to personalize your study plan with Chapter Review Quizzes and Dynamic Study Modules.

LO 10.1 1. The maximum volume of oxygen consumed by the muscles during exercise defines
   a. target heart rate.
   b. muscular strength.
   c. aerobic capacity.
   d. muscular endurance.

LO 10.1 2. Flexibility is the range of motion around
   a. specific bones.
   b. a joint or series of joints.
   c. the tendons.
   d. the muscles.

LO 10.3 3. Theresa wants to lower her ratio of fat to her total body weight. She wants to work on her
   a. flexibility.
   b. muscular endurance.
   c. muscular strength.
   d. body composition.

LO 10.1 4. Miguel is a runner able to sustain moderate-intensity, whole-body activity for an extended time. This ability relates to what component of physical fitness?
   a. Flexibility
   b. Body composition
   c. Cardiorespiratory fitness
   d. Muscular strength and endurance

LO 10.6 5. The "talk test" measures
   a. exercise intensity.
   b. exercise time.
   c. exercise frequency.
   d. exercise duration.

LO 10.6 6. An example of aerobic exercise is
   a. brisk walking.
   b. bench-pressing weights.
   c. stretching exercises.
   d. holding yoga poses.

LO 10.7 7. Isabella has been lifting 95 pounds while doing leg curls. To become stronger, she began lifting 105 pounds while doing leg curls. What principle of strength development does this represent?
   a. Reversibility
   b. Overload
   c. Strain increase
   d. Specificity of training

LO 10.10 8. Which of the following includes sequences of movements specifically designed to increase strength?
   a. Pilates
   b. Ashtanga yoga
   c. Tai chi
   d. Bikram yoga

LO 10.11 9. People with type 2 diabetes
   a. should not engage in physical activity.
   b. should avoid weight-bearing activities.
   c. should limit physical activity to 30 minutes a day or less.
   d. can improve blood glucose levels through physical activity.

LO 10.13 10. Overuse injuries can be prevented by
   a. monitoring quantity and quality of workouts.
   b. engaging in only one type of aerobic training.
   c. working out daily.
   d. working out with a friend.

Answers to these questions can be found on page A-1. If you answered a question incorrectly, review the module identified by the Learning Outcome. For even more study tools, visit MasteringHealth.

CVD, Cancer, and Diabetes 11

An overwhelming percentage of deaths in the United States are due to three major causes: cardiovascular disease, diabetes, and cancer. Nearly 84 million Americans—1 of every 3 adults—suffer from one or more types of **cardiovascular disease (CVD)**, diseases of the heart and blood vessels.[1] CVD has been the leading killer of U.S. adults every year since 1900, with the exception of the flu pandemic of 1918. Growing rates of obesity, hypertension, and diabetes contribute to CVD in the United States and worldwide.

Diabetes is one of the fastest growing health threats in the world today, with over 382 million people classified as diabetic in 2013.[2] Diabetes is the primary cause of death each year for over 71,000 Americans and a contributing factor to over 231,000 deaths from cardiovascular disease, kidney disease, and other diseases.[3]

As recently as 50 years ago, a cancer diagnosis was typically a death sentence. Cancer remains the second leading cause of death in the United States.[4] Although there were nearly 1.7 million *new* cancer diagnoses and over 585,000 deaths in 2014, the good news is that cancer death rates have been declining by over 2 percent per year in the last decades. Early detection and better treatments have dramatically improved the prognosis for many people, particularly for those diagnosed early.[5]

11.1 Understanding the Cardiovascular System

learning outcome

11.1 Identify the elements and functions of the cardiovascular system.

The cardiovascular system is the network of organs and vessels through which blood flows as it carries oxygen and nutrients to all parts of the body. It includes the heart, arteries, arterioles (small arteries), veins, venules (small veins), and capillaries (minute blood vessels).

The Heart: A Mighty Machine

The heart is a muscular, four-chambered pump, roughly the size of your fist. It is a highly efficient, extremely flexible organ that contracts 100,000 times each day and pumps the equivalent of 2,000 gallons of blood to all areas of the body. In a 70-year lifetime, an average human heart beats 2.5 billion times.

The human body contains approximately 6 quarts of blood, which transports nutrients, oxygen, waste products, hormones, and enzymes throughout the body. Blood aids in regulating body temperature, cellular water levels, and acidity levels of body components and helps defend the body against toxins and harmful microorganisms. Adequate blood supply is essential to health.

The heart's four chambers work together to circulate blood constantly throughout the body. The two large upper chambers, **atria**, receive blood from the rest of the body; the two lower chambers, **ventricles**, pump the blood out again. Small valves regulate steady, rhythmic flow of blood and prevent leakage or backflow between chambers.

Flow of Blood through the Heart and Blood Vessels

Heart activity depends on a complex interaction of biochemical, physical, and neurological signals. To understand blood flow through the heart, follow the steps in Figure 11.1, from deoxygenated blood entering the heart to oxygenated blood being pumped into the blood vessels. Different types of blood vessels are required for different parts of this process. **Arteries** carry blood away from the heart. All arteries carry oxygenated blood, *except* for the pulmonary arteries, which carry deoxygenated blood to the lungs, where the blood picks up oxygen and gives up carbon dioxide. The arteries branch off from the heart, then divide into smaller vessels called **arterioles**, then into even smaller **capillaries**. Capillaries have thin walls that permit the exchange of oxygen, carbon dioxide, nutrients, and waste products with body cells. Carbon dioxide and other waste products are transported to the lungs and kidneys through **veins** and **venules** (small veins).

Your heartbeat is governed by an electrical impulse that directs the heart muscle to move, resulting in sequential contraction of the chambers. This signal starts in a small bundle of highly specialized cells in the right atrium, called the **sinoatrial node (SA node)**, that serves as a natural pacemaker. The average adult heart at rest beats 70 to 80 times per minute.

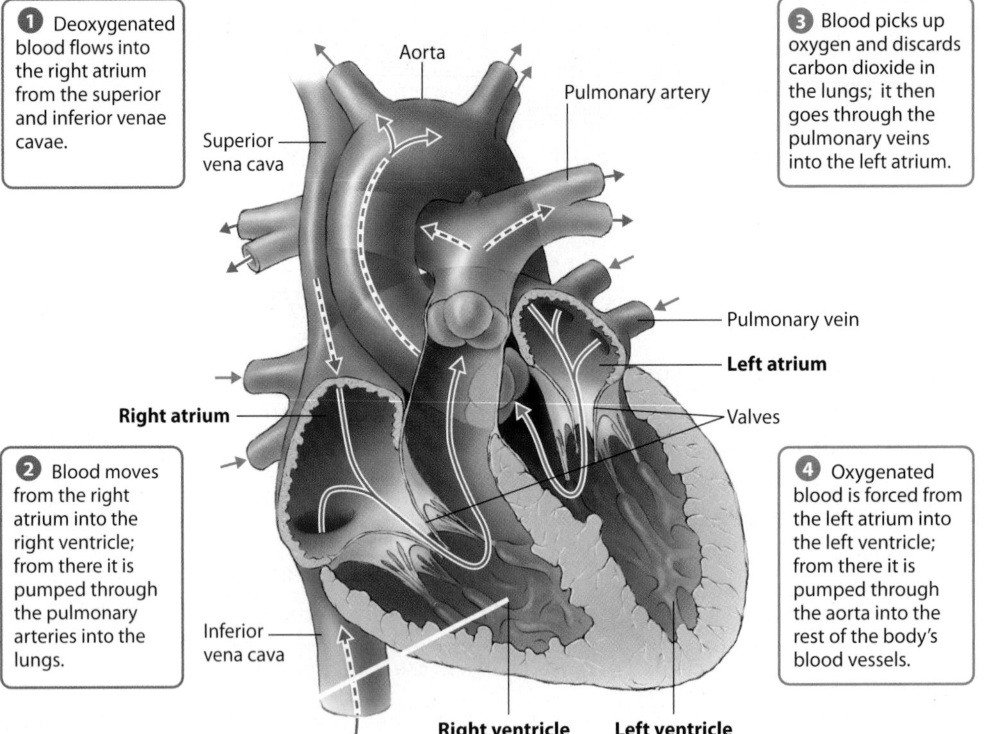

Figure 11.1 Blood Flow within the Heart

check yourself

- **Describe the pathway that blood follows as it circulates through the heart.**

Cardiovascular Disease: An Epidemiological Overview

learning outcome

11.2 Describe patterns in the prevalence of cardiovascular disease relative to gender and ethnicity.

Cardiovascular disease claims more lives each year than the next three leading causes of death combined (cancer, chronic lower respiratory diseases, and accidents), accounting for nearly 33 percent of all deaths in the United States.[6] Consider the following:

- Many CVD-related fatalities are sudden cardiac deaths, an abrupt, profound loss of heart function (cardiac arrest) that causes death either instantly or shortly after symptoms occur. Fifty percent of men and 64 percent of women who die suddenly have had no previous symptoms.[7]
- CVD has claimed the lives of more women than men every year since 1984. Only among people aged 20 to 39 is CVD significantly more prevalent among men than among women (Figure 11.2).[8] Women also have a higher lifetime prevalence of stroke.[9]
- Among women, African Americans and Asian/Pacific Islanders (particularly South Asians) have the highest percentages of CVD deaths, at 34 and 33 percent, respectively.[10]
- Among men, Asian/Pacific Islanders and African Americans have the highest percentages of CVD deaths, at 32.8 percent and 31.7 percent, respectively.[11]
- American Indian and Alaska Natives have the lowest percentages of deaths from CVD.[12]
- Among those aged 20 to 39, 20.3 percent have metabolic syndrome (MetS), a dangerous grouping of key risk factors for CVD. Among those aged 40 to 59, rates jump to 40.8 percent, and for those 60 and over, rates are nearly 52 percent.[13]

Although millions of Americans are living longer with CVD problems, many lack adequate health insurance and fail to obtain screenings and treatments early enough. Large numbers of CVD survivors suffer from physical and emotional disability in the form of fear, depression, and/or inability to perform activities of daily living. While actual death rates have declined, soaring costs for medicines, home health care, rehabilitation services and hospital care, and outpatient tests make recovery challenging. In spite of major improvements in medication, surgery, and other health care procedures, 25 percent of men and 38 percent of women will die within 1 year of having an initial heart attack.[14] The older the age at first heart attack, the greater the risk of dying.[15]

The economic burden of cardiovascular disease on our society is huge—more than $315 billion in direct and indirect costs.[16] Of this amount, nearly $194 billion is direct costs, including physicians and other professionals, hospital services, prescribed medication, and home health care.[17] Indirect costs, attributed to projected losses in future productivity, make up the remainder of the roughly $122 billion in costs.[18] Based on current trends, projections indicate total direct and indirect costs of CVD will surpass $918 billion by 2030.[19] While economic concerns are huge, the effects of CVD on patients, families, communities, and society may be even greater.

With an international trend toward obesity, more and more countries face epidemic CVD rates. The World Health Organization (WHO) estimates CVD accounts for 30 percent of all deaths globally.[20] Unfortunately, over 80 percent of the world's deaths from CVD occur in low- and middle-income countries, places where people have more risks and fewer options for prevention and treatment.[21]

Although death rates are relatively easy to calculate, the short- and long-term psychological problems that occur after a person has a heart attack are harder to measure. Imagine the anxiety caused by wondering if your heart will fail each time you exercise, or fearing that sexual activity might cause another heart attack. Knowing more about your specific CVD risks, your limitations, and what you can do about them is key to taking healthy action.

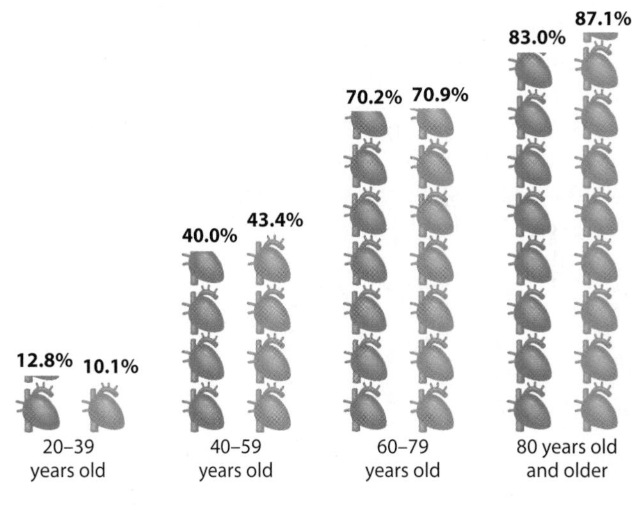

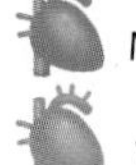

Figure 11.2 Prevalence of Cardiovascular Disease (CVD) in U.S. Adults Aged 20 and Older by Age and Sex

Source: Data from A. S. Go et al., "Heart Disease and Stroke Statistics—2014 Update: A Report from the American Heart Association," *Circulation* 129 (2014): e28-e292.

check yourself

- **What are some patterns in cardiovascular disease relative to gender and ethnicity?**

11.3 Key Cardiovascular Diseases: Hypertension

learning outcome

11.3 Define hypertension and explain how it is measured.

The major cardiovascular diseases include hypertension, atherosclerosis, coronary heart disease, and stroke. Each of these cardiovascular diseases causes deaths and disabilities; their causes and treatments are discussed in the following modules.

Hypertension refers to sustained high blood pressure. In general, the higher your blood pressure, the greater your risk for CVD. Hypertension is known as the silent killer—it often has few overt symptoms, and people often don't know they have it.

The prevalence of hypertension in the United States continues to increase in spite of significant efforts aimed at treatment and control; today more than 1 in 3 U.S. adults has high blood pressure. At nearly 47 percent, African Americans have the highest rate of high blood pressure in the United States.[22] Rates are also much higher among the elderly, men, and those who don't have a high school education.[23]

Blood pressure is measured by two numbers—for example, 110/80 mm HG, stated as "110 over 80 millimeters of mercury." The top number refers to **systolic pressure**, the pressure applied to the walls of the arteries when the heart contracts, pumping blood to the rest of the body. The bottom number is **diastolic pressure**, the pressure applied to the walls of the arteries during the heart's relaxation phase, when blood reenters the chambers of the heart in preparation for the next heartbeat.

2,150

Americans die every day of CVD.

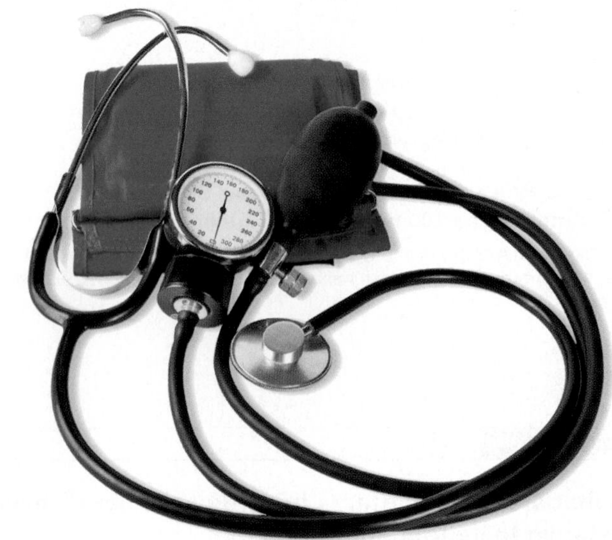

TABLE 11.1 **Blood Pressure Classifications**

Classification	Systolic Reading (mm Hg)		Diastolic Reading (mm Hg)
Normal	Less than 120	And	Less than 80
Prehypertension	120–139	Or	80–89
Hypertension			
Stage 1	140–159	Or	90–99
Stage 2	Greater than or equal to 160	Or	Greater than or equal to 100

Note: If systolic and diastolic readings fall into different categories, treatment is determined by the highest category. Readings are based on the average of two or more properly measured, seated readings on each of two or more health care provider visits.

Source: National Heart, Lung, and Blood Institute, *The Seventh Report of the Joint National Committee on Prevention, Detection, Evaluation, and Treatment of High Blood Pressure*, NIH Publication no. 03-5233, (Bethesda, MD: National Institutes of Health, 2003).

Normal blood pressure varies depending on weight, age, and physical condition. High blood pressure is usually diagnosed when systolic pressure is 140 or above. When only systolic pressure is high, the condition is known as *isolated systolic hypertension* (*ISH*), the most common form of high blood pressure in older Americans. See Table 11.1 for a summary of blood pressure guidelines.

Systolic blood pressure tends to increase with age, whereas diastolic blood pressure increases until age 55 and then declines. Men under the age of 45 are at nearly twice the risk of becoming hypertensive as their female counterparts; however women tend to have higher rates of hypertension after age 65.[24] Over 30 percent of the population are considered to be **prehypertensive**, meaning that their blood pressure is above normal, but not yet in the hypertensive range. These individuals have a significantly greater risk of becoming hypertensive.[25]

Treatment of hypertension can involve dietary changes (reducing sodium and calorie intake), weight loss (when appropriate), use of diuretics and other medications (when prescribed by a physician), regular exercise, treatment of sleep disorders such as sleep apnea, and the practice of relaxation techniques and effective coping and communication skills.

check yourself

- **What is hypertension, and what are its causes and treatments?**

Key Cardiovascular Diseases: Atherosclerosis

learning outcome

11.4 List the major factors contributing to atherosclerosis.

Atherosclerosis comes from the Greek words *athero* (meaning gruel or paste) and *sclerosis* (hardness). In this condition, fatty substances, cholesterol, cellular waste products, calcium, and fibrin (a clotting material in the blood) build up in the inner lining of an artery. *Hyperlipidemia* (an abnormally high blood lipid level) is a key factor in this process, and the resulting buildup is called **plaque**.

As plaque accumulates, vessel walls become narrow and may eventually block blood flow or cause vessels to rupture (Figure 11.3). The pressure buildup is similar to that achieved when putting your thumb over the end of a hose while water is on. Pressure builds within arteries just as pressure builds in the hose. If vessels are weakened and pressure persists, the vessels may burst or the plaque itself may break away from the walls of the vessels and obstruct blood flow. In addition, fluctuation in the blood pressure levels within arteries can damage internal arterial walls, making it even more likely that plaque will stick to injured wall surfaces and accumulate.

Atherosclerosis is often called **coronary artery disease (CAD)** because of the damage to the body's main coronary arteries on the outer surface of the heart. These are the arteries that provide blood supply to the heart muscle itself. Most heart attacks result from blockage of these arteries. Atherosclerosis and other circulatory impairments also often reduce blood flow and limit the heart's blood and oxygen supply, a condition known as **ischemia**.

When atherosclerosis occurs in the lower extremities, such as in the feet, calves, or legs, or in the arms, it is called **peripheral artery disease (PAD)**. Over 8.5 million people—particularly those over 65, non-Hispanic blacks, and women in the United States—have PAD, and many are not receiving treatment because they are asymptomatic or don't recognize subtle symptoms.[26] Most often characterized by pain and aching in the legs, calves, or feet upon walking or exercise (known as *intermittent claudication*), PAD is a leading cause of disability in people over the age of 50. While it strikes both men and women, men, smokers, and diabetics tend to develop it more frequently.[27] In recent years, increased attention has been drawn to PAD's role in subsequent blood clots and resultant heart attacks, particularly among people who sit in cramped airplanes for long distances without getting up and moving. Sometimes PAD in the arms can be caused by trauma, certain diseases, radiation therapy, surgery, repetitive motion syndrome, or a combination of factors. Damage to vessels and threats to health can be severe, with a two- to three-times greater risk of stroke and heart attack among those who have PAD.[28]

Atherosclerosis treatment focuses on lifestyle changes, drugs that reduce the risk of plaque, medical procedures to open vessels, or surgery to open clogged vessels. Millions of Americans take drugs designed to reduce triglycerides and LDL (bad cholesterol) and increase HDL (good cholesterol). Statins are the most commonly prescribed; however they are not without risk. The most common risk is muscle pain that ranges from mild to severe. Other potential side effects include digestive issues, liver damage, increased risk of diabetes, and memory loss. People considering statins should discuss the risks versus the benefits with their doctors.

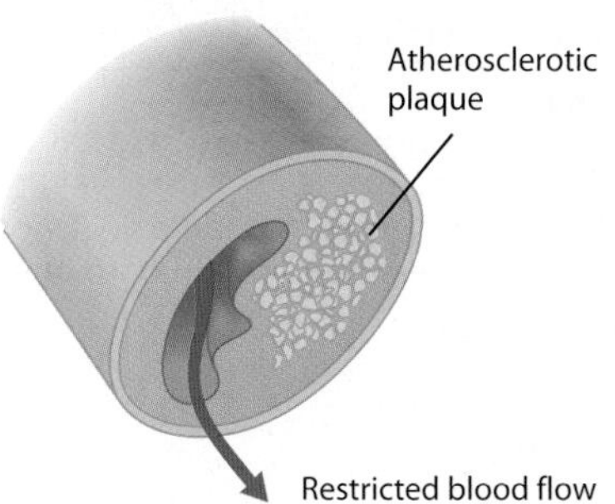

Figure 11.3 Atherosclerosis and Coronary Artery Disease

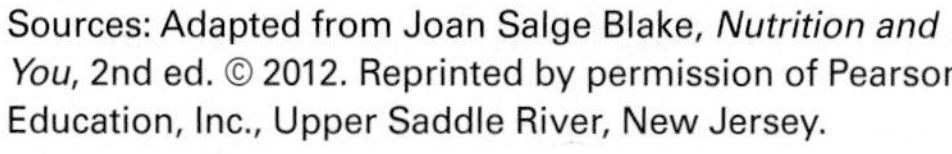

In atherosclerosis, arteries become clogged by a buildup of plaque. When atherosclerosis occurs in coronary arteries, blood flow to the heart muscle is restricted and a heart attack may occur.

Sources: Adapted from Joan Salge Blake, *Nutrition and You*, 2nd ed. © 2012. Reprinted by permission of Pearson Education, Inc., Upper Saddle River, New Jersey.

VIDEO TUTOR
Atherosclerosis and Coronary Artery Disease

check yourself

- **What is atherosclerosis, and what are its causes?**
- **What are the symptoms of peripheral artery disease (PAD)? Who is most at risk?**

11.5

Key Cardiovascular Diseases: Coronary Heart Disease

learning outcome

11.5 List the major factors contributing to a heart attack and the signs of a heart attack.

Of all the major cardiovascular diseases, **coronary heart disease (CHD)** is the greatest killer, accounting for about 1 in 6 deaths in the United States. Nearly 1 million new and recurrent heart attacks occur in the United States each year.[29]

A **myocardial infarction (MI)**, or **heart attack**, involves an area of the heart that suffers permanent damage because its normal blood supply has been blocked. This condition is often brought on by a **coronary thrombosis** (clot) or an atherosclerotic narrowing that blocks a coronary artery (an artery supplying the heart muscle with blood). When a clot, or **thrombus**, becomes dislodged and moves through the circulatory system, it is called an **embolus**. Whenever blood does not flow readily, there is a corresponding decrease in oxygen flow to tissue below the blockage.

If the blockage is extremely minor, an otherwise healthy heart will adapt over time by enlarging existing blood vessels and growing new ones to reroute needed blood through other areas. This system, called **collateral circulation**, is a form of self-preservation that allows an affected heart muscle to cope with damage.

When a heart blockage is more severe, however, the body is unable to adapt on its own, and outside life-saving support is critical. The hour following a heart attack is the most crucial period.

It is important to know and recognize the symptoms of a heart attack so that help can be obtained immediately (Table 11.2). Ignoring symptoms or delays in seeking treatment can have fatal consequences. Be sure to be familiar with heart attack symptoms and know how to summon emergency help at home, work, and school.

Skills for Behavior Change

WHAT TO DO WHEN A HEART ATTACK HITS

People often miss the signs of a heart attack, or they wait too long to seek help, which can have deadly consequences. Knowing what to do in an emergency could save your life or somebody else's.

- **Keep a list of emergency rescue service numbers next to your telephone and in your pocket, wallet, or purse. Be aware of whether your local area has a 9-1-1 emergency service.**
- **Expect the person to deny the possibility of anything as serious as a heart attack, particularly if that person is young and appears to be in good health. If you're with someone who appears to be having a heart attack, don't take no for an answer; insist on taking prompt action.**
- **If you are with someone who suddenly collapses, perform cardiopulmonary resuscitation (CPR). See www.heart.org for information on the new chest-compression-only techniques recommended by the American Heart Association. If you're trained and willing, use conventional CPR methods.**

Sources: Adapted from American Heart Association, "Warning Signs of Heart Attack, Stroke, and Cardiac Arrest," 2012, www.heart.org.

TABLE 11.2 Common Heart Attack Symptoms and Signs

Sign or Symptom	Gender Who Most Commonly Experiences It
Crushing or squeezing chest pain	More common in men
Pain radiating down arm, neck, or jaw	More common in men
Chest discomfort or pressure with shortness of breath, nausea/vomiting, or lightheadedness	Women more likely to feel pressure than pain. Shortness of breath, nausea, and lightheadedness common in both women and men
Shortness of breath without chest pain, discomfort in back, neck, or jaw or in one or both arms	More common in women
Unusual weakness	More common in women
Unusual fatigue	More common in women
Sleep disturbances	More common in women
Indigestion, flulike symptoms	More common in women

Sources: American Heart Association, "Symptoms of Heart Attack in Women," 2012, www.heart.org.

check yourself

- **What is a heart attack, and what are its causes?**
- **What should you do if someone shows signs of a heart attack?**

11.6 Key Cardiovascular Diseases: Stroke

learning outcome

11.6 List the major factors contributing to stroke and the signs of a stroke.

A **stroke** (or *cerebrovascular accident*) occurs when blood supply to the brain is interrupted, killing brain cells, which have little capacity to heal or regenerate.

Strokes may be *ischemic* (caused by plaque or a clot that reduces blood flow) or *hemorrhagic* (due to bulging or rupture of a weakened blood vessel). Figure 11.4 illustrates blood vessel disorders that can lead to a stroke. An **aneurysm** is the most life-threatening hemorrhagic stroke.

Mild strokes cause temporary dizziness, weakness, or numbness. More serious interruptions in blood flow may impair speech, memory, or motor control. Others affect heart and lung function regulation, killing within minutes. Nearly 7 million Americans suffer a stroke every year, and almost 129,000 die as a result.[30] Strokes account for 1 in 19 deaths each year.[31] Even scarier, it is thought that more young people are having strokes than ever before, possibly due to increased obesity and hypertension.[32]

See It! Videos

See how two young women have regained their lives after experiencing a stroke. Watch **Stroke in Young Adults** in the Study Area of MasteringHealth.

Many major strokes are preceded days, weeks, or months earlier by **transient ischemic attacks (TIAs)**, brief interruptions of the brain's blood supply that cause temporary impairment.[33] Symptoms of TIAs include dizziness (particularly on rising), weakness, temporary paralysis or numbness in the face or other regions, temporary memory loss, blurred vision, nausea, headache, and difficulty speaking. Some people experience unexpected falls or have blackouts; others have no obvious symptoms.

The earlier a stroke is recognized and treatment started, the more effective the treatment. One of the great medical successes in recent years is the decline in the death rate from strokes, which in the United States has dropped by one-third since the 1980s.[34] Greater awareness of stroke symptoms, improvements in emergency medicine protocols and medicines, and a greater emphasis on fast rehabilitation and therapy after a stroke have helped many survive.

Despite improved treatments, stroke survivors do not always make a full recovery; often, problems with speech, memory, swallowing, and activities of daily living persist. Depression is also an issue for many survivors.

Skills for Behavior Change

A SIMPLE TEST FOR STROKE

People often ignore, minimize, or misunderstand stroke symptoms. Starting treatment within just a few hours is crucial for the best recovery outcomes. So if you suspect someone is having a stroke, use the tool many emergency teams do to assess what is happening: think FAST.

1. **Facial Droop: Ask the person to smile. It is normal for both sides of the face to move equally, and it is abnormal if one side moves less easily.**
2. **Arm Weakness: Ask the person to raise both arms. It is normal if both arms move equally (or not at all). It is abnormal if one arm drifts or cannot be raised as high as the other.**
3. **Speech Difficulty: Have the patient restate a sentence such as, "You can't teach an old dog new tricks." It is normal if they can say the sentence correctly, and it is abnormal if they use inappropriate words, slur, or cannot speak.**
4. **Time to ACT and call 9-1-1. Don't delay if you note 1 to 3 above. Time is of the essence.**

Source: Cincinnati Prehospital Stroke Scale, adapted from the Uniform Document for Georgia EMS Providers, Department of Public Health, State of Georgia. Available at http://ems.ga.gov.

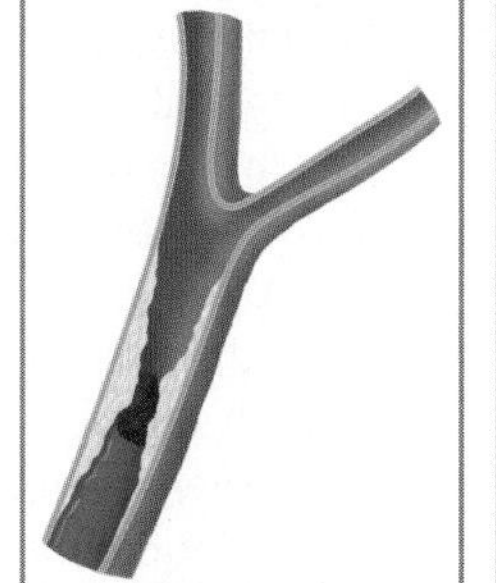

(a) A **thrombus** is a blood clot that forms inside a blood vessel and blocks the flow of blood at its origin.

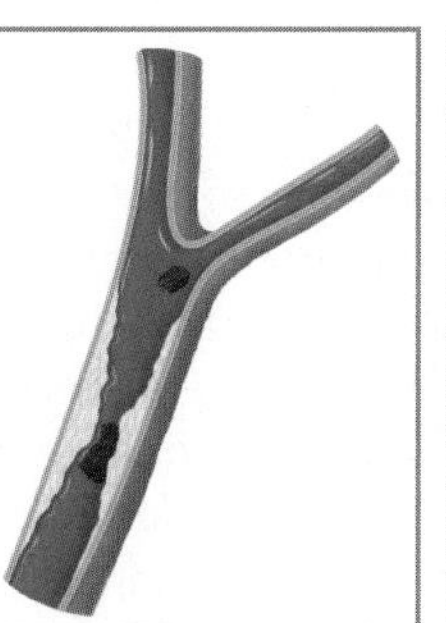

(b) An **embolus** is a blood clot that breaks off from its point of formation and travels in the bloodstream until it lodges in a narrowed vessel and blocks blood flow.

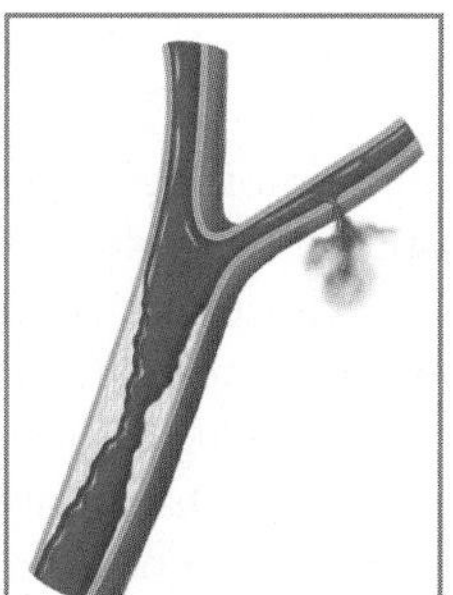

(c) A **hemorrhage** occurs when a blood vessel bursts allowing blood to flow into the surrounding tissue or between tissues.

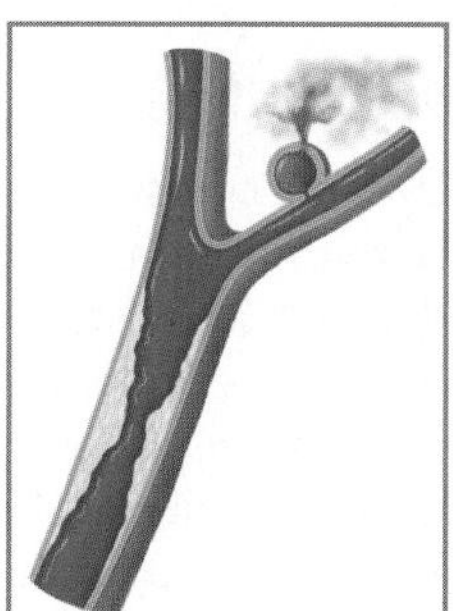

(d) An **aneurysm** is the bulging of a weakened blood vessel wall.

Figure 11.4 Blood Vessel Disorders That Can Lead to Stroke

check yourself

- **What is stroke, and what are its causes?**
- **What should you do if someone shows signs of a stroke?**

11.7 Other Cardiovascular Diseases

learning outcome

11.7 Know the signs and symptoms of angina pectoris, arrhythmias, congestive heart failure, and childhood cardiovascular defects.

Other cardiovascular diseases of concern include angina pectoris, arrhythmias, congestive heart failure, and childhood cardiovascular defects.

Angina Pectoris

Angina pectoris occurs when there is not enough oxygen to supply the heart muscle, resulting in chest pain or pressure. Nearly 8 million people in the U.S. suffer from mild-to-severe symptoms of angina—from indigestion or heartburn-like sensations to chest crushing pain.[35] Generally, the more serious the oxygen deprivation, the more severe the pain. Although angina pectoris is not a heart attack, it does indicate underlying heart disease.

Mild angina cases are treated with rest. Treatments for more severe cases involve drugs that affect either supply of blood to the heart muscle or the heart's demand for oxygen. Pain and discomfort are often relieved with *nitroglycerin*, a drug used to relax (dilate) veins, reducing the amount of blood returning to the heart and so lessening its workload. Patients with angina caused by spasms of the coronary arteries are often given *calcium channel blockers*, which prevent calcium atoms from passing through the arteries and causing the contractions. *Beta blockers* control potential overactivity of the heart muscle.

Arrhythmias

Over the course of a lifetime, most people experience some type of **arrhythmia**, an irregularity in heart rhythm that occurs when the electrical impulses in your heart that coordinate heartbeat don't work properly. A person with a racing heart in the absence of exercise or anxiety may be experiencing *tachycardia*, the medical term for abnormally fast heartbeat. On the other end of the continuum is *bradycardia*, or abnormally slow heartbeat. When a heart goes into **fibrillation**, it beats in a sporadic pattern that causes extreme inefficiency in moving blood through the cardiovascular system. If untreated, fibrillation may be fatal.

Not all arrhythmias are life-threatening. In many instances, excessive caffeine or nicotine consumption can trigger an arrhythmia episode. However, severe cases may require drug therapy or external electrical stimulus to prevent serious complications. When in doubt, it is always best to check with your doctor.

Congestive Heart Failure

When the heart muscle is damaged and can't pump enough blood to supply body tissues, fluids may begin to accumulate in various parts of the body, most notably the lungs, feet, ankles, and legs. Acute shortness of breath and fatigue are often key symptoms of **heart failure (HF)** or **congestive heart failure (CHF)**. Nearly 6.6 million adults age 20 and over in the United States have HF, with cases estimated to rise to nearly 10 million by 2030.[36] Underlying causes of HF may include heart injury that results in damage to heart muscle (**cardiomyopathy**), affects heart valves, or causes problems with heart rhythms. Infectious diseases, such as rheumatic fever, can damage heart valves. Bacteria and viruses can inflame blood vessels, increasing atherosclerotic plaque formation. Uncontrolled high blood pressure, coronary artery disease, diabetes, and other chronic conditions can all lead to heart failure. Certain prescription drugs such as NSAIDS and diabetes medications also increase risks, as do chronic drug and alcohol abuse. In some cases, damage is due to cancer radiation or chemotherapy treatments.

Untreated, HF can be fatal. However, most cases respond well to treatment, which includes *diuretics* (water pills) to relieve fluid accumulation; drugs such as *digitalis* that increase the heart's pumping action; and *vasodilators*, drugs that expand blood vessels and decrease resistance, making the heart's work easier.

Congenital and Rheumatic Heart Disease

Approximately 32,000 children are born in the United States each year with some form of **congenital cardiovascular defect** (*congenital* means the problem is present at birth).[37] These may be relatively minor, such as slight *murmurs* (low-pitched sounds caused by turbulent blood flow through the heart) caused by valve irregularities, which many children outgrow. About 25 percent of those born with congenital heart defects must undergo invasive procedures to correct problems within the first year of life.[38] Underlying causes are unknown but may be related to hereditary factors; maternal diseases, such as rubella, that occurred during fetal development; or a mother's chemical intake (particularly alcohol or methamphetamine) during pregnancy. With advances in pediatric cardiology, the prognosis for children with congenital heart defects is better than ever before.

Rheumatic heart disease is attributed to rheumatic fever, an inflammatory disease caused by an unresolved *streptococcal infection* of the throat (strep throat). Over time, the strep infection can affect connective tissues of the heart, joints, brain, or skin. In some cases, the infection can lead to an immune response in which antibodies attack the heart as well as the bacteria. Many operations on heart valves are related to rheumatic heart disease.

check yourself

- **Name and describe several common cardiovascular diseases.**

11.8

Reducing CVD Risk: Metabolic Syndrome

learning outcome

11.8 List the cluster of factors composing metabolic syndrome.

A large cluster of factors are related to increased risk for cardiovascular disease. Recently, the U.S. Burden of Disease Collaborators determined that the greatest contributor to overall CVD burden was suboptimal diet, followed by tobacco smoking, high body mass index, high blood pressure, high fasting plasma glucose, and physical inactivity.[39] A growing body of research has implicated selected CVD risks and conditions such as obesity and hypertension with an increased risk for impaired cognitive function and an increased risk for Alzheimer's disease.[40] **Cardiometabolic risks** are the combined risks, which indicate physical and biochemical changes that can lead to diseases. Some risks result from choices and behaviors and are modifiable, whereas others are inherited or are intrinsic (such as age and gender) and cannot be changed.

Over the past decade, health professionals have attempted to establish diagnostic cutoff points for a cluster of combined cardiometabolic risks, variably labeled *syndrome X, insulin resistance syndrome,* and most recently, **metabolic syndrome (MetS)**. Historically, MetS is believed to increase risk for atherosclerotic heart disease by as much as three times normal rates. Twenty percent of people age 20 to 39, 41 percent of people age 40 to 59, and nearly 52 percent of those over the age of 60 meet its criteria.[41] Although different professional organizations have slightly different criteria for MetS, that of the National Cholesterol Education Program's Adult Treatment Panel (NCEP/ATPIII) is most commonly used. According to these criteria, for a diagnosis of metabolic syndrome a person would have three or more of the following risks (Figure 11.5):[42]

- Abdominal obesity (waist measurement of more than 40 inches in men or 35 inches in women)
- Elevated blood fat (triglycerides greater than 150 mg/dL)
- Low levels of high-density lipoprotein (HDL; "good" cholesterol) (less than 40 mg/dL in men and less than 50 mg/dL in women)
- Blood pressure greater than 130/85 mm Hg
- Fasting glucose greater than 100 mg/dL (a sign of insulin resistance or glucose intolerance)

The use of the metabolic syndrome classification and other, similar terms has been important in highlighting the relationship between the number of risks a person possesses and that person's likelihood of developing CVD and diabetes. Groups such as the AHA and others are giving increased attention to multiple risks and emphasizing cardiovascular health in lifestyle interventions.

ELEVATED BLOOD TRIGLYCERIDES
• Greater than or equal to 150 mg/dL
REDUCED BLOOD HDL CHOLESTEROL
• Men: Less than 40 mg/dL
• Women: Less than 50 mg/dL
ELEVATED FASTING BLOOD GLUCOSE
• Greater than or equal to 100 mg/dL
ELEVATED BLOOD PRESSURE
• Systolic blood pressure greater than or equal to 130 mm Hg
• Diastolic blood pressure greater than or equal to 85 mm Hg
ELEVATED WAIST CIRCUMFERENCE
• Men: Greater than or equal to 40 inches
• Women: Greater than or equal to 35 inches

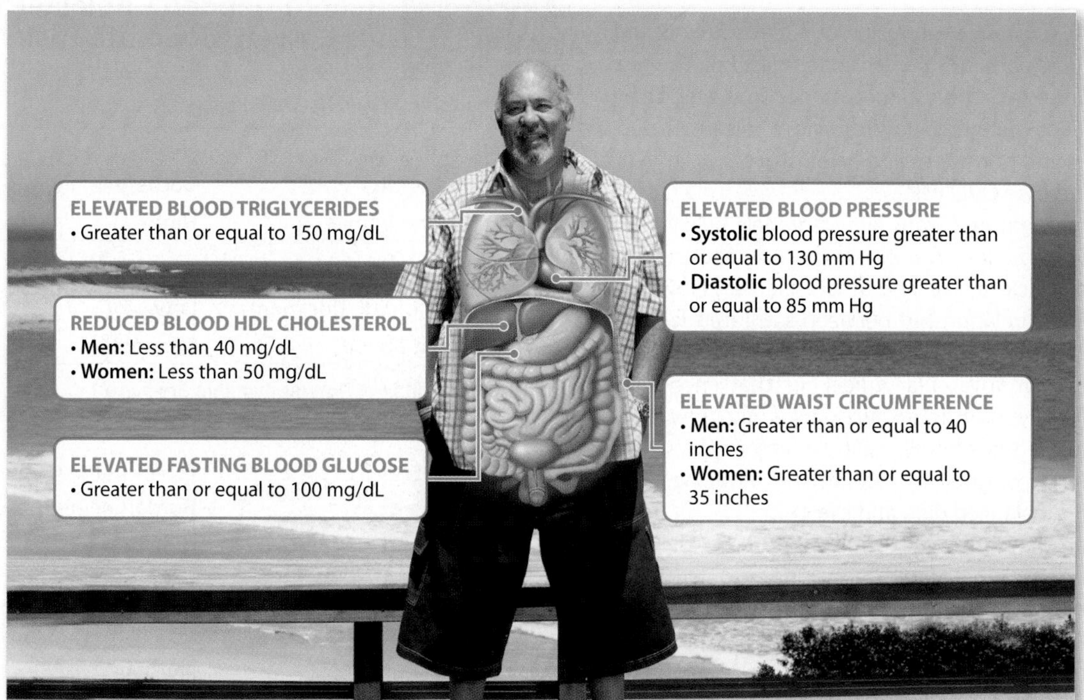

Figure 11.5 Risk Factors Associated with Metabolic Syndrome

check yourself

- **How does metabolic syndrome contribute to the risk of heart disease?**

11.9

Reducing CVD Risk: Modifiable Risks

learning outcome

11.9 Describe modifiable factors affecting CVD risk.

From the first moments of your life, you begin to accumulate risks for CVD. Your past and current lifestyle choices may haunt you as you enter your middle and later years. Behaviors you choose today and over the coming decades can actively reduce or promote your risk for CVD.

Avoid Tobacco Smoke

Cigarette smokers are 2 to 4 times more likely to develop coronary heart disease[43] and more than 10 times as likely to develop peripheral vascular diseases[44] than are nonsmokers. Smoking also doubles a person's risk of stroke.[45] Nonsmokers regularly exposed to secondhand smoke have a 25 to 30 percent increased risk of heart disease, with over 35,000 deaths per year.[46]

The good news is that if you stop smoking, your heart can mend itself. After 1 year, the former smoker's risk of heart disease drops by 50 percent. Between 5 and 15 years after quitting, the risk of stroke and CHD becomes similar to that of nonsmokers. Quitting by age 30 reduces chances of dying prematurely from tobacco-related diseases by more than 90 percent.[47]

Cut Back on Saturated Fat and Cholesterol

Cholesterol is a fat-like substance found in your bloodstream and cells. Your body products about 75 percent of cholesterol; the rest comes from foods in your diet. Cholesterol is carried in the blood by LDL and HDL lipoproteins (defined below); it plays a role in production of cell membranes and hormones and helps process vitamin D. However, high levels increase CVD risk.

Diets high in saturated fat and *trans* fats are widely believed to raise cholesterol levels and make the blood more viscous, which increases risk of heart attack, stroke, and atherosclerosis. However, researchers looking at the relationship between saturated fat and increased risk of CVD recently concluded that current evidence doesn't clearly support cardiovascular guidelines that encourage high consumption of polyunsaturated fatty acids and low consumption of total saturated fats.[48] Still, multiple factors play a role in CVD risk, and experts continue to recommend reducing saturated fats, maintaining a balanced diet, and exercising.

Historically, clinicians have looked at total cholesterol, triglycerides, and high and low-density lipoproteins as being key to determining CVD risks. **Low-density lipoprotein (LDL)**, or "bad" cholesterol, is believed to build up on artery walls; **high-density lipoprotein (HDL)**, or "good" cholesterol, appears to remove such buildup. In theory, if LDL levels get too high or HDL levels too low, cholesterol will accumulate inside arteries and lead to cardiovascular problems. However, new research indicates that raising HDL to prevent negative CVD outcomes may not be as beneficial as once thought.[49]

Other blood lipid factors may increase CVD risk. *Lipoprotein-associated phospholipase A2 (Lp-PLA2)* is an enzyme that circulates in the blood and attaches to LDL; it plays an important role in plaque accumulation and increased risk for stroke and coronary events, particularly in men.[50] *Apolipoprotein B (apo B)* is a primary component of LDL essential for cholesterol delivery to cells. Some researchers believe apo B levels may be more important to heart disease risk than total cholesterol or LDL levels.[51]

When you consume calories, the body converts any extra to **triglycerides**, which are stored in fat cells to provide energy. High counts of blood triglycerides are often found in people who are obese or overweight or who have high cholesterol levels, heart problems, or diabetes. A baseline cholesterol test (lipid panel or lipid profile) measures triglyceride, HDL, LDL, and total cholesterol. It should be taken at age 20, with follow-ups every 5 years, then annually for men over 35 and women over 45. (See Table 11.3 for recommended levels of cholesterol and triglycerides.)

See It! Videos

What habits can you change now to improve your heart health? Watch **Importance of Heart Health** in the Study Area of MasteringHealth.

TABLE 11.3 **Recommended Cholesterol Levels for Lower/Moderate-Risk Adults**

Total Cholesterol Level (lower numbers are better)	
Less than 200 mg/dL	Desirable
200 to 239 mg/dL	Borderline high
240 mg/dL and above	High
HDL Cholesterol Level (higher numbers are better)	
Less than 40 mg/dL (for men)	Low
60 mg/dL and above	Desirable
LDL Cholesterol Level (lower numbers are better)	
Less than 100 mg/dL	Optimal
100 to 129 mg/dL	Near or above optimal
130 to 159 mg/dL	Borderline high
160 to 189 mg/dL	High
190 mg/dL and above	Very high
Triglyceride Level (lower numbers are better)	
Less than 150 mg/dL	Normal
150–199 mg/dL	Borderline high
200–499 mg/dL	High
500 mg/dL and above	Very high

Source: Adapted from ATP III Guidelines At-a-Glance Quick Desk Reference, National Heart, Lung, and Blood Institute, National Institutes of Health. Update on Cholesterol Guidelines, 2004.

How can I improve my cholesterol level?

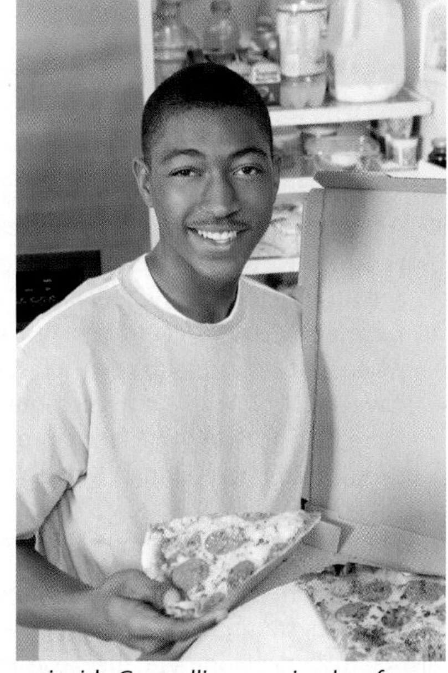

You get cholesterol from two primary sources: from your body (which involves genetic predisposition) and from food. The good news is that the 25 percent of the cholesterol you get from foods is the part where you can make real improvements in overall cholesterol profiles, even if you have a high genetic risk. Controlling your intake of saturated fats and *trans* fats will help you keep your cholesterol level in check.

In spite of all of the education on the dangers of high cholesterol, Americans continue to have higher-than-recommended levels and millions are on cholesterol-lowering drugs. Nearly 44 percent of adults age 20 and over have cholesterol levels at or above 200 mg/dL, and another 14 percent have levels in excess of 240 mg/dL.[52]

Modify Other Dietary Habits

Research continues into dietary modifications that may affect heart health. An overall approach, such as the DASH eating plan from the National Heart, Lung, and Blood Institute, has strong evidence to back up its claims of reducing CVD risk:

- Consume 5 to 10 milligrams per day of soluble fiber from sources such as oat bran, fruits, vegetables, legumes, and psyllium seeds.
- Consume about 2 grams per day of **plant sterols**, which are present in many fruits, vegetables, nuts, seeds, cereals, legumes, vegetable oils, and other plant sources.
- Eat less sodium. Excess sodium has been linked to high blood pressure, which can affect CVD risk.

See It! Videos

Can a way of eating reduce your risk of heart disease? Watch **Mediterranean Diet Could Help Reduce Heart Disease** in the Study Area of MasteringHealth.

Several foods, including fish high in omega-3 fatty acids, olive oil, whole grains, nuts, green tea, and dark chocolate, have been shown to reduce the chances that cholesterol will be absorbed in the cells, reduce levels of LDL cholesterol, or enhance the protective effects of HDL cholesterol.[53]

Maintain a Healthy Weight

Overweight people are more likely to develop heart disease and stroke even if they have no other risk factors. If you're heavy, losing even 5 to 10 pounds can make a significant difference.[54] This is especially true if you're an "apple" (thicker around upper body and waist) rather than a "pear" (thicker around hips and thighs).

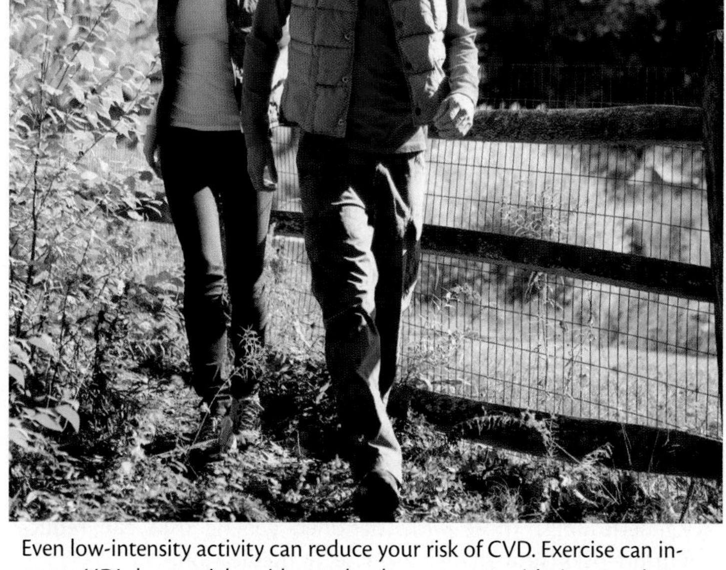

Even low-intensity activity can reduce your risk of CVD. Exercise can increase HDL, lower triglycerides, and reduce coronary risks in several ways.

Exercise Regularly

Inactivity is a definite risk factor for CVD.[55] Even light activity—walking, gardening, housework, dancing—is beneficial if done regularly and over the long term.

Control Diabetes and Blood Pressure

Heart disease death rates among adults with diabetes are two to four times higher than the rates for adults without diabetes. At least 68 percent of people with diabetes die of some form of heart disease or stroke.[56]

Although blood pressure typically creeps up with age, lifestyle changes can dramatically lower CVD risk. Among the most beneficial are losing extra pounds, cutting back on sodium, exercising more, reducing alcohol and caffeine intake, and quitting smoking.

Manage Stress Levels

Stress may trigger cardiac events or even sudden cardiac death, and it increases the risks of hypertension, stroke, and elevated cholesterol levels. Research indicates that everyday, chronic stressors can lead to increased risk of coronary events, HBP, strokes, and sudden cardiac death in much the same way as acute natural disasters do.[57]

check yourself

- **Of the risk factors described, which are of the most concern to you? What kind of changes could you make to improve in these areas?**

11.10

Reducing CVD Risk: Nonmodifiable Risks

learning outcome

11.10 Identify nonmodifiable factors affecting CVD risk.

Some risk factors for CVD cannot be prevented or controlled. Among these factors are the following:

- **Race and Ethnicity.** African Americans tend to have the highest overall rates of CVD and hypertension and the lowest rates of physical activity. The rate of high blood pressure in African Americans is among the highest in the world. Mexican Americans have the highest percentage of adults with cholesterol levels exceeding 200 mg/dL and the highest rates of obesity and overweight.[58] Figure 11.6 summarizes deaths from heart disease and stroke by ethnicity.
- **Heredity.** Family history of heart disease appears to increase CVD risk significantly. Amount of cholesterol produced, tendencies to form plaque, and a host of other factors seem to have genetic links. Those with identified genetic risks can reduce future risks through diet, exercise, or medication.

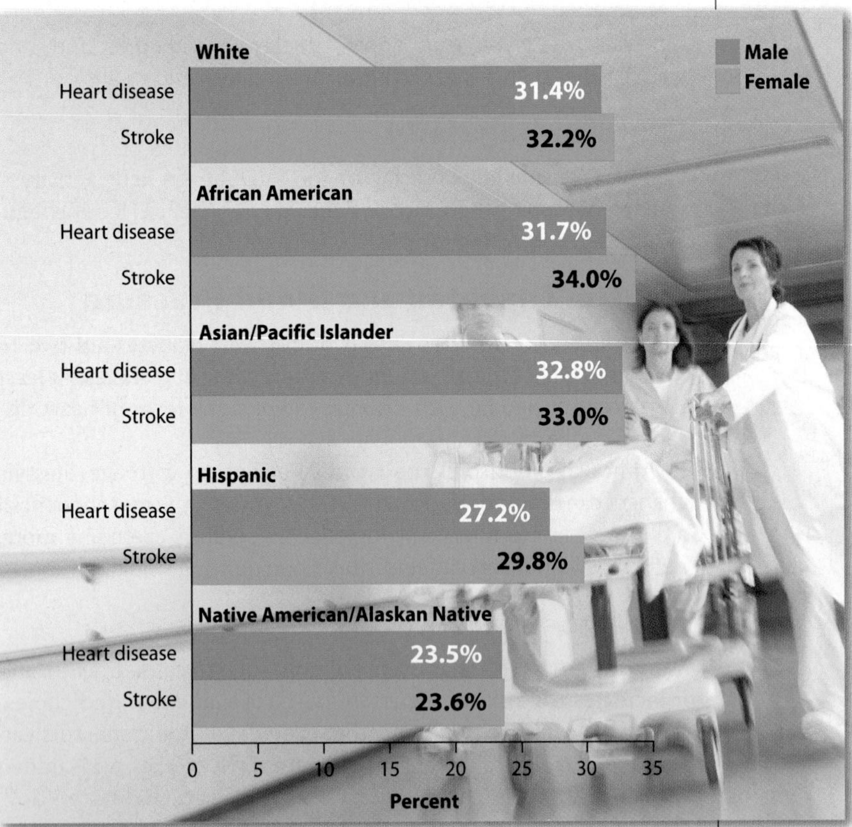

Figure 11.6 Deaths from Heart Disease and Stroke in the United States by Ethnicity

Sources: American Heart Association, "Statistics At a Glance—2014," Population Fact Sheets; A. S. Go et al., "Heart Disease and Stroke Statistics—2014 Update: A Report from the American Heart Association," *Circulation* 129 (2014):: e28–e292, Statistics, 2014, chart 13.8.

- **Age.** Although cardiovascular disease can affect all ages, 82 percent of heart attacks occur in people over age 65.[59] Increasing age ups the risk for CVD for all.
- **Gender.** Men are at greater risk for CVD until about age 60, when women catch up and then surpass them. Women under 35 have a fairly low risk, although oral contraceptives and smoking increase risk. Hormonal factors appear to reduce risk for women, though after menopause, women's LDL levels tend to rise.[60]

Inflammation and C-Reactive Protein

Inflammation—which occurs when tissues are injured, for example by bacteria, trauma, toxins, or heat—may play a major role in atherosclerosis development, because injured vessel walls are more prone to plaque formation. Cigarette smoke, high blood pressure, high LDL cholesterol, diabetes mellitus, certain forms of arthritis, and exposure to toxins have been linked to increased risk of inflammation. However, the greatest risk appears to be from infectious disease pathogens, most notably *Chlamydia pneumoniae* (a common cause of respiratory infections); *Helicobacter pylori* (a bacterium that causes ulcers); herpes simplex virus; and *cytomegalovirus* (another herpes virus infecting most Americans before age 40).

During an inflammatory reaction, C-reactive proteins (CRPs) tend to be present in blood at high levels. A recent meta-analysis shows a strong association between C-reactive proteins in the blood and increased risks for atherosclerosis and CVD.[61] Doctors can test patients using an assay called hs-CRP; if levels are high, action could be taken to prevent progression to reduce inflammation.

Homocysteine

Homocysteine, an amino acid normally present in blood, was thought to be a prelude to coronary heart disease, peripheral artery disease, and increased risk of stroke. Scientists hypothesized that homocysteine inflamed the inner lining of the arterial walls and promoted fat deposits and the development of blood clots.[62] Early studies indicated that folic acid and other B vitamins may help break down homocysteine in the body. However, professional groups such as the American Heart Association do not currently recommend taking folic acid supplements to lower homocysteine levels and prevent CVD; instead they recommend following a healthy diet.[63]

check yourself

- **Of the risk factors described, which is of the most concern to you and why?**

11.11 Diagnosing and Treating CVD

learning outcome

11.11 Describe techniques for diagnosing and treating CVD.

There are many diagnostic, treatment, prevention, and rehabilitation options for cardiovascular disease. Medications can strengthen heartbeat, control arrhythmias, remove fluids, reduce blood pressure, and improve heart function.

CVD Diagnostic Techniques

An **electrocardiogram (ECG)** is a record of the heart's electrical activity. Patients may undergo a *stress test*—exercise on a stationary bike or treadmill with an electrocardiogram—or a *nuclear stress test,* which involves injecting a radioactive dye and taking images of the heart to reveal blood flow problems. In **angiography** (*cardiac catheterization*), a thin tube called a *catheter* is threaded through heart arteries, a dye is injected, and an X-ray is taken to identify blocked areas. A **positron emission tomography (PET) scan** produces three-dimensional images of the heart as blood flows through it. In *magnetic resonance imaging (MRI),* powerful magnets look inside the body to help identify damage, congenital defects, and disease. *Ultrafast computed tomography (CT),* an especially fast heart X-ray, is used to evaluate bypass grafts, diagnose ventricular function, and identify irregularities. *Coronary calcium score* is derived from another type of ultrafast CT used to diagnose calcium levels in heart vessels; high levels increase risk.

Surgical Options

Coronary bypass surgery has helped many patients survive coronary blockages or heart attacks. In a coronary artery bypass graft (CABG, referred to as a "cabbage"), a blood vessel is taken from another site in the patient's body (usually the saphenous vein in the leg or the internal thoracic artery [ITA] in the chest) and implanted to "bypass" blocked coronary arteries and transport blood to heart tissue.

With an **angioplasty** (sometimes called a *balloon angioplasty*), a catheter is threaded through blocked heart arteries. The catheter has a balloon at the tip, which is inflated to flatten fatty deposits against arterial walls, allowing blood to flow more freely. New forms of laser angioplasty and *atherectomy,* a procedure that removes plaque, are done in several clinics.

Many people with heart blockage undergo angioplasty and receive a **stent**, a steel mesh tube inserted to prop open the artery. Although stents are highly effective, inflammation and tissue growth in the area may actually increase after the procedure, and in about 30 percent of patients, the treated arteries become clogged again within 6 months.[64] Newer stents are usually medicated to reduce this risk.

Drug Therapies

Although aspirin has been touted as possibly reducing risks for future heart attacks, the benefits of an aspirin regimen for otherwise healthy adults remains in question. New research indicates an

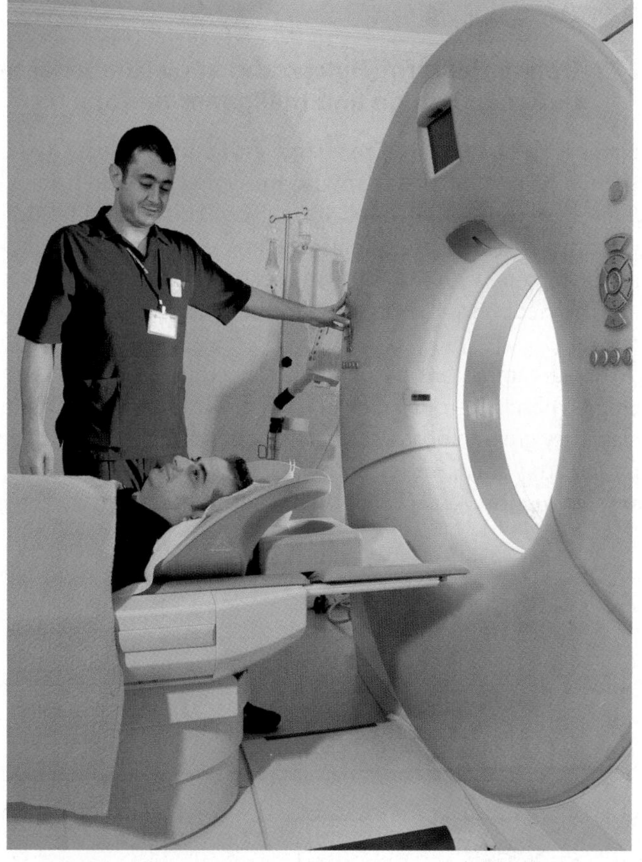

Magnetic resonance imaging is one of several methods used to detect heart damage, abnormalities, or defects.

increased risk of gastrointestinal bleeding and stroke in those who take it daily.[65] Furthermore, once a patient has taken aspirin regularly for possible protection against CHD, stopping this regimen may, in fact, increase his or her risk.[66]

Clot-busting therapy with **thrombolysis** can be performed within the first 1 to 3 hours after an attack. Thrombolysis involves injecting an agent such as *tissue plasminogen activator* (*tPA*) to dissolve the clot and restore some blood flow, thereby reducing the amount of tissue that dies from ischemia.[67]

Cardiac Rehabilitation and Recovery

Every year, more than 1 million Americans survive heart attacks. Millions more have a number of medical interventions to help them survive and thrive. Strategies for rehabilitation may include exercise training and classes on nutrition and CVD risk management. Not all patients choose to participate, due to lack of insurance, fear of another attack due to exercise, or other barriers. However, the benefits of rehabilitation far outweigh the risks.

check yourself

- **How is CVD commonly diagnosed and treated?**

11.12

What Is Cancer?

learning outcome

11.12 Define the term *cancer,* and know the difference between benign and malignant tumors.

Cancer is the name given to a large group of diseases characterized by the uncontrolled growth and spread of abnormal cells. When something interrupts normal cell programming, uncontrolled growth and abnormal cellular development result in a **neoplasm**, a new growth of tissue serving no physiological function. This neoplasmic mass often forms a clump of cells known as a **tumor**.

Not all tumors are **malignant** (cancerous); in fact, most are **benign** (noncancerous). Benign tumors are generally harmless unless they grow to obstruct or crowd out normal tissues. A benign tumor of the brain, for instance, may become life threatening if it grows enough to restrict blood flow and cause a stroke. The only way to determine whether a tumor is malignant is through **biopsy**, or microscopic examination of cell development.

Benign tumors generally consist of ordinary-looking cells enclosed in a fibrous shell or capsule that prevents their spreading to other body areas. In contrast, malignant tumors are usually not enclosed in a protective capsule and can therefore spread to other organs (Figure 11.7). This process, known as **metastasis**, makes some forms of cancer particularly aggressive in their ability to overwhelm bodily defenses. Malignant tumors frequently metastasize throughout the body, making treatment extremely difficult. Unlike benign tumors, which merely expand to take over a given space, malignant cells invade surrounding tissue, emitting clawlike protrusions that disturb the RNA and DNA within normal cells. Disrupting these substances, which control cellular metabolism and reproduction, produces **mutant cells** that differ in form, quality, and function from normal cells.

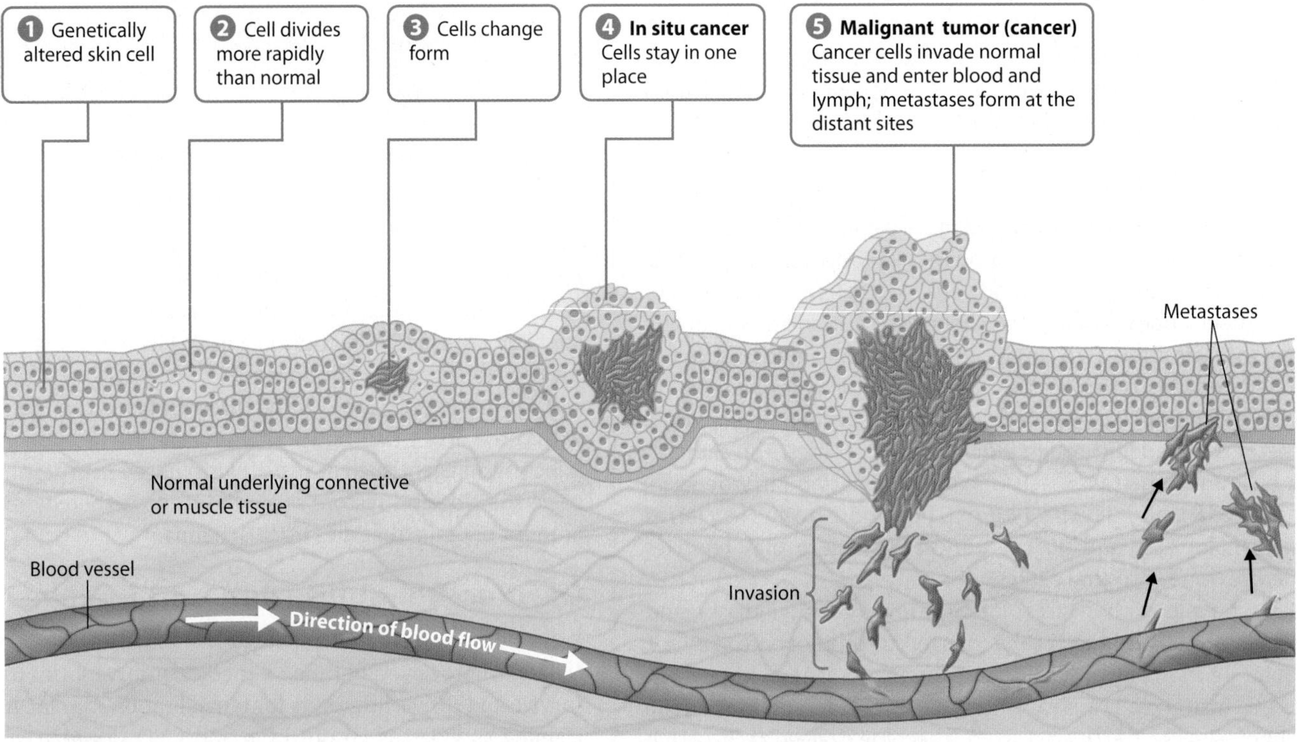

Figure 11.7 Metastasis

A mutation to the genetic material of a skin cell triggers abnormal cell division and changes cell formation, resulting in a cancerous tumor. If the tumor remains localized, it is considered in situ cancer. If the tumor spreads, it is considered a malignant cancer.

VIDEO TUTOR
Metastasis

check yourself

- **What is cancer?**
- **What is the difference between benign and malignant tumors?**

11.13

Types and Sites of Cancer

learning outcome

11.13 List the major types and most common sites of cancer.

The word *cancer* refers not to a single disease, but to hundreds of different diseases. They are grouped into four broad categories based on the type of tissue from which the cancer arises:

- **Carcinomas.** Epithelial tissues (tissues covering body surfaces and lining most body cavities) are the most common sites for cancers; cancers occurring in epithelial tissue are called *carcinomas.* These cancers affect the outer layer of the skin and mouth as well as the mucous membranes. They metastasize initially through the circulatory or lymphatic system and form solid tumors.
- **Sarcomas.** Sarcomas occur in the mesodermal, or middle, layers of tissue—for example, in bones, muscles, and general connective tissue. In the early stages of disease, they metastasize primarily via the blood. These cancers are less common but generally more virulent than carcinomas. They also form solid tumors.
- **Lymphomas.** Lymphomas develop in the lymphatic system—the infection-fighting regions of the body—and metastasize through the lymphatic system. Hodgkin's disease is an example. Lymphomas also form solid tumors.
- **Leukemias.** Cancer of the blood-forming parts of the body, particularly the bone marrow and spleen, is called leukemia. A non-solid tumor, leukemia is characterized by an abnormal increase in the number of white blood cells that the body produces.

Figure 11.8 shows the most common sites of cancer and the estimated number of new cases and deaths from each type in 2011.

Estimated New Cases of Cancer*		Estimated Deaths from Cancer*	
Female	Male	Female	Male
Breast 232,670 (29%)	Prostate 232,670 (29%)	Lung & bronchus 72,330 (26%)	Lung & bronchus 86,930 (28%)
Lung & bronchus 108,210 (13%)	Lung & bronchus 108,210 (13%)	Breast 40,000 (15%)	Prostate 29,480 (10%)
Colon & rectum 65,000 (8%)	Colon & rectum 71,830 (9%)	Colon & rectum 24,040 (9%)	Colon & rectum 26,270 (8%)
Uterine corpus 52,630 (6%)	Urinary bladder 56,390 (7%)	Pancreas 19,420 (7%)	Pancreas 20,170 (7%)
Thyroid 47,790 (6%)	Melanoma of the skin 43,890 (5%)	Ovary 14,270 (5%)	Liver & intrahepatic bile duct 15,870 (5%)
Non-Hodgkin lymphoma 32,530 (4%)	Kidney & renal pelvis 39,140 (5%)	Leukemia 10,050 (4%)	Leukemia 14,040 (5%)
Melanoma of the skin 32,210 (4%)	Non-Hodgkin lymphoma 38,270 (4%)	Uterine corpus 8,590 (3%)	Esophagus 12,450 (4%)
Kidney & renal pelvis 24,780 (3%)	Oral cavity & pharynx 30,220 (4%)	Non-Hodgkin lymphoma 8,520 (3%)	Urinary bladder 11,170 (4%)
Pancreas 22,890 (3%)	Leukemia 30,100 (4%)	Liver & intrahepatic bile duct 7,130 (3%)	Non-Hodgkin lymphoma 10,470 (3%)
Leukemia 22,280 (3%)	Pancreas 22,289 (3%)	Brain & other nervous system 6,230 (2%)	Kidney & renal pelvis 8,900 (3%)
All Sites 810,320 (100%)	All Sites 855,220 (100%)	All Sites 275,370 (100%)	All Sites 310,010 (100%)

*Excludes basal and squamous cell skin cancers and in situ carcinoma except urinary bladder. Percentages may not total 100% due to rounding.

Figure 11.8 Leading Sites of New Cancer Cases and Deaths, 2014 Estimates

Source: Data from Table on page 4, American Cancer Society, *Cancer Facts & Figures 2014* (Atlanta, GA: American Cancer Society, Inc.). Note that percentages do not add up to 100 due to omissions of certain rare cancers as well as rounding of statistics.

check yourself

- **What are the major types of cancer?**
- **What sites are the most common sites of cancer?**

11.14 Risk Factors for Cancer

learning outcome

11.14 List lifestyle, genetic, environmental, and medical risk factors for cancer.

Specific risk factors for cancer fall into two major classes: hereditary risk and acquired (environmental) risk. Hereditary factors cannot be modified, whereas environmental factors are potentially modifiable.

Lifestyle Risks for Cancer

Anyone can develop cancer; however, nearly 77 percent of cancers are diagnosed at age 55 and above.[68] *Lifetime risk* refers to the probability that an individual, over the course of a lifetime, will develop cancer or die from it. In the United States, men have a lifetime risk of about 1 in 2 and women 1 in 3.[69]

Relative risk is a measure of the strength of the relationship between risk factors and a particular cancer. For example, a male smoker's relative risk of getting lung cancer is about twice that of a male nonsmoker.[70]

Tobacco Use Of all the risk factors for cancer, smoking is among the greatest. In the United States, tobacco is responsible for nearly 1 in 5 deaths annually, or about 443,000 premature deaths each year.[71] Smoking is associated with increased risk of at least 15 different cancers, including causal relationships between smoking and liver cancer, colorectal polyps, and colorectal cancer.[72] Smoking accounts for 30 percent of all cancer deaths and 87 percent of all lung cancer deaths in the United States.[73] Chances of developing cancer are 23 times higher among male smokers and 13 times higher among female smokers, compared to nonsmokers.[74]

Of the several lifestyle risk factors for cancer, tobacco use is perhaps the most significant and the most preventable.

Alcohol and Cancer Risk Countless studies have implicated alcohol as a risk factor for cancer. Light to moderate alcohol intake (more than one drink per day) appears to increase risk of breast cancer among women.[75] Moderate alcohol intake (above one drink per day) in women also appears to increase the risk of cancers of the oral cavity and pharynx, esophagus, and larynx, and binge drinking may increase gastric and pancreatic cancer risk.[76] For men, regular heavy consumption of alcohol appears to increase the risk of esophageal and liver cancers more than sevenfold. The risk of colon, stomach, and prostate cancers in men was about 80 percent higher among heavy drinkers, while lung cancer risk rose by almost 60 percent compared to nondrinkers.[77]

Poor Nutrition, Physical Inactivity, and Obesity About one-third of U.S. cancer deaths may be due to lifestyle factors such as overweight or obesity, physical inactivity, and nutrition.[78] Dietary choices and physical activity are the most important modifiable determinants of cancer risk (besides not smoking). Several studies indicate a relationship between high body mass index (BMI) and death rates for cancers of the esophagus, colon, rectum, liver, stomach, kidney, and pancreas, and others.[79] Women who gain 55 pounds or more after age 18 have almost a 50 percent greater risk of breast cancer compared to those who maintain their weight.[80] The relative risk of colon cancer in men is 40 percent higher for obese men than for nonobese men. Numerous other studies support the link between cancer and obesity.[81]

Stress and Psychosocial Risks People who are under chronic, severe stress or who suffer from depression or other persistent emotional problems show higher rates of cancer than their healthy counterparts. Sleep disturbances or an unhealthy diet may weaken the body's immune system, increasing susceptibility to cancer. Another possible contributor to cancer development is poverty and the health disparities associated with low socioeconomic status.

Genetic and Physiological Risks

Scientists believe that about 5 percent of all cancers are strongly hereditary; some people may be more predisposed to the malfunctioning of genes that ultimately cause cancer.[82]

Suspected cancer-causing genes are called **oncogenes**. Though these genes are typically dormant, certain conditions such as age; stress; and exposure to carcinogens, viruses, and radiation may activate them, causing cells to grow and reproduce uncontrollably. Scientists are uncertain whether only people who develop cancer have oncogenes or whether we all have genes that can become oncogenes under certain conditions.

Certain cancers, particularly those of the breast, stomach, colon, prostate, uterus, ovaries, and lungs, appear to run in families. Hodgkin's disease and certain leukemias show similar familial patterns. Can we attribute these patterns to genetic susceptibility or to the fact that people in the same families experience similar environmental risks? The complex interaction of hereditary predisposition, lifestyle, and environment makes it a challenge to determine a single cause. Even among those predisposed to mutations, avoiding risks may decrease chances of cancer development.

Reproductive and Hormonal Factors Increased numbers of fertile years (early menarche, late menopause), not having children or having them later in life, recent use of birth control pills or hormone replacement therapy, and opting not to breast-feed all appear to increase risks of breast cancer.[83] However, although these factors appear to play a significant role in increased risk for non-Hispanic white women, they do not appear to have as strong an influence on Hispanic women.[84] Although earlier studies suggested that hormone therapy may slightly increase the risk of lung cancer, newer research has shown no significant increases due to hormone therapy.[85]

Inflammation Risks

Inflammatory processes in the body are thought to play a significant role in the development of cancer—from initiation and promoting cancer cells to paving the way for them to invade, spread, and weaken the immune response.[86] According to some researchers, 90 percent of cancers are caused by cellular mutations and environmental factors that occur as a result of inflammation. These researchers believe that up to 20 percent of cancers are the result of chronic infections, 30 percent are the result of tobacco smoking and inhaled particulates such as asbestos, and 35 percent are due to dietary factors.[87]

Occupational and Environmental Risks

Though workplace hazards account for only a small percentage of all cancers, several substances are known to cause cancer when exposure levels are high or prolonged. Asbestos, nickel, chromate, benzene, arsenic, and vinyl chloride are **carcinogens** (cancer-causing agents), as are certain dyes and radioactive substances, coal tars, inhalants, and possibly some herbicides and pesticides.

Radiation Ionizing radiation (IR)—radiation from X-rays, radon, cosmic rays, and ultraviolet radiation (primarily UVB radiation)—is the only form of radiation proven to cause human cancer. Virtually any part of the body can be affected by IR, but bone marrow and the thyroid are particularly susceptible. Radon exposure in homes can increase lung cancer risk, especially in cigarette smokers. To reduce the risk of harmful effects, diagnostic medical and dental X-rays are set at the lowest dose levels possible.

Nonionizing radiation produced by radio waves, cell phones, microwaves, computer screens, televisions, electric blankets, and other products has been a topic of great concern in recent years, though research has not proven excess risk to date.

Chemicals in Foods Much of the concern about chemicals in food centers on possible harm from pesticide and herbicide residue. Continued research regarding pesticide and herbicide use is essential, and scientists and consumer groups stress the importance of a balance between chemical use and the production of high-quality food products.

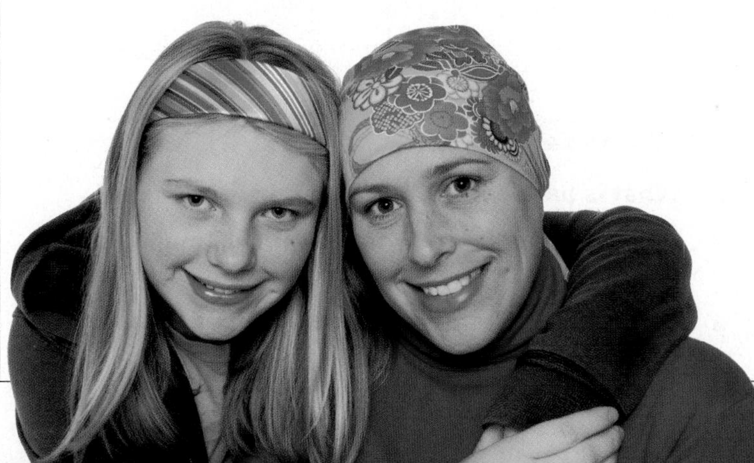

Some forms of cancer have strong genetic bases; daughters of women with breast cancer have an increased risk of developing the disease.

Infectious Disease Risks

Over 10 percent of all cancers in the United States are caused by infectious agents such as viruses, bacteria, or parasites.[88] Worldwide, approximately 15–20 percent of human cancers have been traced to infectious agents.[89] Infections are thought to influence cancer development in several ways, most commonly through chronic inflammation, suppression of the immune system, or chronic stimulation.

Hepatitis B, Hepatitis C, and Liver Cancer Viruses such as the ones that cause chronic forms of hepatitis B (HBV) and C (HCV) chronically inflame liver tissue, which may make it more hospitable for cancer development.

Human Papillomavirus and Cervical Cancer Between 70 and 100 percent of women with cervical cancer have evidence of human papillomavirus (HPV) infection, which is also believed to be a cause of vaginal and vulvar cancers in women and penile cancers in men. A vaccine is available to help protect men and women from becoming infected with HPV. The vaccine seems to be effective in reducing risks of cervical and penile cancer.[90]

***Helicobacter pylori* and Stomach Cancer** *Helicobacter pylori* is a bacterium found in the stomach lining of approximately 30 to 40 percent of Americans. It causes irritation, scarring, and ulcers, damaging the lining of the stomach and leading to cellular changes that may lead to cancer. More than half of all cases of stomach cancer may be linked to *H. pylori* infection, even though most infected people don't develop cancer.[91] Treatment with antibiotics often cures the ulcers, which appears to reduce risk of new stomach cancer.[92]

Medical Factors

Some medical treatments can increase a person's risk for cancer. The use of estrogen for relieving women's menopausal symptoms is now recognized to have contributed to multiple cancer risks; hence prescriptions for estrogen therapy have declined dramatically. Some chemotherapy drugs have been shown to increase risks for other cancers; weighing the benefits versus harms of these treatments is always necessary.

check yourself

- **What are some major lifestyle, genetic, environmental, and medical risk factors for cancer?**
- **What are your risks for cancer? What lifestyle changes can you make to mitigate these risks?**

11.15

Lung Cancer

learning outcome

11.15 Identify the major factors contributing to lung cancer.

Lung cancer is the leading cause of cancer deaths for both men and women in the United States. It killed an estimated 160,000 Americans in 2014, accounting for nearly 27 percent of all cancer deaths.[93] The lifetime risks for males and females getting lung cancer is 1 in 13 and 1 in 16, respectively. Risks begin to rise around age 40 and continue to climb through all age groups thereafter.[94]

Since 1987, more women have died each year from lung cancer than from breast cancer, which over the previous 40 years was the major cause of cancer deaths in women. Although lower smoking rates have boded well for cancer statistics, there is growing concern about the number of young people, particularly women and persons of low income and low educational levels, who continue to pick up the habit.

There is also concern about increase in lung cancers among *never smokers*—people who have never smoked, but nevertheless have as many as 15 percent of all lung cancers. Never smokers' lung cancer is believed to be related to exposure to secondhand smoke, radon gas, asbestos, indoor wood-burning stoves, and aerosolized oils caused by cooking with oil and deep fat frying.[95] Unfortunately, because doctors often don't think of lung cancer when a never smoker presents with a cough, patients are often put on antibiotics or cough suppressants as therapy. By the time they recognize that it's really lung cancer, their cancer is likely to be more advanced and treatment more challenging.

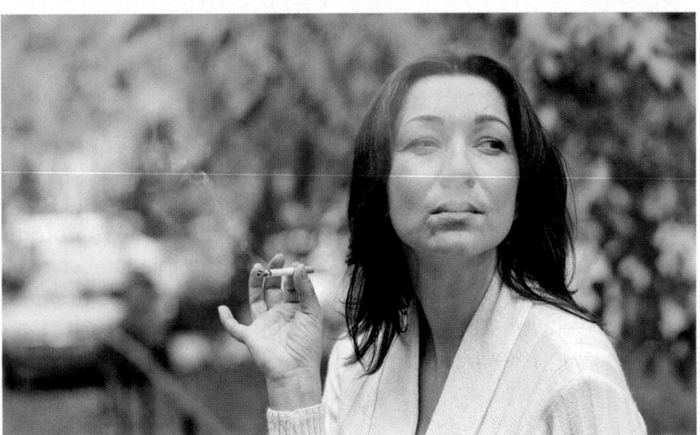

If my mom quits smoking now, will it reduce her risk of cancer, or is it too late?

It's never too late to quit. Stopping smoking at any time will reduce your risk of lung cancer, in addition to the numerous other health benefits that are gained. Studies of women have shown that within 5 years of quitting, their risk of death from lung cancer had decreased by 21 percent, when compared with people who had continued smoking.

90%

of all lung cancers could be avoided if people did not smoke.

Detection, Symptoms, and Treatment

Symptoms of lung cancer include a persistent cough, blood-streaked sputum, voice change, chest pain or back pain, and recurrent attacks of pneumonia or bronchitis. Newer computerized tomography (CT) scans, molecular markers in saliva, and newer biopsy techniques have improved screening accuracy for lung cancer but have a long way to go.

Treatment depends on type and stage of cancer. Surgery, radiation therapy, chemotherapy, and targeted biological therapies are all options. If the cancer is localized, surgery is usually the treatment of choice. If it has spread, surgery is combined with radiation, chemotherapy and other targeted drug treatments. Fewer than 15 percent of lung cancer cases are diagnosed at the early, localized stages. Early stage cancers have a 54 percent 1-year survival rate, falling to 6–18 percent at 5 years after diagnosis.[96]

Risk Factors and Prevention

Risks for cancer increase dramatically based on the quantity of cigarettes smoked and the number of years smoked, often referred to as *pack years*. The greater the number of pack years smoked, the greater the risk of developing cancer. Quitting smoking does reduce the risk of developing lung cancer.[97] Exposure to industrial substances or radiation also highly increases the risk for lung cancer.

check yourself

- **What is lung cancer, and what are its causes?**
- **What can you do to protect yourself against lung cancer?**
- **What are the symptoms and treatment of lung cancer?**

Colon and Rectal Cancers

learning outcome

11.16 Identify the major factors contributing to colorectal cancer.

Colorectal cancers (cancers of the colon and rectum) continue to be the third most commonly diagnosed cancer in both men and women and the third leading cause of cancer deaths, even though death rates are declining.[98] In 2014, there were 96,830 cases of colon cancer and 40,000 cases of rectal cancer diagnosed in the United States, as well as 50,310 deaths.[99] Ninety percent of colorectal cancers occur in individuals who are over the age of 50. From birth to age 49, men have a 1 in 305 risk of developing it, while women have a 1 in 334 chance.[100]

Detection, Symptoms, and Treatment

Because colorectal cancer tends to spread slowly, the prognosis is quite good if it is caught in the early stages. In fact, when caught at an early, localized stage, 5-year survival rates are over 90 percent.[101] But in its early stages, colorectal cancer typically has no symptoms. As the disease progresses, bleeding from the rectum, blood in the stool, and changes in bowel habits are the major warning signals.

An excellent way to catch such cancers early is through testing. Colonoscopies and other screening tests should begin at age 50 for most people. Virtual colonoscopies and fecal DNA testing are newer diagnostic techniques that have shown promise. However, only 10 percent of all Americans over age 50 have had the most basic screening test—the at-home *fecal occult blood* test (FBOT)—in the past year, and slightly over 50 percent have had an endoscopy test.[102] Only 59 percent of those over age 50 who should be screened actually get screened, and Hispanics and non-English-speaking individuals have even lower rates of screening.[103]

Treatment often consists of radiation or surgery. Chemotherapy, although not used extensively in the past, is today a possibility.

Risk Factors and Prevention

Anyone can get colorectal cancer, but people who are older than age 50, who are obese, who have a family history of colon and rectal cancer, who have a personal or family history of polyps (benign growths) in the colon or rectum, or who have inflammatory bowel problems such as colitis run an increased risk. A history of diabetes also seems to increase risk. Other possible risk factors include diets high in fat or low in fiber, high consumption of red and processed meats, smoking, sedentary lifestyle, high alcohol consumption, and low intake of fruits and vegetables. New research shows an alarming increase in colorectal cancer among young adults. If these trends continue, we may see a 90% increase in incidence among those 20–34 years old between 2010 and 2030.[104]

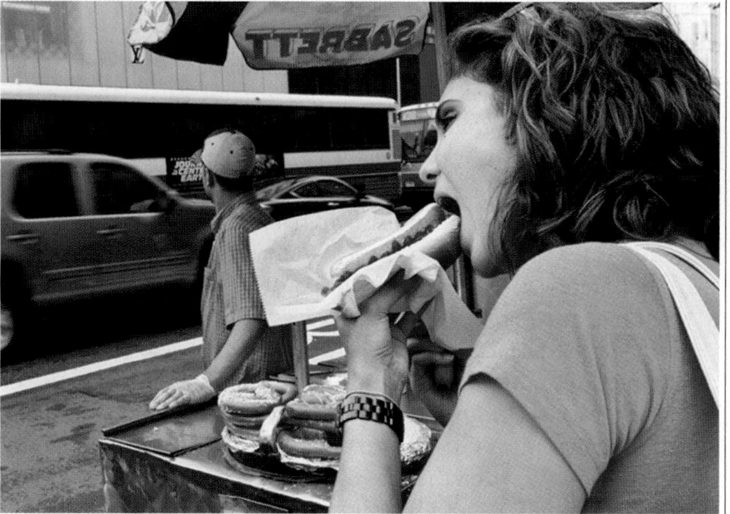

The consumption of red meat and processed meats is a risk factor for colorectal cancer, as is obesity. Food additives, particularly sodium nitrate, are used to preserve and give color to red meat and to protect against pathogens, particularly *Clostridium botulinum*, the bacterium that causes botulism. Concern about the carcinogenic properties of nitrates, which are often used in hot dogs, hams, and luncheon meats, has led to the introduction of meats that are nitrate-free or contain reduced levels of the substance.

Regular exercise, a diet with lots of fruits and other plant foods, a healthy weight, and moderation in alcohol consumption appear to be among the most promising prevention strategies. Consumption of milk and calcium also appears to decrease risks. New research suggests that nonsteroidal anti-inflammatory drugs (NSAIDs) such as aspirin, postmenopausal hormones, folic acid, calcium supplements, selenium, and vitamin E may also help.[105]

check yourself

- **What is colorectal cancer, and what are its causes?**
- **What can you do to protect against colorectal cancer?**

11.17 Breast Cancer

learning outcome

11.17 Identify the major factors contributing to breast cancer.

Breast cancer is a group of diseases that cause uncontrolled cell growth in breast tissue, particularly in the glands that produce milk and the ducts that connect those glands to the nipple. Cancers can also form in the connective and lymphatic tissues of the breast.

In 2014, approximately 232,679 women and 2,360 men in the United States were diagnosed with invasive breast cancer for the first time. In addition, 63,570 new cases of in situ breast cancer, a more localized cancer, were diagnosed. About 40,430 women (and 430 men) died, making breast cancer the second leading cause of cancer death for women.[106] Women have a 1 in 8 lifetime risk of being diagnosed with breast cancer. From birth to age 49, the risk is 1 in 53, but between the ages of 50 and 59, the chance for breast cancer becomes 1 in 43.[107] Most health groups have advocated screening for breast cancer more thoroughly after age 40.

Detection

The earliest signs of breast cancer are usually observable on mammograms, often before lumps can be felt. However, mammograms are not foolproof, and there is debate regarding the optimal age at which women should start regularly receiving them. Hence, regular breast self-examination (BSE) is also important (see below for information on BSE). Although not recommended as a screening tool per se, a newer form of magnetic resonance imaging (MRI) appears to be even more accurate, particularly in women with genetic risks for tumors or those who have suspicious areas of the breast or surrounding tissue that warrant a clearer image. If you are referred for a breast MRI, be sure to go to a facility where they can perform a breast biopsy if there are any areas that need further investigation.[108]

Symptoms

If breast cancer grows large enough, it can produce the following symptoms: a lump in the breast or surrounding lymph nodes, thickening, dimpling, skin irritation, distortion, retraction or scaliness of the nipple, nipple discharge, or tenderness.

Breast Awareness and Self-Exam

Breast self-exam has been recommended by major health organizations as a form of early breast cancer screening for the last two decades (Figure 11.9). However, a 2009 "study of studies" done by the U.S. Preventive Services Task Force determined that breast self-exams did not decrease suffering and death and, in fact, often lead to unnecessary worry, unnecessary tests, and increased health care costs. As a result of this research, several groups have downgraded the recommendation about BSE from "do them and do them regularly" to "learn how to do them, and if you desire, do them to know your body and be able to recognize changes."

To do a breast self-exam, begin by standing in front of a mirror to inspect the breasts, looking for their usual symmetry. Some breasts are not symmetrical, and if this is not a change, it is okay. Raise and lower both arms while checking that the breasts move evenly and freely. Next, inspect the skin, looking for areas of redness, thickening, or dimpling, which might have the appearance of an orange peel. Look for any scaling on the nipple.

To feel for lumps, raise one arm above your head while either standing or lying. This will flatten out the breast, making it easier to feel the tissue. Using the index, middle, and fourth fingers of your opposite hand, gently push down on the breast tissue and move the fingers in small circular motions, varying pressure from light to more firm. Start at

What are some of the challenges facing cancer survivors?

The journey through cancer survivorship is not always smooth. Even after the 5-year benchmark is reached, living a full, positive life in cancer's wake can be a major challenge. There may be physical, emotional, and financial issues to cope with for years after diagnosis and treatment. Survivors may find themselves struggling with access to health insurance and life insurance, financial strains, difficulties with employment, and the toll on personal relationships. Survivors also have to live with the possibility of a recurrence. However, cancer survivors can and do live active, productive lives despite these challenges.

one edge of the breast and move upward and then downward, working your way across the breast until all of the breast tissue has been covered. Often, breast tissue will feel dense and irregular, and this is usually normal. It helps to do regular self-exams to become familiar with what your breast tissue feels like; then, if there is a change, you will notice. Cancers usually feel like a dense or firm little rock and are very different from the normal breast tissue.

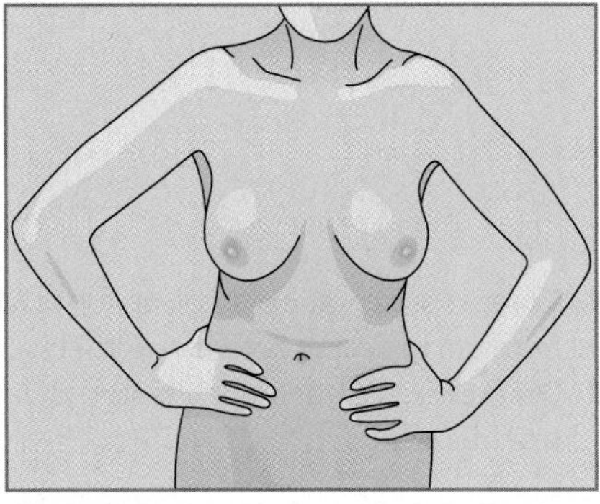

1 Face a mirror and check for changes in symmetry.

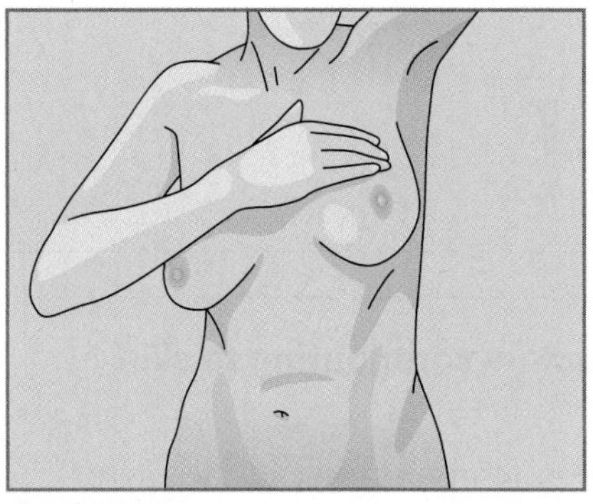

2 Either standing or lying down, use the pads of the three middle fingers to check for lumps. Follow an up and down pattern on the breast to ensure all tissue gets inspected.

Figure 11.9 Breast Self-Examination

Next, lower the arm and reach into the top of the underarm and pull downward with gentle pressure feeling for any enlarged lymph nodes. To complete the exam, squeeze the tissue around the nipple. If you notice discharge from the nipple and you have not recently been breastfeeding, consult your doctor. Likewise, if you notice any asymmetry, skin changes, scaling on the nipple, or new lumps in the breast, you should see your doctor for evaluation.

Treatment

Treatments range from a lumpectomy to radical mastectomy to various combinations of radiation or chemotherapy. Among nonsurgical options, promising results have been noted among women using *selective estrogen-receptor modulators* (*SERMs*) such as tamoxifen and raloxifene, particularly among women whose cancers appear to grow in response to estrogen. These drugs, as well as new *aromatase inhibitors*, work by blocking estrogen. The 5-year survival rate for people with localized breast cancer has risen from 80 percent in the 1950s to 99 percent today.[109] However, these statistics vary dramatically, based on the stage of the cancer when it is first detected and whether it has spread. If the cancer has spread to the lymph nodes or other organs, the 5-year survival rate drops to as low as 24 percent.[110]

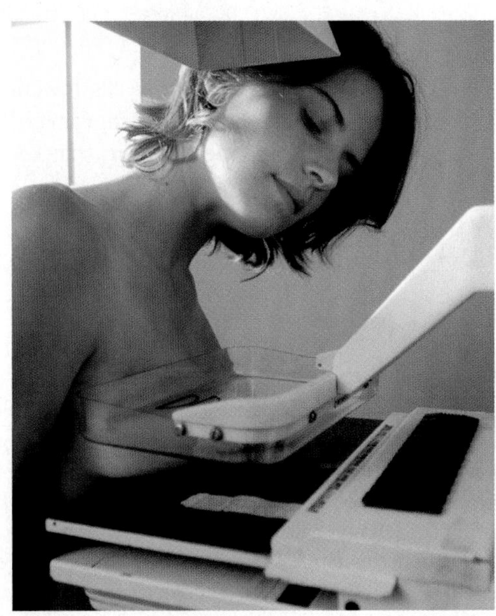

Early detection through mammography and other techniques greatly increase a woman's chance of surviving breast cancer.

Risk Factors and Prevention

The incidence of breast cancer increases with age. Although there are many possible risk factors, those well supported by research include family history of breast cancer, menstrual periods that started early and ended late in life, weight gain after the age of 18, obesity after menopause, recent use of oral contraceptives or postmenopausal hormone therapy, never bearing children or bearing a first child after age 30, consuming two or more drinks of alcohol per day, and physical inactivity. In addition, there is new evidence that heavy smoking, particularly among women who started smoking before their first pregnancy, increases risk. Other factors that increase risk include having dense breasts, type 2 diabetes, high bone mineral density, and exposure to high-dose radiation.[111] Although the *BRCA1* and *BRCA2* gene mutations are rare and occur in less than 1 percent of the population, they account for approximately 5 to 10 percent of all cases of breast cancer.[112] Women who possess these genes have up to an 80 percent risk of developing breast cancer in their lives and tend to develop breast cancer at earlier ages. Because these genes are rare, routine screening for them is not recommended unless there is a strong family history (particularly among younger primary relatives) of breast cancer.[113]

See It! Videos

Could you have inherited breast cancer from a female relative? Watch **Breast Cancer Patients Getting Younger** in the Study Area of MasteringHealth.

International differences in breast cancer incidence correlate with variations in diet, especially fat intake, although a causal role for these dietary factors has not been firmly established. Sudden weight gain has also been implicated. Research also shows that regular exercise can reduce risk.[114] Research indicates if you eat more fiber, breast cancer rates seem to go down, and if you eat less, rates seem to increase.[115]

check yourself

- **What is breast cancer, and what are its causes?**
- **What can you do to protect against breast cancer?**

11.18 Skin Cancer

learning outcome

11.18 Identify the major factors contributing to skin cancer.

Skin cancer is the most common form of cancer in the United States today, with over 3.5 million diagnosed cases in 2014.[116] Millions more remain undiagnosed and untreated, and 1 in 5 people in the United States will be diagnosed in their lifetime. In 2014, an estimated 12,980 deaths from skin cancer will occur, 9,710 from melanoma and 3,370 from other skin cancers.[117]

The two most common types of skin cancer—basal cell and squamous cell carcinomas—are highly curable. **Malignant melanoma**, the third most common form of skin cancer, is the most deadly. The majority of these deaths are in white men over the age of 50, with only rare cases among African Americans. Between 65 and 90 percent of melanomas are caused by exposure to ultraviolet (UV) light or sunlight.[118]

Detection, Symptoms, and Treatment

Basal and squamous cell carcinomas show up most commonly on the face, ears, neck, arms, hands, and legs as warty bumps, colored spots, or scaly patches. Bleeding, itchiness, pain, or oozing are other symptoms that warrant attention. Although surgery may be necessary to remove these, they are seldom life threatening.

In striking contrast is melanoma, an invasive killer that may appear as a skin lesion. Typically, the lesion's size, shape, or color changes and it spreads to regional organs and throughout the body. Malignant melanomas account for over 75 percent of all skin cancer deaths. Figure 11.10 shows melanoma compared to basal cell and squamous cell carcinomas. The *ABCD* rule can help you remember the warning signs of melanoma:

- **Asymmetry.** One half of the mole or lesion does not match the other half.
- **Border irregularity.** The edges are uneven, notched, or scalloped.
- **Color.** Pigmentation is not uniform. Melanomas may vary in color from tan to deeper brown, reddish black, black, or deep bluish black.
- **Diameter.** Diameter is greater than 6 millimeters (about the size of a pea).

Treatment of skin cancer depends on the type of cancer, its stage, and its location. Surgery, laser treatments, topical chemical agents, *electrodessication* (tissue destruction by heat), and *cryosurgery* (tissue destruction by freezing) are common treatments. For melanoma, treatment may involve surgical removal of the regional lymph nodes, radiation, or chemotherapy.

Risk Factors and Prevention

Anyone who overexposes himself or herself to ultraviolet (UV) radiation without adequate protection is at risk for skin cancer. The risk is greatest for people who:

- Have fair skin; blonde, red, or light brown hair; blue, green, or gray eyes
- Always burn before tanning, or burn easily and peel readily
- Don't tan easily but spend lots of time outdoors
- Use no or low-SPF (sun protection factor) sunscreens or expired suntan lotions
- Have had skin cancer or have a family history of skin cancer
- Experienced severe sunburns during childhood

Preventing skin cancer is a matter of limiting exposure to harmful UV rays. Upon exposure, the skin responds by increasing its thickness and the number of pigment cells (melanocytes), which produce the "tan" look. Ultraviolet light damages the skin's immune cells, lowering the normal immune protection of skin and priming it for cancer. Photodamage also causes wrinkling by impairing collagens that keep skin soft and pliable.

See It! Videos

Is there such a thing as a "safe" tan? Watch **Extreme Tanning** in the Study Area of MasteringHealth.

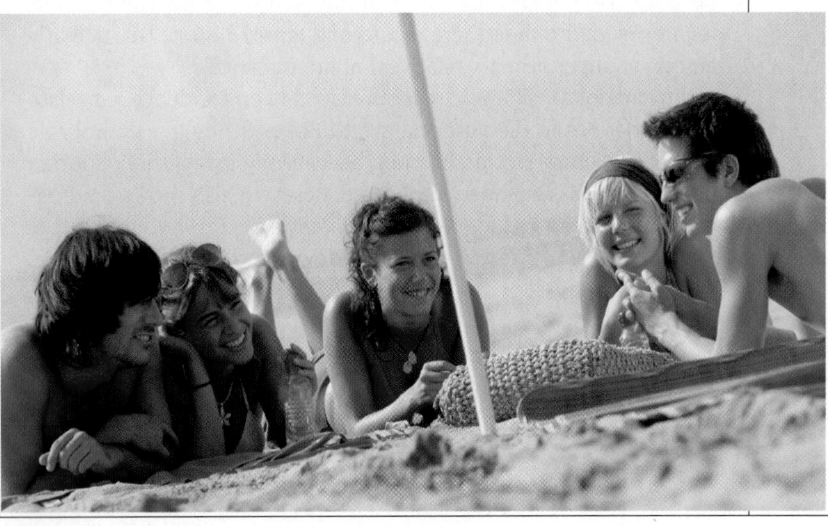

Is there any safe way to get a tan?

Unfortunately, no. There is no such thing as a "safe" tan, because a tan is visible evidence of UV-induced skin damage. The injury accumulated through years of tanning contributes to premature aging, as well as increasing your risk for disfiguring forms of skin cancer, eye problems, and possible death from melanoma. Whether the UV rays causing your tan came from the sun or from a tanning bed, the damage—and the cancer risk—is the same. Nor is an existing "base tan" protective against further damage. According to the American Cancer Society, tanned skin can provide only about the equivalent of sun protection factor (SPF) 4 sunscreen—much too weak to be considered protective.

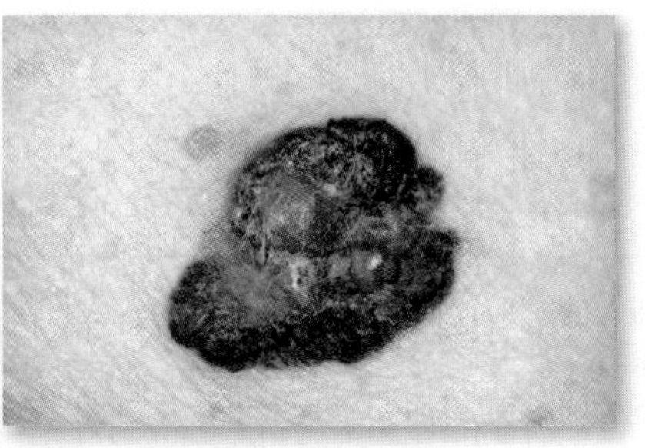
ⓐ Malignant melanoma

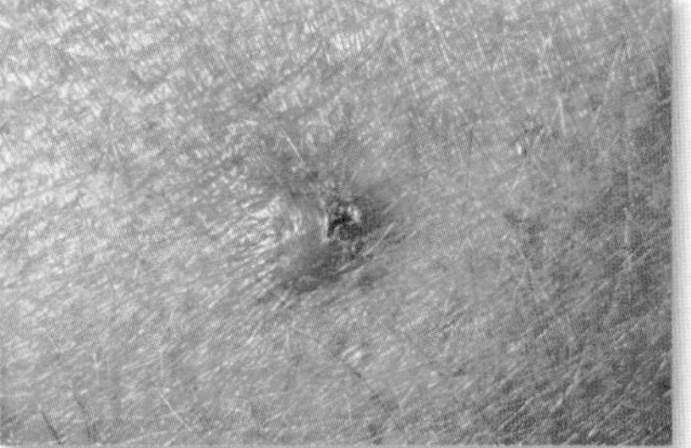
ⓑ Basal cell carcinoma

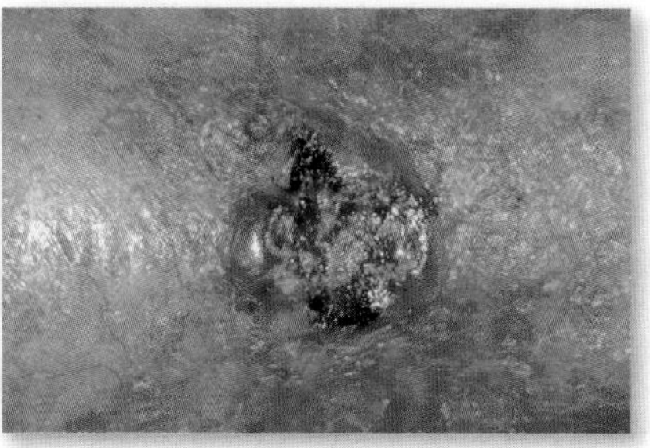
ⓒ Squamous cell carcinoma

Figure 11.10 Types of Skin Cancers
Preventing skin cancer includes keeping a careful watch for any new, pigmented growths and for changes to any moles. The ABCD warning signs of melanoma (a) include *asymmetrical* shapes, irregular *borders, color* variation, and an increase in *diameter*. Basal cell carcinoma (b) and squamous cell carcinoma (c) should be brought to your physician's attention but are not as deadly as melanoma.

Artificial Tans: Sacrificing Health for Beauty

In spite of the risks, many Americans strive for a tan each year, prompting some psychologists to speculate that there might be a form of compulsion to tan termed "*tanorexia*." Tanning is thought to be addictive due to some form of brain response to UVR light, prompting physiological or psychological responses. Recent studies of young adults exposed to indoor tanning suggests a possible link to tanning dependence and activation of the reward system.[119] However, critics argue that this research is preliminary and that large-scale clinical trials are necessary to confirm an association.

In our culture, being tan is equated with being healthy, chic, and attractive. Indoor tanning is a multi-billion-dollar industry. Teens and 20-somethings are the most likely to be users of indoor tanning overall, but users should know that their "glow" comes with a greatly increased cancer risk.

Many people believe—incorrectly—that tanning booths are safer than sitting in the sun. But all tanning lamps emit UVA rays, and most emit UVB rays as well. Both types of light rays cause long-term skin damage and can contribute to cancer. Consider the following:[120]

- There is a 59 percent increased risk of melanoma in those exposed to regular UV radiation from tanning beds. Tanning devices have been listed as carcinogenic for humans.
- People who use tanning beds are 2.5 times more likely to develop squamous cell carcinoma and 1.5 times more likely to develop basal cell carcinoma.
- High-pressure sunlamps used in some salons emit doses of UV radiation that can be as much as 12 times that of the sun.
- Up to 90 percent of visible skin changes commonly blamed on aging are caused by the sun.
- Some tanning facilities don't calibrate the UV output of their tanning bulbs, which can lead to more or less exposure than is paid for.
- Tanning booths and beds pose significant hygiene risks. Don't assume that those little colored water sprayers used to "clean" the inside of the beds are sufficient to kill organisms. The busier the facility, the more likely you'll come into contact with germs that could make you ill.

Skills for Behavior Change

TIPS FOR PROTECTING YOUR SKIN IN THE SUN

Avoid the sun or seek shade from 10 A.M.to 4 P.M., when the sun's rays are strongest. Even on a cloudy day, up to 80 percent of the sun's rays can get through.

- **Apply an SPF 15 or higher sunscreen evenly to all uncovered skin before going outside. Look for a "broad-spectrum" sunscreen that protects against both UVA and UVB radiation. If the label does not specify, apply the sunscreen 15 minutes before going outside.**
- **Know your SPFs. An SPF 15 product typically blocks about 94 percent of UVB rays, while an SPF 30 may block 97 percent. If you pay more for a 70–100 SPF product , you are probably just paying extra for no greater benefit.**
- **Check the expiration date on your sunscreen. Sunscreens lose effectiveness over time.**
- **Remember to apply sunscreen to your eyelids, lips, nose, ears, neck, hands, and feet. If you don't have much hair, apply sunscreen to the top of your head, too.**
- **Reapply sunscreen often. The label will tell you how often you need to do this. If it isn't waterproof, reapply it after swimming, or when sweating a lot.**
- **Wear loose-fitting, light-colored clothing. You can now purchase in most sporting goods stores clothing that has SPF protection. Wear a wide-brimmed, light-colored hat to protect your head and face.**
- **Use sunglasses with 99 to 100 percent UV protection to protect your eyes. Look for polarization in your shades.**
- **Check your skin for cancer, keeping an eye out for changes in birthmarks, moles, or sunspots.**

Source: Based on U.S. Food and Drug Administration, "FDA Sheds Light on Sunscreens," 2013, www.fda.gov.

check yourself

- **What is skin cancer, and what are its causes?**
- **What can you do to protect against skin cancer?**

11.19 Prostate and Testicular Cancer

learning outcome

11.19 Identify the major factors contributing to prostate and testicular cancer.

Prostate Cancer

Prostate cancer is the most frequently diagnosed cancer in American males today, after skin cancer, and it is the second leading cause of cancer deaths in men after lung cancer. In 2014, about 233,000 new cases of prostate cancer were diagnosed in the United States. About 1 in 6 men will be diagnosed with prostate cancer during his lifetime. However, with improved screening and early diagnosis, 5-year survival rates are nearly 100 percent for all but the most advanced cases. Men who are obese and smoke have an increased risk of dying from prostate cancer.[121]

Detection, Symptoms, and Treatment The prostate is a muscular, walnut-sized gland that surrounds part of a man's urethra, the tube that transports urine and sperm out of the body. A part of the reproductive system, its primary function is to produce seminal fluid. Symptoms of prostate cancer may include weak or interrupted urine flow; difficulty starting or stopping urination; feeling the urge to urinate frequently; pain on urination; blood in the urine; or pain in the low back, pelvis, or thighs. Many men have no symptoms in the early stages.

Men over age 40 should have an annual digital rectal prostate examination. Another screening method for prostate cancer is the **prostate-specific antigen (PSA)** test, a blood test that screens for an indicator of prostate cancer. However, the United States Preventive Services Task Force recommends that otherwise asymptomatic men no longer receive the routine PSA test because, overall, it does not save lives and may lead to unnecessary treatments.

Risk Factors and Prevention Increasing age is one of the biggest risks for prostate cancer, as is African ancestry or a family history of prostate cancer. Over 97 percent of all cases occur in men over the age of 50.[122] African American men and Jamaican men of African descent have the highest documented prostate cancer incidence rates in the world and are more likely to be diagnosed at more advanced stages than other racial groups.[123] Having a father or brother with prostate cancer more than doubles a man's risk of getting prostate cancer. Men who have had several relatives with prostate cancer, especially those with relatives who developed prostate cancer at younger ages, are also at higher risk.[124]

Eating more fruits and vegetables, particularly those containing *lycopene*, a pigment found in tomatoes and other red fruits, may lower the risk of prostate cancer death.[125] Diets high in processed meats or dairy and obesity appear to increase risks.[126] The best advice is to follow recommendations for a balanced diet and to maintain a healthy weight.

Testicular Cancer

Testicular cancer is one of the most common types of solid tumors found in young adult men, affecting nearly 8,820 young men in 2014.[127] Over one-half of all cases occur between the ages of 20 and 34.[128] However, with a 95 percent 5-year survival rate, it is one of the most curable forms of cancer, particularly if caught in localized stages. Men with undescended testicles appear to be at greatest risk, and some studies indicate a genetic influence. Risk is also higher if you are white, if you have HIV or AIDS, or if a primary relative (father or brother, in particular) has had testicular cancer.[129]

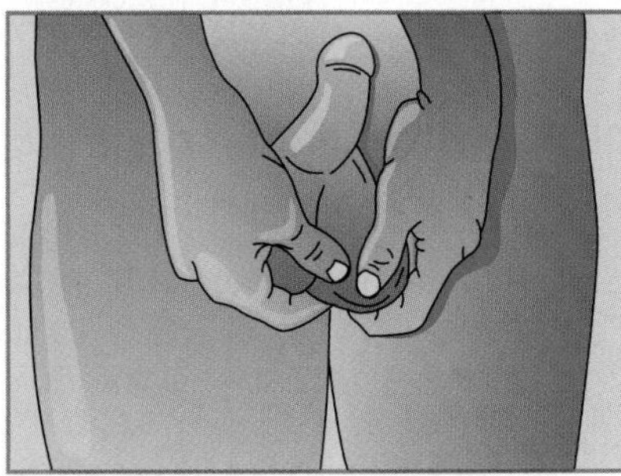

Figure 11.11 Testicular Self-Examination

Testicular Self-Exam

Testicular tumors first appear as an enlargement of the testis or thickening in testicular tissue. Some men report a heavy feeling, dull ache, or pain that extends to the lower abdomen or groin area. Testicular self-exams have long been recommended for teen boys and young men to perform monthly as a means of detecting testicular cancer (Figure 11.11). However, recent studies discovered that findings from monthly self-exams result in testing for noncancerous conditions and thus are not cost-effective. For this reason, the U.S. Preventive Services Task Force has dropped their recommendation for monthly testicular exams. Regardless, most cases of testicular cancer are discovered through self-exam, and there is currently no other screening test for the disease.

How To Examine Your Testicles

The testicular self-exam is best done after a hot shower, which will relax the scrotum and make the exam easier. Standing in front of a mirror, hold the testicle with one hand while gently rolling its surface between the thumb and fingers of your other hand. Feel underneath the scrotum for the tubes of the epididymis and blood vessels that sit close to the body. Repeat with the other testicle. Look for any lump, thickening, or pea-like nodules, paying attention to any areas that may be painful over the entire surface of the scrotum. When done, wash your hands with soap and water. Doing regular self-exams will help you to know what is normal for you and to note any irregularity. Consult a doctor if you note anything that is unusual.

check yourself

- **What are prostate and testicular cancer, and what are their causes?**

Other Cancers

learning **outcome**

11.20 Know the signs and symptoms of ovarian and uterine cancers, leukemia, and lymphoma.

Ovarian Cancer

Ovarian cancer is the fifth leading cause of cancer deaths for women, with about 22,000 women diagnosed in 2012 and 14,270 dying from it.[130] It causes more deaths than any other cancer of the reproductive system; women tend not to discover it until the cancer is at an advanced stage. If detected when localized, 5-year survival rates are 92 percent. If diagnosed at the regional level, rates drop to 72 percent, and if metastasis is diffuse and distant, survival rates drop to 27 percent.[131]

A woman may complain of feeling bloated, having pain in the pelvic area, feeling full quickly, or feeling the need to urinate more frequently. Some may experience persistent digestive disturbances; other symptoms include fatigue, pain during intercourse, unexplained weight loss, unexplained changes in bowel or bladder habits, and incontinence. If these vague symptoms persist for more than a week or two, prompt medical evaluation is a must.

Early-stage treatment typically includes surgery, chemotherapy, and occasionally radiation. Depending on the patient's age and desire to bear children, one or both ovaries, fallopian tubes, and the uterus may be removed.

Primary relatives (mother, daughter, sister) of a woman who has had ovarian cancer are at increased risk. A family or personal history of breast or colon cancer is also associated with increased risk. Women who have never been pregnant are more likely to develop ovarian cancer than those who have given birth to a child; the more children a woman has had, the less risk she faces. The use of estrogen postmenopausal therapy may increase a woman's risk, as will smoking and obesity.[132]

Using birth control pills, adhering to a low-fat diet, having multiple children, and breast-feeding can reduce risk of ovarian cancer.[133]

To protect yourself, get a complete pelvic examination. Women over 40 should have a cancer-related checkup every year. Uterine ultrasound or a blood test is recommended for those with risk factors or unexplained symptoms.

Cervical and Endometrial (Uterine) Cancer

Most uterine cancers develop in the body of the uterus, usually in the endometrium. The rest develop in the cervix, located at the base of the uterus. In 2014, an estimated 12,360 new cases of cervical cancer and 52,630 cases of endometrial cancer were diagnosed in the United States.[134] As more women have regular **Pap test** screenings—a procedure in which cells taken from the cervical region are examined for abnormal activity—rates should decline even further in the future. Pap tests are very effective for detecting early-stage cervical cancer, though less effective for detecting cancers of the uterine lining. Women have a lifetime risk of 1 in 151 for being diagnosed with cervical cancer and a 1 in 37 risk of being diagnosed with uterine corpus cancer.[135] Early warning signs of uterine cancer include bleeding outside the normal menstrual period or after menopause or persistent unusual vaginal discharge.

Risk factors for cervical cancer include early age at first intercourse, multiple sex partners, cigarette smoking, and certain sexually transmitted infections, including HPV (the cause of genital warts) and herpes. For endometrial cancer, age, estrogen, and obesity are strong risk factors. Risks are increased by treatment with tamoxifen for breast cancer, metabolic syndrome, late menopause, never bearing children, history of polyps in the uterus or ovaries, history of other cancers, and race (white women are at higher risk).[136]

See It! Videos

How can you prevent cervical cancer? Watch **Preventing Cervical Cancer** in the Study Area of MasteringHealth.

Leukemia and Lymphoma

Leukemia is a cancer of the blood-forming tissues that leads to proliferation of millions of immature white blood cells. These abnormal cells crowd out normal white blood cells (which fight infection), platelets (which control hemorrhaging), and red blood cells (which carry oxygen to body cells). This results in symptoms such as fatigue, paleness, weight loss, easy bruising, repeated infections, nosebleeds, and other forms of hemorrhaging occur.

Leukemia can be acute or chronic and can strike both sexes and all age groups. An estimated 52,380 new cases were diagnosed in the United States in 2014.[137] Chronic leukemia can develop over several months and have few symptoms. It is usually treated with radiation and chemotherapy. Other methods of treatment include bone marrow and stem cell transplants.

Lymphomas, a group of cancers of the lymphatic system that include Hodgkin's disease and non-Hodgkin lymphoma, are among the fastest growing cancers, with an estimated 79,990 new cases in 2014.[138] Much of this increase has occurred in women. The cause is unknown; however, a weakened immune system is suspected—particularly one exposed to viruses such as HIV, hepatitis C, and Epstein-Barr virus (EBV). Treatment varies by type and stage; chemotherapy and radiotherapy are commonly used.

check yourself

- **What are the signs and symptoms of ovarian and uterine cancers, leukemia, and lymphoma?**

11.21 Cancer Detection and Treatment

learning outcome

11.21 Describe several common cancer detection and treatment options.

Detecting Cancer

Magnetic resonance imaging (MRI) uses a huge electromagnet to detect tumors by mapping the vibrations of atoms in the body on a computer screen. The **computerized axial tomography (CAT) scan** uses X-rays to examine parts of the body. *Prostatic ultrasound* (a rectal probe using ultrasonic waves to produce an image of the prostate) is being investigated as a means to increase early detection of prostate cancer, combined with the PSA blood test. In 2011, the FDA approved the first 3D mammogram machines, which offer significant improvements in imaging and breast cancer detection but deliver nearly double the radiation risk of conventional mammograms. Table 11.4 shows screening recommendations for selected cancers.

Cancer Treatments

Treatments vary according to type and stage of cancer. Surgery to remove the tumor and surrounding tissue may be performed alone or with other treatments. The surgeon may operate using traditional surgical instruments or a laser, laparoscope, or other tools.

Stereotactic radiosurgery, also known as **gamma knife surgery**, uses a targeted dose of gamma radiation to zap tumors without any blood loss. **Radiotherapy** (use of radiation) and **chemotherapy** (use of drugs) that kill cancerous cells are also used. Radiation is most effective in treating localized cancer because it can be targeted to a particular area. Side effects include fatigue, changes to skin in the affected area, and slightly greater chances of developing another type of cancer.

Chemotherapy may be used to shrink a tumor before or after surgery or radiation therapy or on its own. Powerful drugs are administered, usually in cycles so the body can recover from their effects. Side effects, which may include nausea, hair loss, fatigue, increased chance of bleeding, bruising, infection, and anemia, fade after treatment. Other effects, such as loss of fertility, may be permanent. Long-term damage to the cardiovascular and other body systems from radiotherapy and chemotherapy can be significant.

Participation in clinical trials (people-based studies of new drugs or procedures) has provided hope for many. Deciding whether to participate in a clinical trial can be difficult. Despite the risks, which should be carefully considered, thousands of clinical trial participants have benefited from treatments otherwise unavailable to them. Before beginning any form of cancer therapy, be a vigilant and vocal consumer. Read and seek information from cancer support groups. Check the skills of your surgeon, radiation therapist, and doctor in terms of clinical experience and interpersonal interactions. Look at Oncovin and other websites supported by the National Cancer Institute and the American Cancer Society (ACS) to check out clinical trials, reports on treatment effectiveness, experimental therapies, etc. And although you may like and trust your family doctor, it is always a good idea to seek consultation or advice from larger cancer facilities.

77%

of cancers are diagnosed in adults age 55 or older.

New Cancer Treatments

Surgery, chemotherapy, and radiation therapy remain the most common cancer treatments. However, newer techniques may be more effective for certain cancers or certain patients:

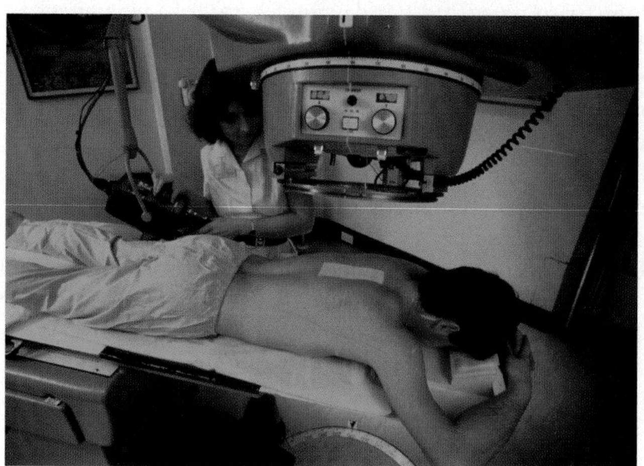

How does radiation therapy work?

Radiation therapy is often used to target and destroy cancerous tumors. The machine in this photograph emits gamma rays, which are typically used to treat localized secondary cancers and also provide pain relief for otherwise untreatable cancers. Gamma rays are less powerful than the X rays emitted from linear accelerators, another machine frequently used in radiation therapy.

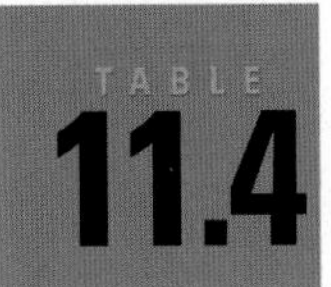

TABLE 11.4 Screening Guidelines for Early Cancer Detection in Average Risk and Asymptomatic People

Cancer Site	Screening Procedure	Age and Frequency of Test
Breast	Mammograms	The National Cancer Institute (NCI) recommends that women in their forties and older have mammograms every 1 to 2 years. Women who are at higher-than-average risk of breast cancer should talk with their health care provider about whether to have mammograms before age 40 and how often to have them.
Cervix	Pap test (Pap smear)	Women should begin having Pap tests 3 years after they begin having sexual intercourse or when they reach age 21 (whichever comes first). Most women should have a Pap test at least once every 3 years.
Colon and rectum	***Fecal occult blood test:*** Sometimes cancer or polyps bleed. This test can detect tiny amounts of blood in the stool. ***Sigmoidoscopy:*** Checks the rectum and lower part of the colon for polyps. ***Colonoscopy:*** Checks the rectum and entire colon for polyps and cancer.	People aged 50 and older should be screened. People who have a higher-than-average risk of cancer of the colon or rectum should talk with their doctor about whether to have screening tests before age 50 and how often to have them.
Prostate	Prostate-specific antigen (PSA) test	Some groups encourage yearly screening for men over age 50, and some advise men who are at a higher risk for prostate cancer to begin screening at age 40 or 45. Others caution against routine screening. Currently, Medicare provides coverage for an annual PSA test for all men age 50 and older.

Sources: National Cancer Institute, National Institutes of Health, "What You Need to Know About Cancer Screening," www.cancer.gov; National Cancer Institute, "Fact Sheet, Prostate-Specific Antigen (PSA) Test," www.cancer.gov.

- **Immunotherapy.** Immunotherapy is designed to enhance the body's disease-fighting systems. Biological response modifiers such as interferon and interleukin-2 are under study.
- **Biological therapies.** *Cancer-fighting vaccines* alert the body's immune defenses to cells gone bad. Rather than preventing disease as other vaccines do, they help people who are already ill.
- **Gene therapies.** Viruses may carry genetic information that makes the cells they infect (such as cancer cells) susceptible to an antiviral drug. Scientists are also looking at ways to transfer genes that increase immune response to the cancerous tumor or that confer drug resistance to bone marrow so higher doses of chemotherapeutic drugs can be given.
- **Angiogenesis inhibitors.** Some compounds may stop tumors from forming new blood vessels, a process called *angiogenesis*. Without adequate blood supply, tumors either die or grow very slowly.
- **Disruption of cancer pathways.** Steps in the *cancer pathway* include oncogene actions, hormone receptors, growth factors, metastasis, and angiogenesis. Preliminary studies are under way to design compounds that inhibit actions at each of these steps.
- **Smart drugs.** *Targeted smart-drug therapies* attack only the cancer cells and not the entire body.
- **Enzyme inhibitors.** An enzyme inhibitor, *TIMP2*, shows promise for slowing metastasis of tumor cells. A metastasis suppressor gene, *NM23*, has also been identified.
- **Neoadjuvant chemotherapy.** This method uses chemotherapy to shrink the tumor before surgically removing it.
- **Stem cell research.** Transplants of stem cells from donor bone marrow are used when a patient's bone marrow has been destroyed by disease, chemotherapy, or radiation.

check yourself

- **What are the screening recommendations for several common cancers?**
- **Have you been screened for any cancers for which you might be at risk? Why or why not?**
- **What are some traditional and new treatments for cancer?**

11.22 What Is Diabetes?

learning outcome

11.22 Explain the development of diabetes and distinguish between type 1 and type 2 diabetes.

Over 382 million people were classified as diabetic in 2013, and cases are expected to rise to 592 million by 2035.[139] While the number of people with diabetes has increased in virtually all countries of the world, 80 percent of those with diabetes live in low- and middle-income countries where access to prevention and treatment may be lacking. Globally, most people with diabetes are between 40 and 59 years of age.[140]

The United States isn't immune to epidemic rates of diabetes. Over the past 2 decades, diabetes rates have increased dramatically.[141] The Centers for Disease Control and Prevention (CDC) estimates that nearly 26 million people—almost 10 percent of the U.S. population—have diabetes.[142] Experts predict more than 1 in 3 Americans will have diabetes by 2050. Diabetes kills more Americans each year than breast cancer and AIDS, and millions suffer the physical and emotional burdens of dealing with this difficult disease.[143]

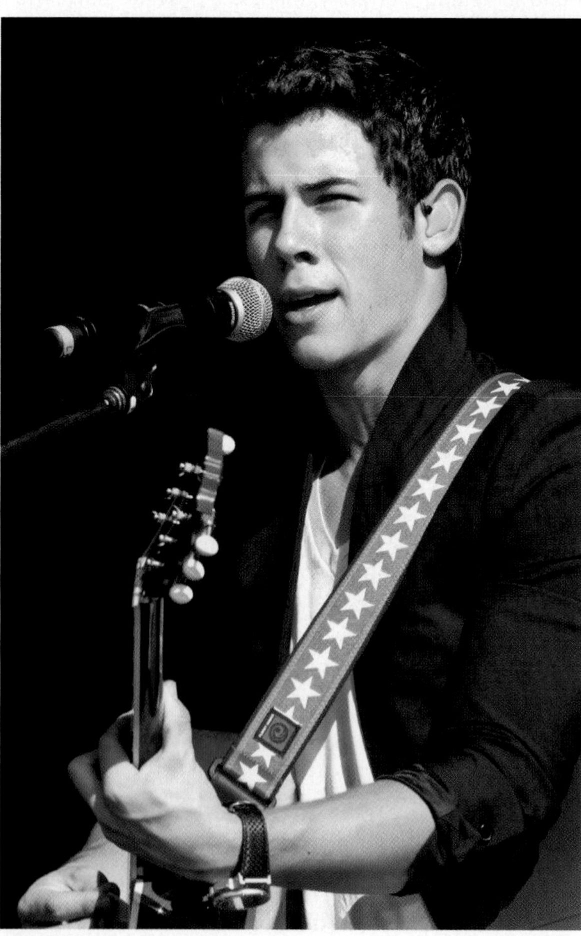

Singer and pop star Nick Jonas is one of the 5 to 10 percent of diabetics diagnosed with type 1.

Diabetes rates climb with age. While they aren't as high for college-age adults, overall rates have increased, even among the youngest populations. Among persons aged 18 to 44, approximately 2.4 percent have diabetes, compared to roughly 12.7 percent of those aged 45 to 65, and over 21 percent of those 65 to 74.[144] Diabetes is the primary cause of death each year for over 71,000 Americans.[145] All told, diabetes contributes to over 231,000 deaths, ravaging the immune system, contributing to CVD, kidney, respiratory, liver, and a host of other problems.[146] Additionally, the costs of diagnosing and treating diabetes are staggering. The younger a person is when he or she develops the disease, the greater the long-term costs.

Diabetes mellitus is actually a group of diseases, each with its own mechanism, but all characterized by a persistently high level of glucose, a type of sugar, in the blood. High blood glucose levels—or **hyperglycemia**—in diabetes can lead to serious health problems and premature death.

In a healthy person, carbohydrates from foods are broken down into a monosaccharide called *glucose*. Red blood cells use only glucose for fuel; brain and other nerve cells prefer glucose over other fuels. Excess glucose is stored as glycogen in the liver and muscles. The average adult has 5 to 6 grams of glucose in the blood at any given time, enough to provide energy for about 15 minutes of activity. Once circulating glucose is used, the body draws upon its glycogen reserves.

See It! Videos

Are diabetes patients getting even younger? Watch **Young Adults and Diabetes** in the Study Area of MasteringHealth.

1 in 3

people in the U.S. will have diabetes by 2050, based on current trends.

8 million people in the U.S. are undiagnosed diabetics.

Whenever a surge of glucose enters the bloodstream, the **pancreas**, an organ just beneath the stomach, secretes a hormone called **insulin**, stimulating cells to take up glucose from the bloodstream and carry it into cells. Conversion of glucose to glycogen for storage in the liver and muscles is also assisted by insulin.

Type 1 Diabetes

Type 1 diabetes (insulin-dependent diabetes) is an autoimmune disease in which the immune system attacks and destroys insulin-making cells in the pancreas, reducing or stopping insulin production. Without insulin, cells cannot take up glucose, and blood glucose levels become permanently elevated.

Type 1 diabetes used to be called *juvenile diabetes* because it most often appears during childhood or adolescence. Only about 5 percent of diabetic cases are type 1.[147] European ancestry, a genetic predisposition, and certain viral infections all increase the risk.[148] People with type 1 diabetes require daily insulin injections or infusions and must carefully monitor their diet and exercise levels.

Type 2 Diabetes

Type 2 diabetes (non-insulin-dependent diabetes) accounts for 90 to 95 percent of all cases.[149] In type 2, either the pancreas does not make sufficient insulin or the body cells become resistant to its effects and don't efficiently use available insulin (Figure 11.12), a condition referred to as **insulin resistance**.

Unlike type 1 diabetes, which can appear suddenly, type 2 usually develops slowly. In early stages, cells begin to resist the effects of insulin. One contributor to insulin resistance is an overabundance of free fatty acids in fat cells (common in obese individuals). These free fatty acids inhibit cells' glucose uptake and diminish the liver's ability to self-regulate conversion of glucose into glycogen.

As blood levels of glucose gradually rise, the pancreas attempts to compensate by producing more insulin. Over time, more and more pancreatic insulin-producing cells sustain damage and become nonfunctional. As insulin output declines, blood glucose levels rise enough to warrant diagnosis of type 2 diabetes.

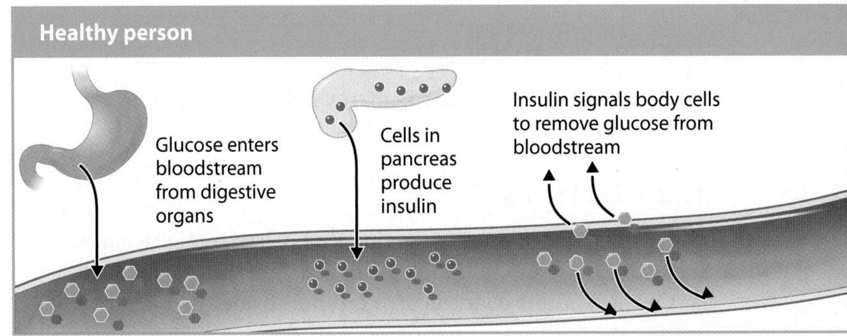

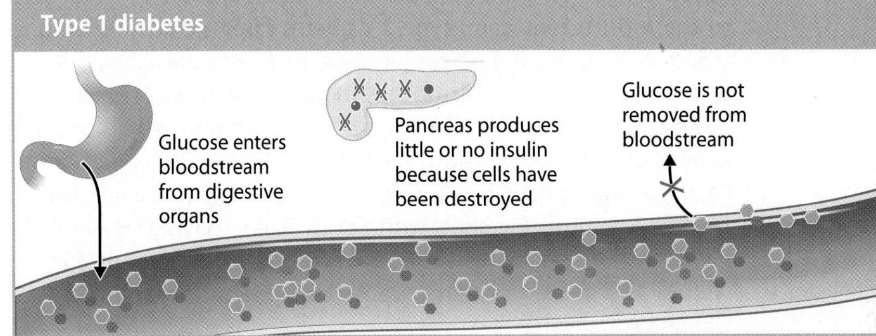

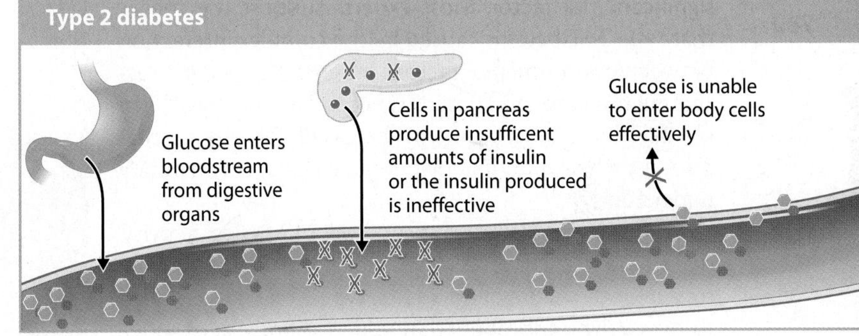

Figure 11.12 Diabetes: What It Is and How It Develops
In a healthy person, a sufficient amount of insulin is produced and released by the pancreas and used efficiently by the cells. In type 1 diabetes, the pancreas makes little or no insulin. In type 2 diabetes, either the pancreas does not make sufficient insulin or cells are resistant to insulin and thus are not able to use it efficiently.

VIDEO TUTOR
How Diabetes Develops

check yourself

- **What is the role of glucose and insulin in diabetes?**
- **What is the difference between type 1 and type 2 diabetes?**
- **Why do you think diabetes rates have increased so dramatically in the United States?**

11.23 Diabetes: Risk Factors, Symptoms, and Complications

learning outcome

11.23 Know the major factors affecting type 2 diabetes.

Risk Factors

Nonmodifiable risk factors include increased age, certain ethnicities, genetic factors, and biological factors.

One in 4 adults over age 65 has type 2 diabetes.[150] In fact, it used to be referred to as *adult-onset diabetes*, but is now being diagnosed at younger ages, even among children and teens. According to the most recent data, type 2 diabetes rates are soaring among U.S. teens—up from 9 percent in 2000 to 23 percent 2009.[151] Rates of youth diabetes have historically increased with age, with females having higher rates than males.[152] Non-Hispanic whites, Native Americans, and black youth have the highest rates, while Asian/Pacific Islanders have the lowest rates.[153] However, recent research points to a surprising shift, with South Asians having significantly higher rates of diabetes (23%) than other ethnic groups (6% in whites, 18% in African Americans, 12.7% in Latinos, and 13% in Chinese Americans).[154]

Having a close relative with type 2 diabetes is another significant risk factor. Most experts support the theory that type 2 diabetes is caused by the complex interaction between environmental factors, lifestyle, and genetic susceptibility. Although numerous potential genes have been identified as likely culprits in increased risk, the mechanisms by which inherited diabetes develops remain poorly understood.[155]

Body weight, dietary choices, level of physical activity, sleep patterns, and stress level are all modifiable risk factors. In both children and adults, type 2 diabetes is linked to overweight and obesity. In adults, a body mass index (BMI) of 25 or greater increases the risk.[156] In particular, excess weight carried around the waistline—a condition called *central adiposity*—and measured by waist circumference is a significant risk factor for older women.[157]

Inadequate sleep may contribute to the development of both obesity and type 2 diabetes—possibly due to the fact that sleep-deprived people tend to engage in less physical activity.[158] There also seems to be a link between the body clock hormone *melatonin* and type 2 diabetes. Melatonin regulates the release of insulin, which adjusts blood sugar levels. Accordingly, body clock disruptions may lead to disruptions in insulin and issues with blood sugar control. People who have genetic defects in receptors for melatonin and have disrupted sleep may increase their risk of type 2 diabetes by six times.[159] Even pulling an "all-nighter" during exams may induce insulin resistance in young, healthy subjects.[160] People who routinely fail to get enough sleep have been shown to be at higher risk for a cluster of risk factors that include poor glucose metabolism.[161]

Recent data from large studies provide evidence of a link between diabetes and psychological or physical stress; however, a recent analysis of studies focused on the role of work-related stress on type 2 diabetes development has shown mixed results, with sleep being more important than stress. Shift workers, in particular, appear to have a greater risk of diabetes, even when BMI and other risks are consider.[162]

A study of young adults with impaired fasting glucose experiencing significant financial stressors showed that physical activity played a key role in reducing stress and blood sugar levels.[163] Research on the effect of chronic stress and lack of sleep on insulin production and diabetes development is in its infancy. To reduce your risks, the best rules to follow are to manage stress and to increase exercise and sleep.[164]

Prediabetes

An estimated 79 million Americans 20 or older—35 percent of the adult population—have a set of symptoms known as **prediabetes**, a condition in which blood glucose levels are higher than normal, but not high enough to be classified as diabetes.[165] If this condition

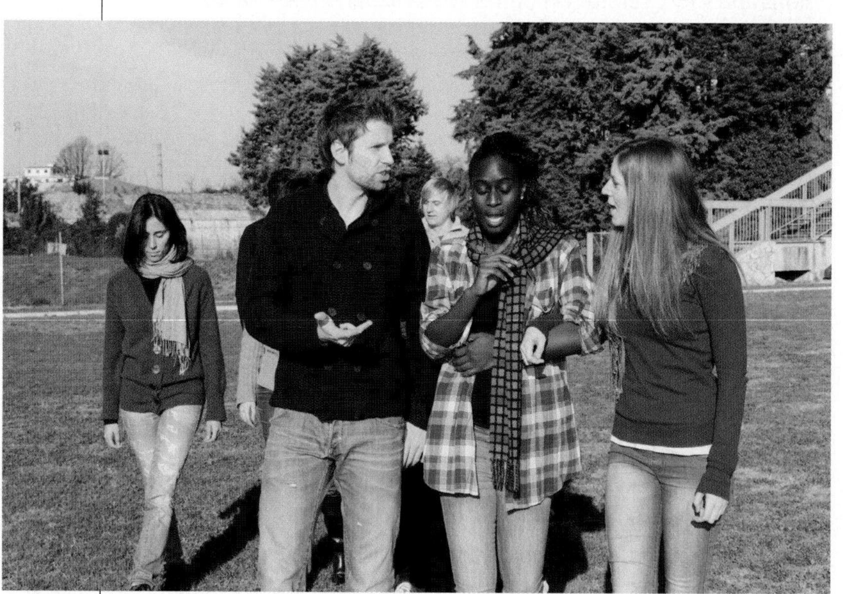

Do college students need to be concerned about diabetes?

Type 2 diabetes used to be almost nonexistent in young people, but in the past decade, cases of type 2 diabetes in people under the age of 20 have risen to the tens of thousands.

is not addressed, diabetes will eventually strike. Prediabetes is one of a cluster of six conditions linked to overweight and obesity that together constitute a dangerous health risk known as metabolic syndrome (MetS) (see Module 11.8). A person with MetS is five times more likely to develop type 2 diabetes than is a person without the syndrome.[166]

If you have already been diagnosed with prediabetes or type 2 diabetes, you can follow the tips in the Skills for Behavior Change box, "Key Steps to Begin Reducing Your Risk for Diabetes," to halt or slow the progression of your condition. Even if you've never had your blood glucose tested, these steps could reduce your risk.

Gestational Diabetes

A third type of diabetes, **gestational diabetes**, is a state of high blood glucose during pregnancy, thought to be associated with metabolic stresses that occur in response to changing hormonal levels. As many as 18 percent of pregnancies are affected by gestational diabetes, posing added risks for the mother and developing fetus.[167] Between 40 and 50 percent of women with gestational diabetes may progress to type 2 diabetes if they fail to make significant lifestyle changes.[168]

Symptoms of Diabetes

Common symptoms of diabetes are similar for type 1 and type 2:

- **Thirst and excessive urination.** Kidneys filter excessive glucose by diluting it with water. This can pull too much water from the body and result in dehydration and increased need to urinate.
- **Weight loss.** Because so many calories are lost in the glucose that passes into urine, a person with diabetes often feels hungry. Despite eating more, he or she typically loses weight.
- **Fatigue.** When glucose cannot enter cells, fatigue and weakness become inevitable.
- **Nerve damage.** High glucose levels damage the smallest blood vessels of the body, leading to numbness and tingling.
- **Blurred vision.** High blood glucose levels can dry out the cornea or damage microvessels in the eye.
- **Poor wound healing and increased infections.** High levels of glucose can affect ability to ward off infection and overall immune function.

Diabetes Complications

Poorly controlled diabetes can lead to a variety of complications:[169]

- **Diabetic coma.** In the absence of glucose, body cells break down stored fat for energy. This produces acidic molecules called *ketones*, excessive amounts of which dangerously elevate blood acid. The diabetic slips into a coma and, without prompt medical intervention, can die.
- **Cardiovascular disease.** More than 68 percent of diabetics have one or more forms of cardiovascular disease, including hypertension, increasing risk of heart attack and stroke significantly. Blood vessels become damaged as glucose-laden blood flows more sluggishly and nutrients and other substances are not transported as effectively.
- **Kidney disease.** Kidneys become scarred by their extraordinary workload and by high blood pressure in their vessels. More than 224,000 Americans are currently living with kidney failure due to diabetes.[170]
- **Amputations.** More than 60 percent of nontraumatic amputations of legs, feet, and toes are due to diabetes. Each year nearly 66,000 nontraumatic lower-limb amputations (180 per day) are performed on people with diabetes.[171]
- **Eye disease and blindness.** Nearly 7.7 million people over the age of 40 have *early-stage retinopathy*, which could lead to blindness without treatment.[172]
- **Infectious diseases.** Persons with diabetes have increased risk of poor wound healing and greater susceptibility to infectious diseases, particularly influenza and pneumonia.
- **Other complications.** Diabetics may have gum and tooth disease, foot neuropathy, and chronic pain that makes walking, driving, and simple tasks more difficult. In addition, persons with diabetes are more likely to suffer from depression, making intervention and treatment more difficult.

Skills for Behavior Change

KEY STEPS TO BEGIN REDUCING YOUR RISK FOR DIABETES

- Maintain a healthy weight, and lose weight if you need to.
- Eat smaller portions and choose foods with less fat, salt, and added sugars. Keep calories equal to energy expended. Eat more fruits, vegetables, and complex carbohydrates, and make sure you consume lean protein
- Get your body moving. Aim for at least 30 minutes of moderate activity 5 days a week.
- Quit smoking; in addition to cancer and heart disease, smoking increases blood glucose levels.
- Reduce or eliminate alcohol consumption. It's high in calories and can interfere with blood glucose regulation.
- Get enough sleep.
- Inoculate yourself against stress. Learn to take yourself less seriously, find time for fun, develop a strong support network, and use relaxation skills.
- If you have a family history, or several risk factors, get regular checkups.

Sources: Centers for Disease Control and Prevention, "National Diabetes Prevention Program," 2014, www.cdc.gov.

check yourself

- **Name three possible complications of poorly controlled diabetes.**
- **What factors put someone at greatest risk for type 2 diabetes?**
- **What are common symptoms of type 1 and type 2 diabetes?**

11.24 Diabetes: Diagnosis and Treatment

learning outcome

11.24 Explain how diabetes is diagnosed and treated.

Diagnosing and Monitoring Diabetes

Generally, a physician orders one of the following blood tests to diagnose prediabetes or diabetes:

- The *fasting plasma glucose (FPG) test* requires the patient to fast overnight; a small sample of blood is then tested for glucose concentration. An FPG level greater than or equal to 100 mg/dL indicates prediabetes, and a level greater than or equal to 126 mg/dL indicates diabetes (Figure 11.13).
- The *oral glucose tolerance test (OGTT)* requires the patient to drink a fluid containing concentrated glucose. Blood is drawn for testing 2 hours later. A reading greater than or equal to 140 mg/dL indicates prediabetes, whereas a reading greater than or equal to 200 mg/dL indicates diabetes.
- The *A1C* or *glycosylated hemoglobin test (HbA1C)* gives the average value of a patient's blood glucose over the past 2 to 3 months, instead of at one moment in time. In general, an A1C of 5.7 to 6.4 means that you are at high risk for diabetes or are prediabetic. If your A1C is 6.5 or higher, diabetes may be diagnosed.[173] *Estimated average glucose (eAG)* shows how AIC numbers correspond to the blood glucose numbers people are used to seeing. For example, someone with an A1C value of 6.1 would be able to look at a chart and see that their average blood glucose was around 128—a high level that should encourage healthy lifestyle modifications.

People with diabetes need to check their blood glucose level several times throughout each day to make sure they stay within their target range. To check blood glucose, diabetics must prick their finger to obtain a drop of blood. A handheld glucose meter is then used to evaluate the blood sample.

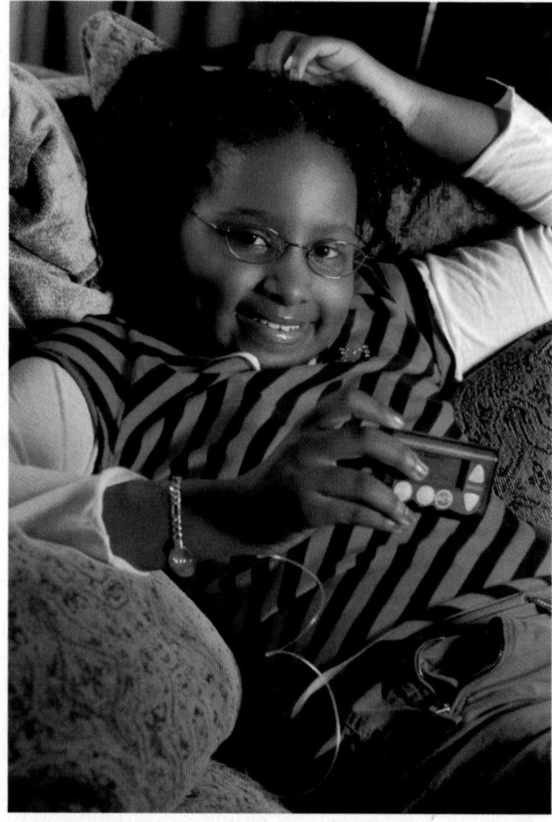

Some type 2 diabetics can control their condition with changes in diet and lifestyle habits or with oral medications. However, some type 2 diabetics and all type 1 diabetics require insulin injections or infusions.

Treating Diabetes

Lifestyle changes can prevent or delay the development of type 2 diabetes by up to 58 percent.[174] For those with type 2 diabetes, such lifestyle changes can prevent or delay need for medication or insulin injections.

Weight loss significantly lowers risk of progressing from prediabetes to diabetes. A loss of as little as 5 to 7 percent of current body weight and regular physical activity significantly lowers the risk of progressing to diabetes.[175]

A low-fat, reduced-calorie diet aids weight loss. Researchers have also studied a variety of foods for their effect on blood glucose levels. A diet high in whole grains reduces risk of type 2 diabetes.[176] Eating high-fiber foods—fruits, vegetables, beans, nuts, and seeds—may reduce diabetes risk.[177] Eating low-carbohydrate diets also appears to reduce overall CVD risks and may have a significant effect on preventing and controlling type 2 diabetes. In addition, consumption of fish high in omega-3 fatty acids is linked with decreased progression of insulin resistance.[178]

It is also important for people with diabetes to prevent surges in blood sugar after they eat. The **glycemic index (GI)** compares foods with the same amount of carbohydrates and determines how quickly and how much each raises blood glucose levels. Foods low on the GI have far less effect on blood glucose than those that are high on the GI. A food's **glycemic load (GL)** is defined as its GI (potential to raise blood glucose) multiplied by the grams of carbohydrates it provides, divided by 100. By learning to combine high- and low-GI foods to avoid surges in blood glucose, diabetics can help control their average blood glucose levels throughout the day. Eating smaller amounts, several times a day, from low GI sources is an important part of glucose control.

At least 30 minutes of physical activity 5 days a week reduces risk of type 2 diabetes.[179] The more muscle mass you have and the

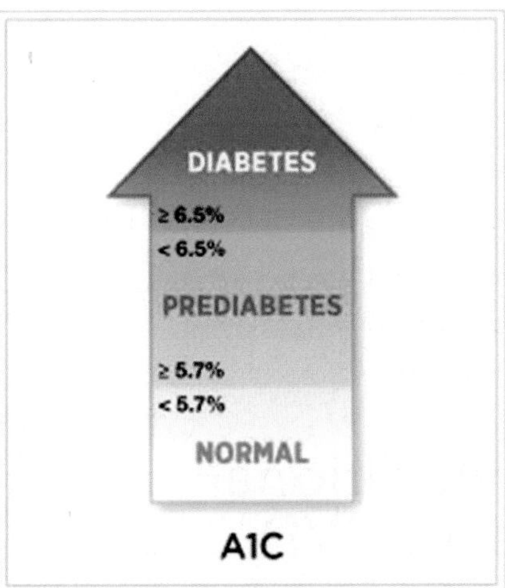

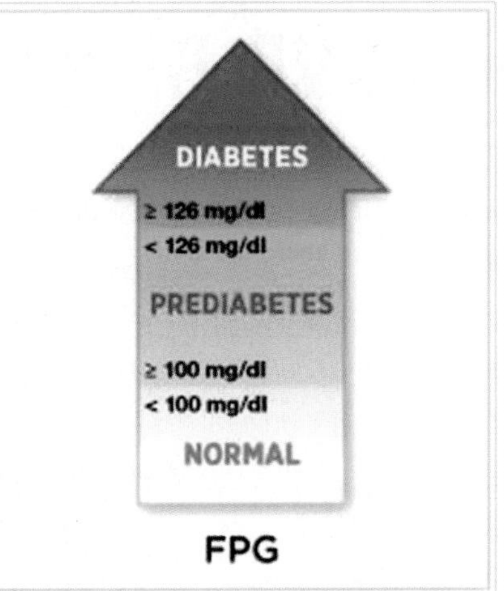

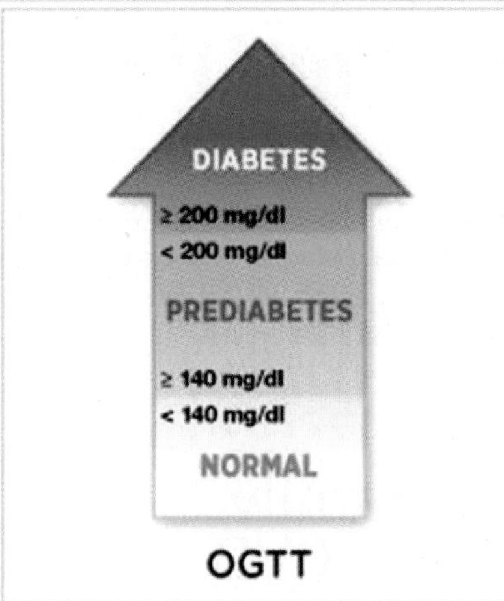

Figure 11.13 Blood Glucose Levels in Prediabetes and Untreated Diabetes
The fasting plasma glucose (FPG) test measures levels of blood glucose after a person fasts overnight. The oral glucose tolerance test (OGTT) measures levels of blood glucose after a person consumes a concentrated amount of glucose. The A1C or glycosylated hemoglobin test (HbA1C) gives the average value of a patient's blood glucose over the past 2 to 3 months.
Source: American Diabetes Association, "Diagnosing Diabetes and Learning about Prediabetes," March 2014, www.diabetes.org.

more you use your muscles, the more efficiently cells use glucose for fuel, meaning there will be less glucose circulating in the bloodstream. For most people, activity of moderate intensity can help keep blood glucose levels under control.

When lifestyle changes fail to control type 2 diabetes, one of several oral medications may be prescribed, each of which influences blood glucose in a different way—reducing the liver's glucose production, slowing absorption of carbohydrates from the small intestine, increasing pancreatic insulin production, or increasing cells' insulin sensitivity.

The newest class of diabetes drugs are known as SGLT2 inhibitors. These drugs cause the kidneys to actually excrete more glucose, which lowers the levels of glucose circulating in the body. All diabetic drugs have side effects and contraindications; however, each person must balance risks of medications with risks of elevated blood glucose.

When lifestyle changes prove challenging and risks are high and increasing, surgery is another option. People who undergo gastric/bariatric surgery for weight loss have shown remarkable reductions in blood glucose and diabetes symptoms for 2–3 years after surgery.[180] Those who combined gastric bypass or sleeve gastrectomy (a surgery where about 80% of the stomach is removed, leaving a small sleeve of stomach tissue connected to the intestines) with intensive medical therapy had similar outcomes.[181] In many cases, former diabetics can stop taking medications for some of their CVD risks and stop diabetes symptoms altogether. Many professional groups are pushing for wider use of these more drastic weight loss methods.[182] Gastric bypass surgeries are not without risks, however, and can include death and serious complications.

With type 1 diabetes, the pancreas cannot produce adequate insulin, making added insulin essential. People with type 2 diabetes whose blood glucose cannot be controlled with other treatments also require insulin. Insulin cannot be taken in pill form because it's a protein, and thus would be digested in the gastrointestinal tract. It must therefore be inserted into the fat layer under the skin, from which it is absorbed into the bloodstream.

Today, many diabetics use an *insulin infusion pump* rather than injections. The pump, small and easily hidden by clothes, delivers insulin in minute amounts throughout the day through a catheter inserted under the skin.

Losing 5%–7% of body weight can cause significant reductions in blood glucose levels and help prevent diabetes.

check yourself

- **What tests are commonly used to diagnose diabetes?**
- **What are some of the treatments for diabetes?**
- **How do people with diabetes monitor their blood glucose level?**

11.25

What's Your Personal CVD Risk?

An interactive version of this assessment is available online in MasteringHealth.

Each of us has a unique level of risk for various diseases, including cardiovascular disease. Answer each of the following questions and total your points in each section.

1 Your Family Risk for CVD

	Yes (1 point)	No (0 points)	Don't Know
1. Do any of your primary relatives (parents, grandparents, siblings) have a history of heart disease or stroke?	○	○	○
2. Do any of your primary relatives have diabetes?	○	○	○
3. Do any of your primary relatives have high blood pressure?	○	○	○
4. Do any of your primary relatives have a history of high cholesterol?	○	○	○
5. Would you say that your family consumed a high-fat diet (lots of red meat, whole dairy, butter/margarine) during your time spent at home?	○	○	○

Total points:__________

2 Your Lifestyle Risk for CVD

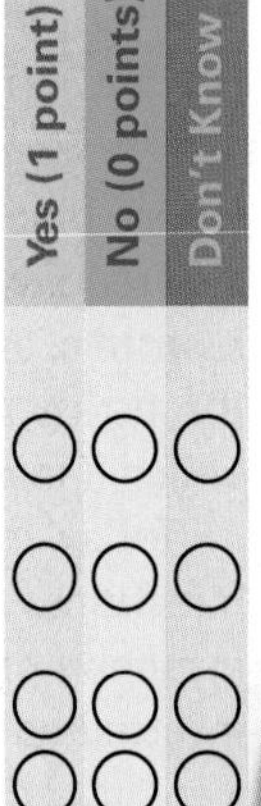

1. **Is your total cholesterol level higher than it should be?**
2. **Do you have high blood pressure?**
3. **Have you been diagnosed as prediabetic or diabetic?**
4. **Do you smoke?**
5. **Would you describe your life as being highly stressful?**

Total points:__________

3 Your Additional Risks for CVD

1. **How would you best describe your current weight?**
   a. **Lower than it should be for my height (0 points)**
   b. **About what it should be for my height (0 points)**
   c. **Higher than it should be for my height (1 point)**
2. **How would you describe the level of exercise that you get each day?**
   a. **Less than I should be exercising each day (1 point)**
   b. **About how much I should be exercising each day (0 points)**
   c. **More than I should be exercising each day (0 points)**
3. **How would you describe your dietary behaviors?**
   a. **Eating only the recommended number of calories each day (0 points)**
   b. **Eating less than the recommended number of calories each day (0 points)**
   c. **Eating more than the recommended number of calories each day (1 point)**
4. **Which of the following statements best describes your typical dietary behavior?**
   a. **I eat from the major food groups, especially trying to get the recommended fruits and vegetables. (0 points)**
   b. **I eat too much red meat and consume too much saturated and *trans* fats from meat, dairy products, and processed foods each day. (1 point)**
   c. **Whenever possible, I try to substitute olive oil or canola oil for other forms of dietary fat. (0 points)**

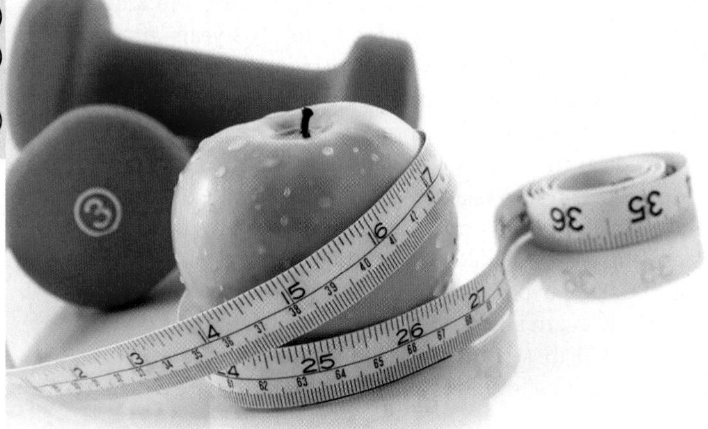

5. Which of the following (if any) describes you?
   a. I watch my sodium intake and try to reduce stress in my life. (0 points)
   b. I have a history of chlamydia infection. (1 point)
   c. I try to eat 5 to 10 milligrams of soluble fiber each day and to substitute a soy product for an animal product in my diet at least once each week. (0 points)

Total points: ___________

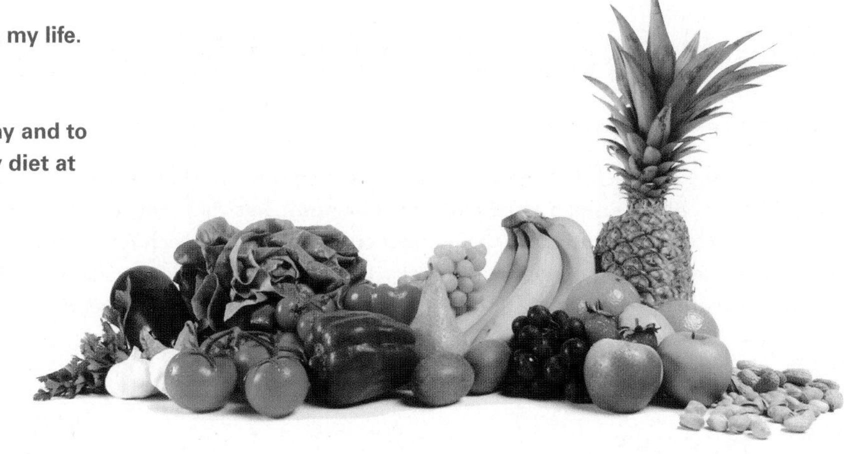

Scoring

If you score between 1 and 5 in any section, consider your risk. The higher the number you've scored, the greater your risk. If you answered "don't know" for any question, talk to your parents or other family members as soon as possible to find out if you have any unknown risks.

Your Plan for Change

The Assess Yourself activity evaluated your risk of heart disease. Based on your results and the advice of your physician, you may need to take steps to reduce your risk of CVD.

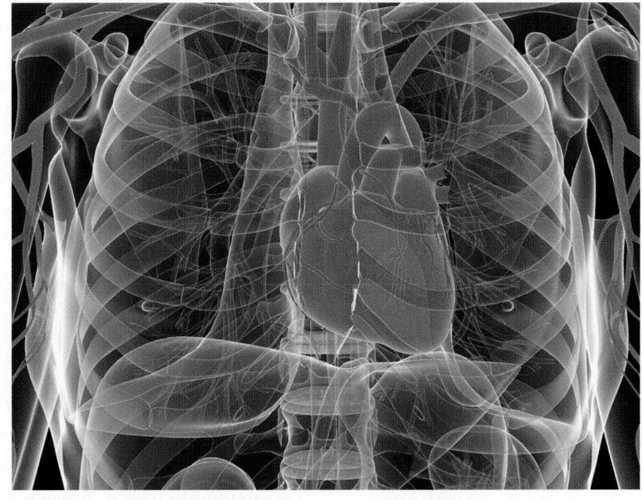

Today, you can:

◯ Get up and move! Take a walk in the evening, use the stairs instead of the escalator, or ride your bike to class. Start thinking of ways you can incorporate more physical activity into your daily routine.

◯ Begin improving your dietary habits by eating a healthier dinner. Replace the meat and processed foods you might normally eat with a serving of fresh fruit or soy-based protein and green leafy vegetables. Think about the amounts of saturated and *trans* fats you consume—which foods contain them, and how can you reduce consumption of these items?

Within the next 2 weeks, you can:

◯ Begin a regular exercise program, even if you start slowly. Set small goals and try to meet them.

◯ Practice a new stress management technique. For example, learn how to meditate.

◯ Get enough rest. Make sure you get at least 8 hours of sleep per night.

By the end of the semester, you can:

◯ Find out your hereditary risk for CVD. Call your parents and find out if your grandparents or aunts or uncles developed CVD. Ask if they know their latest cholesterol LDL/HDL levels. Do you have a family history of diabetes?

◯ Have your own cholesterol and blood pressure levels checked. Once you know your levels, you'll have a better sense of what risk factors to address. If your levels are high, talk to your doctor about how to reduce them.

Assess yourself

11.26

What's Your Personal Risk for Cancer?

An interactive version of this assessment is available online in MasteringHealth.

There are many cancer risk factors that you have the power to change. Once you carefully assess your risks, you can make lifestyle changes and pursue risk-reduction strategies that may lessen your susceptibility to various cancers.

Read each question and circle the number corresponding to each Yes or No. Be honest and accurate to get the most complete understanding of your cancer risks. Individual scores for specific questions should not be interpreted as a precise measure of relative risk, but the totals in each section give a general indication.

1 Breast Cancer

	Yes	No
1. Do you do a monthly breast self-exam?	1	2
2. Do you look at your breasts in the mirror regularly, checking for any irregular indentations/lumps, discharge from the nipples, or other noticeable changes?	1	2
3. Has your mother, sister, or daughter been diagnosed with breast cancer?	2	1
4. Have you ever been pregnant?	1	2
5. Have you had lumps or cysts in your breasts or underarm?	2	1

Total points: __________

2 Skin Cancer

	Yes	No
1. Do you spend a lot of time outdoors, either at work or at play?	2	1
2. Do you use sunscreens with an SPF rating of 15 or more?	1	2
3. Do you use tanning beds or sun booths regularly to maintain a tan?	2	1
4. Do you examine your skin once a month, checking any moles or other irregularities, and using a hand mirror to check hard-to-see areas such as your back, buttocks, genitals, and neck, and under your hair?	1	2
5. Do you purchase and wear sunglasses that filter out harmful sun rays?	1	2

Total points: __________

3 Cancers of the Reproductive System

Men

	Yes	No
1. Do you examine your penis regularly for unusual bumps or growths?	1	2
2. Do you perform regular testicular self-exams?	1	2
3. Do you have a family history of prostate or testicular cancer?	2	1
4. Do you practice safe sex and wear condoms with every sexual encounter?	1	2
5. Do you avoid exposure to harmful environmental hazards such as mercury, coal tars, benzene, chromate, and vinyl chloride?	1	2

Total points: __________

Women

	Yes	No
1. Do you have regularly scheduled Pap tests?	1	2
2. Have you been infected with the human papillomavirus, Epstein-Barr virus, or other viruses believed to increase cancer risk?	2	1
3. Has your mother, sister, or daughter been diagnosed with breast, cervical, endometrial, or ovarian cancer (particularly at a young age)?	2	1
4. Do you practice safe sex and use condoms with every sexual encounter?	1	2
5. Are you obese, taking estrogen, or consuming a diet that is very high in saturated fats?	2	1

Total points: __________

4 Cancers in General

	Question	Yes	No
1.	Do you smoke cigarettes on most days of the week?	2	1
2.	Do you consume a diet that is rich in fruits and vegetables?	1	2
3.	Are you obese, or do you lead a primarily sedentary lifestyle?	2	1
4.	Do you live in an area with high air pollution levels or work in a job where you are exposed to several chemicals on a regular basis?	2	1
5.	Are you careful about the amount of animal fat in your diet, substituting olive oil or canola oil for animal fat whenever possible?	1	2
6.	Do you limit your overall consumption of alcohol?	1	2
7.	Do you eat foods rich in lycopenes (such as tomatoes) and antioxidants?	1	2
8.	Are you "body aware" and alert for changes in your body?	1	2
9.	Do you have a family history of ulcers or of colorectal, stomach, or other digestive-system cancers?	2	1
10.	Do you avoid unnecessary exposure to radiation, cell phone emissions, and microwave emissions?	1	2

Total points: __________

Analyzing Your Scores

Look carefully at each question for which you circled a 2. Are there any areas in which you received mostly 2s? Did you receive total points of 6 or higher in parts 1 through 3? Did you receive total points of 11 or higher in part 4? If so, you have at least one identifiable risk. The higher your score, the more risks you may have.

Your Plan for Change

The Assess Yourself activity identifies certain behaviors that can contribute to increased cancer risks. If you have identified particular risky behaviors, consider steps you can take to change these behaviors and improve your future health.

Today, you can:

○ Perform a breast or testicular self-exam and commit to doing one every month.

○ Take advantage of the salad bar in your dining hall for lunch or dinner and load up on greens, or request veggies such as steamed broccoli or sautéed spinach.

Within the next 2 weeks, you can:

○ Buy a bottle of sunscreen (with SPF 15 or higher) and begin applying it as part of your daily routine. (Be sure to check the expiration date, particularly on sale items!) Also, stay in the shade from 10 A.M. to 2 P.M., as this is when the sun is strongest.

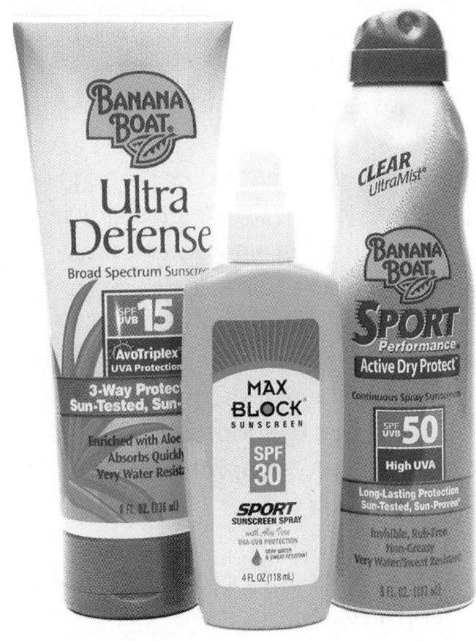

○ Find out your family health history. Talk to your parents, grandparents, or an aunt or uncle to find out if family members have developed cancer. This will help you assess your own genetic risk.

By the end of the semester, you can:

○ Work toward achieving a healthy weight. If you aren't already engaged in a regular exercise program, begin one now. Maintaining a healthy body weight and exercising regularly will lower your risk for cancer.

○ Stop smoking, avoid secondhand smoke, and limit your alcohol intake.

Summary

To hear an MP3 Tutor session, scan here or visit the Study Area in **MasteringHealth**.

LO 11.1 The cardiovascular system consists of the heart and circulatory system, a network of vessels that supplies the body with nutrients and oxygen.

LO 11.2–11.7 Cardiovascular diseases include atherosclerosis, coronary artery disease, peripheral artery disease, coronary heart disease, stroke, hypertension, angina pectoris, arrhythmias, congestive heart failure, and congenital and rheumatic heart disease.

LO 11.8–11.10 Many risk factors for cardiovascular disease can be modified, such as cigarette smoking, high blood cholesterol and triglyceride levels, hypertension, lack of exercise, a diet high in saturated fat, obesity, diabetes, and emotional stress. Some risk factors, such as age, gender, and heredity, cannot be modified.

LO 11.11 Coronary bypass surgery is an established treatment for heart blockage; however, increasing numbers of angioplasty procedures and stents are being used with great success. Drug therapies can be used to prevent and treat CVD.

LO 11.12 Cancer is a group of diseases characterized by uncontrolled growth and spread of abnormal cells. These cells may create tumors.

LO 11.13 Cancers are grouped into four categories: carcinomas, sarcomas, lymphomas, and leukemias.

LO 11.14 Lifestyle factors for cancer include smoking, obesity, poor diet, lack of exercise, and stress. Biological factors include inherited genes, age, and gender. Infectious agents that may cause cancer are chronic hepatitis B and C, human papillomavirus, and genital herpes.

LO 11.15–11.20 There are many different types of cancer. Common cancers include those of the lung, breast, colon and rectum, skin, prostate, testis, ovary, and uterus; leukemia; and lymphomas.

LO 11.21 Early diagnosis improves survival rate. Self-exams for breast, testicular, and skin cancer aid early diagnosis.

LO 11.22 Diabetes mellitus is characterized by a persistently high level of glucose in the blood. In type 1 diabetes, the immune system attacks insulin-making cells in the pancreas, dangerously elevating insulin levels. In type 2 diabetes, the pancreas doesn't make sufficient insulin, or the cells don't use it efficiently.

LO 11.23 Risk factors for diabetes include age, ethnicity, genetics, and lifestyle. Prediabetes will eventually lead to diabetes if health risks are not addressed.

LO 11.24 Treatments for diabetes include improving lifestyle factors, taking medications, undergoing weight-loss surgery, and receiving insulin.

Pop Quiz

Visit MasteringHealth to personalize your study plan with Chapter Review Quizzes and Dynamic Study Modules.

LO 11.6 1. A stroke results
- a. when a heart stops beating.
- b. when cardiopulmonary resuscitation has failed to revive a stopped heart.
- c. when blood flow in the brain has been compromised, either due to blockage or hemorrhage.
- d. when blood pressure rises above 120/80 mm Hg.

LO 11.8 2. Which of the following is *correct* about metabolic syndrome?
- a. It is decreasing among the general population both in the United States and globally.
- b. It lowers your risk of cardiovascular disease.
- c. It includes high fasting blood glucose, obesity, high triglyceride levels, hypertension, and other risks.
- d. It is a nonmodifiable risk factor for CVD.

LO 11.9 3. The "bad" type of cholesterol found in the bloodstream is known as
- a. high-density lipoprotein (HDL).
- b. low-density lipoprotein (LDL).
- c. total cholesterol.
- d. triglycerides.

LO 11.9 4. What does a person's cholesterol level indicate?
- a. The formation of fatty substances, called *plaque,* which can clog the arteries
- b. The level of triglycerides in the blood, which can increase risk of coronary disease
- c. Hypertension, which leads to thickening and hardening of the arteries
- d. The level of *C-reactive proteins* in the blood, indicating inflammation

LO 11.12 5. When cancer cells have *metastasized,*
- a. they have grown into a malignant tumor.
- b. they have spread to other parts of the body.
- c. the cancer is retreating and cancer cells are dying off.
- d. the tumor is localized and considered in situ.

LO 11.12 6. A cancerous *neoplasm* is a
- a. type of biopsy.
- b. form of benign tumor.
- c. type of treatment for a tumor.
- d. malignant group of cells or tumor.

LO 11.14 7. "If you are male and smoke, your chances of getting lung cancer are 23 times greater than those of a nonsmoker." This statement refers to a type of risk assessed statistically, known as
- a. relative risk.
- b. comparable risk.
- c. cancer risk.
- d. genetic predisposition.

LO 11.18 8. The more serious and life-threatening type of skin cancer is
- a. basal cell carcinoma.
- b. squamous cell carcinoma.
- c. melanoma.
- d. lymphoma.

LO 11.22 9. Which of the following is true of type 2 diabetes?
- a. It is an autoimmune disorder.
- b. It is correlated with obesity and sedentary lifestyle.
- c. It usually appears suddenly.
- d. It is also referred to as insulin-dependent diabetes.

LO 11.22 10. By 2050, experts predict more than ____ Americans will have diabetes.
- a. 1 in 3
- b. 1 in 10
- c. 1 in 100
- d. 1 in 200

Answers to these questions can be found on page A-1. If you answered a question incorrectly, review the module identified by the Learning Outcome. For even more study tools, visit MasteringHealth.

12 Infectious Conditions

Disease-causing agents, or **pathogens**, are found throughout our world. New varieties arise constantly; others have existed for as long as there has been life on this planet. Infectious diseases like the common cold are **endemic**, meaning that they are present at expected prevalence rates in virtually all populations on Earth. When the number of cases of a disease suddenly increases with higher than projected endemic numbers, it becomes an **epidemic**; bubonic plague, for example, killed up to one-third of the population of Europe in the 1300s. A **pandemic**, or global epidemic, of influenza killed more than 20 million people in 1918. Today, new, resistant forms of older organisms—such as H1N1 flu and the methicillin-resistant *Staphylococcus aureus*, or MRSA, staph infection—defy current pharmacological weapons.

Despite constant bombardment by pathogens, however, our immune systems are remarkably adept at protecting us. Exposure to invading microorganisms actually helps build resistance to pathogens. Millions of *endogenous microorganisms* live in and on our bodies, usually in peaceful coexistence. *Exogenous microorganisms*, in contrast, are those that don't normally inhabit the body. When they do, they are apt to produce infection or illness. The more easily these pathogens can gain a foothold and sustain themselves, the more **virulent**, or aggressive, they may be in causing disease.

12.1 The Process of Infection

learning outcome

12.1 Explain the process of infection and defenses against pathogens, and list common risk factors for infection.

Most diseases are **multifactorial**, caused by the interaction of several factors inside and outside a person. For a disease to occur, the person, or *host*, must be *susceptible*, which means that the immune system must be in a weakened condition (**immunocompromised**); an *agent* capable of *transmitting* a disease must be present; and the *environment* must be *hospitable* to the pathogen. Although all pathogens pose a threat if they gain entry and begin to grow in the body, the chances that they will do so are actually quite small.

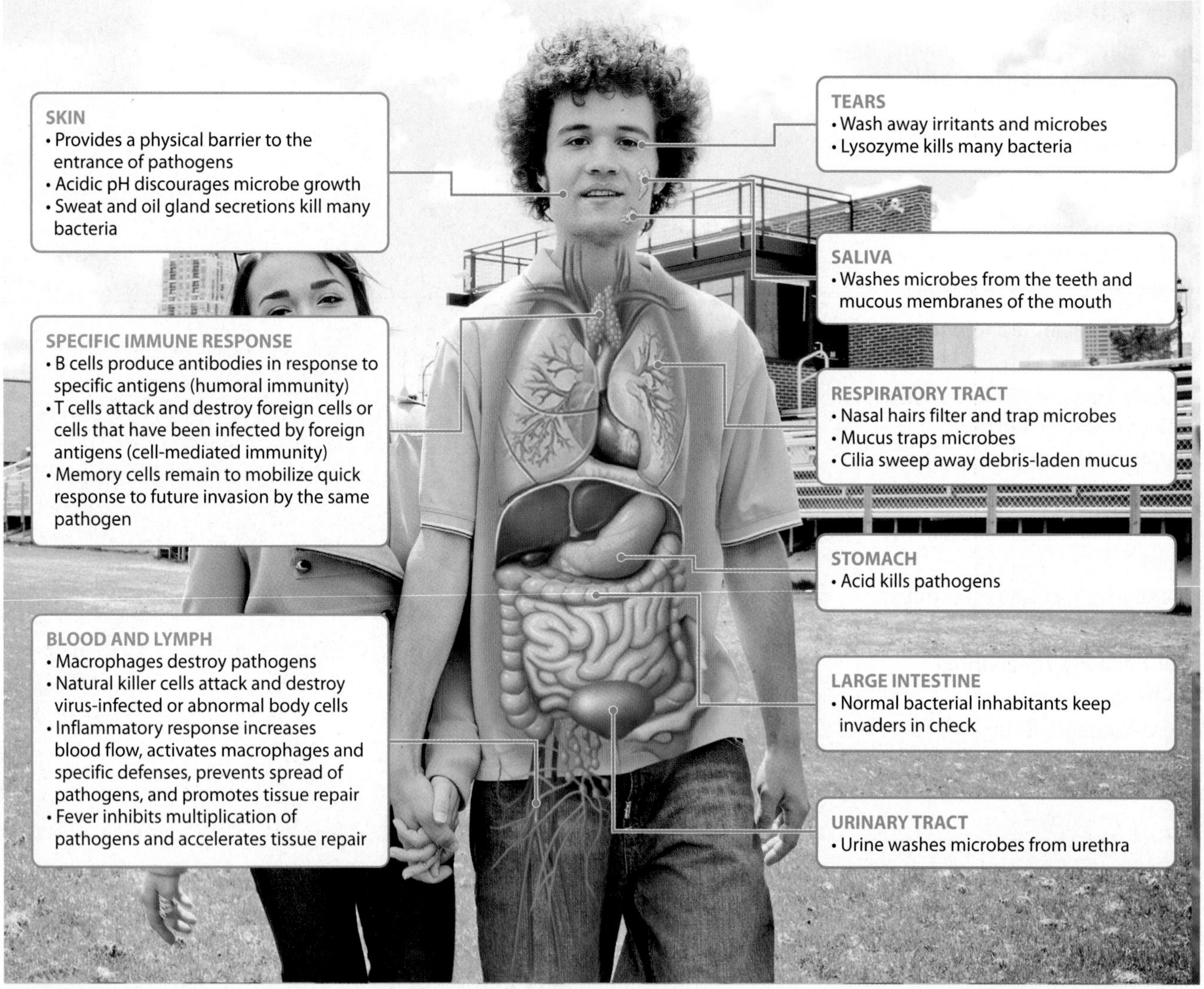

SKIN
- Provides a physical barrier to the entrance of pathogens
- Acidic pH discourages microbe growth
- Sweat and oil gland secretions kill many bacteria

TEARS
- Wash away irritants and microbes
- Lysozyme kills many bacteria

SALIVA
- Washes microbes from the teeth and mucous membranes of the mouth

SPECIFIC IMMUNE RESPONSE
- B cells produce antibodies in response to specific antigens (humoral immunity)
- T cells attack and destroy foreign cells or cells that have been infected by foreign antigens (cell-mediated immunity)
- Memory cells remain to mobilize quick response to future invasion by the same pathogen

RESPIRATORY TRACT
- Nasal hairs filter and trap microbes
- Mucus traps microbes
- Cilia sweep away debris-laden mucus

STOMACH
- Acid kills pathogens

BLOOD AND LYMPH
- Macrophages destroy pathogens
- Natural killer cells attack and destroy virus-infected or abnormal body cells
- Inflammatory response increases blood flow, activates macrophages and specific defenses, prevents spread of pathogens, and promotes tissue repair
- Fever inhibits multiplication of pathogens and accelerates tissue repair

LARGE INTESTINE
- Normal bacterial inhabitants keep invaders in check

URINARY TRACT
- Urine washes microbes from urethra

Figure 12.1 The Body's Defenses against Disease-Causing Pathogens
In addition to the defenses listed, many of the body's defensive secretions and fluids, such as earwax, tears, mucus, and blood, contain enzymes and other proteins that can kill some invading pathogens or prevent or slow their reproduction.

VIDEO TUTOR
Chain of Infection

Preventing Pathogens from Entering the Body

Pathogens can enter the body through several routes of transmission. They may be transmitted by *direct contact* between infected persons, such as during sexual relations, kissing, or touching, or by *indirect contact*, such as by touching an object the infected person has had contact with. You may also **autoinoculate** yourself, or transmit a pathogen from one part of your body to another. For example, you may touch a herpes sore on your lip, then transmit the virus to your eye by touch.

Dogs, cats, livestock, and wild animals can spread **zoonotic diseases** through bites or feces or by carrying infected insects into living areas. Although *interspecies transmission* of diseases (diseases passed from humans to animals and vice versa) is rare, it does occur.

Your body constantly protects against and defends you from pathogens that could make you ill. For pathogens to gain entry into your body, they must overcome barriers that prevent pathogens from entering your body, mechanisms that weaken organisms that breach these barriers, and substances that counteract the threat that these organisms pose. Figure 12.1 summarizes some of the body's defenses against invasion.

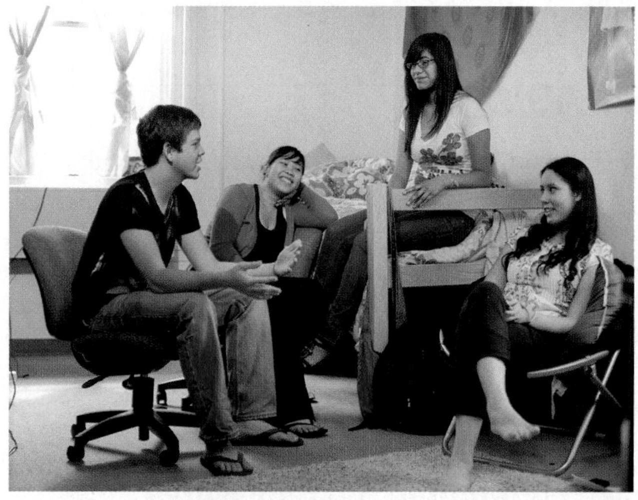

Close quarters, such as college dorms, are prime breeding grounds for contagious diseases such as the flu, colds, and meningitis.

Risk Factors You Can Control

With all these pathogens floating around, how can you avoid getting sick? Fortunately, there are ways to take care of yourself. Too much stress, inadequate nutrition, a low fitness level, lack of sleep, misuse or abuse of legal and illegal drugs, poor personal hygiene, and high-risk behavior significantly increase the risk for many diseases. College students, in particular, often are at higher risk because of many of the above factors, in addition to the fact that alcohol and other drugs, increasing numbers of sexual experiences, and close living conditions all create higher risk for exposure to pathogens. You can make changes in your community to clean up toxins, set policies on contaminant levels, and reduce the likelihood of exposure to pathogens or toxins. The chain of infection between pathogen, environment, and host presents multiple opportunities for individuals and communities to intercede and "break the chain," preventing and controlling disease transmission.

Risk Factors You Typically Cannot Control

Unfortunately, some factors that make you susceptible to a certain disease are either hard to control or completely beyond your control:

- **Heredity.** One of the key factors influencing disease risk is genetics. It is often unclear whether hereditary diseases are due to inherited genetic traits or to inherited insufficiencies in the immune system. Some believe that we may inherit the quality of our immune system, so some people are naturally more resistant to disease and infection.
- **Aging.** People under age 5 and over age 65 are often more vulnerable to infectious diseases because body defenses that we take for granted are either not fully developed or not as effective as they once were. Thinning of the skin, reduced sweating, and other physical changes can make the elderly more vulnerable to disease. In addition, as people age certain **comorbidities** (diseases that occur at the same time) overwhelm the body's ability to ward off enemies and increase the risk of infection. In these situations, **opportunistic infections** can cause illness.
- **Environmental conditions.** A growing body of research points to changes in the climate, where, for example, increases in mosquito populations increase the spread of diseases such as malaria.[1] While temperature change often means more insects and greater chances of infection, dwindling water supplies are more likely to be contaminated. As birds and animals congregate more closely at scarce water sources, they may spread diseases among themselves, potentially threatening each other as well as humans.[2] In addition, long-term exposure to toxic chemicals and catastrophic natural disasters such as earthquakes, floods, and tsunamis are believed to be significant contributors to increasing numbers of infectious diseases.[3]
- **Organism virulence and resistance.** Even tiny amounts of a particularly virulent organism may make the hardiest of us ill. Other organisms have mutated and become resistant to the body's defenses and to medical treatments. **Drug resistance** occurs when pathogens grow and proliferate in the presence of chemicals that would normally slow growth or kill them.

check yourself

- **What are three common routes of infection?**
- **What are some ways your body fights off infection?**
- **List three risk factors for infection that are typically beyond your control.**

12.2 Your Immune System

learning **outcome**

12.2 Explain how the immune system defends against invasion by pathogens.

The immune system is able to quickly recognize and destroy **antigens**—outside or foreign substances capable of causing disease. An antigen can be a virus, a bacterium, a fungus, a parasite, a toxin, or a tissue or cell from another organism. *Immunity* is a condition of being able to resist a particular disease by counteracting the substance that produces the disease.

How the Immune System Works

As soon as an antigen breaches the body's initial defenses, the body responds by forming substances called **antibodies** that are matched to that specific antigen, much as a key is matched to a lock. The body analyzes the antigen, considers its size and shape, verifies that the antigen is not part of the body itself, and then produces a specific antibody to destroy or weaken it. This process is part of a complex system called *humoral immune responses*. **Humoral immunity** is the body's major defense against many bacteria and the poisonous substances, called **toxins**, that they produce.

In **cell-mediated immunity**, specialized white blood cells called **lymphocytes** attack and destroy the foreign invader. Lymphocytes constitute the body's main defense against viruses, fungi, parasites, and some bacteria, and they are found in the blood, lymph nodes, bone marrow, and certain glands. Other key players in this immune response are **macrophages** (a type of phagocytic, or cell-eating, white blood cell).

Two forms of lymphocytes in particular, the *B lymphocytes* (B cells) and *T lymphocytes* (T cells), are involved in the immune response. *Helper T cells* are essential for activating B cells to produce antibodies. They also activate other T cells and macrophages. Another form of T cell, known as the *killer T cell*, directly attacks infected or malignant cells. *Suppressor T cells* turn off or suppress the activity of B cells, killer T cells, and macrophages. After a successful attack on a pathogen, some of the attacker T and B cells are preserved as *memory T* and *B cells*, enabling the body to recognize and respond quickly to subsequent attacks by the same kind of organism.

Once people have survived certain infectious diseases, they become immune to those diseases, meaning that in all probability they will not develop them again. Upon subsequent attack by the same disease-causing microorganisms, their memory T and B cells are quickly activated to come to their defense. Figure 12.2 provides a summary of the cell-mediated immune response.

When the Immune System Misfires: Autoimmune Diseases

Although the immune response generally works in our favor, the body sometimes makes a mistake and targets its own tissue as the enemy, builds up antibodies against that tissue, and attempts to destroy it. This is known as **autoimmune disease** (*auto* means "self"). The National Institutes of Health estimates that over 32 million Americans have *autoantibodies*—proteins made by the immune system that target the body's tissues—that can indicate autoimmunity well before the symptoms of autoimmune diseases begin.[4] Researchers estimate that there are between 80 and 140 different types of autoimmune diseases, many of which are chronic, debilitating, and life threatening. They can affect virtually any part of the body and cause disability and death. Some of the most common include type 1 diabetes, rheumatoid arthritis, multiple sclerosis, celiac disease, and irritable bowel syndrome. Many people do not realize that autoimmune diseases are among the leading causes of death in female children and women under the age of 65 in the United States.[5]

Inflammatory Response, Pain, and Fever If an infection is localized, pus formation, redness, swelling, and irritation often occur. These symptoms are components of the body's inflammatory response, and they indicate that the invading organisms are being fought systemically. The four cardinal signs of inflammation are *redness*, *swelling*, *pain*, and *heat*.

Pain is often one of the earliest signs that an injury or infection has occurred. Pathogens can kill or injure tissue at the site of infection, causing swelling that puts pressure on nerve endings in the area, causing pain. Although pain does not feel good, it plays a valuable role in the body's response to injury or invasion. For example, it can cause a person to avoid activity that may aggravate the injury or site of infection, thereby protecting against further damage.

Another frequent indicator of infection is *fever*, or a body temperature above the average norm of 98.6°F. Fever is frequently caused by toxins secreted by pathogens that interfere with the control of body temperature. Although extremely elevated temperatures are harmful to the body, a mild fever is protective: Raising body temperature by one or two degrees destroys some disease-causing organisms. A fever also stimulates the body to produce more white blood cells, which destroy more invaders. Of course, with fevers beyond 101° or 102°F, risks to the patient outweigh any benefits. In these cases, medical treatment should be obtained.

Vaccines: Bolstering Your Immunity

Recall that once people have been exposed to a specific pathogen, subsequent attacks activate their memory T and B cells, thus giving them immunity. This is the principle on which **vaccination** is based.

A vaccine consists of killed or weakened versions of a disease-causing microorganism or an antigen similar to but less dangerous than the disease antigen. It is administered to stimulate the immune system to produce antibodies against future attacks without actually causing the disease (or by causing a very minor case of it). Vaccines typically are given orally or by injection; this form of immunity is termed *artificially acquired active immunity*, in contrast to *naturally acquired active immunity* (which is obtained by exposure to antigens in the normal course of daily life) or *naturally acquired*

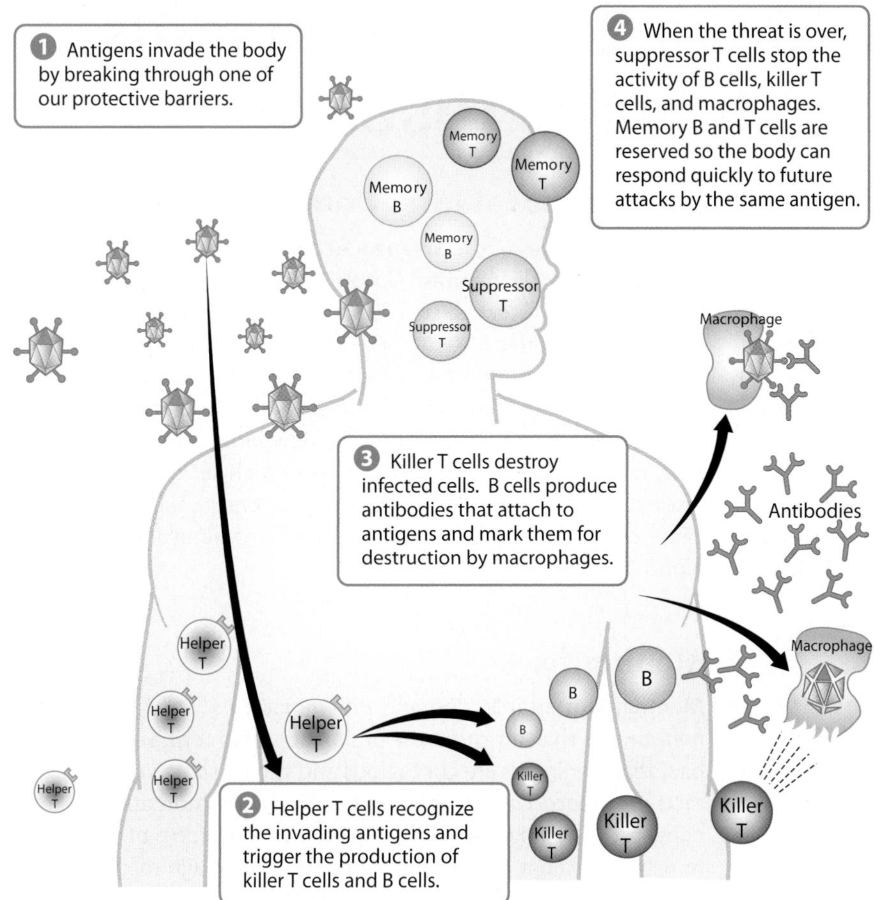

Figure 12.2 The Cell-Mediated Immune Response

passive immunity (as occurs when a mother passes immunity to her fetus via their shared blood supply or to an infant via breast milk). Because of their close living quarters and frequent interactions with other people, college students face a higher than average risk of infection from diseases that are largely preventable. Vaccines that should be a priority among 20-somethings include tetanus-diphtheria-pertussis vaccine (Tdap), meningococcal conjugate vaccine (MCV4), human papillomavirus (HPV), and the influenza vaccine (Table 12.1). Additionally, adults who have not had prior vaccination are recommended to receive measles, mumps, and rubella (MMR) and varicella (chickenpox), and adults with certain health, job, or lifestyle risks are recommended to receive hepatitis A and B and pneumococcal vaccines.[6]

While some advise against vaccinations, avoiding a potentially deadly or disabling disease outweighs any risks. If you develop minor rashes or other symptoms after being immunized, let your doctor know.

TABLE 12.1 Recommended Vaccinations for Adults Aged 19–26 Years Old

- Seasonal flu (influenza) vaccine
- Td or Tdap (tetanus-diphtheria-pertussis) vaccine
- Meningococcal vaccine*
- HPV vaccine series**

Note: *Recommended in some states for students entering colleges and universities due to increased risk among college students living in residential housing.

**Recommended for women up to age 26 years, men up to age 21 years, and men ages 22–26 who have sex with men.

Source: Centers for Disease Control and Prevention, "Adult Vaccinations, What Vaccines Are Recommended for You," Updated March 2014, www.cdc.gov.

Skills for Behavior Change

REDUCE YOUR RISK OF INFECTIOUS DISEASE

- **Limit your exposure to pathogens.** Stay home if you are not feeling well; encourage others to do the same. Don't drag yourself to classes or work and infect others. Don't share utensils or drinking glasses, keep your toothbrush away from those of other people, and wash your hands often. Sneeze or cough into your arm or sleeve rather than your hands. Keep hands away from your mouth, nose, eyes, and other body orifices. Use disposable tissues rather than reusable handkerchiefs. Keep purses and backpacks off of kitchen counters and restroom floors.
- **Exercise regularly.** Regular exercise raises core body temperature, strengthens the immune system, and kills pathogens. Sweat and oil make the skin a hostile environment for many bacteria. Avoid excessive exercise that could overtax the immune system.
- **Get enough sleep.** Sleep allows the body time to refresh itself, produce necessary cells, and reduce inflammation. Even a single night without sleep can increase inflammatory processes and delay wound healing.
- **Stress less.** Rest and relaxation, stress management practices, laughter, and calming music have all been shown to promote healthy cellular activity and bolster immune functioning.
- **Optimize eating.** Enjoy a balanced, healthy diet, including adequate amounts of water, protein, and complex carbohydrates. Eat more omega-3 fatty acids to reduce inflammation, and replace saturated fats with good fats such as olive oil. Antioxidants are believed to be important in immune functioning, so make sure you get your daily fruits and vegetables. Avoid excess alcohol.

check yourself

- **How do vaccines help your body resist viruses?**
- **What are four steps you can take to reduce your overall chances of infection?**

12.3 Bacterial Infections: Staph, Strep, Meningitis, Pneumonia, TB, and Tick-borne Diseases

learning outcome

12.3 List several common bacterial infections.

We can categorize pathogens into six major types: bacteria, viruses, fungi, protozoans, parasitic worms, and prions (see Figure 12.3). Each has a particular route of transmission and characteristic elements that make it unique. In the following pages, we discuss each of these categories and give an overview of some of the diseases that they cause.

Bacteria (singular: *bacterium*) are simple, single-celled microscopic organisms. Although there are several thousand known species of bacteria (and many thousands more that are unknown), just over 100 lead to disease in humans. In many cases, it is not the bacteria themselves that cause disease, but rather the toxins that they produce.

Diseases caused by bacteria can be treated with **antibiotics**. However, today's arsenal of antibiotics is becoming less effective, as strains of bacteria with **antibiotic resistance** become more common. Such "superbugs" can result when successive generations of bacteria mutate to develop an ability to withstand the effects of specific drugs.

Staphylococcal Infections

Staphylococci are normally present on the skin or in the nostrils of most people at any given time and usually present no problems. However, with a cut or break in the *epidermis*, or outer layer of skin, staphylococci may enter the system and cause an **infection**. If you have suffered from acne, boils, styes (infections of the eyelids), or infected wounds, you've probably had a "staph" infection.

Although most of these infections are readily defeated by the immune system, resistant forms of staph are on the rise. One, **methicillin-resistant *Staphylococcus aureus* (MRSA)**, has come under intense scrutiny.[7] Symptoms of MRSA infection often start with a rash or pimple-like skin irritation. Within hours, symptoms may progress to redness, inflammation, pain, and deeper wounds. If untreated, MRSA may invade blood, bones, joints, surgical wounds, heart valves, and lungs; it can be fatal.[8]

Health care–associated or *health care–acquired* MRSA (HA-MRSA) cases arise in settings, such as hospitals or nursing homes, where invasive treatments, infectious pathogens, and weakened immune systems converge. In *community-acquired MRSA* (CA-MRSA), people are infected during normal daily activities. *Linezolid-resistant Staphylococcus aureus*, or LRSA, is a particularly potent and resistant bacterium that has evolved among patients using the antibiotic linezolid to treat MRSA. Questions about what happens when linezolid no longer works and the antibiotic "well" runs dry have raised red flags for health professionals everywhere. People recovering from surgery, those with weakened immune systems, and those with underlying respiratory problems may be at tremendous risk if LRSA remains unchecked.

Streptococcal Infections

At least five types of the **Streptococcus** microorganism are known to cause bacterial infections. Group A streptococci (GAS) cause the most common diseases, such as streptococcal pharyngitis ("strep throat") and scarlet fever.[9] One particularly virulent group of GAS can lead to rare but serious diseases such as *toxic shock syndrome* or *necrotizing fasciitis* (often referred to as "flesh-eating strep").[10] Group B streptococci can cause illness in newborns, pregnant women, older adults, and adults with illnesses such as diabetes or liver disease. A form of resistant *Streptococcus pneumoniae* is a leading cause of bacterial pneumonia, ear infections, sinus infections, and bloodstream infections or "*sepsis*."

Meningitis

Meningitis is an infection and inflammation of the *meninges*, the membranes that surround the brain and spinal cord. Some forms of bacterial meningitis are contagious and can be spread through contact; *pneumococcal meningitis* is the most common and the most dangerous. *Meningococcal meningitis*, a virulent form of meningitis, remains prevalent on college campuses.[11] Although meningitis can occur at any age, adolescents ages 16 to 21 have the highest rates, particularly those living in close quarters such as dormitories.

The signs of meningitis are sudden fever, severe headache, and a stiff neck, particularly causing difficulty touching chin to chest. Persons suspected of having meningitis should receive immediate, aggressive medical treatment. Vaccines are available for some types of meningitis.

Pneumonia

Pneumonia is a general term for a range of conditions that result in inflammation of the lungs and difficulty breathing. It is characterized by chronic cough, chest pain, chills, high fever, fluid accumulation, and eventual respiratory failure.

Bacterial pneumonia responds readily to antibiotic treatment in the early stages, but can be deadly in more advanced stages. Pneumonias caused by viruses, fungi, chemicals, or other substances in the lungs are more difficult to treat. Vulnerable populations include children; the poor; those displaced by war, famine, and natural disasters; older adults; those occupationally exposed to chemicals and particulates that damage the lungs; and those suffering from other illnesses.

Ticks are a vector for several devastating bacterial diseases.

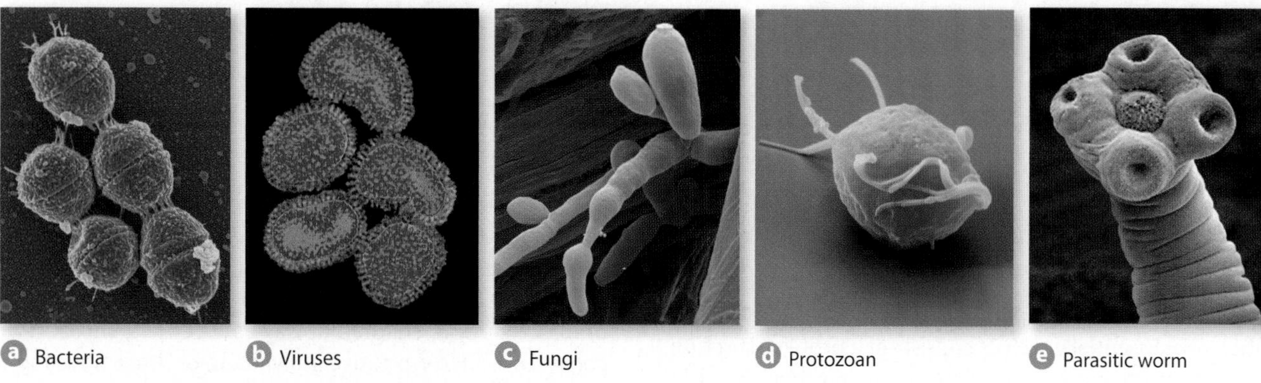

Figure 12.3 Examples of Five Major Types of Pathogens
(a) Color-enhanced scanning electron micrograph (SEM) of *Streptococcus* bacteria, magnified 40,000×. (b) Colored transmission electron micrograph (TEM) of influenza (flu) viruses, magnified 32,000×. (c) Color SEM of *Candida albicans*, a yeast fungus, magnified 50,000×. (d) Color TEM of *Trichomonas vaginalis*, a protozoan, magnified 9,000×. (e) Color-enhanced SEM of a tapeworm, magnified 50×.

Tuberculosis (TB)

With an astounding one-third of the world's population infected and over 1.3 million deaths each year, only HIV/AIDS is a greater global infectious agent killer than **tuberculosis (TB)**.[12] Many health professionals assumed that TB was conquered in the United States, but even though rates have declined in the last two decades, there were still nearly 10,000 cases of TB documented in the United States in 2012.[13] During the past 20 years, overcrowding and poor sanitation in some developing nations kept the disease alive. Failure to isolate active cases of TB and fully treat them, a migration of TB to the United States through immigration and international travel, and a weakened public health infrastructure that funded less screening kept the disease from disappearing in North America.

Most tuberculosis-related deaths occur in developing countries, where it accounts for 26 percent of all preventable deaths.[14] Most TB cases and deaths occur in men; however, TB is among the top three killers of women globally, as well as the leading cause of death among HIV-positive patients.[15]

Symptoms include persistent coughing, weight loss, fever, and spitting up blood. Coughing is the most common mode of transmitting TB, and infected people can be contagious without actually showing any symptoms. Those at highest risk include the poor, especially children, and the chronically ill; people in crowded prisons and homeless shelters who continuously inhale the same contaminated air are also at higher risk, as are persons with compromised immune systems.

The current recommended treatment for TB involves taking four drugs for 6 to 9 months; however, a new 12-dose regimen is available for high-risk populations.[16] The lengthy, difficult treatment, along with barriers to obtaining drugs and care in many developing areas, leads to missed doses and treatments that end before the cure and thus breed drug-resistant bacteria.

Multidrug-resistant TB (MDR-TB) is a form of TB that is resistant to at least two of the best anti-TB drugs. An even more dangerous form, **extensively drug-resistant TB (XDR-TB)**, is extremely difficult to treat. These newer strains of tuberculosis are reaching epidemic proportions in many regions of the world.[17]

Tick-borne Bacterial Diseases

Certain tickborne diseases have become major health threats in the United States. The most noteworthy include two bacterially caused diseases that spike in the summer months in many states. *Lyme disease* is particularly present in the upper Midwest. Symptoms range from none; to a rash or bull's eye lesion and flu-like symptoms; to chronic arthritis, blindness, and long-term disability. *Ehrlichiosis* has flu-like symptoms that may progress quickly to respiratory difficulties and even death. Fortunately, antibiotics given early in the disease course are effective in preventing any serious threats.

How can you protect yourself from a staph infection? Watch **Toxic Staph Outbreak** in the Study Area of MasteringHealth.

Once believed to be closely related to viruses, **rickettsia** are now considered a form of bacteria. They multiply within small blood vessels, causing vascular blockage and tissue death. Rickettsia require an insect vector (carrier) for transmission to humans. Two common forms of human rickettsial disease are *Rocky Mountain spotted fever* (*RMSF*), carried by a tick, and *typhus*, carried by a louse, flea, or tick. These produce similar symptoms, including high fever, weakness, rash, and coma; both can be life threatening.

For all insect-borne diseases, the best protection is to stay indoors at dusk and early morning to avoid high insect activity. If you must go out, wear protective clothing or use bug sprays containing natural oils, pyrethrins, or DEET (diethyl toluamide). If you are traveling where insect-borne diseases are prevalent, bed nets and other protective measures may be necessary.

check yourself

- **List three illnesses or conditions that can result from bacterial infection.**
- **What can you do to reduce your risk of bacterial infections?**

12.4 Viral Infections: Mono, Hepatitis, Herpes, Mumps, Measles, and Rubella

learning outcome

12.4 Identify the causes and symptoms of common viral infections.

Viruses are the smallest known pathogens, approximately 1/500th the size of bacteria. Essentially, a virus consists of a protein structure that contains either *ribonucleic acid* (*RNA*) or *deoxyribonucleic acid* (*DNA*). Viruses are incapable of carrying out any life processes on their own. To reproduce, viruses must invade and inject their own DNA and RNA into a host cell, take it over, and force it to make copies of itself. The new viruses then erupt out of the host cell and seek other cells to invade. While viruses are incapable of carrying out any life processes on their own, hundreds of viruses are known to cause diseases in humans.

Viral diseases can be difficult to treat because many viruses can withstand heat, formaldehyde, and large doses of radiation. Some viruses have **incubation periods** (the length of time required to develop fully and cause symptoms in their hosts) that last for years, which delays diagnosis. Drug treatment for viral infections is also limited. Drugs powerful enough to kill viruses generally kill the host cells, too, although some medications block stages in viral reproduction without damaging the host cells.

Infectious Mononucleosis

Caused primarily by the Epstein-Barr virus, **mononucleosis** is most widespread among people between the ages of 15 and 24, with college students or those living in close quarters among those at highest risk. By adulthood, 90 to 95 percent of people have been infected, many without ever showing symptoms.[18] Because saliva seems to be a key route of transmission, "mono" has often been referred to as the "kissing disease." However, sharing eating utensils, drinking vessels, towels, cosmetics, or even coughing can spread the virus. Body fluids, including blood, genital secretions, and mucus, can also spread the disease. Common symptoms include bone-crushing fatigue, headache, fever, aches and pains, sore throat, rashes, and swollen lymph nodes. Anything that weakens the immune system, such as high stress, lack of sleep, poor diet, or too much alcohol or drug use, can increase risk. A simple blood test can determine whether you have mono. Rest, balanced nutrition, stress management, and healthy lifestyle are the best treatments.

Hepatitis

Hepatitis is a virally caused inflammation of the liver. Symptoms include fever, headache, nausea, loss of appetite, skin rashes, pain in the upper right abdomen, dark yellow-brown urine, and jaundice. Nearly 4.5 million Americans have one of several forms of hepatitis (A, B, C, D, and E), with hepatitis A, B, and C having the highest rates of incidence.[19]

Hepatitis A (HAV) is contracted by eating food or drinking water contaminated with human feces. Since vaccinations became available, U.S. HAV rates have declined dramatically, yet an estimated 2,700 new cases are diagnosed and treated annually.[20] Handlers of infected food, children at day care centers, those having sexual contact with HAV-positive individuals, or those traveling to regions where HAV is endemic are at higher risk, as are those who ingest seafood from contaminated water or use contaminated needles. Fortunately, individuals infected with hepatitis A don't become chronic carriers, and vaccines for the disease are available.

Hepatitis B (HBV) is spread through unprotected sex; sharing needles or accidental needlesticks; or, for newborns, an infected mother. It can lead to chronic liver disease or liver cancer. Numbers of HBV cases have declined rapidly since vaccines became available, and needle exchange programs have helped reduce risks of infection. Still, nearly 40,000 cases are reported each year in the United States, and over 1.4 million are chronic carriers.[21] Globally, HBV infections are on the decline, but over 240 million are chronically infected.[22]

Hepatitis C (HCV) infections are on an epidemic rise, because resistant forms of the virus are emerging. Some cases can be traced to blood transfusions or organ transplants. An estimated 17,000

Why does it matter if people "opt out" of recommended vaccines?

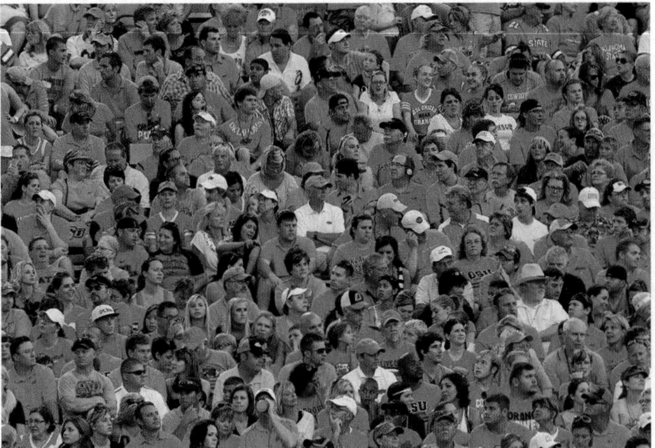

Vaccinations are key in protecting us from infectious diseases, yet many people "opt out" for religious or philosophical reasons. College students and those who live or routinely hang out in crowded areas, ride on public transportation, travel internationally, attend major sporting events or concerts, or spend time in hospitals where sick people congregate are more likely to come in contact with those who are sick. Keeping up-to-date on your vaccines is a big part of being responsible and protecting yourself and others.

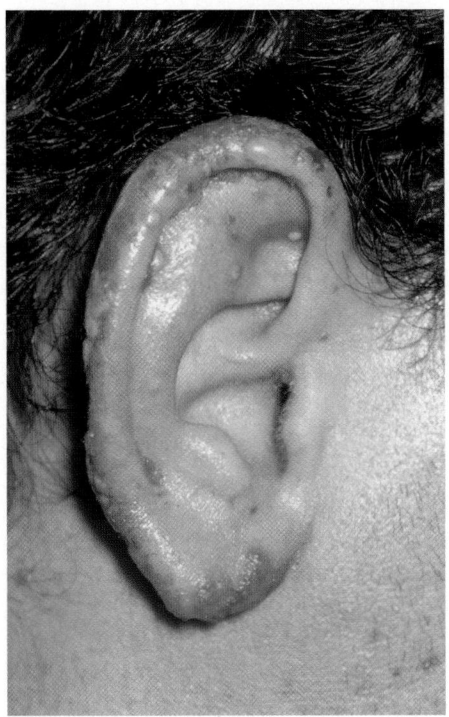

A series of fluid-filled blisters on the face, neck, or torso can be a sign of herpes gladiatorum. This form of herpes is easily spread, especially among athletes.

new cases occur in the United States each year, with approximately 3.2 million people chronically infected.[23] Of those infected, 75–85 percent develop chronic infections; if the infection is left untreated, the person may develop cirrhosis of the liver, liver cancer, or liver failure.[24] Although there is no vaccine for HCV, new drugs have been successful in treating the disease.

To prevent spread of HBV and HCV, use latex condoms every time you have sex; don't share personal-care items that might have blood on them, such as razors or toothbrushes; get a blood test for HBV; never share needles; and if you are having body art done, go only to reputable artists or piercers who follow established sterilization and infection-control protocols.

Herpes Viruses

Herpes viruses are among the more common viruses infecting humans; painful, blistering rashes are hallmarks of these infections. These diseases are easily transmitted via physical contact and can become chronic problems.

Caused by the *herpes varicella zoster virus* (*HVZV*), **chickenpox** produces symptoms of fever and fatigue 13 to 17 days after exposure, followed by skin eruptions that itch, blister, and produce a clear fluid. The virus is present in these blisters for approximately 1 week. Although a vaccine is available, many parents incorrectly assume that the vaccine is not necessary and that contracting the disease will ensure lifelong immunity.

For a small segment of the population, the chickenpox virus reactivates later in life during times of high stress or when the immune system is taxed by other diseases. This painful, blistering rash, accompanied by extreme pain and other possible complications, is called **shingles**; it affects over 1 million people in the United States, most of whom are over the age of 60.[25] The best way to prevent shingles is to get vaccinated.

Herpes gladiatorum is caused by the herpes simplex type 1 virus. It shows itself as a blistered rash on the face, neck, or torso. Herpes gladiatorum is also referred to as "mat pox" or "wrestler's herpes," as it's highly contagious via mats used in a yoga studio or gym or through body-to-body contact.

Herpes infections that are sexually transmitted are discussed later in this chapter.

Mumps

With vaccine introduction, reported cases of **mumps** have declined, but in the last decade, several outbreaks have occurred in the United States and globally, largely attributed to parents' unsubstantiated fears of vaccine complications keeping many school-aged children from being vaccinated.

Approximately one half of all mumps infections produce only minor symptoms, with about one third of infected people never showing any. The most common symptom is the swelling of the parotid (salivary) glands. One of the greatest dangers associated with mumps is the potential for sterility in men who contract the disease in young adulthood. Some victims also suffer hearing loss.

Measles and Rubella

Measles is a highly contagious viral disorder that often affects young children, but it is increasing among young adults today, particularly on college campuses. Many young adults may not have been fully vaccinated in their youth, as their parents may have thought the disease was no longer a problem in the United States. Those who refuse vaccination put the immunocompromised and others at risk, as babies are typically not vaccinated until after 1 year of age. Many regions of the world have large numbers of unvaccinated individuals.[26]

Symptoms include an itchy rash and a high fever. Measles can be life threatening, causing high fever, pneumonia, encephalitis, and other complications. Symptoms tend to be worse for those under 5 and those 20 and over. In 2011, nearly 40 percent of children under the age of 5 with measles had to be hospitalized.[27]

Rubella (German measles) is a milder viral infection that causes rashes, usually on upper extremities, and is believed to be spread by inhalation. Rubella is a threat to the very young and unborn, as it is known to cause blindness, deafness, heart defects, and cognitive impairments in fetuses and newborns. Infections in children not immunized against measles can lead to fever-induced problems such as rheumatic heart disease, kidney damage, and neurological disorders.

check yourself

- **List three illnesses or conditions that can result from viral infection.**
- **What can you do to reduce your risk of viral infections?**

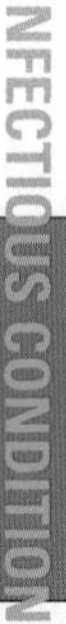

12.5 Viral Infections: The Cold and Flu

learning outcome

12.5 Identify the causes and symptoms of the common cold and influenza.

The Common Cold

Colds can be caused by any number of viruses (there may be over 200), though the rhinovirus is responsible for 30–50 percent of all colds, followed by the coronavirus, at 10–15 percent.[28] Colds are **endemic** (always present to some degree) throughout the world. Otherwise healthy people carry cold viruses in their noses and throats most of the time; these are held in check until the host's resistance is lowered. It is possible to "catch" a cold—from airborne droplets of a sneeze or from skin-to-skin or mucous membrane contact—though the hands are the greatest avenue for virus transmission. Covering your nose and mouth with a tissue or handkerchief when sneezing is better than using your bare hand.

Several strategies for preventing a cold include bolstering your immune system with healthy diet, exercise, stress reduction, sleep, and other behaviors. Washing your hands with regular soap and water and keeping your hands away from your eyes, nose, and mouth are also key. If you have a cold, keep away from others; if others have a cold, avoid close contact and wash your hands often. Throw used tissues in the trash, and disinfect TV remotes and other objects that you have been touching. Contrary to popular belief, you cannot catch a cold from getting a chill, but the chill may lower your immune system's resistance to a pathogenic virus if one is present.

SYMPTOMS	COLD	FLU
Fever	Rare	Usual; high (100–102°F, occasionally higher, especially in children); lasts 3–4 days
Headache	Rare	Common
General aches and pains	Slight	Usual; often severe
Fatigue, weakness	Sometimes	Usual; can last up to 2–3 weeks
Extreme exhaustion	Never	Usual; at the beginning of the illness
Stuffy nose	Common	Sometimes
Sneezing	Usual	Sometimes
Sore throat	Common	Sometimes
Chest discomfort, cough	Common; mild to moderate, hacking cough	Common; can become severe
TREATMENT	Antihistamines, decongestants, nonsteroidal anti-inflammatory medicines	Antiviral medicines—see your doctor
PREVENTION	Wash your hands often with soap and water; avoid close contact with anyone with a cold	Annual vaccination; antiviral medicines—see your doctor
COMPLICATIONS	Sinus congestion, middle ear infection, asthma	Bronchitis, pneumonia; can worsen chronic conditions; can be life threatening

Figure 12.4 Is It a Cold or the Flu?
Source: Adapted from the National Institute of Allergy and Infectious Diseases, "Is It a Cold or the Flu?," 2008, www.niaid.nih.gov.

The evidence that *Echinacea* can prevent or shorten the duration of colds is inconclusive according to summaries of several studies.[29] There is also scant evidence that mega-doses of vitamin C can cure or even reduce symptoms of the cold.[30]

Influenza

In otherwise healthy people, **influenza**, or flu, is usually not life threatening (see Figure 12.4). However, for individuals over 65, under 5, or with respiratory problems or heart disease, it can be very serious. Approximately 200,000 Americans will need hospitalization each year for influenza treatment.[31] Treatment is *palliative*—focused on symptom relief rather than cure.

If you have bad body aches, fatigue, and fever, it is likely that you have the flu. In the absence of these symptoms, but the presence of a stuffy or runny nose, sneezing, a sore throat, and often a cough, over-the-counter medicines targeting symptoms of the common cold may help.[32]

Three varieties of flu virus have been discovered, with many strains within each. The A form of the virus is generally the most virulent, followed by B and C. Immunity to one form doesn't necessarily convey immunity to others.

Flu Vaccine Strains of influenza are constantly changing, so flu vaccines are formulated each year that combine three types of killed flu viruses from the A and B varieties (called trivalent vaccines).[33] The viruses are selected based on forecasting of the strains likely to emerge in various regions of the world. If researchers correctly predict strains, vaccines are between 70 and 90 percent effective in healthy adults for about a year; if the prediction is off, a shot may not totally protect you from the flu; however, symptoms may be less severe.[34] If you have had a severe reaction to past flu shots, have a severe allergy to chicken eggs, are running a fever, or have other issues, consult with your doctor before having a shot. An optional nasal spray flu vaccine is available for healthy people age 1 to 49 who are not pregnant. Flu shots take 2 to 3 weeks to become effective, so people at risk should get these shots in the fall before the flu season begins. Options for low- or no-cost vaccines are campus health centers, local public health departments, local pharmacies and big box stores, and community centers. Compared to the high cost of lost days of work or missed classes, possible hospitalization, and expensive medicines to treat symptoms, the flu vaccine is a sound investment.

If you feel you've been exposed to the flu or have early symptoms, see your doctor, as antiviral sprays, capsules, and powders that can reduce symptoms, prevent complications, and speed your recovery are available.

check yourself

- **What are the causes, symptoms, and treatment for the common cold and influenza?**

Other Pathogens

learning outcome

12.6 Describe how fungi, protozoans, parasitic worms, and prions cause infection.

Bacteria and viruses account for many, but not all, common diseases. Other organisms can also infect a host. Among these are fungi, protozoans, parasitic worms, and prions.

Fungi

Our environment is inhabited by hundreds of species of **fungi**, multi- or unicellular organisms that obtain food by infiltrating the bodies of other organisms, both living and dead. Many fungi, such as edible mushrooms, penicillin, and the yeast used to make bread, are useful to humans, but some species can produce infections. *Candidiasis* (vaginal yeast infection), ringworm, jock itch, and toenail fungus are common fungal diseases.

With most fungal diseases, keeping the affected area clean and dry and treating it promptly with appropriate medications (often available over the counter) will generally bring relief. Fungal diseases typically transmit via physical contact, so avoid going barefoot in public showers, hotel rooms, and other areas where fungus may be present.

Coccidioidomycosis, also known as *valley fever*, is an infection that occurs when humans or pets inhale soil-dwelling fungal spores. In the last decade, rates have soared in desert regions of Mexico, Central and South America, and the southwestern United States.[35] Because early symptoms of headache, aches, and fever are common, cases often go unreported and can quickly progress to pneumonia, meningitis, or other life-threatening complications. As many as 40 percent of cases require hospitalization and have symptoms lasting weeks or months.[36] The best means of prevention is to avoid actions that stir the soil and cause spores to be aerosolized. Staying indoors during dust storms may also help reduce risks.

Protozoans

Protozoans are single-celled organisms that cause diseases such as African sleeping sickness and malaria. Although prevalent in nonindustrialized countries, they are largely controlled in the United States. The most common protozoan disease in the United States is *trichomoniasis*. A common waterborne protozoan disease, *giardiasis*, can cause intestinal pain and discomfort weeks after infection. Protection of water supplies is the key to prevention.

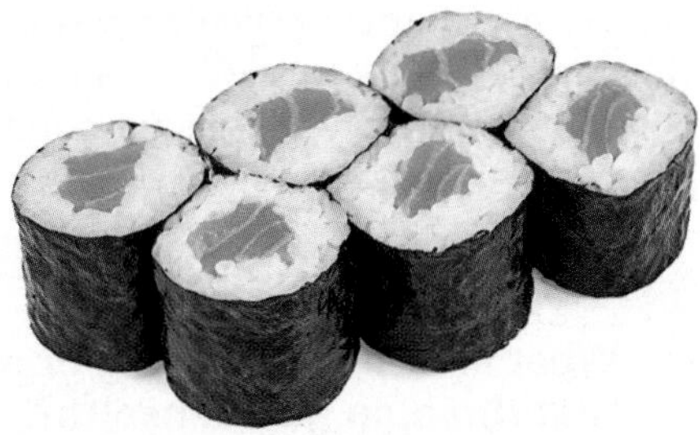

Eating raw fish, such as sushi, can increase your risk of infection from parasitic worms.

Parasitic Worms

Parasitic worms are the largest of the pathogens. Ranging in size from small pinworms to large tapeworms, most are more a nuisance than a threat. Of special note are worm infestations associated with eating raw fish such as sushi. Eating raw fish can lead to infection with herring worms, round worms, and other parasites. Symptoms ranging from nausea and vomiting to severe pain and cramping may occur as worms invade intestines and the immune system fights back. Medicines can be prescribed to kill worms. In severe cases, surgery may be required to remove them. You can prevent worm infestations by cooking fish and other foods to temperatures sufficient to kill the worms and their eggs. Worms can also be contracted through close contact with pets at home and poor pet and human hygiene. Preventive measures include getting your pets checked and wearing shoes in parks or public places where animal feces are present.

Prions

A **prion** is a self-replicating, protein-based agent that can infect humans and animals. One such prion is believed to be the underlying cause of spongiform diseases such as *bovine spongiform encephalopathy (BSE)* or "mad cow disease" found in beef cattle in various regions of the world. If humans eat contaminated meat from cattle with BSE, they may develop a mad cow-like disease known as *variant Creutzfeldt-Jakob disease (vCJD)*. Symptoms of vCJD include loss of memory, tremors, and muscle spasms or "ticks." Within a fairly short time period, depression, difficulty walking, seizures, and severe dementia can ultimately lead to death in both cows and humans.[37] An increasing number of infected cattle have been found in the United States and globally. To date, there have been three cases of vCJD in the United States.[38] Improved surveillance and reporting is necessary to determine if more cases exist. In the meantime, because infected brain and spinal tissue of cattle have been implicated in global infections, these animal parts from high-risk older cattle are restricted from the human food chain.[39]

check yourself

- **What are three illnesses or conditions that can result from fungi, protozoans, parasitic worms, or prions?**
- **What can you do to reduce your risk of these illnesses or conditions?**

12.7 Emerging Diseases

learning outcome

12.7 Explain the problem of emerging and resurgent diseases.

Although our immune systems are adept at responding to challenges, microbes and other pathogens appear to be gaining ground. Rates of infectious diseases have rapidly increased over the past decade, owing to a combination of overpopulation, inadequate health care, increasing poverty, environmental degradation, and drug resistance.[40]

West Nile Virus

Spread by infected mosquitoes, there are several thousand active cases of West Nile virus in the United States every year. Although most people infected have minor flu-like symptoms and fully recover, approximately 1 percent of those infected have neurological symptoms, indicative of a more serious form of *West Nile encephalitis* (inflammation of the brain).[41] Symptoms can include severe neurological complications, including respiratory failure, paralysis, seizures, and death. Survivors often face years of intensive rehabilitation. Those with compromised immune systems or other health problems are more likely to have complications.[42] Today, only Alaska and Hawaii remain free of the disease, and avoiding mosquito bites is the best way to prevent it.[43]

Avian (Bird) Flu

Avian influenza is an infectious disease of birds, with strains capable of crossing the species barrier to cause severe illness in humans who come in contact with bird droppings or fluids. Bird flu appears to have originated in Asia and spread via migrating bird populations.[44] Although the virus has yet to mutate into a form highly infectious to humans, outbreaks in which people contract the disease from birds in rural areas of the world (where people often live in close proximity to poultry and other animals) have occurred. As of March 2013, the World Health Organization (WHO) had recorded 650 cases of bird flu in humans, with 386 deaths.[45]

Many health experts suggest that if this virus becomes transmissible between humans, it is virulent enough to surpass the lethality of the influenza epidemics of 1918 and 1919, which caused millions of deaths. This type of pandemic flu or global epidemic could decimate the world's population.

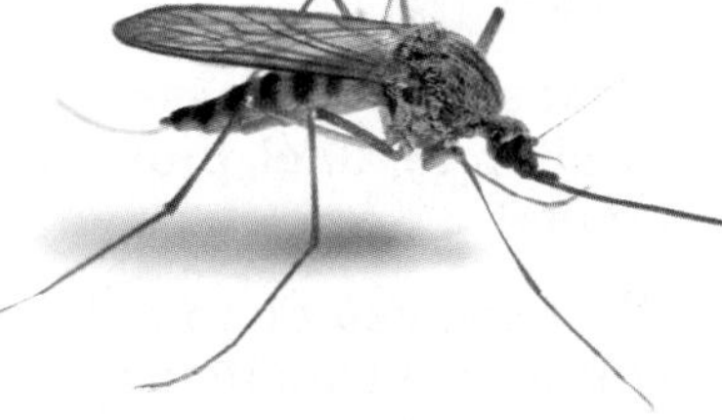

Mosquitoes spread many diseases, including West Nile virus and malaria.

Escherichia coli O157:H7

Escherichia coli O157:H7 is one of over 170 types of *E. coli* bacteria that can infect humans. Most *E. coli* organisms are harmless and live in the intestines of healthy animals and humans. *E. coli* O157:H7, however, produces a lethal toxin and can cause severe illness or death. It can live in the intestines of healthy cattle and then contaminate food products at slaughterhouses. Eating ground beef that is rare or undercooked, drinking unpasteurized milk or juice, or swimming in sewage-contaminated water or public pools can also cause infection.

A symptom of infection is nonbloody diarrhea, usually 2 to 8 days after exposure; however, asymptomatic cases have been noted. Children, older adults, and people with weakened immune systems are particularly vulnerable to serious side effects such as kidney failure, intestinal damage, or death.

Ebola Virus Disease

Ebola virus disease (EVD) is a rare, often fatal, disease that is ravaging parts of Central and West Africa, with over 8,000 cases reported in September 2014 and death rates of 50 to 90 percent. Fruit bats, chimps, and other animals are natural hosts and spread the disease to humans, who spread it to others via contact with infected body fluids or surfaces such as sheets and clothing. Once infected, blood clotting ability diminishes, leading to internal and external bleeding. Without rehydration, organ failure and death can occur. Body rash, vomiting, diarrhea, fever, pain, and headache are early symptoms. Currently no vaccines are available, although two are being tested.

Malaria

Today, approximately 50 percent of the world's population, mostly those living in the poorest countries, are at risk for malaria. The disease is transmitted by mosquitoes carrying a parasite. There were 207 million cases of malaria and an estimated 627,000 to 780,00 deaths in 2012, even though mortality rates have dropped significantly in the last decade.[46] Most deaths occur among poor and vulnerable children and pregnant women in sub-Saharan Africa.[47]

Travelers from malaria-free regions entering areas where there is malaria transmission are highly vulnerable, as they have little or no immunity and often receive a delayed or wrong malaria diagnosis when they return home.[48] Mosquito nets and use of insect repellents are particularly important to prevention, as is removal of standing water in yards. Natural disasters that leave standing water in which mosquitoes can flourish pose increased risks. Resistance to chloroquine, once a widely used and highly effective treatment, is now found in most regions of the world, and other treatments are losing their effectiveness at alarming rates.

check yourself

- **What are three emerging or resurgent diseases that threaten global health?**

Antibiotic Resistance

learning **outcome**

12.8 Explain the phenomenon of antibiotic resistance.

Antibiotics are supposed to wipe out bacteria that are susceptible to them. However, many common antibiotics are becoming ineffective against resistant strains of bacteria. Here's how this happens: Bacteria and other microorganisms that cause infections and diseases can evolve rapidly, developing ways to survive drugs that had once been able to kill or weaken them. Through this process, some of the bacteria and microorganisms are becoming "superbugs" that cannot be stopped with existing medications.

Antibiotic Resistance on the Rise

Antibiotic resistance is a problem today for several reasons:[49]

- **Improper use of antibiotics and resulting growth of superbugs.** When used improperly, antibiotics kill only the weak bacteria, leaving the strongest to thrive and replicate. Bacteria can swap genes with one another under the right conditions, so hardy drug-resistant germs can share their resistance mechanisms with other germs. These germs adapt and mutate, and eventually an entire colony of resistant bugs grows and passes on its resistance traits to new generations of bacteria.

  Over time, most pathogens evolve, but human negligence can speed the resistant ones on their journey. If a patient begins an antibiotic regimen, but stops taking the drug as soon as symptoms abate rather than finishing the course of antibiotics, then the surviving bacteria build immunity to the drugs used to treat them. Doctors who overprescribe antibiotics or give them for virally caused diseases also contribute to antibiotic resistance.
- **Overuse of antibiotics in food production.** About 70 percent of antibiotic production today is used to treat sick animals living in crowded feedlots and to encourage growth in livestock, poultry, and even farmed fish. Many believe that ingesting animal products full of antibiotics may contribute to resistance in humans. In addition, water runoff and sewage from feedlots can contaminate the water in rivers and streams with antibiotics. A growing problem is the use of antibiotics to treat household pets. Many of these prescriptions go unused and are dumped in toilets and garbage, posing a threat to community water systems.
- **Misuse and overuse of antibacterial soaps and other cleaning products.** Preying on the public's fear of germs and disease, the cleaning industry adds antibacterial ingredients to many of its dish soaps, hand cleaners, shower scrubs, surface scrubs, and other household products. Just how much these products contribute to overall resistance is difficult to assess; as with antibiotics, the germs these products do not kill may become stronger than before.

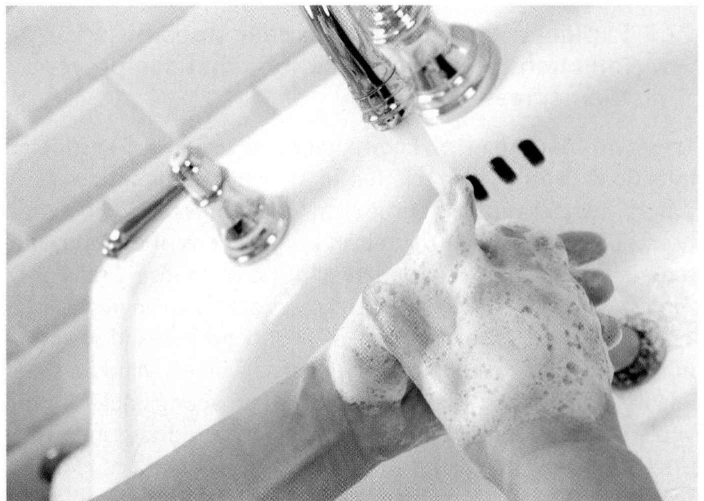

To prevent the spread of infectious disease, wash your hands!

What Can You Do?

You can take the following steps to prevent antibiotic resistance:

- **Get regular vaccinations.** If someone in your house has a resistant bacterial infection, be careful about hand washing and general hygiene. Don't share towels or personal items.
- **Be responsible with medications.** Take medications as prescribed and finish the full course. Talk to your local pharmacist or waste disposal company about how to dispose of unused drugs.
- **Use regular soap, not antibacterial soap, when washing your hands.** Some experts say that antibacterial cleaning products do more harm than good. Research suggests that antibacterial agents contained in soaps actually may kill normal bacteria, thus creating an environment for resistant, mutated bacteria that are impervious to antibacterial cleaners and antibiotics.
- **Avoid food treated with antibiotics.** Buy meat from animals that were not unnecessarily dosed with antibiotics. (Look for that information on the label of meat products.)

check yourself

- **How do bacteria become resistant to antibiotics?**
- **What can you do to prevent antibiotic resistance?**

12.9

Sexually Transmitted Infections

learning outcome

12.9 Explain risk factors for sexually transmitted infections and identify actions that can prevent their spread.

There are more than 20 known types of **sexually transmitted infections (STIs)**. Often referred to as synonymous with sexually transmitted diseases (STDs), the term STI describes a condition that has visible symptoms or that alters key functions of the body; the term is seen as more appropriate and less stigmatizing than STD. Almost half of the newly diagnosed cases of STIs are in people ages 15–24.[50] While STIs affect people of all backgrounds and socioeconomic levels, they disproportionately affect women, minorities, and infants and are most prevalent in teens and young adults.[51] More virulent strains and antibiotic-resistant forms indicate increasing threats to at-risk populations.

Early symptoms of an STI are often mild and unrecognizable. Left untreated, some of these infections can have grave consequences, such as sterility, blindness, central nervous system destruction, disfigurement, and even death. Infants born to mothers carrying the organisms for these infections are at risk for a variety of health problems.

110 million people are living with a STI in the United States.

What's Your Risk?

Several reasons have been proposed to explain the present high rates of STIs. The first relates to the moral and social stigmas associated with these infections. Shame and embarrassment often keep infected people from seeking treatment. Unfortunately, the infected usually continue to be sexually active, thereby infecting unsuspecting partners. People who are uncomfortable discussing sexual issues may also be less likely to use, and ask their partners to use, condoms to protect against STIs and pregnancy.

Another reason proposed for the STI epidemic is our casual attitude about sex. Bombarded by a media that glamorizes sex, many people take sexual partners without considering the consequences. Others are pressured into sexual relationships they don't really want or that they aren't ready for. Generally, the more sexual partners a person has, the greater the risk for contracting an STI.

Ignorance—about the infections, their symptoms, and the fact that someone can be asymptomatic but still infected—is also a factor. A person who is infected but asymptomatic can unknowingly spread an STI to others who also ignore or misinterpret symptoms. By the time either partner seeks medical help, he or she may have infected several others. In addition, many people mistakenly believe that certain sexual practices—oral sex, for example—carry no risk for STIs. In fact, oral sex practices among young adults may be responsible for increases in herpes and other STIs. Figure 12.5 shows the continuum of risk for various sexual behaviors. The **Skills for Behavior Change** offers tips for ways to practice safer sex.

High-risk behaviors	Moderate-risk behaviors	Low-risk behaviors	No-risk behaviors
Unprotected vaginal, anal, and oral sex—any activity that involves direct contact with bodily fluids, such as ejaculate, vaginal secretions, or blood—are high-risk behaviors.	Vaginal, anal, or oral sex with a latex or polyurethane condom and a water-based lubricant used properly and consistently can greatly reduce the risk of STI transmission. Dental dams used during oral sex can also greatly reduce the risk of STI transmission.	Mutual masturbation, if there are no cuts on the hand, penis, or vagina, is very low risk. Rubbing, kissing, and massaging carry low risk, but herpes can be spread by skin-to-skin contact from an infected partner.	Abstinence, phone sex, talking, and fantasy are all no-risk behaviors. 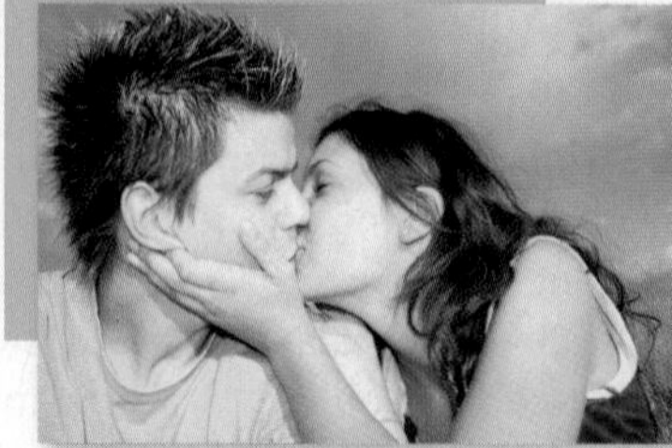

Figure 12.5 Continuum of Risk for Various Sexual Behaviors
Different behaviors have different levels of risk for various sexually transmitted infections (STIs); however, no matter what, any sexual activity involving direct contact with blood, semen, or vaginal secretions is high risk.

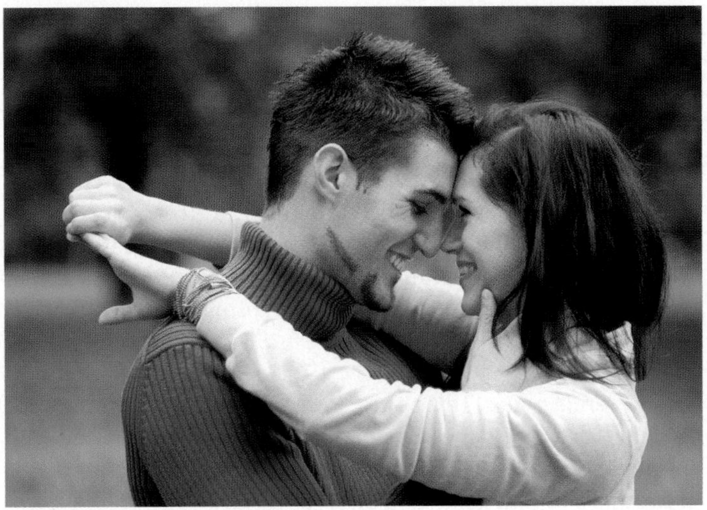

How can I tell if someone I'm dating has an STI?

You can't tell if someone has an STI just by looking at them; it isn't something broadcast on a person's face, and many people with STIs are themselves unaware of the infection because it could be asymptomatic. The only way to know for sure is to go to a clinic and get tested. In addition, partners need to be open and honest with each other about their sexual histories, and practice safer sex.

Routes of Transmission

STIs are generally spread through some form of intimate sexual contact. Vaginal intercourse, oral–genital contact, hand–genital contact, and anal intercourse are the most common modes of transmission. Less likely, but still possible, modes of transmission include mouth-to-mouth contact and contact with fluids from body sores that may be spread by the hands. Although each STI is a different infection caused by a different pathogen, all STI pathogens prefer dark, warm, moist places, especially the mucous membranes lining the reproductive organs. Most of them are susceptible to light and excess heat, cold, and dryness, and many die quickly on exposure to air. Like other communicable infections, STIs have both pathogen-specific *incubation periods* and periods of time during which transmission is most likely, called *periods of communicability*.

Where to Go for Help

If you are concerned about your own risk or that of a friend, arrange a confidential meeting with a health professional at your college health service or community STI clinic. He or she will provide you with the information that you need to decide whether you should be tested for an STI. If the student health service is not an option for you, seek assistance through your local public health department or community STI clinic.

Skills for Behavior Change

SAFE IS SEXY

Practicing the following behaviors will help you reduce your risk of contracting a sexually transmitted infection (STI):

- **Avoid casual sexual partners. All sexually active adults who are not in a lifelong monogamous relationship should practice safer sex.**
- **Always use a condom or a dental dam (a sensitive latex sheet, about the size of a tissue, that can be placed over the female genitals to form a protective layer) during vaginal, oral, or anal sex. Remember that condoms do not provide 100 percent protection against all STIs.**
- **Postpone sexual involvement until you are assured that your partner is not infected; discuss past sexual history, and if necessary, get tested for any potential STIs.**
- **Avoid injury to body tissue during sexual activity. Some pathogens can enter the bloodstream through microscopic tears in anal or vaginal tissues.**
- **Avoid unprotected oral, anal, or vaginal sexual activity in which semen, blood, or vaginal secretions could penetrate mucous membranes or enter through breaks in the skin.**
- **Avoid using drugs and alcohol, which can dull your senses and affect your ability to take responsible precautions with potential sex partners.**
- **Wash your hands before and after sexual encounters. Urinate after sexual relations and, if possible, wash your genitals.**
- **Total abstinence is the only absolute way to prevent the transmission of STIs, but abstinence can be a difficult choice to make. If you have any doubt about the potential risks of having sex, consider other means of intimacy (at least until you can ensure your safety)—massage, dry kissing, hugging, holding and touching, and masturbation (alone or with a partner).**
- **Think about situations ahead of time to avoid risky behaviors, including settings with alcohol and drug use.**
- **If you are worried about your own HIV or STI status, get tested. Don't risk infecting others.**
- **If you contract an STI, ask your health care provider for advice on notifying past or potential partners.**

Sources: American College of Obstetricians and Gynecologists, *How to Prevent Sexually Transmitted Diseases*, ACOG Education Pamphlet AP009 (Washington, DC: American College of Obstetricians and Gynecologists, September 2013), Available at www.acog.org; American Social Health Association, "Sexual Health: Reduce Your Risk," 2014, www.ashastd.org.

check yourself

- **How are STIs transmitted?**
- **What can you do to protect yourself against STIs?**

12.10 Sexually Transmitted Infections: HIV/AIDS

learning outcome

12.10 Define HIV/AIDS and explain its transmittal and treatment.

Acquired immunodeficiency syndrome (AIDS) is a significant global health threat. Since 1981, when AIDS was first recognized, approximately 75 million people worldwide have become infected with **human immunodeficiency virus (HIV)**, the virus that causes AIDS. About 35.3 million people worldwide are living with HIV.[52] In the United States, there are over 1 million people infected with HIV. About 15,000 people die from HIV/AIDS each year.[53]

Initially, people were diagnosed as having AIDS only when they developed blood infections, the cancer known as Kaposi's sarcoma, or other indicator diseases common in male AIDS patients. The Centers for Disease Control and Prevention (CDC) has expanded the indicator list to include pulmonary tuberculosis, recurrent pneumonia, and invasive cervical cancer. Perhaps the most significant indicator today is a drop in the level of the body's master immune cells, CD4 cells (also called helper T cells), to one-fifth the level in a healthy person.

How HIV Is Transmitted

HIV typically enters one person's body via another person's infected body fluids (e.g., semen, vaginal secretions, blood), often through a break in the mucous membranes of the genital organs or the anus. After initial infection, HIV multiplies rapidly, progressively destroying helper T cells (which call the rest of the immune response to action), weakening the body's resistance to disease.

HIV cannot reproduce outside its living host, except in a controlled laboratory environment, and does not survive well in open air. It cannot be transmitted through casual contact.[54] Insect bites do not transmit HIV.[55]

High-Risk Behaviors AIDS is not a disease of gay people or minority groups; rather, it is related to high-risk behaviors such as having unprotected sexual intercourse and sharing needles. People who engage in high-risk behaviors increase their risk for the disease; people who do not have minimal risk. Figure 12.6 shows the breakdown of sources of HIV infection among U.S. men and women.

The majority of HIV infections arise from the following high-risk behaviors:

- **Exchange of body fluids.** The greatest risk factor is the exchange of HIV-infected body fluids during vaginal or anal intercourse. Blood, semen, and vaginal secretions are the major fluids of concern.
- **Injecting drugs.** A significant percentage of AIDS cases in the United States result from sharing or using HIV-contaminated needles and syringes. Although users of illegal drugs are commonly considered the only members of this category, others may also share needles—for example, people with diabetes who inject insulin or athletes who inject steroids.

Mother-to-Child (Perinatal) Transmission This can occur during pregnancy, during labor and delivery, or through breast-feeding. Without antiretroviral treatment, approximately 15 to 45 percent of HIV-positive pregnant women will transmit the virus to their infant.[56]

Body Piercing and Tattooing Body piercing and tattooing can be done safely, but dangerous pathogens can be transmitted with any puncture of the skin. Unsterile needles can transmit staph, HIV, hepatitis B and C, tetanus, and other diseases. If you opt for tattooing or body piercing, take the following safety precautions:[57]

- Look for clean, well-lighted work areas and inquire about sterilization procedures.
- Packaged, sterilized needles should be used once, then discarded. A piercing gun cannot be sterilized properly. Watch that the artist uses new needles and tubes from a sterile package.
- Immediately before piercing or tattooing, the body area should be carefully sterilized. The artist should wash his or her hands and put on new latex gloves for each procedure.
- Leftover tattoo ink should be discarded after each procedure. Do not allow the artist to reuse ink that has been used for other customers. Used needles should be disposed of in a "sharps" container.

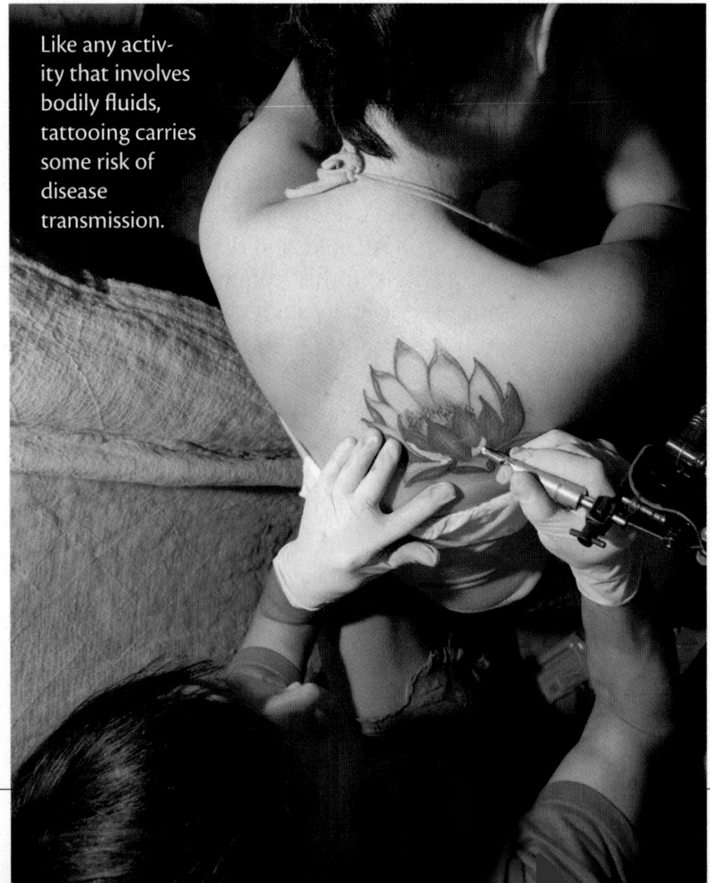

Like any activity that involves bodily fluids, tattooing carries some risk of disease transmission.

Symptoms of HIV/AIDS

A person may go for months or years after infection by HIV before any significant symptoms appear; incubation time varies greatly from person to person. For adults who receive no medical treatment, it takes an average of 8 to 10 years for the virus to cause the slow, degenerative changes in the immune system that are characteristic of AIDS. During this time, the person may experience *opportunistic infections* (infections that gain a foothold when the immune system is not functioning effectively). Colds, sore throats, fever, tiredness, nausea, and night sweats commonly appear. Later symptoms include wasting syndrome, swollen lymph nodes, and neurological problems. As the immune system continues to decline, the body becomes more vulnerable to infection. A diagnosis of AIDS, the final stage of HIV infection, is made when the infected person has either a dangerously low CD4 (helper T) cell count (below 200 cells per cubic milliliter of blood) or has contracted one or more opportunistic infections characteristic of the disease (such as Kaposi's sarcoma or *Pneumocystis carinii* pneumonia).

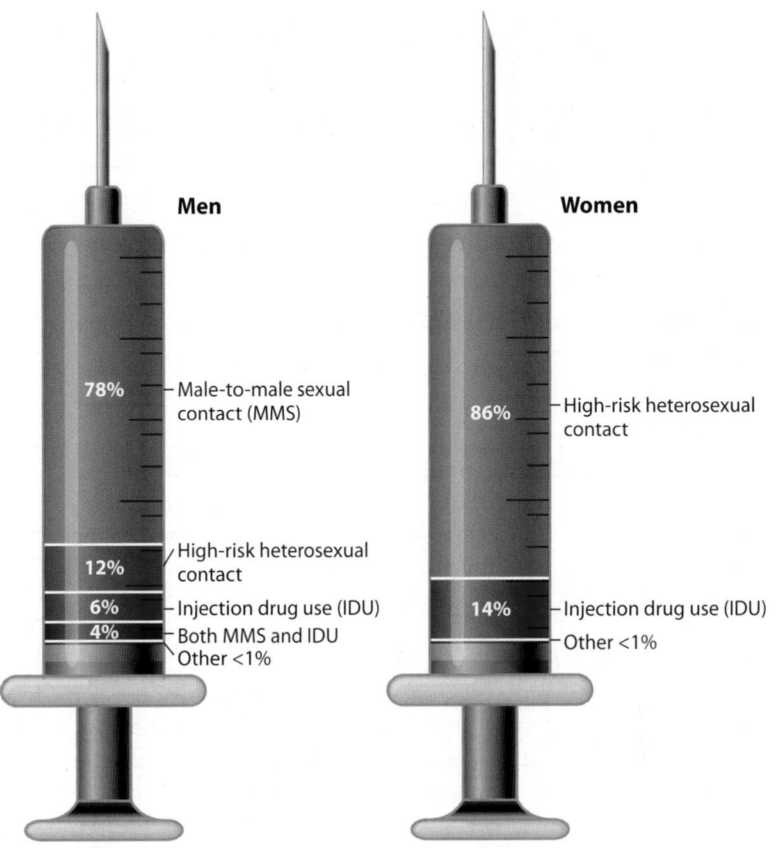

Figure 12.6 Sources of HIV Infection in Men and Women in the United States, 2011

Source: Centers for Disease Control and Prevention, *HIV Surveillance: Epidemiology of HIV Infection (through 2011)*, Updated 2013, www.cdc.gov.

Testing for HIV Antibodies

Once antibodies have formed in reaction to HIV, a blood test known as the *ELISA* (enzyme-linked immunosorbent assay) may detect their presence. It can take 3 to 6 months after initial infection for sufficient antibodies to develop in the body to show a positive test result. Therefore, individuals with negative test results should be retested within 6 months. When a person who previously tested *negative* (no HIV antibodies present) has a subsequent test that is *positive*, seroconversion is said to have occurred. In such a situation, the person would typically take another ELISA test, followed by a more precise test known as the *Western blot*. These are not AIDS tests per se. Rather, they detect antibodies for HIV, indicating the presence of the virus in the person's system.

Health officials distinguish between *reported* and *actual* cases of HIV infection because it is believed that many HIV-positive people avoid being tested. One reason is fear of knowing the truth. Another is the fear of recrimination from employers, insurance companies, and medical staff. However, early detection and reporting are important, because immediate treatment for someone in the early stages of HIV disease is critical.

Treatments and Prevention

New drugs have slowed the progression from HIV to AIDS and prolonged life expectancies for most AIDS patients. Increasing evidence indicates that treating HIV-positive babies within a few hours of birth can dramatically restrict—and perhaps eliminate—infection. A clinical trial is being conducted to study this treatment and to further investigate implications.[58] Antiretroviral therapy (ART), the current treatment method, combines selected drugs, especially protease inhibitors and reverse transcriptase inhibitors. *Protease inhibitors* (e.g., amprenavir, ritonavir, and saquinavir) act to prevent production of the virus in cells HIV has already invaded. Other drugs, such as AZT, ddl, ddC, d4T, and 3TC, inhibit the HIV enzyme *reverse transcriptase* before the virus has invaded the cell, thereby preventing infection of new cells.

Although these drugs provide longer survival rates for people with HIV, we are still a long way from a cure. Newer drugs that held promise are becoming less effective as HIV develops resistance to them. Costs of taking multiple drugs are prohibitive, and side effects are common.

Although scientists have been working on a variety of HIV vaccine trials, no vaccine is currently available. The only way to prevent HIV infection is through the choices you make in sexual behaviors and drug use and by taking responsibility for your own health and the health of your loved ones. So what should you do?

Of course, the simplest answer is abstinence. If you don't exchange body fluids, you won't get the disease. If you do decide to be intimate, the next best option is to use a condom.

check yourself

- **What are three common routes of transmission for HIV?**
- **What can you do to prevent the spread of HIV and to protect yourself against it?**

12.11 Sexually Transmitted Infections: Chlamydia and Gonorrhea

learning outcome

12.11 List the symptoms and treatment of chlamydia and gonorrhea.

Two of the most common sexually transmitted infections are chlamydia and gonorrhea.

Chlamydia

Chlamydia, an infection caused by the bacterium *Chlamydia trachomatis* that often presents no symptoms, is the most commonly reported STI in the United States. Chlamydia infects an estimated 2.8 million Americans annually, the majority of them women.[59] This estimate could be higher, because many cases go unreported.

Signs and Symptoms In men, early symptoms may include painful and difficult urination; frequent urination; and a watery, pus-like discharge from the penis. Symptoms in women may include a yellowish discharge, spotting between periods, and occasional spotting after intercourse. However, many chlamydia victims display no symptoms and therefore do not seek help until the disease has done secondary damage. Women are especially likely to be asymptomatic; many do not realize they have the disease, which can put them at risk for secondary damage.

Complications Men can suffer injury to the prostate gland, seminal vesicles, and bulbourethral glands, and they can suffer from arthritis-like symptoms and inflammatory damage to the blood vessels and heart. Men can also experience *epididymitis*, inflammation of the area near the testicles.

In women, chlamydia-related inflammation can injure the cervix or fallopian tubes, causing sterility, and it can damage the inner pelvic structure, leading to **pelvic inflammatory disease (PID)**. If an infected woman becomes pregnant, she has a high risk for miscarriage and stillbirth. Chlamydia may also be responsible for one type of *conjunctivitis*, an eye infection that affects not only adults but also infants, who can contract the disease from an infected mother during delivery (Figure 12.7). Untreated conjunctivitis can cause blindness.[60]

Women with chlamydia are also at greater risk for **urinary tract infections (UTIs)**. A woman's urethra is much shorter than a man's, making it easier for bacteria to enter the bladder. In addition, a woman's urethra is closer to her anus than is a man's, allowing bacteria to spread into her urethra and cause an infection. Symptoms of a UTI in women include a burning sensation during urination and lower abdominal pain. A UTI can be diagnosed through a urine test and treated by antibiotics.

Men can also get UTIs, although they are rarer. One form most commonly caused by *Chlamydia trachomatis* is *nongonococcal urethritis*. Infections should be taken seriously—if you have a milky penile discharge and/or burning during urination, contact your health care provider.[61]

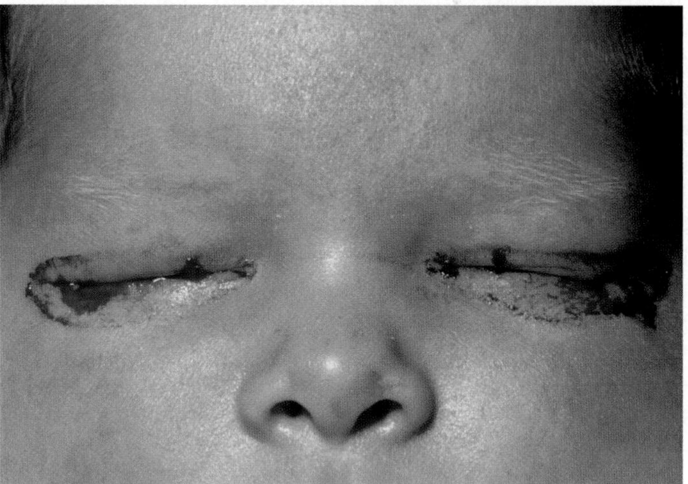

Figure 12.7 Conjunctivitis in a Newborn's Eyes
Untreated chlamydia and gonorrhea in a pregnant woman can be passed to her child during delivery, causing the eye infection conjunctivitis.

Diagnosis and Treatment A sample of urine or fluid from the vagina or penis is collected to identify the presence of the bacteria. Unfortunately, chlamydia tests are not a routine part of many health clinics' testing procedures. If detected early, chlamydia is easily treatable with antibiotics such as tetracycline, doxycycline, or erythromycin.

Gonorrhea

Gonorrhea is one of the most common STIs in the United States, surpassed only by chlamydia in number of cases. The CDC estimates that there are over 820,000 cases per year, plus many more cases that go unreported.[62] Caused by the bacterial pathogen *Neisseria gonorrhoeae*, gonorrhea primarily infects the linings of the urethra, genital tract, pharynx, and rectum. It may spread to the eyes or other body regions by the hands or through body fluids, typically during vaginal, oral, or anal sex. Most cases occur in individuals between the ages of 15 and 24.[63]

Signs and Symptoms In men, a typical symptom is a white, milky discharge from the penis accompanied by painful, burning urination 2 to 9 days after contact (Figure 12.8). Epididymitis can also occur as a symptom of infection. However, some men with gonorrhea are asymptomatic.

In women, the situation is just the opposite: Most women do not experience any symptoms, but if a woman does experience symptoms, they can include vaginal discharge or a burning sensation on urinating.[64] The organism can remain in the woman's vagina, cervix, uterus, or fallopian tubes for long periods with no apparent symptoms other than an occasional slight fever. Thus a woman can be unaware that she has been infected and that she is infecting her sexual partners.

Complications In a man, untreated gonorrhea may spread to the prostate, testicles, urinary tract, kidney, and bladder. Blockage of the vasa deferentia due to scar tissue may cause sterility. In some cases, the penis develops a painful curvature during erection. If the infection goes undetected in a woman, it can spread to the fallopian tubes and ovaries, causing sterility or, at the very least, severe inflammation and PID. The bacteria can also spread up the reproductive tract or, more rarely, through the blood and infect the joints, heart valves, or brain. If an infected woman becomes pregnant, the infection can be transmitted to her baby during delivery, potentially causing blindness, joint infection, or a life-threatening blood infection.

Diagnosis and Treatment Diagnosis of gonorrhea is similar to that of chlamydia, requiring a sample of either urine or fluid from the vagina or penis to detect the presence of the bacteria. If detected early, gonorrhea is treatable with antibiotics, but the *Neisseria gonorrhoeae* bacterium has begun to develop resistance to some antibiotics. Chlamydia and gonorrhea often occur at the same time, though different antibiotics are needed to treat each infection separately.[65]

Complications of STIs: PID in Women, Epididymitis in Men

If left untreated, many STIs can lead to serious complications for both men and women. Pelvic inflammatory disease (PID) can be caused by *Neisseria gonorrhoeae* or *Chlamydia trachomatis*. Pelvic inflammatory disease is a catchall term for a number of infections of the uterus, fallopian tubes, and ovaries that are complications resulting from an untreated STI.

Symptoms of PID vary but generally include lower abdominal pain, fever, unusual vaginal discharge, painful intercourse, painful urination, and irregular menstrual bleeding. The vague symptoms associated with chlamydial and gonococcal PID can cause a delay seeking medical care, thereby increasing the risk of permanent damage and scarring that can lead to infertility and other complications. In the United States, approximately 1 million women develop PID every year. It is estimated that 1 in 8 sexually active adolescent girls will develop PID before the age of 20.[66]

Epididymitis is swelling (inflammation) of the epididymis, and it is most common among young men ages 19 to 35.[67] Epididymitis is most commonly caused by the spread of *Neisseria gonorrhoeae* or *Chlamydia trachomatis* from the urethra or the bladder. Symptoms can include blood in the semen, swollen groin area, discharge from the urethra, discomfort in the lower abdomen or pelvis, and pain during ejaculation or during urination. A physical examination along with other medical tests, including a testicular scan and tests for chlamydia and gonorrhea, can diagnose the condition. Treatment usually involves pain medications and anti-inflammatory medications.

The serious complications that can result from untreated STIs further illustrate the need for early diagnosis and treatment. Regular screening and testing is particularly important because many STIs are often asymptomatic, increasing the risk of complications such as PID and epididymitis.

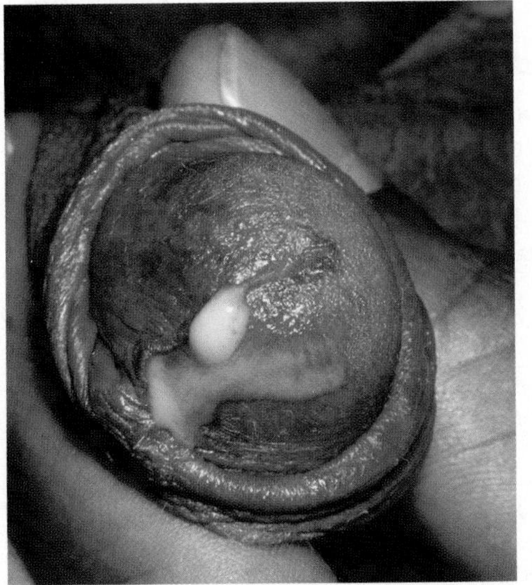

Figure 12.8 Gonorrhea
One common symptom of gonorrhea in men is a milky discharge from the penis, accompanied by burning sensations during urination. Whereas these symptoms will cause most men to seek diagnosis and treatment, women with gonorrhea are often asymptomatic, so they may not be aware they are infected.

Skills for Behavior Change

COMMUNICATING ABOUT SAFER SEX

At no time in your life is it more important to communicate openly than when you are starting an intimate relationship. The following will help you communicate with your partner about potential risks:

- **Plan to talk before you find yourself in an awkward situation.**
- **Select the right moment and place for both of you to discuss safer sex; choose a relaxing environment in a neutral location, free of distractions.**
- **Remember that you have a responsibility to your partner to disclose your own health status. You also have a responsibility to yourself to stay healthy.**
- **Be direct, honest, and determined in talking about sex before you become involved.**
- **Discuss the issues without sounding defensive or accusatory. Reassure your partner that your reasons for desiring abstinence or safer sex arise from respect and not distrust.**
- **Analyze your own beliefs and values ahead of time. Know where you will draw the line on certain actions, and be very clear with your partner about what you expect.**
- **Decide what you will do if your partner does not agree with you. Anticipate potential objections or excuses, and prepare your responses accordingly.**

Source: Adapted from Queensland Health, "Talking to Your Partner about Sex," 2010, www.health.qld.gov.au.

check yourself

- **What are the primary signs of chlamydia? Of gonorrhea?**
- **How does PID affect women? How does epididymitis affect men?**

12.12 Sexually Transmitted Infections: Syphilis

learning outcome

12.12 List the symptoms and treatment of syphilis in men and women.

Syphilis is caused by a bacterium, the spirochete *Treponema pallidum*. The incidence of syphilis is highest in adults aged 20 to 39, and it is particularly high among African Americans and men who have sex with men. Because it is extremely delicate and dies readily on exposure to air, dryness, or cold, the organism is generally transferred only through direct sexual contact or from mother to fetus. The incidence of syphilis in newborns has continued to increase in the United States.[68]

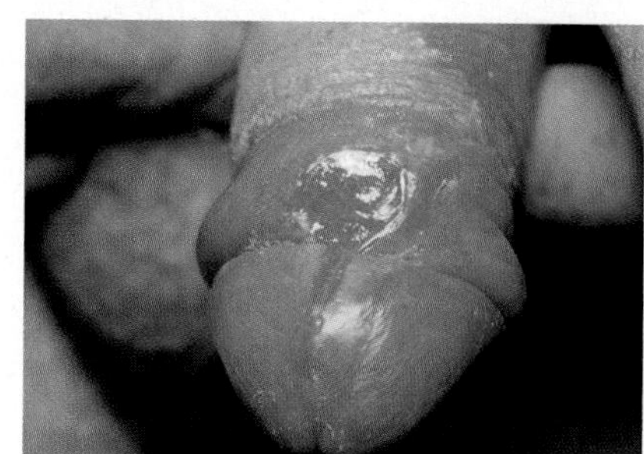

Figure 12.9 Syphilis A chancre on the site of the initial infection is a symptom of primary syphilis.

Signs and Symptoms

Syphilis is known as the "great imitator," because its symptoms resemble those of several other infections. It should be noted, however, that some people experience no symptoms at all. Syphilis can occur in four distinct stages:[69]

- **Primary syphilis.** The first stage of syphilis, particularly for men, is often characterized by the development of a **chancre** (pronounced "shank-er"), a sore located most frequently at the site of initial infection that usually appears 3 to 4 weeks after initial infection (see Figure 12.9). In men, the site of the chancre tends to be the penis or scrotum; in women, the site of infection is often internal, on the vaginal wall or high on the cervix, where the chancre is not readily apparent and the likelihood of detection is not great. Whether or not it is detected, the chancre is oozing with bacteria, ready to infect an unsuspecting partner. In both men and women, the chancre will disappear in 3 to 6 weeks.
- **Secondary syphilis.** If the infection is left untreated, a month to a year after the chancre disappears secondary symptoms may appear, including a rash or white patches on the skin or on the mucous membranes of the mouth, throat, or genitals. Hair loss may occur, lymph nodes may enlarge, and the victim may develop a slight fever or headache. In rare cases, sores develop around the mouth or genitals. As during the active chancre phase, these sores contain infectious bacteria, and contact with them can spread the infection.
- **Latent syphilis.** After the secondary stage, if the infection is left untreated, the syphilis spirochetes begin to invade body organs, causing lesions called *gummas*. The infection now is rarely transmitted to others, except during pregnancy, when it can be passed to the fetus.
- **Tertiary/late syphilis.** Years after syphilis has entered the body, its effects become all too evident if still untreated. Late-stage syphilis indications include heart and central nervous system damage, blindness, deafness, paralysis, premature senility, and, ultimately, dementia.

Complications

Pregnant women with syphilis can experience complications such as premature births, miscarriages, and stillbirths. An infected pregnant woman may transmit the syphilis to her unborn child. The infant will then be born with *congenital syphilis*, which can cause death; severe birth defects such as blindness, deafness, or disfigurement; developmental delays; seizures; and other health problems. Because in most cases the fetus does not become infected until after the first trimester, treatment of the mother during this time will usually prevent infection of the fetus.

Diagnosis and Treatment

Two methods can be used to diagnose syphilis. In the primary stage, a sample from the chancre is collected to identify the bacteria. Another method of diagnosing syphilis is through a blood test. Syphilis can easily be treated with antibiotics, usually penicillin, for all stages except the late stage.

check yourself

- **What are the four stages of untreated syphilis?**
- **How is syphilis diagnosed and treated?**

Sexually Transmitted Infections: Herpes

learning outcome

12.13 List the symptoms and treatment of both types of herpes simplex virus.

Herpes is a general term for a family of infections characterized by sores or eruptions on the skin that are caused by the herpes simplex virus. The herpes family of diseases is not transmitted exclusively by sexual contact; kissing or sharing eating utensils can also transmit the infection.

Herpes infections range from mildly uncomfortable to extremely serious. **Genital herpes** affects approximately 16.2 percent of the population aged 14 to 49 in the United States.[70]

The two types of herpes simplex virus are HSV-1 and HSV-2. Only about 1 in 6 Americans currently has HSV-2; however, about half of adults have HSV-1, usually appearing as cold sores on the mouth.[71] Both herpes simplex types 1 and 2 can infect any area of the body, producing lesions (sores) in and around the vaginal area; on the penis; and around the anal opening, buttocks, thighs, or mouth (see Figure 12.10). Herpes simplex virus remains in nerve cells for life and can flare up when the body's ability to maintain itself is weakened.

People may get genital herpes by having sexual contact with others who don't know they are infected or who are having outbreaks of herpes without any sores. A person with genital herpes can also infect a sexual partner during oral sex. The virus is spread rarely, if at all, by touching objects such as a toilet seat.

Signs and Symptoms

The precursor phase of a herpes infection is characterized by a burning sensation and redness at the site of infection. This phase is quickly followed by the second phase, in which a blister filled with a clear fluid containing the virus forms. If you pick at this blister or otherwise spread this fluid with fingers, lipstick, etc., you can autoinoculate other body parts. Particularly dangerous is the possibility of spreading the infection to your eyes, which can cause blindness.

Over a period of days, the blister will crust over, dry up, and disappear, and the virus will travel to the base of an affected nerve supplying the area and become dormant. Only when the victim becomes overly stressed, when diet and sleep are inadequate, when the immune system is overworked, or when excessive exposure to sunlight or other stressors occur will the virus become reactivated (at the same site) and begin the blistering cycle again. Each time a sore develops, it casts off (sheds) viruses that can be highly infectious. However, a herpes site also can shed the virus when no overt sore is present, particularly during the interval between the earliest symptoms and blistering.

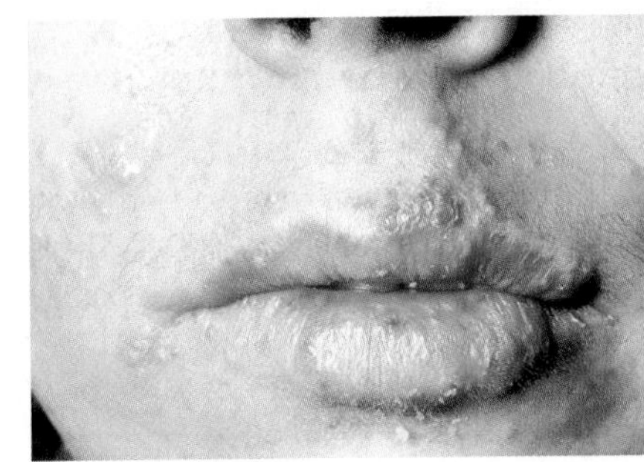

Figure 12.10
Herpes
Both genital and oral herpes can be caused by either herpes simplex virus type 1 or 2.

Complications

Genital herpes is especially serious in pregnant women because the baby can be infected as it passes through the vagina during birth. Many physicians recommend cesarean deliveries for infected women. Additionally, women with a history of genital herpes appear to have a greater risk of developing cervical cancer.

Diagnosis and Treatment

Diagnosis involves a blood test or analyzing a sample from the suspected sore. Although there is no cure for herpes at present, certain drugs can be used to treat symptoms. During the precursor phase, prescription medicines such as acyclovir and over-the-counter medications such as Abreva will often keep the disease from spreading. However, most drugs only seem to work if the infection is confirmed during the first few hours after contact. The effectiveness of other treatments, such as L-lysine, is largely unsubstantiated. Over-the-counter medications may reduce the length of time of sores/symptoms. Other drugs, such as famciclovir (FAMVIR), may reduce viral shedding between outbreaks, possibly reducing risks to sexual partners.[72]

check yourself

- **What are the primary signs of and treatments for herpes?**

12.14 Sexually Transmitted Infections: Human Papillomavirus

learning outcome

12.14 List the various problems caused by human papillomavirus.

Genital warts (*venereal warts* or *condylomas*) are caused by a group of viruses known as **human papillomavirus (HPV)**. There are over 100 different types of HPV; more than 40 types are sexually transmitted and classified as either low risk or high risk.

A person becomes infected when certain types of HPV penetrate the skin and mucous membranes of the genitals or anus. This is among the most common STIs, with 79 million Americans currently infected with genital HPV and approximately 14 million new cases each year.[73]

Signs and Symptoms

Genital HPV appears relatively easy to catch. The typical incubation period is 6 to 8 weeks after contact. People infected with low-risk HPV may develop genital warts, a series of bumps or growths on the genitals (see Figure 12.11).

Complications

Infection with high-risk types of HPV may lead to cervical *dysplasia*, or changes in cells that may lead to a precancerous condition. Exactly how high-risk HPV infection leads to cervical cancer is uncertain. It is known that a Pap test done as routine screening for women aged 21 to 65 years old can help prevent cervical cancer.[74] High-risk types of HPV (16 and 18) are responsible for an estimated 70 percent of cervical cancer cases.[75] In addition, HPV may pose a threat to a fetus exposed to the virus during birth.

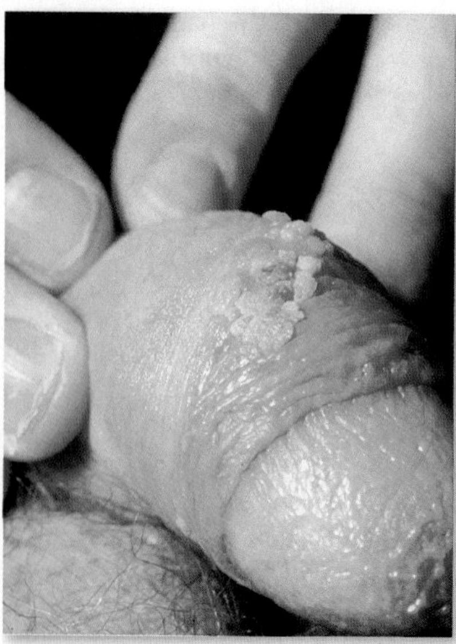

Figure 12.11 Genital Warts
Genital warts are caused by certain types of the human papillomavirus.

Diagnosis and Treatment

Diagnosis of genital warts from low-risk types of HPV is determined through visual examination by a health care provider. High-risk types can be diagnosed in women through microscopic analysis of cells from a Pap smear or by collecting a sample from the cervix to test for HPV DNA. There is currently no HPV DNA test for men.

Treatment is available only for the low-risk forms of HPV that cause genital warts. The warts can be treated with topical medication or frozen with liquid nitrogen and then removed. Large warts may require surgical removal.

HPV Vaccines

Most sexually active people will contract some form of human papillomavirus (HPV) at some time in their lives, though they may never know it. Of the approximately 40 types of sexually transmitted HPV, most cause no symptoms and go away on their own. As discussed previously, low-risk types can cause genital warts, but some high-risk types can cause cervical cancer in women and other less common genital cancers. Currently, two HPV vaccines, Cervarix and Gardasil, can help prevent women from becoming infected with HPV and subsequently developing cervical cancer.

HPV vaccines are recommended for 11- and 12-year-old girls and can also be given to girls 9 or older. It is also recommended for girls and women aged 13 through 26 who have not yet been vaccinated or completed the vaccine series. One of the HPV vaccines, Gardasil, is also licensed for males aged 9 through 26. Only Gardasil protects against low-risk HPV types 6 and 11; because these HPV types cause 90 percent of cases of genital warts in females and males, Gardasil is approved for use with males as well as females.[76]

Note that the vaccines do not protect against all types of HPV, so about 30 percent of cervical cancers will not be prevented by the vaccines.[77] Women should continue getting screened for cervical cancer through regular Pap tests. Also, the vaccines do not prevent other STIs, so it is still important for sexually active persons to lower their risk for other STIs.

check yourself

- **How can women guard themselves against HPV-linked cervical cancer?**

Other Sexually Transmitted Infections

learning outcome

12.15 List the symptoms and treatment of other common STIs.

Several other sexually transmitted infections have less serious effects than infections such as HIV and syphilis, but nevertheless should be avoided.

Candidiasis (Moniliasis)

Most STIs are caused by pathogens that come from outside the body; however, the yeast-like fungus *Candida albicans* is a normal inhabitant of the vaginal tract in most women. (See Figure 12.3 for a micrograph of this fungus.) Only when the normal chemical balance of the vagina is disturbed will these organisms multiply and cause the fungal disease **candidiasis**, also sometimes called *moniliasis* or a *yeast infection*.

Signs and Symptoms Symptoms of candidiasis include severe itching and burning of the vagina and vulva and a white, cheesy vaginal discharge.[78] When this microbe infects the mouth, whitish patches form, and the condition is referred to as *thrush*. Thrush infection can also occur in men and is easily transmitted between sexual partners. Symptoms of candidiasis can be aggravated by contact with soaps, douches, perfumed toilet paper, chlorinated water, and spermicides.

Diagnosis and Treatment Diagnosis of candidiasis is usually made by collecting a vaginal sample and analyzing it to identify the pathogen. Antifungal drugs applied on the surface or by suppository usually cure candidiasis in just a few days.

Trichomoniasis

Unlike many STIs, **trichomoniasis** is caused by a protozoan, *Trichomonas vaginalis*. (See Figure 12.3 for a micrograph of this organism.) An estimated 3.7 million Americans have the infection, but only about one-third of those who contract it experience symptoms.[79] Although usually transmitted by sexual contact, the "trich" organism can also be spread by toilet seats, wet towels, or other items that have discharged fluids on them.

Signs and Symptoms Symptoms among women include a foamy, yellowish, unpleasant-smelling discharge accompanied by a burning sensation, itching, and painful urination. Most men with trichomoniasis do not have any symptoms, though some men experience irritation inside the penis, mild discharge, and a slight burning after urinating.[80]

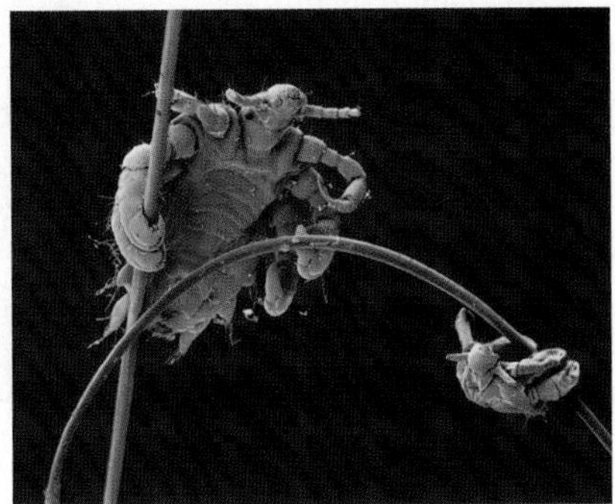

Figure 12.12 Pubic Lice Pubic lice, also known as "crabs," are small, parasitic insects that attach themselves to pubic hair.

Diagnosis and Treatment Diagnosis of trichomoniasis is determined by collecting fluid samples from the penis or vagina to test for the presence of the protozoan. Treatment includes oral metronidazole, usually given to both sexual partners to avoid the possible "ping-pong" effect of repeated cross-infection typical of STIs.

Pubic Lice

Pubic lice, often called "crabs," are small parasitic insects that are usually transmitted during sexual contact (see Figure 12.12). More annoying than dangerous, they move easily from partner to partner during sex. They have an affinity for pubic hair and attach themselves to the base of these hairs, where they deposit their eggs (nits). One to 2 weeks later, the nits develop into adults that lay eggs and migrate to other body parts, thus perpetuating the cycle. Although sexual contact is the most common mode of transmission, you can "catch" pubic lice from lying on sheets or sitting on a toilet seat that an infected person has used.

Signs and Symptoms Symptoms of pubic lice infestation include itchiness in the area covered by pubic hair, bluish-gray skin color in the pubic region, and sores in the genital area.

Diagnosis and Treatment Diagnosis of pubic lice involves an examination by a health care provider to identify the eggs in the genital area. Treatment includes washing clothing, furniture, and linens that may harbor the eggs. It usually takes 2 to 3 weeks to kill all larval forms.

check yourself

- **Describe symptoms and treatment of candidiasis and trichomoniasis.**
- **How are pubic lice transmitted and treated?**

Assess yourself

12.16

STIs: Do You Really Know What You Think You Know?

The following quiz will help you evaluate whether your beliefs and attitudes about sexually transmitted infections (STIs) lead you to behaviors that increase your risk of infection. Indicate whether you believe the following items are true or false, then consult the answer key that follows.

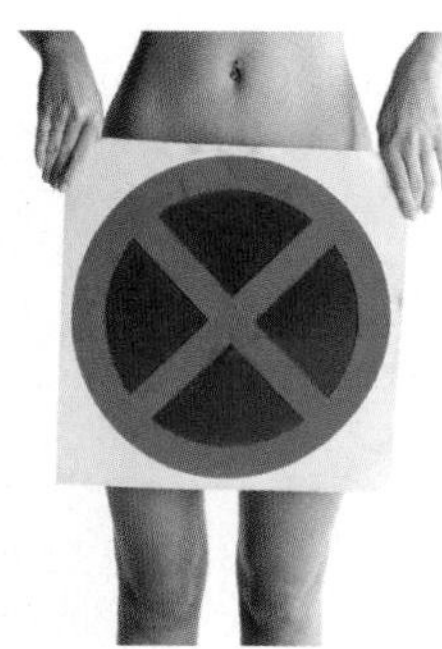

An interactive version of this assessment is available online in MasteringHealth.

	True	False
1. You can always tell when you've got an STI because the symptoms are so obvious.	◯	◯
2. Some STIs can be passed on by skin-to-skin contact in the genital area.	◯	◯
3. Herpes can be transmitted only when a person has visible sores on his or her genitals.	◯	◯
4. Oral sex is safe sex.	◯	◯
5. Condoms reduce your risk of both pregnancy and STIs.	◯	◯
6. As long as you don't have anal intercourse, you can't get HIV.	◯	◯
7. All sexually active females should have a regular Pap smear.	◯	◯
8. Once genital warts have been removed, there is no risk of passing on the virus.	◯	◯
9. You can get several STIs at one time.	◯	◯
10. If the signs of an STI go away, you are cured.	◯	◯
11. People who get STIs have a lot of sex partners.	◯	◯
12. All STIs can be cured.	◯	◯
13. You can get an STI *more than once.*	◯	◯

Answer Key

1. **False.** The unfortunate fact is that many STIs show no symptoms. This has serious implications: (a) you can be passing on the infection without knowing it and (b) the pathogen may be damaging your reproductive organs without you knowing it.
2. **True.** Some viruses can be present on the skin around the genital area. Herpes and genital warts are the main culprits.
3. **False.** Herpes is most easily passed on when the sores and blisters are present, because the fluid in the lesions carries the virus. But the virus is also found on the skin around the genital area. Most people contract herpes this way, unaware that the virus is present.

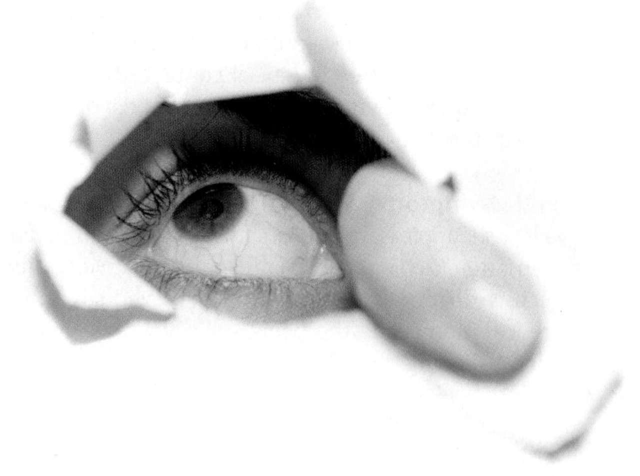

4. **False.** Oral sex is not safe sex. Herpes, genital warts, and chlamydia can all be passed on through oral sex. Condoms should be used on the penis. Dental dams should be placed over the female genitals during oral sex.
5. **True.** Condoms significantly reduce the risk of pregnancy when used correctly. They also reduce the risk of STIs. It is important to point out that abstinence is the only behavior that provides complete protection against pregnancy and STIs.
6. **False.** HIV is present in blood, semen, and vaginal fluid. Any activity that allows for the transfer of these fluids is risky. Anal intercourse is a high-risk activity, especially for the receptive (passive) partner, but other sexual activity is also a risk. When you don't know your partner's sexual history and you're not in a long-term monogamous relationship, condoms are a must.
7. **True.** A Pap smear is a simple procedure involving the scraping of a small amount of tissue from the surface of the cervix (at the upper end of the vagina). The sample is tested for abnormal cells that may indicate cancer. All sexually active women should have regular Pap smears.

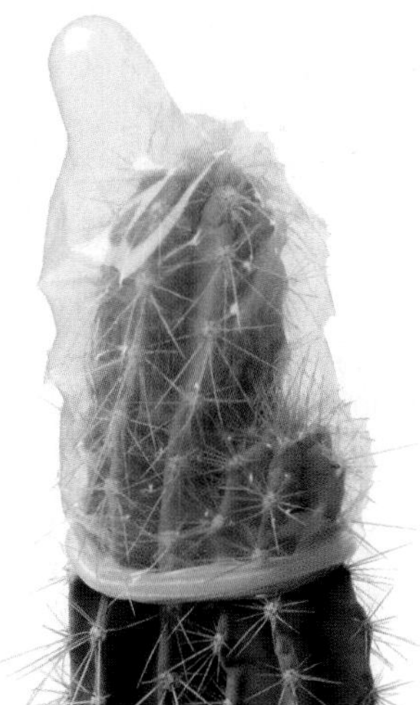

8. **False.** Genital warts, which may be present on the penis, the anus, and inside and outside the vagina, can be removed. However, the virus that caused the warts will always be present in the body and can be passed on to a sexual partner.
9. **True.** It is possible to have many STIs at one time. In fact, having one STI may make it more likely that a person will acquire more STIs. For example, the open sore from herpes creates a place where HIV can easily be transmitted.
10. **False.** The symptoms may go away, but your body is still infected. For example, syphilis is characterized by various stages. In the first stage, a painless sore called a chancre appears for about a week and then goes away.
11. **False.** If you have sex once with an infected partner, you are at risk for an STI.
12. **False.** Some STIs are viruses and therefore cannot be cured. There is no cure at present for herpes, HIV/AIDS, or genital warts. These STIs are treatable (to lessen the pain and irritation of symptoms), but not curable.
13. **True.** Experiencing one infection with an STI does not mean that you can never be infected again. A person can be reinfected many times with the same STI. This is especially true if a person does not get treated for the STI and thus keeps reinfecting his or her partner with the same STI.

Sources: Adapted from Jefferson County Public Health, "STI Quiz," Modified 2013, http://jeffco.us. Used with permission; Adapted from Family Planning Victoria, "Play Safe," Updated July 2005, www.fpv.org.au. © Family Planning Victoria. Used by permission.

Your Plan for Change

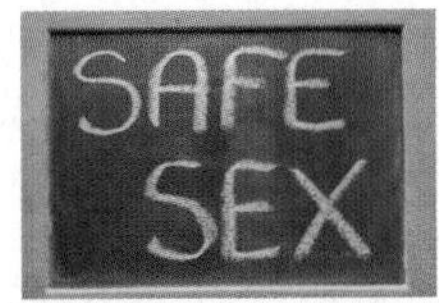

The Assess Yourself activity lets you consider your beliefs and attitudes about STIs and identify possible risks you may be facing. Now that you have considered these results, you can begin to change behaviors that may be putting you at risk for STIs and for infection in general.

Today, you can:

◯ Put together an "emergency" supply of condoms. Outside of abstinence, condoms are your best protection against an STI. If you don't have a supply on hand, visit your local drugstore or health clinic. Remember that both men and women are responsible for preventing the transmission of STIs.

◯ To prevent infections in general, get in the habit of washing your hands regularly. After you cough, sneeze, blow your nose, use the bathroom, or prepare food, find a sink, wet your hands with warm water, and lather up with soap. Scrub your hands for about 20 seconds (count to 20 or recite the alphabet), rinse well, and dry your hands.

Within the next 2 weeks, you can:

◯ Talk with your significant other honestly about your sexual history. Make appointments to get tested if either of you think you may have been exposed to an STI.

◯ Adjust your sleep schedule so that you're getting an adequate amount of rest every night. Being well rested is one key aspect of maintaining a healthy immune system.

By the end of the semester, you can:

◯ Check your immunization schedule and make sure you're current with all recommended vaccinations. Make an appointment with your health care provider if you need a booster or vaccine.

◯ If you are due for an annual pelvic exam, make an appointment. Ask your partner if he or she has had an annual exam and encourage him or her to make an appointment if not.

Summary

To hear an MP3 Tutor session, scan here or visit the Study Area in **MasteringHealth**

LO 12.1–12.2 Your body has several defense systems to keep pathogens from invading. The skin is the body's major protection. The immune system creates antibodies to destroy antigens. Fever and pain play a role in defending the body. Vaccines bolster the body's immune system against specific diseases.

LO 12.3–12.6 The major classes of pathogens are bacteria, viruses, fungi, protozoans, parasitic worms, and prions. Bacterial infections include staphylococcal infections, streptococcal infections, meningitis, pneumonia, tuberculosis, and tick-borne diseases. Major viral infections include the common cold; influenza; hepatitis; the herpes viruses, including chickenpox, shingles, and herpes gladiatorum; mumps; measles; and rubella.

LO 12.7 Emerging and resurgent diseases such as avian flu, West Nile virus, and malaria pose significant threats for future generations. Many factors contribute to these risks. Possible solutions focus on a public health approach to prevention.

LO 12.8 Many bacteria are evolving to become "superbugs" that are resistant to antibiotics. Being responsible with medications and using regular (not antibacterial) soap can prevent antibiotic resistance.

LO 12.9 Sexually transmitted infections (STIs) are spread through sexual intercourse, oral–genital contact, anal sex, hand–genital contact, and sometimes mouth-to-mouth contact.

LO 12.10 Acquired immunodeficiency syndrome (AIDS) is caused by the human immunodeficiency virus (HIV). Globally, HIV/AIDS has become a major threat to the world's population. Anyone can get HIV by engaging in high-risk sexual activities that include exchange of body fluids, by having received a blood transfusion before 1985, and by injecting drugs (or having sex with someone who does). You can reduce your risk for contracting HIV significantly by not engaging in risky sexual activities or IV drug use.

LO 12.11–12.15 STIs include chlamydia, gonorrhea, syphilis, herpes, human papillomavirus (HPV) and genital warts, candidiasis, trichomoniasis, and pubic lice. Sexual transmission may also be involved in some urinary tract infections (UTIs).

Pop Quiz

Visit MasteringHealth to personalize your study plan with Chapter Review Quizzes and Dynamic Study Modules.

LO 12.1 **1.** Jennifer touched her viral herpes sore on her lip and then touched her eye. She ended up with the herpes virus in her eye as well. This is an example of
- a. acquired immunity.
- b. passive spread.
- c. autoinoculation.
- d. self-vaccination.

LO 12.2 **2.** Which of the following do *not* assist the body in fighting disease?
- a. Antigens
- b. Antibodies
- c. Lymphocytes
- d. Macrophages

LO 12.2 **3.** An example of passive immunity is
- a. inoculation with a vaccine containing weakened antigens.
- b. when the body makes its own antibodies to a pathogen.
- c. the antibody-containing part of the vaccine that came from someone else.
- d. when lymphocytes attack and destroy a foreign invader.

LO 12.4 **4.** Which of the following is a *viral* disease?
- a. Hepatitis
- b. Pneumonia
- c. Malaria
- d. Streptococcal infection

LO 12.5 **5.** Because colds are always present to some degree throughout the world, they are said to be
- a. globally acquired.
- b. vector-borne.
- c. endemic.
- d. resistant to antibiotics.

LO 12.6 **6.** Which of the following diseases is caused by a prion?
- a. Shingles
- b. Listeria
- c. Mad cow disease
- d. Trichomoniasis

LO 12.10 **7.** Which of the following is a true statement about HIV?
- a. Drugs can provide longer survival rates for HIV.
- b. An infected mother cannot pass the virus to her baby.
- c. You can get HIV from a public restroom toilet seat.
- d. HIV symptoms usually appear immediately after initial infection.

LO 12.11 **8.** Pelvic inflammatory disease (PID) is a(n)
- a. sexually transmitted infection.
- b. type of urinary tract infection.
- c. infection of a woman's fallopian tubes or uterus.
- d. disease that both men and women can get.

LO 12.11 **9.** The most widespread sexually transmitted bacterium is
- a. gonorrhea.
- b. chlamydia.
- c. syphilis.
- d. chancroid.

LO 12.12 **10.** Which of the following STIs cannot be treated with antibiotics?
- a. Chlamydia
- b. Gonorrhea
- c. Syphilis
- d. Herpes

Answers to these questions can be found on page A-1. If you answered a question incorrectly, review the module identified by the Learning Outcome. For even more study tools, visit MasteringHealth.

13 Violence and Unintentional Injuries

The World Health Organization (WHO) defines **violence** as "the intentional use of physical force or power, threatened or actual, against oneself, another person, or against a group or community, that either results in or has a high likelihood of resulting in injury, death, psychological harm, maldevelopment or deprivation."[1] Today, most experts realize that emotional and psychological forms of violence can be as devastating as physical blows.

The U.S. Public Health Service categorizes violence resulting in injuries into either intentional injuries or unintentional injuries. **Intentional injuries**—those committed with intent to harm—typically include assaults, homicides, and self-directed injuries. **Unintentional injuries** are those committed without intent to harm. Why do we focus attention on violence and injury in an introductory health text for college and university students? The answer is simple: Violent and abusive interactions are common problems for young adults, as are unintentional—and often preventable—injuries. This chapter discusses common instances of both violence and unintentional injuries, identifying steps you can take to reduce your risk as well as strategies for managing a violent or injurious situation should one occur.

13.1 Crime Rates and Causes of Violence

learning outcome

13.1 List individual and social factors contributing to violence.

Violence has been a part of the American landscape since colonial times; however, it wasn't until the 1980s that the U.S. Public Health Service identified violence as a leading cause of death and disability and gave it chronic disease status, indicating that it was a pervasive threat to society.

Statistics from the Federal Bureau of Investigation (FBI) have shown that, after steadily increasing from 1973 to 2006, rates of overall crime and certain types of violent crime have been decreasing over the past few years (Figure 13.1).[2]

Why be so concerned about violence if the major forms of violent crime are on a downward trend? The answer is that *any* violence affects us all. Even if we have never been victimized personally, we all are victimized by violent acts that cause us to be fearful; impinge on our liberty; and damage the reputation of our campus, city, or nation.

Violence on Campus

Campus gun violence has made headline news far too many times in recent years. Whether at Virginia Tech University, where 32 people died in the deadliest mass shooting in U.S. history; at UC Santa Barbara, where 7 people were gunned down and many more injured in 2014; or at Sandy Hook Elementary, where 26 elementary school students and teachers were gunned down by a 20-year-old, campus shootings are on the rise, and no age group is immune. Today, it would be hard to find a campus without a safety plan in place to prevent and respond to this type of violent crime.

Murder
-6.9
Forcible rape
-10.6
Robbery
-1.8
Aggravated assault
-6.6
Burglary
-8.1
Larceny-theft
-4.7
Motor vehicle theft
-3.2
Arson
-15.6

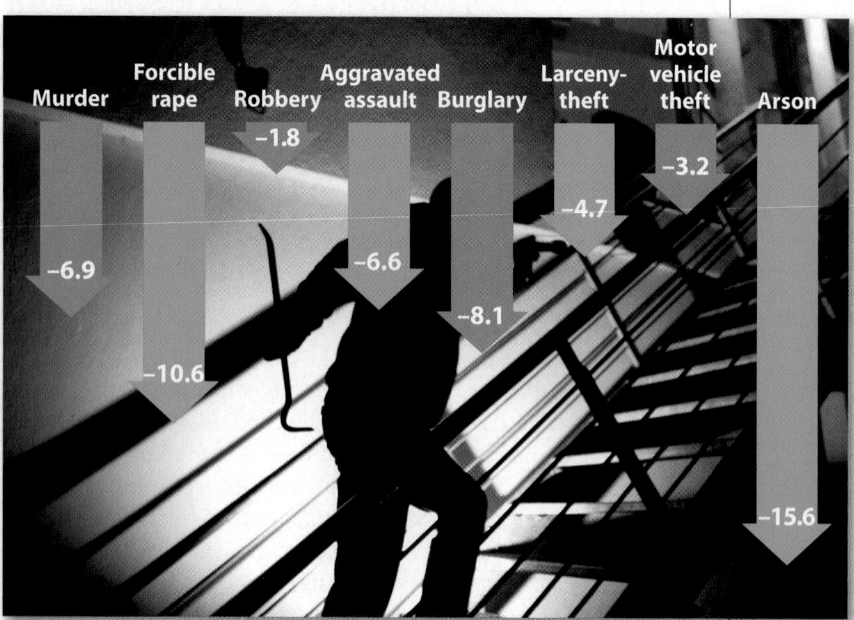

79% of crimes against college students occur at off-campus locations.

Relationship violence is one of the most prevalent problems on college campuses. In the most recent American College Health Association survey, 10.3 percent of women and 6.4 percent of men reported being emotionally abused in the past 12 months by a significant other. Almost 7 percent of women and 3.3 percent of men reported being stalked, and 2 percent of women and 1.8 percent of men reported being involved in a physically abusive relationship. Nearly 1 percent of men and over 2 percent of women reported being in a sexually abusive relationship.[3]

The statistics on reported violence on campus represent only a glimpse of the big picture. It is believed that fewer than 25 percent of campus crimes in general are reported to *any* authority.[4] Even though over 20 percent of college women will be raped or sexually assaulted before they graduate, 95 percent of them never report these crimes.[5] Why do so many never report these assaults? Typical reasons include concerns over privacy, fear of retaliation, embarrassment or shame, lack of support, perception that the crime was too minor or they were somehow at fault, or uncertainty that it was a crime.

Factors Contributing to Violence

Several factors increase the likelihood of violent acts:[6]

- **Community contexts.** Environments where interactions with unsafe neighborhoods, schools, and workplaces predominate increase risks of exposure to drugs, guns, and gangs. Inadequately staffed police and social services add to risks.[7]
- **Societal factors.** Social and cultural norms that support male dominance over women and violence as a means of settling problems increase risks.[8]

Figure 13.1 Declining Crime Rates
FBI statistics show reported violent crimes decreasing in early 2013. Although numbers of violent crimes reported to police have decreased in recent years, surveys of Americans indicate that overall violence rates have increased in the last 2 years, particularly as identity theft, burglaries, theft, simple assaults, and other crimes have increased.
Source: Data from U.S. Department of Justice, Federal Bureau of Investigation, "Crime in the United States, 2013. January to June, 2013," May 2014, www.fbi.gov.

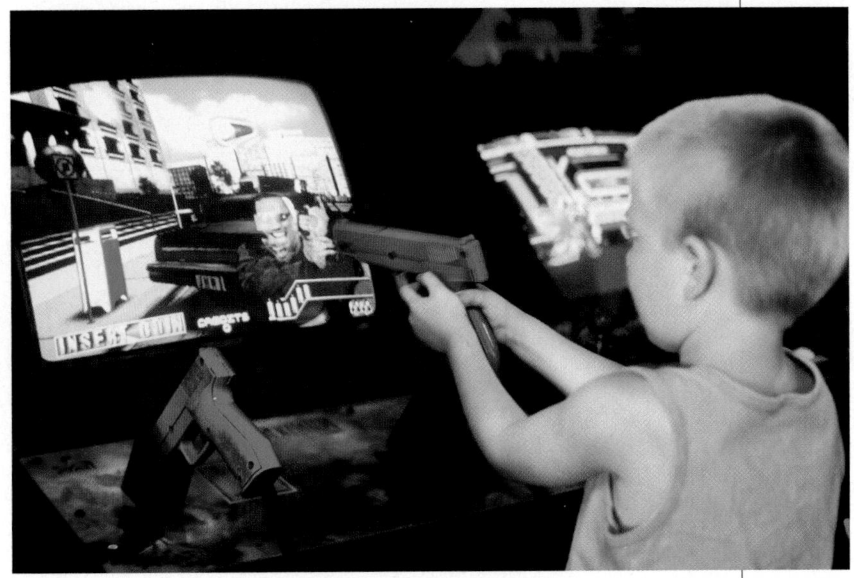

Does violence in the media cause violence in real life?

Evidence of the real-world effects of violence in the media is inconclusive. Arguably, Americans today—especially children—are exposed to more depictions of violence in the news, movies, music, and games than ever before, but research has not shown a clear link between a person's exposure to violent media and his or her propensity to engage in violent acts. Regardless, many people are concerned that children today are being exposed to more violence than they have the emotional or cognitive maturity to handle.

- **Religious beliefs and differences.** Extreme religious beliefs can lead people to think that violence against others is justified.
- **Political differences.** Civil unrest and differences in political party affiliations and beliefs have historically been triggers for violent acts.
- **Breakdowns in the criminal justice system.** Overcrowded prisons, lenient sentences, early releases, and inadequate availability of mental health services can encourage repeat offenses and future violence.
- **Stress.** People who are in crisis or under stress are more apt to be highly reactive, striking out at others, displaying anger, or acting irrationally.[9]

What Makes People Prone to Violence?

Personal factors also can increase risks for violence. The family and home environment may be the greatest contributor to eventual violent behavior among family members.[10] *Anger* tends to be an active, attack-oriented emotion in which people feel powerful and in control for a short period.[11] Anger typically occurs when there is a *triggering event*, or a person has learned that acting out in angry ways can get them what they want. Learning to assess the underlying "self talk" or the beliefs that lead to anger is an important part of prevention.

People who anger quickly often have low tolerance for frustration. The cause may be genetic or physiological; typically, however, anger-prone people come from families that are disruptive, chaotic, and unskilled in emotional expression.[12] Those who have been bullied in school may also be prone to react with violence in future situations.[13]

Aggressive behavior is often a key aspect of violent interactions. **Primary aggression** is goal-directed, hostile self-assertion that is destructive in nature. **Reactive aggression** is more often part of an emotional reaction brought about by frustration.

Substance abuse is also linked to violence.[14] Consumption of alcohol precedes over half of all violent crimes and is a major factor in domestic violence at all levels.[15] Men who are heavier drinkers are the most likely to be violent sexual perpetrators.[16] Alcohol abuse, particularly binge drinking, is associated with physical victimization among males and sexual victimization among females on campuses.[17] Additionally, numbers of suicide attempts and completions are highly correlated to drug and alcohol intake.[18]

How Much Impact Does the Media Have?

While early studies seemed to support a link between excessive exposure to violent media and subsequent violent behavior, much of this research has now been called into question.[19] Although there appears to be an association between celebrity suicide depicted in the media and subsequent increases in fan suicides, it is no stronger than the increase in suicides that occur when a peer suicide occurs.[20]

Despite evidence to the contrary, some continue to believe that viewing violent media somehow numbs people to humanity, allows people to commit violence without empathy or regret, or even triggers violent events.[21] However, critics point out that today's young people are exposed to more media violence—on the Internet and TV, and in movies and video games—than any previous generation, yet rates of violent crime among youth have fallen to 40-year lows.[22] Still, concerns have been raised about those who spend a disproportionate amount of time online instead of interacting in real-time, face-to-face communication. Debate also continues over whether viewers of media violence become desensitized to violence.

check yourself

- **What are three factors that might make a person prone to violence?**

Interpersonal Violence

learning outcome

13.2 Identify and define the various types of interpersonal violence.

Intentional injury can be categorized into three major types: *interpersonal violence, collective violence,* and *self-directed violence*—although there is some degree of overlap among these groups.[23] **Interpersonal violence** includes violence inflicted against one individual by another, or a small group of others; homicide, hate crimes, domestic violence, child abuse, elder abuse, and sexual victimization all fit into this category.

Homicide

Homicide, defined as murder or non-negligent manslaughter, is the fifteenth leading cause of death in the United States but the second leading cause of death for persons aged 15 to 24. It accounts for over 16,000 premature deaths in the United States annually, the majority of which are caused by firearms.[24] Over half of all homicides occur among people who know one another. In two-thirds of these cases, the perpetrator and the victim are friends or acquaintances; in one-third, they belong to the same family.[25]

Homicide rates reveal clear differences across races and ages. Whereas overall homicide rates in the United States have fluctuated minimally, and have even decreased in some populations, those involving young victims and perpetrators, particularly young black males, have surged. Based on the most recent data, homicide rates were nearly 52 per 100,000 for African American males aged 10 to 24, compared with almost 14 per 100,000 for Hispanic males and only 3 per 100,000 for white males.[26]

See It! Videos

What would you do if you saw someone being bullied for being gay? Watch **Teen Bullied for Being Gay** in the Study Area of MasteringHealth.

The rates of homicide in the United States are higher than in many other developed nations (Table 13.1). As Figure 13.2 shows, the number of gun-related homicides in the United States is particularly high; handguns are consistently responsible for more murders than any other single type of weapon.[27] Today, 35 percent of American homes have a gun on the premises, with nearly 300 million privately owned guns registered—and millions more that are unregistered and/or illegal. The presence of a gun in the home triples the risk of a homicide in that location and increases suicide risk more than five times.[28] However, gun-rights advocates say that the problem lies not with guns, but with the people who own them, and point to countries such as Canada, with similar numbers of guns as in the United States, but with much lower gun-related crime rates.

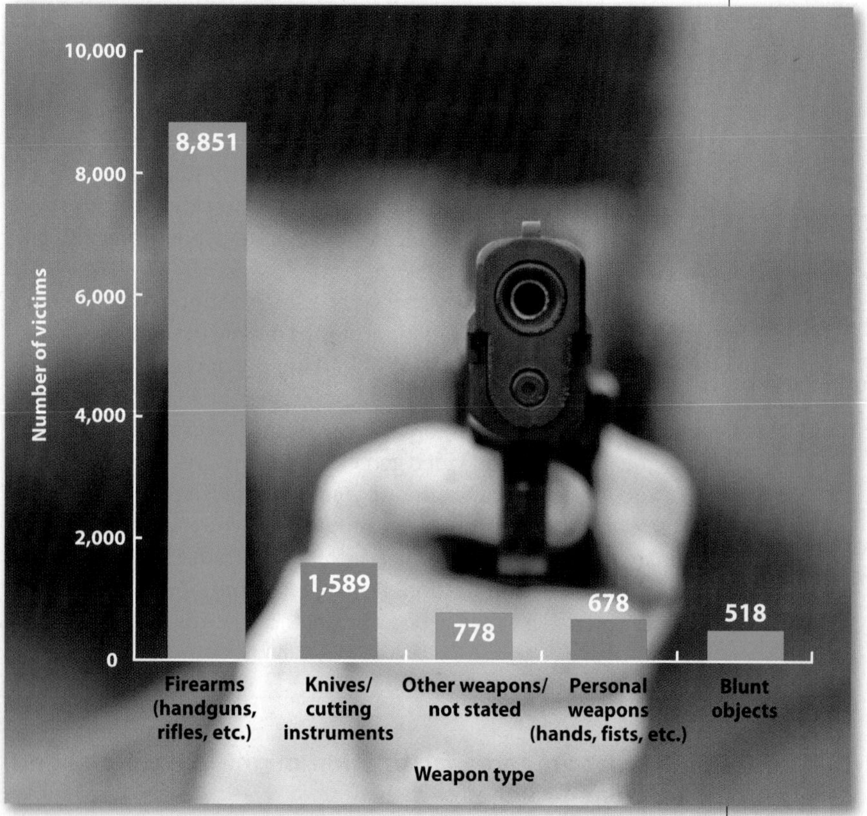

Figure 13.2 Homicide in the United States by Weapon Type, 2012

Sixty-seven percent of murders in the United States are committed using firearms, far outweighing all other weapons combined.

Source: Data from U.S. Department of Justice, Federal Bureau of Investigation, "Crime in the United States, 2012, Expanded Homicide Data," Table 8, www.fbi.gov.

Hate Crimes

A **hate crime** is a crime committed against a person, property, or group of people that is motivated by the offender's bias against a race, religion, disability, sexual orientation, or ethnicity. As a result of national efforts to promote understanding and appreciation of diversity, reports of hate crimes have declined to an all-time low of 5,796 reported incidents in 2012, according to the FBI (Figure 13.3).[29] Of these hate crimes, over 48 percent were a result of bias toward a particular race, nearly 20 percent were motivated by bias based on sexual orientation, 19 percent toward religion, 11.5 percent by ethnicity/national origin bias, and nearly 1.6 percent reflected bias toward disabilities. In 2012, *gender* and *gender identity* were added to hate crime statistics.[30]

In sharp contrast, when a representative sample of Americans completed the anonymous National Crime Victimization Survey, an estimated 294,000 violent and property hate crimes occurred in 2012.[31] Fear of retaliation keeps many hate crimes hidden—60 percent of hate crimes may never be reported, and only about 25 percent of those reported are reported by victims themselves.[32]

Bias-related crime, sometimes referred to as **ethnoviolence,** describes violence based on prejudice and discrimination among ethnic groups in the larger society. **Prejudice** is an irrational attitude of hostility directed against an individual; a group; a race; or the supposed characteristics of an individual, group, or race. **Discrimination** constitutes actions that deny equal treatment or opportunities to a group of people, often based on prejudice. Often prejudice and discrimination stem from a fear of change and a desire to blame others when forces such as the economy and crime seem to be out of control.

Common reasons given to explain bias-related and hate crimes include (1) *thrill seeking* by multiple offenders through a group attack, (2) *feeling threatened* that others will take their jobs or property or best them in some way, (3) *retaliating* for some real or perceived insult or slight, and (4) *fearing the unknown or differences*. For other people, hate crimes are a part of their mission in life, either due to religious zeal or distorted moral beliefs.

Statistics on bias and hate crimes on campus are difficult to find, but increasing media attention has put these issues in the national spotlight. Campuses have responded to reports of hate crimes by offering courses that emphasize diversity, zero tolerance for violations, training faculty appropriately, and developing policies that enforce punishment for hate crimes.

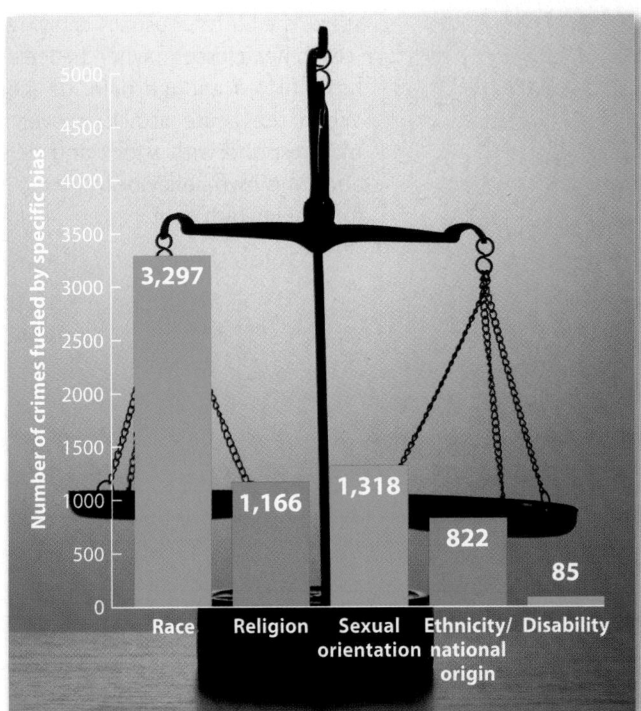

Figure 13.3 Bias-Motivated Crimes, Single-Bias Incidence, 2012
Source: Data from Federal Bureau of Investigation, "Hate Crime Statistics, 2012," Table 1, 2012, www.fbi.gov.

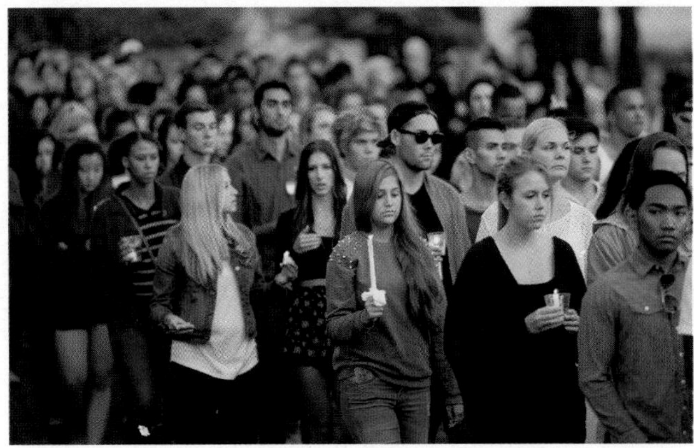

School shootings are becoming all too familiar stories in the news. These students are mourning for victims of a school shooting at UC Santa Barbara. Tragedies like these, in addition to gun violence in other public places, have brought the gun debate to campuses.

TABLE 13.1 Homicide Rates in Selected Nations

Rank	Country	Homicide Rate per 1,000 people
1	Colombia	0.617847
2	South Africa	0.496008
5	Russia	0.201534
6	Mexico	0.130213
16	Zimbabwe	0.0749938
24	United States	0.042802
26	India	0.0344083
40	France	0.0173272
43	Australia	0.0150324
44	Canada	0.0149063
55	Ireland	0.00946215
60	Japan	0.00499933
61	Saudi Arabia	0.00397456

Source: Data from United Nations Office on Drugs and Crime, "UNODC Homicide Statistics," 2014, www.unodc.org.

check yourself

- **What factors are correlated with increased homicide rates in the United States?**
- **List three reasons given to explain hate crimes.**

13.3 Violence in the Family

learning outcome

13.3 Explain how personal and social factors can lead to domestic violence and child and elder abuse.

Sadly, victims of violence and abuse may find that the perpetrators of these crimes are their own spouse, partner, parent, or child. Why do people commit acts of violence against their own loved ones?

Domestic Violence

Domestic violence refers to the use of force to control and maintain power over another person in the home environment. It can occur between parent and child, between spouses or intimate partners, or between siblings or other family members. The violence may involve emotional abuse; verbal abuse; threats of physical harm; and physical violence ranging from slapping and shoving to beatings, rape, and homicide.

Intimate partner violence (IPV) describes physical, sexual, or psychological harm done by a current or former partner or spouse; it can occur among heterosexual or same-sex couples and does not require sexual intimacy. Over the course of a year, millions of women and men are victims of rape, physical and psychological abuse, stalking, and other offenses by an intimate partner. Homicide committed by a current or former intimate partner is the leading cause of death of pregnant women in the United States.[33] In addition, 74 percent of all murder–suicides in the United States involve an intimate partner.[34]

Nearly half of all women and men in the United States have experienced psychological aggression by an intimate partner in their lifetime. Psychological abusers seek to intimidate and debase their partners, thereby gaining control over the partner and the relationship. Those who have experienced this violence are more likely to report depression, difficulty in intimate relationships, frequent headaches, chronic pain, difficulty with sleeping, activity limitations, poor physical health, irritable bowel syndrome, and other health problems.[35]

Have you ever heard of a woman who is repeatedly beaten by her partner and wondered, "Why doesn't she just leave him?" There are many reasons some women find it difficult to break their ties with their abusers. Some, particularly those with small children, are financially dependent on their partners. Others fear retaliation against themselves or their children. Some hope the situation will change with time, and others stay because cultural or religious beliefs forbid divorce. Finally, some women still love the abusive partner and are concerned about what will happen to him if they leave.

In the 1970s, psychologist Lenore Walker developed a theory called the *cycle of violence* that explained predictable, repetitive patterns of psychological and/or physical abuse in abusive relationships.[36] Over the years, Walker's initial work has been criticized for its lack of scientific rigor, anecdotal approach, and seeming overstatement of selected patterns as universal truths. In her most recent book, *The Battered Woman Syndrome*, Walker responds to many of her early critics with improved quantitative analysis, reviews of recent research, and an extensive list of experts in the field of violence.[37]

Today, the cycle of violence continues to be important to understanding why people stay in otherwise unhealthy relationships. The cycle consists of three major phases:

1. **Tension building.** This phase typically occurs prior to the overtly abusive act and includes breakdowns in communication, anger, psychological aggression and violent language, growing tension, and fear.
2. **Incident of acute battering.** At this stage, the batterer usually is trying to "teach her a lesson"; when he feels he has inflicted enough pain, he stops. When the acute attack is over, he may respond with shock and denial about his own behavior or blame her for making him do it.

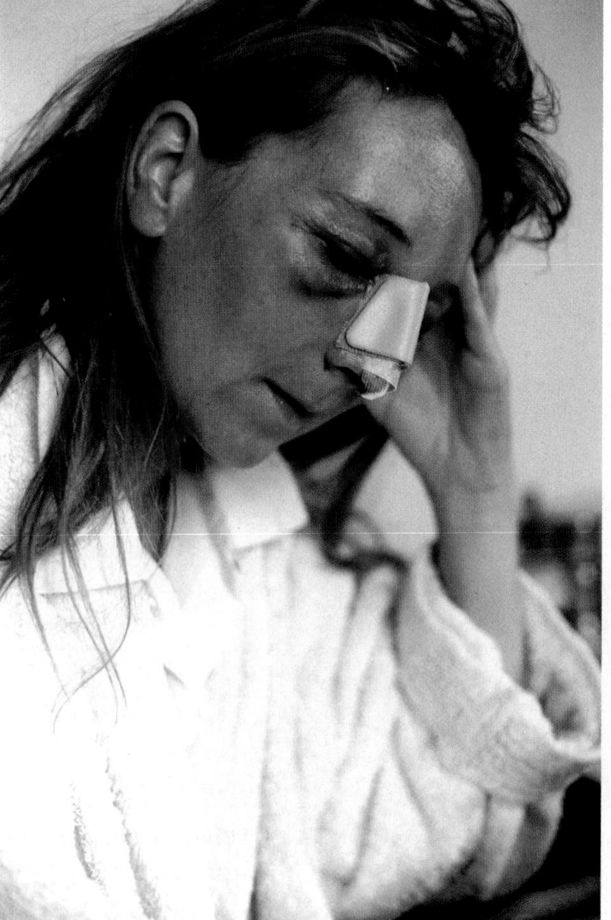

Why do people stay in abusive relationships?

People who stay with their abusers may do so because they are dependent on the abuser, because they fear the abuser, or even because they love the abuser. In some cultures, women may not be free to leave an abusive relationship because of restrictive laws, religious beliefs, or social mores.

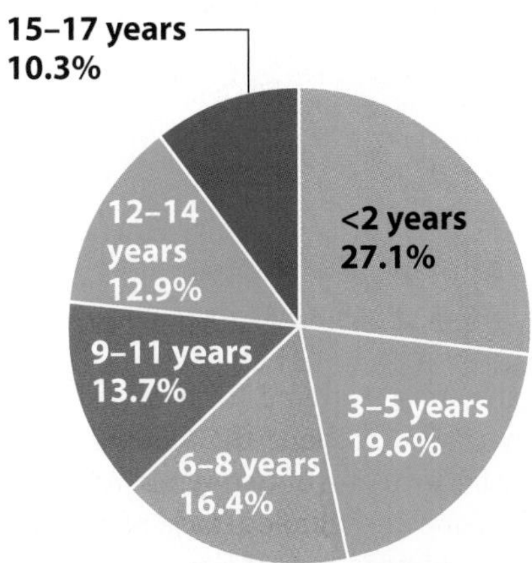

Figure 13.4 Child Abuse and Neglect Victims by Age, 2011
Source: U.S. Department of Health and Human Services, Administration on Children, Youth and Families, *Child Maltreatment 2011* (Washington, DC: U.S. Government Printing Office, 2012).

3. **Remorse/reconciliation.** During this "honeymoon" period, the batterer may be kind, loving, and apologetic, swearing that he will never act violently again and will work to change his behavior. However, when things that triggered past abuse resurface, the cycle starts over.

For a woman caught in this cycle, it is often very hard to summon the resolution to extricate herself. Most need effective outside intervention.

No single reason explains why people tend to be abusive in relationships. Alcohol abuse is often associated with such violence, and marital dissatisfaction is also a predictor. Numerous studies also point to differences in communication patterns between abusive and nonabusive relationships. Stress, mental health issues, economic uncertainty/frustration, jealousy, issues of power/control and gender roles, and issues with self-esteem are among common rationale given for IPV.[38]

Child Abuse and Neglect

Children living in families in which domestic violence or sexual abuse occurs are at great risk for damage to personal health and well-being. **Child maltreatment** is defined as any act or series of acts of commission or omission by a parent or caregiver that results in harm, potential for harm, or threat of harm to a child.[39] **Child abuse** refers to *acts of commission*, which are deliberate or intentional words or actions that cause harm, potential harm, or threat of harm to a child. The abuse may be sexual, psychological, physical, or any combination of these. **Neglect** is an *act of omission*, meaning a failure to provide for a child's basic needs for food, shelter, clothing, medical care, education, or proper supervision. Last year, over 75 percent of reported cases of maltreatment or abuse were for neglect, more than 15 percent were for physical abuse, and nearly 10 percent were for sexual abuse. Although exact figures for child abuse are difficult to obtain, in 2013 an estimated 3.8 million cases of child abuse were reported, involving the alleged maltreatment of approximately 6 million children.[40] Figure 13.4 shows the rates of abuse among children of different ages.

Sexual abuse of children by adults or older children includes sexually suggestive conversations; inappropriate kissing, touching, or petting; oral, anal, or vaginal intercourse; and other kinds of sexual interaction. Recent studies indicate that the rates of sexual abuse in children range from 3 to 32 percent of all children, with girls being at greater risk than young boys, even though young boys are abused in significant numbers.[41]

The shroud of secrecy surrounding this problem makes it likely the number of actual cases are grossly underestimated. Unfortunately, the programs taught in schools today, often with an emphasis on "stranger danger," may give children the false impression that they are more likely to be assaulted by a stranger. In reality, 90 percent of child sexual abuse victims know their perpetrator, with nearly 70 percent of children abused by family members, usually an adult male.[42]

See It! Videos

Should strangers step in to prevent partner abuse? Watch **Will Anyone Confront Abusive Boyfriend?** in the Study Area of MasteringHealth.

People who were abused as children bear spiritual, psychological, and/or physical scars. Studies have shown that child sexual abuse has an impact on later life: Children who experience sexual abuse are at increased risk for anxiety disorders, depression, eating disorders, post-traumatic stress disorder (PTSD), and suicide attempts.[43] Youth who have been sexually abused are 25 percent more likely to experience teen pregnancy, 30 percent more likely to abuse their own children, and are much more likely to have problems with alcohol abuse or drug addiction.[44]

There is no single profile of a child abuser. Frequently, the perpetrator is a young adult in his or her mid-twenties without a high school diploma, living at or below the poverty level, depressed, socially isolated, with a poor self-image, and having difficulty coping with stressful situations. In many instances, the perpetrator has experienced violence and is frustrated by life.

Not all violence against children is physical. Health can be severely affected by psychological violence—assaults on personality, character, competence, independence, or general dignity as a human being. Negative consequences of this kind of victimization can include depression, low self-esteem, and a pervasive fear of offending the abuser.

Elder Abuse

Each year, hundreds of thousands of adults over the age of 60 are abused, neglected, or financially exploited as they enter the later years of life, and these statistics are likely an underestimate.[45] Many victims fail to report because they are embarrassed or because they don't want the abuser to get in trouble or retaliate by putting them in a nursing home or escalating the abuse. Some do not report due to feeling guilty because someone has to take care of them. Others suffer from dementia and may not be aware of the abuse. A variety of social services focus on protecting our seniors, just as we endeavor to protect other vulnerable populations.

check yourself

- **How does the cycle of violence explain why people stay in dangerous or unhealthy relationships?**
- **What steps can be taken to reduce child and elder abuse?**

13.4 Sexual Victimization

learning outcome

13.4 Identify the types and prevalence of rape and sexual assault.

The term *sexual victimization* refers to any situation in which an individual is coerced or forced to comply with or endure another's sexual acts or overtures. It can run the gamut from harassment to stalking to assault and rape. As with all forms of violence, both men and women are susceptible to sexual victimization.

Sexual victimization and violence can have devastating and far-reaching effects on people of any age. Fear, sexual avoidance, sleeplessness, anxiety, and depression are just a few of the long-term consequences for victims of sexual victimization.[46]

Sexual Assault and Rape

Sexual assault is any act in which one person is sexually intimate with another person without that person's consent. This may range from touching to forceful penetration and may include, for example, ignoring indications that intimacy is not wanted, threatening force or other negative consequences, and actually using force.

Although the exact prevalence of sexual violence is not known, a new survey indicates bisexual women have the highest lifetime prevalence of rape by any perpetrator (46.1%), followed by heterosexual women (17.4%) and lesbians (13.1%).[47] Seventy-four percent of bisexual women, 46.4 percent of lesbians, and 43.4 percent of heterosexual women report a lifetime prevalence of sexual violence other than rape. Heterosexual men reported a lifetime prevalence of rape of less than 1 percent (percentages were too small to estimate for gay and bisexual men). For a lifetime prevalence of sexual violence other than rape, the reported rates are 47.4 percent for bisexual men, 40.2 percent for gay men, and 20.8 percent for heterosexual men.

I SHOULD
NOT HA
BE A VI
TO BE
THESE
DEMANDS
ARE
OUR RIGHT
IS THE
URGENCY
PROTECT
OUR
BODIES

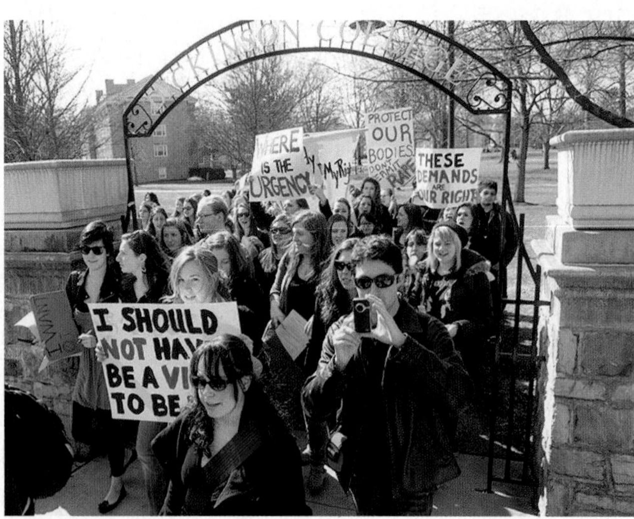

The reluctance to report sexual assault on campus and the difficulty of pursuing criminal proceedings in the campus environment can create turmoil in victims' lives, while too rarely leading to punishment of offenders.

Considered the most extreme form of sexual assault, **rape** is defined as "penetration without the victim's consent." Incidents of rape generally fall into one of two types. An **aggravated rape** is any rape involving one or multiple attackers, strangers, weapons, or physical beatings. A **simple rape** is a rape perpetrated by one person, whom the victim knows, and does not involve a physical beating or use of a weapon. Most rapes are classified as simple rape, but that terminology should not be taken to mean that a simple rape is any less violent or criminal.

Over 20% of undergraduate women have been sexually assaulted one or more times during their undergraduate years.

By most indicators, reported cases of rape appear to have declined in the United States since the early 1990s, even as reports of other forms of sexual assault have increased. This decline is thought to be due to shifts in public awareness and attitudes about rape, combined with tougher crime policies, major educational campaigns, and media attention. These changes enforce the idea that rape is a violent crime and should be treated as such. However, numerous sources indicate that rape is among one of the most underreported crimes, particularly on college campuses.[48]

The terms *date rape* and *acquaintance rape* have been used interchangeably in the past. However, most experts now believe that the term *date rape* is inappropriate because it implies a consensual interaction in an arranged setting and may, in fact, minimize the crime of rape when it occurs. **Acquaintance rape** refers to any rape in which the rapist is known to the victim. Acquaintance rape is more common when drugs or alcohol have been consumed by the offender or victim, making the campus party environment a high-risk venue. Alcohol is frequently involved in rape, as are a growing number of rape-facilitating drugs such as Rohypnol and gamma-hydroxybutyrate (GHB).

Rape on U.S. Campuses In 1992, Congress passed the Campus Sexual Assault Victim's Bill of Rights, known as the *Ramstad Act*, which gave victims the right to call in off-campus authorities to investigate campus crimes and required universities to develop educational programs. More recent provisions of the act specify notification procedures and options for victims, rights of victims and accused perpetrators, and consequences if schools do not comply.[49]

A lot of campus rapes start here.
Whenever there's drinking or drugs, things can get out of hand. So it's no surprise that many campus rapes involve alcohol.
But you should know that under any circumstances, sex without the other person's consent is considered rape. A felony, punishable by prison. And drinking is no excuse.
That's why, when you party, it's good to know what your limits are. You see, a little sobering thought now can save you from a big problem later.

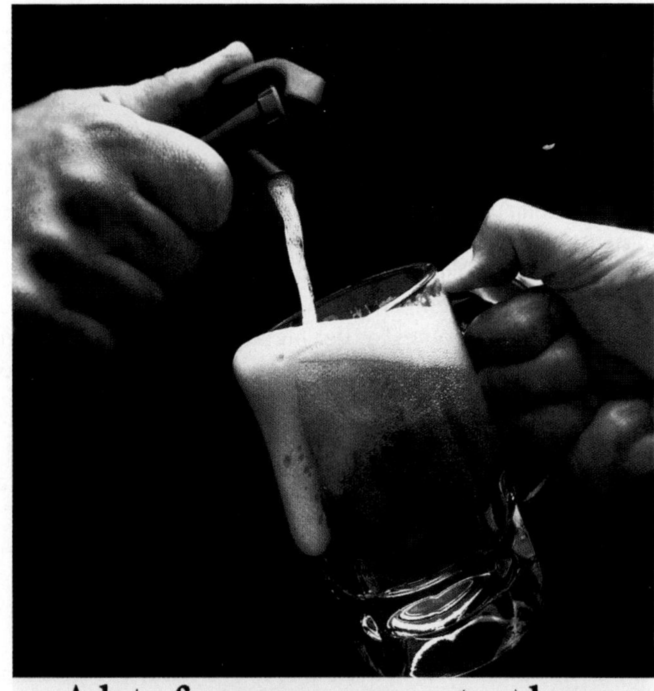

What does *acquaintance rape* mean?

VIDEO TUTOR Acquaintance Rape on Campus

The term *date rape* was formerly applied to a sexual assault occurring in the context of a dating relationship. The term has fallen out of favor because the word *date* implies something reciprocal or arranged, thus minimizing the crime. The term *acquaintance rape* is now more commonly used, referring to any rape in which the rapist is known to the victim, even if only minimally. Acquaintance rape is particularly common on college campuses, where alcohol and drug use can impair young people's judgment and self-control.

Over 20 percent of college students are sexually assaulted as undergraduates.[50] Responding to increased evidence of major issues on college campuses, President Obama formed a national task force to study sexual assault and make recommendations for change. Colleges are being asked to identify and respond to the problem on their campuses, teach the definition of consent and the legal ramifications of any actions that are undertaken without clear consent, and teach "bystander education" to show students how to intervene in potentially harmful situations. Ironically, as campuses improve education and awareness, increase reporting, and call for zero tolerance, the numbers of reported forcible rapes and assaults has increased 49 percent between 2008 and 2012.[51] However, it is likely that these increases indicate an increased willingness of victims to come forward.

Marital Rape Although its legal definition varies within the United States, **marital rape** can be any unwanted intercourse or penetration (vaginal, anal, or oral) obtained by force, threat of force, or when the spouse is unable to consent. This problem has undoubtedly existed since the origin of marriage as a social institution, though it is noteworthy that marital rape did not become a crime in all 50 states until 1993. Even more noteworthy is the fact that 30 states still allow exemptions from marital rape prosecution, meaning that the judicial system may treat it as a lesser crime.[52]

Although research in this area is scarce, it has been estimated that 10–14 percent of married women are raped by their husbands in the United States. About one-third of women report having had "unwanted sex" with their partner.[53] In general, women under 25 and those from lower socioeconomic groups are at highest risk of marital rape. Internationally, women raised in cultures where male dominance is the norm and women are treated as property tend to have higher rates of forced sex within the confines of marriage. Women who are pregnant, ill, separated, or divorced have higher rates, as do women from homes where other forms of domestic violence are common and where there is a high rate of alcoholism or substance abuse.

Social Contributors to Sexual Violence

Certain societal assumptions and traditions can promote sexual violence, including the following:

- **Trivialization.** Many people think that rape committed by a husband or intimate partner doesn't count as rape.
- **Blaming the victim.** In spite of efforts to combat this type of thinking, there is still the belief that a scantily clad woman "asks" for sexual advances.
- **Pressure to be macho.** Males are taught from a young age that showing emotions is a sign of weakness. This portrayal often depicts men as aggressive and predatory and females as passive targets.
- **Male socialization.** Many still believe "boys will be boys." Women are often *objectified* (treated as sexual objects) in the media, which contributes to the idea that it's natural for men to be predatory.
- **Male misperceptions.** With media implying that sex is the focus of life, it's not surprising that some men believe that when a woman says no, she is really asking to be seduced.
- **Situational factors.** Dates in which the male makes all the decisions, pays for everything, and generally controls the entire situation are more likely to end in an aggressive sexual scenario. Alcohol and other drugs increase the risk and severity of assaults.

check yourself

- **What are three types of rape and sexual abuse?**
- **What are two social contributors to sexual violence?**

13.5 Other Forms of Sexual Violence

learning **outcome**

13.5 Explain the definitions of, and ways to address, sexual harassment and stalking.

Sexual harassment and stalking are two common forms of sexual violence, even when they do not involve physical harm.

Sexual Harassment

Sexual harassment is defined as unwelcome sexual conduct that is related to any condition of employment or evaluation of student performance. Unwelcome sexual advances, requests for sexual favors, and other verbal or physical conduct of a sexual nature constitute sexual harassment when any of the following occurs:[54]

- Submission to such conduct is made either explicitly or implicitly a term or condition of an individual's employment or education
- Submission to or rejection of such conduct by an individual is used as the basis for employment or education-related decisions affecting such an individual
- Such conduct is sufficiently severe or pervasive that it has the effect, intended or unintended, of unreasonably interfering with an individual's work or academic performance because it has created an intimidating, hostile, or offensive environment and would have such an effect on a reasonable person of that individual's status.

Commonly, people think of harassment as involving only faculty members or persons in power, where sex is used to exhibit control of a situation. However, peers can harass one another, too. Sexual harassment may include unwanted touching; unwarranted sex-related comments or subtle pressure for sexual favors; deliberate or repeated humiliation or intimidation based on sex; and gratuitous comments, jokes, questions, or remarks about clothing or bodies, sexuality, or past sexual relationships.

17.6% of the sexual harassment charges received by the U.S. Equal Opportunity Commission in 2013 were filed by men.

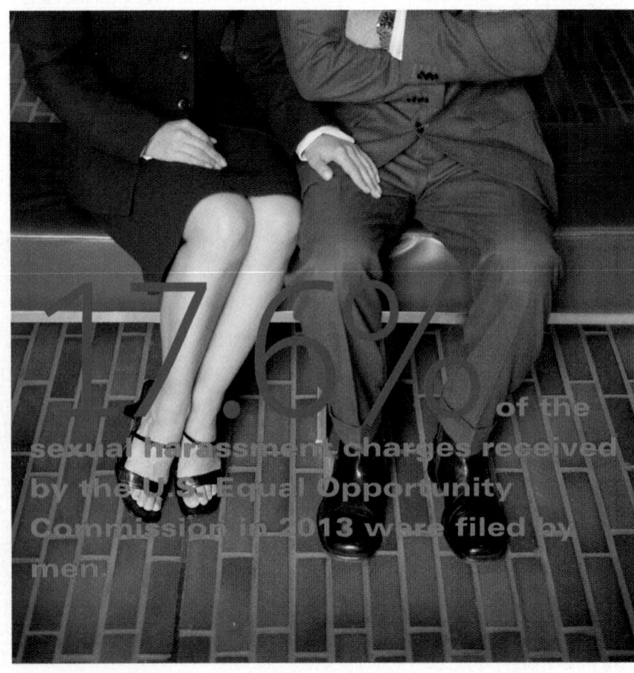

Most schools and companies have sexual harassment policies in place, as well as procedures for dealing with harassment problems. If you feel you are being harassed, the most important thing you can do is be assertive:

- **Tell the harasser to stop.** Be clear and direct. Tell the person if it continues that you will report it. If the harassing is via phone or Internet, block the person.
- **Document the harassment.** Make a record of each incident. If the harassment becomes intolerable, a record of exactly what occurred (and when and where) will help make your case. Save copies of all communication from the harasser.
- **Try to make sure you aren't alone in the harasser's presence.** Witnesses to harassment can ensure appropriate validation of the event.
- **Complain to a higher authority.** Talk to legal authorities or your instructor, adviser, or counseling center psychologist about what happened.
- **Remember that you have not done anything wrong.** You will likely feel awful after being harassed (especially if you have to complain to superiors). However, feel proud that you are not keeping silent.

Stalking

Stalking can be defined as conduct directed at a person that would cause a reasonable person to feel fear. This may include repeated visual or physical proximity, nonconsensual written or verbal communication, and implied or explicit threats.[55] More than 1 in 4 victims report being stalked via some form of technology.[56] The most common stalking behaviors included unwanted phone calls and messages, spreading rumors, spying on the victim, and showing up at the same places as the victim without having a reason to be there.[57]

Millions of women and men are stalked annually in the United States; the vast majority of stalkers are persons involved in relationship breakups or other dating acquaintances.[58] Adults 18 to 24 experience the highest rates of stalking. Like sexual harassment, stalking is an underreported crime. Often students do not think a stalking incident is serious enough to report, or they worry that the police will not take it seriously.

See It! Videos

Is there a hidden culture of sexual harassment on campuses across the country? Watch **Sexual Harassment on Campus** in the Study Area of MasteringHealth.

check yourself

- **How can sexual harassment be prevented and controlled?**

Collective Violence

learning outcome

13.6 List the factors associated with terrorism and gang violence.

Collective violence is violence perpetrated by groups against other groups and includes violent acts related to political, governmental, religious, cultural, or social clashes. Gang violence and terrorism are two forms of collective violence that have become major threats in recent years.

Gang Violence

Gang violence is increasing in many regions of the world; U.S. communities face escalating threats from gang networks engaged in drug trafficking, sex trafficking, shootings, beatings, thefts, carjackings, and the killing of innocent victims caught in the crossfire. Currently, there are over 33,000 gangs in the United States, with membership in excess of 1.4 million.[59] Gangs are believed to be responsible for 48 percent of violent crime overall in the United States, and in some locations, as much as 90 percent.[60]

Why do young people join gangs? Often, gangs give members a sense of self-worth, companionship, security, and excitement. In other cases, gangs provide economic security through drug sales, prostitution, and other types of criminal activity. Friendships with delinquent peers, lack of parental monitoring, negative life events, and alcohol and drug use appear to increase risks for gang affiliation. Other risk factors include low self-esteem, academic problems, low socioeconomic status, alienation from family and society, a history of family violence, and living in gang-controlled neighborhoods.[61] Since it becomes difficult to leave gangs once youth become involved, prevention strategies appear to offer promise.

Terrorism

Numerous terrorist attacks around the world reveal the vulnerability of all nations to domestic and international threats. In the United States, this was particularly apparent on September 11, 2001, when terrorist attacks on the World Trade Center and the Pentagon revealed the vulnerability of our nation to domestic and international threats. More than 15 years later, threats against our airlines, mass transportation systems, cities, national monuments, and our population fuel fears of looming terrorist attacks. Effects on our economy, travel restrictions, additional security measures, and military buildups are but a few of the examples of how terrorist threats have affected our lives. As defined in the U.S. Code of Federal Regulations, **terrorism** is the "unlawful use of force or violence against persons or property to intimidate or coerce a government, the civilian population, or any segment thereof in furtherance of political or social objectives."[62]

Over the past decade, the Centers for Disease Control and Prevention (CDC) established the *Emergency Preparedness and Response Division*. This group monitors potential public health problems such as bioterrorism, chemical emergencies, radiation emergencies, mass casualties, national disaster, and severe weather; develops plans for mobilizing communities in the case of emergency; and provides information about terrorist threats. In addition, the Department of Homeland Security works to prevent future attacks, and the FBI and other government agencies have prepared a set of procedures and guidelines to ensure citizens' health and safety.

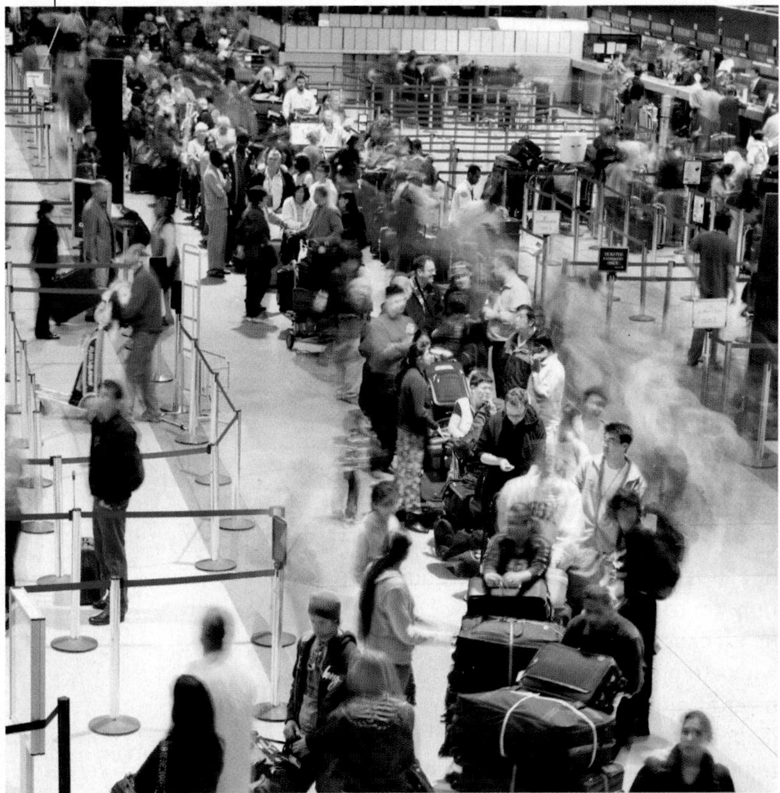

The threat of terrorism has affected many aspects of our daily lives. From increased security at airports to restrictions on public transit, steps taken to protect against terrorism have changed day-to-day activities.

check yourself

- **What is collective violence?**
- **What factors contribute to collective violence?**

13.7 How to Avoid Becoming a Victim of Violence

learning outcome

13.7 List strategies to prevent violence against yourself and others.

After a violent act is committed against someone we know, we may acknowledge the horror of the event, express sympathy, and go on with our lives, but it may take the brutalized person months or years to recover both physically and emotionally. For this reason, preventing a violent act is far better than recovering from it. Both individuals and communities can play important roles in the prevention of violence and intentional injuries. Assaults and threats can arise from in-person encounters, or they may develop from online encounters.

Social Networking Safety

At any given time, millions of people are chatting away on social networking sites with friends, family, and strangers and posting photos and personal information that may be available to people they barely know, sometimes placing them at considerable risk. These sites raise some concerns about potential risks—from stalking and identity theft to embarrassment and defamation.

Posting personal information online, such as your phone number, class schedule, and e-mail address, poses a threat to personal safety and puts you at greater risk for identify theft or even stalking. Additionally, posting negative messages about employers or colleagues can have damaging consequences: Hiring and firing decisions have been influenced by information employees and job applicants made publicly available on Facebook and Twitter. Using social media sites for dating or hookups poses addition risks; in addition to the vulnerabilities involved in exchanging personal information with strangers, underage users may pose as adults, leading to claims of inappropriate sexual contact with minors and other criminal offenses on the part of people interacting with them online.

Although very real threats to health, reputation, financial security, and future employment lie in wait for those who post indiscriminately and unwisely to the Web, social networking sites are far from wholly dangerous. To safely enjoy the benefits and to avoid the risks of social networking sites, you'll need to practice a little caution and use some common sense. The following tips will help you to remain safe, protect your identity, and feel free to express yourself without fear of repercussions:

- Don't post anything on the Web that you wouldn't want someone to pick out of your trash and read. Your address, phone numbers, banking information, calendar, family secrets, and other information should be kept off the sites.
- Don't post compromising pictures, videos, or other things that you wouldn't want your mother or coworkers to see.
- Never meet a stranger in person whom you've met only online without bringing a trusted friend along or, at the very least, notifying a close friend of where you will be and when you will return. Arrange a ride home with a friend in advance and choose a well-established, public place to meet during daylight hours. Don't give your address or traceable phone numbers to the person you are meeting.
- When you get rid of phones or other devices, make sure you wipe them of your data and close all accounts in your name.
- Avoid banking or accessing sensitive personal financial documents when using public WiFi servers. Make sure your cell phone is not posting your location publically.
- Change your passwords and security questions often, and don't write them all down where someone can find them.

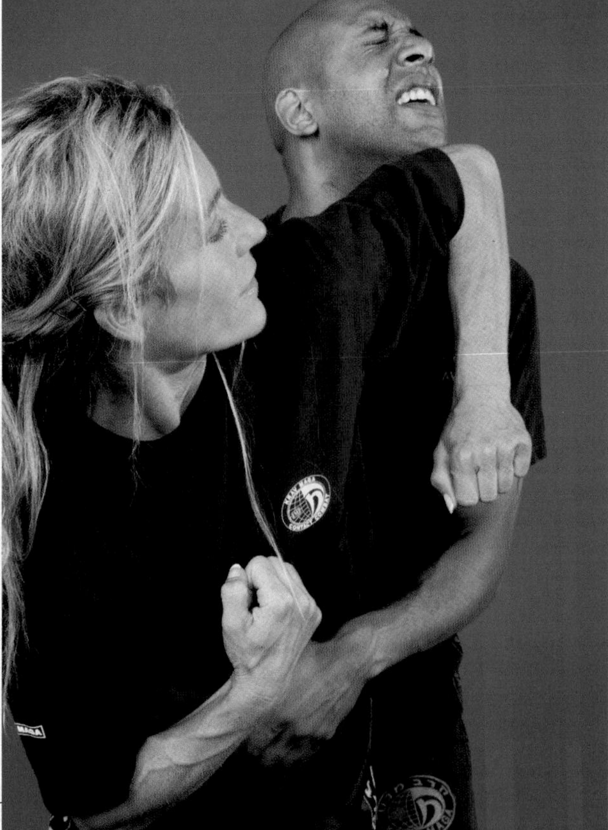

How can I protect myself from becoming a victim of violence?

One of the best ways to protect yourself from violence is to avoid situations or circumstances that could lead to it. Another way to protect yourself is to learn self-defense techniques, such as shown here. College campuses often offer safety workshops and self-defense classes to arm students with the physical and mental skills that may help them to repel or deter an assailant.

Self-Defense against Rape and Personal Assault

Assault can occur no matter what preventive actions you take, but commonsense self-defense tactics can lower the risk. Self-defense is a process that includes increasing your awareness, developing self-protective skills, taking reasonable precautions, and having the judgment necessary to respond quickly to changing situations. Because rape on campus often occurs in social or dating settings, it is important to know ways to avoid and extract yourself from potentially dangerous situations. The **Skills for Behavior Change** box identifies practical tips for preventing dating violence.

Most attacks by unknown assailants are planned in advance. Many rapists use certain ploys to initiate their attacks. Examples include asking for help; offering help; staging a deliberate "accident," such as bumping into you; or posing as a police officer or other authority figure. Sexual assault frequently begins with a casual, friendly conversation.

Listen to your feelings and trust your intuition. Be assertive and direct to someone who is getting out of line or becoming threatening. Stifle your tendency to be nice, and don't fear making a scene. Use the following tips to let a potential assailant know that you mean what you say and are prepared to defend yourself:

- **Speak in a strong voice.** State "Leave me alone!" rather than questions such as, "Will you please leave me alone?" Avoid apologies and excuses. Sound like you mean it.
- **Maintain eye contact with a would-be attacker.** Eye contact keeps you aware of the person's movements and conveys an aura of strength and confidence.
- **Stand up straight, act confident, and remain alert.** Walk as if you own the sidewalk.

If you are attacked, act immediately. Draw attention to yourself and your assailant. Scream, "Fire!" Research has shown that passersby are much more likely to help if they hear the word *fire* rather than just a scream.

What to Do if a Rape Occurs

If you are a rape victim, report the attack. This gives you a sense of control. Follow these steps:

- Call 9-1-1.
- Do not bathe, shower, douche, clean up, or touch anything that the attacker may have touched.
- Save the clothes you were wearing, and do not launder them. They will be needed as evidence. Bring a clean change of clothes to the clinic or hospital.
- Contact the rape assistance hotline in your area, and ask for advice on therapists or counseling if you need additional help or advice.

If a friend is raped, here's how you can help:

- Believe the rape victim. Don't ask questions that may appear to imply that she/he is at a fault in any way for the assault.
- Recognize that rape is a violent act and that the victim was not looking for this to happen.
- Encourage your friend to see a doctor immediately, because she may have medical needs but feel too embarrassed to seek help on her own. Offer to go with her.
- Encourage her to report the crime.
- Be understanding, and let her know you will be there for her.
- Recognize that this is an emotional recovery, and it may take months or years for her to bounce back.
- Encourage your friend to seek counseling.

One of the most important things you can do is to be supportive. Don't put your friend on the defensive with questions such as "Why didn't you leave?" or "What were you thinking by taking that drink?" Better options for questions might be "What happened? What do you feel that you want to do now? Is there anyone in particular you want to call or talk to? Is there anything I can do for you?"

Skills for Behavior Change

REDUCING YOUR RISK OF DATING VIOLENCE

- Prior to your date, think about your values; set personal boundaries before you walk out the door.
- If a situation feels like it is getting out of control, stop and talk, speak directly, and don't worry about hurting feelings. Be firm.
- Watch your alcohol consumption. Drinking might get you into situations you'd otherwise avoid.
- Do not accept beverages or open-container drinks from anyone you do not know well and trust. At a bar or a club, accept drinks only from the bartender or wait staff.
- Never leave a drink or food unattended. If you get up to dance, have someone you trust watch your drink or take it with you.
- Go out with several couples or in groups when dating someone new.
- Stick with your friends. Agree to keep an eye out for one another at parties, and have a plan for leaving together and checking in with one another. Never leave a bar or party alone with a stranger.
- Pay attention to your date's actions. If there is too much teasing and all the decisions are made for you, it could mean trouble. Trust your intuition.
- Practice what you will say to your date if things go in an uncomfortable direction. You have the right to express your feelings, and it is OK to be assertive. Do not be swayed by arguments such as "What about my feelings?," "You were leading me on," and "If you really cared about me, you would."

check yourself

- **What are three things you can do to reduce your risk of personal assault?**
- **How can you support a friend who has been raped or assaulted?**

13.8 Campus and Community Responses to Violence

learning outcome

13.8 Describe how college campuses are responding to the threat of violence.

Increasingly, campuses have become microcosms of the greater society, complete with the risks, hazards, and dangers that people face in the world. Many college administrators have been proactive in establishing violence-prevention policies, programs, and services. Campuses have begun to take a careful look at the aspects of campus culture that promote and tolerate violent acts.

Prevention and Early Response Efforts

Campuses are reviewing the effectiveness of emergency messaging systems, including mobile phone alert systems. The REVERSE 9-1-1 system uses database and geographic information system (GIS) mapping technologies to notify campus police and community members in the event of problems, and other systems allow administrators to send out alerts in text, voice, e-mail, or instant message format. Some schools program the phone numbers, photographs, and basic student information for all incoming first-year students into a university security system so that in the event of a threat students need only hit a button on their phones, whereupon campus police will be notified and tracking devices will pinpoint their location.

Changes in the Campus Environment

Recognizing that they may be liable for not protecting their students, and out of a genuine concern for faculty, staff, and student health, administrators are asking key questions about the safety of the campus environment. Campus lighting, parking lot security, call boxes for emergencies, removal of overgrown shrubbery along bike paths and walking trails, and stepped-up security are increasingly on the radar of campus safety personnel. Buildings themselves are designed with better lighting and more security provisions, and in some cases security cameras have been installed in hallways, classrooms, and public places throughout campus. Safe rides are provided for students who have consumed too much alcohol; campus leaders have become more involved in campus safety issues; and health promotion programs have stepped up their violence prevention efforts through seminars on acquaintance rape, sexual assault, harassment, and other topics.

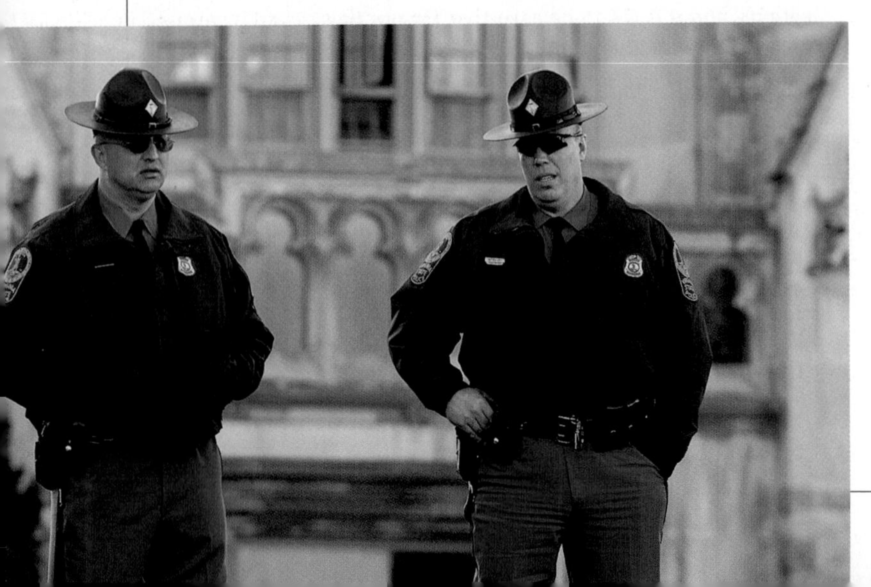

Hazing, which can be defined as "any activity expected of someone joining or participating in a group that humiliates, degrades, abuses, or endangers them regardless of a person's willingness to participate," can contribute to an atmosphere of violence and intimidation on campus.[63] The issue of hazing has become headline news, with several deaths reported over the last few years. Currently, hazing is considered a crime in 39 states. Most institutions have policies against hazing, but few students ever report it.

Typically, hazing involves forcing students to consume excessive alcohol; dress in humiliating garb; undergo forced sleep deprivation; endure verbal abuse from group members; or physical abuse in the form of beatings, heat or cold exposure, or forced sexual acts. According to a national study, 55 percent of college students involved in clubs, teams, and organizations experience hazing, and 9 out of 10 students who experience hazing in college do not realize they've been hazed.[64]

In 95 percent of cases in which students identified their experience as hazing, they did not report the events to campus officials.[65] One reason for this seems to be that more students perceive positive rather than negative outcomes of hazing, for example, feeling a sense of accomplishment or belonging. Students also report that school administrators do little to prevent hazing beyond maintaining a "hazing is not tolerated" stance. If schools are to have an impact on the prevalence of hazing on their campuses, they need to implement broader prevention and intervention efforts and work to educate their campus community on the physical and legal perils of hazing.

Campus Law Enforcement

Campus law enforcement has changed over the years by increasing both numbers of its members and its authority to prosecute student offenders. Campus police are responsible for emergency responses to situations that threaten safety, human resources, the general campus environment, traffic and bicycle riders, and other dangers. They have the power to enforce laws with students in the same way those laws are handled in the general community. In fact, many campuses now hire state troopers or local law enforcement officers to deal with campus issues rather than maintain a separate police staff.

Coping in the Event of Campus Violence

Although schools have worked tirelessly to prevent violence, it can and does still occur. In its aftermath, some may find it difficult to remain on campus as it represents a place of violation and lack of safety; others may experience problems with concentration, studying, and other daily activities. Although there is no "fix" for traumatic events, several strategies can be helpful. In the event of a campus-wide tragedy, members of the campus community should be allowed to mourn. Memorial services and acknowledgment of grief, fear, anger, and other emotions are critical to healing. Students, faculty, and staff should also be involved in planning to prevent future problems—it can help to impart a feeling of control. To cope with emotional trauma, students should seek out resources in their community, such as support groups, therapists, and trusted family members or friends. Journaling or writing about feelings can also help.

Community Strategies for Preventing Violence

You can take a number of steps to ensure your personal safety (see **Skills for Behavior Change**). However, it is also necessary to address issues of violence and safety at a community level. Because the factors that contribute to violence are complex and interrelated, community strategies for prevention must also be multidimensional, focusing on individuals, schools, families, communities, policies, programs, and services designed to reduce risk. The CDC's Injury Response initiatives include interventions designed to prevent violence before it begins:

- Inoculate children against violence in the home. Teaching youth principles of respect and responsibility are fundamental to the health and well-being of future generations.
- Develop policies and laws that prevent violence. Enforce laws so offenders know you mean business in your settings.
- Develop skills-based educational programs that teach the basics of interpersonal communication, elements of healthy relationships, anger management, conflict resolution, appropriate assertiveness, stress management, and other health-based behaviors.
- Involve families, schools, community programs, athletics, music, faith-based organizations, and other community groups in providing experiences that help young people to develop self-esteem and self-efficacy.
- Promote tolerance and acceptance and establish and enforce policies that forbid discrimination. Offer diversity training and mandate involvement.
- Improve community services focused on family planning, mental health services, day care and respite care, and alcohol and substance abuse prevention.
- Make sure walking trails, parking lots, and other public areas are well lit, unobstructed, and patrolled regularly to reduce threats.
- Improve community-based support and treatment for victims and ensure that individuals have choices available when trying to stop violence in their lives.

Skills for Behavior Change

STAY SAFE ON ALL FRONTS

You can take a number of steps to protect yourself from assault. Follow these tips to increase your awareness and reduce your risk of a violent attack.

OUTSIDE ALONE

- **Carry a cell phone and keep it turned on, but stay off it. Be aware of what is happening around you. Don't walk to your car in a dark parking lot while chatting to others. Stay alert.**
- **If you are being followed, don't go home. Head for a location where there are other people. If you decide to run, run fast and scream loudly to attract attention.**
- **Vary your routes; walk or jog with others. Stay close to others.**
- **Park near lights; avoid dark areas where people could hide.**
- **Carry pepper spray or other deterrents. Consider using your campus escort service.**
- **Tell others where you are going and when you expect to be back.**

IN YOUR CAR

- **Lock your doors. Do not open your doors or windows to strangers.**
- **If someone hits your car while you are driving, drive to the nearest gas station or other public place. Call the police or road service for help, and stay in your car until help arrives.**
- **If a car appears to be following you, do not drive home. Drive to the nearest police station.**

IN YOUR HOME

- **Install deadbolts on all doors and locks on all windows. Don't leave a spare key outside. Consider installing a home alarm system.**
- **Lock doors when at home, even during the day. Close blinds and drapes whenever you are away and in the evening when you are home.**
- **Rent apartments that require a security code or clearance to gain entry; avoid easily accessible apartments such as first-floor units. When you move into a new residence, pay a locksmith to change the keys and locks.**
- **Don't let repair people in without asking for identification; have someone with you when repairs are made.**
- **Keep a cell phone near your bed and call 9-1-1 in emergencies. Buy phones that have E911 locators so that emergency personnel can find you even when you can't respond or don't know where you are.**
- **If you return to find your residence has been broken into, don't enter. Call the police. If you encounter an intruder, it is better to give up your money than to fight back.**

check yourself

- **What can schools and communities do to prevent or reduce violence?**

13.9 Reducing Your Risk on the Road

learning outcome

13.9 List the major causes of motor vehicle accidents, and how to stay safe on the road.

Over 33,500 Americans of all ages died in the over 5.6 million motor vehicle accidents (MVAs) in 2012—an average of 92 people per day.[66]

Factors Contributing to MVAs

Factors within your control—distracted driving, impaired driving, speeding, and vehicle safety issues such as failure to wear your seat belt—contribute to the great majority of MVAs.[67]

Distracted Driving Four types of activities constitute distracted driving: looking at something other than the road; hearing something not related to driving; manipulating something other than the steering wheel; and thinking about something other than driving.[68] In 2012, over 3,300 Americans died and over 420,000 were injured in distraction-affected crashes.[69]

Behaviors of greatest concern are texting and talking on a cell phone. Overall, 31 percent of U.S. drivers age 18 to 64 report texting while driving, and 69 percent report that they talk on their cell phone while driving.[70] Texting is particularly deadly: Highway safety experts estimate that the average time a person's eyes are off the road while texting is about 5 seconds. At 55 mph, that's the equivalent of driving the length of a football field blindfolded.[71] Laws regulating cell phone use while driving have been passed in several states: 43 states ban text-messaging for all drivers, and 12 states ban all handheld cell phone use of any kind.[72]

Other common distractions include manipulating handheld devices, adjusting CD players or the radio, looking in the mirror, calling out the window, and eating. Engaging in manual tasks like these triples your risk of getting into a crash.[73] The next time you're tempted to text, make a call, or even swat an insect while driving, pull over. Handle the distraction. Then rejoin traffic when you're ready.

Impaired Driving In 2012, over 10,300 people in the United States died in MVAs that involved an alcohol-impaired driver. This represents an average of one such death every 51 minutes. Viewed another way, 31 percent of all MVA fatalities are due to alcohol impairment.[74] People age 21 through 24 have the highest percentage of alcohol-impaired drivers involved in fatal crashes.[75] Use of drugs other than alcohol is also a significant cause of MVA injury and death.[76] And many researchers contend that driving while sleep deprived is as dangerous as driving drunk.

Public health and law enforcement agencies are cooperating on measures to keep impaired drivers off the road:

- Designated driver programs, including public funding of "safe rides"
- Strict enforcement of laws defining impaired driving and the legal drinking age
- Measures to prevent repeat offenses, including mandatory alcohol or drug abuse treatment, ignition interlock systems that prevent vehicle operation by anyone with a blood alcohol concentration above a specified level, stricter testing for and punishment of those who abuse prescription medicines and/or drive when sleep impaired, and license revocation

Speeding Every day, 25–30 Americans die in speed-related car crashes.[77] Many people speed because they don't perceive it as dangerous. Unfortunately, such attitudes lead to over 10,200 deaths each year.[78]

Vehicle Safety Issues Wearing a safety belt cuts your risk of death or serious injury in a crash by about half.[79] If you're transporting an infant or child, follow state laws governing use and location of age-appropriate safety seats.

Vehicles can include many safety features, from airbags to stability control. Unfortunately, people who don't have the financial resources to drive vehicles with state-of-the-art features—and that often includes college students—are at increased risk during MVAs. Still, the next time you're planning to purchase a car, new or used, look for features recommended by the Insurance Institute for Highway Safety:

1. Does the car have front airbags? Side airbags? (Airbags don't eliminate the need for safety belts.)
2. Does the car have antilock brakes? Traction and stability control?
3. Does the car have impact-absorbing crumple zones?
4. Are there strengthened passenger compartment side walls?
5. Is there a strong roof support? (The center doorpost on four-door models gives you an extra roof pillar.)

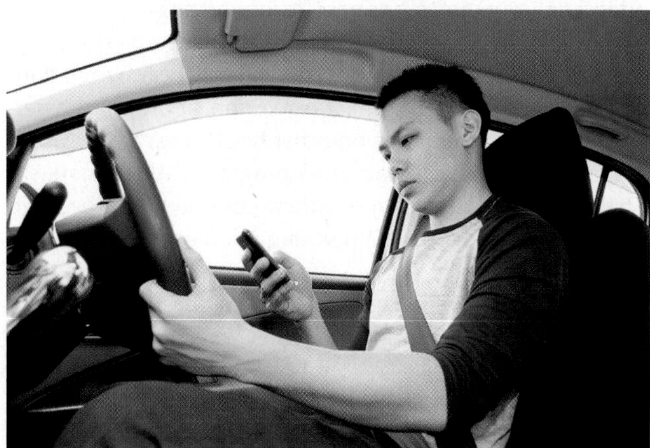

What's wrong with texting while driving?

Texting or talking on a cell phone while driving puts you at a greater risk of being in a motor vehicle accident. It also increases the risk of injury and death to other drivers, passengers, and pedestrians and is illegal in many states.

STAY SOBER
STAY ALIVE
IF YOU MUST DRINK
PLEASE DON'T DRIVE

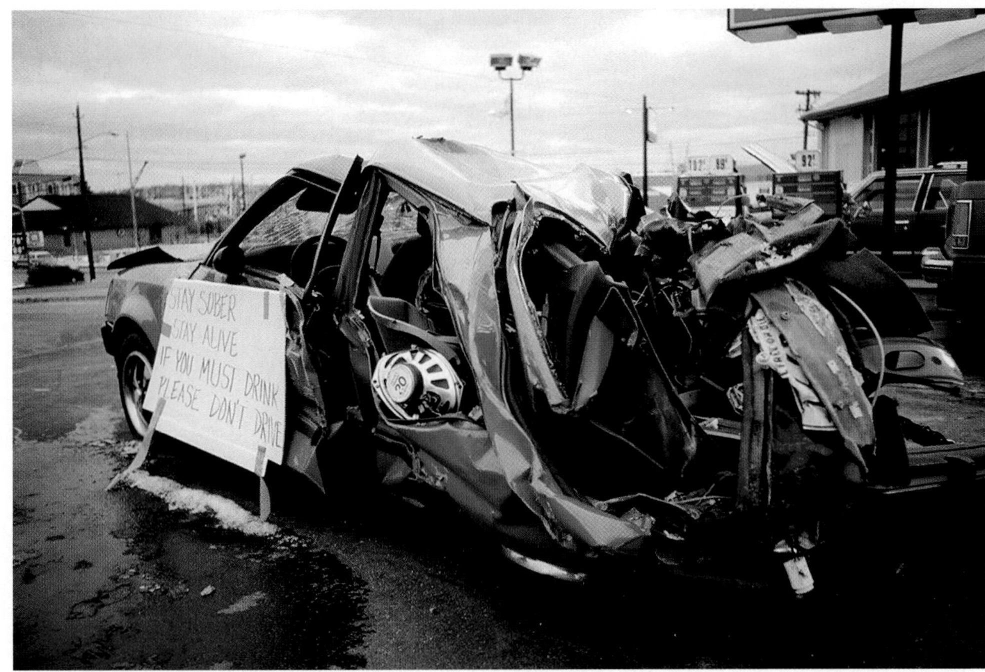

Driving under the influence of alcohol greatly increases the risk of being involved in a motor vehicle crash. Of all drivers between the ages of 21 and 24 involved in fatal crashes, nearly 1 out of 3 were legally drunk.

Another factor is the size of the vehicles involved. All cars sold in the United States must meet U.S. Department of Transportation standards for crash worthiness. However, in 2012 there were nearly four times as many deaths per vehicle among minicars as compared to very large cars, and 23 of the top 26 cars with the lowest rates of driver deaths were midsize or larger.[80] Many college students drive small cars because they are more affordable and use less gas, but the laws of physics make such cars more dangerous.

What about motorcycles? Per vehicle mile traveled, motorcyclists are about 26 times more likely than passenger car occupants to die in an MVA, and 5 times more likely to be injured. In 2012, this translated into over 4,900 motorcyclist deaths and 93,000 injuries.[81]

Many motorcyclists involved in MVAs have avoided severe injuries because they were wearing a helmet. Although the benefits of helmets and protective clothing are well established, only 19 states have full helmet requirements for anyone riding a motorcycle.[82] To find out your state requirements, go to www.iihs.org.

Risk-Management Driving Techniques

Although you can't control what other drivers are doing, you can reduce your risk of injury in an MVA:

- Don't manipulate electronic devices or talk on a cell phone while driving, even if the phone is hands-free.
- Don't drink and drive—take a taxi or arrange for someone to be the designated driver.
- Don't drive when tired or when in a highly emotional or stressed state.
- Never tailgate. The rear bumper of the car ahead of you should be at least 3 seconds worth of distance away, making stopping safely possible. Increase the distance when visibility is reduced, speed is increased, or roads are slick.
- Scan the road ahead of you and to both sides.
- Drive with your low-beam headlights on, *day and night*, to make your car more visible to other drivers.
- Anticipate the actions of others as much as you can; be on the alert for unsignaled lane changes, sudden braking, or other unexpected maneuvers.
- Obey all traffic laws.
- Whether you're the driver or a passenger, always wear a seat belt.

Road Rage

The National Highway Traffic Safety Administration (NHTSA) defines aggressive driving as "the operation of a motor vehicle in a manner that endangers or is likely to endanger persons or property."[83] An extreme version of such behavior is *road rage*, which is believed to be a leading cause of highway deaths. Although you cannot control or predict the behavior of others, there are steps you can take to avoid becoming a victim of road rage:

See It! Videos

Are you at risk of falling asleep at the wheel? Watch **Dozing and Driving: 1 in 24 Asleep at Wheel** in the Study Area of MasteringHealth.

- **Avoid eye contact and engagement.** If you're driving or in public and someone tries to get a reaction from you, avoid confrontation and remove yourself from the situation.
- **Don't antagonize.** Slowing down in traffic to bug someone in an obvious hurry, honking your horn, flashing your high beams, or other passive-aggressive gestures can upset even the most mild-mannered people.
- **If someone follows you after a nasty interaction, either in a car or on foot, do not immediately go home or to your workplace.** Head for the nearest police station or busy area. Never isolate yourself.
- **Take names.** If you don't know the person, try keeping a mental description or get a license plate number. Report offenders, even if you're afraid of getting involved.
- **Stay calm.** Think before opening your mouth, and practice stress management whenever possible.

check yourself

- **What are three factors linked to increased risk of motor vehicle accidents?**
- **What can you do to stay safe on the road?**

13.10 Safe Recreation

learning outcome

13.10 Explain how to stay safe while biking, skateboarding, skiing, snowboarding, swimming, and boating.

Recreational activities among young people that commonly involve injury include biking, skateboarding, snow sports, and swimming and boating. By following some basic guidelines while doing these activities, you can have fun and be safe.

Bike Safety

The NHTSA reports that, in 2011, 677 people died in cycling accidents, and 48,000 were injured. The fatality rate is six times higher for males than females, and males age 45 to 54 had the highest number of cycling-related deaths.[84] Most fatal collisions are due to cyclists' errors, usually failure to yield at intersections. However, alcohol also plays a significant role in bicycle deaths and injuries: In 2011, nearly one-fourth (23%) of cyclists killed were legally drunk, and in 37 percent of all fatal accidents between motor vehicles and bicycles, either the driver or the cyclist was drunk.[85]

All cyclists should wear a properly fitted bicycle helmet every time they ride (Figure 13.5). The NHTSA reports that a helmet is the single most effective way to prevent head injury resulting from a bicycle crash. Moreover, bear in mind that cyclists are considered vehicle operators; they are required to obey the same rules of the road as drivers.

Cyclists should consider the following suggestions:

- Wear a helmet approved by the American National Standards Institute (ANSI) or the Snell Memorial Foundation.
- Watch the road and listen for traffic sounds! Never listen to an MP3 player or talk on a cell phone, even hands free, while cycling.
- Don't drink and ride.
- Follow all traffic laws, signs, and signals.
- Ride with the flow of traffic.
- Wear light or brightly colored, reflective clothing that is easily seen at dawn, dusk, and during full daylight.
- Avoid riding after dark. If you must ride at night, use a front light and a red reflector or flashing rear light, as well as reflective tape or other markings on your bike and clothing.
- Know and use proper hand signals.
- Keep your bicycle in good condition.
- Use bike paths whenever possible.
- Stop at stop signs and traffic lights.

Safe Skateboarding

According to the U.S. Consumer Product Safety Commission (CPSC), skateboard-related injuries are commonly due to riding in traffic, trick riding, excessive speed, and consumption of alcohol. Lack of protective equipment, poor board maintenance, riding on irregular road surfaces, inexperience, and overconfidence also play a role.[86] Skateboard safety tips from the CPSC:[87]

- Wear an approved helmet, padded clothes, special skateboarding gloves, and padding for your knees and other joints. Padding should be snug but loose enough to allow movement.
- Between uses, check your board for loose, broken, sharp, or cracked parts, and have it repaired if necessary.
- Examine the surface where you'll be riding for holes, bumps, and debris.
- Never skateboard in the street.
- Never hitch a ride from a car, bicycle, or other vehicle.
- Practice complicated stunts in specially designed areas, wearing protective padding.
- Don't speed.
- Don't ride alone.
- Don't drink and ride.

Safety in the Snow

The National Ski Areas Association (NSAA) reports that, on average during the past 10 years, there have been about 40 fatalities per year in U.S. ski areas.[88] Severe nonfatal injuries, such as head trauma and spinal cord injury, also occur, but at a similarly low rate. This makes snow sports much safer, overall, than bicycling, swimming, and many others. The rate of injury has also been declining for decades, largely because of shorter skis, improved safety

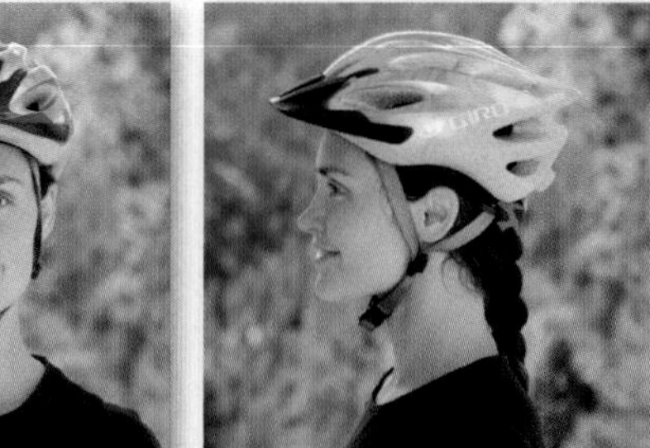

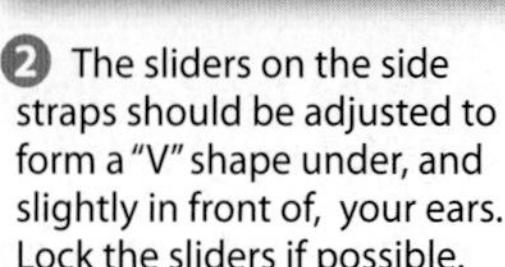

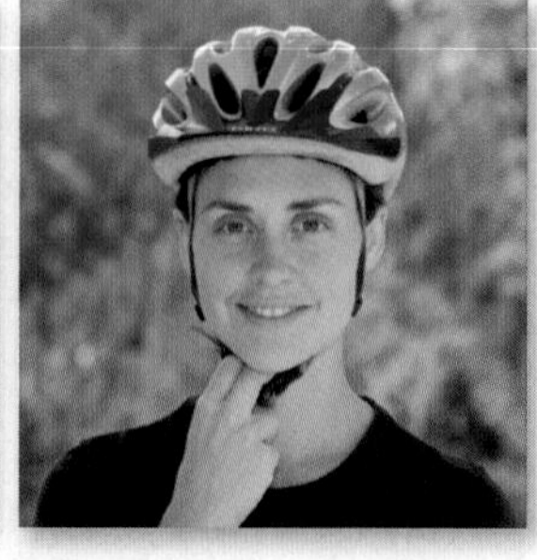

1 The helmet should sit level on your head and low on your forehead—one or two finger-widths above your eyebrows.

2 The sliders on the side straps should be adjusted to form a "V" shape under, and slightly in front of, your ears. Lock the sliders if possible.

3 The chin strap buckle should be centered under your chin. Tighten the strap until it is snug, so that no more than two fingers fit under the strap.

Figure 13.5 Fitting a Bicycle Helmet
When your helmet is fitted correctly, opening your mouth wide in a yawn should cause the helmet to pull down on your head. Also, you should not be able to rock the helmet back more than the width of two fingers above the eyebrows or forward into your eyes.

VIDEO TUTOR
Biking Safety

features on equipment, and increased safety efforts at resorts, such as having more monitors on the slopes, setting aside special family skiing areas, and encouraging helmet use.

One of the most important ways to protect yourself while skiing or snowboarding is to wear an approved helmet; helmet use reduces the risk of any head injury by 30 to 50 percent.[89] It's also important to keep skis and snowboards in good condition and to choose trails according to your ability. Pay attention to the locations of others; if you stop, move to the side of the trail. Observe all posted signs and warnings.

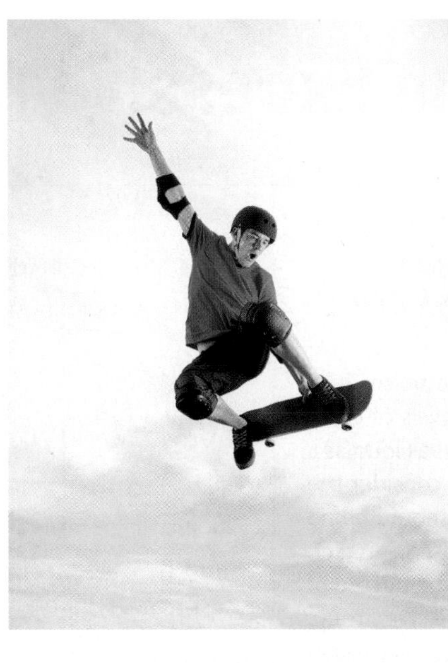

Do I really have to wear a helmet while I'm skateboarding?

The majority of skateboarding injuries occur among people who have been practicing the sport for more than a year, often when they attempt a stunt beyond their level of skill. Wearing a helmet, no matter how experienced a skateboarder you are, will help protect you in case of a fall.

Water Safety

About ten Americans die every day from unintentional drowning, making this the fifth leading cause of unintentional injury death among Americans of all ages. Males are four times more likely than females to die from unintentional drowning, and alcohol plays a significant role in many drownings: Up to 70 percent of all deaths associated with water recreation among adolescents and adults involve alcohol.[90]

Swimming Almost half of adults surveyed say they've had an experience in which they nearly drowned.[91] Most drownings occur during water recreation—swimming, diving, or just simply having fun—in unorganized or unsupervised areas, such as ponds or pools without lifeguards present. Many drowning victims were strong swimmers.

All swimmers should take the following precautions:

- Don't drink alcohol before or while swimming.
- Don't enter the water without a life jacket unless you can swim at least 50 feet unassisted.
- Know your limitations; get out of the water when you start to feel even slightly fatigued.
- Never swim alone, even if you are a skilled swimmer. You never know what might happen.
- Never leave a child unattended, even in extremely shallow water.
- Before entering water, check the depth. Most neck and back injuries result from diving into water that is too shallow.
- Never swim in a river with currents too swift for easy, relaxed swimming.
- Never swim in muddy or dirty water that obstructs your view of the bottom. Water that is discolored and choppy or foamy may indicate a rip current.
- If you're caught in a rip current, swim parallel to the shore. Once you are free of the current, swim toward the shore.
- Learn cardiopulmonary resuscitation (CPR). CPR performed by bystanders has been shown to improve outcomes in drowning victims.[92]

Boating In 2013, the U.S. Coast Guard received reports of 2,620 injured boaters and 560 deaths.[93] About 77 percent of these boating fatalities were drownings, and among those who drowned, 84 percent were not wearing a **personal flotation device**—that is, a lifejacket.[94] Although operator inattention, inexperience, excessive speed, and mechanical failure also contributed to these deaths, alcohol consumption was the leading factor.[95]

About one-third of all boating fatalities involve alcohol.[96] When boat operators are drinking, both collisions with other boats and falls overboard are much more likely. If someone who has been drinking does fall overboard, he or she is more likely to drown or to die of hypothermia. Unfortunately, the "designated driver" concept does not apply to boating—intoxicated passengers often cause or contribute to boating accidents. The U.S. Coast Guard and every state have "Boating under the Influence" (BUI) laws that carry stringent penalties, including fines, license revocation, and even jail time.[97]

Consider the following safety tips from the American Boating Association:[98]

- Before leaving home, let others know where you are going, who will be with you, and when you expect to return.
- Check the weather. Listen to advisories regarding high winds, storms, and other environmental factors.
- Even for short trips, make sure the vessel doesn't leak, has enough fuel (if powered), and has proper safety equipment.
- Make sure you have enough life jackets for all on board; make life jackets easily accessible.
- Carry an emergency radio and cell phone.
- Don't drink alcohol before you leave, and don't bring any aboard.

The U.S. Coast Guard recommends that before setting out, you put on your life jacket. Most modern life jackets are thin and flexible and can be worn comfortably all day. Children must wear a life jacket once the vessel is under way, unless they are below deck. Wear a life jacket not only when sailing or motor boating, but also when canoeing, kayaking, and rafting.

check yourself

- **What are three strategies that can help keep you safe when biking or skateboarding? In the snow? On the water?**

13.11 Avoiding Injury from Excessive Noise

learning outcome

13.11 List factors contributing to noise-induced hearing loss and explain how to protect your hearing.

Our modern society is too often filled with excessive noise. Take a look at Figure 13.6, which shows the decibel (dB) levels of common sounds. In general, noise levels above 85 dB (about as loud as a diesel truck) increase risks for hearing loss. When you consider the many such noises people are exposed to every day, it should be no surprise that hearing loss is becoming increasingly common. In fact, an estimated 48 million U.S. teens and adults have some degree of hearing loss.[99] This represents about 20 percent of this age group. Moreover, because hearing loss becomes more common with each decade we age, the prevalence of hearing loss in the United States is expected to rise as the population ages overall.

Noise-induced hearing loss results when exposure to high-decibel (high-dB) noise, usually over time, damages sensory receptors in the cochlea, or inner ear. One of the highest rates of sudden noise-induced hearing loss is among adults 20 to 29. A recent study of college students who reported having normal hearing revealed that, when tested, 12 percent showed at least moderate hearing loss.[100] The study authors identified a correlation between use of a personal music player and increased risk for hearing loss. Several other studies have also linked hearing loss in young adults to the use of portable listening devices. However, the precise decibel level, frequency, and duration of exposure that might correlate with hearing loss is currently under investigation.[101]

Another source of hearing impairment is frequent concert attendance. Most rock musicians use earplugs when performing or rehearsing, and their audiences would be wise to do the same. Hearing loss may result from one evening in front of huge speakers at a rock concert. Sporting events, such as stock car races and football games, can also be very loud. If you can't hear the person standing next to you at a concert or sporting event, then you should put in earplugs or look for a quieter spot. In addition, you should rest your ears between nights out partying or attending concerts or loud sporting events.

What can you do to avoid hearing loss while still enjoying your music? Keep the volume at or below 80 dB—a level at which you can carry on a conversation—and you won't need to limit time spent listening to music. If a friend nearby can hear your music, it's definitely too loud. And though debate continues over the relative safety of over-the-ear earphones versus ear buds, earphones seem to be safer.[102]

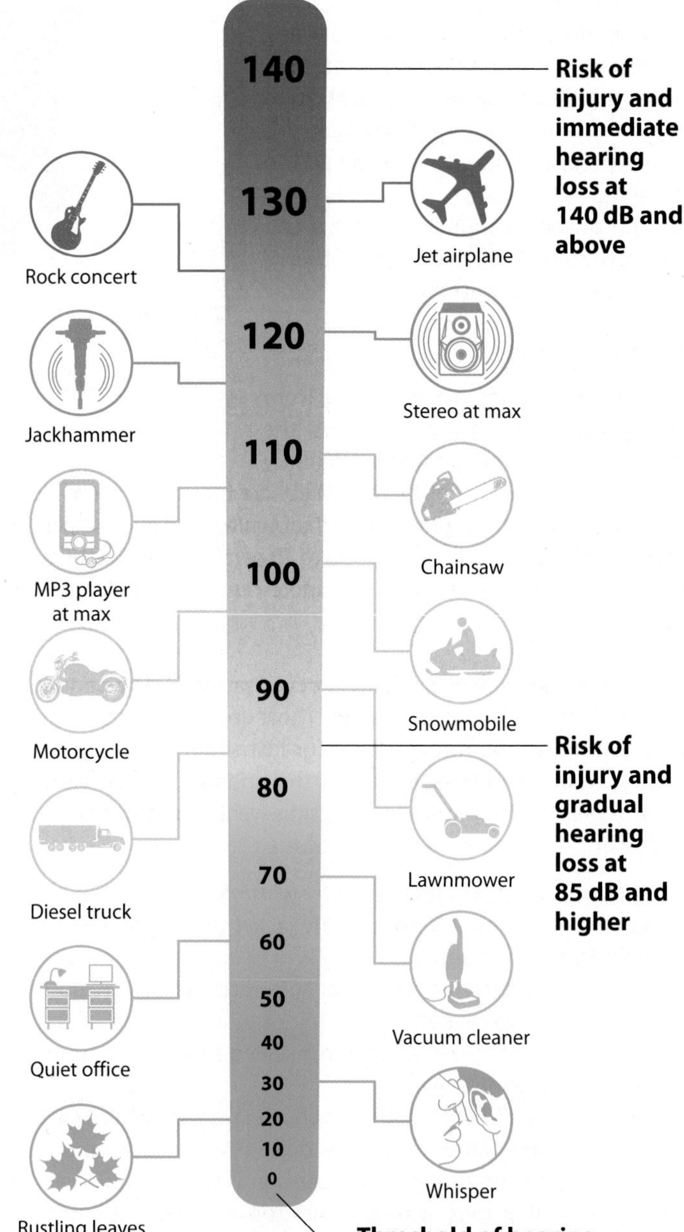

Figure 13.6 Noise Levels of Various Sounds (dB)
Decibels increase logarithmically, so each increase of 10 dB represents a tenfold increase in loudness.

Source: Adapted from National Institute on Deafness and Other Communication Disorders, "How Loud Is Too Loud? Bookmark," Updated July 2011, www.nidcd.nih.gov.

check yourself

- **What are three things you can do to avoid hearing loss?**

Safety at Home

learning outcome

13.12 List steps to take to prevent and address common household safety hazards.

Poisoning

A **poison** is any substance that is harmful when ingested, inhaled, injected, or absorbed through the skin. In 2012, the 57 poison control centers in the United States logged more than 2.2 million calls for assistance with a poisoning.[103] To prevent poisoning:[104]

- Read and follow all usage and warning labels before taking medications or working with chemicals, including household products.
- Never share or sell prescription drugs.
- Never take more than one medication at the same time without the approval of your health care provider. Mixing medications, such as a prescription drug and an OTC remedy, can result in poisoning.
- Never mix household products together; combinations can give off toxic fumes.
- When working with chemicals, wear a protective mask and make sure the area in which you work is well ventilated. Wear gloves and other protective clothing, and eyeglasses or an eye guard if splashing could occur.
- Keep medications, dietary supplements, and alcohol out of sight of children, preferably in a locked cabinet.
- Program the 24-hour national poison control number, 1-800-222-1222, into your phone.

If you suspect you have ingested or inhaled a poison or you are with someone who has collapsed, dial 9-1-1. If the victim is not breathing and you are trained in CPR, provide CPR until paramedics arrive. If the victim is awake and alert, dial the poison control hotline (1-800-222-1222). Follow the instructions given. If you go to a hospital emergency room, bring the suspected poison, if possible.

Falls

Falls are the third most common cause of death from unintentional injury and the most common cause of traumatic brain injury.[105] Although falls are most common among older adults, people of all ages experience them. To reduce your risk of falls:

- Leave nothing lying around on the floor or stairs.
- Avoid using small scatter rugs and mats. Use rubberized liners to secure large rugs to the floor.
- Train pets to stay away from your feet.
- Install slip-proof mats, treads, or decals in showers and tubs and on the stairs.
- If you need to reach something or to change a ceiling light, use an appropriate stool or ladder.
- Wear supportive shoes. Flip-flops and loose shoes can trip you.

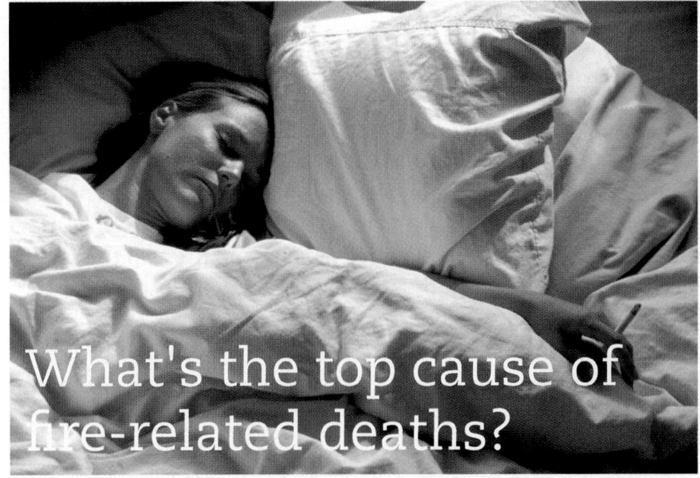

Smoking is the number one cause of fire-related deaths. If you fall asleep with a lit cigarette, bedding and clothing can quickly ignite. If you can't quit, take it outside.

Fire

In 2010, more than 2,600 Americans—not including firefighters—died in a fire.[106] The three main causes of fires in campus housing are cooking, careless smoking, and arson. However, a variety of other factors typically contribute to injuries from dormitory fires: alcohol use, ignoring of fire drills and actual alarms, poorly maintained or vandalized alarm systems, and failure to call 9-1-1.[107] To prevent fires:

- Extinguish cigarettes in ashtrays. Never smoke in bed!
- Set lamps away from drapes, linens, and paper.
- Keep kitchen cloths and sleeves away from stove burners. Use caution when lighting barbecue grills.
- Keep candles away from combustibles. Never leave candles unattended.
- Avoid overloading electrical circuits with appliances and cords.
- Have the proper fire extinguishers ready; replace batteries in smoke alarms and test them periodically.

If a fire breaks out, your priority is to get out *as soon as possible*. First, feel the door handle: If it's hot, don't open the door! Go to a window, open it wide, and call for help. Hang a sheet from the window to alert rescuers. Call 9-1-1. If smoke is entering your room, seal cracks in the door with blankets or towels. Stay low—there's less smoke close to the floor.

If the handle is not hot, open the door cautiously. If the hallway is clear, get out, yelling, "Fire!" and knocking on doors as you leave. If you encounter smoke, stay low—crawl if necessary. If you pass a fire alarm, pull it. Always use stairs, never an elevator. Once you're outside, dial 9-1-1.

check yourself

- **What are two things each that you can do to prevent household poisoning, falls, and fire?**

13.13

Avoiding Workplace Injury

learning outcome

13.13 Identify common workplace injuries and how to avoid them.

American adults spend most of their waking hours on the job. Although most job situations are pleasant and productive, others pose hazards. Transportation incidents make up the largest number of fatal work injuries (more than 40%). Workers in material moving, construction, and extraction (mining), and those in the service industry, are at high risk of fatal injuries. Farmers, fishing workers, and loggers are also at high risk.[108]

Although on-the-job deaths capture media attention, workers may also be seriously injured or disabled at their jobs. Common work injuries include cuts and lacerations, chemical burns, fractures, sprains, and strains (often of the back), and repetitive motion disorders. Because so many work injuries are due to overexertion, poor body mechanics, or repetitive motion, they are largely preventable. We discuss these problems and share some prevention strategies here.

Protect Your Back

Low back pain (LBP), usually as a result of injury, is the major cause of disability for people ages 20 to 45 in the United States; this age groups suffers more frequently and severely from this problem than older people do.[109] It is one of the most commonly experienced chronic ailments among college students. In a recent survey, 12.3 percent of college students reported having seen their doctor in the previous year because of back pain.[110]

Most injuries to the back are in the lumbar spine area (lower back); strengthening core muscle groups and stretching muscles to avoid cramping and spasms reduce risks. Frequently, sports injuries, stress on spinal bones and tissues, the sudden jolt of a car accident, or other obvious causes are the culprits. Other times, sitting too long in the same position or hunching over your computer while pulling an all-nighter can leave you with pain so severe you can't stand up or walk comfortably. Carrying heavy backpacks is another frequent source of LBP.

Avoid typical risks by using common sense when engaging in activities that could injure your back. Get up and stretch intermittently while working in a static position. Good posture can also reduce back problems.

Other measures you can take to reduce the risk of back pain:

- Invest in a high-quality, supportive mattress.
- Avoid high-heeled shoes, which tilt the pelvis forward.
- Control your weight. Extra weight puts increased strain on your knees, hips, and back.
- Warm up and stretch before exercising or lifting heavy objects.
- When lifting something heavy, use proper form (Figure 13.7). Do not bend from the waist or take the weight load on your back.
- Buy a desk chair with good lumbar support.
- Move your car seat forward so your knees are elevated slightly.
- Engage in regular exercise, particularly core exercises that strengthen and stretch abdominal muscles and back muscles.
- Downsize your backpack.

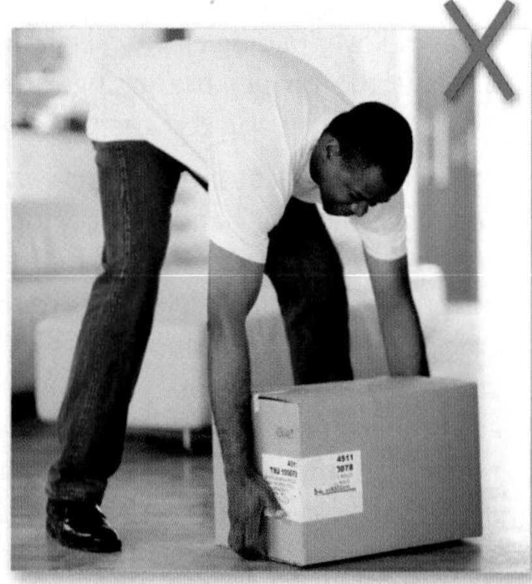

(a) Attempting to lift a heavy object by bending at your waist is a common cause of back injury.

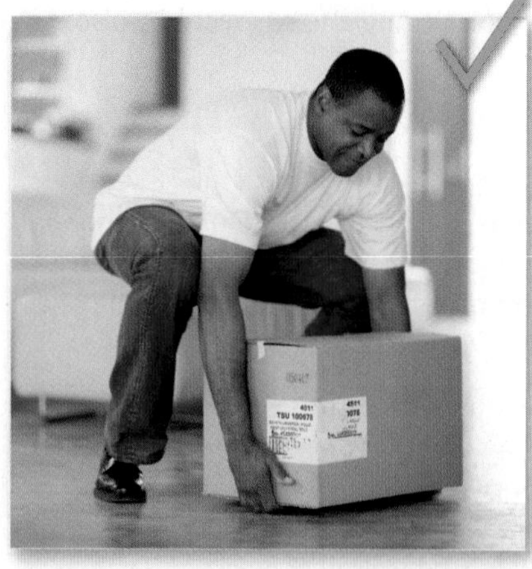

(b) Start as close to the object as possible, with it positioned between your knees as you squat down. Keep your feet parallel, or stagger one foot in front of the other. Keep the object close to your body as you stand, using your legs, not your back, to lift.

Figure 13.7 Lifting a Heavy Object

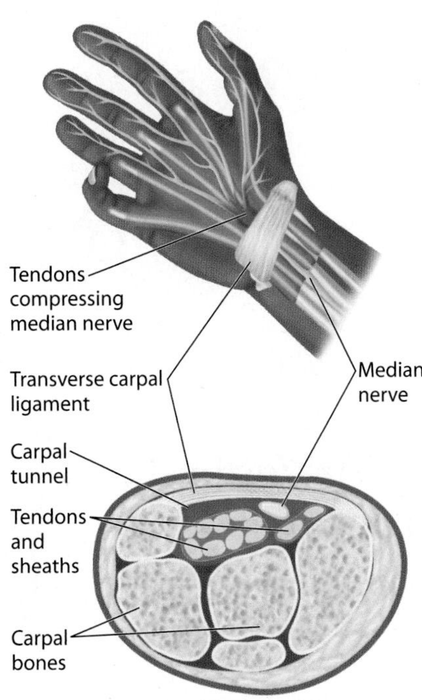

Figure 13.8 Carpal Tunnel Syndrome
The carpal tunnel is a space beneath the transverse carpal ligament and above the carpal bones of the wrist. The median nerve and the tendons that allow you to flex your fingers run through this tunnel. Carpal tunnel syndrome occurs when repetitive use prompts inflammation of the tissues and fluids of the tunnel. This, in turn, compresses the median nerve.

Maintain Alignment while Sitting

Think back over your day: How many hours have you sat glued to a computer or book? Were you slouching, hunched over, or sitting up straight? Your answers are probably reflected in the degree of aching and stiffness you may be feeling right now. So how can you maintain healthy alignment while you work? Try these strategies:

1. Sit comfortably with your feet flat on the floor or on a footrest, and your knees level with your hips. Raise or lower your chair, or move to a different chair, to achieve this position.
2. Your middle back should be firmly against the back of the chair. The small of your back should be supported, too. If you can't feel the chair back supporting your lumbar region, try placing a small cushion or rolled towel behind the curve of your lower back.
3. Keep your shoulders relaxed and straight, not rolled or hunched forward.
4. The angle of your elbows should be 90 degrees to your upper arms. Adjust your position or the position of your device to achieve this angle.
5. Ideally, you should be looking straight ahead, not peering down at the device's screen.

Avoid Repetitive Motion Disorders

It's the end of the term, and you've finished the last of several papers. After hours of nonstop typing, your hands are numb and you feel intense pain that makes the thought of typing one more word unbearable. You may be suffering from one of several **repetitive motion disorders (RMDs)**, sometimes called *overuse syndrome, cumulative trauma disorders*, or *repetitive stress injuries*. These refer to a family of soft tissue injuries that begin with inflammation and gradually become disabling.

Repetitive motion disorders include carpal tunnel syndrome, bursitis, tendonitis, and ganglion cysts, among others. Twisting of the arm or wrist, overexertion, and incorrect posture or position are usually contributors. The areas most likely to be affected are the hands, wrists, elbows, and shoulders, but the neck, back, hips, knees, feet, ankles, and legs can be affected, too. Over time, RMDs can cause permanent damage to nerves, soft tissue, and joints. Usually, RMDs are associated with repeating the same task and gradually irritating the area in question. Certain sports (tennis, golf, and others), gripping the wheel while driving, keyboarding or texting, and a number of technology-driven activities can also result in RMDs.

Because many of these injuries occur in everyday work, play, and athletics, they are often not reported to national agencies that keep track of injury statistics. Nevertheless, cases of "BlackBerry thumb," carpal tunnel syndrome, and other maladies are widespread.

One of the most common RMDs is **carpal tunnel syndrome (CTS)**, an inflammation of the soft tissues and fluids within the "tunnel" through the carpal bones of the wrist (Figure 13.8). This puts pressure on the median nerve, which runs down the forearm through the tunnel. Symptoms include numbness, tingling, and pain in the fingers and hands. Carpal tunnel syndrome typically results from spending hours typing at the computer keyboard, flipping groceries through computerized scanners, or manipulating other objects in jobs "made simpler" by technology. The risk for CTS can be reduced by proper design of workstations, protective wrist pads, and worker training. Physical and occupational therapy is an important part of treatment and recovery.

Strategies for avoiding repetitive motion disorders include:[111]

- If you are doing repetitive motion activities such as taking notes in class by hand, reduce your force and relax your grip. There are pens available that offer oversized grips and free-flowing ink, which lessen the strain on your hand.
- Take frequent breaks to stretch your hands and wrists.
- Keep your hands and fingers warm. A cold environment can lead to stiffness and hand pain. You may need to wear fingerless gloves if you can't control your environment.

check yourself

- **What are two strategies to protect your back?**
- **What workplace factors contribute to repetitive motion disorders?**
- **What can you do to maintain healthy alignment in your study and work areas?**

Assessyourself

13.14

Are You at Risk for Violence or Injury?

An interactive version of this assessment is available online in MasteringHealth.

How often are you at risk for sustaining an intentional or unintentional injury? Answer the questions below to find out.

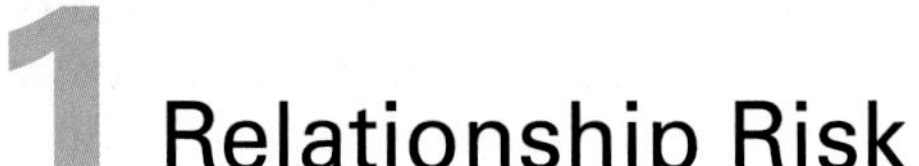

1 Relationship Risk

How often does your partner:

	Never	Sometimes	Often
1. Criticize you for your appearance (weight, dress, hair, etc.)?	○	○	○
2. Embarrass you in front of others by putting you down?	○	○	○
3. Blame you or others for his or her mistakes?	○	○	○
4. Curse at you, shout at you, say mean things, insult, or mock you?	○	○	○
5. Demonstrate uncontrollable anger?	○	○	○
6. Criticize your friends, family, or others who are close to you?	○	○	○
7. Threaten to leave you if you don't behave in a certain way?	○	○	○
8. Manipulate you to prevent you from spending time with friends or family?	○	○	○
9. Express jealousy, distrust, and anger when you spend time with other people?	○	○	○
10. Make all the significant decisions in your relationship?	○	○	○
11. Intimidate or threaten you, making you fearful or anxious?	○	○	○
12. Make threats to harm others you care about, including pets?	○	○	○
13. Control your telephone calls, monitor your messages, or read your e-mail without permission.	○	○	○
14. Punch, hit, slap, or kick you?	○	○	○
15. Make you feel guilty about something?	○	○	○
16. Use money or possessions to control you?	○	○	○
17. Force you to perform sexual acts that make you uncomfortable or embarrassed?	○	○	○
18. Threaten to kill himself or herself if you leave?	○	○	○
19. Follow you, call to check on you, or demonstrate a constant obsession with what you are doing?	○	○	○

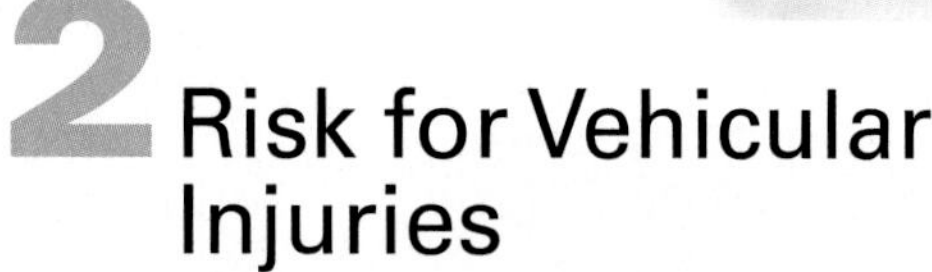

2 Risk for Vehicular Injuries

How often do you:

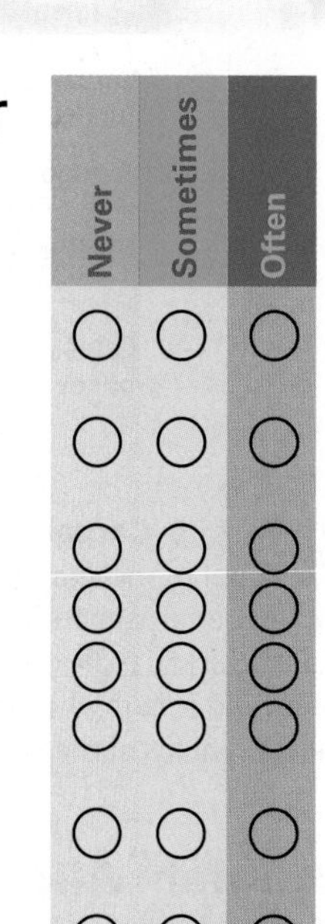

	Never	Sometimes	Often
1. Drive after you have had one or two drinks?	○	○	○
2. Drive after you have had three or more drinks?	○	○	○
3. Drive when you are tired?	○	○	○
4. Drive while you are extremely upset?	○	○	○
5. Drive while using your cell phone?	○	○	○
6. Drive or ride in a car while not wearing a seat belt?	○	○	○
7. Drive faster than the speed limit?	○	○	○
8. Accept rides from friends who have been drinking?	○	○	○

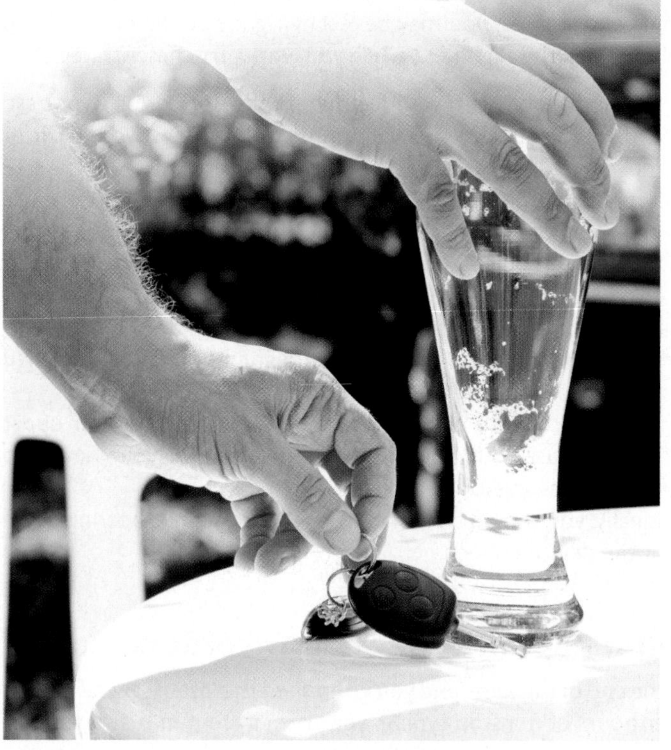

3 Online Safety

How often do you:

	Never	Sometimes	Often
1. Give out your name/address on the Internet?	○	○	○
2. Put personal identifying information on your blog, Facebook, or other websites?	○	○	○
3. Post personal pictures, travel/vacation plans, and other private material on social networking sites?	○	○	○
4. Date people you meet online?	○	○	○
5. Use a shared or public computer to check e-mail without clearing the browser cache?	○	○	○
6. Make financial transactions online without confirming security measures?	○	○	○

4 Risk for Assault or Rape

How often do you:

	Never	Sometimes	Often
1. Drink more than 1 or 2 drinks while out with friends or at a party?	○	○	○
2. Leave your drinks unattended while you get up to dance or go to the bathroom?	○	○	○
3. Accept drinks from strangers while out at a bar or party?	○	○	○
4. Leave parties with people you barely know or just met?	○	○	○
5. Walk alone in poorly lit or unfamiliar places?	○	○	○
6. Open the door to strangers?	○	○	○
7. Leave your car or home door unlocked?	○	○	○
8. Talk on your cell phone, oblivious to your surroundings?	○	○	○

Analyzing Your Responses

Look at your responses to the list of questions in each of these sections. Part 1 focused on relationships—if you answered "sometimes" or "often" to several of these questions, you may need to evaluate your situation. In Parts 2 through 4, if you answered "often" to any question, you may need to adjust your behavior and educate yourself about steps you can take to remain safe.

Your Plan for Change

The Assess Yourself activity gave you a chance to consider symptoms of abuse in your relationships and signs of unsafe behavior in other realms of your life. Now that you are aware of these signs and symptoms, you can work on changing behaviors to reduce your risk.

Today, you can:

○ Pay attention as you walk your normal route around campus and think about whether you are taking the safest route. Is it well lit? Do you walk in areas that receive little foot traffic? Are there any emergency phone boxes along your route? Does campus security patrol the area? If part of your route seems unsafe, look around for alternate routes. Vary your route when possible.

○ Look at your residence's safety features. Is there a secure lock, dead bolt, or keycard entry system on all outer doors? Can windows be shut and locked? Is there a working smoke alarm in every room and hallway? Are the outside areas well lit? If you live in a dorm or apartment building, is there a security guard at the main entrance? If you notice any potential safety hazards, report them to your landlord or campus residential life administrator right away.

Within the next 2 weeks, you can:

○ If you are worried about potentially abusive behavior in a partner or in a friend's partner, visit the campus counseling center and ask about resources on campus or in your community to help you deal with potential relationship abuse. Consider talking to a counselor about your concerns or sitting in on a support group.

○ Next time you attend a party, set limits for yourself in order to remain in control of your behavior and to avoid putting yourself in a dangerous or compromising position. Decide ahead of time on the number of drinks you will have, arrange with a friend to monitor each other's behavior during the party, and be sure you have a reliable, safe way of getting home.

By the end of the semester, you can:

○ Learn ways to protect yourself by signing up for a self-defense workshop or violence prevention class on campus or in the community.

○ Get involved in an on-campus or community group dedicated to promoting safety. You might want to attend a meeting of an antiviolence group, join in a Take Back the Night rally, or volunteer at a local rape crisis center or battered women's shelter.

Summary

To hear an MP3 Tutor session, scan here or visit the Study Area in **MasteringHealth.**

LO 13.1 Factors that lead people to be violent include economic difficulties, parental influence, cultural beliefs, discrimination, political differences, substance abuse, stress, excessive fear, anger, and a history of violence.

LO 13.2–LO 13.5 Interpersonal violence includes homicide, domestic violence, child abuse, elder abuse, and sexual victimization. Each of these causes significant emotional, social, and physical risks to health.

LO 13.6 Forms of collective violence, including gang violence and terrorism, result in fear, anxiety, and issues of discrimination.

LO 13.7 Recognizing how to protect yourself, knowing where to get help, and having honest, straightforward dialogue in dating situations can help reduce the risk of becoming a victim of violence.

LO 13.8 Shootings and extreme acts of violence on campuses have resulted in a groundswell of activities designed to protect students. Preventing violence means community activism; prioritizing mental and emotional health; and skills training in anger management, coping, parenting, and other key areas.

LO 13.9 Distracted driving, impaired driving, and road rage are factors in an overwhelming number of motor vehicle accidents. A well-designed and well-maintained vehicle can reduce the likelihood and severity of accidents, as can simple risk-management techniques.

LO 13.10 Basic safety guidelines—including wearing appropriate safety gear and staying sober—can help people stay safe during sports and recreation.

LO 13.11 High-decibel noise can lead to hearing loss; music listeners should keep earphone volume to a reasonable level and use earplugs or distance themselves from speakers to protect hearing at concerts and similar events.

LO 13.12 To stay safe at home, know how to prevent—and what to do in the event of—poisoning, fire, and injury.

LO 13.13 In the workplace, proper ergonomics can help prevent injuries and repetitive motion disorders.

Pop Quiz

Visit MasteringHealth to personalize your study plan with Chapter Review Quizzes and Dynamic Study Modules.

LO 13.2 1. An example of an *intentional injury* is
a. a car crash.
b. murder.
c. drowning.
d. road rage.

LO 13.3 2. Jack beats his wife Melissa "to teach her a lesson." Afterward, he denies attacking her. The phase of the cycle of violence that this illustrates is
a. acute battering.
b. chronic battering.
c. remorse/reconciliation.
d. tension building.

LO 13.4 3. In a sociology class, students were discussing sexual assault. One student commented that some women dress too provocatively. The social assumption this student made is
a. minimization.
b. trivialization.
c. blaming the victim.
d. "boys will be boys."

LO 13.4 4. Rape by a person the victim knows and that does not involve a physical beating or use of a weapon is called
a. simple rape.
b. sexual assault.
c. simple assault.
d. aggravated rape.

LO 13.5 5. Which of the following is an example of stalking?
a. Making intimate and sexually implied comments to another person
b. Repeated visual, physical, or virtual seeking out of another person
c. Unwelcome sexual conduct by the perpetrator
d. Sexual abuse of a child

LO 13.5 6. When Sofia began her new job with all male coworkers, her supervisor told her that he enjoyed having an attractive woman in the workplace, and he winked at her. His comment constitutes
a. acquaintance rape.
b. sexual assault.
c. sexual harassment.
d. sexual battering.

LO 13.9 7. Which of the following is *not* a good response to another driver's road rage?
a. Avoid eye contact.
b. Remember the person's license plate number.
c. Drive home immediately.
d. Drive to the nearest police station.

LO 13.10 8. The majority of skateboarding accidents happen to riders who
a. are new to the sport.
b. have been riding for more than a year.
c. are trying out new equipment.
d. are skating on public property.

LO 13.11 9. Above what decibel level do risks for hearing loss increase?
a. 70 dB (vacuum cleaner)
b. 85 dB (diesel truck engine)
c. 108 dB (MP3 player at maximum volume)
d. 130 dB (jet airplane engine)

LO 13.13 10. Which of the following is a common factor in repetitive motion disorders?
a. Incorrectly aligned computer workstation setup
b. Keeping a heavy object close to your body when lifting it off the ground
c. Looking straight ahead at a computer screen
d. Keeping hands and fingers too warm when you're typing for long periods

Answers to these questions can be found on page A-1. If you answered a question incorrectly, review the module identified by the Learning Outcome. For even more study tools, visit MasteringHealth.

Environmental Health 14

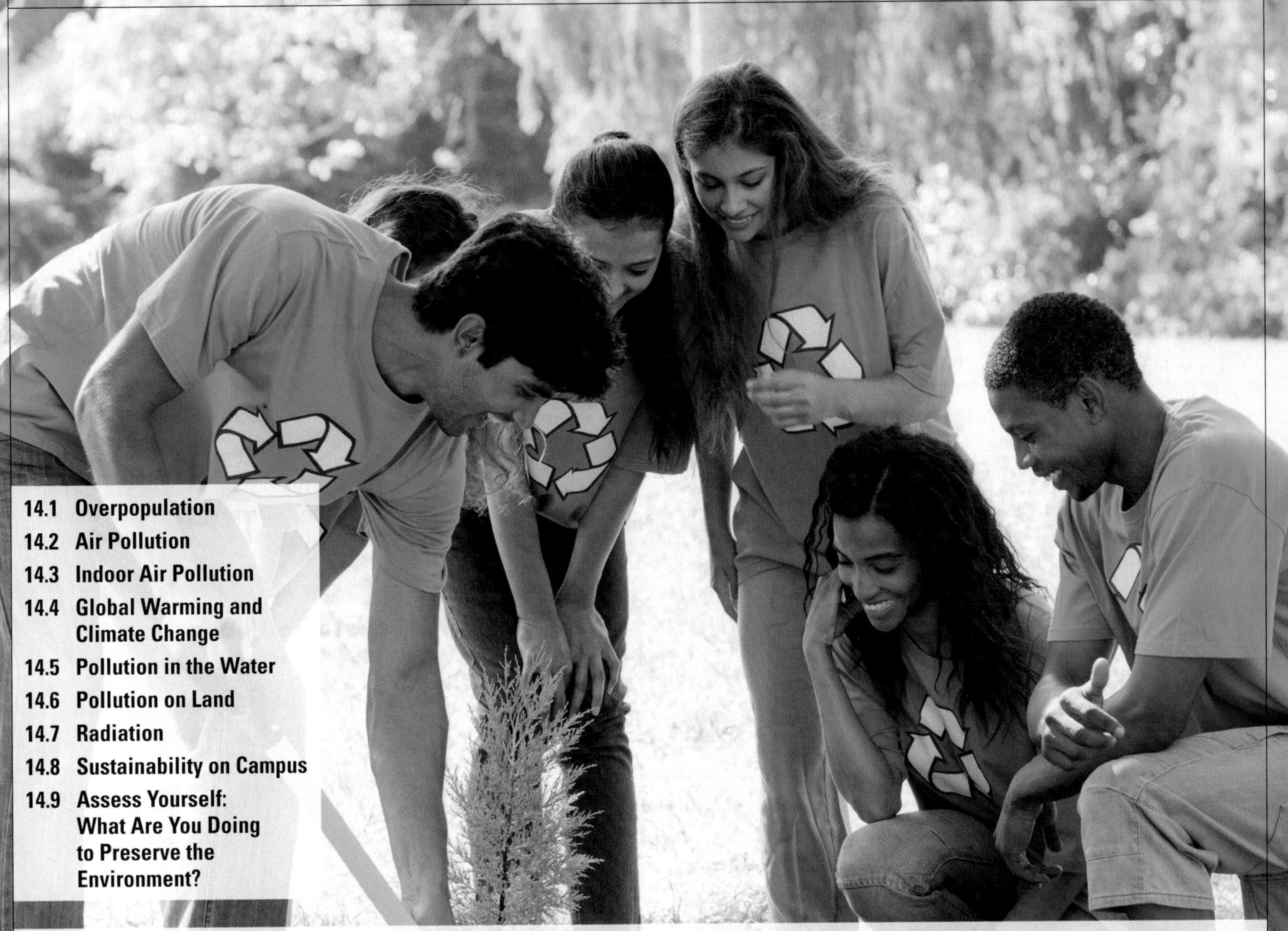

". . . The fact is, the 12 hottest years on record have all come in the last 15. Heat waves, droughts, wildfires, and floods—all are now more frequent and intense. We can choose to believe that Superstorm Sandy, and the most severe drought in decades, and the worst wildfires some states have ever seen were all just a freak coincidence. Or we can choose to believe in the overwhelming judgment of science—and act before it's too late."

—President Barack Obama, 2013 State of the Union address, February 12, 2013.

The global population has grown more in the past 50 years than at any other time in history. Polar ice caps are melting at rates that defy even the direst predictions, and threats of rising sea levels loom. One in 4 existing mammals is threatened with extinction as humans destroy habitat, exacerbate drought and flooding through climate change, and pollute the environment. Clean water is becoming increasingly scarce, fossil fuels are dwindling quickly, and solid and hazardous wastes are growing in proportion to population.

Have we crossed the point at which we will be unable to restore the balance between humans and nature? We must understand the factors that contribute to our global environmental crisis, and know what actions individuals, communities, and political powers need to take to bring the environmental health of planet Earth back into balance. This chapter gives an overview of these factors and actions.

14.1 Overpopulation

learning outcome

14.1 List factors affecting population growth and overpopulation.

Anthropologist Margaret Mead wrote, "Every human society is faced with not one population problem but two: how to beget and rear enough children and how not to beget and rear too many."[1] The United Nations projects that the world population will grow from its current level of 7 billion to 9.3 billion by 2050 and to 10.1 billion by 2100 (Figure 14.1)[2]—assuming a fairly constant **fertility rate**, the average number of births per woman in a specific country or region. Recent data indicate that the fertility rates have increased significantly, particularly in the developing regions of the world, leading many to believe that our population projections may grossly underestimate what may really happen in the next decades.[3] Much of the overall population increase is projected to occur in high-fertility regions such as Africa, as well as countries with large populations such as India, China, Brazil, the Russian Federation, Indonesia, and the United States.[4]

Factors Affecting Population Growth

A number of factors have led to the world population's increase. Key among them are changes in fertility and mortality rates. The global fertility rate in the world has declined to an average of 2.5 births for women. While Europe, the United States, Mexico, China, and others have shown consistent declines in recent years, other countries such as Niger and Somalia continue to have higher fertility rates (see Table 14.1). Today, the U.S. fertility rate is approximately two births per woman, slightly more than "replacement" values necessary to sustain population growth and less than the global rate.[5]

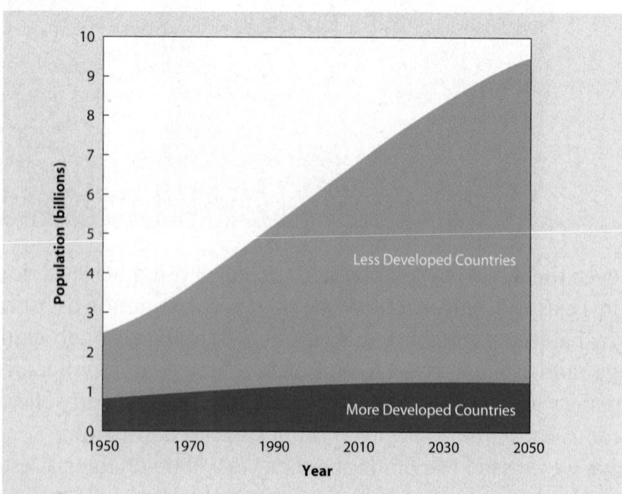

Figure 14.1 Projected World Population Growth, 1950–2300

Source: Population Reference Bureau, *2013 World Population Data Sheet*, 2013, www.prb.org.

Historically, in countries where women have little education and little control over reproductive choices, and where birth control is either not available or frowned upon, pregnancy rates continue to rise. As women become more educated, obtain higher socioeconomic status, work more outside of the home, and have more control over reproduction, fertility rates decline. Many countries have enacted strict population control measures or have encouraged their citizens to limit the size of their families. Proponents of *zero population growth* believe that each couple should produce only two offspring, allowing the population to stabilize.

Mortality rates from chronic and infectious diseases have declined as a result of improved public health infrastructure, increased availability of drugs and vaccines, better disaster preparedness, and other factors. As people live longer, they use more of the Earth's resources, too.

Differing Growth Rates The country projected to have the largest increase in population in coming decades is India, adding another 600 million people by 2050, surpassing China as the most populous nation.[6] With a current population of over 318 million and a net gain of one person every 13 seconds after accounting

TABLE **14.1 Selected Total Fertility Rates Worldwide, 2013**

Country	Number of Children Born per Woman*
Niger	7.58
Chad	7.00
Somalia	6.86
India	2.50
Mexico	2.20
United States	1.97
Australia	1.88
Canada	1.67
China	1.66
Russia	1.53
Germany	1.42
Japan	1.41

*Indicates the average number of children that would be born per woman if all women lived to the end of their childbearing years and bore children according to a given fertility rate at each age.

Source: Data from Population Reference Bureau, "World Population Data Sheet–2013," 2014, www.prb.org.

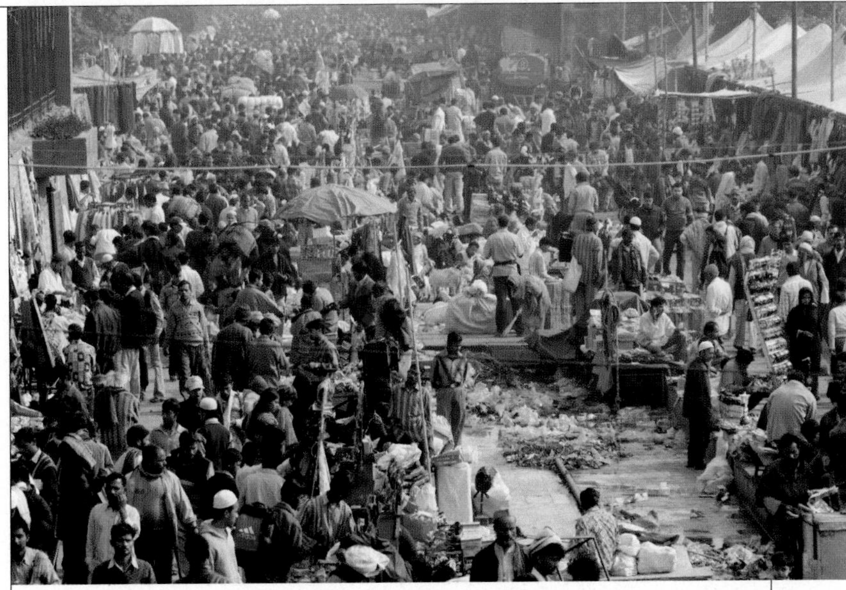

for births, deaths, and international migration into the country, the United States leads most other industrialized nations in growth. It also has one of the largest "ecological footprints," exerting a greater impact on many of the planet's resources than most other nations.[7]

Measuring the Impact of People

Today, experts are analyzing the **carrying capacity of the earth**—the largest population that can be supported indefinitely, given the resources available in the environment. At what point will we be unable to restore the balance between humans and nature? Since 1996, the global demand for natural resources has doubled. It now takes 1.5 years to regenerate the renewable resources used in 1 year by humans. By 2030, one report indicates that it will take the equivalent of two planets to meet the demand for resources.[8] Evidence of the effects of unchecked population growth is everywhere:

- **Impact on other species.** Changes in the **ecosystem** are resulting in mass destruction of many species and their habitats. Rain forests are being depleted, oceans are being polluted, and over half of the world's wetlands have been lost in the last century.[9] Twelve percent of all birds are threatened, more than 100 species of mammals are already extinct, and tiger populations have declined by 95 percent in the last century.[10] In spite of major efforts to stop organized crime's international killing of elephants for ivory, nearly 20,000 African elephants were slaughtered in Africa in 2013, causing many to question their ultimate survival.[11] About a third of amphibians (frogs, toads, and salamanders) are already gone, and many of those that survive have chemically induced ailments or genetic mutations that will hasten their demise. Along with mammals, rapid declines in plant species are reasons for concern.[12]
- **Impact on the food supply.** We are currently fishing the oceans at rates that are 250 percent more than they can regenerate, and scientists project a global collapse of all fish species by 2050.[13]

  Aquatic ecosystems continue to be heavily contaminated by chemical and human waste. Recent reports indicate that our oceans are 30 percent more acidic now than they were just 200 years ago, largely due to human-caused pollutants. Living coral reefs that support aquatic life have declined by over 50 percent in the last 27 years, with virtual dead zones stretching for miles on ocean floors.[14] Other threats such as radiation and invasive species add to contaminants, which hasten the demise of natural sea life and lead to increased fish farms rather than wild fish catches.

  Today, our global quest for enough food means that increasing amounts of the earth's surface are used for agriculture. Because agriculture accounts for over 90 percent of our global water footprint, groundwater withdrawals have tripled in the last 50 years, which puts increased pressure on dwindling water reserves.[15] Drought and erosion and natural disasters make growing food increasingly difficult, and food shortages and famine are occurring in many regions of the world with increasing frequency.
- **Land degradation and contamination of drinking water.** The per capita availability of freshwater is declining rapidly, and contaminated water remains the greatest single environmental cause of human illness. Unsustainable land use and climate change are increasing land degradation, including erosion, toxic chemical infiltration, nutrient depletion, deforestation, and other problems that will inevitably affect human life.
- **Energy consumption.** "Use it *and* lose it" is an apt saying for our use of nonrenewable energy sources in the form of **fossil fuels** (oil, coal, natural gas). Although we are seeing a shift toward renewable energy sources, such as hydropower, solar power, and wind power, the predominant energy sources are still fossil fuels. The United States is the largest consumer of liquid fossil fuels and natural gas,[16] and in many developing regions of the world, movement toward greater industrialization and citizen affluence has also resulted in skyrocketing demand for limited fossil fuels.

Why is population growth an environmental issue?

Every year the global population grows by 90 million, but Earth's resources are not expanding. Population increases are believed responsible for most current environmental stress.

check yourself

- **What are some contributing factors for overpopulation worldwide?**
- **Name three impacts of overpopulation on the environment.**

14.2 Air Pollution

learning outcome

14.2 Identify the major factors contributing to air pollution.

The term *air pollution* refers to the presence of substances (suspended particles and vapors) not found in perfectly clean air. Natural events, living creatures, and toxic by-products have always polluted the environment. What is new is the vast array of **pollutants**, their concentrations, and their potential interactive effects.

Air pollutants are either *naturally occurring* or *anthropogenic* (human caused). Naturally occurring air pollutants include particulate matter, such as ash from volcanic eruptions. Anthropogenic sources include those caused by *stationary sources* (e.g., power plants, factories, and refineries) and *mobile sources* such as vehicles.[17] According to the Environmental Protection Agency (EPA), mobile sources are the major contributors of key air pollutants such as carbon monoxide (CO), sulfur oxide (SO_x), and nitrogen oxide (NO_x). Motor vehicles alone contribute nearly 30 percent of all CO emissions.[18] Mopeds and scooters contribute their share of air pollution too. Whether idling or at full throttle, scientists report that scooters and mopeds emit fine particle aromatic hydrocarbons and other chemicals, which constitute a considerable health risk if you are sitting behind them in traffic or in cities where the air is concentrated with scooter exhaust.[19]

Components of Air Pollution

Concern about air quality prompted Congress to pass the Clean Air Act in 1970 and to amend it several times since then. The goal was to develop standards for six of the most widespread air pollutants that seriously affect health: sulfur dioxide, particulates, carbon monoxide, nitrogen dioxide, ground-level ozone, and lead. There have been major decreases in these six criteria pollutants, even as populations have increased in the United States. However, ozone and particulate matter continue to be present at significant levels.[20]

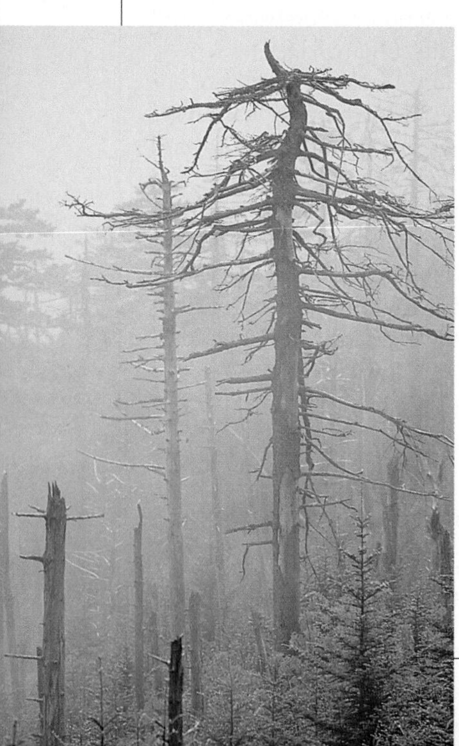

Acid deposition has many harmful effects on the environment. Because its toxins seep into groundwater and enter the food chain, it also poses health hazards to humans.

Photochemical Smog

Smog is a brownish haze produced by the photochemical reaction of sunlight with hydrocarbons, nitrogen compounds, and other gases in vehicle exhaust. It is sometimes called *ozone pollution* because ozone is a main component of smog. Smog tends to form in areas that experience a **temperature inversion**, in which a cool layer of air is trapped under a layer of warmer air, preventing the air from circulating. Smog is more likely to occur in valley areas surrounded by hills or mountains, such as Los Angeles and Mexico City. The most noticeable adverse effects of smog are difficulty breathing, burning eyes, headaches, and nausea. Long-term exposure poses serious health risks, particularly for children, older adults, pregnant women, and people with chronic respiratory disorders.

When the AQI is in this range:	... air quality conditions are	... as symbolized by this color:
0 to 50	Good	Green
51 to 100	Moderate	Yellow
101 to 150	Unhealthy for sensitive groups	Orange
151 to 200	Unhealthy	Red
201 to 300	Very unhealthy	Purple
301 to 500	Hazardous	Maroon

Figure 14.2 Air Quality Index (AQI)
The EPA provides individual AQIs for ground-level ozone, particle pollution, carbon monoxide, sulfur dioxide, and nitrogen dioxide. All AQIs are presented using the general values, categories, and colors of this figure.
Source: U.S. Environmental Protection Agency, "Air Quality Index: A Guide to Air Quality and Your Health," Updated May 2014, http://airnow.gov.

Air Quality Index

The Air Quality Index (AQI) is a measure of how clean or polluted the air is on a given day and if there are any health concerns related to air quality. The AQI focuses on health effects that can happen within a few hours or days after breathing polluted air.

The AQI scale is from 0 to 500: The higher the AQI value, the greater the level of air pollution and associated health risks. An AQI value of 100 generally corresponds to the national air quality standard for the pollutant, which is the level the EPA has set to protect public health. AQI values below 100 are generally considered satisfactory. When AQI values rise above 100, air quality is considered unhealthy at certain levels for specific groups of people and at higher levels for everyone. As shown in Figure 14.2, the EPA has divided the AQI scale into six categories with corresponding color codes. National and local weather reports generally include information on the day's AQI.

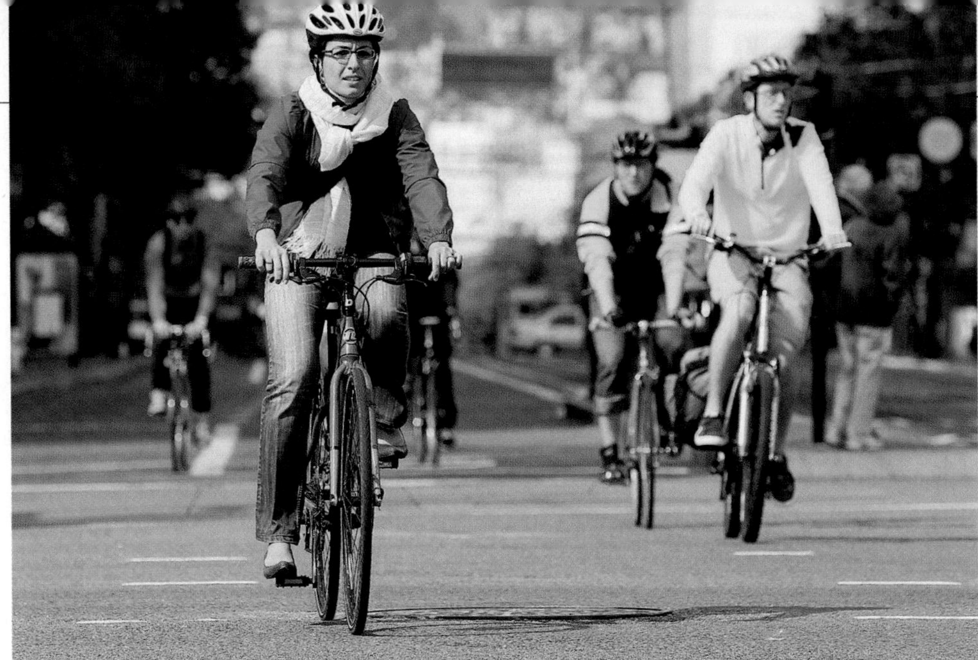

What can I do to reduce air pollution?

Much of the rise in air pollution is directly related to excess carbon dioxide (CO_2) released from burning carbon-containing fossil fuels. When you drive your car, for example, the burning of these fossil fuels emits CO_2 into the atmosphere. Making small changes such as driving less, riding your bike more, taking public transportation, or carpooling can help reduce your contribution to air pollution in the environment.

Acid Deposition and Acid Rain

Acid deposition (replacing the term *acid rain*) refers to the deposition of *wet* (rain, snow, sleet, fog, cloud water, and dew) and *dry* (acidifying particles and gases) acidic components that fall to the earth in dust or smoke.[21] Sulfur dioxide (SO_2) and NO_x cause damage to plants, aquatic animals, forests, and humans over time. In the United States, roughly two-thirds of all sulfur dioxide and one-fourth of all nitrogen oxides come from electric power generation that relies on burning fossil fuels.[22] When coal-powered plants, oil refineries, and other facilities burn these fuels, the sulfur and nitrogen in the emissions combine with oxygen and sunlight to become SO_2 and NO_x. Small acid particles are then carried by the wind and combine with moisture to produce acidic rain or snow.[23]

Acid deposition gradually acidifies ponds, lakes, and other bodies of water. Once the acidity reaches a certain level, plant and animal life cannot survive.[24] Ironically, acidified lakes and ponds become a clear deep blue, giving the illusion of beauty and health. Every year, acid deposition destroys millions of trees; much of the world's forestlands are now experiencing damaging levels of acid deposition.[25]

Acid deposition aggravates and may even cause bronchitis, asthma, and other respiratory problems, and people with emphysema or heart disease may suffer from exposure, as may developing fetuses.[26] Acid deposition can cause metals such as aluminum, cadmium, lead, and mercury to **leach** out of the soil. If these metals make their way into water or food supplies, they can cause cancer in humans.

Although there have been substantial reductions in SO_2 and NO_x emissions from power plants that use the fossil fuels coal, gas, and oil in the last decade, full recovery is still years away. Global pressure to reduce use and invest in technology to dramatically reduce emissions from coal production and burning was a key aspect of 2012 global environmental meetings in Rio de Janeiro and in other parts of the world. Although coal is "cleaner" than it was a decade ago from a production standpoint, the idea of "clean coal" is far from reality.[27]

Ozone Layer Depletion

The ozone layer forms a protective stratum in Earth's stratosphere—the highest level of our atmosphere, 12 to 30 miles above Earth's surface. The ozone layer protects our planet and its inhabitants from ultraviolet B (UVB) radiation, a primary cause of skin cancer. Such radiation damages DNA and weakens immune systems.

In the 1970s, instruments developed to test atmospheric contents indicated that chemicals used on Earth, especially **chlorofluorocarbons** or **CFCs** (used in products such as refrigerants and hair sprays), were contributing to the ozone layer's rapid depletion. When released into the air through spraying or off-gassing, CFCs migrate into the ozone layer, where they decompose and release chlorine atoms. These atoms cause ozone molecules to break apart and ozone levels to be depleted.

The U.S. government banned the use of aerosol sprays containing CFCs in the 1970s. The discovery of an ozone "hole" over Antarctica led to treaties whereby the United States and other nations agreed to further reduce the use of CFCs and other ozone-depleting chemicals. Today, more than 197 United Nations countries have agreed to basic protocols designed to preserve and protect the ozone layer.[28]

check yourself

- **What are four factors contributing to air pollution?**
- **How can you reduce air pollution as an individual? What types of government policy interventions could reduce air pollution?**

14.3 Indoor Air Pollution

learning outcome

14.3 Identify pollutants that affect indoor air quality.

A growing body of evidence indicates that the air *inside* buildings can be much more hazardous than outdoor air even in the most industrialized cities. Potentially dangerous chemical compounds can increase risks of cancer, contribute to respiratory problems, reduce the immune system's ability to fight disease, and increase problems with allergies and allergic reactions.

Age, preexisting medical conditions, and respiratory function can affect your risk of being affected by indoor air pollution.[29] Those with allergies may be particularly vulnerable, as may those living in newer airtight, energy-efficient homes. Health effects may develop over years of exposure or may occur in response to toxic levels of pollutants.

Prevention of indoor air pollution should focus on three main areas: *source control* (eliminating or reducing individual contaminants), *ventilation improvements* (increasing the amount of outdoor air coming indoors), and *air cleaners* (removing particulates from the air).[30]

Sources of Indoor Air Pollution

The main sources of indoor air pollution are as follows.

Environmental Tobacco Smoke Perhaps the greatest source of indoor air pollution is *environmental tobacco smoke* (*ETS*), also known as secondhand smoke, which contains carbon monoxide and cancer-causing particulates. The level of carbon monoxide in cigarette smoke in enclosed spaces has been found to be 4,000 times higher than that allowed in the clean air standard established by the EPA.[31] The only effective way to eliminate ETS is to enact strict no-smoking policies. Many U.S. cities ban smoking in public places, at worksites, and in automobiles where children are present.

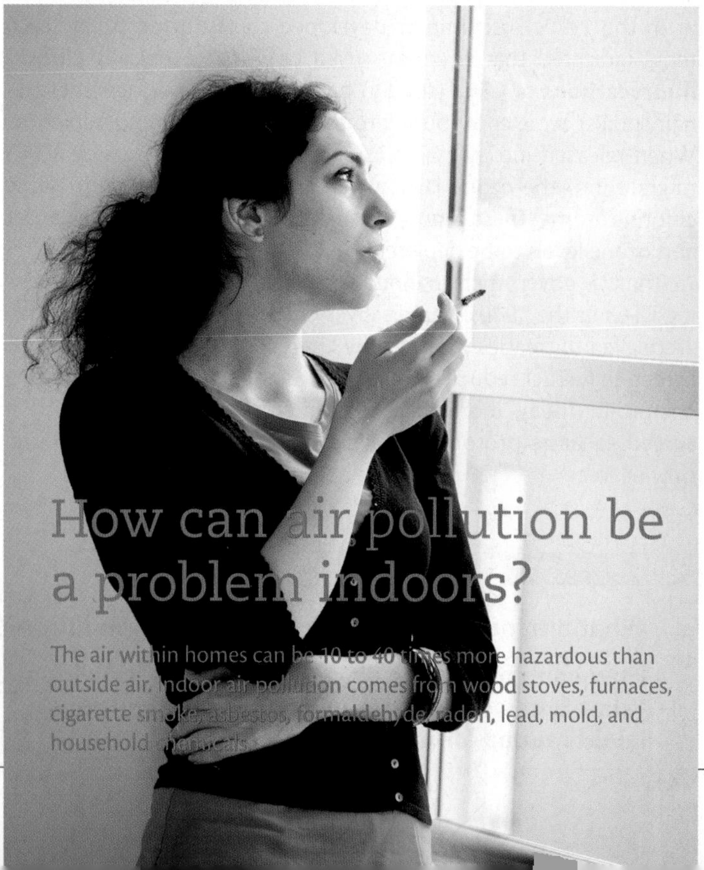

How can air pollution be a problem indoors?

The air within homes can be 10 to 40 times more hazardous than outside air. Indoor air pollution comes from wood stoves, furnaces, cigarette smoke, asbestos, formaldehyde, radon, lead, mold, and household chemicals.

Home Heating If you rely on wood or on oil- or gas-fired furnaces for home heating, make sure your heating appliance is properly installed, vented, and maintained. In wood stoves, burning properly seasoned wood reduces particulates. Thorough cleaning and maintenance can prevent carbon monoxide buildup in the home. Inexpensive home monitors are available to detect high carbon monoxide levels.

Asbestos **Asbestos** is a mineral compound used to insulate vinyl flooring, roofing materials, heating pipe coverings, and many other products in buildings constructed before 1970. When bonded to other materials, asbestos is relatively harmless, but if its tiny fibers become loosened and airborne, they can embed themselves in the lungs, leading to cancer of the lungs, stomach, and chest lining and other life-threatening lung diseases. If asbestos is detected in the home, it must be removed or sealed off by a professional.

Secondhand smoke contains more than **7,000** chemicals, hundreds of which are toxic.

Formaldehyde Formaldehyde is a colorless, strong-smelling gas released from building materials or new carpet in a process called *outgassing*. Outgassing is highest in new products, but the process can continue for many years.

Exposure to formaldehyde can cause respiratory problems, dizziness, fatigue, nausea, and rashes. Long-term exposure can lead to central nervous system disorders and cancer. Ask about the formaldehyde content of products you are considering for your home, and avoid those that contain it.

Radon **Radon** is an odorless, colorless gas found in soil. It can penetrate homes through cracks or other openings in the basement or foundation. Radon is the second leading cause of lung cancer, after smoking.[32]

The EPA estimates that as many as 1 in 3 U.S. homes may have elevated radon levels.[33] Homes below the third floor should be tested for radon, ideally every 2 years or when moving into a new home. Inexpensive test kits are available in hardware stores.

Lead **Lead** is a metal pollutant sometimes found in paint, batteries, soils, drinking water, pipes, dishes, and other items. Recently, toys produced in China have been recalled due to unsafe levels of lead in their paint.

Up to 25 percent of U.S. homes still have lead-based paint hazards, and an estimated 535,000 American children under 5 have unsafe blood lead levels.[34] To reduce lead exposure, keep areas where children play as dust-free as possible, and do not remove lead paint yourself. Many cities have free lead-testing programs.

Mold Molds are fungi that live both indoors and outdoors. They produce tiny reproductive spores that continually waft through air. These spores can irritate lungs and cause other health problems. For ways to reduce mold exposure, see Skills for Behavior Change.

Sick Building Syndrome **Sick building syndrome (SBS)** occurs when occupants of a building experience acute health effects linked to time spent in a building but no specific illness or cause can be identified.[35] Poor ventilation is a primary cause of SBS. Other causes include faulty furnaces; pet dander; mold; volatile organic compounds from products such as hairspray, cleaners, and adhesives; and heavy metals such as lead. Symptoms include eye irritation, sore throat, queasiness, and worsened asthma.

Indoor air pollution and SBS are increasing concerns in the classroom and workplace. Many U.S. schools have unsatisfactory indoor air quality, often due to poor ventilation, construction techniques that block outside air, and the use of synthetic construction materials.[36] Poor air quality can trigger allergies, asthma, and other health problems.[37]

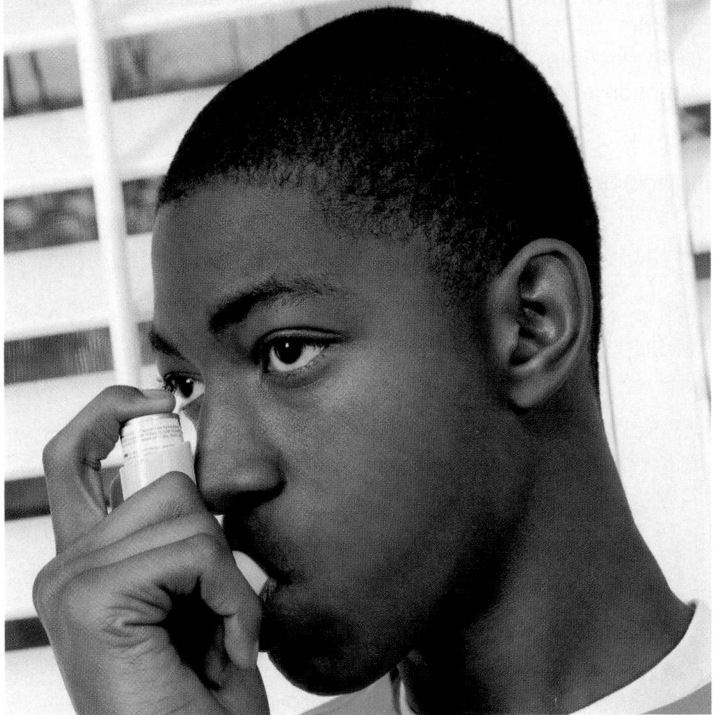

What causes asthma?

Asthma is caused by inflammation of the airways in the lungs, restricting airflow and leading to wheezing, chest tightness, shortness of breath, and coughing. In most people, asthma is brought on by contact with allergens or irritants in the air; some people also have exercise-induced asthma. People with asthma can generally control their symptoms through the use of inhaled medications, and most asthmatics keep a "rescue" inhaler of bronchodilating medication on hand to use in case of a flare-up.

Air Pollution and Asthma

Asthma is a long-term, chronic inflammatory disorder that causes tiny airways in the lung to spasm in response to triggers. Symptoms include wheezing, difficulty breathing, shortness of breath, and coughing. Although most asthma attacks are mild, severe attacks can trigger potentially fatal contractions of the bronchial tubes.

Asthma falls into two types: extrinsic and intrinsic. The more common form, *extrinsic* or *allergic asthma*, is associated with allergic triggers; it tends to run in families and develop in childhood. *Intrinsic* or *nonallergic asthma* may be triggered by anything except an allergy. Several factors can increase your risk of developing asthma—one of the most significant is environmental allergens and irritants.[38]

Asthma rates have increased 30 percent in the last 20 years.[39] Many blame increasing pollution rates, especially in poor and nonwhite communities, as well as triggers such as dust mites in mattresses, chemicals in carpets and furniture, and airtight modern buildings.

Skills for Behavior Change

BE MOLD FREE

- Keep the humidity level in your home between 40 and 60 percent.
- Use a dehumidifier in damp rooms or basements.
- Be sure your home has adequate ventilation, including exhaust fans in the kitchen and bathrooms. If there are no fans, open windows.
- Buy paints with mold-resistant properties or add mold inhibitors.
- In the bathroom, wipe down shower doors, keep surfaces dry, and if necessary, use environmentally safe mold-killing products. Do not carpet bathrooms and basements or other rooms that are routinely damp.
- Many antimold products commonly used in outdoor areas are extremely toxic; pets and wildlife may wander through these after they've been applied. Use them sparingly or not at all.
- Wash rugs used in entryways and other areas where moisture can accumulate.
- Get rid of mattresses and furniture exposed to excessive moisture.
- Dry clothing thoroughly before putting it away.
- When buying a house, don't skimp on mold inspections. Check for mold growth regularly, especially in rental units where landlords may not pay attention to these risks.

check yourself

- **What are four common indoor air pollutants and their sources?**

14.4

Global Warming and Climate Change

learning outcome

14.4 Describe how greenhouse gas buildup contributes to climate change.

Climate change refers to a shift in typical weather patterns across the world. These changes can include fluctuations in seasonal temperatures, rain or snowfall amounts, and the occurrence of catastrophic storms. **Global warming** is a type of climate change where average temperatures increase. Over 97 percent of scientists now agree the planet is warming, and over the last half century, this warming has been driven primarily by human activity—predominantly the burning of fossil fuels.[40] Over the last 100 years, the average temperature of the earth has increased by 1.5°F, with projections of another 2° to 11.5°F rise in the next 100 years.[41]

According to the National Aeronautics and Space Administration (NASA), the National Oceanic and Atmospheric Administration (NOAA), and the National Research Council, climate change poses major risks to lives, and excess **greenhouse gases** are a key culprit.[42] The *greenhouse effect* is a natural phenomenon in which greenhouse gases, such **carbon dioxide (CO_2)**, nitrous oxide, methane, CFCs, and hydrocarbons, form a layer in the atmosphere, allowing solar heat to pass through and trapping some of the heat close to the surface, where it warms the planet (see Figure 14.3). Excess carbon dioxide accounts for 82 percent of greenhouse gases emitted through human activity in the United States.[43]

Scientific Evidence of Climate Change

Climate responds to changes in naturally occurring greenhouse gases as well as solar output and the earth's orbit; however, recent evidence points to unusual changes in climate that go beyond predictable natural causes:[44]

- Global sea levels rose 6.7 inches in the last 100 years, much of it in the last decade. With accelerated glacial and ice sheet melts, this rise is likely to increase dramatically.
- Earth's temperature is rising, with 20 of the warmest years ever since 1981 and all of the 10 warmest years occurring in last 12 years.
- Ice sheets are shrinking; Greenland is losing 36–60 cubic miles of ice per year, whereas Antarctica is losing 36 cubic miles of ice per year. Glaciers are receding at unprecedented and rapid rates in the Alps, Himalayas, Andes, Rockies, Alaska, and Africa.
- Ocean temperatures are rising and becoming more acidic.
- There have been record high temperatures, drought, and flooding in various parts of the United States.

Multiple reconstructions of the earth's climate history show that the amounts of greenhouse gases in the atmosphere went up dramatically around the time of the industrial revolution—when humans began burning fossil fuels on a large scale—and this correlates very closely with temperature increases.[45] Studies also indicate that large changes in climate can occur in decades rather than centuries or thousands of years.[46]

Direct results of climate change, such as rising sea levels, glacier retreat, arctic shrinkage at the poles, altered patterns of agriculture, deforestation, forest fires, drought, extreme weather events, increases in tropical diseases, loss of biological species, and economic devastation, have catastrophic consequences.

Reducing the Threat of Global Warming and Moving Toward Sustainable Development

Climate change problems are largely rooted in our energy, transportation, and industrial practices and fossil fuel burning.[47] However, the problem isn't just one of increased CO_2 production. Rapid deforestation contributes to the rise in greenhouse gases. Trees take in carbon dioxide, transform it, store the carbon for food, and release oxygen into the air. As we lose forests at the rate of hundreds of acres per hour, we lose the capacity to store and dissipate carbon dioxide.

To slow climate change, most experts agree that reducing consumption of fossil fuels, shifting to alternative energy sources, and

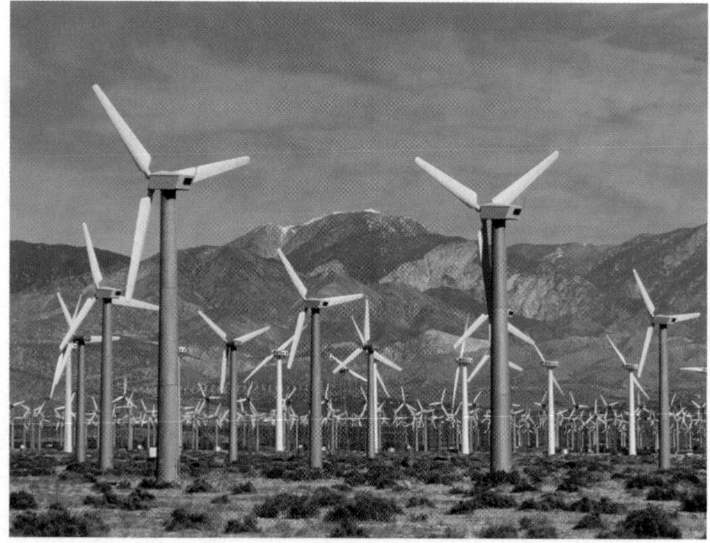

How can I help prevent climate change?

By reducing use of fossil fuels, using high-efficiency vehicles, and supporting increased use of renewable resources such as solar, wind, and water power, you can help combat climate change. For example, the National Renewable Energy Laboratory predicts that, with proper development, wind power could provide 20 percent of U.S. energy needs.

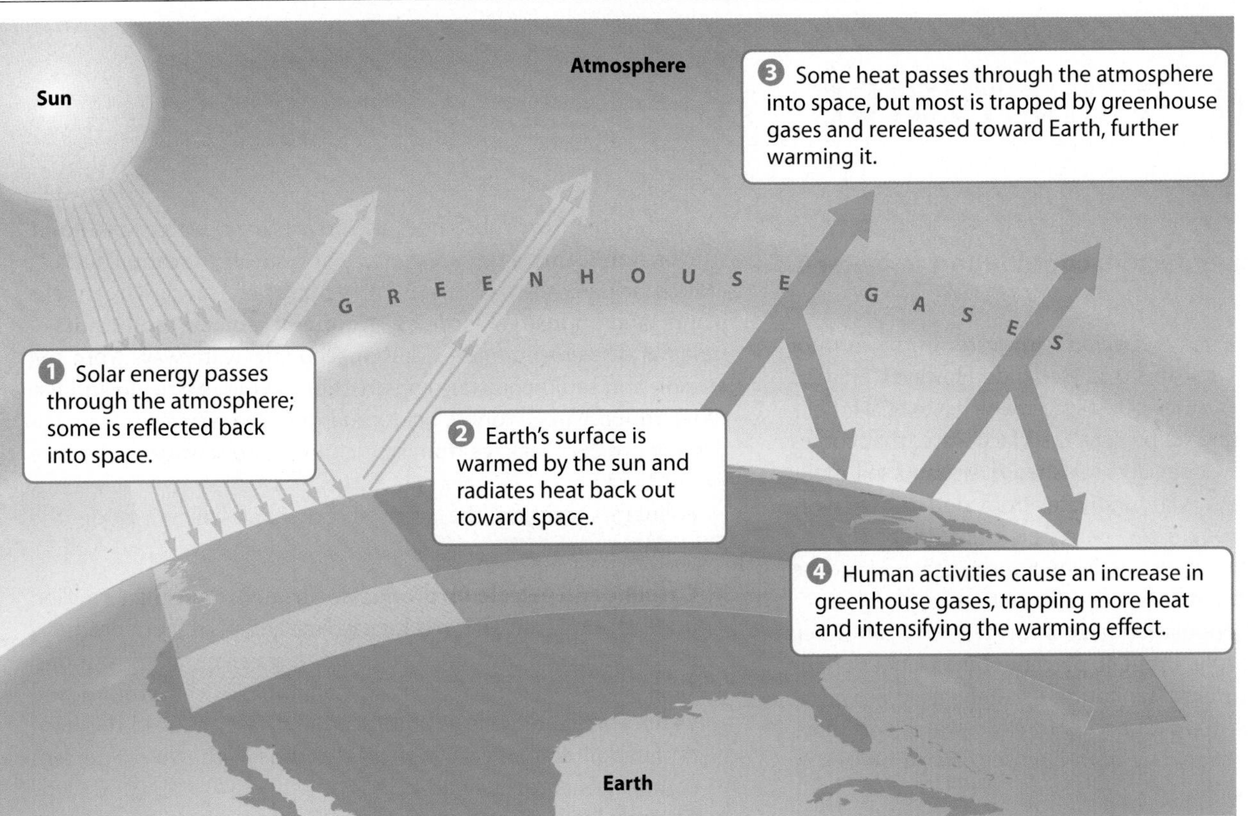

Figure 14.3 The Enhanced Greenhouse Effect

The natural greenhouse effect is responsible for making Earth habitable; it keeps the planet 33°C (60°F) warmer than it would be otherwise. An increase in greenhouse gases resulting from human activities is creating the enhanced greenhouse effect, trapping more heat and causing dangerous global climate change.

VIDEO TUTOR
Enhanced Greenhouse Effect

using mass transportation are all crucial. Clean energy, green factories, improved energy efficiency, and governmental regulation are also key. Several international efforts to reduce human emissions responsible for climate change have taken place. One of the earlier efforts, known as the Kyoto Protocol, outlined an international plan to reduce the human-made emissions responsible for climate change.[48] Although over 160 countries agreed to participate, the United States opted out,[49] ostensibly because of concerns that major developing nations, including India and China, were not required to reduce emissions under the treaty. A major United Nations Conference on Sustainable Development and Environmental concerns (known as RIO+20) took place in 2012 in Rio de Janeiro and outlined a plan for protecting the environment (called "The World We Want") through **sustainable development**—development that meets the needs of the present without compromising the needs of future generations.[50] However, leaders of many nations, including the United States, France, Germany, and the United Kingdom, opted not to attend, and the resulting plan includes a list of general goals to work toward, but without the force necessary to motivate nations to comply with sustainable development needs.

See It! Videos

How is climate change affecting the weather during winter? Watch **Snowstorms in the Forecast** in the Study Area of MasteringHealth.

In 2012, some of the major CO_2 emitting countries contributed to what appears to be a slowing of the CO_2 trend. After years of double digit carbon emission increases, overall emissions increased only about 1.1 percent. Global coal consumption, responsible for almost 40 percent of emissions, grew by less than 1 percent, well below the decade average of 4 percent per year. In 2013, the United States had a 12 percent reduction in coal and a shift to cleaner burning natural gas.[51] More wind, solar, and bioenergy use, reductions in natural gas prices, more strict emission standards, and public concerns about smog and pollution are likely reasons for these improvements in many regions.[52]

Although stricter laws on vehicular carbon emissions and the development of cars that operate on electricity, hydrogen, biodiesel, ethanol, or other alternative energy sources are promising, we have a long way to go to reduce fossil fuel consumption. While hybrid cars often use much less gasoline, in areas where coal is the major source of electricity, issues arise as to whether using coal for electricity rather than gas really makes a car "green." Many communities and campuses have established plans to reduce their carbon footprint. Creating user-friendly bicycle lanes, bike garages to prevent theft, and "bike to work" days motivate students to leave cars at home. Some campuses have raised fees for parking in the hopes of discouraging students from bringing cars to campus. You can participate in this effort by finding ways to reduce your own **carbon footprint**, or the amount of CO_2 emissions you contribute to the atmosphere in your daily life.

check yourself

- **What are some possible effects of uncontained global warming?**

14.5 Pollution in the Water

learning outcome

14.5 Identify the major factors contributing to water pollution.

Seventy-five percent of Earth is covered with water in the form of oceans, seas, lakes, rivers, streams, and wetlands. However, only 2.5 percent of all of the earth's water is freshwater, which is crucial for our survival. Of that freshwater, 1.2 percent is surface water that comes from lakes, ground ice, swamps and marshes, rivers, and soil moisture; another 30.1 percent is groundwater from underwater wells and aquifers; and the remaining 68.7 percent is locked in glaciers and ice caps. We draw our drinking water from groundwater and surface water, but much of it is too polluted or difficult to reach.[53]

Over half the global population faces a shortage of clean water. More than 2.6 billion people, about 40 percent of the planet's population, have no access to basic sanitation or adequate toilet facilities. More than 1 billion have no access to clean water, and more than 4,500 children die every day from illnesses caused by lack of safe water and sanitation.[54]

By 2030, demand for freshwater is projected to exceed the current supply by over 40 percent, increasing competition for scarce reserves and posing a major risk to human survival. Some areas of the world will be at high risk due to extended drought, population increases, and dwindling supply.[55] Poor sanitation, consumer waste, agricultural enterprises, residential and commercial development in areas that are historically arid, and public apathy all add to the burden placed on our water resources.[56]

Water Contamination

Any substance that gets into the soil can enter the water supply. Industrial pollutants and pesticides work their way into soil, then into groundwater. Underground storage tanks containing gasoline may leak. A comprehensive U.S. Geological Survey investigation discovered the presence of low levels of many chemical compounds in a network of 139 streams across the United States. Steroids, pharmaceuticals, personal care products, hormones, insect repellent, and wastewater compounds were all detected.[57]

Tap water in the United States is among the safest in the world. Under the Safe Drinking Water Act (SDWA), the EPA sets standards for drinking water quality. Cities and municipalities have strict policies and procedures governing water treatment, filtration, and disinfection to screen out pathogens and microorganisms. However, their ability to filter out increasing amounts of chemical by-products and other substances is in question. A recent study of over 50 large wastewater sites in the United States revealed that over half of the samples tested positive for at least 25 prescription and over-the-counter drugs. While levels of the drugs are low and appear to pose little risk to humans, they have been shown to have significant effects on aquatic life.[58]

Many other toxic substances also flow into our waterways. **Point source pollutants** enter a waterway at a specific location such as a ditch or pipe; the two major entry points are sewage treatment plants and industrial facilities. **Nonpoint source pollutants**—*runoff* and *sedimentation*—drain or seep into waterways from soil erosion and sedimentation, construction wastes, pesticide and fertilizer runoff, street runoff, acid mine drainage, wastes from engineering projects, leakage from septic tanks, and sewage sludge (see Figure 14.4).

Pollutants causing the greatest potential harm include the following:

- **Gasoline and petroleum products.** There are more than 2 million underground storage tanks for gasoline and petroleum products in the United States, most located at gasoline filling stations. Tank leaks allow petroleum to contaminate the ground and water. Fortunately, clean up procedures have reduced this contamination dramatically in the last decade, with over 70 percent compliance among violators.[59]
- **Chemical contaminants.** *Organic solvents* are chemicals designed to dissolve grease and oil. These extremely toxic substances are used to clean clothing, painting equipment, plastics, and metal parts. Consumers often dump leftover products into the toilet or into street drains. Industries pour leftovers into barrels, which are then buried. Eventually, the chemicals eat through the barrels and leach into groundwater.
- **Polychlorinated biphenyls. Polychlorinated biphenyls (PCBs)** were used for many years as insulating materials in high-voltage electrical equipment. The human body does not excrete ingested PCBs, but rather stores them in fatty tissues and the liver. Exposure to PCBs is associated with birth defects, cancer,

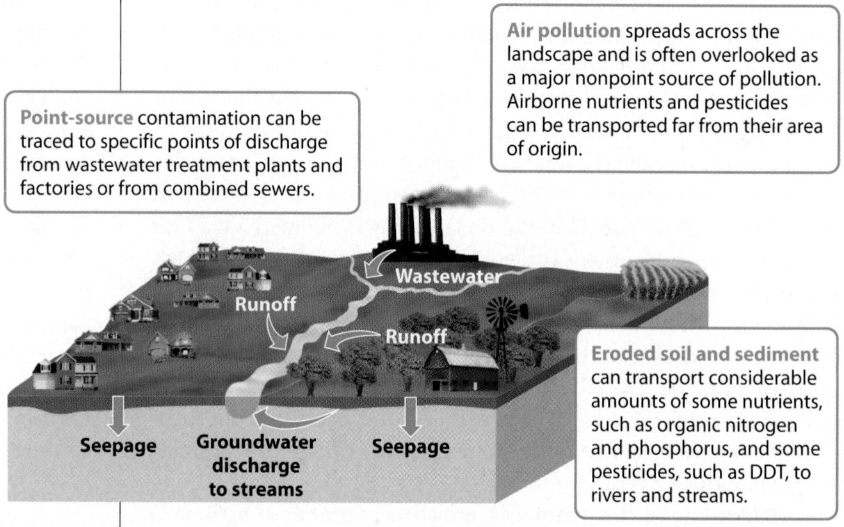

Point-source contamination can be traced to specific points of discharge from wastewater treatment plants and factories or from combined sewers.

Air pollution spreads across the landscape and is often overlooked as a major nonpoint source of pollution. Airborne nutrients and pesticides can be transported far from their area of origin.

Wastewater
Runoff
Runoff
Seepage
Groundwater discharge to streams
Seepage

Eroded soil and sediment can transport considerable amounts of some nutrients, such as organic nitrogen and phosphorus, and some pesticides, such as DDT, to rivers and streams.

Figure 14.4 Potential Sources of Groundwater Contamination

Source: Adapted from U.S. Geological Survey, Wisconsin Water Science Center, "Learn More about Groundwater," 2008, http://wi.water.usgs.gov.

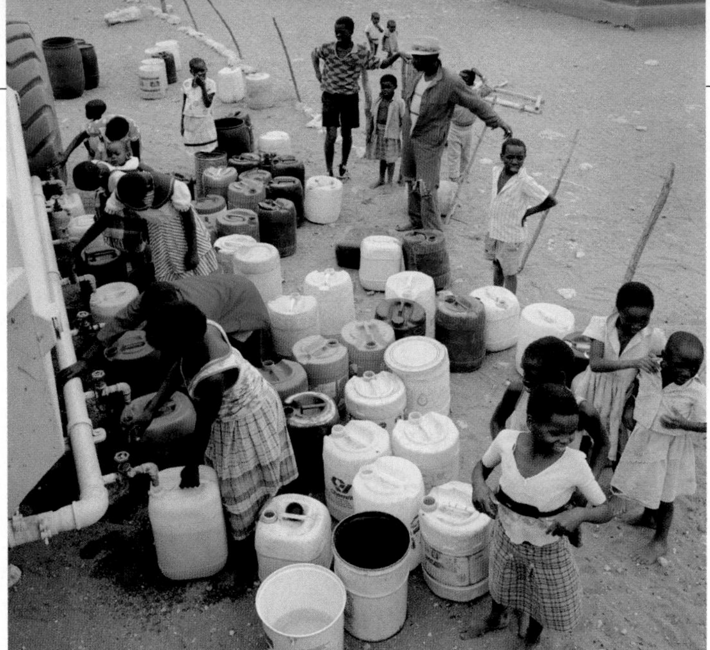

Is there really a water scarcity?

The lack of clean water and sanitation is a major global problem. *Closed basins* are regions where existing water cannot meet the agricultural, industrial, municipal, and environmental needs. The Stockholm International Water Institute estimates that 1.4 billion people live in a closed basin, and the problem is worsening.

and skin problems. The manufacture of PCBs was discontinued in the United States in 1977, but approximately 500 million pounds have been dumped into landfills and waterways, where they continue to pose an environmental threat.[60]

- **Dioxins. Dioxins** are found in herbicides (chemicals used to kill vegetation). They're much more toxic than PCBs; long-term effects include possible immune system damage and increased risk of infections and cancer. Short-term exposure to high concentrations of PCBs or dioxins can have severe consequences, including nausea; vomiting; diarrhea; painful rashes and sores; and chloracne, in which the skin develops painful pimples that may never go away.
- **Pesticides. Pesticides** are chemicals designed to kill insects, rodents, plants, and fungi. Americans use more than a billion pounds of pesticides each year, the majority of which settle on the land and in our air and water.[61] Pesticides evaporate readily and are often dispersed by winds over a large area or carried out to sea. In tropical regions, many farmers use pesticides heavily, and the climate promotes their rapid release into the atmosphere. Pesticide residues cling to fruits and vegetables and can accumulate in the body. Potential hazards associated with exposure to pesticides include birth defects, liver and kidney damage, and nervous system disorders.

Fracking

Hydraulic fracturing of shale (*fracking*) is a method of extracting otherwise inaccessible natural gas from the ground. Most of the natural reserves of gas in North America are trapped in shale beds that have long been inaccessible to cost-effective tapping; according to some experts, these deposits could provide the United States with enough natural gas to power the country for a century.[62] But the process also has many people concerned about the environmental risks to water and airborne pollutants that go with it.

In fracking, underground rock and dense soil are cracked open by pumping highly pressurized fluids into them, creating fissures that allow oil or gas to flow to the surface for extraction. Much of the fracking liquid comes up with the gas or oil and is stored in chemical pools for delivery to treatment plants. However, some scientists and members of the public are concerned that a portion of this toxic, chemical-laden sludge can seep down and contaminate aquifers that supply drinking water to many regions of the country. In addition to potential groundwater contamination, the EPA has noted that fracking causes airborne pollution from methane, sulfur oxide, benzene, and other pollutants, each of which pose significant risks to human health and the environment.[63] At present, fewer regulations exist to control the safe collection of harmful gases from fracking compared with other energy technologies. A recent rash of earthquakes in regions of the country where shale gas is being extracted by fracking has sparked speculation that changing the internal pressures of the earth's surface via deep wells formed by fracking may pose additional risks.[64] The debate continues over the use of fracking and what criteria should be used to regulate it.

See It! Videos

Is bottled water better for you? Watch **Americans' Obsession with Bottled Water** in the Study Area of MasteringHealth.

Skills for Behavior Change

WASTE LESS WATER!

In the Kitchen

- Turn off the tap while washing dishes.
- Check faucets and pipes for leaks. Leaky faucets can waste more than 3,000 gallons of water each year.
- Equip faucets with aerators to reduce water use by 4 percent.
- Wash only full dishwasher loads; use the energy-saving mode.

In the Laundry Room

- Wash only full laundry loads.
- Upgrade to a high-efficiency washing machine.

In the Bathroom

- Detect and fix leaks. A leaky toilet can waste 200 gallons of water every day.
- Install a high-efficiency toilet that uses 60 percent less water.
- Take showers instead of baths; limit showers to the time it takes to lather and rinse.
- Replace old showerheads with efficient models that use 60 percent less water.
- Turn off the tap while brushing your teeth to save up to 8 gallons of water per day.

check yourself

- **What are three major sources of water pollution?**
- **What are four steps that you can take to reduce water waste?**

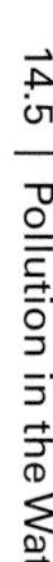

14.6 Pollution on Land

learning outcome

14.6 List the major factors contributing to pollution on land.

Much of the waste that ends up polluting the water starts out polluting the land. A growing population creates more pressure on the land to accommodate increasing amounts of refuse, much of which is nonbiodegradable and some of which is directly harmful to living organisms.

Solid Waste

One of the most common ways that people try to preserve the environment is by participating in recycling programs (Figure 14.5). However, each day, every person in the United States generates nearly 4.4 pounds of municipal solid waste (MSW), more commonly known as trash or garbage—containers and packaging; discarded food; yard debris; and refuse from residential, commercial, institutional, and industrial sources (see Figure 14.6).[65] The total comes to about 251 million tons of MSW each year.[66] Although experts believe that up to 90 percent of our trash is recyclable, we still fall far short of this goal with respect to most types of trash. In the United States, 34.8 percent of all MSW is recovered and recycled or composted, over 14 percent is burned at combustion facilities, and the remaining 54 percent is disposed of in landfills.[67]

Americans are among the worst of the food wasters, wasting over 40 percent of all edible food annually.[68] Big box stores that promote "bigger size is cheaper" entice people to buy more than they can eat before it spoils. Freezers in homes encourage waste as food dries up before it is eaten, while other food sits on shelves until past its expiration date. If weather or insects cause produce to be blemished, we reject it in stores and it is tossed in the trash. The average person in the United States dumps about 20 pounds of food each month, equivalent to between \$28 and \$43 per month. If we cut our food waste by just 15 percent, some estimate 26 million food-insecure people in the United States could be fed.[69]

The number of landfills in the United States has actually decreased in the past decade, but their sheer mass has increased. Many people worry that we are rapidly losing our ability to dispose of all of the waste we create. As communities run out of landfill space, it is becoming common to haul garbage to other states or to dump it illegally in woods, waterways, or oceans, where it contaminates ecosystems, or to ship it to landfills in developing countries, where it becomes someone else's problem. In today's throwaway society, we need to become aware of the amount of waste we generate every day and to look for ways to recycle, reuse, and—most desirable of all—reduce what we consume.

Communities, businesses, and individuals can adopt several strategies to control waste:

- *Source reduction* (*waste prevention*) involves altering the design, manufacture, or use of products and materials to reduce the amount and toxicity of what gets thrown away. The most effective MSW-reducing strategy is to prevent waste from ever being generated in the first place.

  Several communities across the United States have placed a ban or tax on plastic bags to reduce their use in retail stores. Proponents say plastic bags are bad for the environment because they are made from nonbiodegradable petroleum, are infrequently recycled, and are commonly littered, ending up in waterways where they become a wildlife hazard.
- *Recycling* involves sorting, collecting, and processing materials to be reused in the manufacture of new products. This process diverts items such as paper, glass, plastics, and metals from the waste stream.
- *E-recycling* involves properly disposing of trashed computers, televisions, cell phones, and other electronic devices. The global burden of electronic waste has skyrocketed in recent years as we struggle to find sources for disposal and e-recycling. Visit www.epa.gov and www.ecyclingcentral.com to find information about locations for electronic waste recycling in your state and to learn how to reduce electronic waste in your MSW. Although there are many avenues for disposing of items like cell phones, the best way to avoid electronic waste is not succumb to the "latest and greatest" craze in the first place—hang on to your TV, phone, or device for as long as possible.

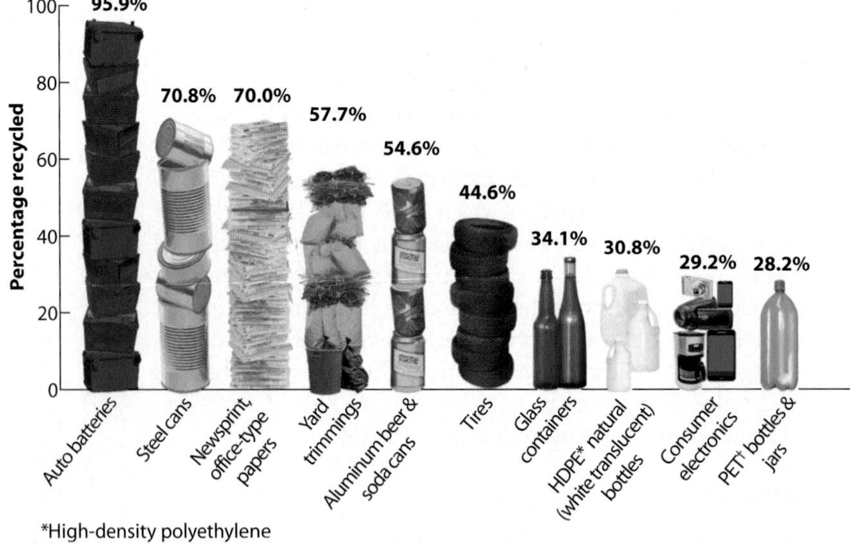

Figure 14.5 How Much Do We Recycle?

Source: Data from U.S. Environmental Protection Agency, *Municipal Solid Waste Generation, Recycling, and Disposal in the United States: Facts and Figures for 2012*, February 2014, epa-530-F-14-001, www.epa.gov.

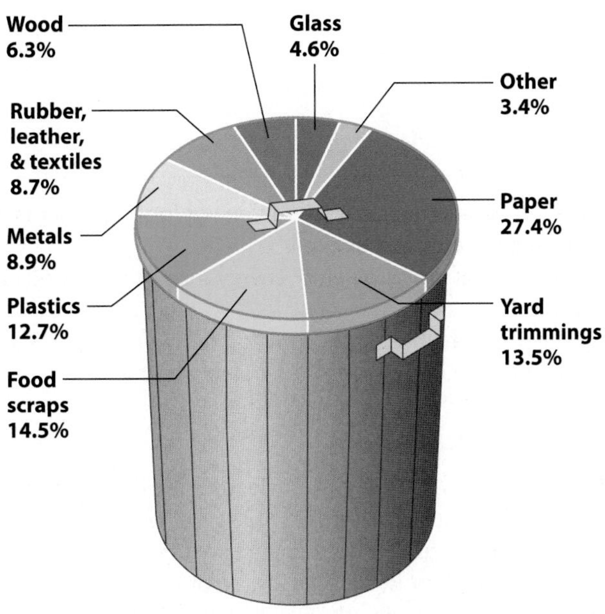

Figure 14.6 What's in Our Trash?

Source: Data from U.S. Environmental Protection Agency, *Municipal Solid Waste Generation, Recycling, and Disposal in the United States: Facts and Figures for 2012*, February 2014, epa-530-F-14-001, www.epa.gov.

- *Composting* involves collecting organic waste, such as food scraps and yard trimmings, and allowing it to decompose with the help of microorganisms (mainly bacteria and fungi). This process produces a nutrient-rich substance used to fertilize gardens and for soil enhancement. Many communities now have yard carts that allow you to mix your food scraps in with yard trimmings.
- *Combustion with energy recovery* typically involves the use of boilers and industrial furnaces to incinerate waste and use the burning process to generate energy.

Hazardous Waste

Hazardous waste is defined as waste with properties that make it capable of harming human health or the environment. In 1980, the Comprehensive Environmental Response, Compensation, and Liability Act, or **Superfund**, was enacted to provide funds for cleaning up what are typically "abandoned" hazardous waste dump sites. This fund is financed through taxes on the chemical and petroleum industries, payments by those responsible for dumping waste, and federal tax revenues. Over the past three decades, the Superfund has located and assessed tens of thousands of hazardous waste sites, worked to protect people and the environment from contamination at the worst sites, and involved affected communities, states and other groups in cleanup. The vast majority of sites have been cleared or "recovered."[70]

The large number of hazardous waste dump sites in the United States indicates the severity of our toxic chemical problem. American manufacturers generate more than 1 ton of chemical waste per person per year (275 million tons annually).[71] Many wastes are now banned from land disposal or are treated to reduce their toxicity before they become part of land disposal sites. The EPA has developed protective requirements for land disposal facilities, such as double liners, detection systems for substances that may leach into groundwater, and groundwater monitoring systems.

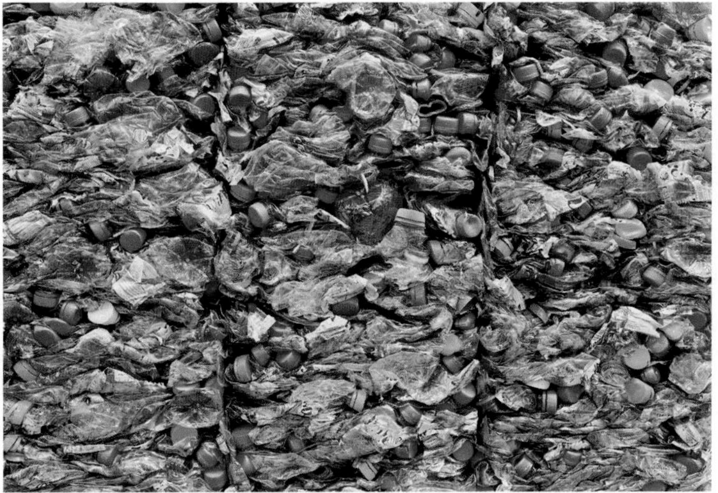

38.6%

of the plastic from plastic water bottles was recycled in 2012, more than double that which was recycled in 2005.

It's likely that you have hazardous waste sitting on a garage shelf or under a kitchen or bathroom sink. Pesticides, paints and paint thinners, solvents, moss killers, batteries, old gasoline cans, many cleaning products, glues, and adhesives as well as paint and stain removers and hot tub or pool chemicals are all examples of potential hazardous wastes.

To be a thoughtful consumer, read the labels on products before buying them. Whenever possible, substitute less toxic, natural products for hazardous ones. Remember to never pour old pesticides, cleaning agents, gasoline, or solvents down the drain or dump them on the ground.

See It! Videos

What do those numbers on the bottoms of plastic bottles mean? Watch **Crack Those Recycling Codes** in the Study Area of MasteringHealth.

There are many effective substitutes for harsh cleaning products:

- To get out laundry or carpet stains, use club soda.
- To get rid of moths in your pantry or clothes, use cedar shavings or lavender.
- To clean dirty windows and surfaces, mix water with vinegar or ammonia.
- To clean your showers, sinks, and tubs, skip the toxic chemical sprays. Use a vinegar/water solution or baking soda. Wipe surfaces dry after showering to avoid buildup.

check yourself

- **How can we reduce the amount of municipal solid waste generated?**
- **What is hazardous waste, and what are its dangers?**

14.7 Radiation

learning outcome

14.7 Explain the environmental and personal risks associated with radiation.

Radiation is energy that travels in waves or particles. Many different types of radiation make up the electromagnetic spectrum. Exposure to radiation is an inescapable part of life on this planet, and only some of it poses a threat to human health.

Nonionizing Radiation

Nonionizing radiation is radiation at the lower end of the electromagnetic spectrum. This radiation moves in relatively long wavelengths and has enough energy to move atoms but not enough to remove electrons or alter molecular structure. Examples of nonionizing radiation are radio waves, TV signals, microwaves, infrared waves, and visible light.

Although many believe that *electromagnetic fields* (*EMFs*) generated by electric power delivery systems increase one's risk for cancer, reproductive dysfunction, and other ailments, others point to major inconsistencies in the research and little resulting hazard to health. However, one particular form of EMF—radio frequency (RF) energy emitted by cell phones—is currently the subject of much debate and research. Cell phones emit RF energy when turned on, and in theory, all of that RF energy has the potential to penetrate the skull, neck, and upper torso. For the very young whose skulls have not yet sufficiently hardened, the risk may be even greater.

Many countries, including the United States, use standards set by the Federal Communications Commission (FCC) for radio frequency energy based on research by several scientific groups. These groups identified a whole-body *specific absorption rate* (*SAR*) value for exposure to RF energy. Four watts per kilogram was identified as a level above which harmful biological effects may occur. The FCC requires wireless phones to comply with a limit of 1.6 watts per kilogram. (To find the SAR level for your phone, go to www.fcc.gov.)

After over a decade of research trying to prove a solid link to cell phone use and some type of disease, we've come up with very little conclusive evidence. However, much of the available research was done before cell phones were regularly used for hours each day to play games, browse the Internet, and check up on social media sites in addition to talking and texting. The U.S. Food and Drug Administration, the World Health Organization, and other major health agencies suggest a need for more research since no long-term studies exist. A new European Cohort Study of Mobile phone use (COSMOS) will follow 250,000 people for the next 20 years to determine increased risks and should provide much needed insight.[72]

In the meantime, a few small changes in behavior can greatly reduce the amount of RF energy your body absorbs:

- Limit the amount of time you spend talking on the phone. When you do make calls, use a hands-free device that keeps the phone away from your head.
- Because wireless earpieces also emit energy, only use them when you are actively engaged in a call.
- Buy a phone that emits lower RF energy than others based on its SAR level.
- Keep the phone further away from you during the night, such as on a side table or dresser, so it's off of your pillow.

Ionizing Radiation

Ionizing radiation is caused by the release of particles and electromagnetic rays from atomic nuclei during the normal process of disintegration. Some naturally occurring elements, such as uranium, emit radiation. The sun is another source of ionizing radiation, in the form of high-frequency ultraviolet rays—those against which the ozone layer protects us.

Exposure is measured in **radiation absorbed doses (rads)**, also called *roentgens*. Harm can occur with dosages as low as 100 to 200 rads, including nausea, diarrhea, fatigue, anemia, sore throat, and hair loss. At 350 to 500 rads, symptoms become more severe, and death may result because the radiation hinders bone marrow production of white blood cells that protect us from disease. Dosages above 600 to 700 rads are fatal.

Recommended maximum "safe" dosages range from 0.5 to 5 rads per year.[73] Approximately 50 percent of the radiation to which we are exposed comes from natural sources, including radon gas in the air and cosmic radiation. Another 45 percent comes from medical and dental X-rays. The remaining 5 percent is nonionizing radiation from such sources as computer monitors, microwave ovens, televisions, and radar screens.[74] Most of us are exposed to far less radiation than the safe maximum dosage per year. The effects of long-term exposure to relatively low levels of radiation are unknown.

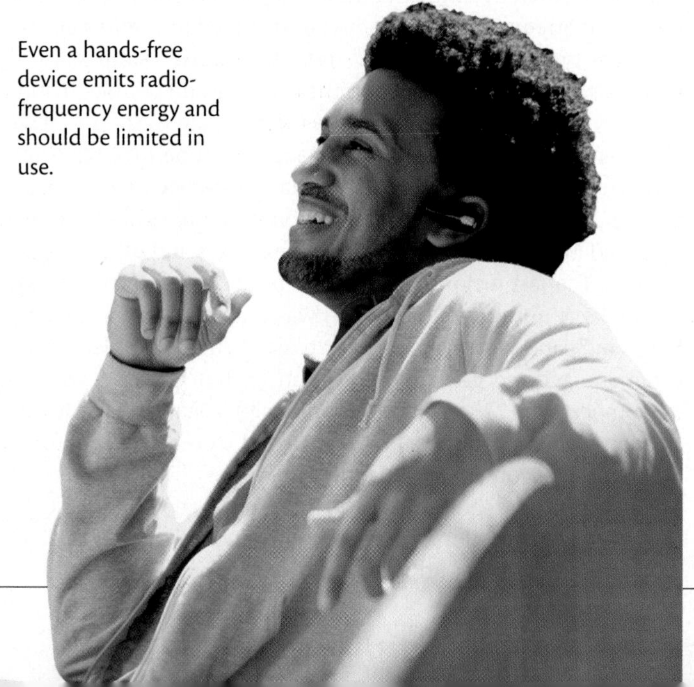

Even a hands-free device emits radiofrequency energy and should be limited in use.

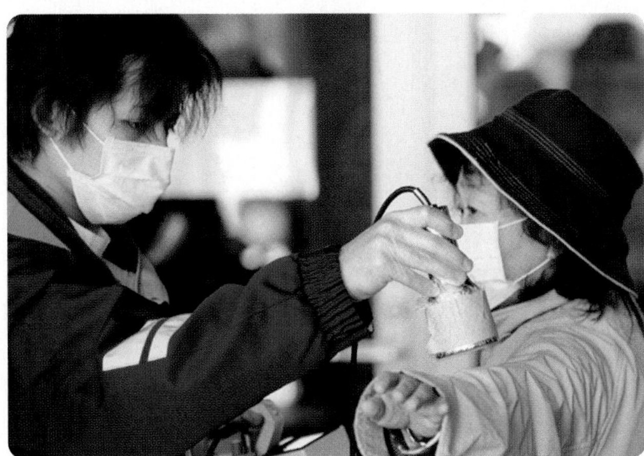

Testing a resident for radiation in Fukushima, Japan.

Nuclear Power Plants

Currently, nuclear power plants account for less than 1 percent of the total radiation to which we are exposed; however, the number of U.S. plants may increase in the next decade, so exposure levels may also increase. Proponents of nuclear energy believe that it is a safe and efficient way to generate electricity. Initial costs of building nuclear power plants are high, but actual power generation is relatively inexpensive. A 1,000-megawatt reactor produces enough energy for 650,000 homes and saves 420 million gallons of fossil fuels each year. In some areas where nuclear power plants were decommissioned, electricity bills tripled when power companies turned to hydroelectric or fossil fuel sources to generate electricity. Nuclear reactors discharge fewer carbon oxides into the air than do fossil fuel–powered generators. Advocates believe that converting to nuclear power could help slow global warming.

The advantages of nuclear energy must be weighed against the disadvantages. Disposal of nuclear waste is extremely problematic. In addition, a reactor core meltdown could pose serious threats to the immediate environment and to the world in general. A **nuclear meltdown** occurs when the temperature in the core of a nuclear reactor increases enough to melt the nuclear fuel and breach the containment vessel. Most modern facilities seal the reactors and containment vessels in concrete buildings with pools of cold water on the bottom. If a meltdown occurs, the building and the pool are supposed to prevent radiation from escaping.

The International Atomic Energy Agency ranks nuclear and radiological accidents and incidents by severity on a scale of 1 to 7. To date, we have had two major nuclear disasters that resulted in a 7, the highest severity rating, meaning that there was a major release of radioactive material with widespread health and environmental consequences. The first was the 1986 reactor core fire and explosion at the Chernobyl nuclear power plant in Ukraine, which has led to conservative estimates of 2,000 to as many as 724,000 deaths. Many regions surrounding the area may be uninhabitable for decades.[75]

The damage to the Fukushima Daiichi Nuclear Power Station in northern Japan caused by the March 2011 earthquake and tsunami was also listed as a level 7 nuclear disaster, the worst since Chernobyl, and has awakened worldwide fears about nuclear power. The Fukushima Daiichi Nuclear Power Station, positioned in the region hardest hit by the tsunami, suffered several explosions, multiple fires,

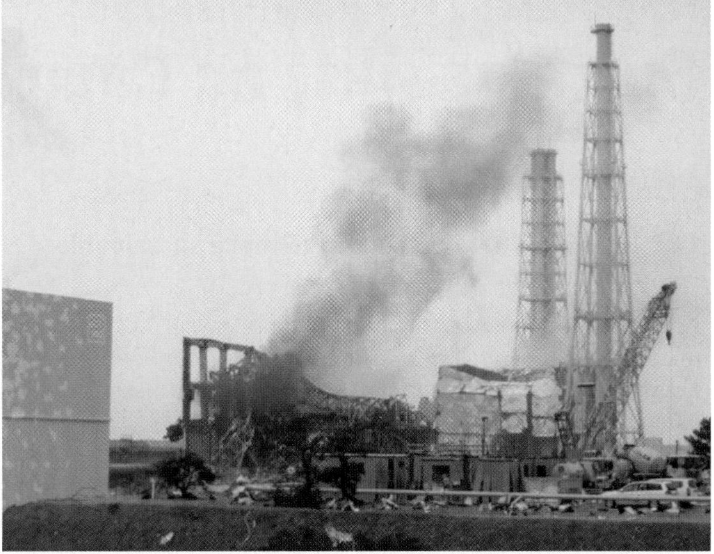

The 2011 accident at the Fukushima Daiichi plant in Japan, following an earthquake and tsunami, raised new questions about the safety of nuclear power.

radioactive gas leaks, and a partial meltdown in three of its reactors. Despite continued exposure to toxic radioactive material and risk to their lives, nuclear plant workers labored for weeks to stave off a full-scale meltdown and to minimize the destruction to the public and surrounding region by attempting to cool and repair the damaged reactors.

Of all the hundreds of dangerous radioactive chemicals released during the Fukushima Daiichi nuclear emergency, scientists expressed the most concern about the levels of iodine, plutonium, cesium, and strontium in the atmosphere, water, and food supplies. According to reports of tests on food and drinking water samples made in late March 2011, iodine and cesium were detected, but the majority of measurements remained below regulation values. Additionally, small amounts of plutonium were found in the soil outside the plant, though not enough to pose a significant health risk.[76] Long-term health outcomes associated with the Fukushima Daiichi nuclear emergency will be closely monitored by Japanese officials as well as by officials globally. This emergency has spurred Japan and other nations to reconsider the safety of nuclear power plants and the policies necessary to protect the environment and public health. Some research suggests that there may be as many as 400,000 additional cancer patients and over 40,000 deaths from thyroid cancer alone among those within 200 kilometers of the Fukushima Daiichi plant; however, exact information is difficult to obtain.[77]

Even with the looming possibility of nuclear disasters, the use of nuclear power worldwide is expected to double in the next 20 to 25 years.[78]

check yourself

- **What is the difference between ionizing and nonionizing radiation?**
- **What are some benefits and drawbacks to the use of nuclear power?**

14.8 Sustainability on Campus

learning outcome

14.8 Identify what you can do to make sustainable choices in college.

As a college student, your actions and those of your friends, roommates, and school can have a lasting impact on your health and the health of the environment. College is a great time to make a positive difference and minimize your ecological footprint.

According to a recent survey, almost 40 percent of college freshman indicated that adopting green practices to protect the environment are essential or very important.[79] You do not need to be an environmental science major or a self-proclaimed "hippie" to make a difference. Making sustainable choices can be a goal for your apartment, your sorority or fraternity, your team, or your residence hall.

Small choices you make beginning today can make a difference. Start making a positive impact by turning off lights when you leave a room or restroom. See if your residence has a way of minimizing the amount of lights used on a floor. Sometimes lights are connected through several outlets; turning off a strand might still provide enough light but minimize the amount of energy consumed. Find out whether your administration supports the use of CFLs—compact fluorescent lights—longer-lasting, energy-conserving bulbs that give off the same amount of light as an incandescent bulb at a fraction of the energy used. Next time you go to the store, buy a couple for your lighting fixtures and start making a positive impact.

Making Green Electronic Choices

When buying a new appliance, look for the Energy Star logo, indicating that the appliance meets energy-efficiency standards set by the EPA and U.S. Department of Energy. Adjust the controls on your new appliances so that they do not run at full power all the time. This will help curb unnecessary energy usage and lower the cost of your monthly energy bills. Better yet, consider unplugging items such as MP3 players, tablets, TVs, computers, hair dryers, coffee pots, power strips, and cell phones, all of which still consume energy when not in use.

What about your computer? While in school, you will probably use it for everything from social networking to writing papers. Fortunately, you have many options to help you make better energy-conserving choices when it comes to computer use. When buying a computer, always look for the Energy Star logo. If every home office product in the U.S. met Energy Star requirements, we could prevent 1.4 billion greenhouse gases per year.[80] Also make sure to set your computer to sleep, hibernate, or low-power mode when not in use.

When you look for a printer, choose one that prints double-sided (or print double-sided yourself by manually flipping the pages), which will help reduce the amount of paper you use. Do not print unnecessary documents, and make sure you recycle used paper; don't just throw it away! Turn off your printer (or better yet, unplug it) when not in use.

Cable and satellite TV boxes are another source of energy drain on the environment—and potentially your bank account. You may be surprised to find out that even while you're *not* watching TV, your cable box is using more electricity than almost any appliance in your house, except for your air conditioner. A recent report indicates that a set-top cable or satellite box can consume as much as 35 watts of power and can cost around $8.00 a month (depending on energy costs in your area).[81] When the almost quarter of a million cable boxes in U.S. homes are taken together, it is estimated that they use as much electricity as is generated by *four* nuclear power plants. While you can buy Energy Star rated appliances, cable boxes are still among the worst electronics in energy efficiency, and manufacturers have been slow to respond to pressure to make costly, energy-saving changes. Unfortunately, shutting off the boxes does little to help, as they consume power even when turned off as hard drives keep running, downloading, and updating. While unplugging the cable boxes can stop that, it may cause other problems and require a long reboot when you want to use the system. What can you do to reduce the massive amounts of energy associated with your cable box? Consider limiting the amount of cable boxes in your home or do more streaming on lower energy use devices such as laptops. Another option is to take action by writing your congressional representative and to get involved in pushing for changes.

In addition to your cable box, also consider the energy consumption of your television. In general, the bigger the screen, the greater the power consumption; moving from a 36-inch to a 60-inch set can make for a major hit on your electric bill and the amount of electricity consumed. In addition, LCD and plasma sets often use more electricity than comparable sized LED sets. There are several online resources for comparing energy consumption levels. Sets purchased after 2010 have to meet even more stringent qualifications for an Energy Star rating due to changes in regulations.

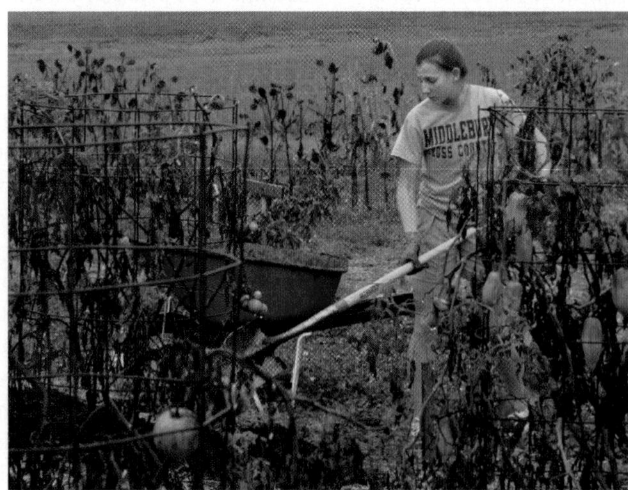

Schools can "go green" by supporting organic gardens and other sustainable activities.

Does receiving support, such as plentiful bicycle racks, for alternative forms of transportation around campus make it more likely that you can contribute to a greener environment?

If you must have a 40-inch or larger set, there are things you can do to reduce your energy use:

- Adjust your brightness and contrast controls downward. Most people don't need the standard brightness settings that make sets "pop" in the showroom.
- Buy one size down from what you think you need.
- Pay careful attention to Energy Star ratings. Newer sets have better ratings overall, with old tube sets being the worst culprits of all.

Choosing a Green Location

While you can make smart consumer choices to reduce your ecological footprint, another issue to think about is the physical location of your campus and where you live. A recent report from the American Lung Association rated the cleanest and dirtiest U.S. cities in terms of air pollution.[82] Among the top 10 in ozone pollution were Los Angeles, Sacramento, and Houston; Bakersfield, Los Angeles, and Pittsburgh were all high in particle pollution. The cleanest in ozone pollution included Honolulu, Fargo (North Dakota), and Gainesville (Florida); the lowest in particle pollution included Cheyenne (Wyoming), Santa Fe (New Mexico), and Tucson. In the future, will students consider air pollution and other environmental factors when making their choices about schooling? Would you consider moving to or from a given urban environment based on air quality and other "green" issues?

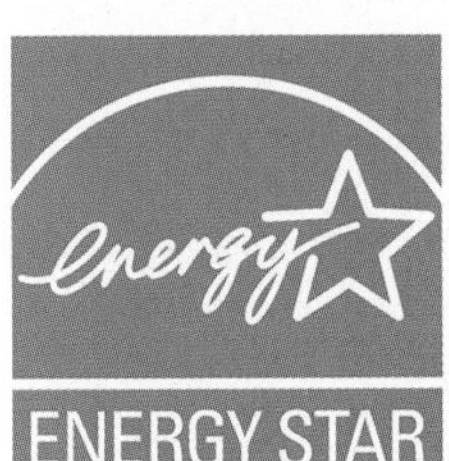

The Energy Star logo signals that an appliance meets energy conservation standards.

According to *Sierra* magazine, of the nation's most sustainable colleges, 91 percent have organic gardens, 90 percent serve protein-rich meat-free meals daily, and 64 percent maintain bike-sharing programs.[83] These "green" colleges also have programs to protect wildlife on their property, include courses focused on sustainability in their curriculum, and take measures to divert their waste from landfills. Consider researching and getting involved with the measures toward sustainability at your school.

Skills for **Behavior Change**

SHOPPING TO SAVE THE PLANET

Home Goods

- **Look for products with less packaging or with refillable, reusable, or recyclable containers.**
- **Do not use caustic cleansers. Simple vinegar or a dilute mixture of water and bleach is usually just as effective and less harsh on your home and the environment.**
- **Buy laundry products that are free of dyes, fragrances, and sulfates.**
- **Use soap and water to clean surfaces, not disposable cleaning cloths and spray-on shower cleaners. Avoid antibacterial soaps and cleaners because they contribute to microbial resistance.**
- **Buy recycled paper products when you can.**
- **Purchase bed linens and bath towels that are made from bamboo, hemp, or organic cotton.**
- **Use reusable mugs, plates, napkins, and silverware rather than disposable products. Wash and reuse plastic silverware.**

Electronics

- **Purchase appliances with the Energy Star logo. Remember that your big-screen TV may be a huge energy drain, along with your old refrigerator. Replace outdated appliances when you can, and watch those energy levels.**
- **Buy CFLs instead of less energy-efficient incandescent bulbs. Use caution when installing and removing CFLs and avoid breakage—CFLs contain mercury. Clear the room for at least 30 minutes after any accidental breakage.**

Groceries

- **Bring your own reusable, washable grocery bags to the store. (Be sure to wash bags after carrying meat in them.)**
- **Be a better food planner. Make a list when shopping and only buy what you will use.**
- **Buy foods that are produced sustainably or organically or foods produced with fewer chemicals and pesticides.**
- **Purchase locally produced foods to reduce pollutants associated with transporting food long distances.**
- **Eat lower on the food chain. By eating more vegetables and nuts, legumes, and other food crops, and reducing consumption of meat, dairy, and animal products, you have a smaller footprint stomping on the planet.**
- **Don't be picky. Buy fruit and vegetables even if they don't have a perfect shape, and eat them before they rot. Consider using fruits that are slightly bruised or a little too soft for baked goods or blending them into smoothies.**
- **Do not buy plastic bottles of water. Purchase a hard plastic or stainless steel water bottle and fill it from a filtered source. Wash it regularly.**

check yourself

- **What are three changes you can make now to help the environment?**
- **What, if any, are reasons that prevent you from making choices that are environmentally aware?**

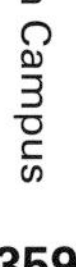

14.9

What Are You Doing to Preserve the Environment?

Environmental problems often seem too big for one person to make a difference. Each day, though, there are things you can do that contribute to the planet's health. For each statement below, indicate how often you follow the described behavior.

An interactive version of this assessment is available online in MasteringHealth.

	Always	Usually	Sometimes	Never
1. Whenever possible, I walk or ride my bicycle rather than drive a car.	1	2	3	4
2. I carpool with others to school or work.	1	2	3	4
3. I have my car tuned up and inspected every year.	1	2	3	4
4. When I change the oil in my car, I make sure the oil is properly recycled, rather than dumped on the ground or into a floor drain.	1	2	3	4
5. I avoid using the air conditioner except during extreme conditions.	1	2	3	4
6. I turn off the lights when a room is not being used.	1	2	3	4
7. I take a shower rather than a bath most of the time.	1	2	3	4
8. I have water-saving devices installed on my shower, toilet, and sinks.	1	2	3	4
9. I make sure faucets and toilets in my home do not leak.	1	2	3	4
10. I use my bath towels more than once before putting them in the wash.	1	2	3	4
11. I wear my clothes more than once between washings when possible.	1	2	3	4
12. I make sure that the washing machine is full before I wash a load of clothes.	1	2	3	4
13. I purchase biodegradable soaps and detergents.	1	2	3	4
14. I use biodegradable trash bags.	1	2	3	4
15. At home, I use dishes and silverware rather than disposable products.	1	2	3	4
16. When I buy prepackaged foods, I choose the ones with the least packaging.	1	2	3	4
17. I do not subscribe to newspapers and magazines that I can view online.	1	2	3	4
18. I do not use a hair dryer.	1	2	3	4
19. I bring reusable bags to the grocery store.	1	2	3	4
20. I don't run water continuously when washing the dishes, shaving, or brushing my teeth.	1	2	3	4
21. I use unbleached or recycled paper.	1	2	3	4
22. I use both sides of printer paper and other paper when possible.	1	2	3	4
23. If I have items I do not want to use anymore, I donate them to charity so someone else can use them.	1	2	3	4
24. I carry a reusable mug for my coffee or tea and have it filled, rather than using a new paper cup each time I buy a hot beverage.	1	2	3	4
25. I carry and use a refillable water bottle rather than frequently buying bottled water.	1	2	3	4
26. I clean up after myself while enjoying the outdoors (picnicking, camping, etc.).	1	2	3	4
27. I volunteer for cleanup days in the community in which I live.	1	2	3	4
28. I consider candidates' positions on environmental issues before casting my vote.	1	2	3	4

For Further Thought

Review your scores. Are your responses mostly 1s and 2s? If not, what actions can you take to become more environmentally responsible? Are there ways to help the environment on this list that you had not thought of before? Are there behaviors not on the list that you are already doing?

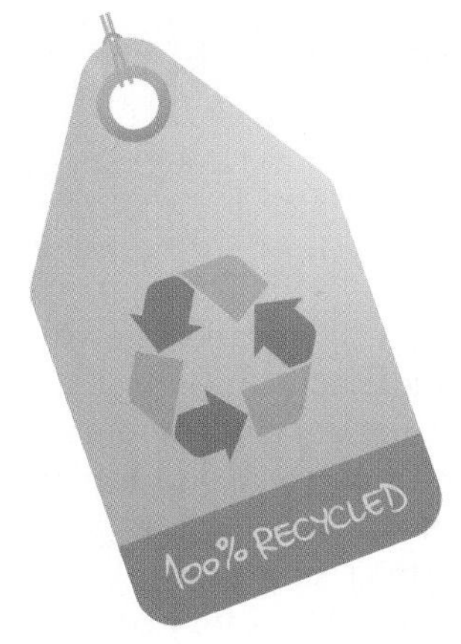

Your Plan for Change

The Assess Yourself activity gave you the chance to look at your behavior and consider ways to conserve energy, save water, reduce waste, and otherwise help protect the planet. Now that you have considered these results, you can take steps to become more environmentally responsible.

Today, you can:

◯ Find out how much energy you are using. Visit http://footprint.wwf.org.uk to find out what your carbon footprint is and how your behaviors would affect the planet if others lived like you. Learn about what you can do to change your carbon footprint.

◯ Reduce the amount of paper waste in your mailbox. You can stop junk mail, such as credit card offers and unwanted catalogs, by visiting the Direct Marketing Association's Mail Preference Service site at www.dmachoice.org. You can also call 1-888-5 OPT OUT to put an end to unwanted mail. In addition, the website www.catalogchoice.org is a free service that lets you decline paper catalogs you no longer want to receive.

Within the next 2 weeks, you can:

◯ Look into joining a local environmental group, attending a campus environmental event, or taking an environmental science course.

◯ Take part in a local cleanup day or recycling drive. These can be fun opportunities to meet like-minded people while benefiting the planet.

By the end of the semester, you can:

◯ Interview and talk with your campus's dining hall director about initiating a compost recycling program. The EPA provides information on setting up an indoor compost bin at www.epa.gov.

◯ Make a habit of recycling everything you can. Find out what items can be recycled in your neighborhood and designate a box or bin to hold recyclable materials—cans, bottles, plastic, newspapers, junk mail, and so on—until you can transport them to a curbside bin or drop-off center.

◯ Work to influence the environment on a larger scale. Take part in an environmental activism group on campus or in your community. Listen carefully to what political candidates say about the environment. Let your legislators know how you feel about environmental issues and that you will vote according to their record on the issues.

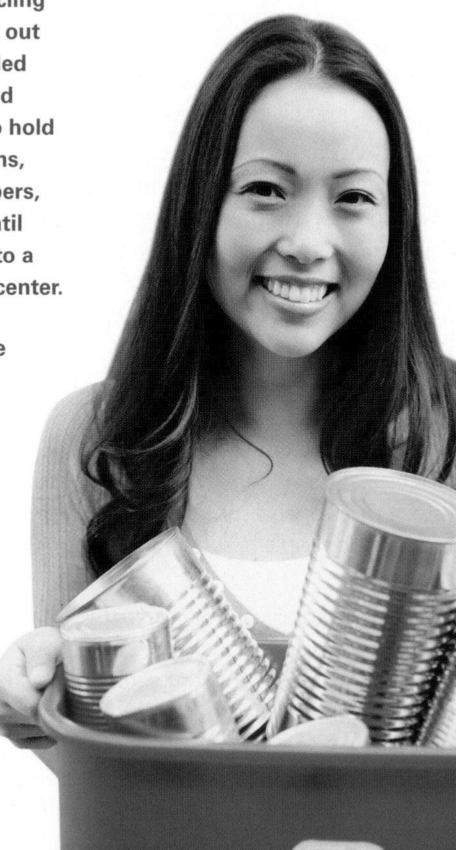

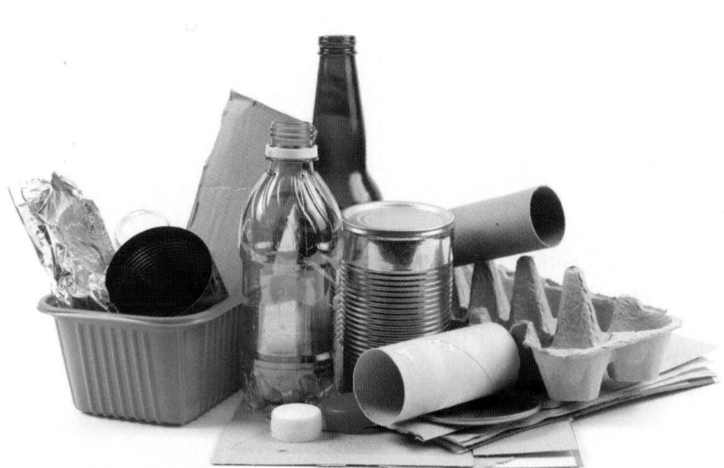

Summary

To hear an MP3 Tutor session, scan here or visit the Study Area in **MasteringHealth.**

LO 14.1 Population growth is the single largest factor affecting the environment. Demand for more food, water, and energy—as well as places to dispose of waste—places great strain on Earth's resources. The United States is among the greatest consumers of natural resources per person of any nation in the world. We can do more to reduce, reuse, and recycle.

LO 14.2 The primary constituents of air pollution are sulfur dioxide, particulate matter, carbon monoxide, nitrogen dioxide, ground level ozone, lead, carbon dioxide, and hydrocarbons.

LO 14.3 Indoor air pollution is caused primarily by tobacco smoke, woodstove smoke, furnace emissions, asbestos, formaldehyde, radon, lead, and mold.

LO 14.4 Pollution is depleting Earth's protective ozone layer and contributing to global warming, a type of climate change, by enhancing the greenhouse effect.

LO 14.5 Water pollution can be caused by either point sources (direct entry) or nonpoint sources (runoff or seepage). Major contributors to water pollution include petroleum products, organic solvents, polychlorinated biphenyls (PCBs), dioxins, pesticides, and lead.

LO 14.6 Solid waste pollution includes household trash, plastics, glass, metal products, and paper. Limited landfill space creates problems. Hazardous waste is toxic; improper disposal creates health hazards for people in surrounding communities.

LO 14.7 Nonionizing radiation comes from electromagnetic fields, such as those around power lines. Ionizing radiation results from the natural erosion of atomic nuclei. The disposal and storage of radioactive waste from nuclear power plants pose potential problems for public health.

LO 14.8 Living sustainably includes making smart consumer choices and reducing the amount of resources you use in daily life.

Pop Quiz

Visit MasteringHealth to personalize your study plan with Chapter Review Quizzes and Dynamic Study Modules.

LO 14.1 **1.** The largest population that can be supported indefinitely given the resources available is known as the earth's
a. maximum fertility rate.
b. fertility capacity.
c. maximum population growth.
d. carrying capacity.

LO 14.2 **2.**The phenomenon that creates a barrier to protect us from the sun's harmful ultraviolet radiation rays is
a. photochemical smog.
b. the ozone layer.
c. gray air smog.
d. the greenhouse effect.

LO 14.2 **3.** The air pollutant that originates primarily from motor vehicle emissions is
a. particulates.
b. nitrogen dioxide.
c. sulfur dioxide.
d. carbon monoxide.

LO 14.3 **4.** One possible source of indoor air pollution is a gas present in some carpets and home furnishings called
a. lead.
b. asbestos.
c. radon.
d. formaldehyde.

LO 14.3 **5.** Which of the following substances separates into tiny fibers that can become embedded in the lungs?
a. Asbestos
b. Particulate matter
c. Radon
d. Formaldehyde

LO 14.5 **6.** Some herbicides contain toxic substances called
a. THMs.
b. PCPs.
c. dioxins.
d. PCBs.

LO 14.5 **7.** The terms *point source* and *nonpoint source* are used to describe the two general sources of
a. water pollution.
b. air pollution.
c. noise pollution.
d. ozone depletion.

LO 14.6 **8.** A DVD you recently purchased came with less packaging than DVDs once had. This is an example of controlling municipal solid waste via
a. source reduction.
b. recycling.
c. composting.
d. incineration.

LO 14.7 **9.** Which gas is considered radioactive and could become cancer causing when it seeps into a home?
a. Carbon monoxide
b. Radon
c. Hydrogen sulfide
d. Natural gas

LO 14.7 **10.** What is the recommended safe level of rad exposure per year?
a. 0.5 to 5 rads
b. 5 to 100 rads
c. 100 to 200 rads
d. 200 to 350 rads

Answers to these questions can be found on page A-1. If you answered a question incorrectly, review the module identified by the Learning Outcome. For even more study tools, visit MasteringHealth.

Consumerism and Complementary and Alternative Medicine

15

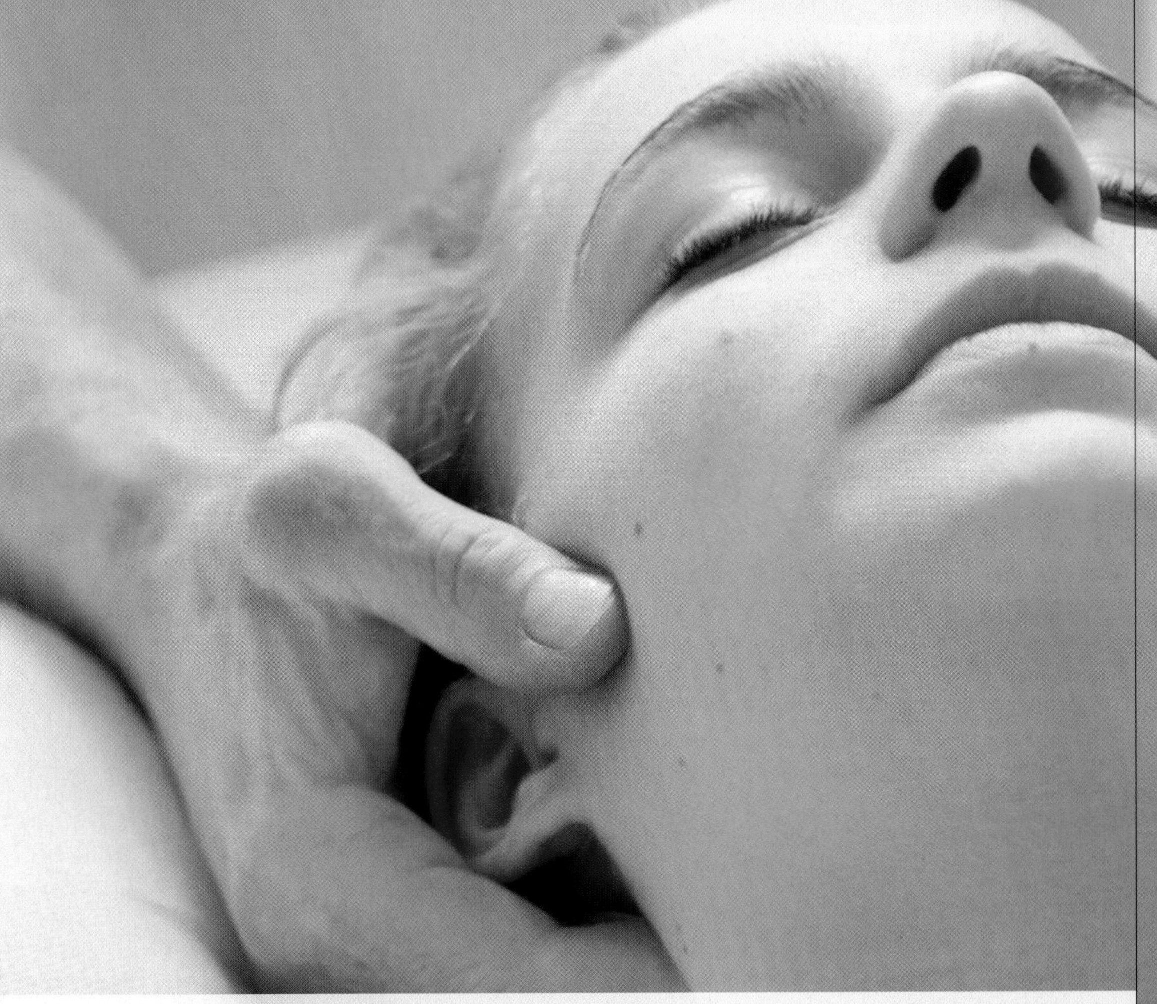

Have there been times when you wondered whether you were sick enough to go to your campus health clinic? Have you left medical visits feeling that you didn't get a thorough exam, or with more questions than when you arrived? Have you wondered about, or successfully used, alternative medical care? Have you ever had to help a loved one make health care decisions?

There are many reasons for you to learn to make better decisions about your health and health care. Most important, you only have one body. If you don't treat it with care, you will pay a major price in terms of monetary costs and consequences to your health. Doing everything you can to stay healthy and to recover rapidly when you do get sick will enhance every other part of your life. Throughout this book we have emphasized the importance of healthy preventive behaviors. Learning when and how to navigate the health care system are important parts of taking charge of your health.

15.1 Taking Responsibility for Your Health Care

learning outcome

15.1 Explain how to use the medical system and when to seek medical help.

As the health care industry has become more sophisticated in seeking your business, so must you become more sophisticated in purchasing its products and services. Acting responsibly in times of illness can be difficult, but the person best able to act on your behalf is you.

If you are not feeling well, you must first decide whether you need to seek medical advice. Not seeking treatment, whether because of high costs or limited coverage, or trying to medicate yourself when more rigorous methods of treatment are needed is potentially dangerous. Understanding the benefits and limits of self-care is critical for responsible consumerism.

Self-Care

Individuals can practice behaviors that promote health, prevent disease, and minimize reliance on the formal medical system. Minor afflictions can often be treated without professional help. Self-care consists of knowing your body, paying attention to its signals, and taking appropriate action to stop the progression of illness or injury. Common forms of self-care include the following:

- Diagnosing symptoms or conditions that occur frequently but may not require physician visits (e.g., the common cold, minor abrasions)
- Using over-the-counter remedies to treat minor infrequent pains, scrapes, or symptoms
- Performing monthly breast or testicular self-examinations
- Learning first aid for common, uncomplicated injuries and conditions
- Checking blood pressure, pulse, and temperature
- Doing periodic checks for blood cholesterol level
- Learning from reliable self-help books, websites, and DVDs
- Benefiting from nutrition, rest, exercise, and meditation and other relaxation techniques

In addition, a vast array of at-home diagnostic kits are now available to test for pregnancy, allergies, HIV, genetic disorders, and many other conditions. Caution is in order here: diagnoses from these devices and kits may not always be accurate—or you may not have the ability to understand the ramifications of what you learn without professional interpretation. Home health tests are not substitutes for regular, complete examinations by a trained practitioner.

Using self-care methods appropriately takes education and effort. Taking prescription drugs used for a previous illness to treat your current illness, using unproven self-treatment methods, or using other people's medications are examples of inappropriate self-care.

When to Seek Help

Effective self-care means paying attention to your body's warning signs and understanding when to seek medical attention. Deciding which conditions warrant professional advice is not always easy. Generally, you should consult a physician if you experience *any* of the following:

- A serious accident or injury
- Sudden or severe chest pains, especially if they cause breathing difficulties
- Trauma to the head or spine accompanied by persistent headache, blurred vision, loss of consciousness, vomiting, convulsions, or paralysis
- Sudden high fever or recurring high temperature (over 102°F for children and 103°F for adults) and/or sweats
- Tingling sensation in the arm accompanied by slurred speech or impaired thought processes
- Adverse reactions to a drug or insect bite (shortness of breath, severe swelling, dizziness)
- Unexplained bleeding or loss of fluid from any body opening
- Unexplained sudden weight loss
- Persistent or recurrent diarrhea or vomiting
- Blue-colored lips, eyelids, or nail beds

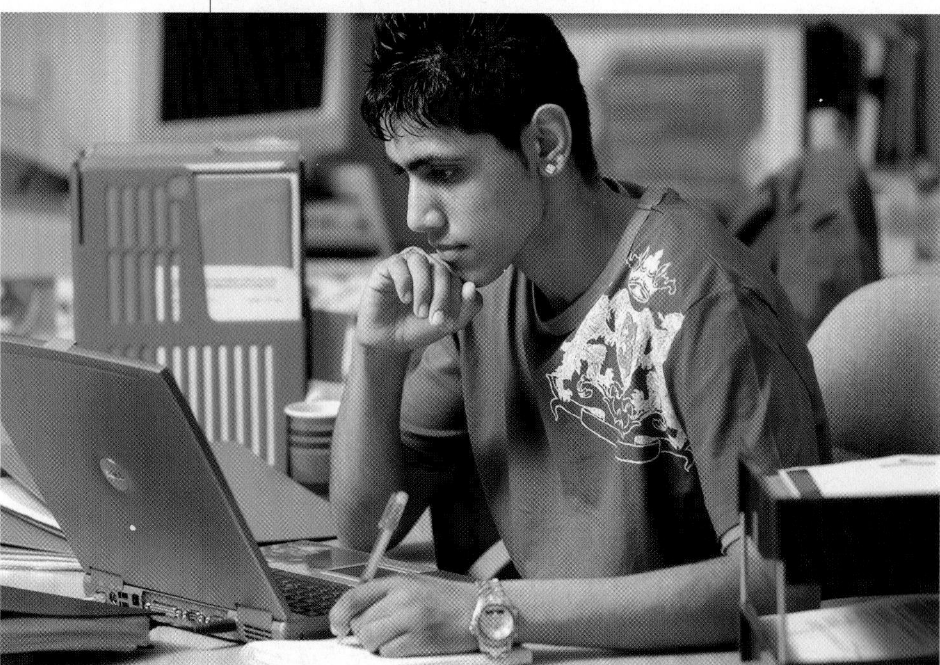

Deciding when to contact a physician can be difficult. Most people first research symptoms online and try to diagnose and treat a condition themselves.

- Any lump, swelling, thickness, or sore that does not subside or that grows for over a month
- Any marked change or pain in bowel or bladder habits
- Yellowing of the skin or the whites of the eyes
- Any symptom that is unusual and recurs over time
- Pregnancy

The Placebo Effect

The *placebo effect* is an apparent cure or improved state of health brought about by a substance, product, or procedure that has no generally recognized therapeutic value. Patients often report improvements in a condition based on what they expect, desire, or were told would happen after receiving a treatment, even though that treatment was, for example, simple sugar pills instead of powerful drugs.

There is also a *nocebo* effect, in which a practitioner's negative assessment of a patient's symptoms leads to a worsening of the condition, such as increased anxiety and pain. Similarly, a negative assessment of a treatment's potential efficacy induces a failure to respond to that treatment.

Researchers are investigating how and why expectation appears to change physiology. Evidence from pain studies suggests that use of a placebo for pain control causes the brain to release the same endogenous (natural) opioids it releases when the study participant uses a pain medication with an active ingredient.[1] But pain is not the only factor to respond to expectation: A study of resting tremor (such as involuntary finger-tapping) in patients with Parkinson's disease found that positive or negative expectations of a treatment's effectiveness reduced or increased patient tremor when they were given the same valid medication or the same placebo.[2] Similar chemical changes on brain imaging tests were seen with placebos in studies of depression and alcohol dependency treatment.[3]

See It! Videos

How do you avoid misdiagnosed medical advice online? Watch **Misdiagnosis on the Web** in the Study Area of MasteringHealth.

See It! Videos

Knowing your medical history can keep you informed of health risks. Watch **Your Medical History** in the Study Area of MasteringHealth.

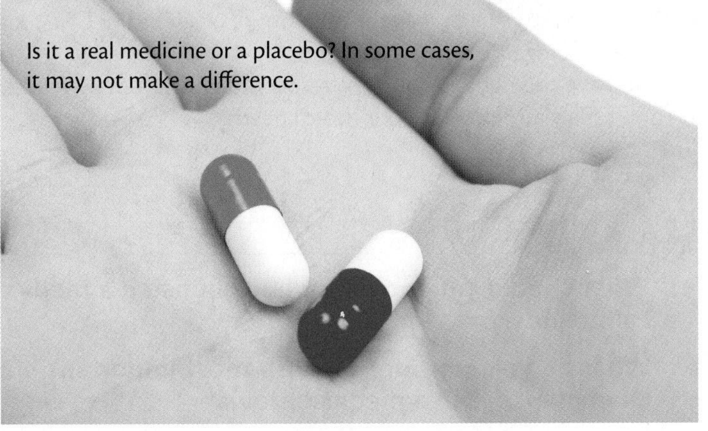
Is it a real medicine or a placebo? In some cases, it may not make a difference.

People who unknowingly use placebos when medical treatment is needed increase their risk for health problems. However, what we learn from the ways in which placebos work may someday help us harness the mind's power to treat certain diseases and conditions.

Skills for Behavior Change

BE PROACTIVE IN YOUR HEALTH CARE

Here are some tips for getting the most out of doctor visits and being proactive in your health care:

- **Keep records of your own and your family's medical histories.**
- **Research your condition—causes, physiological effects, possible treatments, and prognosis. Don't rely on your health care provider for this information.**
- **If you use a complementary and alternative medicine (CAM) therapy such as acupuncture, choose a practitioner with care. Your insurer may also cover such services.**
- **Bring a friend or relative along to medical visits to help you review what the doctor says. If you go alone, take notes. Write down what happened and what was said.**
- **Ask the practitioner to explain the problem and possible treatments, tests, and drugs in a clear and understandable way. If you don't understand something, ask for clarification.**
- **If a health care provider prescribes any medications, ask whether you can take generic equivalents that cost less.**
- **Ask for a written summary of the results of your visit and any lab tests.**
- **Find out what studies have been done on the safety and effectiveness of any treatment in which you are interested. Consult only reliable sources—texts, journals, and government resources. Start with the websites listed at the end of this text.**
- **If you have any doubt about a recommended treatment, get a second opinion.**
- **Decisions regarding treatment should be made in consultation with your health care provider and based on your condition and needs.**
- **If you use any CAM therapy, inform your primary health care provider. It is particularly important to talk with your provider if you are thinking about replacing your prescribed treatment with one or more supplements, are currently taking a prescription drug, have a chronic medical condition, are planning to have surgery, are pregnant or nursing, or are thinking about giving supplements to children.**
- **When filling prescriptions, ask the pharmacist to show you the package inserts that list medical considerations. Request detailed information about potential drug and food interactions.**
- **Remember that *natural* and *safe* are not necessarily the same. You can become seriously ill from seemingly harmless "natural" products. Be cautious about combining herbal medications, just as you would about combining other drugs. Seek help if you notice any unusual side effects.**

check yourself

- **What are four instances in which you should seek medical help?**

15.2 Assessing Health Professionals

learning outcome

15.2 List factors to consider when choosing a medical provider.

The most satisfied patients are those who feel their health care provider explains diagnosis and treatment options thoroughly and communicates competency and caring.[4] When evaluating health care providers, consider the following questions:

- Does the provider listen to you and give you time to ask questions? Does the provider return your calls? Is he or she available to answer questions between visits?
- What professional education and training has the provider had? What license or board certification(s) does he or she hold? Note that *board-certified* indicates that a physician has passed the national board examination for his or her specialty (e.g., pediatrics) and has been certified as competent in that specialty; *board-eligible* means that the physician is eligible to take a specialty board's exam, but not necessarily that he or she has passed it.
- Is the provider a specialist in family or internal medicine, or does the provider have another specialty? Is this right for you?
- Is the provider affiliated with an accredited medical facility or institution? The Joint Commission is an independent nonprofit organization that evaluates and accredits more than 15,000 health care organizations and programs in the United States. Accreditation requires that these institutions verify all education, licensing, and training claims of affiliated practitioners.
- Is the provider open to complementary or alternative strategies? Would he or she refer you for different treatments if appropriate?
- Does the provider indicate clearly how long a given treatment may last, what side effects you might expect, and what problems you should watch for?
- Who will be responsible for your care when your provider is on vacation or off call?
- Are professional reviews and information on any lawsuits involving the provider available online?
- If you have health insurance, is the provider in-network? You will most likely end up paying less out of pocket with an in-network doctor.

Ask yourself the following questions about the quality of care you are receiving:

- Did your health care provider take a thorough health history and ask for any recent updates to it? Was your examination thorough?
- Did your provider listen to you?
- Did you feel comfortable asking questions? Did your provider answer thoroughly, in a way that was easy to understand?

Asking the right questions at the right time may save you suffering and expense. Many patients find that writing their questions down before an appointment helps.

Active participation in your treatment is the only sensible course in a health care environment that encourages **defensive medicine**, or the use of medical practices designed to avert the possibility of malpractice suits. In a recent survey of physicians, 58 percent indicated that they have ordered a test or procedure for primarily defensive medicine reasons.[5] Unwarranted treatment such as the overuse of antibiotics and use of diagnostic tests to protect against malpractice exposure are driving up the cost of medicine.[6]

In addition to asking the suggested questions above, being proactive in your health care also means that you should be aware of your rights as a patient:[7]

1. The right of informed consent means that before receiving any care you should be fully informed of what is planned, the risks and potential benefits, and possible alternative forms of treatment, including the option to refuse treatment. Your consent must be voluntary and without any form of coercion. It is critical that you read any consent forms carefully and amend them as necessary before signing.
2. You have the right to know whether the treatment you are receiving is standard or experimental. In experimental conditions, you have the legal and ethical right to know if any drug is being used in the research project for a purpose not approved by the Food and Drug Administration (FDA) and whether the study is one in which some people receive treatment while others receive a placebo.
3. You have the right to make decisions regarding the health care that is recommended by the physician.
4. You have the right to confidentiality. This means that you do not have an obligation to reveal the source of payment for your treatment. It also means you have the right to make personal decisions concerning all reproductive matters.
5. You have the right to receive adequate health care, as well as to refuse treatment and to cease treatment at any time.
6. You are entitled to have access to all of your medical records and to have those records remain confidential.
7. You have the right to continuity of health care.
8. You have the right to seek the opinions of other health care professionals regarding your condition.
9. You have the right to courtesy, respect, dignity, responsiveness, and timely attention to your health needs.

check yourself

- **What should you look for when choosing a medical provider?**
- **What do you consider the four most important characteristics in a medical provider?**

15.3 Types of Allopathic Health Care Providers

learning outcome

15.3 Identify the main types of allopathic health care providers.

Conventional health care, also called **allopathic medicine,** mainstream medicine, or traditional Western medical practice, is based on the premise that illness is a result of exposure to harmful environmental agents, such as infectious microorganisms and pollutants or organic changes in the body. The prevention of disease and the restoration of health involve vaccines, drugs, surgery, and other treatments.

Allopathic health care providers use **evidence-based medicine,** in which decisions regarding patient care are based on a combination of clinical expertise, patient values, and current best scientific evidence.

Selecting a **primary care practitioner (PCP)**—a medical practitioner you can visit for routine ailments, preventive care, general medical advice, and referrals—is not easy. The PCP for most people is a family practitioner, internist, pediatrician, or obstetrician-gynecologist (ob-gyn). Some people see nurse practitioners or physician assistants who work for individual doctors or medical groups, whereas others use nontraditional providers as their primary source of care. As a college student, you may opt to visit a PCP at your campus health center.

Doctors undergo rigorous training before they can begin practicing. After 4 years of undergraduate work, students typically spend 4 years studying for the medical degree (MD). Some students then choose a specialty, such as pediatrics, cardiology, or surgery, spending a 1-year internship and several years in residency with that emphasis.

Specialists include **osteopaths,** general practitioners who receive training similar to that of MDs, but who place special emphasis on the skeletal and muscular systems. Their treatments may involve manipulation of muscles and joints. Osteopaths receive the degree of doctor of osteopathy (DO) rather than MD.

Eye care specialists can be either ophthalmologists or optometrists. An **ophthalmologist** holds a medical degree and can perform surgery and prescribe medications. An **optometrist** typically evaluates visual problems and fits glasses but is not a trained physician. If you have an eye infection, glaucoma, or other eye condition that requires diagnosis and treatment, you need to see an ophthalmologist.

Dentists are specialists who diagnose and treat diseases of the teeth, gums, and oral cavity. They attend dental school for 4 years and receive the title of doctor of dental surgery (DDS) or doctor of medical dentistry (DMD). *Orthodontists* specialize in the alignment of teeth. *Oral surgeons* perform surgical procedures to correct problems of the mouth, face, and jaw.

Nurses are highly trained and strictly regulated health professionals who provide a wide range of services, including patient education, counseling, community health and disease prevention information, and administration of medications. Registered nurses (RNs) in the United States complete either a 4-year program leading to a bachelor of science in nursing (BSN) degree or a 2-year associate degree program. Lower-level licensed practical or vocational nurses (LPNs or LVNs) complete a 1- to 2-year training program based in a community college or a hospital.

Nurse practitioners (NPs) are nurses with advanced training obtained through either a master's degree program or a specialized nurse practitioner program. Nurse practitioners have the training and authority to conduct diagnostic tests and prescribe medications (in some states).

Physician assistants (PAs) examine and diagnose patients, offer treatment, and write prescriptions under a physician's supervision. Unlike an NP, a PA must practice under a physician's supervision.

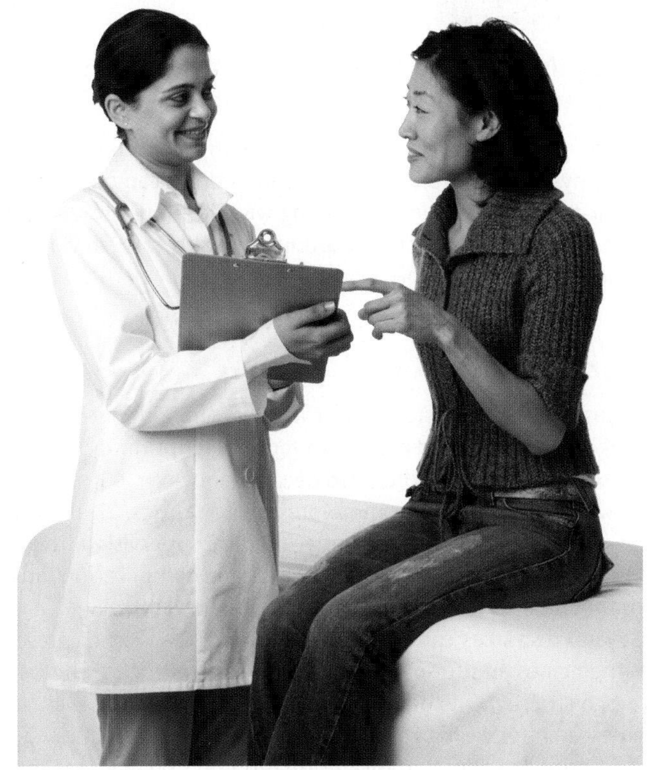

Understanding the differences among different types of health care providers is important. In some cases, you may need to see a doctor with a particular specialty; in other cases, a nurse practitioner or physician assistant may be satisfactory.

check yourself

- **What is allopathic medicine?**
- **What are some of the major types of allopathic health care providers?**

15.4 Choosing Health Products: Prescription and OTC Drugs

learning outcome

15.4 Explain how to determine the risks and benefits of prescription and over-the-counter medicines.

Prescription drugs can be obtained only with a written prescription from a physician, whereas over-the-counter drugs can be purchased without a prescription. Just as making wise decisions about providers is an important aspect of responsible health care, so is making wise decisions about medications.

Prescription Drugs

In about 3 out of 4 doctor visits, the physician administers or prescribes at least one medication.[8] In fact, prescription drug use has increased steadily over the past decade, and over 68 percent of Americans now use one or more prescription drugs.[9] Even though these drugs are administered under medical supervision, the wise consumer still takes precautions. Hazards and complications arising from the use of prescription drugs are common.

Several resources can help you determine the risks of prescription medicines and to make educated decisions about whether to take a given drug. One of the best is the Center for Drug Evaluation and Research (www.fda.gov). This consumer-specific section of the FDA website provides current information on risks and benefits of prescription drugs.

Generic drugs, medications sold under a chemical name rather than a brand name, contain the same active ingredients as brand-name drugs but are less expensive. If your doctor prescribes a drug, always ask if a generic equivalent exists and if it would be safe and effective for you to try. There is some controversy about effectiveness of generic drugs: Substitutions sometimes are made in minor ingredients that can affect the way the drug is absorbed, potentially causing discomfort or even allergic reactions in some patients.[10] Tell your doctor about any reactions you have to medications.

Medications Online: Buyer Beware Consumers may choose to have prescriptions filled online for convenience and to save money. Although many websites operate legally and observe the traditional safeguards for dispensing drugs, be wary of rogue websites that sell unapproved or counterfeit drugs or that sidestep practices meant to protect consumers.

The Verified Internet Pharmacy Practice Sites (VIPPS) seal is given to online pharmacy sites that meet state licensure requirements. Follow these tips to protect yourself from fraudulent sites:[11]

- Buy only from state-licensed pharmacy sites based in the United States (preferably from VIPPS-certified sites).
- Don't buy from sites that sell prescription drugs without a prescription or that offer to prescribe a medication for the first time without a physical exam by your doctor or by answering an online questionnaire.
- Use legitimate websites that have a licensed pharmacist to answer your questions.
- Don't provide personal information, such as a Social Security number, credit card information, or medical or health history, unless you are sure the website will keep your information safe and private.

48.5% of Americans report taking at least one prescription drug in the past month; 21.7% report taking three or more such drugs.

Be very cautious if you consider ordering medications from an online pharmacy.

Over-the-Counter (OTC) Drugs

Over-the-counter (OTC) drugs are nonprescription substances used for self-medication. American consumers spend billions of dollars yearly on OTC preparations for relief of everything from runny noses to ingrown toenails. Despite a common belief that OTC products are safe and effective, indiscriminate use and abuse can occur with these drugs as with all others. For example, people who frequently drop medication into their eyes to "get the red out" or pop antacids after every meal are likely to become dependent on these remedies. Many experience adverse side effects because they ignore or don't read the warnings on OTC drug labels. The FDA has developed a standard label that appears on most OTC products (Figure 15.1).

Understanding the actions and side effects of OTC drugs is part of being a smart consumer. *Pain relievers* can be useful for counteracting localized or general pain and for reducing fever. They exist in several general formulations (common brand names follow each): *aspirin* (Bayer, Bufferin), *acetaminophen* (Tylenol), *ibuprofen* (Advil, Motrin), and *naproxen sodium* (Aleve, Naprosyn). Possible side effects include stomach problems ranging from simple stomach upset to worsening of ulcers; overdose or prolonged overuse can cause liver damage. Aspirin and ibuprofen also

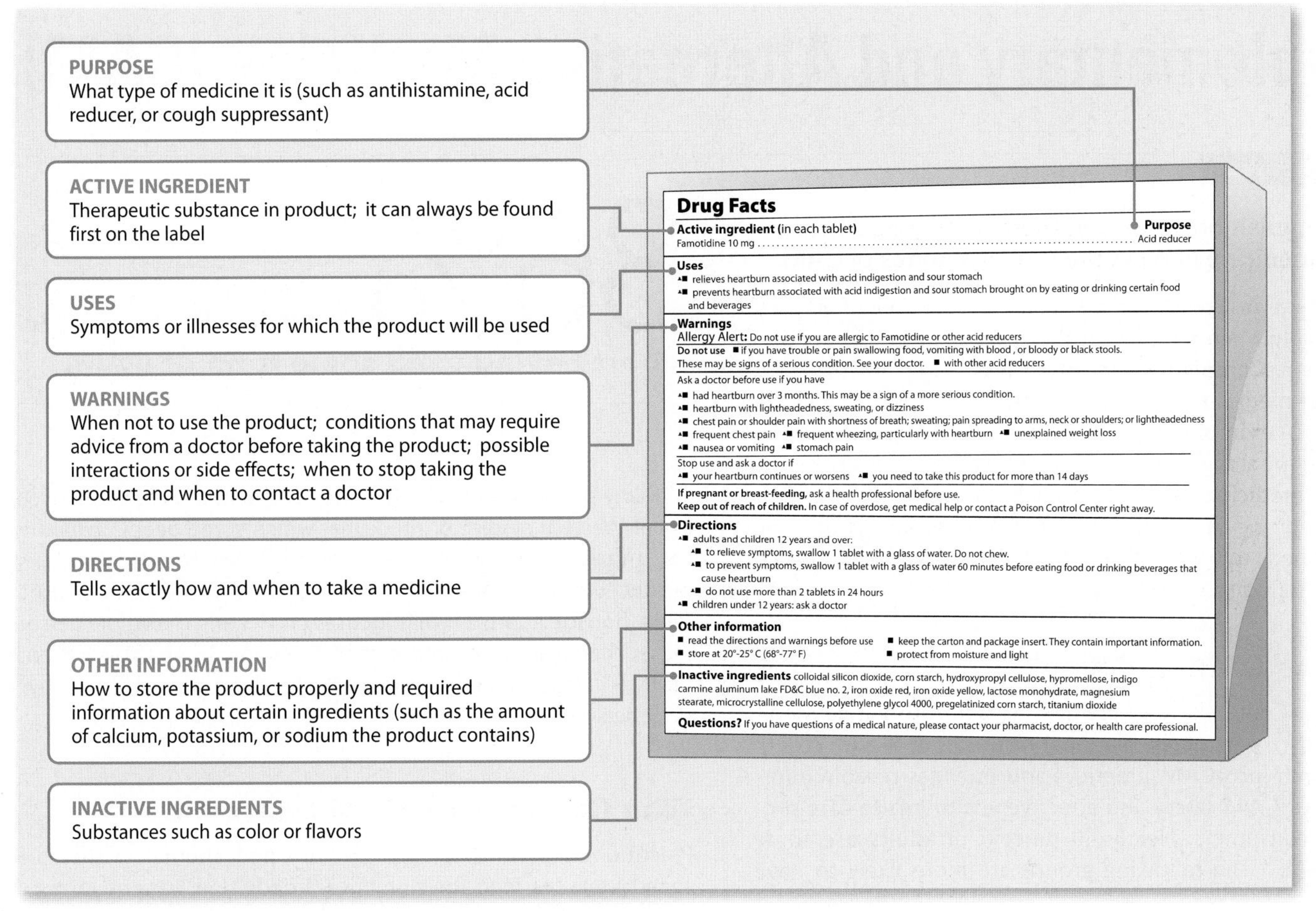

Figure 15.1 The Over-the-Counter Medicine Label

Source: Consumer Healthcare Products Association, OTC Label, www.otcsafety.org. Used with permission.

VIDEO TUTOR
Being a Good Health Care Consumer

reduce blood clotting ability (which can be a problem for those taking anticlotting medications) and, for a few users, can trigger severe allergic reactions. Finally, aspirin should not be taken by anyone under 18, because it has been associated with Reye's syndrome in children and teenagers.

Cold and allergy medicines mask (but don't eliminate) symptoms in a variety of ways. *Antihistamines* (Claritin, Benadryl, Xyzal) dry runny noses, clear postnasal drip and sinus congestion, and reduce tears. They are mild central nervous system depressants and, as such, can cause drowsiness, dizziness, and disturbed coordination in many people. *Decongestants* (Sudafed, DayQuil, Allermed) reduce nasal stuffiness due to colds. In terms of side effects, different people react differently to these medications: Some may exhibit nervousness, restlessness, and sleep problems, whereas others may feel drowsy or nauseated.

Antacids (Tums, Maalox) relieve "heartburn," usually by combating stomach acid with a chemical base such as calcium or aluminum. Occasional use is safe, but chronic use can lead to reduced mineral absorption from food; possible concealment of ulcer; reduced effectiveness of anticlotting medications; interference with the function of certain antibiotics (for antacids that contain aluminum); worsened high blood pressure (for antacids that contain sodium); and aggravated kidney problems.

Laxatives (Ex-lax, Citrucel) are designed to relieve constipation. Although safe with limited and occasional use, long-term regular use can lead to reduced absorption of minerals from food, dehydration, and even dependency (the user's body becoming dependent on the drug for regular bowel movement).

Sleep aids and relaxants (Nytol, Sleep-Eze, Sominex) are designed to help relieve occasional sleeplessness. Short-term side effects include drowsiness and reduced mental alertness, dry mouth and throat, constipation, dizziness, and lack of coordination. Long-term use can lead to dependency.

check yourself

- **What factors should you consider when ordering prescription drugs online?**
- **What are the benefits and potential side effects for three OTC drugs that you use or might use in the future?**

15.5 Complementary and Alternative Medicine (CAM)

learning outcome

15.5 Distinguish between complementary and alternative medicine and list the four categories of CAM.

Although the terms *complementary* and *alternative* are often used interchangeably when referring to therapies, there is a distinction between them. **Complementary medicine** is used *together with* conventional medicine as part of a modern integrative-medicine approach.[12] An example of complementary medicine is the use of massage therapy along with prescription medicine to treat anxiety. **Alternative medicine** has traditionally been used *in place of* conventional medicine—for example, following a special diet or using an herbal remedy to treat cancer *instead* of using radiation, surgery, or other conventional treatments.

Who Uses CAM and Why?

The National Center for Complementary and Alternative Medicine (NCCAM), part of the National Institutes of Health (NIH), funds research into CAM practices and provides reliable information about CAM safety and effectiveness to health care providers and consumers. Nearly 40 percent of adults use some form of CAM.[13] The following groups are more likely to have used CAM:

- More women than men
- People with higher educational levels
- People who have been hospitalized in the past year
- Former smokers (compared with current smokers or those who have never smoked)
- People with back, neck, head, or joint aches or other painful conditions
- People with gastrointestinal disorders or sleeping problems

36% of 18- to 29-year-olds report having used some form of CAM.

Many people seek CAM therapies as alternatives to the conventional Western system of medicine, which some people regard as too invasive, too high-tech, and too toxic in terms of laboratory-produced medications. In contrast, most CAM therapies incorporate a **holistic** approach that focuses on treating the whole person, rather than just an isolated part of the body. Some CAM patients believe that alternative practices will give them greater control over their health care.

Who Can Provide CAM Treatments?

Practitioners of most complementary and alternative therapies spend years learning their practice. In addition, various forms of CAM are increasingly being taught in U.S. medical schools. Similar to conventional medicine, there is no national training, certification, or licensure standard for CAM practitioners, and state regulations differ. Whereas practitioners of conventional medicine have graduated from U.S.-sanctioned schools of medicine or are licensed medical practitioners recognized by the American Medical Association (AMA)—the governing body for all physicians—each CAM domain has a different set of training standards, guidelines for practice, and licensure procedures.

Figure 15.2 The Ten Most Common Complementary and Alternative Medicine (CAM) Therapies among U.S. Adults

Source: Data from P. M. Barnes, B. Bloom, and R. Nahin, "Complementary and Alternative Medicine Use among Adults and Children: United States, 2007," *CDC National Health Statistics Report*, no. 12 (December 2008).

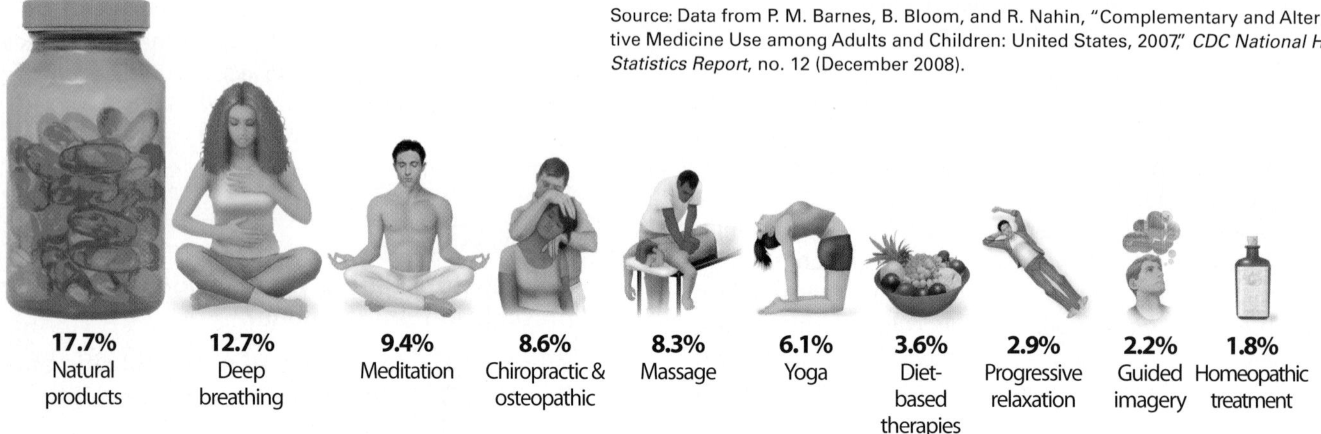

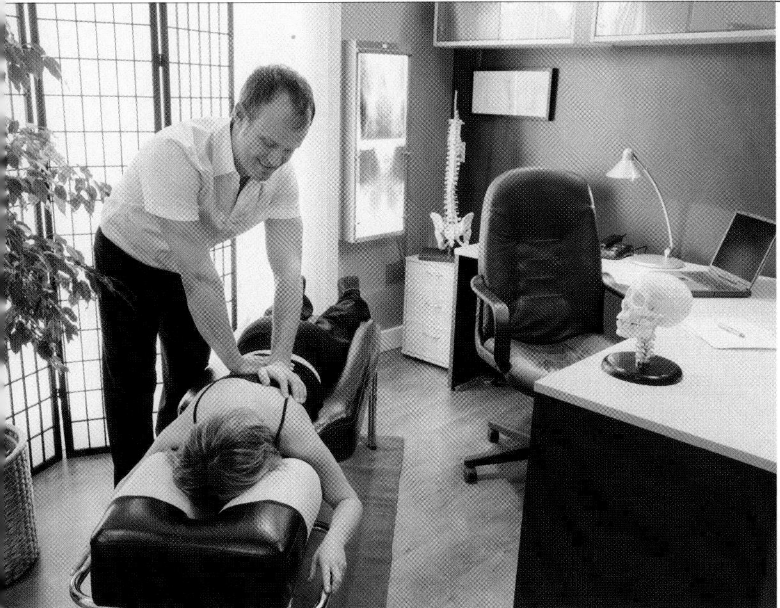

Why are so many people using alternative medicine?

People use alternative medicine for multiple reasons, and many treatments can benefit a variety of physical and mental ailments. For example, chiropractic medicine has shown positive results among people with back and neck pain and headaches.

Nearly all health insurance providers cover at least one form of CAM, with acupuncture, chiropractic, and massage therapy being the most common. However, people who choose CAM often must pay the full cost of services themselves.

What Are the Major Therapies and Categories of CAM?

The ten most common CAM therapies are identified in Figure 15.2. CAM therapies vary widely in terms of the nature and extent of the treatment and the types of problems for which they offer help. They also vary in effectiveness. Research has shown some to be effective for specific conditions, whereas others simply have not been adequately studied or research indicates they are not effective for any specific condition.[14]

Before considering any treatments, consult reliable resources to thoroughly evaluate risks, the scientific basis of claimed benefits, and any contraindications to using the product or service. Avoid practitioners who promote their treatments as a cure-all for every health problem or who seem to promise remedies for ailments that have thus far defied the best scientific efforts of mainstream medicine. In short, apply the same strategies to researching CAM as you would to choosing allopathic care.

The NCCAM has grouped the many varieties of CAM into five general domains of practice, recognizing that domains may overlap (Figure 15.3).

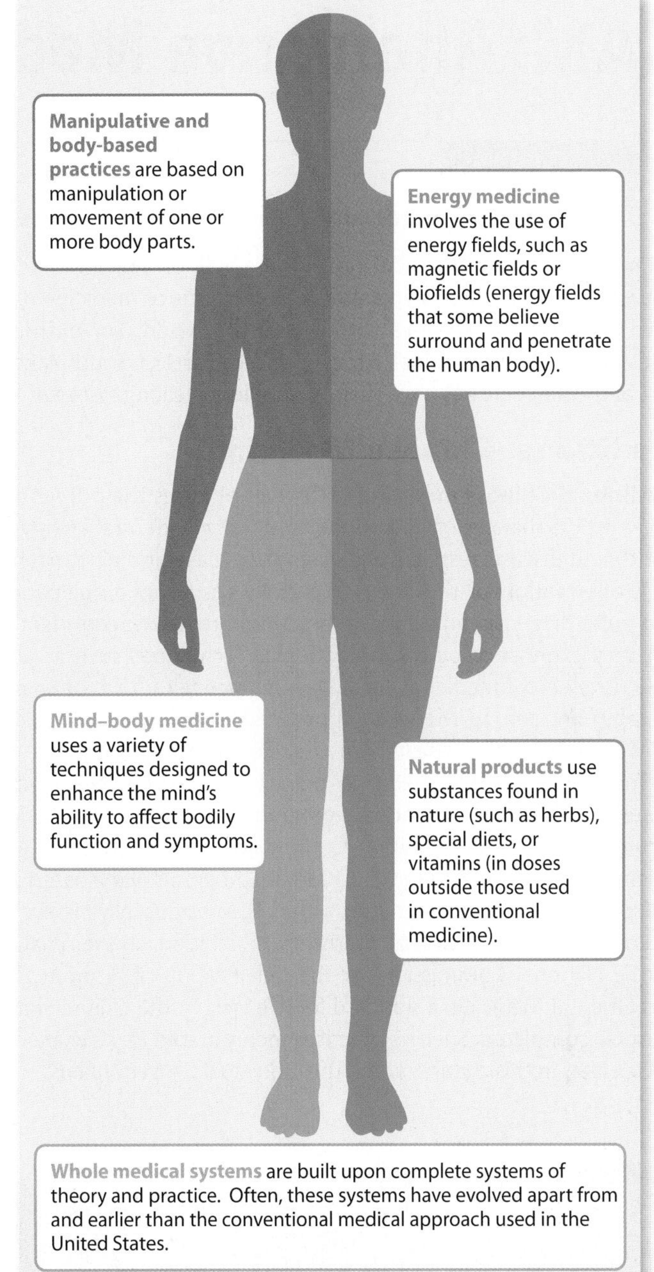

Figure 15.3 The Categories of Complementary and Alternative Medicine (CAM)

NCCAM groups CAM practices into four types, recognizing that there can be some overlap. In addition, NCCAM studies entire CAM medical systems, which cut across all categories.

Source: National Center for Complementary and Alternative Medicine, "The Use of Complementary and Alternative Medicine in the United States," NCCAM Publication no. D434, 2010.

VIDEO TUTOR
CAM: Risks vs. Benefits

check yourself

- **What is the difference between complementary and alternative medicine?**
- **What are the five categories of CAM?**

15.6 CAM: Alternative Medical Systems

learning outcome

15.6 Describe the major alternative medical systems.

Alternative (whole) medical systems are built on specific systems of theory and practice. Many alternative systems of medicine have been practiced by cultures throughout the world. For example, Native American, aboriginal, African, Middle Eastern, South American, and Asian cultures have their own unique healing systems.

Traditional Chinese Medicine

Traditional Chinese medicine (TCM) emphasizes the proper balance or disturbances of **qi** (pronounced "chee"), or vital energy, in health and disease, respectively. Diagnosis is based on personal history, observation of the body (especially the tongue), palpation, and pulse diagnosis, an elaborate procedure requiring considerable skill and experience by the practitioner. Techniques such as acupuncture, herbal medicine, massage, and *qigong* (a form of energy therapy) are among the TCM approaches to health and healing. TCM is complex, and research into its effectiveness is limited.[15]

Traditional Chinese medicine practitioners within the United States must complete a graduate program at a college or university approved by the Accreditation Commission for Acupuncture and Oriental Medicine (ACAOM). Graduate programs vary based on the specific area of concentration within TCM but usually involve an extensive 3- or 4-year clinical internship. In addition, an examination by the National Commission for the Certification of Acupuncture and Oriental Medicine, a standard for licensing in the United States, must be completed. Specific practices incorporated in TCM are discussed later in this chapter under the individual CAM domains.

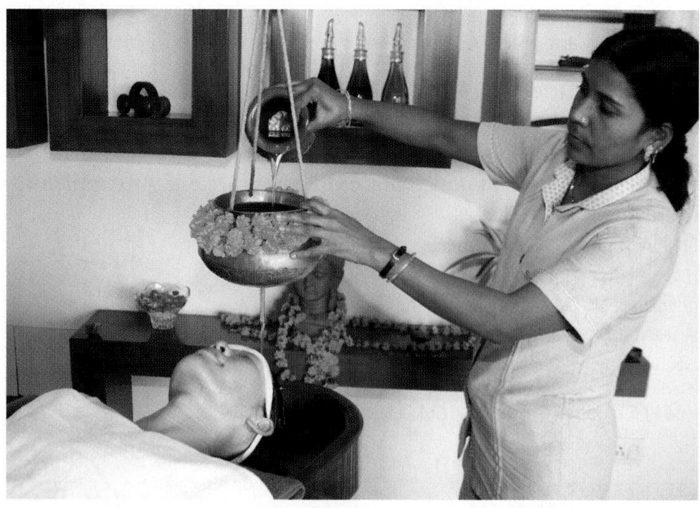

Shirodhara—a traditional Ayurvedic treatment in which warm herbalized oil is poured over the forehead in guided rhythmic patterns—is said to relieve stress and anxiety, treat insomnia and chronic headaches, and improve memory.

Ayurveda

Ayurveda (Ayurvedic medicine) relates to the "science of life," an alternative medical system that began and evolved over thousands of years in India. Ayurveda seeks to integrate and balance the body, mind, and spirit and to restore harmony in the individual.[16] Ayurvedic practitioners use various techniques, including questioning, observing, and touching patients and classifying patients into one of three body types, or *doshas*, before establishing a treatment plan. They then establish a treatment plan to bring the doshas into balance, thereby reducing the patient's symptoms. Dietary modification and herbal remedies drawn from the botanical wealth of the Indian subcontinent are common. Treatments may also include certain yoga postures, meditation, massage, steam baths, changes in sleep patterns and sun exposure, and controlled breathing. Research into Ayurveda is limited, but studies have shown some of the herbal remedies to be effective.[17]

Training of Ayurvedic practitioners varies. At present, no national standard exists for certifying or training Ayurvedic practitioners, although professional groups are working toward creating licensing guidelines.

Homeopathy

Homeopathic medicine, developed in Germany in the late 1700s, is an unconventional Western system based on the principle that "like cures like"—in other words, the same substance that in large doses produces the symptoms of an illness will in very small doses cure the illness. Many homeopathic remedies are derived from toxic substances such as arsenic and belladonna; however, the preparation of the remedy may be so diluted that no actual molecules of the original substance remain.[18] Little evidence supports homeopathy being effective in terms of treating any specific condition.[19]

Homeopathic training varies considerably and is offered through diploma programs, certificate programs, short courses, and correspondence courses. Laws that detail requirements to practice vary from state to state.

Naturopathy

Naturopathic medicine views disease as a manifestation of the body's effort to ward off impurities and harmful substances from the environment. Naturopathic physicians emphasize restoring health rather than curing disease. They employ an array of healing practices, including nutrition; homeopathy; acupuncture; herbal medicine; spinal and soft-tissue manipulation; physical therapies involving electric currents, ultrasound, water, magnets, and light therapy; therapeutic counseling; and pharmacology.

Several major naturopathic schools in the United States and Canada provide training, conferring the *naturopathic doctor* (*ND*) degree on students who have completed a 4-year graduate program that emphasizes humanistically oriented family medicine.

check yourself

- **Describe three alternative medical systems.**

CAM: Manipulative and Body-Based Practices

learning outcome

15.7 Describe major manipulative and body-based CAM practices.

The CAM category of **manipulative and body-based practices** includes methods based on manipulation or movement of the body.

Chiropractic Medicine

Chiropractic medicine has been practiced for more than 100 years and focuses on manipulation of the spine and other neuromuscular structures.[20] The goals of chiropractic medicine are to correct alignment problems, alleviate pain, and support the body's self-healing abilities. Today, many health care organizations work closely with chiropractors, and many insurance companies pay for chiropractic treatment, particularly if it is recommended by a medical doctor.

Chiropractic medicine is based on the idea that a life-giving energy flows through the spine by way of the nervous system. If the spine is partly misaligned, that force is disrupted. Chiropractors use a variety of techniques to manipulate the spine into proper alignment so energy can flow unimpeded. Therapies may combine spinal adjustments with treatments such as heat and ice, electrical stimulation, exercise, and relaxation techniques. Chiropractic treatment can be effective for back pain, neck pain, and headaches.[21]

The average chiropractic training program requires 4 years of intensive courses in biochemistry, anatomy, physiology, diagnostics, pathology, nutrition, and related topics, plus hands-on clinical training. Many chiropractors then obtain certification in neurology, geriatrics, or pediatrics. Although states vary, increasing numbers require a 4-year undergraduate degree prior to entrance into a 4-year chiropractic program. Applicants must then pass an examination given by the National Board of Chiropractic Examiners. Chiropractic practice is licensed and regulated in all 50 states.[22]

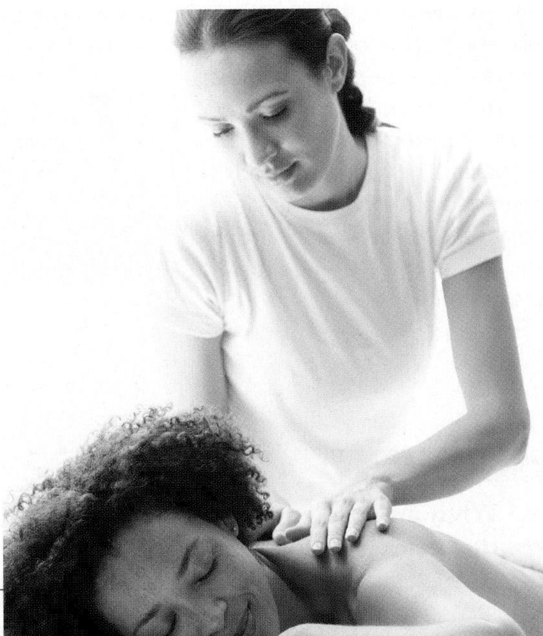

Oh, my aching back? Try massage!

Massage Therapy

Massage therapy is soft tissue manipulation by trained therapists for relaxation and healing. Therapists manipulate the patient's muscles and connective tissues to loosen the fibers and break up adhesions, improve the body's circulation, and remove waste products. Massage is used to treat painful conditions, promote relaxation, reduce stress and anxiety, and relieve depression. Some of the more popular types of massage therapy are the following:

- *Swedish massage* uses long strokes, kneading, and friction on the muscles and moves the joints to aid flexibility.
- *Deep tissue massage* uses strokes and pressure on areas where muscles are tight or knotted, focusing on layers of muscle deep under the skin.
- *Sports massage* is performed to prevent athletic injury and keep the body flexible. It is also used to help athletes recover from injuries.
- *Trigger point massage* (or *pressure point massage*) applies deep, focused pressure on myofascial trigger points—"knots" that can form in the muscles, are painful when pressed, and can cause symptoms throughout the body.
- *Shiatsu massage* uses varying, rhythmic pressure on parts of the body believed important for the flow of vital energy.

The course of study in massage schools typically covers sciences such as anatomy and physiology as well as massage techniques and business, ethical, and legal considerations.[23] The programs vary in length, quality, and whether they are accredited. For licensing, many states require a minimum of 500 hours of training and a passing grade on a national certification exam. Massage therapists work in private studios and health spas, as well as in medical and chiropractic offices, studios, hospitals, nursing homes, and fitness centers.[24]

Bodywork

CAM encompasses a broad range of movement-based approaches used to promote physical, emotional, mental, and spiritual well-being. The *Alexander Technique* is a movement education method designed to release harmful tension in the body to improve ease of movement, balance, and coordination. The *Feldenkrais method* is a system of gentle movements and exercises. It is designed to improve movement, flexibility, coordination, and overall functioning through techniques that enhance awareness and retrain the nervous system. *Pilates* is a popular exercise method focused on improving flexibility, strength, and body awareness. It involves a series of controlled movements, some of which are performed using special equipment.

check yourself

- **What are two manipulative and body-based CAM practices? What treatments do they involve?**

15.8 CAM: Energy Medicine

learning outcome

15.8 Describe major energy-based CAM practices.

Energy medicine therapies focus either on energy fields thought to originate within the body (biofields) or on fields from other sources (electromagnetic fields). The existence of these fields has not been experimentally proven. Some forms of energy therapy manipulate biofields by applying pressure and/or manipulating the body by placing the hands in, or through, these fields.[25] Popular examples of biofield therapy include acupuncture, acupressure, qigong, Reiki, and therapeutic touch.

Acupuncture and Acupressure

Acupuncture, one of the oldest forms of traditional Chinese medicine (and one of the most popular among Americans), is sought for a wide variety of health conditions, including musculoskeletal dysfunction, mood enhancement, and wellness promotion. It describes a family of procedures that involve stimulating anatomical points of the body with a series of precisely placed needles. The placement and manipulation of acupuncture needles is based on traditional Chinese theories of life-force energy (*qi*) flow through *meridians*, or energy pathways, in the body.

Following acupuncture, most participants in clinical studies report high levels of satisfaction with the treatment and improvement in their condition; however, extensive research has been inconclusive, and there is significant controversy over whether or not such results are simply a placebo response.[26] A 2012 study provided further evidence of a modest but significant reduction in chronic pain among people receiving acupuncture, particularly when they believe it will work and when needles are used in a specific way.[27]

Most U.S. acupuncturists are state licensed; however, licensing requirements vary by state. Many have completed a 2- to 3-year postgraduate program to obtain a master of traditional Oriental medicine (MTOM) degree. In addition, many conventional physicians and dentists practice acupuncture.[28]

Acupressure is based on the same principles of energy flow as acupuncture. Instead of inserting needles, however, the therapist applies pressure to points critical to balancing *yin* and *yang*, the two complementary principles that influence overall harmony (health) of the body. The goal of the therapy is for *qi* to be evenly distributed and flow freely throughout the body. Practitioners must have the same basic training and understanding of meridians and acupuncture points as do acupuncturists.

Other Forms of Energy Therapy

Qigong, a traditional Chinese medicine technique, brings together movement, meditation, and regulation of breathing to increase the flow of *qi*, enhance blood circulation, and improve immune function. Recent research shows that qigong, and the related practice *tai chi*, are effective for promoting bone health, cardiopulmonary fitness, and balance.[29]

Reiki is a hands-on energy therapy that originated in Japan. The name is derived from the Japanese words representing "universal" and "vital energy," or *ki*. Reiki is based on the belief that by channeling *ki* to the patient, the practitioner facilitates healing. In two related therapies, *therapeutic touch* and *healing touch*, the therapist attempts to perceive, through his or her hands held just above the patient's body, imbalances in the patient's energy. The therapist promotes healing by increasing the flow of the body's energies and bringing them into balance. Research supporting the effectiveness of these therapies is limited.[30]

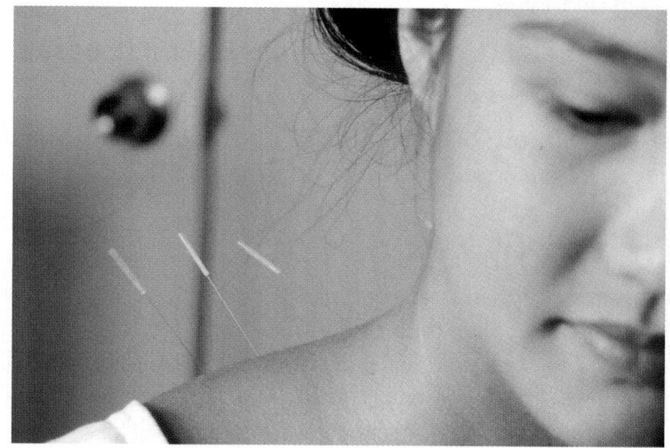

How does acupuncture work?

In acupuncture, long, thin needles are inserted into specific points along the body. This is thought to increase the flow of life-force energy, providing many physical and mental benefits.

See It! Videos

Is acupuncture right for you? Watch **Health Benefits of Acupuncture** in the Study Area of MasteringHealth.

check yourself

- **What are two energy-based CAM practices? What do their treatments involve?**

15.9

Other CAM Practices

learning outcome

15.9 Describe several mind–body and biologically based CAM practices.

Mind–Body Medicine

Mind–body medicine employs a variety of techniques designed to facilitate the mind's capacity to affect bodily functions and symptoms. At present, mind-body techniques include deep breathing, meditation, yoga, progressive relaxation, and guided imagery—all commonly used CAM therapies in the United States.

Research on **psychoneuroimmunology (PNI)** supports the effectiveness of mind–body therapies. PNI studies the interrelationships among behavioral, neural, endocrine, and immune processes.[31] Scientists are exploring how relaxation, biofeedback, meditation, yoga, laughter, exercise, and activities that involve mind "quieting" may counteract negative stressors and increase immune function.

A recent review study of PNI found that psychological support—including relaxation therapies—can improve wound healing,[32] whereas inflammatory molecules such as C-reactive protein, which is a risk factor for heart disease, were found to be reduced in older adults after 16 weeks of **tai chi**.[33]

Dietary Products

Dietary products, including specially formulated foods and dietary supplements, are perhaps the most controversial domain of CAM therapies because of the sheer number of options available and the many claims that are made about their effects. Many of these claims have not been thoroughly investigated, and many of the products are not currently regulated.

CAM therapies commonly involve increased intake of certain *functional foods*—foods said to improve some aspect of physical or mental functioning beyond the contribution of their specific nutrients. Both whole foods, such as broccoli and nuts, and modified foods, such as an energy bar said to enhance memory, are classified as functional foods.[34] Food producers sometimes refer to their functional foods as **nutraceuticals** to emphasize their combined nutritional and pharmaceutical benefits. For example, the label on a package of cocoa may state that the product provides antioxidants. The claim is backed up by research: Cocoa contains antioxidant phytochemicals called flavonoids, which have been shown to modestly reduce blood pressure.[35] The FDA regulates claims made on food labels; however, the FDA does not test functional foods prior to their coming to market and can only remove a product from the market if it is found to be unsafe.

Other common functional foods and their benefits include the following:

- **Plant stanols/sterols.** Reduces "bad" low-density lipoprotein (LDL) cholesterol.
- **Oat fiber.** Can lower LDL cholesterol; serves as a natural soother of nerves; stabilizes blood sugar levels.

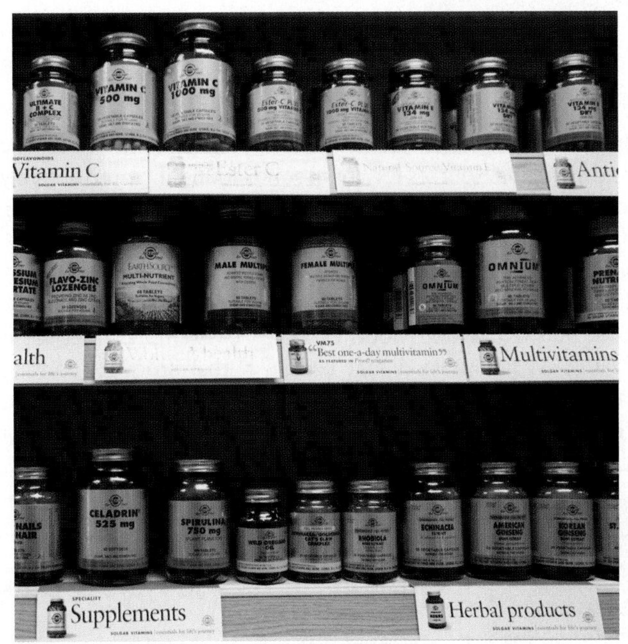

Do herbal remedies have any risks or side effects?

Herbs do have the potential to cause negative side effects. St. John's wort, for example, has potentially dangerous interactions with some prescription antidepressants and should never be taken with them. Other herbs, such as kava, can have negative effects even when taken alone.

- **Soy protein.** May lower heart disease risk by reducing LDL cholesterol and triglycerides.
- **Garlic.** Lowers cholesterol and reduces clotting tendency of blood; lowers blood pressure; may serve as a form of antibiotic.
- **Ginger.** May prevent motion sickness, stomach pain, and stomach upset; discourages blood clots; may relieve rheumatism.
- **Probiotics.** Yogurt and other fermented dairy foods that are labeled "Live and Active Cultures" contain active, friendly bacteria called *probiotics*. Normal residents of the large intestine, probiotics in foods are thought to reduce the risk for certain types of infections, including opportunistic yeast infections and those associated with acute diarrhea. The National Institutes of Health (NIH) is currently funding extensive research into the therapeutic effects of probiotics on human health.[36]

check yourself

- **What are several mind–body practices used in complementary medicine?**
- **What are functional foods?**

15.10 Herbal Remedies and Supplements

learning outcome

15.10 Describe how to evaluate the safety and efficacy of herbal remedies and supplements.

People have been using herbal remedies for thousands of years. Herbs were the original sources for compounds found in approximately 25 percent of the pharmaceutical drugs we use today, including aspirin (white willow bark), the heart medication digitalis (foxglove), and the cancer treatment Taxol (Pacific yew).

It's tempting to assume herbal remedies are safe because they are natural, but natural does not mean safe. For example, in recent years the NCCAM has warned that certain herbal products containing kava may be associated with severe liver damage.[37] Even rigorously tested products can be risky. Many plants are poisonous, and some can be toxic if ingested in high doses. Others may be dangerous when combined with prescription or over-the-counter drugs, could disrupt the normal action of the drugs, or could cause unusual side effects.[38] Table 15.1 gives an overview of some of the most common herbal supplements on the market.

In general, herbal medicines tend to be milder than synthetic medications and produce their effects more slowly. But too much of any herb, particularly from nonstandardized extracts, can cause problems.

Not all the supplements on the market today are directly derived from plant sources. In recent years, there have been increasing media claims on the health benefits of various hormones, enzymes, and other biological and synthetic compounds. Although a few products have been widely studied, there is little quality research to support the claims of many others. Table 15.2 lists popular nonherbal supplements and their risks and benefits.

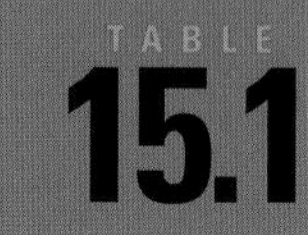

TABLE 15.1 Common Herbs and Herbal Supplements: Benefits, Research, and Risks

Herb	Claims of Benefits	Research Findings	Potential Risks
Echinacea (purple coneflower, *Echinacea purpurea, E. angustifolia, E. pallida*)	Stimulates the immune system and helps fight infection. Used to both prevent and treat colds and flu.	Some studies have provided preliminary evidence of its effectiveness in treating respiratory infections, but two recent studies found no benefit either for prevention or treatment.	Allergic reactions, including rashes, increased asthma, gastrointestinal problems, and anaphylaxis (a life-threatening allergic reaction).
Flaxseed (*Linum usitatissimum*) and flaxseed oil	Used as a laxative and for hot flashes and breast pain, as well as to reduce cholesterol levels and risk of heart disease and cancer.	Flaxseed contains soluble fiber and may have a laxative effect. Study results are mixed on whether flaxseed decreases hot flashes. Insufficient data is available on the effect of flaxseed on cholesterol levels, heart disease, or cancer risks.	Delays absorption of medicines, but otherwise has few side effects. Oil taken in excess could cause diarrhea. Should be taken with plenty of water.
Ginkgo (*Ginkgo biloba*)	Popularly used to prevent cognitive decline, dementia, and Alzheimer's disease, and general vascular disease.	Although some small studies have had promising results, the large Ginkgo Evaluation of Memory study found ginkgo did not reduce Alzheimer's disease or dementia, slow cognitive decline, or reduce blood pressure.	Gastric irritation, headache, nausea, dizziness, difficulty thinking, memory loss, and allergic reactions. Ginkgo seeds are highly toxic; only products made from leaf extracts should be used.
Ginseng (*Panax ginseng*)	Claimed to increase resistance to stress, boost the immune system, lower blood glucose and blood pressure, and improve stamina and sex drive.	Some studies suggest that ginseng may improve immune function and lower blood glucose; however, research overall is inconclusive.	Headaches, insomnia, and gastrointestinal problems are the most commonly reported adverse effects.
Green tea (*Camellia sinensis*)	Useful for lowering cholesterol and risk of some cancers, protecting the skin from sun damage, bolstering mental alertness, and boosting heart health.	Although some studies have shown promising links between green and white tea consumption and cancer prevention, recent research questions the ability of tea to significantly reduce the risk of breast, lung, or prostate cancer.	Insomnia, liver problems, anxiety, irritability, upset stomach, nausea, diarrhea, or frequent urination.

Sources: National Center for Complementary and Alternative Medicine, "Herbs at a Glance," January 2014, http://nccam.nih.gov; American Cancer Society, "Green Tea," May 2012, www.cancer.org.

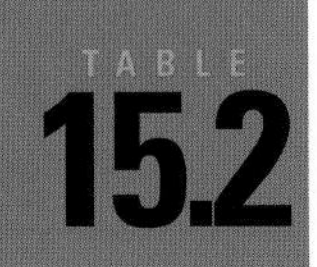

TABLE 15.2 Common Nonherbal Supplements: Benefits, Research, and Risks

Supplement	Claims	Research Findings	Potential Risks
Coenzyme Q10 (antioxidant enzyme found in the heart, liver, kidneys, and pancreas)	Used to improve heart function and reduce blood pressure; also used to increase male fertility and to prevent cancer.	Appears to improve heart function in patients with heart failure. Research on blood-pressure reduction is mixed. May improve sperm quality and count. No proven cancer-prevention benefits.	Does not appear to be associated with serious side effects. Some common side effects include nausea, headaches, insomnia, and heartburn. May reduce effectiveness of anticoagulant medications.
Vitamin E	Claimed to reduce risk of heart disease and age-related vision impairment and slow cognitive decline.	Research into the role of vitamin E in heart disease and vision loss is mixed. There is no evidence supporting its use for improving brain function.	High doses cause bleeding when taken with blood thinners.
Glucosamine (biological substance that helps the body grow cartilage)	Used to relieve pain and inflammation in arthritis and related degenerative joint diseases.	Research shows no significant difference in effectiveness between glucosamine and a placebo. For moderate-to-severe joint pain, glucosamine may be effective when taken with chondroitin sulfate.	Few side effects noted.
Carnitine (amino acid derivative)	Used to improve athletic performance and slow cognitive decline.	Extensive research finds no evidence it improves performance in healthy athletes. Limited evidence suggests that it may enhance mental function in older adults with mild cognitive impairment.	Interacts with some drugs. Common side effects include nausea, vomiting, abdominal cramps, diarrhea, "fishy" body odor. Some evidence of increased risk for cardiovascular disease.
Melatonin (hormone)	Used to regulate circadian rhythms (to prevent jet lag) and treat insomnia; claims of antiaging benefits.	Some evidence supports its usefulness in regulating sleep patterns. No scientific support for antiaging claims.	Nausea, headaches, dizziness, blood vessel constriction; possibly a danger for people with high blood pressure or other cardiovascular problems.
SAMe (pronounced "sammy") (biological compound that aids over 40 functions in the body)	Used in treatment of mild to moderate depression and in treatment of arthritis pain.	Studies have supported its usefulness in treating depression and arthritis pain.	Fewer side effects than prescription antidepressants, but questions remain over correct dosage, form, and long-term side effects.
Zinc (mineral)	Supports immune system; lozenges used to lessen duration and severity of cold symptoms.	Some research suggests that zinc lozenges can reduce the severity and duration of a cold if taken within 24 hours of onset of symptoms.	Use of zinc lozenges can cause nausea. Excessive use can reduce immune function.

Source: Office of Dietary Supplements, National Institutes of Health, "Dietary Supplement Fact Sheets," April 2014, http://ods.od.nih.gov.

Strategies to Protect Supplement Consumers' Health

The burgeoning popularity of functional foods and dietary supplements concerns many scientists and consumers. It is important to gather whatever information you can on both the safety and efficacy of any CAM treatment you are considering. In the case of functional foods and dietary supplements, start your own research with NCCAM (www.nccam.nih.gov) and the Cochrane Collaboration's review on complementary and alternative medicine (www.cochrane.org).

Dietary supplements can currently be sold without FDA approval. This raises issues of consumer safety. Even when products are dispensed by CAM practitioners, the situation can be risky. Products sold in "health food" stores and over the Internet may have varying levels of the active ingredient or may contain additives to which the consumer may have an adverse reaction.

As a result of such concerns, pressure has mounted to establish an approval process for dietary supplements similar to the process the FDA uses for drugs. In the meantime, if you're considering purchasing a dietary supplement, look for the USP Verified Mark on the label (Figure 15.4). The USP (United States Pharmacopeia) is a nonprofit, scientific organization. It does not regulate or determine the safety of medications, foods, or dietary supplements, but it does offer verification services to manufacturers of dietary supplement products. Dietary supplement products must meet stringent quality and manufacturing criteria to earn the USP Verified Mark.[39]

Figure 15.4 The U.S. Pharmacopeia Verified Mark

Source: Used with permission of The United States Pharmacopeial Convention, 12601 Twinbrook Parkway, Rockville, MD 20857.

check yourself

- **What factors should you consider when evaluating herbs or supplements?**

15.11 Health Insurance

learning outcome

15.11 Outline the structure of the U.S. health insurance system.

Whether you're visiting your regular doctor, consulting a specialist, or preparing for a hospital stay, chances are you'll be using some form of health insurance to pay for your care. The fundamental principle of insurance underwriting is that the cost of health care can be predicted for large populations, with the total resulting cost determining health care premiums (payments). Policyholders pay **premiums** into a pool, which is held in reserve until needed. When you are sick or injured, the insurance company pays out of the pool, regardless of your total contribution. Depending on circumstances, you may never pay for what your medical care costs, or you may pay much more. The idea is that you pay affordable premiums so that you never have to face catastrophic bills.

In today's profit-oriented system, insurers prefer to have healthy people in their plans who pour money into risk pools without taking money out. Unfortunately, not everyone has health insurance. In total, about 31 million Americans—15.8 percent—are *uninsured*; that is, they have no private health insurance and are not eligible for Medicare, Medicaid, or other subsidized government health programs.[40] The vast majority of the uninsured work or are dependents of employed people.

Not having health insurance has been associated with individuals delaying health care, as well as increased mortality. *Underinsurance*—the inability to pay for expenses despite being covered—can also cause poor health outcomes. In a 2013 national survey of college students, 6 percent of respondents said they did not have health insurance.[41] However, those who are covered only under their school's health care plan—18.9 percent according to the same survey—may not realize that such plans are usually short term and have a low upper limit of benefits, which would be problematic if the student were to have a severe illness or injury. Few students buy higher-level catastrophic plans.

Racial and ethnic minorities are overly represented in the number of uninsured Americans. Almost a third of all Hispanic Americans are uninsured compared to 18.7 percent of African Americans and 11.5 percent of whites.[42] Issues such as citizenship and language barriers contribute to some of the disparities in access to health insurance for many in our country.

Why should all Americans be concerned about those who are uninsured and underinsured? People without adequate health care coverage are less likely than other Americans to have their children immunized, seek early prenatal care, obtain annual blood pressure checks and other screenings, and seek attention for symptoms of health problems. Experts believe that this ultimately leads to higher system costs because their conditions go undetected at their earliest, most treatable stage, deteriorating to a more debilitating and costly stage before they are forced to seek help, often in an emergency room. Because emergency care is far more expensive than clinic care, uninsured and underinsured patients are often unable to pay, and the cost is absorbed by "the system" in the form of higher hospital costs, insurance premiums, and taxes.

Private Health Insurance

Originally, health insurance consisted solely of coverage for hospital costs (it was called *major medical*), but gradually it was extended to cover routine treatment and other areas, such as dental services and pharmaceuticals. These payment mechanisms, which provided no incentive to contain costs, laid the groundwork for today's steadily rising health care costs. At the same time, because most insurance did not cover routine or preventive services, consumers were encouraged to wait until illness developed to seek care instead of seeking preventive care. Consumers were also free to choose any provider or service, including inappropriate—and often very expensive—care.

To limit potential losses, private insurance companies began increasingly employing several mechanisms: cost sharing (in the form of deductibles, co-payments, and coinsurance), waiting periods, exclusions, "preexisting condition" clauses, and upper limits on payments:

- *Deductibles* are payments (commonly about $1,000 annually) you make for health care before insurance coverage kicks in to pay for eligible services.

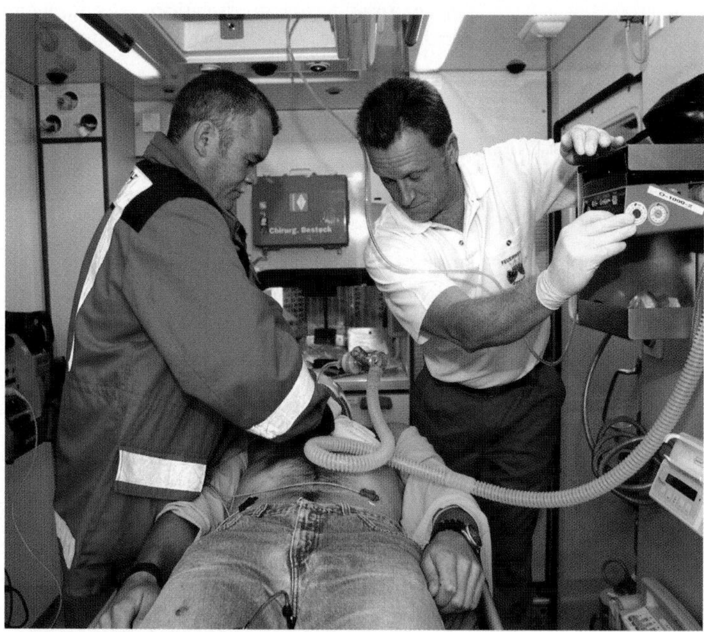

People without insurance can't gain access to preventive care, so they seek care only in an emergency or crisis. Because emergency care is extraordinarily expensive, they often are unable to pay, and the cost is absorbed by those who can pay—the insured or taxpayers.

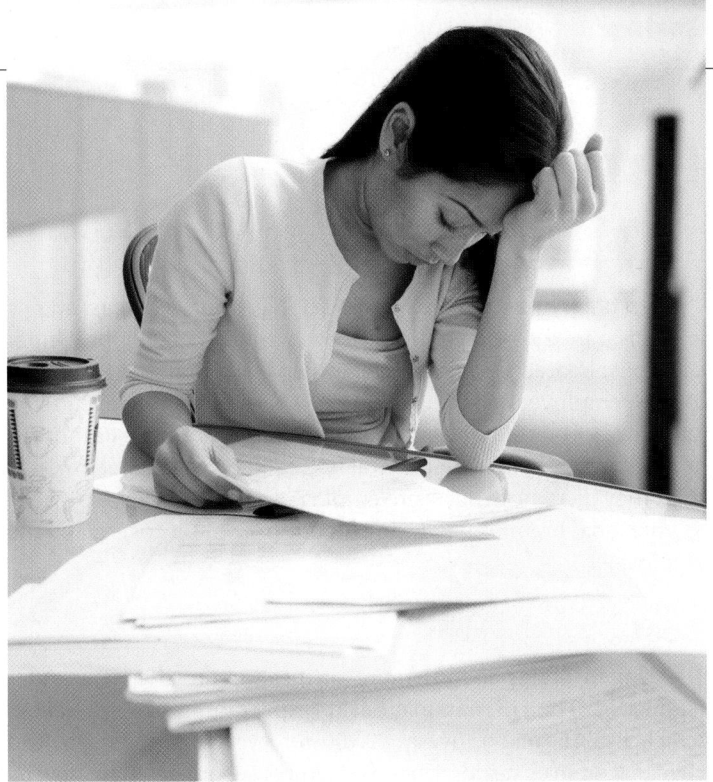

What should I consider when choosing health insurance?

Choosing a health insurance plan can be confusing. Some things to think about include how comprehensive your coverage needs to be, how convenient your care must be, how much you are willing to spend on premiums and co-payments, what the overall cost will be, and whether the services of the plan meet your needs.

- *Co-payments* are set amounts that you pay per service or product received, regardless of the total cost (e.g., $20 per doctor visit or per prescription filled).
- *Coinsurance* is the percentage of costs that you must pay based on the terms of the policy (e.g., 20% of the total bill).
- Some group plans specify a *waiting period* that cannot exceed 90 days before they will provide coverage. Waiting periods do not apply to plans purchased by individuals.
- All insurers set some limits on the types of *covered services* (e.g., most exclude cosmetic surgery, private rooms, and experimental procedures).
- *Preexisting condition clauses* once limited the insurance company's liability for medical conditions that a consumer had before obtaining coverage. For example, if a person applying for insurance had cancer, the insurer could deny the application entirely, or agree to cover the applicant, but only for conditions unrelated to the cancer. Under the 2010 Patient Protection and Affordable Care Act (ACA) no one can be discriminated against because of a preexisting condition.
- Some insurance plans also imposed an *annual upper limit* or *lifetime limit*, after which coverage would end. The ACA makes this practice illegal.

Managed Care

Managed care describes a health care delivery system consisting of a network of providers and facilities linked contractually to deliver health benefits within a set annual budget, sharing economic risk, with membership rules for participating patients. More than 73 million Americans are enrolled in health maintenance organizations (HMOs), the most common type.[43] Managed care plans have grown steadily over the past decade—indemnity insurance, which pays providers on a fee-for-service basis, has become unaffordable or unavailable for most Americans.

Health maintenance organizations provide a range of covered benefits (e.g., checkups, surgery, lab tests) for a fixed prepaid amount. This is both the least expensive form of managed care and the most restrictive—patients are typically required to use the plan's doctors and hospitals and to see a PCP for treatment and referrals.

Preferred provider organizations (PPOs) are networks of independent doctors and hospitals. Members may see doctors not on the preferred list, for an additional cost.

In point of service (POS) plans—offered by many HMOs—a patient selects a PCP from a list of participating providers; this physician becomes the patient's "point of service." If referrals are made outside the network, the patient is still partially covered.

Medicare and Medicaid

The government, through programs such as Medicare and Medicaid, currently funds 45 percent of total U.S. health care spending.[44]

Medicare covers 99 percent of Americans over age 65, all totally and permanently disabled people (after a waiting period), and all people with end-stage kidney failure—together, these groups comprise over 60 million people, or 1 in 6 Americans.[45] As the costs of care have soared, Medicare has placed limits on provider reimbursements. As a result, some physicians and managed care programs have stopped accepting Medicare patients.

To control hospital costs, in 1983 the federal government set up a Medicare payment system based on *diagnosis-related groups (DRGs)*. Nearly 500 groupings of diagnoses were created to establish how much a hospital would be reimbursed for a particular patient. This system motivates hospitals to discharge patients quickly, to provide more ambulatory care, and to admit patients classified into the most favorable (profitable) DRGs. Many private health insurance companies have also adopted reimbursement rates based on DRGs.

Medicaid is a federal–state welfare program covering approximately 62 million people defined as low income, including many who are blind, disabled, elderly, pregnant, or eligible for Temporary Assistance for Needy Families (TANF). Because each state determines eligibility and payments to providers, the way Medicaid operates from state to state varies widely.

check yourself

- **What are four common barriers to adequate health insurance?**
- **What structures and limits do private insurers use to control costs?**

15.12 Issues Facing the Health Care System

learning outcome

15.12 Identify the major challenges facing the U.S. health care system.

In recent decades, the number of Americans without health insurance increased dramatically as costs and restrictions on eligibility for coverage rose. In 2010, Congress passed the Patient Protection and Affordable Care Act (ACA) to provide a means for these and all Americans to obtain affordable heath care. In addition to increasing access to care, the ACA is expected to address America's high cost of care and to improve the overall quality of care.

Access

Access to care is one of the challenges facing the U.S. health care system. In 2012, there were almost 700,000 physicians in the United States.[46] However, there is an oversupply of higher-paid specialists and a shortage of lower-paid primary care physicians (family practitioners, internists, pediatricians, etc.). Likewise, of the nearly 5,000 non-federal hospitals in the United States, over 60 percent serve urban areas, leaving many rural communities without readily accessible care.[47]

Managed care health plans determine access on the basis of participating providers, health plan benefits, and administrative rules. Often this means that consumers do not have the freedom to choose specialists, facilities, or treatment options beyond those contracted with the health plan and recommended by their primary care provider, even if care providers and facilities are only a few miles away. Quality of the patient's health insurance plan matters, too: patients with excellent insurance coverage may be encouraged to undergo expensive tests and treatments, whereas patients with poor insurance may not be informed of the full variety of diagnostic and treatment options.[48]

Key provisions in the ACA aim to increase access to quality health insurance among Americans:

- Insurers are now required to cover several preventive services, such as health screenings for cancer and counseling on topics such as losing weight, quitting smoking, and reducing alcohol use.
- Insurers are required to cover young adults on a parent's plan through age 26.
- Coverage is required for prescription medications, including psychotropic medications.
- Americans with preexisting conditions cannot be denied coverage.
- No annual and lifetime limits on benefits are allowed.
- Affordable Insurance Exchanges (AIEs) facilitate consumer shopping and enrollment in plans with the same kinds of choices that members of Congress have.
- Small businesses, which typically paid as much as 18 percent more than large businesses for health insurance coverage for their employees, now qualify for special tax credits to help fund insurance plans.

Even before passage of the ACA, Congress provided assistance with insurance coverage for employees who change jobs. Under the Consolidated Omnibus Budget Reconciliation Act (COBRA), former employees, retirees, and their spouses and dependents have the option to continue their insurance for up to 18 months at group rates. People who enroll in COBRA pay a higher amount than they did when they were employed, as they're covering both the personal premium and the amount previously covered by the employer.

Cost

The United States spends more on health care than any other nation. In 2014, U.S. national health expenditures were projected to reach \$3.1 trillion, nearly \$9,700 for every man, woman, and child.[49] Moreover, health care expenditures are projected to grow by 5.8 percent each year, reaching over \$5 trillion annually by 2022—nearly 20 percent of our projected gross domestic product (GDP; see Figure 15.5).[50]

Why are America's health care costs so high? Many factors are involved: a for-profit health industry; excess administrative costs; duplication of services; an aging population; growing rates of obesity, inactivity, and related health problems; demand for new medical technologies; an emphasis on crisis-oriented care instead of prevention; and inappropriate use of services.

Our system's more than 2,000 health insurance companies prevents *economies of scale* (bulk purchasing at a reduced cost) and administrative efficiency realized in countries with single-payer systems. Commercial insurance companies commonly experience administrative costs greater than 12 percent of the total health care insurance premium.[51] These administrative expenses contribute to the high cost of

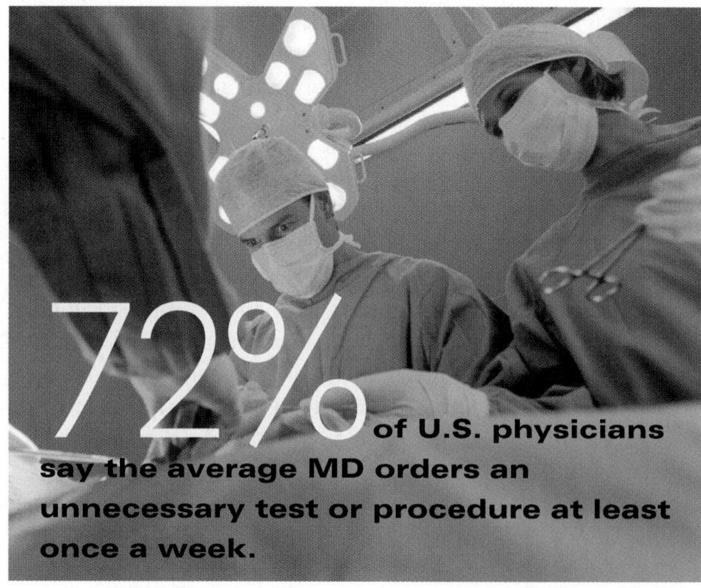

health care and are largely passed on to consumers in the form of higher prices for goods and services.

The ACA mandates the following cost-control measures:

- Insurance companies that spend less than 80 percent of premium dollars on medical care in a given year have to send enrollees a rebate.
- All insurance companies have to publicly justify their actions if they plan to raise rates by 10 percent or more.
- Tougher screening procedures and penalties are helping to reduce health care fraud.

2014 estimated total expenditures = $3.1 trillion

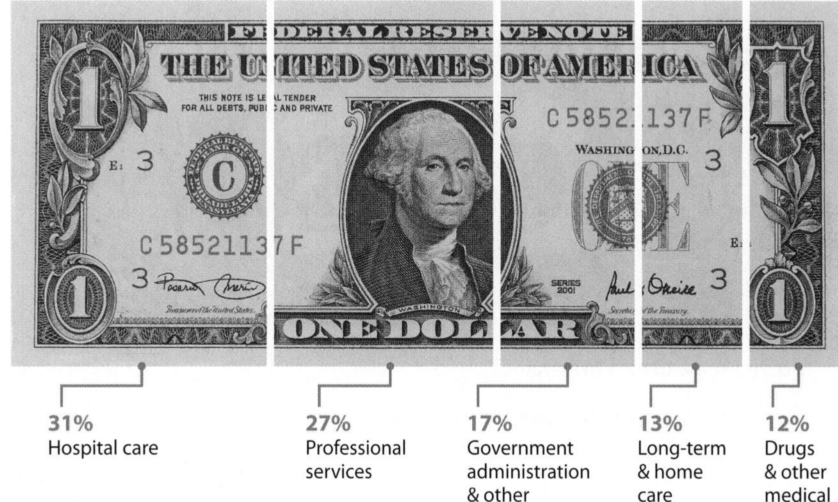

Figure 15.5 Where Do We Spend Our Health Care Dollars?

Source: Data are from Centers for Medicare & Medicaid Services, "National Health Expenditure Projections 2012–2022: Forecast Summary," November 2013, www.cms.gov.

The Debate over Universal Coverage

Whether universal health care coverage will—or should—be achieved in the United States and through what mechanism remain hotly debated topics. Proponents of reform argue that health care is a basic human right and should be available and affordable for everyone. Opponents of health care reform feel that health care is not a right, but a commodity. They contend that the high cost of changing the system is more than the United States can afford and that the government should not interfere in what has been largely a free-market industry. In addition, lobbying efforts by the insurance industry, pharmaceutical manufacturers, and special interest groups have all played a role in thwarting comprehensive reform.

The ACA does not provide for a system of national health care but is merely a set of initial steps toward increasing the number of insured Americans. Although it has reduced the number of uninsured Americans by an estimated 9 million, it has been subjected to intense and often rancorous debate. The reforms mandated by the ACA are currently being implemented, and their actual effects are uncertain.

Debate continues over the goal of universal coverage. Arguments for national health insurance include the following:[52]

- Health care is a human right. The United Nations Universal Declaration of Human Rights states that "everyone has the right to a standard of living adequate for the health and well-being of oneself and one's family, including ... medical care."[53]
- Americans would be more likely to engage in preventive health behaviors and clinicians would be encouraged to practice preventive medicine; people who are underinsured and uninsured often avoid preventive care checkups because of the cost.
- A national system of health care would further increase economic prosperity by enabling Americans to live longer and healthier lives, thus increasing their contributions to society.

Arguments against national health insurance include the following:[54]

- Health care is not a right, because it is not in the Bill of Rights in the U.S. Constitution, which lists rights the government cannot infringe upon, not services the government must ensure.
- It is the individual's responsibility to ensure personal health. Diseases and health problems can often be prevented by choosing to live healthier lifestyles.
- Expenses for health care would have to be paid for with higher taxes or spending cuts in other areas.
- Profit motives, competition, and ingenuity lead to cost control and effectiveness. These concepts should be brought to health care reform.

Quality

The U.S. health care system has several mechanisms for ensuring quality: education, licensure, certification/registration, accreditation, peer review, and malpractice litigation. Some of these are mandatory before a professional or organization may provide care; others are voluntary. Insurance companies and government payers may link payment to whether a practitioner is board certified or a facility is accredited by an appropriate agency. In addition, most insurance plans require prior authorization and/or second opinions, not only to reduce costs, but also to improve quality of care.

Although our health care spending far exceeds that of any other nation, we rank far below many other nations in key indicators of quality. In 2011, the Department of Health and Human Services released to Congress a National Strategy for Quality Improvement in Health Care. Its priorities include a new emphasis on promoting the safest, most preventive, and most effective care, increasing communication and coordination among providers, and ensuring that patients and families are engaged as partners in their care.[55]

check yourself

- **What are two arguments for and two against universal health care coverage?**
- **What are three challenges faced by the U.S. health care system?**

Assess yourself

Are You a Smart Health Care Consumer?

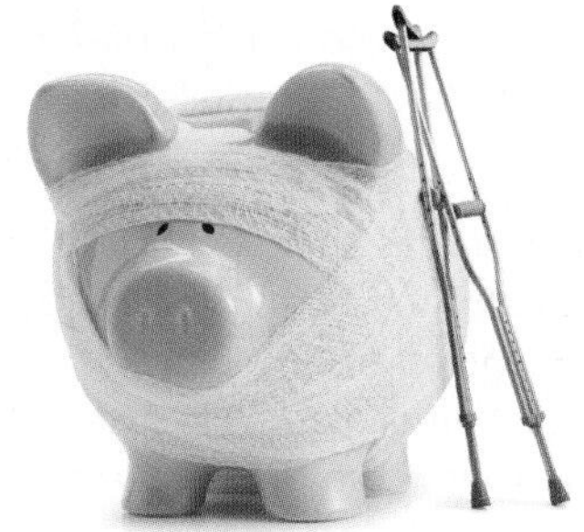

An interactive version of this assessment is available online in MasteringHealth.

Answer the following questions to determine what you might do to become a better health care consumer.

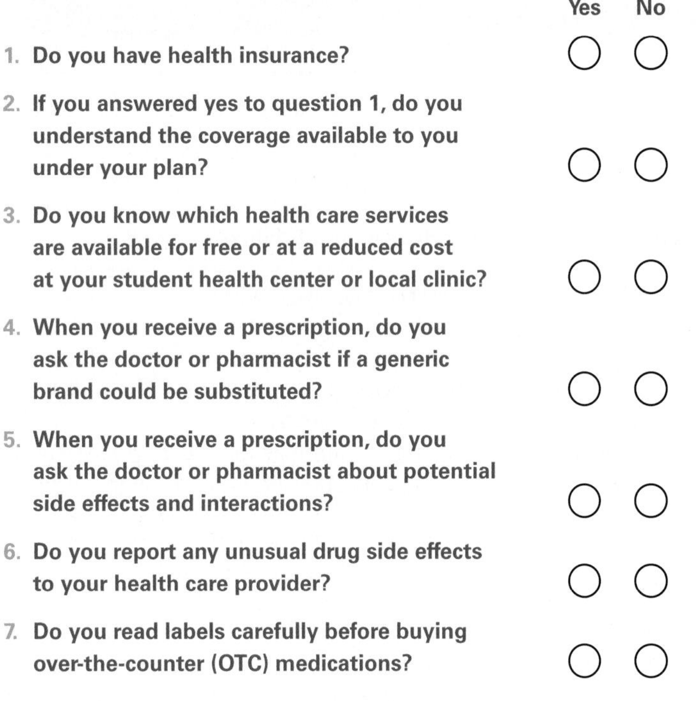

	Yes	No
1. Do you have health insurance?	◯	◯
2. If you answered yes to question 1, do you understand the coverage available to you under your plan?	◯	◯
3. Do you know which health care services are available for free or at a reduced cost at your student health center or local clinic?	◯	◯
4. When you receive a prescription, do you ask the doctor or pharmacist if a generic brand could be substituted?	◯	◯
5. When you receive a prescription, do you ask the doctor or pharmacist about potential side effects and interactions?	◯	◯
6. Do you report any unusual drug side effects to your health care provider?	◯	◯
7. Do you read labels carefully before buying over-the-counter (OTC) medications?	◯	◯
8. Do you take medication as directed?	◯	◯
9. When you receive a diagnosis, do you seek more information about the diagnosis and treatment?	◯	◯
10. When considering a CAM technique, do you research and identify scientific findings about the specific CAM therapy?	◯	◯
11. Do you research the credentials of your practitioner before receiving treatment?	◯	◯
12. Do you inform new practitioners of all the treatments you are currently receiving, including all CAM and traditional therapies?	◯	◯
13. Do you choose only supplements with the USP (United States Pharmacopeia) seal on their labels?	◯	◯
14. Do you consult a physician before taking a supplement?	◯	◯

Your Plan for Change

Once you have considered your responses to the Assess Yourself questions, you may want to change or improve certain behaviors in order to get the best treatment from your health care provider and the health care system.

Today, you can:

◯ Research your insurance plan. Find out which health care providers and hospitals you can visit, the amounts of co-payments and premiums you are responsible for, and the drug coverage offered.

◯ Update your medicine cabinet. Dispose properly of any expired prescriptions or OTC medications. Keep on hand a supply of basic items, such as pain relievers, antiseptic cream, bandages, cough suppressants, and throat lozenges.

Within the next 2 weeks, you can:

◯ Find a regular health care provider if you do not already have one and make an appointment for a general checkup.

◯ Check with your insurance provider and see what CAM practitioners and therapies are covered.

◯ Find out what alternative therapies your college's health clinic offers.

By the end of the semester, you can:

◯ Become an advocate for others' health. Write to your congressperson or state legislature to express your interest in health care reform.

◯ Make relaxation and mind–body stress-reducing techniques a part of your everyday life. This can simply mean practicing meditation or deep breathing, or even taking long walks in nature. You don't need to visit a CAM practitioner or follow a specific therapeutic practice to benefit from methods of relaxation, meditation, and spiritual awakening.

Summary

To hear an MP3 Tutor session, scan here or visit the Study Area in **MasteringHealth.**

LO 15.1 Self-care and individual responsibility are key factors in reducing rising health care costs and improving health status. Planning can help you navigate health care treatment in unfamiliar situations or emergencies.

LO 15.2 Evaluate health professionals by considering their qualifications, their record of treating similar problems, and their ability to work with you.

LO 15.3 Conventional Western (allopathic) medicine is based on scientifically validated methods and procedures. Medical doctors, specialists of various kinds, nurses, and physician assistants practice allopathic medicine.

LO 15.4 Consumers need to understand the risks and benefits of prescription drugs and over-the-counter (OTC) medications. Regulations governing drug labels help ensure that information about these products is available.

LO 15.5 People are using complementary and alternative medicine (CAM) in increasing numbers.

LO 15.6 Alternative medical systems include traditional Chinese medicine (TCM), Ayurveda, homeopathy, and naturopathy.

LO 15.7–LO 15.9 CAM also includes manipulative and body-based practices, energy medicine, mind–body medicine, and biologically based practices.

LO 15.10 The FDA does not study and approve dietary supplements before they are brought to market; thus there is no guarantee of their safety or effectiveness. However, the USP Verified Mark indicates that a supplement has met certain criteria for product purity and manufacturing standards.

LO 15.11 Health insurance is based on the concept of spreading risk. Insurance is provided by private insurance companies (which charge premiums) and government Medicare and Medicaid programs (which are funded by taxes). Managed care attempts to control costs by streamlining administration and stressing preventive care.

LO 15.12 Concerns about the U.S. health care system include access, cost, and quality. The Patient Protection and Affordable Care Act was passed by Congress in 2010 to address these issues.

Pop Quiz

Visit MasteringHealth to personalize your study plan with Chapter Review Quizzes and Dynamic Study Modules.

LO 15.1 **1.** Of the following conditions, which would be appropriately managed by self-care?
a. A persistent temperature of 104°F or higher
b. Sudden weight loss of more than a few pounds without changes in diet or exercise patterns
c. A sore throat, runny nose, and cough that persist for a few days
d. Yellowing of the skin or the whites of the eyes

LO 15.3 **2.** What medical practice is based on procedures whose objective is to heal by countering the patient's symptoms?
a. Allopathic medicine
b. Nonallopathic medicine
c. Osteopathic medicine
d. Chiropractic medicine

LO 15.5 **3.** CAM therapies focus on treating both the mind and the whole body, which makes them part of a
a. natural approach.
b. psychological approach.
c. holistic approach.
d. gentle approach.

LO 15.6 **4.** What type of medicine addresses imbalances of *qi*?
a. Chiropractic medicine
b. Naturopathic medicine
c. Traditional Chinese medicine
d. Homeopathic medicine

LO 15.6 **5.** The alternative system of medicine based on the principle that "like cures like" is
a. naturopathic medicine.
b. homeopathic medicine.
c. Ayurvedic medicine.
d. chiropractic medicine.

LO 15.9 **6.** The use of techniques to improve the psychoneuroimmunology of the human body is called
a. acupressure.
b. mind–body medicine.
c. Reiki.
d. bodywork.

LO 15.6 **7.** What system places equal emphasis on body, mind, and spirit and strives to restore the innate harmony of the individual?
a. Ayurvedic medicine
b. Homeopathic medicine
c. Naturopathic medicine
d. Traditional Chinese medicine

LO 15.10 **8.** The "USP Dietary Supplement Verified" seal indicates that a supplement is
a. safe and pure.
b. effective.
c. low cost.
d. child safe.

LO 15.11 **9.** What mechanism used by private insurance companies requires that the subscriber pay a certain amount directly to the provider before the insurance company will begin paying for services?
a. Coinsurance
b. Cost sharing
c. Co-payments
d. Deductibles

LO 15.11 **10.** Andrea, 28, is a single parent on welfare. Her medical bills are paid by a federal health insurance program for the poor. This program is
a. an HMO.
b. Social Security.
c. Medicaid.
d. Medicare.

Answers to these questions can be found on page A-1. If you answered a question incorrectly, review the module identified by the Learning Outcome. For even more study tools, visit MasteringHealth.

Answers to Pop Quiz Questions

Chapter 1

1. b; 2. a; 3. b; 4. a; 5. c; 6. d; 7. a; 8. c; 9. a; 10. a

Chapter 2

1. c; 2. a; 3. b; 4. a; 5. b; 6. b; 7. b; 8. b; 9. c; 10. c

Chapter 3

1. c; 2. c; 3. d; 4. b; 5. c; 6. d; 7. c; 8. c; 9. d; 10. c

Chapter 4

1. b; 2. c; 3. c; 4. d; 5. d; 6. c; 7. c; 8. a; 9. b; 10. b

Chapter 5

1. b; 2. c; 3. b; 4. b; 5. c; 6. a; 7. b; 8. d; 9. a; 10. a

Chapter 6

1. b; 2. d; 3. a; 4. c; 5. c; 6. c; 7. a; 8. c; 9. b; 10. c

Chapter 7

1. d; 2. d; 3. c; 4. a; 5. b; 6. c; 7. d; 8. c; 9. b; 10. c

Chapter 8

1. a; 2. b; 3. b; 4. a; 5. d; 6. c; 7. b; 8. d; 9. a; 10. d

Chapter 9

1. a; 2. c; 3. b; 4. b; 5. c; 6. b; 7. a; 8. a; 9. b; 10. b

Chapter 10

1. c; 2. b; 3. d; 4. c; 5. a; 6. a; 7. b; 8. a; 9. d; 10. a

Chapter 11

1. c; 2. c; 3. b; 4. a; 5. b; 6. d; 7. a; 8. c; 9. b; 10. a

Chapter 12

1. c; 2. a; 3. c; 4. a; 5. c; 6. c; 7. a; 8. c; 9. b; 10. d

Chapter 13

1. b; 2. a; 3. c; 4. a; 5. b; 6. c; 7. c; 8. b; 9. b; 10. a

Chapter 14

1. d; 2. b; 3. d; 4. d; 5. a; 6. c; 7. a; 8. a; 9. b; 10. a

Chapter 15

1. c; 2. a; 3. c; 4. c; 5. b; 6. b; 7. a; 8. a; 9. d; 10. c

Glossary

abortion The termination of a pregnancy by expulsion or removal of an embryo or fetus from the uterus.
abstinence Refraining from a behavior.
accountability Accepting responsibility for personal decisions, choices, and actions.
acid deposition The acidification process that occurs when pollutants are deposited by precipitation, clouds, or directly on the land.
acquaintance rape A rape in which the rapist is known to the victim (replaces the formerly used term *date rape*).
acquired immunodeficiency syndrome (AIDS) A disease caused by a retrovirus, the human immunodeficiency virus (HIV), that attacks the immune system, reducing the number of helper T cells and leaving the victim vulnerable to infections, malignancies, and neurological disorders.
acupressure Technique of traditional Chinese medicine related to acupuncture that uses the application of pressure to selected points along the meridians to balance energy.
acupuncture Branch of traditional Chinese medicine that uses the insertion of long, thin needles to affect flow of energy (*qi*) along energy pathways (meridians) within the body.
acute stress The short-term physiological response to an immediate perceived threat.
adaptive response Form of adjustment in which the body attempts to restore homeostasis.
adaptive thermogenesis Theoretical mechanism by which the brain regulates metabolic activity according to caloric intake.
addiction Persistent, compulsive dependence on a behavior or substance, including mood-altering behaviors or activities, despite ongoing negative consequences.
aerobic capacity (or power) The functional status of the cardiorespiratory system; refers specifically to the volume of oxygen the muscles consume during exercise.
aerobic exercise Any type of exercise that requires oxygen to make energy for activity.
aggravated rape Rape that involves one or multiple attackers, strangers, weapons, or physical beating.
alcohol abuse Use of alcohol that interferes with work, school, or personal relationships or that entails violations of the law.
alcohol poisoning A potentially lethal blood alcohol concentration that inhibits the brain's ability to control consciousness, respiration, and heart rate; usually occurs as a result of drinking a large amount of alcohol in a short period of time. Also known as *acute alcohol intoxication.*
alcoholic hepatitis A condition resulting from prolonged use of alcohol in which the liver is inflamed; can be fatal.
Alcoholics Anonymous (AA) An organization whose goal is to help alcoholics stop drinking; includes auxiliary branches such as Al-Anon and Alateen.
alcoholism (alcohol dependency) Condition in which personal and health problems related to alcohol use are severe and stopping alcohol use results in withdrawal symptoms.
allopathic medicine Conventional, Western medical practice; in theory, based on scientifically validated methods and procedures.
allostatic load Wear and tear on the body caused by prolonged or excessive stress responses.
alternative (whole) medical systems Specific theories of health and balance that have developed outside the influence of conventional medicine.
alternative insemination A fertilization procedure accomplished by depositing semen from a partner or donor into a woman's vagina via a thin tube.
alternative medicine Treatment used in place of conventional medicine.
altruism The giving of oneself out of genuine concern for others.
Alzheimer's disease (AD) A chronic condition involving changes in nerve fibers of the brain that results in mental deterioration.
amino acids The nitrogen-containing building blocks of protein.
amniocentesis A medical test in which a small amount of fluid is drawn from the amniotic sac to test for Down syndrome and other genetic diseases.
amniotic sac The protective pouch surrounding the fetus.
amphetamines A large and varied group of synthetic agents that stimulate the central nervous system.
anabolic steroids Artificial forms of the hormone testosterone that promote muscle growth and strength.
anal intercourse The insertion of the penis into the anus.
androgyny High levels of traditional masculine and feminine traits in a single person.
aneurysm A weakened blood vessel that may bulge under pressure and, in severe cases, burst.
angina pectoris Chest pain occurring as a result of reduced oxygen flow to the heart.
angiography A technique for examining blockages in heart arteries.
angioplasty A technique in which a catheter with a balloon at the tip is inserted into a clogged artery; the balloon is inflated to flatten fatty deposits against artery walls and a stent is typically inserted to keep the artery open.
anorexia nervosa An eating disorder characterized by deliberate food restriction, self-starvation or extreme exercising to achieve weight loss, and an extremely distorted body image.
antagonism A drug interaction in which two drugs compete for the same available receptors, potentially blocking each other's actions.
antibiotic resistance The ability of bacteria or other microbes to withstand the effects of an antibiotic.
antibiotics Medicines used to kill microorganisms, such as bacteria.
antibodies Substances produced by the body that are individually matched to specific antigens.
antigen Substance capable of triggering an immune response.
antioxidants Substances believed to protect against oxidative stress and resultant tissue damage at the cellular level.
anxiety disorders Mental illnesses characterized by persistent feelings of threat and worry in coping with everyday problems.
appetite The desire to eat; normally accompanies hunger but is more psychological than physiological.
appraisal The interpretation and evaluation of information provided to the brain by the senses.
arrhythmia An irregularity in heartbeat.
arteries Vessels that carry blood away from the heart to other regions of the body.
arterioles Branches of the arteries.
asbestos A mineral compound that separates into stringy fibers and lodges in the lungs, where it can cause various diseases.
asthma A long-term, chronic inflammatory disorder that causes tiny airways in the lung to spasm in response to triggers. Many cases of asthma are triggered by environmental pollutants.

atherosclerosis Condition characterized by deposits of fatty substances (plaque) on the inner lining of an artery.

atria (singular: *atrium*) The heart's two upper chambers, which receive blood.

attention-deficit/hyperactivity disorder (ADHD) A learning disability characterized by hyperactivity and distraction.

autism spectrum disorder (ASD) A neurodevelopmental disorder characterized by difficulty mastering communication and social behavior skills.

autoerotic behaviors Sexual self-stimulation.

autoimmune disease Disease caused by an overactive immune response against the body's own cells.

autoinoculate Transmission of a pathogen from one part of your body to another part.

autonomic nervous system (ANS) The portion of the central nervous system regulating body functions that a person does not normally consciously control.

Ayurveda (Ayurvedic medicine) A comprehensive system of medicine, derived largely from ancient India, that places equal emphasis on the body, mind, and spirit, and strives to restore the body's innate harmony through diet, exercise, meditation, herbs, massage, exposure to sunlight, and controlled breathing.

background distressors Environmental stressors of which people are often unaware.

bacteria (singular: *bacterium*) Simple, single-celled microscopic organisms; about 100 known species of bacteria cause disease in humans.

barbiturates Drugs that depress the central nervous system and have sedating, hypnotic, and anesthetic effects.

barrier methods Contraceptive methods that block the meeting of egg and sperm by means of a physical barrier (such as condom, diaphragm, or cervical cap), a chemical barrier (such as spermicide), or both.

basal metabolic rate (BMR) The rate of energy expenditure by a body at complete rest in a neutral environment.

belief Appraisal of the relationship between some object, action, or idea and some attribute of that object, action, or idea.

benign Harmless; refers to a noncancerous tumor.

benzodiazepines A class of central nervous system depressant drugs with sedative, hypnotic, and muscle relaxant effects.

bereavement The loss or deprivation experienced by a survivor when a loved one dies.

bidis Hand-rolled flavored cigarettes.

binge drinking A *binge* is a pattern of drinking alcohol that brings blood alcohol concentration (BAC) to 0.08 gram-percent or above; for a typical adult, this pattern corresponds to consuming five or more drinks (male) or four or more drinks (female) in about 2 hours.

binge-eating disorder A type of eating disorder characterized by gorging on food once a week or more, but not typically followed by a purge.

biofeedback A technique using a machine to self-monitor physical responses to stress.

biopsy Removal and examination of a tissue sample to determine if a cancer is present.

biopsychosocial model of addiction Theory of the relationship between an addict's biological (genetic) nature and psychological and environmental influences.

bipolar disorder A form of mood disorder characterized by alternating mania and depression; also called *manic depression*.

bisexual Experiencing attraction to and preference for sexual activity with people of both sexes.

blood alcohol concentration (BAC) The ratio of alcohol to total blood volume; the factor used to measure the physiological and behavioral effects of alcohol.

body composition Describes the relative proportions of fat and fat-free (muscle, bone, water, organs) tissues in the body.

body dysmorphic disorder (BDD) A psychological disorder characterized by an obsession with one's appearance and a distorted view of one's body or with a minor or imagined flaw in appearance.

body image How you see yourself in your mind, what you believe about your appearance, and how you feel about your body.

body mass index (BMI) A number calculated from a person's weight and height that is used to assess risk for possible present or future health problems.

bulimia nervosa An eating disorder characterized by binge eating followed by inappropriate purging measures or compensatory behavior, such as vomiting or excessive exercise, to prevent weight gain.

caffeine A stimulant drug that is legal in the United States and found in many coffees, teas, chocolates, energy drinks, and certain medication.

calorie A unit of measure that indicates the amount of energy obtained from a particular food.

cancer A large group of diseases characterized by the uncontrolled growth and spread of abnormal cells.

candidiasis Yeast-like fungal infection often transmitted sexually; also called moniliasis or yeast infection.

capillaries Minute blood vessels that branch out from the arterioles and venules; their thin walls permit exchange of oxygen, carbon dioxide, nutrients, and waste products among body cells.

carbohydrates Basic nutrients that supply the body with glucose, the energy form most commonly used to sustain normal activity.

carbon dioxide (CO_2) Gas created by the combustion of fossil fuels, exhaled by animals, and used by plants for photosynthesis; the primary greenhouse gas in Earth's atmosphere.

carbon footprint The amount of greenhouse gases produced by an individual, nation, or other entity, usually expressed in equivalent tons of carbon dioxide emissions.

carbon monoxide A gas found in cigarette smoke that binds at oxygen receptor sites in the blood.

carcinogens Cancer-causing agents.

cardiometabolic risks Physical and biochemical changes that are risk factors for the development of cardiovascular disease and type 2 diabetes.

cardiorespiratory fitness The ability of the heart, lungs, and blood vessels to supply oxygen to skeletal muscles during sustained physical activity.

cardiovascular disease (CVD) Diseases of the heart and blood vessels.

cardiovascular system Organ system, consisting of the heart and blood vessels, that transports nutrients, oxygen, hormones, metabolic wastes, and enzymes throughout the body.

carotenoids Fat-soluble plant pigments with antioxidant properties.

carpal tunnel syndrome (CTS) A common occupational injury in which the median nerve in the wrist becomes irritated, causing numbness, tingling, and pain in the fingers and hands.

carrying capacity of the earth The largest population that can be supported indefinitely given the resources available in the environment.

celiac disease An inherited autoimmune disorder affecting the digestive process of the small intestine and triggered by the consumption of gluten.

celibacy State of abstaining from sexual activity.

cell-mediated immunity Aspect of immunity that is mediated by specialized white blood cells that attack pathogens and antigens directly.

cervical cap A small cup made of latex or silicone that is designed to fit snugly over the entire cervix.

cervix Lower end of the uterus that opens into the vagina.

cesarean section (C-section) Surgical birthing procedure in which a baby is removed through an incision made in the mother's abdominal wall and uterus.

chancre Sore often found at the site of syphilis infection.

chemotherapy The use of drugs to kill cancerous cells.

chewing tobacco A stringy type of tobacco that is placed in the mouth and then sucked or chewed.

chickenpox A highly infectious disease caused by the herpes varicella zoster virus.

child abuse Deliberate, intentional words or actions that cause harm, potential for harm, or threat of harm to a child.

child maltreatment Any act or series of acts of commission or omission by a parent or caregiver that results in harm, potential for harm, or threat of harm to a child.

chiropractic medicine Manipulation of the spine and neuromuscular structure to promote proper energy flow.

chlamydia Bacterially caused STI of the urogenital tract; most commonly reported STI in the United States.

chlorofluorocarbons (CFCs) Chemicals that contribute to the depletion of the atmospheric ozone layer.

cholesterol A form of fat circulating in the blood that can accumulate on the inner walls of arteries, causing a narrowing of the channel through which blood flows.

chorionic villus sampling (CVS) A prenatal test that involves snipping tissue from the fetal sac to be analyzed for genetic defects.

chronic disease A disease that typically begins slowly, progresses, and persists, with a variety of signs and symptoms that can be treated but not cured by medication.

chronic mood disorder Experience of persistent emotional states, such as sadness, despair, and hopelessness.

chronic stress An ongoing state of physiological arousal in response to ongoing or numerous perceived threats.

cirrhosis The last stage of liver disease associated with chronic heavy alcohol use, during which liver cells die and damage becomes permanent.

climate change A shift in typical weather patterns that includes fluctuations in seasonal temperatures, rain or snowfall amounts, and the occurrence of catastrophic storms.

clitoris A pea-sized nodule of tissue located at the top of the labia minora; central to sexual arousal in women.

club drugs Synthetic analogs (drugs that produce similar effects) of existing illicit drugs.

codependence A self-defeating relationship pattern in which a person is controlled by an addict's addictive behavior.

cognitive restructuring The modification of thoughts, ideas, and beliefs that contribute to stress.

cohabitation Living together without being married.

collateral circulation Adaptation of the heart to partial damage accomplished by rerouting needed blood through unused or underused blood vessels while the damaged heart muscle heals.

collective violence Violence perpetrated by groups against other groups.

common-law marriage Cohabitation lasting a designated period of time (usually 7 years) that is considered legally binding in some states.

comorbidities The presence of one or more diseases at the same time.

complementary medicine Treatment used in conjunction with conventional medicine.

complete (high-quality) proteins Proteins that contain all nine of the essential amino acids.

complex carbohydrates A major type of carbohydrate that provides sustained energy.

compulsion Preoccupation with a behavior and an overwhelming need to perform it.

compulsive buying disorder People who are preoccupied with shopping and spending.

compulsive exercise Disorder characterized by a compulsion to engage in excessive amounts of exercise and feelings of guilt and anxiety if the level of exercise is perceived as inadequate.

compulsive shoppers People who are preoccupied with shopping and spending.

computerized axial tomography (CAT) scan A scan by a machine that uses radiation to view internal organs not normally visible in X-rays.

conception The fertilization of an ovum by a sperm.

conflict An emotional state that arises when the behavior of one person interferes with the behavior of another.

conflict resolution A concerted effort by all parties to constructively resolve points of contention.

congeners Forms of alcohol that are metabolized more slowly than ethanol and produce toxic by-products.

congenital cardiovascular defect Cardiovascular problem that is present at birth.

congestive heart failure (CHF) or heart failure (HF) An abnormal cardiovascular condition that reflects impaired cardiac pumping and blood flow; pooling blood leads to congestion in body tissues.

consummate love A relationship that combines intimacy, compassion, and commitment.

contemplation A practice of concentrating the mind on a spiritual or ethical question or subject, a view of the natural world, or an icon or other image representative of divinity.

contraception (birth control) Methods of preventing conception.

contraceptive sponge Contraceptive device, made of polyurethane foam and containing nonoxynol-9, that fits over the cervix to create a barrier against sperm.

coping Managing events or conditions to lessen the physical or psychological effects of excess stress.

core strength Strength in the body's core muscles, including deep back and abdominal muscles that attach to the spine and pelvis.

coronary artery disease (CAD) A narrowing or blockage of coronary arteries, usually caused by atherosclerotic plaque buildup.

coronary bypass surgery A surgical technique whereby a blood vessel taken from another part of the body is implanted to bypass a clogged coronary artery.

coronary heart disease (CHD) A narrowing of the small blood vessels that supply blood to the heart.

coronary thrombosis A blood clot occurring in a coronary artery.

corpus luteum A body of cells that forms from the remains of the graafian follicle following ovulation; it secretes estrogen and progesterone during the second half of the menstrual cycle.

cortisol Hormone released by the adrenal glands that makes stored nutrients more readily available to meet energy demands.

countering Substituting a desired behavior for an undesirable one.

Cowper's glands Glands that secrete a fluid that lubricates the urethra and neutralizes any acid remaining in the urethra after urination.

cross-tolerance Development of a physiological tolerance to one drug that reduces the effects of another, similar drug.

cunnilingus Oral stimulation of a woman's genitals.

Daily Values (DVs) Percentages listed as "% DV" on food and supplement labels; made up of the RDIs and DRVs together.

defensive medicine The use of medical practices designed to avert the possibility of malpractice suits in the future.

dehydration Abnormal depletion of body fluids; a result of lack of water.

delirium tremens (DTs) A state of confusion brought on by withdrawal from alcohol; symptoms include hallucinations, anxiety, and trembling.

dementias Progressive brain impairments that interfere with memory and normal intellectual functioning.

denial Inability to perceive or accurately interpret the self-destructive effects of the addictive behavior.

dentist Specialist who diagnoses and treats diseases of the teeth, gums, and oral cavity.

Depo-Provera, Depo-subQ Provera Injectable method of birth control that lasts for 3 months.
depressants Drugs that slow down the activity of the central nervous and muscular systems and cause sleepiness or calmness.
determinants of health The range of personal, social, economic, and environmental factors that influence health status.
detoxification The early abstinence period during which an addict adjusts physically and cognitively to being free from the influences of the addiction.
diabetes mellitus A group of diseases characterized by elevated blood glucose levels.
diaphragm A latex, cup-shaped device designed to cover the cervix and block access to the uterus; should always be used with spermicide.
diastolic blood pressure The lower number in the fraction that measures blood pressure, indicating pressure on arterial walls during the relaxation phase of heart activity.
dietary supplements Vitamins and minerals taken by mouth that are intended to supplement existing diets.
digestive process The process by which the body breaks down foods and either absorbs or excretes them.
dilation and evacuation (D&E) An abortion technique that uses a combination of instruments and vacuum aspiration.
dioxins Highly toxic chlorinated hydrocarbons found in herbicides and produced during certain industrial processes.
dipping Placing a small amount of chewing tobacco between the front lip and teeth for rapid nicotine absorption.
disaccharides Combinations of two monosaccharides.
discrimination Actions that deny equal treatment or opportunities to a group, often based on prejudice.
disease prevention Actions or behaviors designed to keep people from getting sick.
disordered eating A pattern of atypical eating behaviors that is used to achieve or maintain a lower body weight.
gambling disorder Compulsive gambling that cannot be controlled.
distillation The process whereby mash is subjected to high temperatures to release alcohol vapors, which are then condensed and mixed with water to make the final product.
distress Stress that can have a detrimental effect on health; negative stress.
domestic violence The use of force to control and maintain power over another person in the home environment, including both actual harm and the threat of harm.
downshifting Taking a step back and simplifying a lifestyle that has become focused on trying to keep up, is hectic, and is packed with pressure and stress; also known as voluntary simplicity.
drug abuse Excessive use of a drug.
drug misuse Use of a drug for a purpose for which it was not intended.
drug resistance That which occurs when microbes, such as bacteria, viruses, or other pathogens, grow and proliferate in the presence of chemicals that would normally kill them or slow their growth.
dysfunctional families Families in which there is violence; physical, emotional, or sexual abuse; parental discord; or other negative family interactions.
dysmenorrhea Condition of pain or discomfort in the lower abdomen just before or after menstruation.
dyslexia A language-based learning disorder characterized by reading, writing, and spelling problems.
dyspareunia Pain experienced by women during intercourse.
dysthymic disorder (dysthymia) A type of depression that is milder and harder to recognize than major depression; chronic and often characterized by fatigue, pessimism, or a short temper.
eating disorder A psychiatric disorder characterized by severe disturbances in body image and eating behaviors.
ecological or public health model A view of health in which diseases and other negative health events are seen as the result of an individual's interaction with his or her social and physical environment.
ecosystem The collection of physical (nonliving) and biological (living) components of an environment and the relationships between them.
ectopic pregnancy Dangerous condition that results from the implantation of a fertilized egg outside the uterus, usually in a fallopian tube.
ejaculation The propulsion of semen from the penis.
ejaculatory duct Tube formed by the junction of the seminal vesicle and the vas deferens that carries semen to the urethra.
electrocardiogram (ECG) A record of the electrical activity of the heart; may be measured during a stress test.
embolus A blood clot that becomes dislodged from a blood vessel wall and moves through the circulatory system.
embryo The fertilized egg from conception through the eighth week of development.
emergency contraceptive pills (ECPs) Drugs taken within 3 to 5 days after unprotected intercourse to prevent fertilization or implantation.
emotional health The feeling part of psychosocial health; includes your emotional reactions to life.
emotional intelligence A person's ability to identify, understand, use, and manage emotional states effectively and interact positively with others in relationships.
emotions Intensified feelings or complex patterns of feelings.
emphysema A chronic lung disease in which the tiny air sacs in the lungs are destroyed, making breathing difficult.
enablers People who knowingly or unknowingly protect addicts from the natural consequences of their behavior.
endemic Describing a disease that is always present to some degree.
endometriosis Disorder in which endometrial tissue establishes itself outside the uterus.
endometrium Soft, spongy matter that makes up the uterine lining.
endorphins Opioid-like hormones that are manufactured in the human body and contribute to natural feelings of well-being.
energy medicine Therapies using energy fields, such as magnetic fields or biofields.
enhanced greenhouse effect The warming of Earth's surface as a direct result of human activities that release greenhouse gases into the atmosphere, trapping more of the sun's radiation than is normal.
environmental stewardship A responsibility for environmental quality shared by all those whose actions affect the environment.
environmental tobacco smoke (ETS) Smoke from tobacco products, including sidestream and mainstream smoke; commonly called *secondhand smoke.*
epidemic Disease outbreak that affects many people in a community or region at the same time.
epididymis The duct system atop the testis where sperm mature.
epinephrine Also called *adrenaline,* a hormone that stimulates body systems in response to stress.
episodic acute stress The state of regularly reacting with wild, acute stress about one thing or another.
erectile dysfunction (ED) Difficulty in achieving or maintaining a penile erection sufficient for intercourse.
ergogenic drug Substance believed to enhance athletic performance.
erogenous zones Areas of the body that, when touched, lead to sexual arousal.
essential amino acids Nine of the basic nitrogen-containing building blocks of protein, which must be obtained from foods to ensure health.
estrogens Hormones secreted by the ovaries that control the menstrual cycle.

ethnoviolence Violence directed at persons affiliated with a particular ethnic group.

ethyl alcohol (ethanol) An addictive drug produced by fermentation and found in many beverages.

eustress Stress that presents opportunities for personal growth; positive stress.

evidence-based medicine Decisions regarding patient care based on clinical expertise, patient values, and current best scientific evidence.

exercise Planned, structured, and repetitive bodily movement done to improve or maintain one or more components of physical fitness.

exercise addicts People who exercise compulsively to try to meet needs of nurturance, intimacy, self-esteem, and self-competency.

exercise metabolic rate (EMR) The energy expenditure that occurs during exercise.

extensively drug-resistant TB (XDR-TB) Form of TB that is resistant to nearly all existing antibiotics.

fallopian tubes (oviducts) Tubes that extend from near the ovaries to the uterus; site of fertilization and passageway for fertilized eggs.

family of origin People present in the household during a child's first years of life—usually parents and siblings.

fats Basic nutrients composed of carbon and hydrogen atoms; needed for the proper functioning of cells, insulation of body organs against shock, maintenance of body temperature, and healthy skin and hair.

fellatio Oral stimulation of a man's genitals.

female athlete triad A syndrome of three interrelated health problems seen in some female athletes: disordered eating, amenorrhea, and poor bone density.

female condom A single-use polyurethane sheath for internal use during vaginal or anal intercourse to catch semen on ejaculation.

female orgasmic disorder A woman's inability to achieve orgasm.

fermentation The process whereby yeast organisms break down plant sugars to yield ethanol.

fertility A person's ability to reproduce.

fertility awareness methods (FAMs) Several types of birth control that require alteration of sexual behavior rather than chemical or physical intervention in the reproductive process.

fertility rate Average number of births a female in a certain population has during her reproductive years.

fetal alcohol syndrome (FAS) A pattern of birth defects, learning, and behavioral problems in a child caused by the mother's alcohol consumption during pregnancy.

fetus A developing human from the ninth week until birth.

fiber The indigestible portion of plant foods that helps move food through the digestive system and softens stools by absorbing water.

fibrillation A sporadic, quivering pattern of heartbeat that results in extreme inefficiency in moving blood through the cardiovascular system.

fight-or-flight response Physiological arousal response in which the body prepares to combat or escape a real or perceived threat.

FITT Acronym for **F**requency, **I**ntensity, **T**ime, and **T**ype; the terms that describe the essential components of a program or plan to improve a health-related component of physical fitness.

flexibility The range of motion, or the amount of movement possible, at a particular joint or series of joints.

foams Spermicide packaged in aerosol cans and inserted into the vagina with an applicator.

food allergy Overreaction by the body to normally harmless proteins, which are perceived as allergens. In response, the body produces antibodies, triggering allergic symptoms.

food intolerance Adverse effects resulting when people who lack the digestive chemicals needed to break down certain substances eat those substances.

food irradiation Treating foods with gamma radiation from radioactive cobalt, cesium, or other sources of X-rays to kill microorganisms.

formaldehyde A colorless, strong-smelling gas released through off-gassing; causes respiratory and other health problems.

fossil fuels Carbon-based material used for energy; includes oil, coal, and natural gas.

frequency As part of the FITT prescription, refers to how many days per week a person should exercise to improve a component of physical fitness.

functional foods Foods believed to have specific health benefits and/or to prevent disease.

fungi A group of multicellular and unicellular organisms that obtain their food by infiltrating the bodies of other organisms, both living and dead; several microscopic varieties are pathogenic.

gay Sexual orientation involving primary attraction to people of the same sex.

gender The psychological condition of being feminine or masculine as defined by the society in which one lives.

gender identity Personal sense or awareness of being masculine or feminine, a male or a female.

gender roles Expressions of maleness or femaleness in everyday life.

gender-role stereotypes Generalizations concerning how men and women should express themselves and the characteristics each possesses.

gene Discrete segment of DNA in a chromosome that stores the code for assembling a particular body protein.

general adaptation syndrome (GAS) The pattern followed in the physiological response to stress, consisting of the alarm, resistance, and exhaustion phases.

generalized anxiety disorder (GAD) A constant sense of worry that may cause restlessness, difficulty in concentrating, tension, and other symptoms.

generic drugs Medications sold under chemical names rather than brand names.

genetically modified (GM) foods Foods derived from organisms whose DNA has been altered using genetic engineering techniques.

genital herpes STI caused by the herpes simplex virus.

genital warts Warts that appear in the genital area or the anus; caused by the human papillomavirus (HPV).

gestational diabetes Form of diabetes mellitus in which women who have never had diabetes before have high blood sugar (glucose) levels during pregnancy.

global warming A type of climate change in which average temperatures increase.

globesity High number of countries and large percentages of populations within countries who are classified as obese.

glycemic index (GI) Compares foods with the same amount of carbohydrates and determines how much each raises blood glucose levels.

glycemic load (GL) A food's glycemic index (potential to raise blood glucose) multiplied by the grams of carbohydrates it provides, divided by 100.

glycogen The polysaccharide form in which glucose is stored in the liver and, to a lesser extent, in muscles.

gonads The reproductive organs in a male (testes) or female (ovaries) that produce sperm (male), eggs (female), and sex hormones.

gonorrhea Second most common bacterial STI in the United States; if untreated, may cause sterility.

graafian follicle Mature ovarian follicle that contains a fully developed ovum, or egg.

greenhouse gases Gases that accumulate in the atmosphere, where they contribute to global warming by trapping heat near Earth's surface.

grief An individual's reaction to significant loss, including one's own impending death, the death of a loved one, or a quasi-death experience; grief can involve mental, physical, social, or emotional responses.

habit A repeated behavior in which the repetition may be unconscious.
hallucinogens Substances capable of creating auditory or visual distortions and unusual changes in mood, thoughts, and feelings.
hangover The physiological reaction to excessive drinking, including headache, upset stomach, anxiety, depression, diarrhea, and thirst.
hate crime A crime targeted against a particular societal group and motivated by bias against that group.
hazardous waste Waste that, due to its toxic properties, poses a hazard to humans or to the environment.
health The ever-changing process of achieving individual potential in the physical, social, emotional, mental, spiritual, and environmental dimensions.
health belief model (HBM) Model for explaining how beliefs may influence behaviors.
health disparities Differences in the incidence, prevalence, mortality, and burden of diseases and other health conditions among specific population groups.
health promotion The combined educational, organizational, procedural, environmental, social, and financial supports that help individuals and groups reduce negative health behaviors and promote positive change.
healthy life expectancy Expected number of years of full health remaining at a given age, such as at birth.
healthy weight Having a BMI of 18.5 to 24.9, the range of lowest statistical health risk.
heat cramps Involuntary and forcible muscle contractions that occur during or following exercise in hot and/or humid weather.
heat exhaustion A heat stress illness caused by significant dehydration resulting from exercise in hot and/or humid conditions.
heatstroke A deadly heat stress illness resulting from dehydration and overexertion in hot and/or humid conditions.
hepatitis A viral disease in which the liver becomes inflamed, producing symptoms such as fever, headache, and possibly jaundice.
herpes A general term for infections characterized by sores or eruptions on the skin caused by the herpes simplex virus.
herpes gladiatorum A skin infection caused by the herpes simplex type 1 virus and seen among athletes participating in contact sports.
heterosexual Experiencing primary attraction to and preference for sexual activity with people of the opposite sex.
high-density lipoproteins (HDLs) Compounds that facilitate the transport of cholesterol in the blood to the liver for metabolism and elimination from the body.
holistic Relating to or concerned with the whole body and the interactions of systems, rather than treatment of individual parts.
homeopathic medicine Unconventional Western system of medicine based on the principle that "like cures like."
homeostasis A balanced physiological state in which all the body's systems function smoothly.
homicide Death that results from intent to injure or kill.
homosexual Experiencing primary attraction to and preference for sexual activity with people of the same sex.
hormonal contraception Contraceptive methods that introduce synthetic hormones into the woman's system to prevent ovulation, thicken cervical mucus, or prevent a fertilized egg from implanting.
hormone replacement therapy or menopausal hormone therapy Use of synthetic or animal estrogens and progesterone to compensate for decreases in estrogens in a woman's body during menopause.
hostility Cognitive, affective, and behavioral tendencies toward anger and cynicism.
human chorionic gonadotropin (HCG) Hormone detectable in blood or urine samples of a mother within the first few weeks of pregnancy.
human immunodeficiency virus (HIV) The virus that causes AIDS by infecting helper T cells.
human papillomavirus (HPV) A group of viruses, many of which are transmitted sexually; some types of HPV can cause genital warts or cervical cancer.
humoral immunity Aspect of immunity that is mediated by antibodies secreted by white blood cells.
hunger The physiological impulse to seek food, prompted by the lack or shortage of basic foods needed to provide the energy and nutrients that support health.
hymen Thin tissue covering the vaginal opening in some women.
hyperglycemia Elevated blood glucose level.
hyperplasia A condition characterized by an excessive number of fat cells.
hypertension Sustained elevated blood pressure.
hypertrophy The act of swelling or increasing in size, as with cells.
hypnosis A trancelike state that allows people to become unusually responsive to suggestion.
hyponatremia or water intoxication The overconsumption of water, which leads to a dilution of sodium concentration in the blood with potentially fatal results.
hypothalamus An area of the brain located near the pituitary gland; works in conjunction with the pituitary gland to control reproductive functions. It also controls the sympathetic nervous system and directs the stress response.
hypothermia Potentially fatal condition caused by abnormally low body core temperature.
hysterectomy Surgical removal of the uterus.
hysterotomy The surgical removal of the fetus from the uterus.
imagined rehearsal Practicing, through mental imagery, to become better able to perform an event in actuality.
immunocompetence The ability of the immune system to respond to attack.
immunocompromised Having an immune system that is impaired.
Nexplanon (Implanon) A plastic capsule inserted in a woman's upper arm that releases a low dose of progestin to prevent pregnancy.
in vitro fertilization Fertilization of an egg in a nutrient medium and subsequent transfer back to the mother's body.
incomplete proteins Proteins that lack one or more of the essential amino acids.
incubation period The time between exposure to a disease and the appearance of symptoms.
induction abortion An abortion technique in which chemicals are injected into the uterus through the uterine wall; labor begins, and the woman delivers a dead fetus.
infection The state of pathogens being established in or on a host and causing disease.
infertility Inability to conceive after a year or more of trying.
influenza A common viral disease of the respiratory tract.
inhalants Products that are sniffed or inhaled in order to produce highs.
inhalation The introduction of drugs through the respiratory tract via sniffing, smoking, or inhaling.
inhibited sexual desire Lack of sexual appetite or lack of interest and pleasure in sexual activity.
inhibition A drug interaction in which the effects of one drug are eliminated or reduced by the presence of another drug at the same receptor site.
injection The introduction of drugs into the body via a hypodermic needle.
insulin Hormone secreted by the pancreas and required by body cells for the uptake and storage of glucose.
insulin resistance State in which body cells fail to respond to the effects of insulin; obesity increases the risk that cells will become insulin resistant.
intact dilation and extraction (D&X) A late-term abortion procedure in which the body of the fetus is extracted up to the head and then the contents of the cranium are aspirated.

intensity As part of the FITT prescription, refers to how hard or how much effort is needed when a person exercises to improve a component of physical fitness.

intentional injuries Injury, death, or psychological harm inflicted with the intent to harm.

Internet addiction The compulsive use of the computer, personal digital device, cell phone, or other forms of technology to access the Internet for activities such as e-mail, games, shopping, social networking, or blogging.

interpersonal violence Violence inflicted against one individual by another, or by a small group of others.

intersex General term for a variety of conditions in which a person is born with reproductive or sexual anatomy that doesn't seem to fit the typical definitions of female or male. Also termed disorders of sexual development (DSDs).

intervention A planned process of confronting an addict carried out by close family, friends, and a professional counselor.

intimate partner violence (IPV) Violent behavior, including physical violence, sexual violence, threats, and emotional abuse, occurring between current or former spouses or dating partners.

intimate relationships Relationships with family members, friends, and romantic partners, characterized by behavioral interdependence, need fulfillment, emotional attachment, and emotional availability.

intolerance A drug interaction in which the combination of two or more drugs in the body produces extremely uncomfortable reactions.

intrauterine device (IUD) A device, often T-shaped, that is implanted in the uterus to prevent pregnancy.

ionizing radiation Electromagnetic waves and particles having short wavelengths and energy high enough to ionize atoms.

ischemia Reduced oxygen supply to a body part or organ.

jealousy An aversive reaction evoked by a real or imagined relationship involving a person's partner and a third person.

jellies and creams Spermicide packaged in tubes and inserted into the vagina with an applicator.

labia majora "Outer lips," or folds of tissue covering the female sexual organs.

labia minora "Inner lips," or folds of tissue just inside the labia majora.

leach To dissolve and filter through soil.

lead A highly toxic metal found in emissions from lead smelters and processing plants; also sometimes found in pipes or paint in older houses.

learned helplessness Pattern of responding to situations by giving up because of repeated failure in the past.

learned optimism Teaching oneself to think positively.

lesbian Sexual orientation involving attraction of women to other women.

leukoplakia A condition characterized by leathery white patches inside the mouth; produced by contact with irritants in tobacco juice.

libido Sexual drive or desire.

life expectancy Expected number of years of life remaining at a given age, such as at birth.

locavore A person who primarily eats food grown or produced locally.

locus of control The location, *external* (outside oneself) or *internal* (within oneself), that an individual perceives as the source and underlying cause of events in his or her life.

loss of control Inability to reliably predict whether a particular instance of involvement with the addictive substance or behavior will be healthy or damaging.

low-density lipoproteins (LDLs) Compounds that facilitate the transport of cholesterol in the blood to the body's cells and cause the cholesterol to build up on artery walls.

low sperm count A sperm count below 20 million sperm per milliliter of semen.

lymphocyte A type of white blood cell involved in the immune response.

macrominerals Minerals that the body needs in fairly large amounts.

macrophage A type of white blood cell that ingests foreign material.

magnetic resonance imaging (MRI) A device that uses magnetic fields, radio waves, and computers to generate an image of internal tissues of the body for diagnostic purposes without the use of radiation.

mainstream smoke Smoke that is drawn through tobacco while inhaling.

major depression Severe depressive disorder that entails chronic mood disorder, physical effects such as sleep disturbance and exhaustion, and mental effects such as the inability to concentrate; also called *clinical depression*.

male condom A single-use sheath of thin latex or other material designed to fit over an erect penis and to catch semen upon ejaculation.

malignant Very dangerous or harmful; refers to a cancerous tumor.

malignant melanoma A virulent cancer of the melanocytes (pigment-producing cells) of the skin.

managed care Cost-control procedures used by health insurers to coordinate treatment.

manipulative and body-based practices Treatments involving manipulation or movement of one or more body parts.

marijuana Chopped leaves and flowers of *Cannabis indica* or *Cannabis sativa* (hemp); a psychoactive stimulant.

marital rape Any unwanted intercourse or penetration obtained by force, threat of force, or when the spouse is unable to consent.

massage therapy Soft tissue manipulation by trained therapists for relaxation and healing.

masturbation Self-stimulation of genitals.

measles A viral disease that produces symptoms such as an itchy rash and a high fever.

Medicaid A federal-state matching funds program that provides health insurance to low-income people.

Medicare A federal health insurance program that covers people age 65 and older, the permanently disabled, and people with end-stage kidney disease.

medical abortion The termination of a pregnancy during its first 9 weeks using hormonal medications that cause the embryo to be expelled from the uterus.

medical model A view of health in which health status focuses primarily on the individual and a biological or diseased organ perspective.

meditation A relaxation technique that involves concentrated focus to quiet the mind and increase awareness of the present moment.

menarche The first menstrual period.

meningitis An infection of the meninges, the membranes that surround the brain and spinal cord.

menopause The permanent cessation of menstruation, generally between the ages of 40 and 60.

mental health The thinking part of psychosocial health; includes your values, attitudes, and beliefs.

mental illnesses Disorders that disrupt thinking, feeling, moods, and behaviors, and that impair daily functioning.

metabolic syndrome (MetS) A group of metabolic conditions occurring together that increase a person's risk of heart disease, stroke, and diabetes.

metastasis Process by which cancer spreads from one area to different areas of the body.

methicillin-resistant *Staphylococcus aureus* (MRSA) Highly resistant form of staph infection that is growing in international prevalence.

migraine A condition characterized by localized headaches that possibly result from alternating dilation and constriction of blood vessels.

mind-body medicine Techniques designed to enhance the mind's ability to affect bodily functions and symptoms.

mindfulness A practice of purposeful, nonjudgmental observation in which we are fully present in the moment.

minerals Inorganic, indestructible elements that aid physiological processes.

miscarriage Loss of the fetus before it is viable; also called *spontaneous abortion*.

modeling Learning specific behaviors by watching others perform them.
monogamy Exclusive sexual involvement with one partner.
mononucleosis A viral disease that causes pervasive fatigue and other long-lasting symptoms.
monosaccharides Simple sugars that contain only one molecule of sugar.
mons pubis Fatty tissue covering the pubic bone in females; in physically mature women, the mons is covered with coarse hair.
morbidly obese Having a body weight 100 percent or more above healthy recommended levels; in an adult, having a BMI of 40 or more.
mortality The proportion of deaths to the total population, within a given period of time.
motivation A social, cognitive, and emotional force that directs human behavior.
multidrug-resistant TB (MDR-TB) Form of TB that is resistant to at least two of the best antibiotics available.
multifactorial disease Disease caused by interactions of several factors.
mumps A once common viral disease that is controllable by vaccination.
municipal solid waste (MSW) Solid wastes such as durable goods; nondurable goods; containers and packaging; food waste; yard waste; and miscellaneous wastes from residential, commercial, institutional, and industrial sources.
muscle dysmorphia Body image disorder in which men believe that their body is insufficiently lean or muscular.
muscular endurance A muscle's ability to exert force repeatedly without fatiguing or the ability to sustain a muscular contraction for a length of time.
muscular strength The amount of force that a muscle is capable of exerting in one contraction.
mutant cells Cells that differ in form, quality, or function from normal cells.
myocardial infarction (MI) or heart attack A blockage of normal blood supply to an area in the heart.
natural products Treatments using substances found in nature, such as herbs, special diets, or vitamin megadoses.
naturopathy (naturopathic medicine) System of medicine in which practitioners work with nature to restore people's health.
negative consequences Severe problems associated with addiction, such as physical damage, legal trouble, financial problems, academic failure, or family dissolution.
neglect Failure to provide for a child's basic needs such as food, shelter, medical care, and clothing.
neoplasm A new growth of tissue that results from uncontrolled, abnormal cellular development and serves no physiological function.
neurotransmitters Chemicals that relay messages between nerve cells or from nerve cells to other body cells.
nicotine The primary stimulant chemical in tobacco products; nicotine is highly addictive.
nicotine poisoning Symptoms often experienced by beginning smokers, including dizziness, diarrhea, lightheadedness, rapid and erratic pulse, clammy skin, nausea, and vomiting.
nicotine withdrawal Symptoms, including nausea, headaches, irritability, and intense tobacco cravings, suffered by addicted smokers who stop using tobacco.
nonionizing radiation Electromagnetic waves having relatively long wavelengths and enough energy to move atoms around or cause them to vibrate.
nonpoint source pollutants Pollutants that run off or seep into waterways from broad areas of land.
nonverbal communication All unwritten and unspoken messages, both intentional and unintentional.
nuclear meltdown An accident that results when the temperature in the core of a nuclear reactor increases enough to melt the nuclear fuel and the containment vessel housing it.
nurse Health professional who provides many services for patients and who may work in a variety of settings.
nurse practitioner (NP) Professional nurse with advanced training obtained through either a master's degree program or a specialized nurse practitioner program.
nutraceuticals Food or food-based supplements that have combined nutritional and pharmaceutical benefits; used interchangeably with the term *functional foods.*
nutrients The constituents of food that sustain humans physiologically: proteins, carbohydrates, fats, vitamins, minerals, and water.
nutrition The science that investigates the relationship between physiological function and the essential elements of foods eaten.
NuvaRing A soft, flexible ring inserted into the vagina that releases hormones, preventing pregnancy.
obesity A body weight more than 20 percent above healthy recommended levels; in an adult, a BMI of 30 or more.
obesogenic Characterized by environments that promote increased food intake, nonhealthful foods, and physical inactivity; refers to conditions that lead people to become excessively fat.
obsession Excessive preoccupation with an addictive object or behavior.
obsessive-compulsive disorder (OCD) A form of anxiety disorder characterized by recurrent, unwanted thoughts and repetitive behaviors.
oncogenes Suspected cancer-causing genes present on chromosomes.
one repetition maximum (1 RM) The amount of weight or resistance that can be lifted or moved only once.
open relationship A relationship in which partners agree that sexual involvement can occur outside the relationship.
ophthalmologist Physician who specializes in the medical and surgical care of the eyes, including prescriptions for glasses.
opioids Drugs that induce sleep and relieve pain; includes derivatives of opium and synthetics with similar chemical properties; also called *narcotics.*
opium The parent drug of the opioids; made from the seedpod resin of the opium poppy.
opportunistic infections Infections that occur when the immune system is weakened or compromised.
optometrist Eye specialist whose practice is limited to prescribing and fitting lenses.
oral contraceptives Pills containing synthetic hormones that prevent ovulation by regulating hormones.
oral ingestion Intake of drugs through the mouth.
organic Grown without use of pesticides, chemicals, or hormones.
Ortho Evra A patch that releases hormones similar to those in oral contraceptives; each patch is worn for 1 week.
osteopath General practitioner who receives training similar to a medical doctor's but with an emphasis on the skeletal and muscular systems; often uses spinal manipulation as part of treatment.
other specified feeding or eating disorder (OSFED) Eating disorders that are a true psychiatric illness but that do not fit the strict diagnostic criteria for anorexia nervosa, bulimia nervosa, or binge-eating disorder.
ovarian follicles Areas within the ovary in which individual eggs develop.
ovaries Almond-sized organs that house developing eggs and produce hormones.
overload A condition in which a person feels overly pressured by demands.
overuse injuries Injuries that result from the cumulative effects of day-after-day stresses placed on tendons, muscles, and joints.
overweight Having a body weight more than 10 percent above healthy recommended levels; in an adult, having a BMI of 25 to 29.
ovulation The point of the menstrual cycle at which a mature egg ruptures through the ovarian wall.
ovum A single mature egg cell.

pancreas Organ that secretes digestive enzymes into the small intestine, and hormones, including insulin, into the bloodstream.
pandemic Global epidemic of a disease that occurs in several countries at the same time.
panic attack Severe anxiety reaction in which a particular situation, often for unknown reasons, causes terror.
Pap test A procedure in which cells taken from the cervical region are examined for abnormal cellular activity.
parasitic worms The largest of the pathogens, most of which are more a nuisance than they are a threat.
parasympathetic nervous system Branch of the autonomic nervous system responsible for slowing systems stimulated by the stress response.
pathogen A disease-causing agent.
pelvic inflammatory disease (PID) Term used to describe various infections of the female reproductive tract; can be caused by chlamydia or gonorrhea.
penis Male sexual organ that releases sperm.
peptic ulcer Damage to the stomach or intestinal lining, usually caused by digestive juices; most ulcers result from infection by the bacterium *Helicobacter pylori.*
perfect-use failure rate The number of pregnancies (per 100 users) that are likely to occur in the first year of use of a particular birth control method if the method is used consistently and correctly.
perineum Tissue that forms the "floor" of the pelvic region in both men and women.
peripheral artery disease (PAD) Atherosclerosis occurring in the lower extremities, such as in the feet, calves, or legs, or in the arms.
personal flotation device A device worn to provide buoyancy and keep the wearer, conscious or unconscious, afloat with the nose and mouth out of the water; also known as a life jacket.
personality disorders A class of mental disorders that are characterized by inflexible patterns of thought and beliefs that lead to socially distressing behavior.
pesticides Chemicals that kill pests such as insects, weeds, and rodents.
phobia A deep and persistent fear of a specific object, activity, or situation that results in a compelling desire to avoid the source of the fear.
smog Brownish haze that is a form of pollution produced by the photochemical reaction of sunlight with hydrocarbons, nitrogen compounds, and other gases in vehicle exhaust.
physical activity Refers to all body movements produced by skeletal muscles resulting in substantial increases in energy expenditure, but generally refers to movement of the large muscle groups.
physical fitness Refers to a set of attributes that allow you to perform moderate- to vigorous-intensity physical activities on a regular basis without getting too tired and with energy left over to handle physical or mental emergencies.
physician assistant (PA) A midlevel practitioner trained to handle most standard cases of care under the supervision of a physician.
physiological dependence The adaptive state that occurs with regular addictive behavior and results in withdrawal syndrome.
pituitary gland The endocrine gland that controls the release of hormones from the gonads.
placenta The network of blood vessels connected to the umbilical cord that transports oxygen and nutrients to a developing fetus and carries away fetal wastes.
plant sterols Essential components of plant membranes that, when consumed in the diet, appear to help lower cholesterol levels.
plaque Buildup of deposits in the arteries.
platelet adhesiveness Stickiness of red blood cells associated with blood clots.
pneumonia Inflammatory disease of the lungs characterized by chronic cough, chest pain, chills, high fever, and fluid accumulation; may be caused by bacteria, viruses, fungi, chemicals, or other substances.
point source pollutants Pollutants that enter waterways at a specific location.
poison Any substance harmful to the body when ingested, inhaled, injected, or absorbed through the skin.
pollutant A substance that contaminates some aspect of the environment and causes potential harm to living organisms.
polychlorinated biphenyls (PCBs) Toxic chemicals that were once used as insulating materials in high-voltage electrical equipment.
polydrug use Taking several medications, vitamins, recreational drugs, or illegal drugs simultaneously.
polysaccharides Complex carbohydrates formed by the combination of long chains of monosaccharides.
positive reinforcement Presenting something positive following a behavior that is being reinforced.
positron emission tomography (PET) scan Method for measuring heart activity by injecting a patient with a radioactive tracer that is scanned electronically to produce a three-dimensional image of the heart and arteries.
postpartum depression A mood disorder experienced by women who have given birth; involves depression, fatigue, and other symptoms and may last for weeks or months.
post-traumatic stress disorder (PTSD) A collection of symptoms that may occur as a delayed response to a serious trauma.
power The ability to make and implement decisions.
prayer Communication with a transcendent Presence.
preconception care Medical care received prior to becoming pregnant that helps a woman assess and address potential maternal health issues.
prediabetes Condition in which blood glucose levels are higher than normal, but not high enough to be classified as diabetes.
preeclampsia A pregnancy complication characterized by high blood pressure, protein in the urine, and edema.
pre-gaming A strategy of drinking heavily at home before going out to an event or other location.
prehypertensive Blood pressure is above normal, but not yet in the hypertensive range.
prejudice A negative evaluation of an entire group of people that is typically based on unfavorable and often wrong ideas about the group.
premature ejaculation Ejaculation that occurs prior to or almost immediately following penile penetration of the vagina.
premenstrual dysphoric disorder (PMDD) Collective name for a group of negative symptoms similar to but more severe than PMS, including severe mood disturbances.
premenstrual syndrome (PMS) Comprises the mood changes and physical symptoms that occur in some women during the 1 or 2 weeks prior to menstruation.
premium Payment made to an insurance carrier, usually in monthly installments, that covers the cost of an insurance policy.
primary aggression Goal-directed, hostile self-assertion that is destructive in character.
primary care practitioner (PCP) A medical practitioner who treats routine ailments, advises on preventive care, gives general medical advice, and makes appropriate referrals when necessary.
prion A recently identified self-replicating, protein-based pathogen.
process addictions Behaviors such as disordered gambling, compulsive buying, compulsive Internet or technology use, work addiction, compulsive exercise, and sexual addiction that are known to be addictive because they are mood altering.
procrastinate To intentionally put off doing something.
progesterone Hormone secreted by the ovaries; helps the endometrium develop and helps maintain pregnancy.

proof A measure of the percentage of alcohol in a beverage.

prostate gland Gland that secretes nutrients and neutralizing fluids into the semen.

prostate-specific antigen (PSA) An antigen found in prostate cancer patients.

proteins The essential constituents of nearly all body cells; necessary for the development and repair of bone, muscle, skin, and blood; the key elements of antibodies, enzymes, and hormones.

protozoans Microscopic single-celled organisms that can be pathogenic.

psychoactive drugs Drugs that have the potential to alter mood or behavior.

psychological hardiness A personality trait characterized by control, commitment, and the embrace of challenge.

psychological resilience The process of adapting well in the face of adversity, trauma, tragedy, threats, or significant sources of stress, such as family and relationship problems, serious health problems, or workplace and financial stressors.

psychological health The mental, emotional, social, and spiritual dimensions of health.

psychoneuroimmunology (PNI) The study of the interrelationship between the mind and body on immune system functioning.

puberty The period of sexual maturation.

pubic lice Parasitic insects that can inhabit various body areas, especially the genitals.

qi Element of traditional Chinese medicine that refers to the vital energy force that courses through the body; when *qi* is in balance, health is restored.

radiation absorbed doses (rads) Units that measure exposure to radiation.

radiotherapy The use of radiation to kill cancerous cells.

radon A naturally occurring radioactive gas resulting from the decay of certain radioactive elements.

rape Sexual penetration without the victim's consent.

reactive aggression Hostile emotional reaction brought about by frustrating life experiences.

receptor sites Specialized areas of cells and organs where chemicals, enzymes, and other substances interact.

relapse The tendency to return to the addictive behavior after a period of abstinence.

religion A system of beliefs, practices, rituals, and symbols designed to facilitate closeness to the sacred or transcendent.

repetitive motion disorder (RMD) An injury to soft tissue, tendons, muscles, nerves, or joints due to the physical stress of repeated motions; sometimes called *overuse syndrome*, *cumulative trauma disorders*, or *repetitive stress injuries*.

resiliency The ability to adapt to change and stressful events in healthy and flexible ways.

resting metabolic rate (RMR) The energy expenditure of the body under BMR conditions plus other daily sedentary activities.

rheumatic heart disease A heart disease caused by untreated streptococcal infection of the throat.

RICE Acronym for the standard first aid treatment for virtually all traumatic and overuse injuries: **r**est, **i**ce, **c**ompression, and **e**levation.

rickettsia A small form of bacteria that live inside other living cells.

risk behaviors Actions that increase susceptibility to negative health outcomes.

rubella (German measles) A milder form of measles that causes a rash and mild fever in children and may damage a fetus or a newborn baby.

satiety The feeling of fullness or satisfaction at the end of a meal.

saturated fats Fats that are unable to hold any more hydrogen in their chemical structure; derived mostly from animal sources; solid at room temperature.

schizophrenia A mental illness with biological origins that is characterized by irrational behavior, severe alterations of the senses, and often an inability to function in society.

scrotum External sac of tissue that encloses the testes.

seasonal affective disorder (SAD) A type of depression that occurs in the winter months, when sunlight levels are low.

secondary sex characteristics Characteristics associated with sex but not directly related to reproduction, such as vocal pitch, degree of body hair, and location of fat deposits.

self-disclosure Sharing personal feelings or information with others.

self-efficacy Describes a person's belief about whether he or she can successfully engage in and execute a specific behavior.

self-esteem Refers to one's realistic sense of self-respect or self-worth.

self-injury Intentionally causing injury to one's own body in an attempt to cope with overwhelming negative emotions; also called *self-mutilation*, *self-harm*, or *nonsuicidal self-injury* (NSSI).

self-nurturance Developing individual potential through a balanced and realistic appreciation of self-worth and ability.

self-talk The customary manner of thinking and talking to yourself, which can affect your self-image.

semen Fluid containing sperm and nutrients that increase sperm viability and neutralize vaginal acid.

seminal vesicles Glandular ducts that secrete nutrients for the semen.

serial monogamy A series of monogamous sexual relationships.

set point theory Theory that a form of internal thermostat controls our weight and fights to maintain this weight around a narrowly set range.

sexual abuse of children Sexual interaction between a child and an adult or older child.

sexual addiction Compulsive involvement in sexual activity.

sexual assault Any act in which one person is sexually intimate with another without that person's consent.

sexual aversion disorder Desire dysfunction characterized by sexual phobias and anxiety about sexual contact.

sexual dysfunction Problems associated with achieving sexual satisfaction.

sexual fantasies Sexually arousing thoughts and dreams.

sexual harassment Any form of unwanted sexual attention related to any condition of employment, education, or performance evaluation.

sexual identity Recognition of oneself as a sexual being; a composite of biological sex characteristics, gender identity, gender roles, and sexual orientation.

sexual orientation A person's enduring emotional, romantic, sexual, or affectionate attraction to other persons.

sexual performance anxiety A condition of sexual difficulties caused by anticipating some sort of problem with the sex act.

sexual prejudice Negative attitudes and hostile actions directed at sexually identified social groups; also referred to as sexual bias.

sexuality All the thoughts, feelings, and behaviors associated with being male or female, experiencing attraction, being in love, and being in relationships that include sexual intimacy and activity.

sexually transmitted infections (STIs) Infectious diseases caused by pathogens transmitted through some form of intimate, usually sexual, contact.

shaping Using a series of small steps to gradually achieve a particular goal.

shift and persist A strategy of reframing appraisals of current stressors and focusing on a meaningful future that protects a person from the negative effects of too much stress.

shingles A disease characterized by a painful rash that occurs when the chickenpox virus is reactivated.

sick building syndrome (SBS) Occurs when occupants of a building experience acute health effects linked to time spent in a building, but no specific illness or cause can be identified; symptoms diminish when occupants are away from the building.

sidestream smoke The cigarette, pipe, or cigar smoke breathed by nonsmokers.

simple carbohydrates A major type of carbohydrate that provides short-term energy; also called *simple sugars*.

simple rape Rape by one person, usually known to the victim, that does not involve physical beating or use of a weapon.

sinoatrial node (SA node) Cluster of electric pulse-generating cells that serves as a natural pacemaker for the heart.

situational inducement Attempt to influence a behavior through situations and occasions that are structured to exert control over that behavior.

sleep debt The difference between the number of hours of sleep an individual needed in a given time period and the number of hours he or she actually slept.

snuff A powdered form of tobacco that is sniffed or absorbed through the mucous membranes in the nose or placed inside the cheek and sucked.

social bonds The level of closeness and attachment with other individuals.

social cognitive model (SCM) Model of behavior change emphasizing the role of social factors and thought processes (cognition) in behavior change.

social health Aspect of psychosocial health that includes interactions with others, ability to use social supports, and ability to adapt to various situations.

social learning theory Theory that people learn behaviors by watching role models—parents, caregivers, and significant others.

social phobia A phobia characterized by fear and avoidance of social situations; also called *social anxiety disorder*.

social physique anxiety (SPA) A desire to look good that has a destructive effect on a person's ability to function well in social interactions and relationships.

social support Network of people and services with whom you share ties and from whom you get support.

socialization Process by which a society communicates behavioral expectations to its individual members.

spermatogenesis The development of sperm.

spermicides Substances designed to kill sperm.

spiritual health The aspect of psychosocial health that relates to having a sense of meaning and purpose to one's life, as well as a feeling of connection with others and with nature.

spiritual intelligence (SI) The ability to access higher meanings, values, abiding purposes, and unconscious aspects of the self, a characteristic that helps us find a moral and ethical path to guide us through life.

spirituality An individual's sense of purpose and meaning in life, beyond material values.

stalking The willful, repeated, and malicious following, harassing, or threatening of another person.

standard drink The amount of any beverage that contains about 14 grams of pure alcohol (about 0.6 fluid ounce or 1.2 tablespoons).

staphylococci A group of round bacteria, usually found in clusters, that cause a variety of diseases in humans and other animals.

starch Polysaccharide that is the storage form of glucose in plants.

static stretching Stretching techniques that slowly and gradually lengthen a muscle or group of muscles and their tendons.

stent A stainless steel, mesh-like tube that is inserted to prop open the artery.

sterilization Permanent fertility control achieved through surgical procedures.

stereotactic radiosurgery A type of radiation therapy that can be used to zap tumors; also known as gamma knife surgery.

stillbirth A fetus that is dead at birth.

stimulants Drugs that increase activity of the central nervous system.

Streptococcus A round bacterium, usually found in chain formation.

stress A series of mental and physiological responses and adaptations to a real or perceived threat to one's well-being.

stress inoculation A stress-management technique in which a person consciously anticipates and prepares for potential stressors.

stressor A physical, social, or psychological event or condition that upsets homeostasis and produces a stress response.

stroke A condition occurring when the brain is damaged by disrupted blood supply; also called *cerebrovascular accident*.

subjective well-being An uplifting feeling of inner peace.

suction curettage An abortion technique that uses gentle suction to remove fetal tissue from the uterus.

sudden cardiac death Death that occurs as a result of abrupt, profound loss of heart function.

sudden infant death syndrome (SIDS) The sudden death of an infant under 1 year of age for no apparent reason.

suicidal ideation A desire to die and thoughts about suicide.

Superfund Fund established under the Comprehensive Environmental Response, Compensation, and Liability Act to be used for cleaning up toxic waste dumps.

suppositories Waxy capsules that are inserted deep into the vagina, where they melt and release a spermicide.

sustainable development Development that meets the needs of the present without compromising the ability of future generations to meet their own needs.

sympathetic nervous system Branch of the autonomic nervous system responsible for stress arousal.

sympathomimetics Food substances that can produce stresslike physiological responses.

synergism The interaction of two or more drugs that produce more profound effects than would be expected if the drugs were taken separately; also called *potentiation*.

syphilis One of the most widespread bacterial STIs; characterized by distinct phases and potentially serious results.

systolic blood pressure The upper number in the fraction that measures blood pressure, indicating pressure on the walls of the arteries when the heart contracts.

tar A thick, brownish substance condensed from particulate matter in smoked tobacco.

target heart rate The heart rate range of aerobic exercise that leads to improved cardiorespiratory fitness (i.e., 64% to 96% of maximal heart rate).

temperature inversion A weather condition occurring when a layer of cool air is trapped under a layer of warmer air, preventing the air from circulating.

teratogenic Causing birth defects; may refer to drugs, environmental chemicals, radiation, or diseases.

terrorism The unlawful use of force or violence against persons or property to intimidate or coerce a government, the civilian population, or any segment thereof in furtherance of political or social objectives.

testes Male sex organs that manufacture sperm and produce hormones.

testosterone The male sex hormone manufactured in the testes.

tetrahydrocannabinol (THC) The chemical name for the active ingredient in marijuana.

thrombolysis Injection of an agent to dissolve clots and restore some blood flow, thereby reducing the amount of tissue that dies from ischemia.

thrombus Blood clot attached to a blood vessel's wall.

time As part of the FITT prescription, refers to how long a person needs to exercise each time to improve a component of physical fitness.

tolerance Phenomenon in which progressively larger doses of a drug or more intense involvement in a behavior is needed to produce the desired effects.

toxic shock syndrome (TSS) A potentially life-threatening disease that occurs when specific bacterial toxins multiply and spread to the bloodstream, most commonly through improper use of tampons or diaphragms.

toxins Poisonous substances produced by certain microorganisms that cause various diseases.

toxoplasmosis A disease caused by an organism found in cat feces that, when contracted by a pregnant woman, may result in stillbirth or an infant with mental retardation or birth defects.

trace minerals Minerals that the body needs in only very small amounts.
traditional Chinese medicine (TCM) Ancient comprehensive system of healing that uses herbs, acupuncture, and massage to bring vital energy, *qi*, into balance and to remove blockages of qi that lead to disease.
trans fats (trans fatty acids) Fatty acids that are produced when polyunsaturated oils are hydrogenated to make them more solid.
transdermal The introduction of drugs through the skin.
transgendered Having a gender identity that does not match one's biological sex.
transient ischemic attack (TIA) Brief interruption of the blood supply to the brain that causes only temporary impairment; often an indicator of impending major stroke.
transsexual A person who is psychologically of one sex but physically of the other.
transtheoretical model Model of behavior change that identifies six distinct stages people go through in altering behavior patterns; also called the *stages of change model*.
traumatic injuries Injuries that are accidental and occur suddenly and violently.
traumatic stress A physiological and mental response that occurs for a prolonged period of time after a major accident, war, assault, natural disaster, or an event in which one may be seriously hurt, or killed, or witness horrible things.
trichomoniasis Protozoan STI characterized by foamy, yellowish discharge and unpleasant odor.
triglycerides The most common form of fat in the body; excess calories consumed are converted into triglycerides and stored as body fat.
trimester A 3-month segment of pregnancy; used to describe specific developmental changes that occur in the embryo or fetus.
triple marker screen (TMS) A common maternal blood test that can be used to identify fetuses with certain birth defects and genetic abnormalities.
tubal ligation Sterilization of the woman that involves the cutting and tying off or cauterizing of the fallopian tubes.
tuberculosis (TB) A disease caused by bacterial infiltration of the respiratory system.
tumor A neoplasmic mass that grows more rapidly than surrounding tissue.
type As part of the FITT prescription, refers to what kind of exercises a person needs to do to improve a component of physical fitness.
type 1 diabetes Form of diabetes mellitus in which the pancreas is not able to make insulin and therefore blood glucose cannot enter the cells to be used for energy.
type 2 diabetes Form of diabetes mellitus in which the pancreas does not make enough insulin or the body is unable to use insulin correctly.
typical-use failure rate The number of pregnancies (per 100 users) that are likely to occur in the first year of use of a particular birth control method if the method's use is not consistent or always correct.
ultrasonography (ultrasound) A common prenatal test that uses high-frequency sound waves to create a visual image of the fetus.
underweight Having a body weight more than 10 percent below healthy recommended levels; in an adult, having a BMI below 18.5.
unintentional injuries Injury, death, or psychological harm caused unintentionally or without premeditation.
unsaturated fats Fats that have room for more hydrogen in their chemical structure; derived mostly from plants; liquid at room temperature.
urethral opening The opening through which urine is expelled.
urinary tract infection (UTI) Infection, more common among women than men, of the urinary tract; causes include untreated STIs.
uterus (womb) Hollow, pear-shaped muscular organ whose function is to contain the developing fetus.
vaccination Inoculation with killed or weakened pathogens or similar, less dangerous antigens in order to prevent or lessen the effects of a disease.
vagina The passage in females leading from the vulva into the uterus.
vaginal intercourse The insertion of the penis into the vagina.
vaginismus A state in which the vaginal muscles contract so forcefully that penetration cannot occur.
values Principles that influence our thoughts and emotions and guide the choices we make in our lives.
variant sexual behavior A sexual behavior that is not practiced by most people.
vas deferens Tube that transports sperm from the epididymis to the ejaculatory duct.
vasectomy Sterilization of the man that involves the cutting and tying off of both vasa deferentia.
vasocongestion The engorgement of the genital organs with blood.
vegetarian A person who follows a diet that excludes some or all animal products.
veins Vessels that transport waste and carry blood back to the heart from other regions of the body.
ventricles The heart's two lower chambers, which pump blood through the blood vessels.
venules Branches of the veins.
very-low-calorie diets (VLCDs) Diets with a daily caloric value of 400 to 700 calories.
violence Aggressive behaviors that produce injuries and can result in death.
virulent Strong enough to overcome host resistance and cause disease.
viruses Pathogens that invade and inject their own DNA or RNA into a host cell, take it over, and force it to make copies of the pathogen.
visualization The creation of mental images to promote relaxation.
vitamins Essential organic compounds that promote growth and reproduction and help maintain life and health.
vulva Collective term for the external female genitalia.
waist-to-hip ratio Waist circumference divided by hip circumference; a high ratio indicates increased health risks due to unhealthy fat distribution.
wellness The achievement of the highest level of health possible in each of several dimensions.
whole grains Grains that are milled in their complete form, and thus include the bran, germ, and endosperm, with only the husk removed.
withdrawal 1 A method of contraception that involves withdrawing the penis from the vagina before ejaculation; also called coitus interruptus.
withdrawal 2 A series of temporary physical and biopsychosocial symptoms that occurs when an addict abruptly abstains from an addictive chemical or behavior.
work addiction The compulsive use of work and the work persona to fulfill needs for intimacy, power, and success.
yoga A system of physical and mental training involving controlled breathing, physical postures (*asanas*), meditation, chanting, and other practices that are believed to cultivate unity with the *Atman*, or spiritual life principle of the universe.
yo-yo diets Cycles in which people diet and regain weight.
zoonotic diseases Diseases of animals that may be transmitted to humans.

References

Chapter 1

1. World Health Organization (WHO), "Constitution of the World Health Organization," *Chronicles of the World Health Organization* (Geneva: WHO, 1947), Available at www.who.int/governance/eb/constitution/en/index.html
2. R. Dubos, *So Human an Animal: How We Are Shaped by Surroundings and Events* (New York: Scribner, 1968), 15.
3. The Brookings Institution, "Obesity, Prevention, and Health Care Costs," May 2012, www.brookings.edu/research/papers/2012/05/04-health-care-hammond
4. Centers for Disease Control and Prevention, "Table A," *National Vital Statistics Report* 61, no. 6 (2012), Available at www.cdc.gov/nchs/data/nvsr/nvsr61/nvsr61_06.pdf
5. Centers for Disease Control and Prevention, "Achievements in Public Health, 1900–1999: Control of Infectious Diseases," *MMWR* 48, no. 29 (1999): 621–29, Available at www.cdc.gov/mmwr/preview/mmwrhtml/mm4829a1.htm
6. H. L. Walls et al., "Obesity and Trends in Life Expectancy," *Journal of Obesity* 2012 (2012), Article ID 107989, DOI:10.1155/2012/107989
7. Organization for Economic Cooperation and Development, *Health at a Glance 2013: OECD Indicators* (Paris: OECD Publishing, 2013), DOI: 10.1787/health_glance-2013-en
8. M. Heron, "Deaths: Leading Causes for 2010, Table 1," *National Vital Statistics Reports* 62, no. 6 (2013): 17–18 Available at www.cdc.gov/nchs/data/nvsr/nvsr62/nvsr62_06.pdf
9. U.S. Department of Health and Human Services, "*Healthy People 2020: About Healthy People*," Updated December 17, 2012, Available at www.healthypeople.gov/HP2020
10. U.S. Department of Health and Human Services, "*Healthy People 2020: 2020 Topics and Objectives*," Updated November 13, 2013, Available at http://healthypeople.gov/2020/topicsobjectives2020/default.aspx
11. U.S. Department of Health and Human Services, "*Healthy People 2020: Leading Health Indicators*," Updated July 30, 2013, http://healthypeople.gov/2020/LHI/default.aspx
12. U.S. Department of Health and Human Services, "*Healthy People 2020: About Healthy People*," 2012.
13. U.S. Department of Health and Human Services, *Healthy People 2020* (Washington, DC: U.S. Government Printing Office, 2011), Available at www.healthypeople.gov/2020/about/DOHAbout.aspx
14. Centers for Disease Control and Prevention, "Chronic Disease Prevention and Health Promotion," August 2012, www.cdc.gov/chronicdisease/overview/index.htm#2
15. Ibid.
16. U.S. Burden of Disease Collaborators, "The State of US Health, 1990-2010: Burden of Diseases, Injuries, and Risk Factors," *JAMA* 310, no. 6 (2013): 591–606, Available at http://jama.jamanetwork.com/article.aspx?articleid=1710486
17. Ibid.
18. Centers for Disease Control and Prevention, "Alcohol Use and Health Fact Sheets," December 2013, www.cdc.gov/alcohol/fact-sheets/alcohol-use.htm
19. Centers for Disease Control and Prevention, "Smoking and Tobacco Use Fast Facts," February 2014, www.cdc.gov/tobacco/data_statistics/fact_sheets/fast_facts/
20. U.S. Department of Health and Human Services, "*Healthy People 2020: Determinants of Health*," Updated September 20, 2012, www.healthypeople.gov
21. U.S. Burden of Disease Collaborators, "The State of US Health, 1990–2010," 2013.
22. D. Ding et al. "Neighborhood Environment and Physical Activity among Youth: A Review," *American Journal of Preventive Medicine* 41, no. 4 (2011): 442–55; J. Sallis et al., "Role of Built Environments in Physical Activity, Obesity, and Cardiovascular Disease." *Circulation* 125 (2012): 729–37, Available at https://circ.ahajournals.org/content/125/5/729.full
23. M. J. Trowbridge and T.L. Schmid, "Built Environment and Physical Activity Promotion: Place-Based Obesity Prevention Strategies" in "Weight of the Nation," supplement, *Journal of Law, Medicine & Ethics*, Winter 2013, 46–51, Available at www.aslme.org/media/downloadable/files/links/j/l/jlme-41-4-supp_trowbridge.pdf; S. Cummins, E. Flint, and S. A. Matthews, "New Neighborhood Grocery Store Increased Awareness of Food Access but Did Not Alter Dietary Habits or Obesity," *Health Affairs* 33 no. 2 (2014): 283–91.
24. U.S. Department of Health and Human Services, "*Healthy People 2020: Determinants of Health*," 2012.
25. L. Holst, "7.1 Million Americans Have Enrolled in Private Health Coverage under the Affordable Care Act," *The White House Blog*, April 1, 2014, www.whitehouse.gov/blog/2014/04/01/more-7-million-americans-have-enrolled-private-health-coverage-under-affordable-care
26. Centers for Disease Control and Prevention, "CDC Health Disparities and Inequalities Report—United States, 2013," *Morbidity and Mortality Weekly Report* 62, no. 3, Supplement (2013): 1–187, Available at www.cdc.gov/mmwr/preview/ind2013_su.html#HealthDisparities2013; Centers for Disease Control and Prevention, "State-Specific Healthy Life Expectancy at Age 65 Years—United States, 2007–2009," *Morbidity and Mortality Weekly Report* 62, no 28 (2013): 561–66.
27. I. Rosenstock, "Historical Origins of the Health Belief Model," *Health Education Monographs* 2, no. 4 (1974): 328–35.
28. J. O. Prochaska and C. C. DiClemente, "Stages and Processes of Self-Change of Smoking: Toward an Integrative Model of Change," *Journal of Consulting and Clinical Psychology* 51 (1983): 390–95.
29. A. Ellis and M. Benard, *Clinical Application of Rational Emotive Therapy* (New York: Plenum, 1985).

Chapter 2

1. A. H. Maslow, *Motivation and Personality*, 2nd ed. (New York: Harper and Row, 1970).
2. U.S. Department of Health and Human Services, *Mental Health: A Report of the Surgeon General—Executive Summary* (Rockville, MD: U.S. Department of Health and Human Services, Substance Abuse and Mental Health Services Administration, National Institute of Mental Health, 1999), Available at www.surgeongeneral.gov/library/mentalhealth/summary.html.
3. D. Goleman, R. Boyatzis, and A. McKee, *Primal Leadership: Unleashing the Power of Emotional Intelligence* (Boston: Harvard Business Review Press, 2013); M. A. Brackett, S. E. Rivers, and P. Salovey, "Emotional Intelligence: Implications for Personal, Social, Academic, and Workplace Success," *Social and Personality Psychology Compass* 5, no. 1 (2011): 88–103.
4. J. Holt-Lunstad et al., "Social Relationships and Mortality Risks: A Meta-Analytic Review," *PLoS Medicine* 7, no. 7 (2010): e1000316, DOI: 10.1371/journal.pmed.1000316; N. I. Eisenberger and S. W. Cole, "Social Neuroscience and Health: Neurophysiological Mechanisms Linking Social Ties with Physical Health," *Nature Neuroscience* 15 (2012): 669–74, DOI:10.1038/nn.3086; Y. Luo et al., "Loneliness, Health, and Mortality in Old Age: A National Longitudinal Study," *Social Science & Medicine* 74, no. 6 (2012): 907–14.
5. K. Karren et al., *Mind/Body Health: The Effects of Attitudes, Emotions, and Relationships*, 5th ed. (San Francisco: Benjamin Cummings, 2013).
6. National Cancer Institute, "Spirituality in Cancer Care," Revised 2012, www.cancer.gov/cancertopics/pdq/supportivecare/spirituality/patient.
7. C. Carter, *Raising Happiness: 10 Simple Steps for More Joyful Kids and Happier Parents* (New York: Ballantine Publishing, 2010).
8. W. Cheng, W. Ickes, and L. Verhofstadt, "How Is Family Support Related to Students' GPA scores? A Longitudinal Study," *Higher Education* 64, no. 3 (2012): 399–420; L. Rice et al., "The Role of Social Support in Students' Perceived Abilities and Attitudes toward Math and Science," *Journal of Youth and Adolescence* 42, no. 7 (2013): 1028–40; J. Cullum et al., "Ignoring Norms with a Little Help from My Friends: Social Support Reduces Normative Influence on Drinking Behavior," *Journal of Social & Clinical Psychology* 32, no. 1 (2013): 17–33; J. Hirsch and A. Barton, "Positive Social Support, Negative Social Exchanges, and Suicidal Behavior in College Students," *Journal of American College Health* 59, no. 5 (2011): 393–98; I. Yalcin, "Social Support and Optimism as Predictors of Life Satisfaction of College Students," *International Journal for the Advancement of Counseling* 33, no. 2 (2011): 79–87.
9. M. Seligman, *Helplessness: On Depression, Development, and Death* (New York: W. H. Freeman, 1975).
10. P. L. Hill et al., "Examining Concurrent and Longitudinal Relations between Personality Traits and Social Well-Being in Adulthood," *Social Psychological and Personality Science* 3 (2012): 698–705.
11. K. Huffman and C. A. Sanderson, *Real World Psychology* (Hoboken, NJ: Wiley, 2014).
12. S. Rimer, Harvard School of Public Health, "The Biology of Emotion—And What It May Teach Us about Helping People to Live Longer," 2012, www.hsph.harvard.edu/news/hphr/chronic-disease-prevention/happiness-stress-heart-disease
13. Ibid.

14. Ibid; E. A. Wheeler, "Amusing Ourselves to Health: A Selected Review of Lab Findings" in *Positive Psychology: Advances in Understanding Adult Motivation*, ed. J. D. Sinnott (New York: Springer, 2013).
15. R. I. Dunbar et al., "Social Laughter Is Correlated with an Elevated Pain Threshold," *Proceedings of the Royal Society*, September 14, 2011, DOI: 10.1098/rspb.2011.1373.
16. M. Seligman, *Flourish: A Visionary New Understanding of Happiness and Well-Being*, (New York: Free Press, 2011).
17. J. H Pryor et al., *The American Freshman: National Norms Fall 2012* (Los Angeles: Higher Education Research Institute, UCLA), Available at http://heri.ucla.edu/monographs/TheAmericanFreshman2012.pdf.
18. Ibid.
19. Ibid.
20. National Cancer Institute, "General Information on Spirituality," Modified June 2012, www.cancer.gov/cancertopics/pdq/supportivecare/spirituality/Patient/page1
21. H. G. Koenig, "Religion, Spirituality and Health: The Research and Clinical Implications," *ISRN Psychiatry* 2012 (2012), DOI: 10.5402/2012/27830.
22. Ibid.
23. Pew Research Center, "The Global Religious Landscape: A Report on the Size and Distribution of the World's Major Religious Groups as of 2010," December 2012, www.pewforum.org/files/2014/01/global-religion-full.pdf.
24. Ibid.
25. B. L. Seaward, *Managing Stress: Principles and Strategies for Health and Well Being*, 7th ed. (Sudbury, MA: Jones and Bartlett, 2012).
26. DanahZohar.com, "Learn the Qs," Accessed January 2014, http://dzohar.com/?page_id=622.
27. National Institutes of Health, National Center for Complementary and Alternative Medicine, "Exploring the Science of Complementary and Alternative Medicine: Third Strategic Plan: 2011–2015," NIH Publication No. 11-7643, D458, February 2011, http://nccam.nih.gov/about/plans/2011/objective1.htm.
28. Ibid.
29. Ibid.
30. B. C. Bock et al., "Yoga as a Complementary Treatment for Smoking Cessation in Women," *Journal of Women's Health* 21, no. 2 (2012): 240–48; L. Carim-Todd, S. H. Mitchell, and B. S. Oken, "Mind-Body Practices: An Alternative, Drug-Free Treatment For Smoking Cessation? A Systematic Review of the Literature," *Drug and Alcohol Dependence* 132, no. 3 (2013): 399–410; V. Conn, "The Power of Being Present: The Value of Mindfulness Interventions in Improving Health and Well-Being," *Western Journal of Nursing Research* 33 (2011): 993–95; Y. Matchim, J. Armer, and B. Stewart, "Effects of Mindfulness-Based Stress Reduction on Health Among Breast Cancer Survivors," *Western Journal of Nursing Research* 33, no. 8 (2011): 996–1016.
31. D. M. Davis and J. Hayes, "What Are the Benefits of Mindfulness?," *Monitor on Psychology. American Psychological Association* 43, no. 7 (2012): 64, Available at www.apa.org/monitor/2012/07-08/ce-corner.aspx; B. K. Hölzel et al., "Mindfulness Practice Leads to Increases in Regional Brain Gray Matter Density," *Psychiatry Research: Neuroimaging* 191, (2011): 36–43, DOI: 10.1016/j.pscychresns.2010.08.006.
32. NCCAM, "Research Spotlight," 2013; A. Chiesa and A. Serretti, "Mindfulness-Based Stress Reduction for Stress Management in Healthy People A Review and Meta-Analysis," *Journal of Alternative and Complementary Medicine* 15, no. (2009): 593–600; N. Y. Winbush, C. R. Gross, and M. J. Kreitzer, "The Effects of Mindfulness-Based Stress Reduction on Sleep Disturbance: A Systematic Review," *EXPLORE: The Journal of Science and Healing* 3, no. 6 (2007): 585–91; N. E. Morone et al., 'I Felt Like a New Person.' The Effects of Mindfulness Meditation on Older Adults with Chronic Pain: Qualitative Narrative Analysis of Diary Entries," *Journal of Pain*, no. 9 (2008): 841–48. Y. Matchim, "Breast Cancer Survivors Benefit," 2011.
33. Ibid.
34. National Cancer Institute (NCI), "Spirituality in Cancer Care," November 2012, www.cancer.gov/cancertopics/pdq/supportivecare/spirituality/HealthProfessional.
35. C. Lysne and A. Wachholtz, "Pain, Spirituality and Meaning Making: What Can We Learn from the Literature?" *Religions*, no. 2 (2011): 1–16, DOI: 10.3390/rel2010001; H. Koenig and A. Bussing, "Spiritual Needs of Patients with Chronic Diseases," *Religions* 1, no. 1 (2010): 18–27.
36. ClinicalTrials.gov, "Mind–Body Interventions in Cardiac Patients," January 2011, Available at http://clinicaltrials.gov/ct2/show/NCT01270568.
37. G. Lucchetti, A. Lucchetti, and H. Koenig, "Impact of Spirituality/Religiosity on Mortality: Comparison with Other Health Interventions," *The Journal of Science and Healing* 7, no. 4 (2011): 234–38.
38. National Cancer Institute (NCI), "Spirituality in Cancer Care," September 2012, www.cancer.gov/cancertopics/pdq/supportivecare/spirituality/HealthProfessional.
39. National Center for Complementary and Alternative Medicine (NCCAM), "Research Spotlight: Meditation May Increase Empathy," Modified January 2012, http://nccam.nih.gov/research/results/spotlight/060608.htm.
40. G. Desbordes et al., "Effects of Mindful-Attention and Compassion Meditation Training on Amygdala Response to Emotional Stimuli in an Ordinary, Non-Meditative State," *Frontiers in Human Neuroscience* 6, no. 292 (2012), DOI: 10.3389/fnhum.2012.00292.
41. C. Carter, *Raising Happiness: 10 Simple Steps for More Joyful Kids and Happier Parents* (New York: Ballantine Publishing, 2010); R. I. Dunbar et al., "Social Laughter Is Correlated with an Elevated Pain Threshold," *Proceedings of the Royal Society*, September 14, 2011, DOI: 10.1098/rspb.2011.1373.39%.
42. National Center for Complementary and Alternative Medicine (NCCAM), "Prayer and Spirituality in Health: Ancient Practices, Modern Science," *CAM at the NIH* 12 no. 1 (2005): 1–4; National Cancer Institute (NCI), "Spirituality in Cancer Care," September 2012, www.cancer.gov.
43. G. G. Ano and E. B. Vasconcelles, "Religious Coping and Psychological Adjustment to Stress: A Meta-Analysis," *Journal of Clinical Psychology* 61, no. 4 (2005): 461–80; U. Winter et al., "The Psychological Outcome of Religious Coping with Stressful Life Events in a Swiss Sample of Church Attendees," *Psychotherapy and Psychosomatics* 78, no. 4 (2009): 240–44; G. Lucchetti, "Impact of Spirituality/Religiosity," 2011; Y. Matchim, "Breast Cancer Survivors Benefit," 2011.
44. A. Chiesa and A. Serretti, "Mindfulness-Based Stress Reduction for Stress Management in Healthy People: A Review and Meta-Analysis," *Journal of Alternative and Complementary Medicine* 15, no. (2009): 593–600. G. Lucchetti, "Impact of Spirituality/Religiosity," 2011; Y. Matchim, "Breast Cancer Survivors Benefit," 2011.
45. D. R. Vago and D. A. Silbersweig, "Self-Awareness, Self-Regulation, and Self-Transcendence (S-ART): A Framework for Understanding the Neurobiological Mechanisms of Mindfulness," *Human Neuroscience* 6, no. 269 (2012), Available at www.ncbi.nlm.nih.gov/pmc/articles/PMC3480633.
46. G. Desbordes et al., "Effects of Mindful-Attention and Compassion Meditation Training," 2012.
47. Mayo Clinic Staff, MayoClinic.com, "Mental Illness: Causes," September 2012, www.mayoclinic.org/diseases-conditions/mental-illness/basics/causes/con-20033813.
48. Ibid.
49. Substance Abuse and Mental Health Services Administration, *Results from the 2012 National Survey on Drug Use and Health: Mental Health Findings*, NSDUH Series H-47, HHS Publication no. (SMA) 13-4805 (Rockville, MD: Substance Abuse and Mental Health Services Administration, 2013); R. C. Kessler et al., "Twelve-Month and Lifetime Prevalence and Lifetime Morbid Risk of Anxiety and Mood Disorders in the United States," *International Journal of Methods in Psychiatric Research* 21, no. 3 (2012): 169–84, DOI: 10.1002/mpr.1359.
50. Ibid.
51. H. A. Whiteford et al., "Global Burden of Disease Attributable to Mental and Substance Use Disorders: Findings from the Global Burden of Disease Study 2010," *The Lancet* 382, no. 9904 (2013): 1575–86; T. L. Mark et al., "Changes in U.S. Spending on Mental Health and Substance Abuse Treatment, 1986–2005, and Implications for Policy," *Health Affairs* 30, no. 2 (2011): 284–92.
52. R. P. Gallagher, *National Survey of College Counseling 2012* (Pittsburg, PA: The American College Counseling Association, 2012), Available at www.iacsinc.org/NSCCD%202012.pdf.
53. The American Psychological Association. "College Students' Mental Health Is a Growing Concern, Survey Finds." 2013. 44(6), p.13.) http://www.apa.org/monitor/2013/06/college-students.aspx
54. American College Health Association, *American College Health Association–National College Health Assessment II (ACHA–NCHA II): Reference Group Data Report Fall 2013* (Hanover, MD: American College Health Association, 2014), Available at www.acha-ncha.org/reports_ACHA-NCHAII.html.
55. American College Health Association, *American College Health Association-National College Health Assessment II: Reference Group Executive Summary Fall 2013* (Hanover, MD: American College Health Association; 2014).
56. Ibid.
57. R. C. Kessler, et al., "Twelve-Month and Lifetime Prevalence and Lifetime Morbid Risk of Anxiety and Mood Disorders," 2012.
58. American College Health Association, *ACHA–NCHA II: Reference Group Data Report Fall 2013*, 2014.
59. National Institute of Mental Health, "Generalized Anxiety Disorder, GAD," Accessed February 2014, www.nimh.nih.gov/health/publications/anxiety-disorders/generalized-anxiety-disorder-gad.shtml.
60. R. C. Kessler et al., "Twelve-Month and Lifetime Prevalence and Lifetime Morbid Risk of Anxiety and Mood Disorders," 2012,
61. Mayo Clinic Staff, MayoClinic.com, "Panic Attacks and Panic Disorder: Symptoms," May 2012, www.mayoclinic.org/diseases-conditions/panic-attacks/basics/symptoms/con-20020825.

62. R. C. Kessler et al., "Twelve-Month and Lifetime Prevalence and Lifetime Morbid Risk of Anxiety and Mood Disorders," 2012.
63. Ibid.
64. R. C. Kessler et al., "Twelve-Month and Lifetime Prevalence and Lifetime Morbid Risk of Anxiety and Mood Disorders," 2012.
65. R. H. Pietrzak et al., "Prevalence and Axis I Comorbidity of Full and Partial PTSD in the U.S.: Results from Wave 2 of the National Epidemiologic Survey on Alcohol and Related Conditions," *Journal of Anxiety Disorders* 25, no. 3 (2011): 456–65; J. Gradus, United States Department of Veterans Affairs, National Center for PTSD, "Epidemiology of PTSD," January 2014, www.ptsd.va.gov/professional/PTSD-overview/epidemiological-facts-ptsd.asp; S. Staggs, PsychCentral, ""Myths and Facts about PTSD," February 2014, http://psychcentral.com/lib/myths-and-facts-about-ptsd.
66. R. C. Kessler et al., "Twelve-Month and Lifetime Prevalence and Lifetime Morbid Risk of Anxiety and Mood Disorders," 2012; R. H. Pietrzak et al., "Prevalence and Axis I Comorbidity of Full and Partial PTSD in the U.S.," 2011.
67. Ibid.
68. Mayo Clinic Staff, Mayo Clinic.com, "Generalized Anxiety Disorder: Causes," September 2011, www.mayoclinic.org/diseases-conditions/generalized-anxiety-disorder/basics/causes/con-20024562.
69. R. C. Kessler, et al., "Twelve-Month and Lifetime Prevalence and Lifetime Morbid Risk of Anxiety and Mood Disorders," 2012.
70. Ibid.
71. National Institute of Mental Health, "Depression," Revised 2011, www.nimh.nih.gov/health/publications/depression/index.shtml.
72. American College Health Association, *American College Health Association–National College Health Assessment II (ACHA–NCHA II): Reference Group Data Report, Fall 2013* (Hanover, MD: American College Health Association, 2014), Available at www.acha-ncha.org/reports_ACHA-NCHAII.html.
73. C. Blanco et al., "The Epidemiology of Chronic Major Depressive Disorder and Dysthymic Disorder: Results from the National Epidemiologic Survey on Alcohol and Related Conditions," *Journal of Clinical Psychiatry* 71, no. 12 (2010): 1645–56, DOI: 10.4088/JCP.09m05663gry.
74. R. C. Kessler, et al., "Twelve-Month and Lifetime Prevalence and Lifetime Morbid Risk of Anxiety and Mood Disorders," 2012.
75. WebMD, "Seasonal Depression (Seasonal Affective Disorder)," 2012, www.webmd.com/depression/guide/seasonal-affective-disorder.
76. Mayo Clinic Staff, MayoClinic.com, "Depression: Causes," 2013, www.mayoclinic.org/diseases-conditions/depression/basics/causes/con-20032977
77. Mayo Clinic, MayoClinic.com, "Depression in Women: Understanding the Gender Gap", January 2013, www.mayoclinic.org/diseases-conditions/depression/in-depth/depression/art-20047725.
78. HelpGuide.org, "Depression in Men," 2014, www.helpguide.org/mental/depression_men_male.htm.
79. American Psychiatric Association (APA), Mental Health. "Children," Accessed February 2014, www.psychiatry.org/mental-health/people/children.
80. APA, Mental Health. "Seniors," Accessed February 2014, www.psychiatry.org/mental-health/people/seniors.
81. CDC, "An Estimated 1 in 10 U.S. Adults Report Depression," March 31, 2011, www.cdc.gov/features/dsdepression/; A. Akincigil, "Racial and Ethnic Disparities in Depression Care in Community-Dwelling Elderly in the United States," *American Journal of Public Health* 102, no. 2 (2012): 319–28.
82. American Psychiatric Association, *Diagnostic and Statistical Manual of Mental Disorders (DSM-5)*, 5th ed. (Washington, DC: American Psychiatric Association, 2013).
83. R. A. Sansone and L. A. Sansone, "Personality Disorders: A Nation-Based Perspective on Prevalence," *Innovations in Clinical Neuroscience* 8, no. 4 (2011): 13–18.
84. Mayo Clinic Staff, MayoClinic.com, "Borderline Personality Disorder," August 2012, www.mayoclinic.com/health/borderline-personality-disorder/DS00442.
85. M. C. Zanarini et al., "Reasons for Self-Mutilation Reported by Borderline Patients Over 16 Years of Prospective Follow-Up," *Journal of Personality Disorders* 27, no. 6 (2013): 783–94, DOI: 10.1521/pedi_2013_27_115
86. American College Health Association, *ACHA–NCHA II: Reference Group Data Report, Fall 2013*, 2014; M. J. Sornberger et al., "Nonsuicidal Self-Injury and Gender: Patterns of Prevalence, Methods, and Locations among Adolescents," *Suicide and Life-Threatening Behavior* 42, no. 3: 266–78; J. Whitlock et al., "Nonsuicidal Self-Injury in a College Population: General Trends and Sex Differences," *Journal of American College Health* 59, no. 8 (2011): 691–98; M. Smith and J. Segal, HelpGuide.org, "Cutting and Self-Harm," Updated February 2014, www.helpguide.org/mental/self_injury.htm.
87. National Institute of Mental Health, "Schizophrenia," Reviewed February 2013, www.nimh.nih.gov/health/topics/schizophrenia/index.shtml.
88. Ibid.
89. Ibid.
90. Alzheimer's Association, "2012 Alzheimer's Disease Facts and Figures," 2012, www.alz.org.
91. Ibid.
92. Alzheimer's Association, "What Is Alzheimer's?" 2011, www.alz.org.
93. D. L. Hoyert and J. Xu, "Deaths: Preliminary Data for 2011, Table 7," *National Vital Statistics Reports* 61, no. 6 (2012), Available at www.cdc.gov/nchs/data/nvsr/nvsr61/nvsr61_06.pdf.
94. J. C. Turner, "Leading Causes of Mortality among American College Students at 4-year Institutions." Poster presented at the American Public Health Association 139th Annual Conference, October 2011, https://apha.confex.com/apha/139am/webprogram/Paper241696.html.
95. Ibid.; Centers for Disease Control and Prevention, "National Suicide Statistics at a Glance," January 2014, www.cdc.gov/violenceprevention/suicide/statistics/index.html.
96. I. H. Rockett et al., "Leading Causes of Unintentional and Intentional Injury Mortality: United States, 2000–2009," *American Journal of Public Health* 102, no. 11 (2012): e84–e92, DOI: 10.2105/ajph.2012.300960.
97. D. L. Hoyert and J. Xu, "Deaths: Preliminary Data for 2011, Table 7," 2012.
98. Centers for Disease Control and Prevention, "National Suicide Statistics at a Glance," January 2014, www.cdc.gov/violenceprevention/suicide/statistics/mechanism02.html.
99. American Foundation for Suicide Prevention, "Warning Signs of Suicide," Accessed February 2014, www.afsp.org/preventing-suicide/risk-factors-and-warning-signs.
100. Ibid.
101. Ibid.
102. Substance Abuse and Mental Health Services Administration, "Results from the 2012 National Survey on Drug Use and Health: Mental Health Findings," 2013.
103. A. Lasalvia et al., "Global Pattern of Experienced and Anticipated Discrimination Reported by People with Major Depressive Disorder: A Cross-Sectional Survey," *The Lancet* 381, no. 9860 (2013): 55–62, DOI:10.1016/S0140-6736(12)61379-8.
104. U.S. Food and Drug Administration, "Antidepressant Use in Children, Adolescents, and Adults," August 2010, www.fda.gov/Drugs/DrugSafety/InformationbyDrugClass/UCM096273.

Pulled Statistic

page 30, Higher Education Research Institute, "Attending to Student's Inner Lives," April 2011, Available at http://spirituality.ucla.edu/docs/white%20paper/white%20paper%20final.pdf.

Chapter 3

1. American Psychological Association, "Stress in America: Missing the Health Care Connection," February 2013, www.apa.org/news/press/releases/stress/2012/full-report.pdf; S. Bethune, "Health-care Falls Short on Stress Management," *Monitor on Psychology* 44, no. 4 (2013): 22.
2. American Psychological Association, "Stress in America," 2013; S. Bethune, "Health-care Falls Short on Stress Management," 2013; American Psychological Association, *Stress in America 2010, Key Findings*, 2010, www.apa.org/news/press/releases/stress/key-findings.pdf.
3. B. Vanaelst et al. "The Association between Childhood Stress and Body Composition, and the Role of Stress-Related Lifestyle Factors—Cross-Sectional Findings from the Baseline ChiBS Survey," *International Journal of Behavioral Medicine*, (2013), DOI: 10.1007/s12529-013-9294-1. (Epub ahead of print.); S. M.Wilson and A. F. Sato, "Stress and Paediatric Obesity: What We Know and Where To Go," *Stress and Health* 30, no. 2 (2014):91–102, DOI: 10.1002/smi.2501.
4. B. L. Seaward, *Managing Stress: Principles and Strategies for Health and Well-Being*, 8th ed. (Sudbury, MA: Jones & Bartlett, 2013), 8; National Institute of Mental Health (NIMH), "Stress Fact Sheet," Accessed January 2014, www.nimh.nih.gov/health/publications/stress/stress_factsheet_ln.pdf.
5. American Psychological Association, "Stress in America," 2013.
6. Ibid.
7. S. Cohen and D. Janicki-Deverts, "Who's Stressed? Distributions of Psychological Stress in the United States in Probability Samples from 1983, 2006, and 2009," *Journal of Applied Social Psychology* 42, no. 6 (2012): 1320–34, DOI: 10.1111/j.1559-1816.2012.00900.x.
8. H. Selye, *Stress without Distress* (New York: Lippincott Williams & Wilkins, 1974), 28–29.
9. W. B. Cannon, *The Wisdom of the Body* (New York: Norton, 1932).
10. M. P. Picard and D. M. Turnbull, "Linking the Metabolic State and Mitochonrial DNA in Chronic Disease, Health and Aging," *Diabetes* 62, no. 3 (2013), Available at http://diabetes.diabetesjournals.org/content/62/3/672.full; S. Cohen et al., "Chronic Stress, Glucocorticoid Receptor Resistance, Inflammation and Disease Risk," *Proceedings of the National Academy of Sciences of the United States of America* 109, no. 16 (2012): 5995–99, DOI: 10.1073/pnas.1118355109.
11. S. Taylor, *The Tending Instinct: Women, Men and the Biology of Our Relationships* (New York: Henry Holt and Company, 2002).

12. A. Crum, P. Salovey, and S. Achor, "Rethinking Stress: The Role of Mindsets in Determining the Stress Response," *Journal of Personality and Social Psychology* 104, no. 4 (2013): 716–33.
13. P. Thoits, "Stress and Health: Major Findings and Policy Implications," *Journal of Health and Social Behavior*, no. 51 (2010): 554–55, DOI: 10.1177/0022146510383499; K. M. Scott et al., "Associations between Lifetime Traumatic Events and Subsequent Chronic Physical Conditions: A Cross-National, Cross-Sectional Study," *PLoS One* 8, no. 11 (2013): DOI: 10.1371/journal.pone.0080573.
14. A. Steptoe and M. Kivimaki, "Stress and Cardiovascular Disease: An Update on Current Knowledge," *Annual Review of Public Health* 34 (2013): 337–54; E. Backe et al., "The Role of Psychosocial Stress at Work for the Development of Cardiovascular Disease: A Systematic Review," *International Archives of Occupational and Environmental Health* 85, no. 1 (2011): 67–79; A. Steptoe, A. Rosengren, and P. Hjemdahl, "Introduction to Cardiovascular Disease, Stress, and Adaptation" in *Stress and Cardiovascular Disease*, eds. A. Steptoe, A. Rosengren, and P. Hjemdahl (New York: Springer, 2012), 1–14.
15. A. Steptoe and Mike Kivimaki."Stress and Cardiovascular Disease," 2013; S. Richardson et al., "Meta-Analysis of Perceived Stress and Its Association with Incident Coronary Heart Disease," *American Journal of Cardiology* 110, no. 12 (2012): 1711–17.
16. T. Lang et al. "Social Determinants of Cardiovascular Diseases," *Public Health Reviews* 33, no. 2 (2012): 601–22; M. Kivimaki et al., "Job Strain as a Risk Factor for Coronary Heart Disease: A Collaborative Meta-Analysis of Individual Participants," *The Lancet* 380, no. 9852 (2012): 1491–97; E. Mostofsky et al., "Risk of Acute Myocardial Infarction After the Death of a Significant Person on One's Life. The Determinants of Myocardial Infarction Onset Study," *Circulation* 125, no. 3 (2012): 491–96, DOI: 10.1161/CIRCULATIONAHA.111.061770.
17. K. Scott, S. Melhorn, and R. Sakai, "Effects of Chronic Social Stress on Obesity," *Current Obesity Reports Online First*, Accessed January 12, 2012, DOI: 10.1007/s13679-011-0006-3; F. Ippoliti, N. Canitano, and R. Businare, "Stress and Obesity as Risk Factors in Cardiovascular Diseases: A Neuroimmune Perspective, *Journal of Neuroimmune Pharmacology* 8, no. 1 (2013): 212–26; S. Pagota et al., "Association of Post-Traumatic Stress Disorder and Obesity in a Nationally Representative Sample," *Obesity* 20, no. 1 (2012): 200–205.
18. N. Ribertim et al., "Corticotropin Releasing Factor-Induced Amygdala Gamma Aminobutyric Acid Release Plays a Key Role in Alcohol Dependence," *Biological Psychiatry* 67, no. 9 (2010): 831–39; E. P. Zorrilla et al., "Behavioral, Biological, and Chemical Perspectives on Targeting CRF(1) Receptor Antagonists to Treat Alcoholism," *Drug and Alcohol Dependence* 128, no. 3 (2013): 175–86.
19. Mayo Clinic, "Stress and Hair Loss: Are They Related?," January 2014, www.mayoclinic.com/health/stress-and-hair-loss/AN01442.
20. American Diabetes Association, "How Stress Affects Diabetes," 2013, www.diabetes.org/living-with-diabetes/complications/mental-health/stress.html; A. Pandy et al., "Alternative Therapies Useful in the Management of Diabetes: A Systematic Review," *Journal of Bioallied Science* 3, no. 4 (2011): 504–12.
21. National Digestive Diseases Information Clearinghouse (NDDIC), "Irritable Bowel Syndrome: How Does Stress Affect IBS?," October 2013, http://digestive.niddk.nih.gov/ddiseases/pubs/ibs/#stress.
22. H. F. Herlong, "Digestive Disorders 2013," *The Johns Hopkins White Papers* (2013) www.johnshopkinshealthalerts.com.
23. G. Marshall, ed., "Stress and Immune-Based Diseases," *Immunology and Allergy Clinics of North America* 31, no. 1 (2011): 1–148; L. Christian, "Psychoneuroimmunology in Pregnancy: Immune Pathways Linking Stress with Maternal Health, Adverse Birth Outcomes and Fetal Development," *Neuroscience and Biobehavioral Reviews* 36, no. 1 (2012): 350–61, DOI: 10.1016/j.neubiorev.2011.07.005; A. Pedersen, R. Zachariae, and D. Bovbjerb, "Influence of Psychological Stress on Upper Respiratory Infection: A Meta-Analysis of Prospective Studies," *Psychosomatic Medicine* 7 (2010): 823–32.
24. American College Health Association (ACHA), *American College Health Association–National College Health Assessment II (ACHA-NCHA II): Reference Group Data Report, Fall 2013* (Hanover, MD: American College Health Association, 2014).
25. M. Marin et al., "Chronic Stress, Cognitive Functioning and Mental Health," *Neurobiology of Learning and Memory* 96, no. 4 (2011): 583–95; R. M. Shansky and J. Lipps, "Stress-Induced Cognitive Dysfunction: Hormone-Neurotransmitter Interactions in the Prefrontal Cortex," *Neuroscience and Biobehavioral Reviews* 7 (2013): 123, Available at www.ncbi.nlm.nih.gov/pmc/articles/PMC3617365.
26. E. Dias-Ferreira et al., "Chronic Stress Causes Frontostriatal Reorganization and Affects Decision-Making," *Science* 325, no. 5940 (2009): 621–25; D. de Quervan et al., "Glucocorticoids and the Regulation of Memory in Health and Disease," *Frontiers in Neuroendocrinology* 30, no. 3 (2009): 358–70.
27. L. Johansson, "Can Stress Increase Alzheimer's Disease Risk in Women?," *Expert Review of Neurotherapeutics* 14, no. 2 (2014): 123–25, DOI: 10.1586/14737175.2014.878651.
28. T. Frodi and V. O'Keane, "How Does the Brain Deal with Cumulative Stress? A Review with Focus on Developmental Stress, HPA Axis Function and Hippocampal Structure in Humans," *Neurobiology of Disease* 52 (2013): 24–37; P. S. Nurius, E. Uehara, and D. F. Zatzick, "Intersection of Stress, Social Disadvantage, and Life Course Processes: Reframing Trauma and Mental Health," *American Journal of Psychiatric Rehabilitation* 16 (2013): 91–114; K. Scott et al., "Association of Childhood Adversities and Early-Onset Mental Disorders with Adult-Onset Chronic Physical Conditions," *Archives of General Psychiatry* 68, no. 8 (2011): 833–44.
29. National Headache Foundation, "Press Kits: Categories of Headache," 2013, www.headaches.org/press/NHF_Press_Kits/Press_Kits_-_Categories_Of_Headache
30. Mayo Clinic, "Tension Headache: Symptoms," July 2013, www.mayoclinic.org/diseases-conditions/tension-headache/basics/symptoms/con-20014295.
31. WebMD, "Migraines and Headache Health Center: Tension Headaches," 2013, www.webmd.com.
32. National Headache Foundation, "Migraine," Accessed 2014, www.headaches.org/education/Headache_Topic_Sheets/Migraine.
33. Ibid.
34. Ibid.
35. Ibid.
36. National Headache Foundation, "Cluster Headaches," 2013, www.headaches.org
37. American College Health Association, *National College Health Assessment II: Reference Group Data Report, Fall 2013*, 2014.
38. J. Gaultney, "The Prevalence of Sleep Disorders in College Students: Impact on Academic Performance," *Journal of American College Health* 59, no. 2 (2010): 91–97; K. Ahrberg et al., "Interaction between Sleep Quality and Academic Performance," *Journal of Psychiatric Research* 46, no. 12 (2012): 1618–22.
39. K. M. Orzech et al., "Sleep Patterns Are Associated with Common Illness in Adolescents," *Journal of Sleep Research* (2013), DOI: 10.1111/jsr.12096. (Epub ahead of print.); J. M. Krueger and J. A. Majde, "Sleep and Host Defense," in *Principles and Practice of Sleep Medicine*, eds. M. H. Kryger, T. Roth, and W. C. Dement (St. Louis, MO: Saunders, 2011), 261–90; M. Manzer and M. Hussein, "Sleep-Immune System Interaction: Advantages and Challenges of Human Sleep Loss Model," *Frontiers of Neurology* 3, no. 2 (2012): DOI: 10.3389/fneur.2012.00002.
40. X. Yu et al., "TH17 Cell Differentiation Is Regulated by Circadian Clock," *Science* 342, no. 6159 (2013): 727–30; T. Bollinger et al., "Sleep, Immunity and Circadian Clocks: A Mechanistic Model," *Gerontology* 56, no. 6 (2010): 574–80, DOI: 10.1159/000281827.
41. R. Lanfranchi, F. Prince, D. Filipini, and J. Carrier, "Sleep Deprivation Increases Blood Pressure in Healthy Normotensive Elderly and Attenuates the Blood Pressure Response to Orthostatic Challenges," *Sleep* 34, no. 3 (2010): 335–39; F. Cappuccio, D. Cooper, and D. Lanfranco, "Sleep Duration Predicts Cardiovascular Outcomes: A Systematic Review and Meta-Analysis of Prospective Studies," *European Heart Journal* 32 (2011): 1484–92, DOI: 10.1093/eurheartj/ehr007.
42. M. A. Miller and F. P. Cappuccio, "Biomarkers of Cardiovascular Risk in Sleep Deprived People," *Journal of Human Hypertension* 27 (2013): 583–8; F. P. Cappuccio et al., "Sleep Duration Predicts Cardiovascular Outcomes,"2011; S. Agarwal, N. Bajaj, and C. Bae, "Association between Sleep Duration and Cardiovascular Disease: Results from the National Health and Nutrition Examination Survey (NHANES 2005–2008), supplement 1, *Journal of the American College of Cardiology* 59, no. 13 (2012), E1514; F. Sofi et al., "Insomnia and Risk of Cardiovascular Disease: A Meta-analysis," *European Journal of Preventive Cardiology* 21, no. 1 (2014): 51–67.
43. National Institutes of Health, "Information about Sleep," 2011, http://science.education.nih.gov/supplements/nih3/sleep/guide/info-sleep.htm; C. Peri and M. Smith, "What Lack of Sleep Does to Your Mind," WebMD, Accessed January 20, 2012, www.webmd.com/sleep-disorders/excessive-sleepiness-10/emotions-cognitive.
44. E. Fortier-Brochu et al., "Insomnia and Daytime Cognitive Performance: A Meta-Analysis," *Sleep Medicine Reviews* 16, no. 1 (2011), DOI: 10-1016/j.smrv.2011.03.008; W. Klemm, "How Sleep Helps Memory," *Psychology Today*, March 11, 2011, www.psychologytoday.com/blog/memory-medic/201103/how-sleep-helps-memory; M. A. Miller et al., "Chapter: Sleep and Cognition," in *Sleep Disorders* (2014), in press.
45. Z. Terpening et al., "The Contributors of Nocturnal Sleep to the Consolidation of Motor Skill Learning in Healthy Aging and Parkinson's Disease," *Journal of Sleep Research* 22, no. 4 (2013): 398–405; L. Genzel et al., "Complex Motor Sequence Skills Profit from Sleep," *Neuropsychobiology* 66, no. 4 (2012): 237–43, DOI: 10.1159/000341878.

46. Centers for Disease Control and Prevention, "Drowsy Driving: Asleep at the Wheel," January 2014, www.cdc.gov/features/dsdrowsydriving.
47. Centers for Disease Control and Prevention, "Insufficient Sleep Is a Public Health Epidemic," January 2014, www.cdc.gov/features/dssleep/; F. Cappuccio et al. "Sleep Duration and All-Cause Mortality: Systematic Review," *Sleep* 33, no. 5 (2010): 585–92.
48. National Sleep Foundation, "Caffeine and Sleep," 2011, Accessed February, 2014, www.sleepfoundation.org/article/sleep-topics/caffeine-and-sleep.
49. R. Lazarus, "The Trivialization of Distress," in *Preventing Health Risk Behaviors and Promoting Coping with Illness*, eds. J. Rosen and L. Solomon (Hanover, NH: University Press of New England, 1985), 279–98.
50. D. Hellhammer, A. Stone, J. Hellhammer, and J. Broderick, "Measuring Stress," *Encyclopedia of Behavioral Neurosciences* 2 (2010): 186–91.
51. L. D. Rosen et al., "Is Facebook Creating "iDisorders"? The Link between Clinical Symptoms of Psychiatric Disorders and Technology Use, Attitudes and Anxiety," *Computers in Human Behavior* 29, no. 3 (2013): 1243–54, Available at http://dx.doi.org/10.1016/j.chb.2012.11.012.
52. NIH Medline Plus, "Avid Cellphone Use by College Kids Tied to Anxiety, Lower Grades," December 2013, www.nlm.nih.gov/;medlineplus/news/fullstory_143389.html; S. Deatherage et al., "Stress, Coping and the Internet Use of College Students," *Journal of American Health* 62, no. 1 (2014): 40–46, DOI: 10.1080/07448481.2013.843536.
53. S. Schwartz et al., "Acculturation and Well-Being among College Students from Immigrant Families," *Journal of Clinical Psychology* (2012), DOI: 10.1002/jclp21847. (Epub ahead of print.); A. Pieterse, R. Carter, S. Evans, and R. Walter, "An Exploratory Examination of the Associations among Racial and Ethnic Discrimination, Racial Climate, and Trauma-Related Symptoms in a College Student Population," *Journal of Counseling Psychology* 57, no. 3 (2010): 255–63; A. McAleavey, L. Castonguay, and B. Locke, "Sexual Orientation Minorities in College Counseling: Prevalence, Distress, and Symptom Profiles," *Journal of College Counseling* 14, no. 2 (2011): 127–42.
54. K. Cokley et al., "An Examination of the Impact of Minority Status Stress and Imposter Feelings on the Mental Health of Diverse Ethnic Minority College Students," *Journal of Multicultural Counseling and Development* 41, no. 2 (2013): 82–95; D. Iwamoto, L. Kenji, and W. Ming, "The Impact of Racial Identity, Ethnic Identity, Asian Values and Race-Related Stress on Asian Americans and Asian International College Students' Psychological Well-Being," *Journal of Counseling Psychology* 57, no. 1 (2010): 79–91.
55. E. Brondolo et al. "Racism and Hypertension: A Review of the Empirical Evidence and Implications for Clinical Practice," *American Journal of Hypertension* 24, no. 5 (2011): 518–24; F. Fuchs, "Editorial: Why Do Black Americans Have Higher Prevalence of Hypertension?," *Hypertension* 57 (2011): 370–80.
56. P. Hoffman, *Examining Factors of Acculturative Stress on International Students as They Affect Utilization of Campus-Based Health and Counseling Services at Four-Year Public Universities in Ohio*, Doctoral Dissertation, Bowling Green State University, Higher Education Administration, 2010; S. Sumer, *International Students' Psychological and Sociocultural Adaptation in the United States*, Doctoral Dissertation, Georgia State University, 2009.
57. K. Karren et al., *Mind/Body Health: The Effects of Attitudes, Emotions, and Relationships*, 4th ed. (San Francisco: Benjamin Cummings, 2010).
58. B. L. Seaward, *Managing Stress*, 2012.
59. K. Brown, *Predictors of Suicide Ideation and the Moderating Effects of Suicide Attitudes*, masters thesis, University of Ohio, 2011, http://etd.ohiolink.edu/view.cgi?acc_num=tolego1301765761; J. Gomez, R. Miranda, and L. Polanco, "Acculturative Stress, Perceived Discrimination and Vulnerability to Suicide Attempts among Emerging Adults," *Journal of Youth and Adolescence* 40, no. 11 (2011): 1465–76.
60. K. Glanz, B. Rimer, and F. Levis, eds., *Health Behavior and Health Education: Theory, Research, and Practice*, 4th ed. (San Francisco: Jossey-Bass, 2008).
61. S. Abraham, "Relationship between Stress and Perceived Self-Efficacy among Nurses in India," *International Conference on Technology and Business Management*, March 2012, www.icmis.net/ictbm/ictbm12/ICTBM12CD/pdf/D2144-done.pdf; B. L. Seaward, *Managing Stress: Principles and Strategies for Health and Well-Being*, 2012.
62. M. Friedman and R. H. Rosenman, *Type A Behavior and Your Heart* (New York: Knopf, 1974).
63. M. Whooley and J. Wong, "Hostility and Cardiovascular Disease," *Journal of the American College of Cardiology* 58, no. 12 (2011): 1228–30; J. Newman et al. "Observed Hostility and the Risk of Incident Ischemic Heart Disease: A Perspective Population Study from the 1995 Canadian Nova Scotia Health Survey," *Journal of the American College of Cardiology* 58, no. 12 (2011): 1222–28.
64. G. Mate, *When the Body Says No: Understanding the Stress-Disease Connection*, (Hoboken, NJ: John Wiley & Sons, 2011).
65. H. Versteeg, V. Spek, and S. Pedersen, "Type D Personality and Health Status in Cardiovascular Disease Populations: A Meta-Analysis of Prospective Studies," *European Journal of Cardiovascular Prevention and Rehabilitation* (2011), DOI: 10.1177/1741826711425338. (Epub ahead of print.); F. Mols and F. J. Denollet, "Type D Personality in the General Population: A Systematic Review of Health Status, Mechanisms of Disease and Work-Related Problems," *Health and Quality of Life Outcomes* 8, no. 9 (2010): 1–10, Available at www.hqlo.com/content/8/1/9
66. S. Kobasa, "Stressful Life Events, Personality, and Health: An Inquiry into Hardiness," *Journal of Personality and Social Psychology* 37 (1979): 1–11.
67. C. D. Schetter and C. Dolbier, "Resilience in the Context of Chronic Stress and Health in Adults," *Social and Personality Psychology Compass* 5 (2011): 634–52, DOI: 10.1111/j.1751-9004.2011.00379.x.
68. C. Ryff et al., "Psychological Resilience in Adulthood and Later Life: Implications for Health," *Annual Review of Gerontology and Geriatrics* 32, no. 1 (2012): 73–92.
69. E. Chen et al., "Protective Factors for Adults from Low-Childhood Socioeconomic Circumstances: The Benefits of Shift-and-Persist for Allostatic Load," *Psychosomatic Medicine* 74, no. 2 (2012): 178–86, DOI:10.1097/PSY. 0B013e31824206fd.
70. B. L. Seaward, *Managing Stress*," 2012.
71. M. E. P. Seligman, *Flourishing: A Visionary New Understanding of Happiness and Well-Being* (New York: Free Press/Simon and Schuster, 2011); M. E. P. Seligman, *Authentic Happiness: Using the New Positive Psychology to Realize Your Potential for Lasting Fulfillment* (New York: Free Press/Simon and Schuster, 2002).
72. L. Poole et al., "Associations of Objectively Measured Physical Activity with Daily Mood Ratings and Psychophysiological Stress Responses in Women," *Psychophysiology* 48 (2011): 1165–72, DOI: 10.1111/j.1469-8986.2011.01184.x; D. A. Girdano, D. E. Dusek, and G. S. Everly, *Controlling Stress and Tension*, 9th ed. (San Francisco: Benjamin Cummings, 2012), 375.
73. G. Colom et al., "Study of the Effect of Positive Humour as a Variable That Reduces Stress. Relationship of Humour with Personality and Performance Variables," *Psychology in Spain* 15, no. 1 (2011): 9–21.
74. B. L. Seaward, *Managing Stress*, 2012.
75. C. Stern et al. "Effects of Implementation Intention on Anxiety, Perceived Proximity and Motor Performance," *Personality and Social Psychology Bulletin* 39, no. 5 (2013): 623–35; M. A. Adriaanse et al., "Breaking Habits with Implementation Intentions: A Test of Underlying Processes," *Personality and Social Psychology Bulletin* 37, no. 4 (2011): 502–13; A. Dalton and S. Spiller, "Too Much of a Good Thing: The Benefits of Implementation Intentions Depend on the Number of Specific Goals," *Journal of Consumer Research* 39, no. 3 (2012): 600–614.
76. American College Health Association (ACHA), *National College Health Assessment II: Reference Group Data Report, Fall 2013*, 2014.
77. *Yoga Journal*, "Yoga in America," Accessed February 2014, www.yogajournal.com/press/yoga_in_america?print=1.
78. NIH Medline Plus, "What Yoga Can and Can't Do for You," December 2013, www.nlm.nih.gov/medlineplus/news/fullstory_143813.html; J. Kiecolt-Glaser et al., "Stress, Inflammation, and Yoga Practice," *Psychosomatic Medicine* 72, no. 2 (2010): 113–21.
79. V. Barnes and D. Orme-Johnson, "Prevention and Treatment of Cardiovascular Disease in Adolescents through the Transcendental Meditation Program," *Current Hypertension Reviews* 8, no. 3 (2012): 1573–1621.

Pulled Statistics

page 46, American College Health Association (ACHA), *American College Health Association–National College Health Assessment II (ACHA-NCHA II): Reference Group Data Report, Fall 2013* (Hanover, MD: American College Health Association, 2014).

page 51, American Psychological Association, "Stress in America: Missing the Health Care Connection," February 2013, Available at: http://www.apa.org/news/press/releases/stress/2012/full-report.pdf.

page 53, National Sleep Foundation, "2011 Sleep in America Poll: Communications Technology and Sleep," March 2011. Available at: http://www.sleepfoundation.org/article/sleep-america-polls/2011-communications-technology-use-and-sleep.

Chapter 4

1. Y. Luo et al., "Loneliness, Health, and Mortality in Old Age: A National Longitudinal Study," *Social Science and Medicine* 74, no. 6 (2012): 907N14; N. I. Eisenberger and S. W. Cole, "Social Neuroscience and Health: Neurophysiological Mechanisms Linking Social Ties with Physical Health," *Nature Neuroscience* 15, no. 5 (2012): 669–74, DOI:10.1038/nn.3086.
2. R. Sternberg, "A Triangular Theory of Love," *Psychological Review* 93 (1986): 119–35.
3. H. Fisher, *Why We Love* (New York: Henry Holt, 2004); H. Fisher, et al., "Defining the Brain System of Lust, Romantic Attraction, and Attachment,"

Archives of Sexual Behavior* 31, no. 5 (2002): 413–19.
4. Ibid.
5. Ibid.
6. S. Levay and J. Baldwin, *Human Sexuality*, 4th ed. (Sunderland, MA: Sinauer Associates, 2012).
7. M. A. Monto and A. Carey, "A New Standard of Sexual Behavior? Are Claims Associated with the 'Hookup Culture' Supported by Nationally Representative Data?," American Sociological Association Conference (August 2013); R. L. Fielder, K. B. Carey, and M. P. Carey, "Are Hookups Replacing Romantic Relationships? A Longitudinal Study of First-Year Female College Students," *Journal of Adolescent Health* 52, no. 5 (2012): 657–59.
8. Ibid.
9. M. Gatzeva and A. Paik, "Emotional and Physical Satisfaction in Noncohabiting, Cohabiting, and Marital Relationships: The Importance of Jealous Conflict," *Journal of Sex Research* 48, no 1 (2011): 29–42, DOI: 10.1080/00224490903370602; B. Sagarin et al., "Sex Differences in Jealousy: A Meta-Analytic Examination," *Evolution & Human Behavior* 33, no. 6 (2012): 595–14.
10. I. Gershon, *The Breakup 2.0: Disconnecting over New Media* (Syracuse, NY: Cornell University Press, 2012).
11. J. A. Hall, "First Comes Social Networking, Then Comes Marriage? Characteristics of Americans Married 2005–2012 Who Met Through Social Networking Sites," *Cyberpsychology, Behavior, and Social Networking* (March 10, 2014). [Epub ahead of print].
12. A. Smith and M. Duggan, "Online Dating & Relationships," *Pew Research Internet Project*, October 21, 2013, www.pewinternet.org/2013/10/21/online-dating-relationships/
13. C. R. Rogers, "Interpersonal Relationship: The Core of Guidance" in *Person to Person: The Problem of Being Human*, eds. C. R. Rogers and B. Stevens (Lafayette, CA: Real People Press, 1967).
14. N. Evans, "Back to Face the Music? Prince Harry Flies Home After Las Vegas Naked Photos Scandal," *Mirror News* Online, August 22, 2012, www.mirror.co.uk; G. Fowler, "When the Most Personal Secrets Get Outed on Facebook," *The Wall Street Journal*, October 13, 2012, http://online.wsj.com
15. N. Messieh, "Survey: 37% of Your Prospective Employers Are Looking You up on Facebook," News: Social Media, *The Next Web* (blog), April 18, 2012, http://thenextweb.com
16. B. Johnson, "Privacy No Longer a Social Norm, Says Facebook Founder," *The Guardian*, January 10, 2010, www.guardian.co.uk
17. C. Burggraf Torppa, Family and Consumer Sciences, Ohio State University Extension, "Gender Issues: Communication Differences in Interpersonal Relationships," 2010, http://ohioline.osu.edu/flm02/pdf/fs04.pdf; J. Wood, *Gendered Lives: Communication, Gender, and Culture*, 10th ed. (Belmont, CA: Cengage, 2013).
18. J. Wood, *Interpersonal Communication: Everyday Encounters*, 7th ed. (Belmont, CA: Cengage, 2012).
19. Ibid.
20. F. Newport and J. Wilke, "Most in U.S. Want Marriage, but Its Importance Has Dropped," Gallup, August 2, 2013, www.gallup.com/poll/163802/marriage-importance-dropped.aspx
21. Ibid.
22. U.S. Census Bureau, "Families and Living Arrangements: 2013, Table MS-2 Estimated Median Age at First Marriage, by Sex: 1890 to the Present," Accessed April 2014, www.census.gov/hhes/families/data/marital.html
23. I. Siegler et al., "Consistency and Timing of Marital Transitions and Survival During Midlife: The Role of Personality and Health Risk Behaviors," *Annals of Behavioral Medicine* 45, no. 3 (2013): 338–47, DOI: 10.1007/s12160-012-9457-3; A. A. Aizer et al., "Marital Status and Survival in Patients with Cancer," *Journal of Clinical Oncology* 31, no. 31 (2013): 3869–76, DOI: 10.1200/JCO.2013.49.6489.
24. U.S. Department of Health and Human Services, Vital and Health Statistics, "Health Behaviors of Adults: United States, 2008–2010," *DHHS Pub* 10, no. 257 (2013): 7–78, www.cdc.gov/nchs/data/series/sr_10/sr10_257.pdf; C. A. Schoenborn, "Marital Status and Health: United States, 1999–2002," *Advance Data from Vital and Health Statistics*, no. 351, DHHS Publication No. 2005-1250 (Hyattsville, MD: National Center for Health Statistics, 2004), Available at www.cdc.gov/nchs/products/ad.htm
25. Ibid.
26. Ibid.
27. U.S. Census Bureau, "Table C2. Household Relationship And Living Arrangements Of Children Under 18 Years, By Age And Sex: 2012," *America's Families and Living Arrangements: 2012*, November 2013, www.census.gov/hhes/families/data/cps2012.html
28. M. Lino, *Expenditures on Children by Families, 2012* (Alexandria, VA: U.S. Department of Agriculture, Center for Nutrition Policy and Promotion, 2013), www.cnpp.usda.gov/Publications/CRC/crc2012.pdf
29. U.S. Department of Health and Human Services, Division of Vital Statistics, " First Premartical Cohabitation in the United States: 2006–2010 National Survey of Family Growth," *National Health Statistics Report* 64 (2013), www.cdc.gov/nchs/data/nhsr/nhsr064.pdf
30. A. Kuperberg, "Age at Co-Residence, Premarital Cohabitation and Marriage Dissolution: 1985–2009," *Journal of Marriage and Family* 76, no. 2 (2014), DOI: 10.1111/jomf.12092.
31. U.S. Census Bureau, "Frequently Asked Questions about Same-Sex Couple Households," 2013, www.census.gov/hhes/samesex/files/SScplfactsheet_final.pdf
32. National Gay and Lesbian Task Force, "Relationship Recognition Map for Same-Sex Couples in the U.S.," January 2014, www.thetaskforce.org/downloads/reports/issue_maps/rel_recog_1_6_14_color.pdf
33. D. Masci et al., "Gay Marriage Around the World," *Pew Research Religion and Public Life Project*, February 5, 2014, www.pewforum.org/2013/12/19/gay-marriage-around-the-world-2013/#allow
34. U.S. Census Bureau, "Marital Status: 2007-2011 American Community Survey, 5-year Estimates, Table S1201," Accessed April 2014, http://factfinder2.census.gov/faces/tableservices/jsf/pages/productview.xhtml?src=bkmk
35. K. Heller, "The Myth of the High Rate of Divorce," *Psych Central*, April 2, 2014, http://psychcentral.com/lib/2012/the-myth-of-the-high-rate-of-divorce
36. Ibid.
37. R. M. Kreider and R. Ellis, "Number, Timing, and Duration of Marriages and Divorces: 2009," *Current Population Reports, P70-125* (Washington, DC: U.S. Census Bureau, 2011), Available at https://www.census.gov/prod/2011pubs/p70-125.pdf
38. Ibid.
39. The Gottman Institute, "Research FAQs," Accessed April, 2014, www.gottman.com/research/research-faqs/
40. Federal Bureau of Investigation, "Hate Crime Statistics, 2011," December 10, 2012, www.fbi.gov/about-us/cjis/ucr/hate-crime/2011
41. I. A. Hughes, C. Hook, S. F. Ahmed, and P. A. Lee, "Consensus Statement on Management of Intersex Disorders," *Archives of Disease in Childhood* 91, no. 7 (2006): 554–563.
42. P. A. Lee et al., "Consensus Statement on Management of Intersex Disorders," *Pediatrics* 118 (2006): e488–e500.
43. F. M. Biro et al., "Onset of Breast Development in a Longitudinal Cohort," *Pediatrics* 132, no. 6 (2013): 1019–7.
44. Mayo Clinic Staff, "Menstrual Cramps," 2011, www.mayoclinic.com/Health/Menstrual-Cramps/Ds00506
45. NHLBI, "WHI Follow-Up Study Confirms Risk of Long-Term Combination Hormone Therapy Outweigh Benefits for Postmenopausal Women," news release, March 4, 2008, public.nhlbi.nih.gov/newsroom/home/GetPressRelease.aspx?id=2554; NHLBI, "WHI Study Data Confirm Short-Term Health Disease Risks of Combination Hormone Therapy for Postmenopausal Women," news release, February 15, 2010, www.nih.gov/news/health/feb2010/nhlbi-15.htm
46. M. Owings and S. Uddin, "Trends in Circumcision for Male Newborns in U.S. Hospitals: 1979–2010," National Center for Health Statistics (2013), www.cdc.gov/nchs/data/hestat/circumcision_2013/circumcision_2013.htm; Mayo Clinic Staff, "Circumcision (Male): Why It's Done," September 2012, www.mayoclinic.com; American Academy of Pediatrics, "2012 Technical Report, Male Circumcision," *Pediatrics* 130, no. 3 (2012): e756–e785, DOI: 10.1542/peds.2012-1990.
47. Mayo Clinic Staff, "Male Menopause: Myth or Reality?," 2011, Available at www.mayoclinic.com/health/male-menopause/MC00058
48. Ibid.
49. G. F. Kelly, *Sexuality Today*, 10th ed. (New York, NY: McGraw-Hill, 2010).
50. Ibid.
51. J. A. Higgins, J. Trussell, N. B. Moore, and J. K. Davidson, "Young Adult Sexual Health: Current and Prior Sexual Behaviours among Non-Hispanic White U.S. College Students," *Sexual Health* 7, no. 1 (2010): 35–43.
52. American College Health Association, *American College Health Association—National College Health Assessment II (ACHA-NCHA II) Reference Group Data Report, Fall 2013* (Hanover, MD: American College Health Association, 2014), Available at www.acha-ncha.org/reports_ACHA-NCHAII.html.
53. Ibid.
54. Ibid.
55. Mayo Clinic Staff, "Antidepressants: Get Tips to Cope with Side Effects," July 2013, http://www.mayoclinic.org/diseases-conditions/depression/in-depth/antidepressants/art-20049305.
56. Mayo Clinic Staff, "Erectile Dysfunction," February 2012, Available at www.mayoclinic.com/health/erectile-dysfunction/DS00162
57. National Kidney and Urological Diseases Information Clearinghouse, "Erectile Dysfunction," 2012, Available at http://kidney.niddk.nih.gov/KUDiseases/pubs/ED/index.aspx
58. S. G. Deem et al., "Premature Ejaculation," (2013), http://emedicine.medscape.com/article/435884-overview
59. Medline Plus, "Sexual Problems Overview: Medline PlusMen's Health: Sexual Problems," Updated May January 2011, http://womenshealth.gov/mens-health/sexual-health-for-men/sexual-problems.html; J. A. Simon, "Problems of Sexual Function in Menopausal Women," *Menopausal Medicine* 20, no. 4 (2012): S1–S6.

60. A. Mullens, R. Young, M. Dunne, and G. Norton, "The Amyl Nitrite Expectancy Questionnaire for Men Who Have Sex with Men (AEQ-MSM): A Measure of Substance-Related Beliefs," *Substance Use & Misuse* 46, no. 13 (2011): 1642–50.

Pulled Statistics

page 74, CareerBuilder, "Thirty-seven percent of companies use social networks to research potential job candidates, according to new CareerBuilder Survey," 2012, http://www.careerbuilder.com/share/aboutus/pressreleasesdetail.aspx?id=pr691&sd=4%2F18%2F2012&ed=4%2F18%2F2099.

page 79, W. Wang and P. Taylor, "For Millennials, Parenthood Trumps Marriage," Pew Research (2011), http://www.pewsocialtrends.org/2011/03/09/for-millennials-parenthood-trumps-marriage/.

page 91, Data from American College Health Association, *American College Health Association—National College Health Assessment II: Undergraduate Students Reference Group Data Report, Fall 2013* (Hanover, MD: American College Health Association; 2014). Available at www.acha-ncha.org/reports_ACHA-NCHAII.html.

Chapter 5

1. American College Health Association, *American College Health Association—National College Health Assessment II (ACHA-NCHA II): Reference Group Data Report, Fall 2013* (Hanover, MD: American College Health Association, 2014), Available at www.acha-ncha.org/reports_ACHA-NCHAII.html.
2. J. Trussell, "Contraceptive Efficacy," in *Contraceptive Technology*, 20th rev ed. R. A. Hatcher et al. (New York, NY: Ardent Media, 2011).
3. Ibid.
4. Ibid.
5. Ibid.
6. Ibid.
7. World Health Organization, Media Centre, "Nonoxynol-9 Ineffective in Preventing HIV Infection," Accessed May 2014, www.who.int/mediacentre/news/notes/release55/en/
8. J. Trussell, "Contraceptive Efficacy," 2011.
9. Ibid.
10. J. Trussell, "Contraceptive Efficacy," 2011.
11. Ibid.
12. Ibid.
13. American College Health Association, *American College Health Association—National College Health Assessment II: Reference Group Data, Fall 2013* (Hanover, MD: American College Health Association, 2014).
14. Drug Information Online, Drugs.com, "Seasonale," October 2013, www.drugs.com/seasonale.html; Drug Information Online Drugs.Com, "Seasonique," October 2013, www.drugs.com/seasonique.html
15. J. Trussell, "Contraceptive Efficacy," 2011.
16. Ibid.
17. O. Lidegaard et al., "Thrombotic Stroke and Myocardial Infarction with Hormonal Contraception," *New England Journal of Medicine* 366, no. 24 (2012): 2257–66, DOI: 10.1056/NEJMoa1111840.
18. J. Trussell, "Contraceptive Efficacy," 2011.
19. Janssen Pharmaceuticals, "OrthoEvra," October 2012, www.orthoevra.com
20. J. Trussell, "Contraceptive Efficacy," 2011.
21. Janssen Pharmaceuticals, "Important Safety Update for U.S. Health Care Professionals ORTHO EVRA," March 2011, www.orthoevra.com/isi-hcp.html
22. J. Trussell, "Contraceptive Efficacy," 2011.
23. Ibid.
24. Pfizer, "Depo-subQ Provera," September 2013, www.depo-subqprovera104.com/
25. J. Trussell, "Contraceptive Efficacy," 2011.
26. Merck & Co., Inc., "Nexplanon," March 2014, www.merck.com/product/usa/pi_circulars/n/nexplanon/nexplanon_pi.pdf
27. Buhlig, K.Z. et al. "Worldwide Use of Intrauterine Contraception: A Review," *Contraception*, 2014. 89(3):162.
28. The American Congress of Obstetricians and Gynecologists, "ACOG Committee Opinion-Adolescents and Long-Acting Reversible Contraception: Implants and Intrauterine Devices, Number 539," October 2012, www.acog.org/Resources_And_Publications/Committee_Opinions/Committee_on_Adolescent_Health_Care/Adolescents_and_Long-Acting_Reversible_Contraception
29. J. Trussell, "Contraceptive Efficacy," 2011.
30. Office of Population Research & Association of Reproductive Health Professionals, The Emergency Contraception Website, "Answers to Frequently Asked Questions about Effectiveness," Updated April 2014, http://ec.princeton.edu/questions/eceffect.html
31. J. Jacobson, "Court Orders FDA to Make Emergency Contraception Available Over-the-Counter for All Ages," *RH Reality Check*, April, 5 2013, http://rhrealitycheck.org/article/2013/04/05/court-orders-fda-to-make-emergency-contraception-available-over-the-counter-for-all-ages/
32. American College Health Association, *American College Health Association—National College Health Assessment II (ACHA-NCHA II): Reference Group Data Report, Fall 2013* (Hanover, MD: American College Health Association, 2014), Available at www.acha-ncha.org/reports_ACHA-NCHAII.html.
33. J. Trussell, "Contraceptive Efficacy," 2011.
34. Ibid.
35. J. Jones, W. Mosher, and K. Daniels, "Current Contraceptive Use in the United States, 2006–2010, and Changes in Patterns of Use since 1995," *National Health Statistics Reports*, no. 60 (Hyattsville, MD: National Center for Health Statistics, 2012).
36. J. Trussell, "Contraceptive Efficacy," 2011.
37. Ibid.
38. Guttmacher Institute, "Fact Sheet: Induced Abortion in the United States," February 2014, www.guttmacher.org/pubs/fb_induced_abortion.html
39. American Psychological Association, Task Force on Mental Health and Abortion, *Report of the Task Force on Mental Health and Abortion* (Washington, DC: American Psychological Association, 2008), www.apa.org/pi/wpo/mental-health-abortion-report.pdf
40. Boston Women's Health Collective, *Our Bodies, Ourselves: A New Edition for a New Era* (New York: Simon & Schuster, 2005).
41. L. Saad, "Abortion," *Gallup Politics* (blog), January 22, 2013, www.gallup.com/poll/160058/majority-americans-support-roe-wade-decision.aspx
42. H. D. Boonstra and E. Nash, "A Surge of State Abortion Restrictions Puts Providers and the Women They Serve in the Crosshairs," *Guttmacher Policy Review* 17, no. 1 (2014), www.guttmacher.org/pubs/gpr/17/1/gpr170109.pdf
43. S. Singh and J. E. Darroch, "Adding It Up: Costs and Benefits of Contraceptive Services—Estimates for 2012" (New York, NY: Guttmacher Institute and United Nations Population Fund, 2012); Guttmacher Institute, "In Brief: Facts on Induced Abortion Worldwide," January 2012, www.guttmacher.org/pubs/fb_IAW.html
44. S. Singh and J. E. Darroch, "Adding It Up," 2012; Guttmacher Institute, "In Brief: Facts on Induced Abortion Worldwide," 2012.
45. APA, *Report of the Task Force*, 2008; J. R. Steinberg, C. E. McCulloch, and N. E. Adler, "Abortion and Mental Health: Findings From the National Comorbidity Survey-Replication," *Obstetrics & Gynecology* 123, no. 2 (2014): 263–70.
46. Ibid.
47. Ibid.
48. Guttmacher Institute, "Fact Sheet: Induced Abortion in the United States," 2014.
49. Ibid.
50. Ibid.
51. Planned Parenthood, "The Abortion Pill (Medication Abortion)," Accessed May 2014, www.plannedparenthood.org/health-topics/abortion/abortion-pill-medication-abortion-4354.asp
52. K. Cleland et al., "Significant Adverse Events and Outcomes After Medical Abortion," *Obstetrics and Gynecology* 121, no. 1 (2013): 166–71.
53. Ibid.
54. Centers for Disease Control and Prevention, "Preconception Care and Health Care: Women," July 2013, www.cdc.gov/preconception/women.html
55. Centers for Disease Control and Prevention, "Preconception Care and Health Care: Women," July 2014, www.cdc.gov/preconception/women.html
56. J. A. Martin et al., U.S. Department of Health and Human Services, National Center for Health Statistics, "Births: Final Data for 2012," *National Vital Statistics Reports* 62, no. 9 (2013), Available at www.cdc.gov/nchs/data/nvsr/nvsr62/nvsr62_09.pdf#table01
57. American Pregnancy Association, "Miscarriage," Updated November 2011, http://americanpregnancy.org/pregnancycomplications/miscarriage.html.
58. S. M. Schrader and K. L. Marlow, "Assessing the Reproductive Health of Men with Occupational Exposures," *Asian Journal of Andrology* 16, no. 1 (2014): 23–30.
59. Truven Health Analytics, "The Cost of Having a Baby in the United States," January 2013, http://transform.childbirthconnection.org/wp-content/uploads/2013/01/Cost-of-Having-a-Baby1.pdf
60. M. Lino, *Expenditures on Children by Families, 2012* (Alexandria, VA: U.S. Department of Agriculture, Center for Nutrition Policy and Promotion, 2013), www.cnpp.usda.gov/ExpendituresonChildrenbyFamilies.htm
61. National Association of Child Care Resource and Referral Agencies, "Parents and the High Cost of Child Care, 2013 Report," August 2013, www.naccrra.org/sites/default/files/child_care_aware_of_america_annual_report_0.pdf
62. Planned Parenthood, "Pregnancy Tests," Accessed May 2014, www.plannedparenthood.org/health-topics/pregnancy/pregnancy-test-21227.asp
63. Committee on Obstetric Practice, "Committee Opinion no. 548, American Congress of Obstetricians and Gynecologists: Weight Gain During Pregnancy," *Obstetrics and Gynecology* 121, no. 1 (2013): 210–12, DOI: 10.1097/01.AOG.0000425668.87506.4c
64. The American Congress of Obstetricians and Gynecologists, "Tobacco, Alcohol, Drugs, and Pregnancy," December 2013, www.acog.org/~/media/For%20Patients/faq170.pdf?dmc=1&ts=20140516T2242271513

65. National Center for Chronic Disease Prevention and Health Promotion, "Tobacco Use and Pregnancy," *Reproductive Health*, Updated January 2014; The American Congress of Obstetricians and Gynecologists, "Tobacco, Alcohol, Drugs, and Pregnancy," December 2013, www.acog.org/~/media/For%20Patients/faq170.pdf?dmc=1&ts=20140516T2242271513
66. J. A. Martin et al., U.S. Department of Health and Human Services, National Center for Health Statistics, "Births: Final Data for 2012," *National Vital Statistics Reports* 62, no. 9 (2013), Available at www.cdc.gov/nchs/data/nvsr/nvsr62/nvsr62_09.pdf#table01
67. V. P. Sepilian et al., "Ectopic Pregnancy," *Medscape Reference*, Updated May 2014, http://emedicine.medscape.com/article/2041923-overview
68. E. Puscheck, "Early Pregnancy Loss," *Medscape Reference: Drugs, Diseases & Procedures*, Updated October 2014, http://reference.medscape.com/article/266317-overview
69. What To Expect, "Stillbirth," Accessed May 2014, www.whattoexpect.com/pregnancy/pregnancy-health/complications/stillbirth.aspx
70. K. L. Wisner et al., "Onset Timing, Thoughts of Self-Harm, and Diagnoses in Postpartum Women with Screen-Positive Depression Findings," *JAMA Psychiatry* 70, no. 5 (2013): 1–9, DOI:10.1001/jamapsychiatry.2013.87.
71. American Academy of Pediatrics, "Benefits of Breastfeeding for Mom," Updated May 2013, www.healthychildren.org/English/ages-stages/baby/breastfeeding/pages/Benefits-of-Breastfeeding-for-Mom.aspx
72. Centers for Disease Control and Prevention, "Sudden Unexpected Infant Death and Sudden Infant Death Syndrome," May 2014, www.cdc.gov/sids/
73. Ibid.
74. MayoClinic.com, "Infertility: Causes," July 2013, www.mayoclinic.com/health/infertility/DS00310/DSECTION=causes
75. U.S. Department of Health and Human Services, "Polycystic Ovary Syndrome (PCOS) Fact Sheet," July 2012, www.womenshealth.gov/publications/our-publications/fact-sheet/polycystic-ovary-syndrome.html
76. Centers for Disease Control and Prevention (CDC), "Pelvic Inflammatory Disease CDC Fact Sheet," *Sexually Transmitted Diseases*, Updated March 2014, www.cdc.gov/std/PID/STDFact-PID.htm
77. Centers for Disease Control and Prevention (CDC), "Assisted Reproductive Technology, (ART)," Updated June 2013, www.cdc.gov/reproductivehealth/infertility/
78. Ibid.
79. Ibid.
80. WebMD Medical Reference, "Fertility Drugs," July 2012, www.webmd.com/infertility-and-reproduction/guide/fertility-drugs
81. American Society for Reproductive Medicine, "Fertility Drugs and the Risk for Multiple Births," Accessed May 2014, Available at www.asrm.org/uploadedFiles/ASRM_Content/Resources/Patient_Resources/Fact_Sheets_and_Info_Booklets/fertilitydrugs_multiplebirths.pdf
82. R. M. Kreider and D. A. Loftquist, "Adopted Children and Stepchildren: 2010," U.S. Census Bureau, April 2014, www.census.gov/content/dam/Census/library/publications/2014/demo/p20-572.pdf

Pulled Statistic

page 105, W. D. Mosher and J. Jones, "Use of Contraception in the United States: 1982–2008," *Vital and Health Statistics* 23, no. 29 (Hyattsville, MD: National Center for Health Statistics, 2010), www.cdc.gov.

Chapter 6

1. Substance Abuse and Mental Health Services Administration, *Results from the 2011 National Survey on Drug Use and Health: Summary of National Findings*, NSDUH Series H-44, HHS Publication No. (SMA) 12-4713 (Rockville, MD: Substance Abuse and Mental Health Services Administration, 2012).
2. J. Swendsen et al., "Use and Abuse of Alcohol and Illicit Drugs in the US Adolescents: Results of the National Comorbidity Survey–Adolescent Supplement," *Archives of General Psychiatry* 69, no. 4 (2012): 390–98.
3. L. D. Johnston et al., *Monitoring the Future National Results on Drug Use: 2012 Overview, Key Findings on Adolescent Drug Use* (Ann Arbor, MI: Institute for Social Research, The University of Michigan, 2013).
4. S. S. Alavi et al., "Behavioral Addiction versus Substance Addiction: Correspondence of Psychiatric and Psychological Views," *International Journal of Preventive Medicine* 3 no. 4 (2012): 290–94.
5. J. Grant et al., "Introduction to Behavioral Addictions," *American Journal of Behavioral Addictions* 36, no. 5 (2010): 233–41.
6. American Society of Addiction Medicine, "Definition of Addiction," April 2011, www.asam.org/for-the-public/definition-of-addiction
7. H. J. Edenberg, "Genes Contributing to the Development of Alcoholism," *Alcohol Research: Current Reviews* 34, no. 3 (2012): 336–38.
8. T. Foroud et al., "Genetic Research: Who Is at Risk for Alcoholism?" *Alcohol Research & Health* 33, no. 1 and 2 (2010): 64–75; A. Agrawal et al., "Linkage Scan for Quantitative Traits Identifies New Regions of Interest," *Drug Alcohol Depend* 93, no. 1 and 2 (2008): 12–20; American Society of Addiction Medicine, "Definition of Addiction," 2011.
9. J. Kinney, *Loosening the Grip: A Handbook of Alcohol Information*, 10th ed. (Boston, MA: McGraw-Hill, 2012), 175.
10. G. Hanson and P. Venturelli, *Drugs and Society*, 11th ed. (Sudbury, MA: Jones and Bartlett, 2011), 49.
11. Ibid., 4.
12. J. Grant et al., "Introduction to Behavioral Addictions," 2010; National Institute on Drug Abuse, National Institutes of Health, U.S. Department of Health and Human Services, *Drugs, Brains, and Behavior: The Science of Addiction*, NIH Publication no. 07-5605 (Bethesda, MD: National Institute on Drug Abuse, Revised 2010), Available at www.nida.nih.gov/scienceofaddiction
13. National Council on Problem Gambling, "FAQs—Problem Gamblers," Accessed May 2014, www.ncpgambling.org/i4a/pages/index.cfm?pageid=3390
14. American Psychiatric Association, *Diagnostic and Statistical Manual of Mental Disorders*, 5th ed. (Arlington, VA: American Psychiatric Publishing, 2013), 585.
15. C. Holden, "Behavioral Addictions Debut in Proposed DSM-5," *Science* 347, no. 5968 (2010): 935.
16. H. Hatfield, "Shopping Spree or Addiction?" *WebMD*, 2014, www.webmd.com/mental-health/features/shopping-spree-addiction; M. Lejoyeux and A. Weinstein, "Compulsive Buying," *The American Journal of Drug and Alcohol Issues* 36, no. 5 (2010): 248–53.
17. Ibid.
18. A. Alexander, "Internet Addiction Statistics 2012," April 24, 2012, http://ansonalex.com/infographics/internet-addiction-statistics-2012-infographic
19. American College Health Association, *American College Health Association—National College Health Assessment II: Reference Group Data Report, Fall 2013* (Hanover, MD: American College Health Association, 2014).
20. S. Sussman, "Workaholism: A Review," *Journal of Addiction Research and Therapy* 10, no. 6 (2012): 4120, www.ncbi.nlm.nih.gov/pmc/articles/PMC3835604
21. M. Clark et al., "All Work and No Play? A Meta-Analytic Examination of the Correlates and Outcomes of Workaholism," *Journal of Management*, February 28, 2014: 1–38.
22. Ibid.
23. K. Berczik et al., "Exercise Addiction: Symptoms, Diagnosis, Epidemiology and Etiology," *Substance Use and Misuse* 47 (2012): 403–17.
24. R. Weiss, "Hypersexuality: Symptoms of Sexual Addiction," *Psych Central*, March 2014, http://psychcentral.com/lib/hypersexuality-symptoms-of-sexual-addiction/
25. Substance Abuse and Mental Health Services Administration, Center for Behavioral Health Statistics and Quality, "Treatment Episode Data Set (TEDS): 2000–2010; National Admissions to Substance Abuse Treatment Services," 2012, DASIS Series S-61, HHS Publication No. (SMA) 12-4701 (Rockville, MD: Substance Abuse and Mental Health Services Administration), Available at www.samhsa.gov/data/2k12/TEDS2010N/TEDS2010NWeb.pdf
26. Centers for Disease Control and Prevention, National Center for Health Statistics, Office of Analysis and Epidemiology, "Table 99: Prescription Drug Use in the Past 30 Days, by Sex, Age, Race and Hispanic Origin: United States Selected Years 1988–1994 through 2007–2010," Health, United States, 2011, www.cdc.gov
27. Consumer Health Care Products Association, "The Value of OTC Medicine to the United States," January 2012, Available at www.chpa.org/ValueofOTCMeds2012.aspx
28. Ibid.
29. L. D. Johnston et al., *Monitoring the Future National Results on Drug Use: 2012 Overview, Key Findings on Adolescent Drug Use* (Ann Arbor, MI: Institute for Social Research, The University of Michigan, 2013).
30. Erowid Vault, " DXM," 2012, www.erowid.org/chemicals/dxm/dxm.shtml
31. U.S. Food and Drug Administration,"GAO Report Assesses State Approaches to Control Pseudoephedrine," *The Law* (blog), February 26, 2013, www.fdalawblog.net/fda_law_blog_hyman_phelps/2013/02/gao-report-assesses-state-approaches-to-control-pseudoephedrine.html
32. Substance Abuse and Mental Health Services Administration, *Results from the 2012 National Survey*, October 2013, Available at www.samhsa.gov/data/NSDUH/2012SummNatFindDetTables/Index.aspx
33. Ibid.
34. Ibid.
35. L. D. Johnston et al., *Monitoring the Future National Results on Drug Use: 2012 Overview, Key Findings on Adolescent Drug Use* (Ann Arbor, MI: Institute for Social Research, The University of Michigan, 2013).
36. Centers for Disease Control and Prevention, "Prescription Pain Killer Overdoses at Epidemic Levels," November 2011, www.cdc.gov/media/releases/2011/p1101_flu_pain_killer_overdose.html
37. American College Health Association, *American College Health Association–National College Health Assessment, Fall 2013* (Baltimore, MD: American College Health Association, 2014), Available at www.acha-ncha.org/reports_ACHA-NCHAII.html.
38. Ibid.
39. Ibid.

40. Ibid.
41. L. M. Garnier-Dykstra et al., "Nonmedical Use of Prescription Stimulants During College: Four-Year Trends in Exposure Opportunity, Use, Motives, and Sources," *Journal of American College Health* 60, no. 3 (2012): 226–34.
42. Substance Abuse and Mental Health Services Administration, "Results from the 2012 National Survey," 2013.
43. Ibid.
44. L. D. Johnston et al., *Monitoring the Future National Survey Results on Drug Use, 1975–2008, Volume II, College Students and Adults Ages 19–50*, NIH Publication no. 09-7403 (Bethesda, MD: National Institute on Drug Abuse, 2009), Available at http://monitoringthefuture.org/pubs.html
45. L. D. Johnston et al., *Monitoring the Future National Survey Results on Drug Use, 1975–2012*, 2013.
46. A. Arria et al., "Drug Use Patterns and Continuous Enrollment in College: Results from a Longitudinal Study," *Journal of Studies on Alcohol and Drugs* 74, no. 1 (2013): 71–83.
47. Substance Abuse and Mental Health Services Administration, "Results from the 2012 National Survey," 2013.
48. National Center on Addiction and Substance Abuse at Columbia University, *Wasting the Best and the Brightest: Substance Abuse at America's Colleges and Universities* (New York, NY: National Center on Addiction and Substance Abuse at Columbia University, 2007), Available at www .casacolumbia.org/addiction-research/reports/ wasting-best-brightest-substance-abuse-americas-colleges-universitys
49. Substance Abuse and Mental Health Services Administration, "Results from the 2012 National Survey," 2013.
50. L. D. Johnston et al., *Monitoring the Future National Results on Drug Use: 2012 Overview, Key Findings on Adolescent Drug Use* (Ann Arbor, MI: Institute for Social Research, The University of Michigan, 2013).
51. CPDD Community Website, "Methamphetamine Abuse and Parkinson's Disease," July 2011, www .cpddblog.com/2011/07/methamphetamine-abuse-and-parkinsons.html
52. Food Manufacturing, "Consumer Trends: 83 Percent of Americans Drink Coffee," April 2013, www .foodmanufacturing.com/news/2013/04/consumer-trends-83-percent-americans-drink-coffee
53. Harvard Health Letter, "What Is It About Coffee?" January 2012, www.health.harvard.edu/press_ releases/what-is-it-about-coffee
54. Substance Abuse and Mental Health Services Administration, *Results from the 2012 National Survey on Drug Use and Health: Detailed Tables*, NSDUH Series H-44, HHS Publication No. (SMA) 12-4713 (Rockville, MD: Substance Abuse and Mental Health Services Administration, 2013).
55. Ibid.
56. National Institute on Drug Abuse, " Drug Facts: Marijuana," January 2014, www.drugabuse.gov/ publications/drugfacts/marijuana
57. National Institute on Drug Abuse, *Research Report: Marijuana Abuse*, NIH Publication no. 05-3859, 2005, Available at www.drugabuse.gov/ ResearchReports/Marijuana; National Institute on Drug Abuse, "NIDA InfoFacts: Drugged Driving," 2009, Available at www.nida.nih.gov/infofacts/ driving.html
58. M. Asbridge et al., "Acute Cannabis Consumption and Motor Vehicle Collision Risk: Systematic Review of Observational Studies and Meta-analysis," *British Medical Journal* 344 (2012): 1–9.
59. National Institute on Drug Abuse, "Drug Facts: Marijuana," January 2014, www.drugabuse.gov/ publications/drugfacts/marijuana
60. Ibid.
61. S. Lev-Ran et al., "The Association between Cannabis Use and Depression: A Systematic Review and Meta-Analysis of Longitudinal Studies," *Psychological Medicine* 24 (2013); L. R. Pacek et al., "The Bidirectional Relationships between Alcohol, Cannabis, Co-occurring Alcohol and Cannabis Use Disorders with Major Depressive Disorder: Results from a National Sample," *Journal of Affect Disorders* 148, no. 2 (2013): 188–95, DOI: 10.1016/j.jad.2012.11.059.
62. L. R. Pacek et al., "The Bidirectional Relationships between Alcohol, Cannabis, Co-occurring Alcohol and Cannabis Use Disorders with Major Depressive Disorder: Results from a National Sample," *Journal of Affect Disorders* 148, no. 2 (2013): 188–95, DOI: 10.1016/j.jad.2012.11.059.
63. L. Degenhardt et al., "The Persistence of the Association between Adolescent Cannabis Use and Common Mental Disorders into Young Adulthood," *Addiction* 108, no. 1 (2013): 124–33.
64. J. Copeland, "Changes in Cannabis Use among Young People: Impact on Mental Health," *Current Opinion in Psychiatry* 26, no. 4 (2013): 325–29.
65. National Institute on Drug Abuse, "Marijuana: Facts for Teens," October 2013, www.drugabuse.gov/ publications/marijuana-facts-teens; Science Daily, "Marijuana Use Prior to Pregnancy Doubles Risk of Premature Birth," July 17, 2012, www.sciencedaily .com/eleases/2012/07/120717182953.htm
66. National Institute on Drug Abuse "Drug Facts: Is Marijuana Medicine," April 2014, www.drugabuse. gov/publications/drugfacts/marijuana-medicine
67. DrugRehab.us, "Pros and Cons of Legalizing Recreational Marijuana," April 2014, www.drugrehab. us/news/pros-cons-legalizing-recreational-marijuana/
68. Ibid.
69. National Institutes of Health, National Institute on Drug Abuse, "Drug Facts: Spice," December 2012, www.drugabuse.gov/publications/drugfacts/ spice-synthetic-marijuana
70. Ibid.; L. D. Johnston et al., *Monitoring the Future National Survey Results on Drug Use, 1975–2012: Volume I, Secondary School Students* (Ann Arbor, MI: Institute for Social Research, The University of Michigan, 2013).
71. National Institutes of Health, National Institute on Drug Abuse, "Drug Facts: Spice," 2012.
72. The Partnership at Drugfree.org, "GHB," Accessed May 2014, www.drugfree.org/drug-guide/ghb
73. L. D. Johnston et al., *Monitoring the Future: National Survey Results on Drug Use, 1975–2012*, 2013.
74. Substance Abuse and Mental Health Services Administration, "Results from the 2012 National Survey," October 2013, Available at www.samhsa. gov/data/NSDUH/2012SummNatFindDetTables/ Index.aspx
75. Ibid.
76. L. D. Johnston et al., *Monitoring the Future National Survey Results on Drug Use, 1975–2012*, 2013.
77. National Institute on Drug Abuse, "NIDA InfoFacts: MDMA (Ecstasy)," September 2013, www .drugabuse.gov/infofacts/ecstasy.html
78. The Partnership at DrugFree.org, "Experts: People Who Think They Are Taking 'Molly' Don't Know What They Are Getting," June 24, 2013, www .drugfree.org/join-together/drugs/experts-people-who-think-they-are-taking-molly-dont-know-what-theyre-getting
79. The National Collegiate Athletic Association, "Substance Use: National Study of Substance Use Trends among NCAA College Student-Athletes," 2012, Available at www.ncaapublications.com/ productdownloads/SAHS09.pdf
80. H. G. Pope et al., "The Lifetime Prevalence of Anabolic-Androgenic Steroid Use and Dependence in Americans: Current Best Estimates," *American Journal on Addictions* 23, no. 4 (2013), 371–77, DOI: 10.1111/j.1521-0391.2013.12118.x
81. Ibid.
82. Substance Abuse and Mental Health Services Administration, "Results from the 2012 National Survey," October 2013, Available at www.samhsa. gov/data/NSDUH/2012SummNatFindDetTables/ Index.aspx
83. Office of National Drug Control Policy, "How Illicit Drug Use Affects Business and the Economy," Executive Office of the President, www.white-house.gov/ondcp/ondcp-fact-sheets/how-illicit-drug-use-affects-business-and-the-economy

Pulled Statistics

page 127, Center for Personal Finance Editors, "Tough Times Serics: It Was Such a Bargain: Help for Compulsive Shoppers," 2014, http://hffo.cuna. org/12433/article/353/html

page 137, Substance Abuse and Mental Health Services Administration, *Results from the 2012 National Survey on Drug Use and Health: Summary of National Findings*, NSDUH Series H-44, HHS Publication No. (SMA) 12-4713 (Rockville, MD: Substance Abuse and Mental Health Services Administration, 2013).

Chapter 7

1. National Center for Health Statistics, "Summary Health Statistics for U.S. Adults: National Health Interview Survey, 2012," *Vital and Health Statistics* 10, no. 260 (2014): 34.
2. M. Davalos et al., "Easing the Pain of an Economic Downturn: Macroeconomic Conditions and Excessive Alcohol Consumption," *Health Economics* 21 no. 11 (2012): 1318–35.
3. National Institute on Alcohol Abuse and Alcoholism, "Apparent per Capita Alcohol Consumption: National, State and Regional Trends, 1977–2010," August 2012, http://pubs.niaaa.nih.gov/publications/Surveillance95/CONS10.htm
4. U.S. Department of Health and Human Services, *The Health Consequences of Smoking—50 Years of Progress: A Report of the Surgeon General* (Atlanta: U.S. Department of Health and Human Services, Centers for Disease Control and Prevention, National Center for Chronic Disease Prevention and Health Promotion, Office on Smoking and Health, 2014), Available at www.surgeongeneral. gov/library/reports/50-years-of-progress/exec-summary.pdf
5. Ibid.; Campaign for Tobacco Free Kids, "The Toll of Tobacco Use in the USA," July 2013, www.tobaccofreekids.org/research/factsheets/pdf/0072.pdf
6. American College Health Association, *American College Health Association—National College Health Assessment II: Reference Group Executive Summary, Fall 2013* (Hanover, MD: American College Health Association, 2014), Available at www.acha-ncha.org/reports_ACHA-NCHAII.html.
7. Substance Abuse and Mental Health Services Administration, *Results from the 2011 National Survey on Drug Use and Health: Volume I. Summary of National Findings*, NSDUH Series H-44, DHHS Publication no. (SMA) 12-4713. Findings (Rockville,

MD: Office of Applied Studies, U.S. Department of Health and Human Services, 2012).

8. U.S. Department of Health and Human Services, National Institute on Alcohol Abuse and Alcoholism, "Moderate and Binge Drinking," 2012, www.niaaa.nih.gov/alcohol-health/overview-alcohol-consumption/moderate-binge-drinking
9. American College Health Association, *National College Health Assessment II: Reference Group Data Report, Fall 2013*, 2014.
10. Ibid.
11. R. Hingson et al., "Magnitude of Alcohol-Related Mortality and Morbidity among U.S. College Students Ages 18–24: Changes from 1998 to 2005," *Journal of Studies on Alcohol and Drugs* 16 (2009): 12–20.
12. C. C. Abar, "Examining the Relationship between Parenting Types and Patterns of Student Alcohol-Related Behavior during Transition to College," *Psychology of Addictive Behaviors* 26, no. 1 (2012): 20; L. Varvil-Weld, "Parents' and Students' Reports of Parenting: Which Are More Reliably Associated with College Student Drinking?," *Addictive Behaviors* 38, no. 3 (2013): 1699–1703.
13. L. D. Johnston, *Monitoring the Future: National Survey Results on Drug Use, 1975–2012: Volume II, College Students and Adults Ages 19–50* (Ann Arbor, MI: Institute for Social Research, The University of Michigan, 2013), Available at www.monitoringthefuture.org/pubs/monographs/mtf-vol2_2012.pdf
14. C. Foster et al., "National College Health Assessment Measuring Negative Alcohol-Related Consequences among College Students," *American Journal of Public Health Research* 2, no. 1 (2014): 1–5.
15. J. W. LaBrie et al., "Are They All the Same? An Exploratory, Categorical Analysis of Drinking Game Types," *Addictive Behaviors* 38, no. 5 (2013): 2133–39; N. P. Barnett et al., "Predictors and Consequences of Pregaming Using Day and Week-Level Measures," *Psychology of Addictive Behaviors* 27, no. 4 (2013): 921.
16. C. Neighbors et al., "Event Specific Drinking among College Students," *Psychology of Addictive Behaviors* 25, no. 4 (2011), 702–707, DOI: 10.1037/a0024051.
17. M. A. Lewis et al., "Use of Protective Behavioral Strategies and Their Association to 21st Birthday Alcohol Consumption and Related Negative Consequences: A between and within Person Evaluation," *Psychology of Addictive Behaviors* 26, no. 2 (2012), 179–86, DOI: 10.1037/a0023797.
18. J. Alfonso et al., "Do Drinking Games Matter? An Examination by Game Type and Gender in a Mandated Student Sample," *The American Journal of Drug and Alcohol Abuse* 39, no. 5 (2013): 312–19.
19. A. Barry et al., "Drunkorexia: Understanding the Co-occurrence of Alcohol Consumption and Eating/Exercise Weight Management Behaviors," *Journal of American College Health Association* 60, no. 3 (2012): 236–43.
20. R. Hingson et al., "Magnitude of Alcohol-Related Mortality and Morbidity among U.S. College Students Ages 18–24," 2009.
21. Ibid.
22. American College Health Association, *National College Health Assessment II: Reference Group Data Report, Fall 2013*, 2014.
23. D. L. Thombs et al., "Event-Level Analyses of Energy Drink Consumption and Alcohol Intoxication in Bar Patrons," *Addictive Behaviors* 35, no. 4 (2010): 325–30; A. Peacock et al., "Patterns of Use and Motivations for Consuming Alcohol Mixed with Energy Drinks," *Psychology of Addictive Behaviors* 27, no. 1 (2013): 202–6; J. Howland et al., "Risks of Energy Drinks with Alcohol," *JAMA* 309, no. 3 (2013): 245–46; A. M. Arria et al., "Energy Drink Consumption and Increased Risk for Alcohol Dependence," *Alcoholism: Clinical and Experimental Research* 35, no. 2 (2011): 365–75; W. I. William et al., "Energy Drinks: Psychological Effects and Impact on Well-Being and Quality of Life: A Literature Review," *Innovations in Clinical Neuroscience* 9, no. 1 (2012): 25–34.
24. D. J. Rohsenow et al., "Hangover Sensitivity after Controlled Alcohol Administration as Predictor of Post-College Drinking," *Journal of Abnormal Psychology* 121, no. 1 (2012): 270–75.
25. M. A. White et al., "Hospitalizations for Alcohol and Drug Overdoses in Young Adults Ages 18–24 in the United States, 1999–2008: Results from the Nationwide Inpatient Sample," *Journal of Studies on Alcohol and Drugs* 72, no. 5 (2011): 774–876.
26. National Institute on Alcohol Abuse and Alcoholism, "Drinking Can Put a Chill on Your Summer Fun," May 2012, http://pubs.niaaa.nih.gov/publications/SummerSafety/SummerSafety.htm; Centers for Disease Control and Prevention, " Unintentional Drowning: Get the Facts," November 2012, www.cdc.gov/HomeandRecreationalSafety/Water-Safety/waterinjuries-factsheet.html
27. Centers for Disease Control and Prevention, "Injury Prevention and Control: Home and Recreational Safety: Fire Deaths and Injuries: Fact Sheet," October 2011, www.cdc.gov/HomeandRecreationalSafety/Fire-Prevention/fires-factsheet.html
28. U.S. Department of Health and Human Services (HHS) Office of the Surgeon General and National Action Alliance for Suicide Prevention, "2012 National Strategy for Suicide Prevention: Goals and Objectives for Action," September 2012, www.surgeongeneral.gov/library/reports/national-strategy-suicide-prevention/full-report.pdf
29. Bureau of Justice Statistics, "Criminal Victimization in the United States, 2008 Table 32, Percent Distribution of Victimizations by Perceived Drug or Alcohol Use by Offender, 2008," May 2011, www.bjs.gov/content/pub/pdf/cvus0802.pdf
30. S. Lawyer et al., "Forcible, Drug-Facilitated, and Incapacitated Rape and Sexual Assault among Undergraduate Women," *Journal of American College Health* 58, no. 5 (2010): 453–60.
31. S. J. Nielsen et al., "Calories Consumed from Alcoholic Beverages by U.S. Adults, 2007–2010," *NCHS Data Brief*, no. 110 (2012), Available at www.cdc.gov
32. M. Silveri, "Adolescent Brain Development and Underage Drinking in the United States: Identifying Risks of Alcohol Use in College Populations," *Harvard Review of Psychiatry* 20, no. 4 (2012): 189–200.
33. Ibid.
34. L. Arriola et al., "Alcohol Intake and the Risk of Coronary Heart Disease in Spanish EPIC Cohort Study," *Heart* 96, no. 10 (2010): 124–30; T. Wilson et al., eds., "Should Moderate Alcohol Consumption Be Promoted?," *Nutrition and Health: Nutrition Guide for Physicians* (New York, NY: Humana Press, 2010); The American Heart Association, "Alcohol and Cardiovascular Disease," 2011, www.heart.org/HEARTORG/Conditions/Alcohol-and-Cardiovascular-Disease_UCM_305173_Article.jsp
35. H. K. Seitz and P. Becker, "Alcohol Metabolism and Cancer Risk," *Alcohol Research and Health* 30, no. 1 (2007): 38–47, Available at http://pubs.niaaa.nih.gov/publications/arh301/38-47.htm.
36. W. Y. Chen et al., "Moderate Alcohol Consumption during Adult Life, Drinking Patterns, and Breast Cancer Risk," *Journal of the American Medical Association* 306, no. 17 (2011): 1884–90.
37. C. S. Berkey et al., "Prospective Study of Adolescent Alcohol Consumption and Risk of Benign Breast Disease in Young Women," *Pediatrics* 125, no. 5 (2010): e1081–87.
38. Centers for Disease Control and Prevention, "Alcohol Use and Binge Drinking among Women of Childbearing Age–United States, 2006–2010," *Morbidity and Mortality Weekly* 61, no. 28 (2012): 534–38, Available at www.cdc.gov/mmwr/preview/mmwrhtml/mm6128a4.htm; Y. Liu et al., "Alcohol Intake between Menarche and First Pregnancy: Prospective Study of Breast Cancer Risk," *Journal of the National Cancer Institute* 105, no. 20 (2013): 1571–78, Available at http://jnci.oxfordjournals.org/content/early/2013/08/24/jnci.djt213.full
39. Centers for Disease Control and Prevention, "Fetal Alcohol Spectrum Disorders (FASDs) Data and Statistics," Updated August 2012, www.cdc.gov/ncbddd/fasd/data.html
40. Fetal Alcohol Spectrum Disorders (FASD) Center for Excellence, "What Is FASD?," March 2014, www.Fasdcenter.samhsa.gov
41. Centers for Disease Control and Prevention, "Ten Leading Causes of Death by Age Group," August 2013, www.cdc.gov/injury/wisqars/leadingcauses.html
42. Centers for Disease Control and Prevention (CDC), "Vital Signs: Drinking and Driving, a Threat to Everyone—October 2011" October 2013, www.cdc.gov/vitalsigns/drinkinganddriving
43. Ibid.
44. National Highway Traffic Safety Administration, "Traffic Safety Facts: 2010 Data Alcohol-Impaired Driving," April 2012, www-nrd.nhtsa.dot.gov/Pubs/811606.pdf
45. Centers for Disease Control and Prevention (CDC), "Vital Signs: Drinking and Driving," 2013.
46. American College Health Association, *National College Health Assessment II: Reference Group Data Report, Fall 2013*, 2014.
47. Insurance Institute for Highway Safety, "Alcohol-Impaired Driving," 2013, www.iihs.org/iihs/topics/t/alcohol-impaired-driving/fatalityfacts/alcohol-impaired-driving/2012#When-alcohol-impaired-crashes-occur.
48. Ibid.
49. Ibid.
50. Medline Plus, "Alcoholism and Alcohol Abuse," February 2014, www.nlm.nih.gov/medlineplus/ency/article/000944.htm
51. Center of Behavioral Health Statistics and Quality, "Nearly Half of College Student Treatment Admissions Were for Primary Alcohol Abuse," *Data Spotlight* (2012), www.samhsa.gov/data/spotlight/Spotlight054College2012.pdf
52. A. Arria, "College Student Success: The Impact of Health Concerns and Substance Abuse," Lecture presented at NASPA Alcohol and Mental Health Conference (Fort Worth, TX: January 19, 2013).
53. M. Waldron et al., "Parental Separation and Early Substance Involvement: Results from Children of Alcoholic and Cannabis Twins," *Drug and Alcohol Dependence* 134 (2014): 78–84.
54. D. Stacey, "RASGRF2 Regulates Alcohol-Induced Reinforcement by Influencing Mesolimbic Dopamine Neuron Activity and Dopamine Release," *Proceedings of the National Academy of Sciences* 109, no. 51 (2012): 21128–33, DOI: 10.1073/pnas.1211844110.
55. J. Niels Rosenquist et al., "The Spread of Alcohol Consumption Behavior in a Large Social Network,"

Annals of Internal Medicine 152, no. 7 (2010): 426–33.
56. Centers for Disease Control and Prevention, Fact Sheet, "Excessive Alcohol Use and Risks to Women's Health: 2010," www.cdc.gov/alcohol/fact-sheets/womens-health.htm
57. K. Keyes et al., "The Role of Race/Ethnicity in Alcohol-Attributable Injury in the United States," *Epidemiologic Reviews* 34, no. 1 (2012): 89–102.
58. T. Zaploski et al., "Less Drinking, yet More Problems: Understanding African American Drinking and Related Problems," *Psychological Bulletin* 140, no. 1 (2013): 188–223.
59. National Institute on Alcohol Abuse and Alcoholism, "Alcohol and the Hispanic Community," July 2013, http://pubs.niaaa.nih.gov/publications/HispanicFact/hispanicFact.htm
60. Substance Abuse and Mental Health Services Administration, *Results from the 2011 National Survey on Drug Use and Health: National Findings*, 2012, www.samhsa.gov/data/NSDUH/2k11Results/NSDUHresults2011.htm
61. Ibid.
62. J. Otto et al., "Association of the ALDHA1*2 Promoter Polymorphism with Alcohol Phenotypes in Young Adults with or without ALDH2*2," *Alcoholism Clinical and Experimental Research* 37, no. 1 (2013): 164–69.
63. Join Together Staff, "7.5 Million Children in the U.S. Live with Alcoholic Parent," February 16, 2012, www.drugfree.org/join-together/alcohol/7-5-million-children-in-u-s-live-with-alcoholic-parent
64. Centers for Disease Control and Prevention, "The High Cost of Excessive Drinking to States," August 19, 2013, www.cdc.gov/features/CostsOfDrinking/
65. Ibid.
66. Underage Drinking Enforcement Training Center, Underage Drinking Costs, "Underage Drinking," September 2011, www.udetc.org/UnderageDrinkingCosts.asp.
67. Ibid.
68. Substance Abuse and Mental Health Services Administration, "The NSDUH Report—Alcohol Treatment: Need, Utilization, and Barriers," April 2009, www.samhsa.gov/data/2k9/AlcTX/AlcTX.htm
69. Substance Abuse and Mental Health Services Administration, *Results from the 2012 National Survey on Drug Use and Health: Summary of National Findings*, U.S. Department of Health and Human Services Series H-46, No. (SMA) 13-4795 (Rockville, MD: Substance Abuse and Mental Health Services Administration, 2013), Available at www.samhsa.gov/data/NSDUH/2012SummNatFindDetTables/NationalFindings/NSDUHresults2012.pdf
70. Centers for Disease Control and Prevention, "50th Anniversary of the First Surgeon General's Report on Smoking and Health," January 2014, www.cdc.gov/mmwr/preview/mmwrhtml/mm6302a1.htm?s_cid=mm6302a1_w
71. CDC, "Smoking and Tobacco Use: Fast Facts," April 2014, www.cdc.gov/tobacco/data_statistics/fact_sheets/fast_facts/
72. Centers for Disease Control and Prevention, "Adult Cigarette Smoking in the United States: Current Estimates," February 2014, www.cdc.gov/tobacco/data_statistics/fact_sheets/adult_data/cig_smoking/; American Cancer Society, "Smokeless Tobacco," December 2013, www.cancer.org/cancer/cancercauses/tobaccocancer/smokeless-tobacco; Centers for Disease Control and Prevention, "Smoking and Tobacco Use: Cigars," November 2013, www.cdc.gov/tobacco/data_statistics/fact_sheets/tobacco_industry/cigars/
73. C. A. Wassenaar et al., "Relationship between CYP2A6 and CHRNA5-CHRNA3-CHRNB4 Variation and Smoking Behaviors and Lung Cancer Risk," *JNCI Journal of the National Cancer Institute* 103, no. 17 (2011): 1342–46, DOI: 10.1093/jnci/djr237; F. Ducci et al., "TTC12-ANKK1-DRD2 and CHRNA5-CHRNA3-CHRNB4 Influence Different Pathways Leading to Smoking Behavior from Adolescence to Mid-Adulthood," *Biological Psychiatry* 69, no. 7 (2011): 650–60; C. Amos, M. Spitz, and P. Cinciripini, "Chipping Away at the Genetics of Smoking Behavior," *Nature Genetics* 42, no. 5 (2010): 366–68.
74. F. Ducci et al., "TTC12-ANKK1-DRD2 and CHRNA5-CHRNA3-CHRNB4 Influence Different Pathways, 2011; T. Korhonen and J. Kaprio, "Genetic Epidemiology of Smoking Behaviour and Nicotine Dependence," 2011, eLS.
75. Ibid.
76. C. Amos, M. Spitz, and P. Cinciripini, "Chipping Away at the Genetics of Smoking Behavior," *Nature Genetics* 42, no. 5 (2010): 366–68.
77. Campaign for Tobacco-Free Kids, "Toll of Tobacco in the United States of America," February 2014, www.tobaccofreekids.org/research/factsheets/pdf/0072.pdf?utm_source=factsheets_finder&utm_medium=link&utm_campaign=analytics
78. American Lung Association, "General Smoking Facts," June 2011, www.lung.org/stop-smoking/about-smoking/facts-figures/general-smoking-facts.html
79. Tobacco Free Providence, "Sweet Deceit Survey Results," January 2012, www.tobaccofreeprovidence.org/2012-01-27-sweet-deceit-survey-results/
80. American Cancer Society, "Cancer Facts & Figures 2014," Accessed April 2014, www.cancer.org/research/cancerfactsstatistics/cancerfactsfigures2014/
81. U.S. Department of Health and Human Services, *The Health Consequences of Smoking—50 Years of Progress*, 2014.
82. Campaign for Tobacco-Free Kids, "State Cigarette Excise Tax Rates & Rankings," December 2013, www.tobaccofreekids.org/research/factsheets/pdf/0097.pdf
83. American College Health Association, *American College Health Association–National College Health Assessment II: Reference Group Data Report, Fall 2013* (Hanover, MD: American College Health Association, 2014), Available at www.acha-ncha.org/reports_ACHA-NCHAII.html.
84. Ibid.
85. Substance Abuse and Mental Health Services Administration, "Results from the 2012 National Survey on Drug Use and Health: Summary of National Findings," 2013.
86. Y. Choi et al., "I Smoke but I Am Not a Smoker": Phantom Smokers and the Discrepancy between Self-Identity and Behavior," *Journal of American College Health* 59, no. 2 (2011): 117–25.
87. E. Sutfin et al., "Tobacco Use by College Students: A Comparison of Daily and Nondaily Smokers," *American Journal of Health Behavior* 36, no. 2 (2012): 218–29.
88. American Cancer Society, "Light Smoking as Risky as a Pack a Day?," January 2013, www.cancer.org/cancer/news/expertvoices/post/2013/01/02/light-smoking-as-risky-as-a-pack-a-day.aspx; L. Stoner et al., "Occasional Cigarette Smoking Chronically Affects Arterial Function," *Ultrasound in Medicine and Biology* 34, no. 12 (2008): 1885–92.
89. L. An et al., "Symptoms of Cough and Shortness of Breath among Occasional Young Adult Smokers," *Nicotine & Tobacco Research* 11, no. 2 (2009): 126–33.
90. Stop Smoking!, "Smoking and Birth Control Pills Are Not Made for Each Other," Retrieved March 6, 2012, www.stop-smoking-updates.com/quitsmoking/smoking-factsheet/facts/smoking-and-birth-control-pills-are-not-made-for-each-other.htm
91. U.S. Department of Health and Human Services, *The Health Consequences of Smoking—50 Years of Progress*, 2014; U.S. Department of Health and Human Services, "How Tobacco Smoke Causes Disease: The Biology and Behavioral Basis for Smoking Attributable Disease: A Report of the Surgeon General," Office of the Surgeon General, 2010, www.surgeongeneral.gov
92. American Cancer Society, "Cancer Facts & Figures 2013," 2013, Available at www.cancer.org
93. K. Sterling et al., "Factors Associated with Small Cigar Use among College Students," *American Journal of Health Behavior* 37, no. 3 (2013): 325–33.
94. American Cancer Society, "Questions about Smoking, Tobacco, and Health: What about More Exotic Forms of Smoking Tobacco, Such as Clove Cigarettes, Bidis, and Hookahs?" February 2014, www.cancer.org/cancer/cancercauses/tobaccocancer/questionsaboutsmokingtobaccoandhealth/questions-about-smoking-tobacco-and-health-other-forms-of-smoking
95. Centers for Disease Control and Prevention, "Smoking and Tobacco Use: Bidis and Kreteks," Updated July 2013, www.cdc.gov/tobacco/data_statistics/fact_sheets/tobacco_industry/bidis_kreteks
96. Ibid.
97. Centers for Disease Control and Prevention, "Youth and Tobacco Use," February 2014, www.cdc.gov/tobacco/data_statistics/fact_sheets/youth_data/tobacco_use/
98. Centers for Disease Control and Prevention, "Tobacco Product Use among Middle and High School Students—United States, 2011 and 2012," *Morbidity and Mortality Weekly Report* 62, no. 45 (2013): 893–97.
99. L. M. Dutra and S. A. Glanz, "Electronic Cigarettes and Conventional Cigarette Use Among US Adolescents. A Cross-sectional Study," *JAMA Pediatrics* (March 6, 2014), DOI:10.1001/jamapediatrics.2013.5488. (Epub ahead of print.)
100. M. Hug, "Health-Related Effects Reported by Electronic Cigarette Users in Online Forums," Journal of Medical Internet Research 15, no. 4, 2014: e59; U.S. Food and Drug Administration, "FDA and Public Health Experts Warn About Electronic Cigarettes," 2010, www.fda.gov/newsevents/newsroom/pressannouncements/ucm173222.htm; L. Dale, Mayo Clinic, "Electronic Cigarettes: A Safe Way to Light Up?," 2011, www.mayoclinic.com/health/electronic-cigarettes/AN02025
101. K. Chatham-Stephens et al., "Notes from the Field: Calls to Poison Centers for Exposures to Electronic Cigarettes—United States, September 2010–February 2014," Morbidity and Mortality Weekly 63, no. 13 (2014): 292–93.
102. Campaign for Tobacco Free Kids, "Toll of Tobacco in the United States of America," 2014.
103. National Cancer Institute, "Lung Cancer Prevention," February 2014, www.cancer.gov/cancertopics/pdq/prevention/lung/HealthProfessional/page2
104. American Cancer Society, "Cancer Facts & Figures 2014," 2014.
105. Ibid.
106. American Cancer Society, "What Are Oral Cavity and Oropharyngeal Cancers?" February 2014,

www.cancer.org/cancer/oralcavityandoropharyngealcancer/detailedguide/oral-cavity-and-oropharyngeal-cancer-what-is-oral-cavity-cancer

107. American Cancer Society, "Cancer Facts & Figures 2014," 2014.
108. American Heart Association, Heart Disease and Stroke Statistics—2014 Update (Dallas, TX: American Heart Association, 2014), Available at http://circ.ahajournals.org/content/129/3/e28
109. Ibid.
110. Ibid.
111. American Heart Association, "Stroke Risk Factors," October 2012, www.strokeassociation.org/STROKEORG/AboutStroke/UnderstandingRisk/Understanding-Risk_UCM_308539_SubHomePage.jsp; Center for Disease Control and Prevention, "Health Effects of Cigarette Smoking," February 2014, www.cdc.gov/tobacco/data_statistics/fact_sheets/health_effects/effects_cig_smoking/
112. American Lung Association, "Benefits of Quitting," March 2012, www.lungusa.org/stop-smoking/how-to-quit/why-quit/benefits-of-quitting
113. U.S. Department of Health and Human Services, *The Health Consequences of Smoking—50 Years of Progress*, 2014.
114. John Hopkins Health Alerts, "Emphysema: Symptoms and Remedies," Accessed March 2012, www.johnshopkinshealthalerts.com/symptoms_remedies/emphysema/96-1.html
115. C. B. Harte et al., "Association between Cigarette Smoking and Erectile Tumescence: The Mediating Role of Heart Rate Variability," *International Journal of Impotence Research* 25, no. 4 (2013): 155–59, DOI: 10.1038/ijir.2012.43.
116. Centers for Disease Control and Prevention, "Tobacco Use and Pregnancy," Modified January 2014, www.cdc.gov/reproductivehealth/TobaccoUsePregnancy/
117. Ibid.
118. American Academy of Periodontology, "Gum Disease Risk Factors," Accessed April 2014, www.perio.org/consumer/risk-factors
119. I. Moreno-Gonzalez, et al., "Smoking Exacerbates Amyloid Pathology in a Mouse Model of Alzheimer's Disease," Nature Communications 4, no. 1495 (2013); J. Cataldo et al., "Cigarette Smoking Is a Risk Factor of Alzheimer's Disease: An Analysis Controlling for Tobacco Industry Affiliation," *Journal of Alzheimer's Disease* 19, no. 2 (2010): 465–80.
120. American Cancer Society, "Secondhand Smoke," Revised February 2014, www.cancer.org/cancer/cancercauses/tobaccocancer/secondhand-smoke
121. Centers for Disease Control and Prevention, "Smoking and Tobacco Use Facts: Secondhand Smoke," April 2014, www.cdc.gov/tobacco/data_statistics/fact_sheets/secondhand_smoke/general_facts/
122. Ibid.
123. National Cancer Institute, "Secondhand Smoke and Cancer," January 2011, www.cancer.gov/cancertopics/factsheet/Tobacco/ETS
124. U.S. Department of Health and Human Services, *The Health Consequences of Involuntary Exposure to Tobacco Smoke*, November 2011; Centers for Disease Control and Prevention, "Smoking and Tobacco Use Fact Sheet," 2014.
125. Centers for Disease Control and Prevention, "Smoking and Tobacco Use: Secondhand Smoke Facts," 2014.
126. Ibid.
127. U.S. Department of Health and Human Services, *The Health Consequences of Involuntary Exposure to Tobacco Smoke*, 2011.
128. Z. Kabir, G. Connolly, and H. Alpert, "Secondhand Smoke Exposure and Neurobehavioral Disorders among Children in the United States," *Pediatrics* (2011), DOI: 10.1542/peds.2011-00232011-0023. (Epub ahead of print.)
129. Ibid.
130. O. Shafey, M. Eriksen, H. Ross, and J. Mackay, "Secondhand Smoking," in *The Tobacco Atlas*, 3d ed. (Atlanta, GA: American Cancer Society, 2009), Available at www.cancer.org/aboutus/GlobalHealth/CancerandTobaccoControlResources/the-tobacco-atlas-3rd-edition
131. U.S. Department of Health and Human Services, *The Health Consequences of Smoking—50 Years of Progress*, 2014
132. Tobacco-Free Kids, "1998 State Tobacco Settlement 15 Years Later," February 2014, www.tobaccofreekids.org/what_we_do/state_local/tobacco_settlement/
133. Family Smoking Prevention and Tobacco Control Act of 2009, HR 1256, 111th Congress of the United States of America, Available at www.govtrack.us/congress/billtext.xpd?bill=h111-1256
134. L. Weber et al., "E-Cigarette Rise Poses Quandary for Employers," *The Wall Street Journal*, January 16, 2014, 41–42.
135. Centers for Disease Control and Prevention, "Tobacco Use: Smoking Cessation," February 2014, www.cdc.gov/tobacco/data_statistics/fact_sheets/cessation/quitting/index.htm#quitting
136. N. Hopper, "What a Pack of Cigarettes Costs Now, State by State," *The Awl*, July 12, 2013, www.theawl.com/2013/07/what-a-pack-of-cigarettes-costs-now-state-by-state
137. American Cancer Society, "Guide to Quitting Smoking: A Word about Quitting Success Rates," February 2014, www.cancer.org/Healthy/StayAwayfromTobacco/GuidetoQuittingSmoking/guide-to-quitting-smoking-success-rates
138. U.S. Food and Drug Administration, "Public Health Advisory: FDA Requires New Boxed Warnings for the Smoking Cessation Drugs Chantix and Zyban," July 1, 2009, www.fda.gov/Drugs/DrugSafety/DrugSafetyPodcasts/ucm170906.htm

Pulled Statistics

page 155, California Department of Alcohol and Drug Programs, "Frequently Asked Questions: General," 2012, http://www.adp.ca.gov/Criminal_Justice/DUI/faqs.shtml
page 164, American Lung Association, "General Smoking Facts," June 2011, http://www.lung.org/stop-smoking/about-smoking/facts-figures/general-smoking-facts.html

Chapter 8

1. U.S. Department of Agriculture, Economic Research Service, "U.S. Per Capita Loss-Adjusted Food Availability: Total Calories," Updated April 2010, www.ers.usda.gov/Data/FoodConsumption/app/reports/displayCommodities.aspx?reportName=Total+Calories&id=36#startForm; U.S. Department of Agriculture, Economic Research Service, "Summary Findings," *Food Availability (Per Capita) Data System*, updated August 2012, www.ers.usda.gov/data-products/food-availability-%28per-capita%29-data-system/summary-findings.aspx#.UYLNPcphris.
2. D. Grotto and E. Zied, "The Standard American Diet and Its Relationship to the Health Status of Americans," *Nutrition in Clinical Practice* 25, no. 6 (2010): 603–12, DOI: 10.1177/0884533610386234.
3. Institute of Medicine of the National Academies, Food and Nutrition Board, *Dietary Reference Intakes for Water, Potassium, Sodium, Chloride, and Sulfate* (Washington, DC: The National Academies Press, 2004), Available at http://iom.edu/Reports/2004/Dietary-Reference-Intakes-Water-Potassium-Sodium-Chloride-and-Sulfate.aspx.
4. Institute of Medicine of the National Academies, Food and Nutrition Board, *Dietary References for Water, Potassium, Sodium, Chloride, and Sulfate* (Washington, DC: The National Academies Press, 2005), Available at www.nal.usda.gov/fnic/DRI/DRI_Water/water_full_report.pdf.
5. American College of Sports Medicine (ACSM), "Selecting and Effectively Using Hydration for Fitness," 2011, Available at www.acsm.org/docs/brochures/selecting-and-effectively-using-hydration-for-fitness.pdf.
6. U.S. Department of Agriculture, Agricultural Research Service, Beltsville Human Nutrition Research Center, Food Surveys Research Group (Beltsville, MD) and U.S. Department of Health and Human Services, Centers for Disease Control and Prevention, National Center for Health Statistics (Hyattsville, MD), *What We Eat in America, NHANES 2009–2010 Data: Table 1. Nutrient Intakes from Food: Mean Amounts Consumed per Individual by Gender and Age, in the United States, 2009–2010*, www.ars.usda.gov/SP2UserFiles/Place/12355000/pdf/0910/tables_1-40_2009-2010.pdf.
7. Food and Nutrition Board, Institute of Medicine, *Dietary Reference Intakes for Energy, Carbohydrate, Fiber, Fat, Fatty Acids, Cholesterol, Protein, and Amino Acids (Macronutrients)* (Washington, DC: National Academies Press, 2005), Available at www.nap.edu/openbook.php?isbn=0309085373.
8. S. M. Phillips and L. J. C. van Loon, "Dietary Protein for Athletes: From Requirements to Optimum Adaptation," *Journal of Sports Science* 29, S1 (2011): S29–S38.
9. Institute of Medicine of the National Academies, "Dietary, Functional, and Total Fiber," in *Dietary Reference Intakes for Energy, Carbohydrate, Fiber, Fat, Fatty Acids, Cholesterol, Protein, and Amino Acids* (Washington, DC: The National Academies Press, 2005), 339–421, www.nap.edu/openbook.php?isbn=0309085373.
10. Ibid.
11. Q. Ben et al., "Dietary Fiber Intake Reduces Risk for Colorectal Adenoma: A Meta-Analysis," *Gastroenterology* 146, no. 3 (2014): 689–99.
12. K. Maki et al., "Whole-Grain Ready-to-Eat Oat Cereal, as Part of a Dietary Program for Weight Loss, Reduces Low-Density Lipoprotein Cholesterol in Adults with Overweight and Obesity More than a Dietary Program Including Low-Fiber Control Foods," *Journal of the American Dietetic Association* 110, no. 2 (2010): 205–14.
13. B. Yao et al., "Dietary Fiber Intake and Risk of Type 2 Diabetes: A Dose-Response Analysis of Prospective Studies," *European Journal of Epidemioly* 29, no. 2 (2014): 79–78, DOI: 10.1007/s10654-013-9876-x.
14. Institute of Medicine of the National Academies, "Dietary, Functional, and Total Fiber," in *Dietary Reference Intakes for Energy, Carbohydrate, Fiber, Fat, Fatty Acids, Cholesterol, Protein, and Amino Acids* (Washington, DC: The National Academies Press, 2005), 339–421, www.nap.edu/openbook.php?isbn=0309085373.
15. C. E. Ramsden et al., "Use of Dietary Linoleic Acid for Secondary Prevention of Coronary Heart Disease and Death: Evaluation of Recovered Data from the Sydney Diet Heart Study and Updated Meta-Analysis," *British Medical Journal* 346 (2013): e8707, DOI: http://dx.doi.org/10.1136/bmj.e8707; L. Gillingham, S. Harris-Janz, and P. Jones, "Dietary Monounsaturated Fatty Acids Are Protective against Metabolic Syndrome and Cardiovascular

Disease Risk Factors," *Lipids* 46, no. 3 (2011): 209–28, DOI: 10.1007/s11745-010-3524-y.

16. W. Willet, "Dietary Fats and Coronary Heart Disease," *Journal of Internal Medicine* 272, no. 1 (2012): 13–24; N. Bendson et al., "Consumption of Industrial and Ruminant Trans Fatty Acids and Risk of CHD: A Systemic Review and Meta-Analysis of Cohort Studies," *European Journal of Clinical Nutrition* 65, no. 7 (2011): 773–83.
17. U.S. Food and Drug Administration, "FDA Targets Trans Fats in Processed Foods," *FDA Consumer Updates*, December 2013, www.fda.gov/ForConsumers/ConsumerUpdates/ucm372915.htm.
18. Ibid.
19. H. J. Silver et al., "Consuming a Balanced High Fat Diet for 16 Weeks Improves Body Composition, Inflammation and Vascular Function Parameters in Obese Premenopausal Women," *Metabolism* 63, no. 4 (2014): 562–73, DOI: 10.1016/j.metabol.2014.01.004; Z. Shadman, "Association of High Carbohydrate versus High Fat Diet with Glycated Hemoglobin in High Calorie Consuming Type 2 Diabetics," *Journal of Diabetes and Metabolic Disorders* 12, no. 1 (2013): 27.
20. Food and Nutrition Board, Institute of Medicine, *Dietary Reference Intakes for Energy*, 2005.
21. National Institutes of Health Office of Dietary Supplements, "Dietary Supplement Fact Sheet: Vitamin D," Reviewed June 2011, http://ods.od.nih.gov/factsheets/VitaminD-HealthProfessional.
22. U.S. Department of Agriculture, *What We Eat in America*, NHANES 2009-2010, Data: Table 1, 2010, www.ars.usda.gov/Services/docs.htm?docid=18349; C. Ayala et al., "Application of Lower Sodium Intake Recommendations to Adults—United States, 1999–2006," *Morbidity and Mortality Weekly* (*MMWR*) 58, no. 11 (2009): 281–83.
23. U.S. Department of Agriculture, *What We Eat in America*, Data: Table 1, 2010.
24. R. L. Bailey et al., "Estimation of Total Usual Calcium and Vitamin D Intakes in the United States," *Journal of Nutrition* 140, no. 4 (2010): 817–22, DOI: 10.3945/jn.109.118539.
25. Academy of Nutrition and Dietetics, "Position of the Academy of Nutrition and Dietetics: Functional Foods." *Journal of the Academy of Nutrition and Dietetics* 113, no. 8 (2013): 1096–103, DOI: 10.1016/j.jand.2013.06.002.
26. Ibid.
27. Ibid.
28. M.E. Obrenovich, et al., "Antioxidants in Health, Disease, and Aging," *CNS Neurol Disord Drug Targets* 10, no. 2 (2011):192–207; V. Ergin, R. E. Hariry, and C. Karasu, "Carbonyl Stress in Aging Process: Role of Vitamins and Phytochemicals as Redox Regulators," *Aging and Disease* 4, no. 5 (2013): 276–94, DOI: 10.14336/AD.2013.0400276.
29. Academy of Nutrition and Dietetics, "Position of the Academy of Nutrition and Dietetics: Functional Foods," 2013; G. M. Cole and S. A. Frautschy, "DHA May Reduce Age-Related Dementia," *Journal of Nutrition* 140, no. 4 (2010): 869–74; D. Swanson, R. Block, and S. A. Mousa, "Omega-3 Fatty Acids EPA and DHA: Health Benefits Throughout Life," *Advanced Nutrition* 3, no.1 (2012): 1–7.
30. P. Hemarajata and J. Versalovic, "Effects of Probiotics on Gut Microbiota: Mechanisms of Intestinal Immunomodulation and Neuromodulation," *Therapeutic Advances in Gastroenterology* 6, no. 1 (2013): 39–51; R. Krajmalnik-Brown et al., "Effects of Gut Microbes on Nutrient Absorption and Energy Regulation," *Nutrition Clinical Practice* 27, no. 2 (2012): 201–14.
31. L. Hooper et al., "Effects of Chocolate, Cocoa, and Flavan-3-ols on Cardiovascular Health: A Systematic Review and Meta-Analysis of Randomized Trials," *American Journal of Clinical Nutrition* 95, no. 3, (2012): 740–53, DOI: 10.3945/ajcn.111.023457; D. Grassi et al., "Protective Effects of Flavanol-Rich Dark Chocolate on Endothelial Function and Wave Reflection during Acute Hyperglycemia," *Hypertension* 60, no. 3 (2012): 827–32, DOI: 10.1161/HYPERTENSIONAHA.112.193995; S. Ramos-Romero et al., "Effect of a Cocoa Flavonoid-Enriched Diet on Experimental Autoimmune Arthritis," *British Journal of Nutrition* 107, no. 4 (2012): 523–32, DOI: 10.1017/S000711451100328X.
32. U.S. Food and Drug Administration, "Nutrition Facts Label: Proposed Changes Aim to Better Inform Food Choices," February 2014, www.fda.gov/ForConsumers/ConsumerUpdates/ucm387114.htm.
33. U.S. Department of Agriculture and U.S. Department of Health and Human Services, *Dietary Guidelines for Americans, 2010,* 7th ed. (Washington, DC: U.S. Government Printing Office, 2010), www.cnpp.usda.gov/publications/dietaryguidelines/2010/policydoc/policydoc.pdf.
34. U.S. Department of Agriculture, "Empty Calories: How Do I Count the Empty Calories I Eat?," Updated June 4, 2011, www.choosemyplate.gov/foodgroups/emptycalories_count_table.html.
35. U.S. Department of Agriculture, *Eating Healthy on a Budget: The Consumer Economics Perspective*, September 2011, www.choosemyplate.gov/food-groups/downloads/ConsumerEconomicsPerspective.pdf; U.S. Department of Agriculture, *Smart Shopping for Veggies and Fruits,* Center for Nutrition Policy and Promotion, September 2011, www.choosemyplate.gov/food-groups/downloads/TenTips/DGTipsheet9SmartShopping.pdf; U.S. Centers for Disease Control and Prevention, *30 Ways in 30 Days to Stretch Your Fruit and Vegetable Budget,* Fruits and Veggies: More Matters, September 2011, www.fruitsandveggiesmatter.gov/downloads/Stretch_FV_Budget.pdf.
36. The Vegetarian Resource Group, "How Often Do Americans Eat Vegetarian Meals? And How Many Adults in the U.S. Are Vegetarian?," *Vegetarian Resource Group Blog*, May 2012, www.vrg.org/blog/2012/05/18/how-often-do-americans-eat-vegetarian-meals-and-how-many-adults-in-the-u-s-are-vegetarian.
37. C. G. Lee et al., "Vegetarianism as a Protective Factor for Colorectal Adenoma and Advanced Adenoma in Asians," *Digestive Diseases and Science* 59, no. 5 (2013): 1025–35, DOI 10.1007/s10620-013-2974-5.
38. Office of Dietary Supplements, "Frequently Asked Questions," July 2013, http://ods.od.nih.gov/Health_Information/ODS_Frequently_Asked_Questions.aspx#; V. A. Moyer, "Vitamin, Mineral, and Multivitamin Supplements for the Primary Prevention of Cardiovascular Disease and Cancer: U.S. Preventive Services Task Force Recommendation Statement," *Annals of Internal Medicine*, 2014, DOI:10.7326/M14-0198.
39. Office of Dietary Supplements, "Vitamin A Fact Sheet for Consumers," June 2013, http://ods.od.nih.gov/factsheets/VitaminA-QuickFacts/; Office of Dietary Supplements, "Vitamin E Fact Sheet for Consumers," June 2013, http://ods.od.nih.gov/factsheets/list-all/VitaminE-QuickFacts/; Office of Dietary Supplements, "Vitamin D Fact Sheet for Consumers," June 2013, http://ods.od.nih.gov/factsheets/VitaminD-QuickFacts/
40. Academy of Nutrition and Dietetics, "It's About Eating Right: Dietary Supplements," January 2013, www.eatright.org/public/content.aspx?id=7918.
41. The Organic Trade Association, "Eight in Ten U.S. Parents Report They Purchase Organic Products," April 2013, http://www.ota.com/organic-consumers/consumersurvey2013.html.
42. The Organic Trade Organization, "Consumer-Driven U.S. Organic Market Surpasses $31 Billion in 2011," 2012, www.organicnewsroom.com/2012/04/us_consumerdriven_organic_mark.html.
43. Mayo Clinic, "Organic Food: Is It More Nutritious?," September 2012, www.mayoclinic.org/healthy-living/nutrition-and-healthy-eating/in-depth/organic-food/art-20043880?pg=2.
44. K. Brandt et al., "Agroecosystem Management and Nutritional Quality of Plant Foods: The Case of Organic Fruits and Vegetables," *Critical Reviews in Plant Sciences* 30, no. 1–2 (2011): 177–97; C. Smith-Spangler et al., "Are Organic Foods Safer or Healthier Than Conventional Alternatives? A Systematic Review," *Annals of Internal Medicine* 157, no. 5 (2012): 348–66, DOI: 10.7326/0003-4819-157-5-201209040-00007.
45. U.S. Environmental Protection Agency, "Pesticides and Foods: Health Problems Pesticides May Pose," May 2012, www.epa.gov/pesticides/food/risks.htm.
46. U.S. Department of Agriculture, Pesticide Data Program: 21st Annual Summary, Calendar Year 2011, Agricultural Marketing Service, February 2013, from www.ams.usda.gov/AMSv1.0/getfile?dDocName=stelprdc5102692.
47. U.S. Food and Drug Administration, "Food Irradiation: What You Need to Know," March 2014, www.fda.gov/Food/ResourcesForYou/Consumers/ucm261680.htm.
48. U.S. Department of Agriculture, Economic Research Service, "Adoption of Genetically Engineered Crops in the U.S.," July 2013, www.ers.usda.gov/data-products/adoption-of-genetically-engineered-crops-in-the-us.aspx.
49. Center for Food Safety, "About Genetically Engineered Foods," Accessed March 2014, www.centerforfoodsafety.org/issues/311/ge-foods/about-ge-foods.
50. Union of Concerned Scientists, "Genetic Engineering Risks and Impacts," November 2013, www.ucsusa.org/food_and_agriculture/our-failing-food-system/genetic-engineering/risks-of-genetic-engineering.html.
51. L. P. Brower et al., "Decline of Monarch Butterflies Overwintering in Mexico: Is the Migratory Phenomenon at Risk?," *Insect Conservation and Diversity* 5, no. 2 (2012): 95–100.
52. Union of Concerned Scientists, "Genetic Engineering Risks and Impacts," November 2013, www.ucsusa.org/food_and_agriculture/our-failing-food-system/genetic-engineering/risks-of-genetic-engineering.html.
53. G. Pinholster, "AAAS Board of Directors: Legally Mandating GM Food Labels Could 'Mislead and Falsely Alarm Consumers,'" *AAAS News*, October 2012, www.aaas.org/news/aaas-board-directors-legally-mandating-gm-food-labels-could-mislead-and-falsely-alarm; World Health Organization, "20 Questions on Genetically Modified Foods," Accessed March 2014, www.who.int/foodsafety/publications/biotech/20questions/en.
54. National Institute of Allergy and Infectious Diseases, "Food Allergy," August 2013, www.niaid.nih.gov/topics/foodallergy/Pages/default.aspx.
55. R. S. Gupta et al., "The Prevalence, Severity, and Distribution of Childhood Food Allergy in the

United States," *Journal of Pediatrics* 128, no. 1 (2011): e9–e17, DOI: 10.1542/peds.2011-0204.
56. National Institute of Allergy and Infectious Diseases, "Food Allergy," 2013.
57. U.S. Food and Drug Administration, "Food Allergies: What You Need to Know," April 2013, www.fda.gov/food/resourcesforyou/consumers/ucm079311.htm.
58. J. N. Keith et al., "The Prevalence of Self-Reported Lactose Intolerance and the Consumption of Dairy Foods among African American Adults Less than Expected," *Journal of the National Medical Association* 103 (2011): 36–45.
59. A. Rubio-Tapia et al., "The Prevalence of Celiac Disease in the United States," *American Journal of Gastroenterology* 107, no. 10 (2012): 1538–44, DOI: 10.1038/ajg.2012.219.
60. U.S. Department of Health and Human Services, "Food Safety Modernization Act (FSMA)," November 2013, www.fda.gov/Food/Guidance-Regulation/FSMA/ucm304045.htm.
61. Centers for Disease Control and Prevention, "Estimates of Food-Borne Illnesses in the United States," January 2014, www.cdc.gov/foodborne-burden/index.html.
62. Centers for Disease Control and Prevention, "Trends in Foodborne Illness in the United States, 2012," April 2013, www.cdc.gov/features/dsfood-net2012.
63. Centers for Disease Control and Prevention, Estimates of Foodborne Illness in the United States, CDC 2011 Estimates: Findings, Updated January 8, 2014, from www.cdc.gov/foodborneburden/2011-foodborne-estimates.html.
64. R. Johnson, "The U.S. Trade Situation for Fruit and Vegetable Products," *Congressional Research Service*, January 2014, Available at www.fas.org/sgp/crs/misc/RL34468.pdf.
65. S. Clark et al., "Frequency of US Emergency Department Visits for Food-Related Acute Allergic Reactions," *Journal of Allergy Clinical Immunology* 127, no. 3 (2011): 682–83, DOI: 10.1016/j.jaci.2010.10.040.

Pulled Statistics

page 179, D. King, A. Mainous, C. Lambourne, "Trends in Dietary Fiber Intake in the United States, 1999–2008," *Journal of the Academy of Nutrition and Dietetics* 112, no. 5 (2012): 642–48, DOI: 10.1016/j.jand.2012.01.019.

page 191, K. Heidal, et al., "Cost and Calorie Analysis of Fast Food Consumption in College Students," Food and Nutrition Sciences 3, no. 7 (2012): 942–46, DOI:10.4236/fns.2012.37124.

Chapter 9

1. D. Spruijt-Metz, "Etiology, Treatment, and Prevention of Obesity in Childhood and Adolescence: A Decade in Review," *Journal of Research on Adolescence* 21 (2011): 129–52, DOI: 10.1111/j.1532-7795.2010.00719.x; S. A. Affenito et al., "Behavioral Determinants of Obesity: Research Findings and Policy Implications," *Journal of Obesity* 2012 (2012), http://dx.doi.org/10.1155/2012/150732.
2. S. A. Affenito et al., "Behavioral Determinants of Obesity: Research Findings and Policy Implications," 2012.
3. C. L. Ogden et al., "Prevalence of Childhood and Adult Obesity in the United States, 2011–2012," *Journal of the American Medical Association* 311, no. 8 (2014): 806–14, DOI:10.1001/jama.2014.732; C. L. Ogden et al, "Prevalence of Obesity Among Adults: United States, 2011–2012," *NCHS Data Brief* 131 (2013), www.cdc.gov/nchs/data/databriefs/db131.htm.
4. U.S. Department of Health and Human Services, *The Surgeon General's Vision for a Healthy and Fit Nation* (Rockville, MD: U.S. Department of Health and Human Services, Office of the Surgeon General, 2010), Available at www.surgeongeneral.gov/library/obesityvision.
5. C. L. Ogden et al., "Prevalence of Childhood and Adult Obesity in the United States, 2011–2012," 2014.
6. A. Go et al., "AHA Statistical Update Heart Disease and Stroke Statistics—2014 Update: A Report from the American Heart Association," *Circulation* 129 (2014): 399–410.
7. C. L. Ogden et al., "Prevalence of Childhood and Adult Obesity in the United States, 2011–2012," 2014.
8. A. Go et al., "AHA Statistical Update Heart Disease and Stroke Statistics—2014 Update," 2014.
9. Ibid.
10. World Health Organization, "Obesity and Overweight Fact Sheet," March 2013, www.who.int/mediacentre/factsheets/fs311/en.
11. Ibid.; International Obesity Taskforce, "Obesity—The Global Epidemic," 2014, www.iaso.org/iotf/obesity/obesitytheglobalepidemic.
12. American Diabetes Association, "Statistics About Diabetes," January 2011, www.diabetes.org/diabetes-basics/statistics
13. J. Cawley and C. Meyerhoefer, "The Medical Care Costs of Obesity: An Instrumental Variables Approach," *Journal of Health Economics* 31, no. 1 (2012): 219, DOI: 10.1016/j.jhealeco.2011.10.003; J. P. Moriarty et al., "The Effects of Incremental Costs of Smoking and Obesity on Health Care Costs among Adults," *Journal of Occupational and Environmental Medicine* 54, no. 3 (2012): 286, DOI: 10.1097/JOM.0b013e318246f1f4.
14. C. Murtaugh et al., "Lifetime Risk and Duration of Chronic Diseases and Disability," *Journal of Aging and Health* 23, no. 3 (2011): 554–77.
15. World Health Organization, "Obesity and Overweight Fact Sheet," March 2013.
16. T. Tanaka, J. S. Ngwa, and F. J. van Rooij, "Genome-wide Meta-Analysis of Observational Studies Shows Common Genetic Variants Associated with Macronutrient Intake," *American Journal of Clinical Nutrition* 97, no. 6 (2013): 1395–402; M. M. Hetherington and J. E. Cecil, "Gene-Environment Interactions in Obesity," *Forum Nutrition* 63 (2010): 195–203; M. Graff, J. S. Ngwa, and T. Workalemahu, "Genome-wide Analysis of BMI in Adolescents and Young Adults Reveals Additional Insights into the Effects of the Genetic Loci over the Life Course," *Human Molecular Genetics* 22, no. 17 (2013): 3597–607; K. Silventoinen et al., "The Genetic and Environmental Influences on Childhood Obesity: A Systematic Review of Twin and Adoption Studies," *International Journal of Obesity* 34, no. 1 (2010): 29–40.
17. T. O. Kilpelainen et al., "Physical Activity Attenuates the Influence of *FTO* Variants on Obesity Risk: A Meta-Analysis of 218,166 Adults and 19,268 Children," *PLoS Medicine* 8, no. 11 (2012), e1001116, DOI:10.1371/journal.pmed.1001116; A. S. Richardson et al., "Moderate to Vigorous Physical Activity Interactions with Genetic Variants and Body Mass Index in a Large US Ethnically Diverse Cohort," *Pediatric Obesity* 9, no. 2 (2013): e35n46, DOI: 10.1111/j.2047-6310.2013.00152.
18. J. C. Wells. "The Evolution of Human Adiposity and Obesity: Where Did It All Go Wrong?," *Disease Models and Mechanisms* 5, no. 5 (2012): 595–607, DOI: 10.1242/dmm.009613; J. R. Speakman et al., "Evolutionary Perspectives on the Obesity Epidemic: Adaptive, Maladaptive, and Neutral Viewpoints," *Annual Review of Nutrition* 33 (2013): 289–317.
19. A. Tremblay et al., "Adaptive Thermogenesis Can Make a Difference in the Ability of Obese Individuals to Lose Body Weight," *International Journal of Obesity* 37 (2013): 759–64.
20. A. Tremblay et al., "Adaptive Thermogenesis Can Make a Difference in the Ability of Obese Individuals to Lose Body Weight," 2013.
21. M. Rotondi, F. Magri, and L. Chiovato, "Thyroid and Obesity: Not a One Way Interaction," *The Journal of Clinical Endocrinology and Metabolism* 96, no. 2 (2011): 344–56.
22. D. E. Cummings et al., "Plasma Ghrelin Levels after Diet-Induced Weight Loss or Gastric Bypass Surgery," *New England Journal of Medicine* 346, no. 21 (2002): 1623–30.
23. M. Khatib et al., "Effect of Ghrelin on Regulation of Growth Hormone Release: A Review," *The Health Agenda* 2, no. 1 (2014); C. DeVriese et al., "Focus on the Short- and Long-Term Effects of Ghrelin on Energy Homeostasis," *Nutrition* 26, no. 6 (2010): 579–84; T. Castaneda et al., "Ghrelin in the Regulation of Body Weight and Metabolism," *Frontiers in Neuroendocrinology* 31, no. 1 (2010): 44–60.
24. P. Marzullo et al. "Investigations of Thyroid Hormones and Antibodies in Obesity: Leptin Levels Are Associated with Thyroid Autoimmunity Independent of Bioanthropometric, Hormonal and Weight-Related Determinants," *The Journal of Clinical Endocrinology and Metabolism* 95, no. 8 (2010): 3965–72;. H. Feng et al., "Review: The Role of Leptin in Obesity and the Potential for Leptin Replacement Therapy," *Endocrine* 44 (2013): 33–39.
25. L. K. Mahan and S. Escott-Stump, *Krause's Food, Nutrition, and Diet Therapy*, 13th ed. (New York, NY: W. B. Saunders, 2012).
26. L. Poston, L. F. Harthoorn, and E. M Van Der Beek, "Obesity in Pregnancy: Implications for the Mother and Lifelong Health of the Child–A Consensus Statement," *Pediatric Research* 69, no. 2 (2011): 175–80; K. L. Connor et al., "Nature, Nurture or Nutrition? Impact of Maternal Nutrition on Maternal Care, Offspring Development and Reproductive Function," *Journal of Physiology* 590, no. 9 (2012): 2167–80.
27. M. A. Schuster et al. "Racial and Ethnic Health Disparities among Fifth-Graders in Three Cities," *The New England Journal of Medicine* 367, no. 8 (2012): 735–45; C. L. Odgen et al., "Prevalence of Obesity and Trends in Body Mass Index among U.S. Children and Adolescents. 1999–2010," *Journal of the American Medical Association* 307 (2012): 483–90.
28. C. Gillespie et al., "The Growing Concern of Poverty in the United States: An Exploration of Food Prices and Poverty on Obesity Rates for Low-Income Citizens," *Undergraduate Economic Review* 8, no. 1 (2012): 1–38.
29. J. F. Sallis et al., "Role of Built Environments in Physical Activity, Obesity and Cardiovascular Disease," *Circulation* 125, no. 5 (2012): 729–737; F. Li et al., "Built Environment, Adiposity, and Physical Activity in Adults Aged 50–75," *American Journal of Preventive Medicine* 35, no. 1 (2008): 38–46.
30. U.S. Department of Health and Human Services, "Summary Health Statistics for U.S. Adults: National Health Interview Survey, 2012," *Vital and Health Statistics* 10, no. 260 (2014), Available at www.cdc.gov/nchs/data/series/sr_10/sr10_260.pdf.
31. Centers for Disease Control and Prevention, "Prevalence of Underweight among Adults Aged

20 years and Over: United States 1960–1962 and 2007–2010," September 2012, www.cdc.gov/nchs/data/hestat/underweight_adult_07_10/underweight_adult_07_10.htm; Centers for Disease Control and Prevention, "Prevalence of Underweight among Children and Adolescents Aged 2–19 Years: United States, 1963–1965 through 2007–2010, www.cdc.gov/nchs/data/hestat/underweight_child_07_10/underweight_child_07_10.htm.

32. Centers for Disease Control and Prevention, "About BMI for Adults," September 2011, www.cdc.gov/healthyweight/assessing/bmi/adult_bmi/index.html.
33. J. I. Mechanick et al., "Clinical Practice Guidelines for the Perioperative Nutritional, Metabolic and Nonsurgical Support of the Bariatric Surgery Patient—2013 Update," *Endocrine Practice* 19, no. 2 (2013): e1–36, www.aace.com/files/publish-ahead-of-print-final-version.pdf.
34. K. M. Flegal et al., "Prevalence and Trends in Obesity among U.S. Adults, 1999–2010," *Journal of the American Medical Association* 307, no. 5 (2012): 491–97.
35. R. Puhl, "Weight Stigmatization toward Youth: A Significant Problem in Need of Societal Solutions," *Childhood Obesity* 7, no. 5 (2011): 359–63; S. A. Mustillo, K. Budd, and K. Hendrix, "Obesity, Labeling, and Psychological Distress in Late-Childhood and Adolescent Black and White Girls: The Distal Effects of Stigma," *Social Psychology Quarterly* 76, no. 3 (2013): 268–89.
36. M. Bombelli et al., "Impact of Body Mass Index and Waist Circumference on the Long Term Risk of Diabetes Mellitus, Hypertension and Cardiac Organ Damage," *Hypertension* 58, no. 6 (2011): 1029–1035; S. Czernichow et al., "Body Mass Index, Waist Circumference and Waist-Hip Ratio: Which Is the Better Discriminator of Cardiovascular Disease Mortality Risk? Evidence from an Individual-Participant Meta-Analysis of 82,864 Participants from Nine Cohort Studies," *Obesity Reviews* 12, no. 9 (2011): 1467–78.
37. National Heart, Lung, and Blood Institute, "Classification of Overweight and Obesity by BMI, Waist Circumference and Associated Disease Risks," 2012, www.nhlbi.nih.gov/health/public/heart/obesity/lose_wt/bmi_dis.htm.
38. University of Maryland Medical Center, Rush University, "Waist to Hip Ratio Calculator," Accessed March 2014, www.healthcalculators.org/calculators/waist_hip.asp
39. World Health Organization, "Waist Circumference and Waist-Hip Ratio: Report of WHO Expert Consultation," 2011, http://whqlibdoc.who.int/publications/2011/9789241501491_eng.pdf.
40. E. Stice et al., "Risk Factors and Prodomal Eating Pathology," *Journal of Child Psychology and Psychiatry* 51, no. 4 (2010): 518–25.
41. S. N. Bleich, J. A. Wolfson, and S. Vine, "Diet-Beverage Consumption and Caloric Intake among US Adults, Overall and by Body Weight," *American Journal of Public Health* 104, no. 3 (2014): e72–78.
42. L. Gray, N. Cooper, A. Dunkley et al., "A Systematic Review and Mixed Treatment Comparison of Pharmacological Interventions for the Treatment of Obesity," *Obesity Reviews* 13, no. 6 (2012): 483–98.
43. Federal Drug Administration, "FDA Consumer Updates: HCG Diet Products are Illegal," March 2014, www.fda.gov/forconsumers/consumerupdates/ucm281333.htm
44. Federal Drug Administration, "Questions and Answers about FDA's Initiative against Contaminated Weight Loss Products," September 2013, www.fda.gov/drugs/resourcesforyou/consumers/questionsanswers/ucm136187.htm; U.S. Food and Drug Administration, "Follow-Up to the November 2009 Early Communication about an Ongoing Safety Review of Sibutramine, Marketed as Meridia," January 2010, www.fda.gov/Drugs/DrugSafety/stmarketDrugSafetyInformationforPatientsandProviders/DrugSafetyInformationforHeathcareProfessionals/ucm198206.htm.
45. ConsumerSearch, "Diet Pills: Reviews," 2012, www.consumersearch.com/diet-pills
46. F. Rubino et al., "Metabolic Surgery to Treat Type 2 Diabetes: Clinical Outcomes and Mechanisms of Action," *Annual Review of Medicine* 61 (2010): 393–411; S. Brethauer et al., "Can Diabetes Be Surgically Cured? Long-term Metabolic Effects of Bariatric Surgery in Obese Patients with Type 2 Diabetes Mellitus," *Annals of Surgery* 258, no. 4 (2013): 628–37.
47. D. E. Arterburn et al., "A Multi-Site Study of Long Term Remission and Relapse of Type 2 Diabetes Mellitus Following Gastric Bypass Obesity Surgery," *Obesity Surgery* 23, no. 1 (2013): 93–102; C. D. Still et al., "Preoperative Prediction of Type 2 Diabetes Remission after Roux-en-Y Gastric Bypass Surgery: A Retrospective Cohort Study," *The Lancet Diabetes & Endocrinology* 2, no. 1 (2014): 38–45.
48. J. S. Blake, *Nutrition and You*, 2nd ed. (San Francisco, CA, Pearson Education, 2011).
49. University of the West of England, "30% of Women Would Trade at Least One Year of Their Life to Achieve Their Ideal Body Weight and Shape," March 2011, http://info.uwe.ac.uk/news/UWENews/news.aspx?id=1949.
50. University of Minnesota Health Talk, "Social Media May Inspire Unhealthy Body Image," May 2013, www.healthtalk.umn.edu/2013/05/15/thigh-gap-and-social-media.
51. Ibid.
52. Centers for Disease Control and Prevention, "FASTSTATS: Obesity and Overweight," November 2013, www.cdc.gov/nchs/fastats/overwt.htm.
53. J. B. Webb et al., "Do You See What I See?: An Exploration of Inter-Ethnic Ideal Body Size Comparisons among College Women," *Body Image* 10, no. 3 (2013): 369–79.
54. Mayo Clinic Staff, "Body Dysmorphic Disorder," May 2013, www.mayoclinic.com/health/body-dysmorphic-disorder/DS00559.
55. J. D. Feusner et al., "Abnormalities of Object Visual Processing in Body Dysmorphic Disorder," *Psychological Medicine* 41, no. 11 (2011): 2385–97, DOI: 10.1017/S0033291711000572.
56. Body Image Health, "The Model for Healthy Body Image and Weight," Accessed May 2014, http://bodyimagehealth.org/model-for-healthy-body-image.
57. I. Ahmed et al., "Body Dysmorphic Disorder," Medscape Reference, Updated January 2014, http://emedicine.medscape.com/article/291182-overview.
58. Mayo Clinic Staff, "Body Dysmorphic Disorder," 2013; KidsHealth, "Body Dysmorphic Disorder," May 2013, http://kidshealth.org/parent/emotions/feelings/bdd.html.
59. I. Ahmed et al., "Body Dysmorphic Disorder," Medscape Reference, Updated January 2014, http://emedicine.medscape.com/article/291182-overview.
60. J. Reel, *Eating Disorders: An Encyclopedia of Causes, Treatment and Prevention*, Portsmouth, NH: Greenwood Publishing, 2013); A. Taheri et al., "The Relationship between Social Physique Anxiety and Anthropometric Characteristics of the Nonathletic Female Students," *Annals of Biological Research* 3, no. 6 (2012): 2727–29; A. Sicilia et al, "Exercise Motivation and Social Physique Anxiety in Adolescents," *Psychologica Belgica* 54, no. 1 (2014): 111–29, DOI: http://dx.doi.org/10.5334/pb.ai.
61. American Psychiatric Association, *Diagnostic and Statistical Manual of Mental Disorders*, 5th ed. (Washington, DC: American Psychiatric Association, 2013).
62. Academy for Eating Disorders, "Prevalence of Eating Disorders," 2014, www.aedweb.org/Prevalence_of_ED.htm.
63. American College Health Association, *National College Health Assessment II: Reference Group Executive Summary, Fall 2013* (Hanover, MD: American College Health Association, 2014), Available at www.acha-ncha.org/reports_ACHA-NCHAII.html.
64. L. M. Gottschlich, "Female Athlete Triad," Medscape Reference, Drugs, Diseases & Procedures, January 25, 2012, http://emedicine.medscape.com/article/89260-overview#a0156.
65. Alliance for Eating Disorders, What Are Eating Disorders?, 2013, www.allianceforeatingdisorders.com/portal/what-are-eating-disorders#.Uycs4_Pn9lY.
66. Ibid.
67. S. A. Swanson, et al., "Prevalence and Correlates of Eating Disorders in Adolescents: Results from the National Comorbidity Survey Replication Adolescent Supplement," *Archives of General Psychiatry* 68, no. 7 (2011): 714–23, DOI: 10.1001/archgenpsychiatry.2011.22.
68. American Psychiatric Association, *Diagnostic and Statistical Manual of Mental Disorders*, 2013.
69. National Eating Disorders Association, "Anorexia Nervosa," www.nationaleatingdisorders.org/anorexia-nervosa.
70. P. Crocker et al., "Body-Related State Shame and Guilt in Women: Do Causal Attributions Mediate the Influence of Physical Self-Concept and Shame and Guilt Proneness," *Body Image* 11, no. 1 (2013): 19–26; A. R. Smith, T. E. Joiner, and D. R. Dodd, "Examining Implicit Attitudes Toward Emaciation and Thinness in Anorexia Nervosa," *International Journal of Eating Disorders* 47, no. 2 (2013): 138–47; R. N. Carey, N. Donaghue, and P. Broderick, "Concern among Australian Adolescent Girls: The Role of Body Comparisons with Models and Peers," *Body Image* 11, no. 1 (2014): 81–84.
71. A.D.A.M. Medical Encyclopedia, U.S. National Library of Medicine, "Anorexia Nervosa," February 2013, www.ncbi.nlm.nih.gov/pubmedhealth/PMH0001401; B. Suchan et al., "Reduced Connectivity between the Left Fusiform Body Area and the Extrastriate Body Area in Anorexia Nervosa Is Associated with Body Image Distortion," *Behavioural Brain Research* 241 (2013): 80–85, DOI: 10.1016/j.bbr.2012.12.002; G. Frank et al., "Altered Temporal Difference Learning in Bulimia Nervosa," *Biological Psychiatry* 70, no. 8 (2011): 728–35, DOI: 10.1016/j.biopsych.2011.05.011.
72. R. Kessler et al., "The Prevalence and Correlates of Binge Eating Disorder in the World Health Organization World Mental Health Surveys," *Biological Psychiatry* 73, no. 9 (2013): 904–14, DOI: 10.1016/j.biopsych.2012.11.020.
73. American Psychiatric Association, "DSM-5 Feeding and Eating Disorders," 2013 www.dsm5.org/documents/eating%20disorders%20fact%20sheet.pdf
74. National Institute of Mental Health, "Eating Disorders," January 2013, www.nimh.nih.gov/health/topics/eating-disorders/index.shtml.
75. T. A. Oberndorfer et al., "Altered Insula Response to Sweet Taste Processing after Recovery from Anorexia and Bulimia Nervosa," *American Journal of Psychiatry* 170, no.10 (2013): 1143–51.

76. Mayo Clinic, "Binge–Eating Disorder," April 2012, www.mayoclinic.com/health/binge-eating-disorder/DS00608.
77. R. Kessler et al., "The Prevalence and Correlates of Binge Eating Disorder in the World Health Organization World Mental Health Surveys," 2013.
78. Castlewood Treatment Center for Eating Disorders, "Binge Eating Disorder DSM-V," January 2012, www.castlewoodtc.com.
79. K. N. Franco, Cleveland Clinic Center for Continuing Education, "Eating Disorders," 2011, www.clevelandclinicmeded.com/medicalpubs/diseasemanagement/psychiatry-psychology/eating-disorders; Mirasol Eating Disorder Recovery Centers, "Eating Disorder Statistics," Accessed March 2014, www.mirasol.net/eating-disorders/information/eating-disorder-statistics.php.
80. H. Goodwin, E. Haycraft, and C. Meyer, "The Relationship between Compulsive Exercise and Emotion Regulation in Adolescents," *British Journal of Health Psychology* 17, no. 4, (2012): 699–10.
81. J. J. Waldron, "When Building Muscle Turns into Muscle Dysmorphia," *Association for Sport Applied Psychology*, Accessed March 2014, www.appliedsportpsych.org/resource-center/health-fitness-resources/when-building-muscle-turns-into-muscle-dysmorphia.
82. M. Silverman, "What Is Muscle Dysmorphia?," Massachusetts General Hospital, February 18, 2011, https://mghocd.org/what-is-muscle-dysmorphia/; J. J. Waldron, "When Building Muscle Turns into Muscle Dysmorphia," 2014.
83. L. M. Gottschlich et al., "Female Athlete Triad," *Medscape Reference*, Accessed March 2014, http://emedicine.medscape.com/article/89260-overview.

Pulled Statistic

page 206, C. D. Fryar and R. B. Ervin, "Caloric Intake from Fast Food among Adults: United States, 2007–2010," NCHS Data Brief, no. 114 (2013), www.cdc.gov

Chapter 10

1. Centers for Disease Control and Prevention, " Behavioral Risk Factor Surveillance System Prevalence and Trends Data," Accessed March 2014, http://apps.nccd.cdc.gov/BRFSS/display.asp?yr=2012&state=US&qkey=8041&grp=0&SUBMIT3=Go.
2. C. E. Garber et al., "American College of Sports Medicine Position Stand: Quantity and Quality of Exercise for Developing and Maintaining Cardiorespiratory, Musculoskeletal and Neuromotor Fitness in Apparently Healthy Adults: Guidance for Prescribing Exercise," *Medicine and Science in Sports and Exercise* 33, no. 7 (2011): 1334–59, DOI: 10.1249/MSS.0b013e318213fefb.
3. American College Health Association, *American College Health Association-National College Health Assessment II (ACHA-NCHA II) Reference Group Executive Summary, Fall 2013* (Hanover, MD: American College Health Association, 2014), Available at www.acha-ncha.org/reports_ACHA-NCHAII.html.
4. National Heart, Lung, and Blood Institute, U.S. Department of Health and Human Services, National Institutes of Health, "What Is Physical Activity," Updated September 2011, www.nhlbi.nih.gov/health/health-topics/topics/phys/; Office of Disease Prevention and Health Promotion, *2008 Physical Activity Guidelines for Americans, 2008*, Available at www.health.gov/paguidelines.
5. P. Kokkinos, H. Sheriff, and R. Kheirbek, "Physical Inactivity and Mortality Risk," *Cardiology Research and Practice*, 11 (2011): 924–49. www.hindawi.com/journals/crp/2011/924945. (Epub ahead of print.)
6. I. Lee et al., "Impact of Physical Inactivity on the World's Major Non-communicable Diseases," *Lancet* 380, no. 9838 (2012): 219–29.
7. S. Plowman and D. Smith, *Exercise Physiology for Health, Fitness, and Performance*, 3rd ed. (Philadelphia, PA: Lippincott Williams & Wilkins, 2011).
8. S. Grover et al., "Estimating the Benefits of Patient and Physician Adherence to Cardiovascular Prevention Guidelines: The MyHealthCheckup Survey," *Canadian Journal of Cardiology* 27, no. 2 (2011): 159–66.
9. American Heart Association, "About Cholesterol," Updated May 2013, www.heart.org/HEARTORG/Conditions/Cholesterol/AboutCholesterol/AboutCholesterol_UCM_001220_Article.jsp.
10. L. Montesi et al., "Physical Activity for the Prevention and Treatment of Metabolic Disorders," *Internal and Emergency Medicine* 8, no. 8 (2013): 655–66.
11. Ibid.
12. D. C. Lee et al. "Changes in Fitness and Fatness on the Development of Cardiovascular Disease Risk Factors Hypertension, Metabolic Syndrome, and Hypercholesterolemia," *Journal of the American College of Cardiology* 59, no. 7 (2012): 665–72.
13. M. Uusitupa, J. Tuomilehto, and P. Puska, "Are We Really Active in the Prevention of Obesity and Type 2 Diabetes at the Community Level?," *Nutrition and Metabolism in Cardiovascular Diseases* 21, no. 5 (2011): 380–89, DOI: 10.1016/j.numecd.2010.12.007.
14. National Diabetes Information Clearinghouse, U.S. Department of Health and Human Services, *Diabetes Prevention Program (DPP)*, NIH Publication no. 09–5099 (Bethesda, MD: National Diabetes Information Clearinghouse, 2008), Available at http://diabetes.niddk.nih.gov/dm/pubs/preventionprogram.
15. N. Magné et al., "Recommendations for a Lifestyle Which Could Prevent Breast Cancer and Its Relapse: Physical Activity and Dietetic Aspects," *Critical Reviews in Oncology and Hematology* 80, no. 3 (2011): 450–59, DOI: 10.1016/j.critrevonc.2011.01.013.
16. L. H. Kushi et al., "American Cancer Society Guidelines on Nutrition and Physical Activity for Cancer Prevention," *CA: A Cancer Journal for Clinicians* 62, no. 1 (2012): 30–67.
17. World Cancer Research Fund/American Institute for Cancer Research, Policy and Action for Cancer Prevention, "Food, Nutrition, and Physical Activity: A Global Perspective" (Washington DC: AICR, 2009); A. Shibata, K. Ishii, and K. Oka, "Psychological, Social, and Environmental Factors of Meeting Recommended Physical Activity Levels for Colon Cancer Prevention among Japanese Adults," *Journal of Science and Medicine in Sport* 12, no. 2 (2010): e155–56; K. Y. Wolin et al., "Physical Activity and Colon Cancer Prevention: A Meta-Analysis," *British Journal of Cancer* 100, no. 4 (2009): 611–16.
18. C. M. Friedenreich and A. E. Cust, "Physical Activity and Breast Cancer Risk: Impact of Timing, Type, and Dose of Activity and Population Subgroup Effects," *British Journal of Sports Medicine* 42, no. 8 (2008): 636–47.
19. M. Nilsson et al., "Increased Physical Activity Is Associated with Enhanced Development of Peak Bone Mass in Men: A Five Year Longitudinal Study," *Journal of Bone and Mineral Research* 27, no. 5 (2012): 1206–14, DOI: 10.1002/jbmr.1549; M. Callréus et al., "Self-Reported Recreational Exercise Combining Regularity and Impact Is Necessary to Maximize Bone Mineral Density in Young Adult Women: A Population-Based Study of 1,061 Women 25 Years of Age," *Osteoporosis International* 23, no. 10 (2012): 2517–26, DOI: 10.1007/s00198-011-1886-5.
20. R. Rizzoli, C. A. Abraham, and M. L. Brandi, "Nutrition and Bone Health: Turning Knowledge and Beliefs in Healthy Behavior," *Current Medical Research & Opinion* 30, no. 1 (2014): 131–41.
21. V. A. Catenacci et al., "Physical Activity Patterns Using Accelerometry in the National Weight Control Registry," *Obesity* 19, no. 6 (2011): 1163N70, DOI: 10.1038/oby.2010.264.
22. T. L. Gillum et al., "A Review of Sex Differences in Immune Function after Aerobic Exercise," *Exercise Immunology Review* 17 (2011): 104–20.
23. MedLine Plus, National Institutes of Health, "Exercise and Immunity," May 2012, www.nlm.nih.gov/medlineplus/ency/article/007165.htm.
24. N. P. Walsh et al., "Position Statement. Part Two: Maintaining Immune Health," *Exercise and Immunology Review* 17 (2011): 64–103.
25. T. L. Gillum et al., "A Review of Sex Differences in Immune Function after Aerobic Exercise," *Exercise Immunology Review* 17 (2011): 104–20.
26. C. Huang et al., "Cardiovascular Reactivity, Stress, and Physical Activity," *Frontiers in Physiology* 4(2013): 1–13, DOI:10.3389/fphys.201300314.
27. T. M. Burkhalter and C. H. Hillman, "A Narrative Review of Physical Activity, Nutrition, and Obesity to Cognitive and Scholastic Performance across the Human Lifespan," *Advances in Nutrition: An International Review Journal* 2, no. 2 (2011): 201S–206S.
28. J. E. Ashlskog, Y. E. Geda, N. R. Graff-Radford, and R. C. Petersen, "Physical Exercise as a Preventive or Disease-Modifying Treatment of Dementia and Brain Aging," *Mayo Clinic Proceedings* 86, no. 9 (2011): 876–84.
29. J. Berry et al., "Lifetime Risks for Cardiovascular Disease Mortality by Cardiorespiratory Fitness Levels Measured at Ages 45, 55, and 65 Years in Men: The Cooper Center Longitudinal Study," *Journal of the American College of Cardiology* 57, no. 15 (2011): 1604–10; J. Woodcock et al., "Non-Vigorous Physical Activity and All-Cause Mortality: Systematic Review and Meta-Analysis of Cohort Studies," *International Journal of Epidemiology* 40, no. 1 (2011): 121–38.
30. C. E. Garber et al., "American College of Sports Medicine Position Stand," 2011.
31. Ibid.
32. T. Gotschi and K. Mills, *Active Transportation for America: The Case for Increased Federal Investment in Bicycling and Walking* (Washington, DC: Rails to Trails Conservancy, 2008), Available at www.railstotrails.org/ourwork/advocacy/activetransportation/makingthecase; D. Shinkle and A. Teigens, *Encouraging Bicycling and Walking: The State Legislative Role* (Washington, DC: National Conference of State Legislatures, 2008), Updated April 2009, Available at www.americantrails.org/resources/trans/Encourage-Bicycling-Walking-State-Legislative-Role.html.
33. Ibid; U.S. Environmental Protection Agency, "Climate Change: What You Can Do—On the Road," Updated September 2013, www.epa.gov/climatechange/wycd/road.html.
34. C. E. Garber et al., "American College of Sports Medicine Position Stand," 2011.
35. American College of Sports Medicine, *ACSM's Resource Manual for Guidelines for Exercise Testing and Prescription* (Philadelphia, PA: Lippincott Williams & Wilkins, 2014).

36. W. Micheo, L. Baerga, and G. Miranda, "Basic Principles Regarding Strength, Flexibility, Flexibility, and Stability Exercises," *Physical Medicine & Rehabilitation* 4, no. 11 (2012): 805–11, DOI: 10.1016/j.pmrj.2012.09.583; C. E. Garber et al., "American College of Sports Medicine Position Stand," 2011.
37. C. E. Garber et al., "American College of Sports Medicine Position Stand," 2011.
38. Ibid.
39. D. G. Behm and A. Chaouachi, "A Review of the Acute Effects of Static and Dynamic Stretching on Performance," *European Journal of Applied Physiology*, March 4, 2011, 21373870. (Epub ahead of print.)
40. K. C. Huxel Bliven and B. E. Anderson, "Core Stability Training for Injury Prevention," *Sports Health: A Multidisciplinary Approach* 5, no. 6 (2013): 514–22.
41. V. Baltzpoulos, "Isokinetic Dynamometry," in *Biomechanical Evaluation of Movement in Sport and Exercise: The British Association of Sport and Exercise Sciences Guidelines*, eds. C. Payton and R. Bartlett (New York, NY: Routledge, 2008), 105.
42. D. G. Behm and J. C. Colao Sanchez, "Instability Resistance Training across the Exercise Continuum," *Sports Health: A Multidisciplinary Approach* 5, no. 6 (2013): 500–503.
43. Ibid.
44. P. Williamson, *Exercise for Special Populations* (Philadelphia, PA: Lippincott Williams & Wilkins, 2011).
45. Ibid.
46. Ibid.
47. Ibid.
48. W. J. Chodzko-Zajko et al., "American College of Sports Medicine Position Stand: Exercise and Physical Activity for Older Adults," *Medicine and Science in Sports and Exercise* 41, no. 7 (2009): 1510–30.
49. M. N. Sawka et al., "American College of Sports Medicine Position Stand: Exercise and Fluid Replacement," *Medicine and Science in Sports and Exercise* 39, no. 2 (2007): 377–90.
50. Ibid.
51. S. Cutts, N. Obi, C. Pasapula, and W. Chan, "Plantar Fasciitis," *Annals of the Royal College of Surgeons of England* 94, no.8 (2012): 539–42.
52. P. Newman et al., "Risk Factors Associated with Medial Tibial Stress Syndrome in Runners: A Systematic Review and Meta-analysis," *Open Access Journal of Sports Medicine* 4 (2013): 229–41.
53. J. A. Rixe et al., "A Review of the Management of Patellofemoral Pain Syndrome," *The Physician and Sports Medicine* 41, no. 3 (2013): 19–28.
54. K. B. Fields et al., "Prevention of Running Injuries," *Current Sports Medicine Reports* 9, no. 3 (2010): 176–82.
55. American Academy of Ophthalmology, "Eye Health in Sports and Recreation," March 2014, www.aao.org/eyesmart/injuries/eyewear.cfm.
56. Ibid.
57. Bicycle Helmet Safety Institute, "Helmet-Related Statistics from Many Sources," January 2014, www.helmets.org/stats.htm.
58. American College Health Association, *American College Health Association-National College Health Assessment II: Reference Group Executive Summary, Fall 2013*, 2014.
59. Bicycle Helmet Safety Institute, "Helmet-Related Statistics from Many Sources," January 2014, www.helmets.org/stats.htm.
60. N. G. Nelson et al., "Exertional Heat-Related Injuries Treated in Emergency Departments in the U.S., 1997–2006," *American Journal of Preventive Medicine* 40, no. 1 (2011): 54–60.
61. L. E. Armstrong et al., "The American Football Uniform: Uncompensable Heat Stress and Hyperthermic Exhaustion," *Journal of Athletic Training* 45, no. 2 (2010): 117–27.
62. E. E. Turk, "Hypothermia," *Forensic Science Medical Pathology* 6, no. 2 (2010): 106–15.
63. Ibid.

Pulled Statistic

page 230, C. E. Garber et al., "American College of Sports Medicine Position Stand: Quantity and Quality of Exercise for Developing and Maintaining Cardiorespiratory, Musculoskeletal and Neuromotor Fitness in Apparently Healthy Adults: Guidance for Prescribing Exercise," *Medicine and Science in Sports and Exercise* 43, no. 7 (2011): 1334–59.

Chapter 11

1. A. S. Go et al., "Heart Disease and Stroke Statistics—2014 Update: A Report from the American Heart Association," *Circulation* (2014) 129:e28-e292.
2. The International Diabetes Federation, *Diabetes Atlas*, 6th ed. 2014, Available at www.idf.org/diabetesatlas.
3. American Diabetes Association, "Fast Facts: Data and Statistics about Diabetes," March 2013, http://professional.diabetes.org/admin/UserFiles/0%20-%20Sean/FastFacts%20March%202013.pdf.
4. American Cancer Society, "Cancer Facts and Figures," Accessed May 2014, Available at www.cancer.org/research/cancerfactsstatistics/cancerfactsfigures2014/index.
5. American Cancer Society, "Cancer Facts and Figures," 2014.
6. A .S. Go et al., "Heart Disease and Stroke Statistics—2014 Update, 2014.
7. Ibid.
8. Ibid.
9. Ibid.
10. Ibid.
11. Ibid.
12. Ibid.
13. Ibid.
14. Ibid.
15. Ibid.
16. Ibid.
17. Ibid.
18. Ibid.
19. Ibid.
20. World Health Organization, "Cardiovascular Diseases (CVDs)—Key Facts," Accessed April 2014, www.who.int/mediacentre/factsheets/fs317/en/#.
21. Ibid.
22. A. S. Go et al., "Heart Disease and Stroke Statistics—2014 Update," 2014.
23. Centers for Disease Control and Prevention, Media Relations, *MMWR–Morbidity and Mortality Weekly Report*, News Synopsis for April 4, 2013, April 2013, www.cdc.gov/media/mmwrnews/2013/0404.html.
24. A. S. Go et al., "Heart Disease and Stroke Statistics—2014 Update," 2014.
25. Centers for Disease Control and Prevention, "High Blood Pressure Facts," March 2014, www.cdc.gov/bloodpressure/facts.htm.
26. A. S. Go et al., "Heart Disease and Stroke Statistics—2014 Update," 2014.
27. American Heart Association, "Peripheral Artery Disease: Undertreated and Understudied in Women," 2012, http://newsroom.heart.org/pr/aha/peripheral-artery-disease-undertreated-228645.aspx; A. S. Go et al., "Heart Disease and Stroke Statistics—2014 Update," 2014.
28. American Heart Association, "Peripheral Artery Disease: Undertreated and Understudied in Women," 2012, http://newsroom.heart.org/pr/aha/peripheral-artery-disease-undertreated-228645.aspx.
29. A.S. Go et al., "Heart Disease and Stroke Statistics—2014 Update," 2014.
30. Ibid.
31. Ibid.
32. B. M. Kissela et al., "Age at Stroke: Temporal Trends in Stroke Incidence in a Large, Biracial Population," *Neurology* 79, no. 17 (2012): 1781–87.
33. A. S. Go et al., "Heart Disease and Stroke Statistics—2014 Update," 2014.
34. Ibid.
35. Ibid.
36. Ibid.
37. Ibid.
38. Ibid.
39. C. J. L Murray et al., "The State of US Health, 1990–2010 Burden of Diseases, Injuries, and Risk Factors," *Journal of the American Medical Association* 310, no. 6 (2013): 591–608.
40. S. Gardener et al., "Dietary Patterns Associated with Alzheimer's Disease and Related Chronic Disease Risk: A Review," *Journal of Alzheimer's Disease and Parkinsonism* S10 (2013): 2161–460; S. Sharp et al., "Hypertension Is a Potential Risk Factor for Vascular Dementia: Systematic Review," *International Journal of Geriatric Psychiatry* 26, no. 7 (2011): 661–69; F. Testai and P. Gorelick, "Vascular Cognitive Impairment and Alzheimer's Disease: Are These Disorders Linked to Hypertension and Other Cardiovascular Risk Factors?," *Clinical Hypertension and Vascular Diseases*, Part 4 (2011): 195–210.
41. A. S. Go et al., "Heart Disease and Stroke Statistics—2014 Update," 2014.
42. S. Grundy et al., "Definition of Metabolic Syndrome. Report of the National Heart, Lung, and Blood Institute/American Heart Association Conference on Scientific Issues Related to Definition," *Circulation* 109, no. 2 (2011): 433–39.
43. A. S. Go et al., "Heart Disease and Stroke Statistics—2014 Update," 2014.
44. Ibid.
45. Ibid.
46. Ibid.
47. National Cancer Institute, "Fact Sheet: Harms of Smoking and Benefits of Quitting," January 2011, www.cancer.gov/cancertopics/factsheet/tobacco/cessation.
48. R. Chowdhury et al., "Association of Dietary, Circulating, and Supplement Fatty Acids with Coronary Risk: A Systematic Review and Meta-Analysis," *Annals of Internal Medicine* 160, no. 6 (2014): 398–406.
49. G. Schwarts et al., "Effects of Dalcetrapib in Patients with a Recent Acute Coronary Syndrome," *New England Journal of Medicine* 367, no. 22 (2012): 2089–2099; C. Zheng and M. Aikawa, "High Density Lipoproteins: From Function to Therapy," *American College of Cardiology* 60, no. 23 (2012): 2380–83.
50. K. M. Moon et al., "Lipoprotein-Associated Phospholipase A2 Is Associated with Atherosclerotic Stroke Risk: The Northern Manhattan Study," *PLoS ONE* 9, no. 1 (2014): e83393, DOI:10.1371/journal.pone.0083393; C. A. Garza et al., "The Association between Lipoprotein-Associated Phospholipse A2 and Cardiovascular Disease: A Systematic Review," *Mayo Clinic Proceedings* 82, no. 2 (2007): 159–65.

51. B. M. Sondermeijer et al., "Non-HDL Cholesterol vs. Apo B for Risk of Coronary Heart Disease in Healthy Individuals: The EPIC-Norfolk Prospective Population Study," *European Journal of Clinical Investigation* 43, no. 10 (2013): 1009–1015.
52. A. S. Go et al., "Heart Disease and Stroke Statistics—2014 Update," 2014.
53. Z. Wang et al., "Black and Green Tea Consumption and the Risk of Coronary Artery Disease: A Meta Analysis," *American Journal of Clinical Nutrition* 93, no. 3 (2011): 506–15; L. Hooper et al., "Effects of Chocolate, Cocoa, and Flavan-3-ols on Cardiovascular Health: A Systematic Review and Meta-analysis of Randomized Trials," *American Journal of Clinical Nutrition* 95, no. 3 (2012): 740–51.
54. Mayo Clinic, "Top 5 Lifestyle Changes to Reduce Cholesterol," September 2012, www.mayoclinic.org/diseases-conditions/high-blood-cholesterol/in-depth/reduce-cholesterol/art-20045935.
55. A. S. Go et al., "Heart Disease and Stroke Statistics—2014 Update,"2014.
56. Ibid.
57. A. Steptoe and M. Kivimaki, "Stress and Cardiovascular Disease: An Update on Current Knowledge," *Annual Review of Public Health* 34 (2013): 337–54; R. C. Thurston, M. Rewak, and L. D. Kubzansky, "An Anxious Heart: Anxiety and the Onset of Cardiovascular Diseases," *Progress in Cardiovascular Diseases* 55, no. 6: 524–37.
58. A. S. Go et al., "Heart Disease and Stroke Statistics—2014 Update," 2014.
59. American Heart Association, "Understand Your Risk of Heart Attack," October 2012, www.heart.org/HEARTORG/Conditions/HeartAttack/UnderstandYourRiskofHeartAttack/Understand-Your-Risk-of-Heart-Attack_UCM_002040_Article.jsp.
60. Ibid.
61. The Emerging Risk Factors Collaboration, "C-Reactive Protein, Fibrinogen and CVD Prediction," *New England Journal of Medicine* 367, no. 14 (2012): 1310–20.
62. D. Wald, J. Morris, and N. Wald, "Reconciling the Evidence on Serum Homocysteine and Ischemic Heart Disease: A Meta-Analysis," *PLoS ONE* 6, no. 2 (2011): e16473; J. Abraham and L. Cho, "The Homocysteine Hypothesis: Still Relevant to the Prevention and Treatment of Cardiovascular Disease?," *Cleveland Clinic Journal of Medicine* 77, no. 12 (2010): 911–18.
63. American Heart Association, "Homocysteine, Folic Acid, and Cardiovascular Disease," January 2012, www.heart.org/HEARTORG/GettingHealthy/NutritionCenter/Homocysteine-Folic-Acid-and-Cardiovascular-Disease_UCM_305997_article.jsptsite.com/html/stent.html.
64. Heartsite, "Coronary Stents," Available at http://www.heartsite.com/html/stent.html.
65. C. M. Rembold, "Review: Aspirin Does Not Reduce CHD or Cancer Mortality But Increases Bleeding," *Annals of Internal Medicine* 156, no. 12 (2012): JC6–3; C. Ling et al., "Aspirin to Prevent Incident Cardiovascular Disease: Is It Causing More Damage Than It Prevents?," *Clinical Practice* 9, no. 3 (2012): 223–25.
66. American Heart Association, "Prevention and Treatment of Heart Attack," January 2013, www.heart.org/HEARTORG/Conditions/HeartAttack/PreventionTreatmentofHeartAttack/Prevention-and-Treatment-of-Heart-Attack_UCM_002042_Article.jsp .
67. A. S. Go et al., "Heart Disease and Stroke Statistics—2014 Update," 2014.
68. American Cancer Society, "Cancer Facts and Figures 2014," 2014, www.cancer.org/research/cancerfactsstatistics/cancerfactsfigures2014/index.
69. Ibid.
70. Ibid.
71. Ibid.
72. U.S. Surgeon General, "The Health Consequences of Smoking—50 Years of Progress: A Report of the Surgeon General, 2014," 2014, www.surgeongeneral.gov/library/reports/50-years-of-progress/index.html.
73. Ibid; American Cancer Society, "Cancer Facts and Figures 2014," 2014, www.cancer.org/research/cancerfactsstatistics/cancerfactsfigures2014/index; Centers for Disease Control and Prevention, "Tobacco Use: Targeting the Nation's Leading Killer—At-a-Glance 2011," Accessed May 2014, www.cdc.gov/chronicdisease/resources/publications/aag/pdf/2011/tobacco_aag_2011_508.pdf.
74. American Cancer Society, "Cancer Facts and Figures 2014," 2014.
75. W. Chen et al., "Moderate Alcohol Consumption During the Adult Life, Drinking Patterns and Breast Cancer Risk," *Journal of the American Medical Association* 306, no. 17 (2011): 1884–90; S.Y. Park et al., "Alcohol Consumption and Breast Cancer Risk among Women from Five Ethnic Groups with Light to Moderate Intake: The Multiethnic Cohort Study," *International Journal of Cancer* 134, no. 6 (2014): 1504–10.
76. American Cancer Society, "Cancer Facts and Figures 2014," 2014; D. Parkin, "Cancers Attributable to Consumption of Alcohol in the UK in 2010," *British Journal of Cancer* 105 (2011): S14–S18, DOI:10:10.1038/bjc.2011.476; National Cancer Institute, "Alcohol and Cancer Risk Sheet," Accessed May 2014, www.cancer.gov/cancertopics/factsheet/Risk/alcohol; I. Tramacere et al., "A Meta-Analysis on Alcohol Drinking and Gastric Cancer Risk," *Annals of Oncology* 23, no. 1 (2012): 28–36; S. Gupta et al., "Risk of Pancreatic Cancer by Alcohol Dose, Duration, and Pattern of Consumption, Including Binge Drinking: A Population-Based Study," *Cancer Causes & Control* 21, no. 7 (2010): 1047–59.
77. M. Jin et al., "Alcohol Drinking and All Cancer Mortality: A Meta-analysis," *Annals of Oncology* 24, no. 3 (2013): 807–16.
78. American Cancer Society, "Cancer Facts and Figures 2014," 2014.
79. C. Eheman et al., "Annual Report to the Nation on the Status of Cancer, 1975–2008, Featuring Cancers Associated with Excess Weight and Lack of Sufficient Physical Activity," *Cancer* 118, no. 9 (2012): 2338–66, DOI: 10.1002/cncr.27514/full; American Cancer Society, "Cancer Facts and Figures 2014," 2014.
80. H. R. Harris et al., "Body Fat Distribution and Risk of Premenopausal Breast Cancer in the Nurses' Health Study II," Journal of the National Cancer Institute 103, no. 3 (2011): 373–78.
81. American Cancer Society, "The Obesity-Cancer Connection and What We Can Do About it," February 2013, www.cancer.org/cancer/news/expertvoices/post/2013/02/28/the-obesity-cancer-connection-and-what-we-can-do-about-it.aspx; C. Eheman et al., "Annual Report to the Nation on the Status of Cancer, 1975–2008, Featuring Cancers Associated with Excess Weight and Lack of Sufficient Physical Activity," *Cancer* 118, no. 9 (2012): 2338–66, DOI: 10.1002/cncr.27514/full.
82. American Cancer Society, Cancer Facts and Figures 2014, 2014.
83. American Cancer Society, "Breast Cancer Overview: What Causes Breast Cancer?" January 2014, www.cancer.org/Cancer/BreastCancer/DetailedGuide/breast-cancer-what-causes.
84. American Cancer Society, "Cancer Facts and Figures for Hispanic/Latinos, 2012–2014," 2014, Available at www.cancer.org/acs/groups/content/@epidemiologysurveilance/documents/document/acspc-034778.pdf; M. Banegas et al., "The Risk of Developing Invasive Breast Cancer in Hispanic Women," *Cancer* 119, no. 7 (2013): 1373–80.
85. American Cancer Society, "Menopausal Hormone Therapy and Cancer Risk," 2013, www.cancer.org/Cancer/CancerCauses/OtherCarcinogens/MedicalTreatments/menopausal-hormone-replacement-therapy-and-cancer-risk; J. Manson et al., "Menopausal Hormone Therapy and Health Outcomes During the Intervention and Extended Poststopping Phases of the Women's Health Initiative Randomized Trials," *JAMA* 310, no. 13 (2013): 1353–68; A. Pesatori et al., "Reproductive and Hormonal Factors and Risk of Lung Cancer: The EAGLE Study," *International Journal of Cancer* 132, no. 11 (2013): 2630–39.
86. Y. Guo et al., "Association between C-reactive Protein and Risk of Cancer: A Meta-Analysis of Prospective Cohort Studies," *Asian Pacific Journal of Cancer Prevention* 14 (2013), DOI: http://dx.doi.org/10.7314/APJCP.2013.14.1.243.
87. S. Grivennikov, F. Gretan, and M. Karin, "Immunity, Inflammation, and Cancer," *Cell* 140, no. 6 (2010): 883–99, DOI: 10.1016/j.cell.2010.01.025.
88. American Cancer Society, "Infectious Agents and Cancer," March 2014, www.cancer.org/Cancer/CancerCauses/OtherCarcinogens/InfectiousAgents/InfectiousAgentsandCancer/infectious-agents-and-cancer-intro.
89. American Cancer Society, "Expert Voices: Viruses, Bacteria and Cancer, or It's Not All Smoke and Sunlight," March 2012, www.cancer.org/cancer/news/expertvoices/post/2012/03/04/viruses-bacteria-and-cancer-or-ite28099s-not-all-smoke-and-sunlight.aspx; American Cancer Society, "Cancer Facts and Figures," 2014.
90. Centers for Disease Control and Prevention, "Human Papillomavirus Vaccination Coverage among Adolescent Girls, 2007-2012, and Postlicensure Vaccine Safety Monitoring, 2006-2013-–United States," July 2013, www.cdc.gov/mmwr/preview/mmwrhtml/mm6229a4.htm; American Cancer Society, "Cancer Facts and Figures," 2014; National Cancer Institute, "Fact Sheet–HPV and Cancer," 2012, www.cancer.gov/cancertopics/factsheet/Risk/HPV.
91. American Cancer Society, "Cancer Facts and Figures," 2014.
92. American Cancer Society, "Infectious Agents and Cancer," Accessed May 2014, www.cancer.org/cancer/cancercauses/othercarcinogens/infectiousagents/infectiousagentsandcancer/infectious-agents-and-cancer-toc.
93. American Cancer Society, "Cancer Facts and Figures," 2014.
94. Ibid.
95. American Cancer Society, "Why Lung Cancer Strikes Nonsmokers," October 2013, www.cancer.org/cancer/news/why-lung-cancer-strikes-nonsmokers.
96. American Cancer Society, "Cancer Facts and Figures," Accessed May 2014, Available at http://www.cancer.org/research/cancerfactsstatistics/cancerfactsfigures2014/index.
97. Centers for Disease Control and Prevention, "Smoking and Tobacco Use: Quitting Smoking,"

February 2014, www.cdc.gov/tobacco/data_statistics/fact_sheets/cessation/quitting/index.htm?utm_source=feedburner&utm_medium=feed&utm_campaign=Feed%3A+CdcSmokingAndTobaccoUseFactSheets+(CDC+-+Smoking+and+Tobacco+Use+-+Fact+Sheets).
98. American Cancer Society, "Colorectal Cancer Facts and Figures, 2014–2016," Accessed May 2014, Available at www.cancer.org/acs/groups/content/documents/document/acspc-042280.pdf; American Cancer Society, "Cancer Facts and Figures," 2014.
99. American Cancer Society, "Cancer Facts and Figures 2014," 2014.
100. Ibid.
101. American Cancer Society, "Colorectal Cancer Facts and Figures, 2014-2016," 2014, www.cancer.org/acs/groups/content/documents/document/acspc-042280.pdf.
102. Ibid; American Cancer Society, "Cancer Facts and Figures 2014," 2014.
103. American Cancer Society, "Colorectal Cancer Facts and Figures, 2014-2016," 2014, www.cancer.org/acs/groups/content/documents/document/acspc-042280.pdf.
104 S. London. "Colorectal Cancer Incidence rises sharply in younger adults." Oncology Practice. January. 2014. http://www.oncologypractice.com/single-view/colorectal-cancer-incidence-rising-sharply-among-younger-adults/a00ffbf510248b815e386d354d058b4b.html.
105. American Cancer Society, "Colorectal Cancer Facts and Figures, 2014-2016," 2014; American Cancer Society, "Cancer Facts and Figures 2014," 2014.
106. Ibid.
107. American Cancer Society, "Cancer Facts and Figures," 2014.
108. American Cancer Society, "Magnetic Resonance Imaging," January 2014, www.cancer.org/cancer/breastcancer/moreinformation/breastcancerearlydetection/breast-cancer-early-detection-a-c-s-recs-m-r-i.
109. American Cancer Society, "Cancer Facts and Figures," 2014.
110. Ibid.
111. Ibid.
112. Ibid.
113. Breast Cancer.org, "Genetics," April 2014, www.breastcancer.org/risk/factors/genetics.
114. Y. Wu, D. Zhang, and S. Kang, "Physical Activity and Risk of Breast Cancer: A Meta-Analysis of Prospective Studies," *Breast Cancer Research and Treatment* 137, no. 3 (2013): 869–82.
115. J. Dong et al., "Dietary Fiber Intake and Risk of Breast Cancer: A Meta-Analysis of Prospective Cohort Studies," *American Journal of Clinical Nutrition* 94, no. 3 (2011): 900–905; D. Aune et al. "Dietary Fiber and Breast Cancer Risks: A Systematic Review and Meta Analysis of Prospective Studies," *Annals of Oncology*, 2012: DOI:10.1093/annuls/mdr589.
116. American Cancer Society, "Cancer Facts and Figures 2014," 2014.
117. Ibid.
118. Ibid.
119. C. Heckman et al., "Psychiatric and Addictive Symptoms of Young Adult Female Indoor Tanners," *American Journal of Health Promotion* 28, no. 3 (2014): 168–74; C. Harrington et al., "Activation of the Mesostriatal Reward Pathway with Exposure to Ultraviolet Radiation (UVR) vs. Sham UVR in Frequent Tanners: A Pilot Study," *Addictive Biology* 17, no. 3 (2012): 680–86.
120. NCSL, "Indoor Tanning Restrictions for Minors—A State-by-State Comparison," May 2014, www.ncsl.org/research/health/indoor-tanning-restrictions.aspx; American College of Dermatology, "The Dangers of Indoor Tanning Beds," 2014, www.aad.org/spot-skin-cancer/understanding-skin-cancer/dangers-of-indoor-tanning; D. Lazovich et al., "Indoor Tanning and Risk of Melanoma: A Case-Control Study in a Highly Exposed Population," *Cancer Epidemiology Biomarkers and Prevention* 19, no. 6 (2010): 1557–68, DOI:10.1158/1055-9965.EPI-09-1249; National Cancer Institute, "Tanning Bed Study Shows Strongest Evidence Yet of Increased Melanoma Risk," *NCI Cancer Bulletin*, 2010, www.cancer.gov/ncicancerbulletin/060110/page2; Skin Cancer Foundation, "Skin Cancer Facts," 2012, www.skincancer.org/skin-cancer-information/skin-cancer-facts.
121. American Cancer Society, "Cancer Facts and Figures," 2014.
122. Ibid.
123. Ibid.
124. Ibid.
125. K. Zu et al. "Dietary Lycopene, Angiogenesis, and Prostate Cancer: A Prospective Study in the Prostate-Specific Antigen Era," *Journal of the National Cancer Institute* 106, no. 2 (2014): 1093–97 .
126. American Cancer Society, "Cancer Facts and Figures 2014," 2014.
127. American Cancer Society, "Cancer Facts and Figures 2014," 2014.
128. Ibid.
129. American Cancer Society, "Testicular Cancer," February 2014, www.cancer.org/cancer/testicularcancer/detailedguide/testicular-cancer-risk-factors; National Cancer Institute, "General Information about Testicular Cancer," December 2013, www.cancer.gov/cancertopics/pdq/treatment/testicular/Patient/page1#Keypoint2.
130. American Cancer Society, "Cancer Facts and Figures 2014," 2014.
131. Ibid.
132. Ibid.
133. Ibid.
134. Ibid.
135. Ibid.
136. National Cancer Institute, "Endometrial Cancer," 2012, www.cancer.gov/cancertopics/types/endometrial.
137. American Cancer Society, "Cancer Facts and Figures 2014," 2014.
138. Ibid.
139. The International Diabetes Federation, *Diabetes Atlas*, 6th ed., 2014.
140. Ibid.
141. E. Selvin et al., "Trends in Prevalence and Control of Diabetes in the United States, 1988–1994 and 1999–2010," *Annals of Internal Medicine* 160, no. 8 (2014): 517–25.
142. Ibid.
143. American Diabetes Association, "Fast Facts: Data and Statistics about Diabetes," 2013.
144. Centers for Disease Control and Prevention, "Summary Health Statistics for U.S. Adults: National Health Interview Survey, 2012," *Vital and Health Statistics* 10, no. 260 (2014), Available at www.cdc.gov/nchs/products/series/series10.htm.
145. American Diabetes Association, "Fast Facts: Data and Statistics about Diabetes," 2013.
146. Ibid.
147. American Diabetes Association, "Diabetes Basics: Type 1," Accessed May 2014, www.diabetes.org/diabetes-basics/type-1.
148. Ibid.
149. The National Diabetes Information Clearinghouse (NDIC), "National Diabetes Statistics: 2011," September 2013, http://diabetes.niddk.nih.gov/dm/pubs/statistics/#fast.
150. Centers for Disease Control and Prevention, "National Diabetes Fact Sheet: 2011," January 2014, www.cdc.gov/diabetes/pubs/factsheet11.htm.
151. D. Dabelea et al., "Is Prevalence of Type 2 Diabetes Increasing in Youth? The SEARCH for Diabetes in Youth Study," American Diabetes Association 72nd Scientific Sessions (Philadelphia, PA: June 8–12, 2012).
152. D. J. Pettitt et al., "Prevalence of Diabetes in U.S. Youth in 2009: The Search for Diabetes in Youth Study," *Diabetes Care* 37, no. 2 (2014): 402–408.
153. Ibid.
154. A. M. Kanaya et al., "Understanding the High Prevalence of Diabetes in U.S. South Asians Compared with Four Racial/Ethnic Groups: The MASALA and MESA Studies," *Diabetes Care* (2014), DOI:10.2337/dc13-2656; American Heart Association, "Statistical Fact Sheet, 2013 Update: Diabetes," 2013, Available at www.heart.org/idc/groups/heart-public/@wcm/@sop/@smd/documents/downloadable/ucm_319585.pdf.
155. R. Mihaescu et al., "Genetic Risk Profiling for Prediction of Type 2 Diabetes," *PLoS Currents* 3 (2011): DOI: 10.1371/currents.RRN1208; E. Ntzani, K. Evangelia, and F. Kavvoura, "Genetic Risk Factors for Type 2 Diabetes: Insights from the Emerging Genomic Evidence," *Current Vascular Pharmacology* 10, no. 2 (2012): 147–55.
156. J. Logue et al., "Association between BMI Measured within a Year After Diagnosis of Type 2 Diabetes and Mortality," *Diabetes Care* 36, no. 4 (2013): 887–93; M. Ashwell, P. Gunn, and S. Gibson, "Waist-to-Height Ratio Is a Better Screening Tool Than Waist Circumference and BMI for Adult Cardiometabolic Risk Factors: Systematic Review and Meta-Analysis," *Obesity Reviews* 13, no. 3 (2012): 275–86.
157. M. Schulze et al., "Body Adiposity Index, Body Fat Content and Incidence of Type 2 Diabetes," *Diabetologia* (2012), DOI. 10.1007/s00125-012-2499-z.
158. L. Bromley et al., "Sleep Restriction Decreases the Physical Activity of Adults at Risk for Type 2 Diabetes," *Sleep* 35, no. 7 (2012): 977–84, DOI:10.5665/sleep.1964.
159. S. Reutrakul and E. V. Cauter, "Interactions between Sleep, Circadian Function, and Glucose Metabolism: Implications for Risk and Severity of Diabetes," *Annals of the New York Academy of Sciences* 1311, no. 1 (2014): 151–73, DOI: 10.1111/nyas.12355A; A. Bonnefond et al., "Rare MTNRIB Variants Impairing Melatonin Receptor 1B Function Contribute to Type 2 Diabetes," *Nature Genetics* (2012), DOI: 10.1038/ng.1053; F. Cappuccio et al., "Quantity and Quality of Sleep and Incidence of Type 2 Diabetes: A Systematic Review and Meta-Analysis," *Diabetes Care* 33, no. 2 (2010): 414–20; R. Hancox and C. Landlus, "Association between Sleep Duration and Haemoglobin A1c in Young Adults," *Journal of Epidemiology & Community Health* (2011), DOI: 10.1136/jech-2011-200217. (Epub ahead of print.)
160. E. Donga et al., "A Single Night of Partial Sleep Deprivation Induces Insulin Resistance in Multiple Metabolic Pathways in Healthy Subjects," *Journal of Clinical Endocrinology and Metabolism* 95, no. 6 (2010): 2963–8, doi: 10.1210/jc.2009-2430; J. P. Chaput et al., "Short Sleep Duration as a Risk Factor for Development of the Metabolic Syndrome in Adults," *Preventive Medicine* 57, no. 6 (2013): 872–77; R. Hancox and C. Landlus,

"Associations between Sleep Duration and Haemoglobin," 2011.

161. E. Feracioli-Oda, A Qawasmi, and M. Bloch, "Meta-Analysis: Melatonin for the Treatment of Primary Sleep Disorders." *PLoS ONE* 8 no. 5 (2013): e63773; J. P. Chaput, J. McNeil, and J. P. Depres et al., "Short Sleep Duration," 2013; F. Cappuccio et al., "Quantity and Quality of Sleep," 2010.
162. M. Cosgrove, L. Sargeant, R. Caleyachetty and S. Griffin, "Work Related Stress and Type 2 Diabetes: A Systematic Review and Meta-Analysis," *Occupational Medicine* (2012), DOI: 10.1093/occmed/kqs002. (Epub ahead of print); T. Monk and D. J. Buysse, "Exposure to Shiftwork as a Risk Factor for Diabetes," *Journal of Biological Rhythms* 28, no. 5 (2013): 356–59; M. Novak et al., "Perceived Stress and Incidence of Type 2 Diabetes: A 35 Year Followup Study of Middle Aged Swedish Men," *Diabetic Medicine* 30, no. 1 (2013): e8–e16.
163. E. Puterman, N. Adler, K., Matthews and E. Epel, "Financial Strain and Impaired Fasting Glucose: The Moderating Role of Physical Activity in the Coronary Artery Risk Development in Young Adults Study," *Psychosomatic Medicine* 74, no. 2 (2012): 187–92.
164. P. Puustinen et al., "Psychological Distress Predicts the Development of Metabolic Syndrome: A Prospective Population-Based Study," *Psychosomatic Medicine* 73 (2011): 158–65.
165. Centers for Disease Control and Prevention, "National Diabetes Fact Sheet: 2011," January 2014, Available at www.cdc.gov/diabetes/pubs/factsheet11.htm.
166. National Heart Lung and Blood Institute, "What Is Metabolic Syndrome?," November 2011, www.nhlbi.nih.gov/health/dci/Diseases/ms/ms_whatis.html.
167. American Diabetes Association, "What is Gestational Diabetes?," March 2014, www.diabetes.org/diabetes-basics/gestational/what-is-gestational-diabetes.html.
168. Ibid.; C. Kim et al., "Gestational Diabetes and the Incidence of Type 2 Diabetes: A Systematic Review," *Diabetes Care* 25, no. 10 (2002): 1862–68; G. Chodick et al., "The Risk of Overt Diabetes Mellitus among Women with Gestational Diabetes: A Population-Based Study," *Diabetic Medicine* 27, no. 7 (2010): 779–85.
169. American Diabetes Association, "Fast Facts: Data and Statistics about Diabetes," March 2013, http://professional.diabetes.org/admin/UserFiles/0%20-%20Sean/FastFacts%20March%202013.pdf; American Diabetes Association, "Living with Diabetes: Complications," Accessed May 2014, www.diabetes.org/living-with-diabetes/complications/; K. Weinspach et al., "Level of Information about the Relationship between Diabetes Mellitus and Periodontitis—Results from a Nationwide Diabetes Information Program," *European Journal of Medical Research* 18, no. 1 (2013): 6, DOI: 10.1186/2047-783X-18-6.
170. National Kidney Foundation, "Fast Facts," January 2014, www.kidney.org/news/newsroom/factsheets/FastFacts.cfm.
171. American Diabetes Association, "Fast Facts: Data and Statistics about Diabetes," 2013.
172. Prevent Blindness America, "Diabetic Retinopathy Prevalence by Age," Accessed May 2014, www.visionproblemsus.org/diabetic-retinopathy/diabetic-retinopathy-by-age.html.
173. K. Behan, "New ADA Guidelines for Diagnosis, Screening of Diabetes," *Advance Laboratory* 20, no. 1 (2011): 22, Available at http://laboratory-manager.advanceweb.com.
174. American Diabetes Association, "Diagnosing Diabetes and Learning about Prediabetes," March 2014, www.diabetes.org/diabetes-basics/diagnosis.
175. Diabetes Prevention Program Research Group, "Reduction in the Incidence of Type 2 Diabetes in the Incidence of Type 2 Diabetes with Lifestyle Intervention or Metformin," *New England Journal of Medicine* 345 (2002): 393–403.
176. S. Jonnalagadda et al., "Putting the Whole Grain Puzzle Together: Health Benefits Associated with Whole Grains—Summary of American Society for Nutrition 2010 Satellite Symposium," *Journal of Nutrition* 41, no. 5 (2011): 10115–25.
177. R. Post et al., "Dietary Fiber for the Treatment of Type 2 Diabetes Mellitus: A Meta-Analysis," *Journal of the American Board of Family Medicine* 25, no. 1 (2012): 16–23; S. Bhupathiraju et al., "Glycemic Index, Glycemic Load and Risk of Type 2 Diabetes: Results from 3 Large US Cohorts and an Updated Meta-Analysis," *Circulation* 129, Supplement 1 (2014): AP140-AP140; A. Olubukola, P. English, and J. Pinkney, "Systematic Review and Meta-Analysis of Different Dietary Approaches to the Management of Type 2 Diabetes," *The American Journal of Clinical Nutrition* 97, no. 3 (2013): 505–16.
178. A. Wallin et al. "Fish Consumption, Dietary Long-Chain N-3 Fatty Acids, and the Risk of Type 2 Diabetes: Systematic Review and Meta Analysis of Prospective Studies," *Diabetes Care* 35, no. 4 (2012): 918–29; L. Djousse et al., "Dietary Omega-3 Fatty Acids and Fish Consumption and Risk of Type 2 Diabetes," *American Journal of Clinical Nutrition* 93, no. 1 (2011): 113–50.
179. American Diabetes Association, "What We Recommend," December 2013, www.diabetes.org/food-and-fitness/fitness/types-of-activity/what-we-recommend.html; National Diabetes Information Clearing House, "Diabetes Prevention Program," September 2013, http://diabetes.niddk.nih.gov/dm/pubs/preventionprogram/index.aspx.
180. S. R. Kashyap et al., "Metabolic Effects of Bariatric Surgery in Patients with Moderate Obesity and Type 2 Diabetes," *Diabetes Care* 36, no. 8 (2013): 2175–82.
181. P. R. Schauer et al., "Bariatric Surgery versus Intensive Medical Therapy for Diabetes-3 Year Outcomes," *New England Journal of Medicine* 2014, DOI:10.1056/NEJMoa1401329.
182. P. Poirier et al. on Behalf of the American Heart Association Obesity Committee of the Council on Nutrition, Physical Activity, and Metabolism, "Bariatric Surgery and Cardiovascular Risk Factors: A Scientific Statement from the American Heart Association," *Circulation* (March 2011), DOI:10.1161/CIR.0b013e3182149099. (Epub ahead of print.)

Pulled Statistics

page 256, A. S. Go et al., "Heart Disease and Stroke Statistics.—2014 Update: A Report from the American Heart Association," *Circulation*, (2014) 129:e28-e292.

page 270 , Centers for Disease Control and Prevention, "Lung Cancer Risk Factors," February 2013, www.cdc.gov.

page 278, American Cancer Society, "Cancer Facts and Figures 2014," May 2014, Available at http://www.cancer.org/research/cancerfactsstatistics/cancerfactsfigures2014/index.

page 280, American Diabetes Association, "Diabetes Fast facts," 2013, http://www.diabetes.org/diabetes-basics/diabetes-statistics.

page 281, Centers for Disease Control and Prevention. National Diabetes Statistics Report: Estimates of Diabetes and Its Burden in the United States, 2014. Atlanta, GA: U.S. Department of Health and Human Services; 2014.

page 285, Diabetes Prevention Program Research Group, "Reduction in the Incidence of Type 2 Diabetes in the Incidence of Type 2 Diabetes with Lifestyle Intervention or Metformin," New England Journal of Medicine 345 (2002): 393–403.

Chapter 12

1. S. Altizer et al., "Climate Change and Infectious Diseases: From Evidence to a Predictive Framework," *Science* 341, no. 6145 (2013): 514–19; WHO, "Climate Change and Infectious Disease," Accessed March 2014, www.who.int/globalchange/climate/en/chapter6.pdf.
2. Ibid; J. Remais et al., "Convergence of Non-communicable and Infectious Diseases in Low- and Middle-Income Countries," *International Journal of Epidemiology* 42, no. 1 (2013): 221–27, DOI:10.1093/ije/dys135; Environmental Protection Agency, "Climate Impacts on Human Health," April 2013, www.epa.gov/climatechange/effects/health.html; E. Shuman, "Global Climate Change and Infectious Diseases," *New England Journal of Medicine* 362 (2010): 1061–63.
3. B. T. Kerridge et al., "Conflict and Diarrheal and Related Diseases: A Global Analysis," *Journal of Epidemiology and Global Health* 3, no. 4 (2013): 269–77; K. F. Cann et al., "Extreme Water-Related Weather Events and Waterborne Disease," *Epidemiology and Infection* 141, no. 4 (2013): 671–86.
4. National Institute of Environmental Health Sciences, "NIH News—New Study Shows 32 Million Americans Have Autoantibodies That Target Their Own Tissues," 2012, www.nih.gov/news/health/jan2012/niehs-13.htm; National Institute of Arthritis and Musculoskeletal and Skin Diseases, "Understanding Autoimmune Diseases," October 2012, www.niams.nih.gov/Health_Info/Autoimmune/default.asp.
5. American Autoimmune Related Diseases Association, "Autoimmune Statistics," 2014, www.aarda.org/autoimmune_statistics.php; National Institute of Arthritis and Musculoskeletal and Skin Diseases, "Understanding Autoimmune Diseases," October 2012, www.niams.nih.gov/Health_Info/Autoimmune/default.asp.
6. Centers for Disease Control and Prevention, "2014 Recommended Immunizations for Adults by Age," 2014, www.cdc.gov/vaccines/schedules/downloads/adult/adult-schedule-easy-read.pdf; CDC, "Adult Vaccination, What Vaccines Are Recommended for You," Updated March 2014, www.cdc.gov/vaccines/adults/rec-vac.
7. Centers for Disease Control and Prevention, "Antibiotic Resistance Threats in the United States, 2013," April 2013, www.cdc.gov/drugresistance/threat-report-2013/pdf/ar-threats-2013-508.pdf; S. Stefani et al., "Methicillin-Resistant *Staphylococcus aureus* (MRSA): Global Epidemiology and Harmonization of Typing Methods," *International Journal of Antimicrobial Agents* 39, no. 4 (2012): 273–82, DOI: 10.1016/j.ijantimicag.2011.09.030; Centers for Disease Control and Prevention, "MRSA Fact Sheet," March 2014, www.cdc.gov/mrsa/pdf/MRSA_ConsumerFactSheet_F.pdf.
8. Centers for Disease Control and Prevention, "Antibiotic Resistance Threats in the United States, 2013," 2013; W. Jarvis, "Prevention and Control of Methicillin-Resistant *Staphylococcus aureus*: Dealing with Reality, Resistance, and Resistance to Reality," *Clinical Infectious Diseases* 50, no. 2 (2010): 218–20.
9. Centers for Disease Control and Prevention, "Scarlet Fever: A Group A Streptococcal

Infection," January 2014, www.cdc.gov/features/scarletfever.
10. Ibid.
11. Centers for Disease Control and Prevention, "Meningitis," April 2014, www.cdc.gov/meningitis/index.html; Centers for Disease Control and Prevention, "Meningococcal Disease: Technical and Clinical Information," April 2014, www.cdc.gov/vaccines/vpd-vac/mening/vac-mening-fs.htm.
12. World Health Organization, "Tuberculosis Fact Sheet," February 2013, www.who.int/mediacentre/factsheets/fs104/en/index.html; Centers for Disease Control and Prevention, "Tuberculosis (TB): Data and Statistics," March 2014, www.cdc.gov/tb/statistics/default.htm.
13. Centers for Disease Control and Prevention, "Tuberculosis (TB): Data and Statistics," 2014; Centers for Disease Control and Prevention, "Trends in Tuberculosis, 2012," September 2013, www.cdc.gov/tb/publications/factsheets/statistics/TBTrends.htm.
14. World Health Organization, "WHO Global Tuberculosis Report 2013: Executive Summary," Accessed April 2014, www.who.int/tb/publications/global_report/gtbr13_executive_summary.pdf?ua=1.
15. Ibid.
16. Centers for Disease Control and Prevention, "Tuberculosis," March 2014, www.cdc.gov/tb.
17. World Health Organization, "WHO Global Tuberculosis Report 2013," 2014.
18. S. Doerr, "Mononucleosis," 2012, www.emedicinehealth.com/script/main/art.asp?articlekey=58850&pf=3; Centers for Disease Control and Prevention, "Epstein-Barr Virus and Infectious Mononucleosis," 2012, www.cdc.gov/ncidod/diseases/ebv.htm.
19. Centers for Disease Control and Prevention, "Viral Hepatitis," March 2014, www.cdc.gov/hepatitis.
20. Centers for Disease Control and Prevention, "Reported Cases of Acute Hepatitis A, by State, United States, 2007–2011," August 2013, www.cdc.gov/hepatitis/Statistics/2011Surveillance/Table2.1.htm.
21. Centers for Disease Control and Prevention, "Viral Hepatitis Statistics and Surveillance—2011," August 2013, www.cdc.gov/hepatitis/Statistics/2011Surveillance/Commentary.htm#hepB; World Health Organization, "Global Report on Prevention and Control of Viral Hepatitis in WHO Member States," July 2013, www.who.int/csr/disease/hepatitis/global_report/en.
22. Ibid.
23. Centers for Disease Control and Prevention, "Hepatitis C FAQs for Health Professionals," Updated February 2014, www.cdc.gov/hepatitis/HCV/HCVfaq.htm.
24. Ibid.
25. Centers for Disease Control and Prevention, "Shingles Vaccination: What You Need to Know," November 2013, www.cdc.gov/vaccines/vpd-vac/shingles/vacc-need-know.htm#notGet-vaccine.
26. Centers for Disease Control and Prevention, "Measles: Make Sure Your Child Is Fully Immunized," March 2014, www.cdc.gov/features/measles.
27. Ibid.
28. National Institute of Allergy and Infectious Diseases, "Common Cold," May 2011, www.niaid.nih.gov/topics/commonCold/Pages/cause.aspx.
29. National Center for Complementary and Alternative Medicine, "Echinacea," April 2013, http://nccam.nih.gov/health/echinacea.
30. National Institute of Allergy and Infectious Diseases, "Common Cold: Prevention," April 2011, www.niaid.nih.gov/topics/commoncold/Pages/prevention.aspx.
31. Centers for Disease Control and Prevention, "Seasonal Influenza: Key Facts about Influenza (Flu) and Flu Vaccine," September 2013, www.cdc.gov/flu/keyfacts.htm.
32. Centers for Disease Control and Prevention, "Cold vs Flu?," September 2013, www.cdc.gov/flu/about/qa/coldflu.htm.
33. Centers for Disease Control and Prevention, "Types of Influenza Viruses," January 2014, www.cdc.gov/flu/about/viruses/types.htm.
34. Centers for Disease Control and Prevention, "Selecting the Viruses in the Seasonal Influenza (Flu) Vaccine," February 2014, www.cdc.gov/flu/about/season/vaccine-selection.htm.
35. Centers for Disease Control and Prevention, "Valley Fever Increasing in Some Southwestern States," March 2013, www.cdc.gov/media/releases/2013/p0328_valley_fever.html.
36. Ibid.
37. Centers for Disease Control and Prevention, "vCJD Factsheet (Variant Creutzfeldt-Jakob Disease)," February 2013, www.cdc.gov/ncidod/dvrd/vcjd/factsheet_nvcjd.htm.
38. Ibid.
39. Ibid.
40. Centers for Disease Control and Prevention, "Antibiotic Resistance Threats in the United States, 2013," April 2013, www.cdc.gov/drugresistance/threat-report-2013/pdf/ar-threats-2013-508.pdf; Centers for Disease Control and Prevention, "Get Smart: Know When Antibiotics Work: Fast Facts," November 2014, www.cdc.gov/getsmart/antibiotic-use/fast-facts.html.
41. Centers for Disease Control and Prevention, "West Nile Virus (WNV): Preliminary Maps and Data for 2013," January 2014, www.cdc.gov/westnile/statsMaps/preliminaryMapsData/index.html.
42. Ibid.
43. Ibid.
44. World Health Organization, "Cumulative Number of Confirmed Human Cases of Avian Influenza A (H5N1) Reported to WHO," January 2014, www.who.int/influenza/human_animal_interface/H5N1_cumulative_table_archives/en/index.html.
45. Ibid.
46. World Health Organization, "Factsheet on the World Malaria Report 2013," December 2013, www.who.int/malaria/media/world_malaria_report_2013.
47. Ibid.
48. Ibid.
49. CDC, "Antibiotic Resistance Threats in the United States, 2013," September 2013, www.cdc.gov/features/antibioticresistancethreats/; D. Meeker et al., "Nudging Guideline-Concordant Antibiotic Prescribing: A Randomized Clinical Trial," JAMA Internal Medicine 174, no 3 (2014): 425–31; Association for Professionals in Infection Control and Epidemiology, "Responsible Use of Antibiotics," 2013, www.apic.org; Association for Professionals in Infection Control and Epidemiology, "Antibiotics, Preserving Them for the Future," 2012, www.apic.org; Centers for Disease Control and Prevention, National Center for Emerging and Zoonotic Infectious Diseases, Division of Healthcare Quality Promotion, "Diseases/Pathogens Associated with Antimicrobial Resistance," Updated January 2013, www.cdc.gov/drugresistance/diseasesconnectedar.html; Centers for Disease Control and Prevention, National Center for Immunization and Respiratory Diseases, Division of Bacterial Diseases, "Antibiotic Resistance Questions & Answers," Updated November 2011, www.cdc.gov/getsmart/antibiotic-use/anitbiotic-resistance-faqs.html.
50. Planned Parenthood, 2014, Sexually Transmitted Diseases, www.plannedparenthood.org/health-topics/stds-hiv-safer-sex-101.htm.
51. Centers for Disease Control and Prevention, "Sexually Transmitted Disease Surveillance, 2012," March 2014, www.cdc.gov/std/stats12/default.htm.
52. Joint United Nations Programme on HIV/AIDS (UNAIDS) and World Health Organization (WHO), 2013 UNAIDS Report on the Global AIDS Epidemic (Geneva: UNAIDS, 2013), Available at www.unaids.org/en/resources/publications/2013/name,85053,en.asp.
53. Centers for Disease Control and Prevention, "Today's HIV/AIDS Epidemic," December 2013, www.cdc.gov/nchhstp/newsroom/docs/hivfactsheets/todaysepidemic-508.pdf.
54. AVERT, "Can You Get HIV From ...?," Updated 2012, www.avert.org/can-you-get-hiv-aids.htm.
55. Ibid.
56. World Health Organization, "Mother to Child Transmission of HIV," Accessed April 2014, www.who.int/hiv/topics/mtct/en.
57. Mayo Clinic Staff, "Tattoos: Understand Risks and Precautions," March 2012, www.mayoclinic.com/health/tattoos-and-piercings/MC00020.
58. M. Smith, "Researchers Report Treatment Clears HIV in Second Baby," MedPage Today, March 6, 2014, www.medpagetoday.com/MeetingCoverage/CROI/44630.
59. Centers for Disease Control and Prevention, "Chlamydia—CDC Fact Sheet, Detailed Version," January 2014, www.cdc.gov/std/chlamydia/STDFact-chlamydia-detailed.htm.
60. Centers for Disease Control and Prevention, "Conjunctivitis (Pink Eye) in Newborns," January 2014, www.cdc.gov/conjunctivitis/newborns.html.
61. MedlinePlus, "Pelvic Inflammatory Disease (PID)," Updated February 2014, www.nlm.nih.gov/medlineplus/ency/article/000888.htm; Mayo Clinic Staff, "Urinary Tract Infection: Risk Factors," August 2012, www.mayoclinic.com/health/urinary-tract-infection/DS00286/DSECTION=risk-factors.
62. Centers for Disease Control and Prevention, "Gonorrhea: CDC Fact Sheet," January 2014, www.cdc.gov/std/gonorrhea/stdfact-gonorrhea.htm.
63. Centers for Disease Control and Prevention, "Sexually Transmitted Disease Surveillance, 2012," March 2014, www.cdc.gov/std/stats12/default.htm.
64. Centers for Disease Control and Prevention, "Gonorrhea: CDC Fact Sheet," January 2014, www.cdc.gov/std/gonorrhea/stdfact-gonorrhea.htm.
65. Ibid.
66. MedlinePlus, "Pelvic Inflammatory Disease (PID)," Updated 2011, www.nlm.nih.gov; Mayo Clinic Staff, "Urinary Tract Infection: Risk Factors," 2012; Centers for Disease Control and Prevention, Division of STD Prevention, National Center for HIV/AIDS, Viral Hepatitis, STD, and TB Prevention, "Sexually Transmitted Diseases Surveillance, 2011: STDs in Women and Infants," Updated 2012, www.cdc.gov.
67. U.S. National Library of Medicine, "Epididymitis," Last review August 2012, www.ncbi.nlm.nih.gov; Centers for Disease Control and Prevention, "STD Treatment Guidelines 2010: Epididymitis," Updated January 2011, www.cdc.gov.
68. Centers for Disease Control and Prevention, "Syphilis—CDC Detailed Fact Sheet," January 2014, www.cdc.gov/std/syphilis/STDFact-Syphilis-detailed.htm.
69. Ibid.

70. Centers for Disease Control and Prevention, "Genital Herpes—CDC Fact Sheet, Detailed Fact Sheet," Modified February 2013, www.cdc.gov/std/herpes/stdfact-herpes-detailed.htm.
71. American Sexual Health Association, "Learn about Herpes: Fast Facts," 2014, www.ashastd.org/std-sti/Herpes/learn-about-herpes.html.
72. Ibid.
73. Centers for Disease Control and Prevention, "Genital HPV Infection—CDC Fact Sheet," March 2014, www.cdc.gov/std/HPV/STDFact-HPV.htm; American Sexual Health Association, "Overview and Fast Stats," Accessed April 2014, www.ashastd.org/std-sti/hpv/overview-and-fast-facts.html; Centers for Disease Control and Prevention, "What is HPV?," February 2013, www.cdc.gov/hpv/whatishpv.html.
74. Centers for Disease Control and Prevention, "What Is HPV?," 2013; Centers for Disease Control and Prevention, March 2014, "What Should I Know About Screening?," www.cdc.gov/cancer/cervical/basic_info/screening.htm; Centers for Disease Control and Prevention, "Cervical Cancer," March 2014, www.cdc.gov/cancer/cervical.
75. National Institute of Cancer, "HPV and Cancer," March 2012, www.cancer.gov/cancertopics/factsheet/Risk/HPV.
76. Centers for Disease Control and Prevention, "Vaccines and Preventable Diseases: HPV Vaccine—Questions & Answers," Reviewed July 2012, www.cdc.gov/vaccines/vpd-vac/hpv/vac-faqs.htm; American Cancer Society, 2014, "Human Papillomavirus (HPV), Cancer and HPV Vaccines—Frequently Asked Questions," Revised 2014, www.cancer.org/cancer/cancercauses/othercarcinogens/infectiousagents/hpv/humanpapillomavirusandhpvvaccinesfaq/index.
77. Ibid.
78. Centers for Disease Control and Prevention, "Genital/Vulvovaginal Candidiasis," February 2014, www.cdc.gov/fungal/diseases/candidiasis/genital/index.html.
79. Centers for Disease Control and Prevention, "Trichomoniasis: CDC Fact Sheet," August 2012, www.cdc.gov/std/trichomonas/STDFact-Trichomoniasis.htm.
80. Ibid.

Pulled Statistic

page 304, Centers for Disease Control and Prevention, "Incidence, Prevalence and Cost of Sexually Transmitted Infections in the United States," 2013, http://www.cdc.gov/std/stats/sti-estimates-fact-sheet-feb-2013.pdf

Chapter 13

1. World Health Organization, *World Report on Violence and Health* (Geneva, Switzerland: World Health Organization, 2002), Available at www.who.int/violence_injury_prevention/violence/world_report/en.
2. U.S. Department of Justice, Federal Bureau of Investigation, "Crime in the United States, Preliminary Semiannual Uniform Crime Report for January–June 2013," May 2014, www.fbi.gov/about-us/cjis/ucr/crime-in-the-u.s/2013/preliminary-semiannual-uniform-crime-report-january-june-2013.
3. American College Health Association, *American College Health Association—National College Health Assessment II: Reference Group Data Report, Fall 2013* (Hanover, MD: American College Health Association, 2014), Available at www.acha-ncha.org/reports_ACHA-NCHAII.html.
4. National Criminal Justice Reference Service, "Section 6: Statistical Overviews," *NCVRW Resource Guide*, 2012, http://bjs.ojp.usdoj.gov.
5. Center for Public Integrity, "Sexual Assault on Campus: A Frustrating Search for Justice," Updated February 2013, www.publicintegrity.org/accountability/education/sexual-assault-campus.
6. World Health Organization Violence Prevention Alliance, "The Ecological Framework," Accessed June 2014, www.who.int/violenceprevention/approach/ecology/en/index.html; Centers for Disease Control and Prevention, National Center for Injury Prevention and Control, "Understanding School Violence: Fact Sheet–2012," Accessed June 2014, www.cdc.gov/violenceprevention/pdf/schoolviolence_factsheet-a.pdf.
7. R. Felner and M. DeVries, " Poverty in Childhood and Adolescence: A Transectional–Ecological Approach to Understanding and Enhancing Resilience in Contexts of Disadvantage and Developmental Risks," *Handbook of Resilience in Children* (New York, NY: 2013): 105–26; American Psychological Association, "Violence and Socioeconomic Status," Accessed June 2014, www.apa.org/pi/ses/resources/publications/factsheet-violence.aspx.
8. World Health Organization Violence Prevention Alliance, "The Ecological Framework," 2014; J. H. Derzon, "The Correspondence of Family Features with Problem, Aggressive, Criminal and Violent Behaviors: A Meta-Analysis," *Journal of Experimental Criminology* 6, no. 3 (2010): 263–92, DOI: 10.1007/s11292-010-9098-0; L. Kiss et al., "Gender-based Violence and Socioeconomic Inequalities: Does Living in More Deprived Neighborhoods Increase Women's Risk of Intimate Partner Violence?" *Social Science and Medicine* 74, no. 8 (2012): 1172–79.
9. M. L. Hunt, A. W. Hughey, and M. G. Burke, "Stress and Violence in the Workplace and on Campus: A Growing Problem for Business, Industry and Academia," *Industry and Higher Education* 26, no. 1 (2012): 43–51.
10. T. Dishion, "A Developmental Model of Aggression and Violence: Microsocial and Macrosocial Dynamic within an Ecological Framework," *Handbook of Developmental Psychology* (New York: Springer US, 2014), 449–465.
11. R. Puff and J. Segher, *The Everything Guide to Anger Management: Proven Techniques to Understand and Control Anger* (Avon, MA: Adams Media, Inc. A Division of F. and W. Media, 2014).
12. C. J. Ferguson, "Genetic Contributions to Antisocial Personality and Behavior: a Meta-Analytic Review from an Evolutionary Perspective," *The Journal of Social Psychology* 150, no. 2 (2010): 160–80; D. Boisvert and J. Vaske, "Genetic Theories of Criminal Behavior," *The Encyclopedia of Criminology and Criminal Justice* (2014): 1–6.
13. W. Gunter and B. Newby, "From Bullied to Deviant: The Victim-Offender-Overlap among Bullying Victims," *Youth Violence and Juvenile Justice* (2014), DOI: 10.1177/1541204014521250 (Epub ahead of print.); M. M. Ttofi, D. P. Farrington, and F. Lösel, "School Bullying as a Predictor of Violence Later in Life: A Systematic Review and Meta-Analysis of Prospective Longitudinal Studies," *Aggression and Violent Behavior* 17, no. 5 (2012): 405–18.
14. K. M. Devries, J. C. Child, and L. J. Bacchus et al., "Intimate Partner Violence Victimization and Alcohol Consumption in Women: A Systematic Review and Meta-Analysis," *Addiction* 109 (2014): 379–391, DOI: 10.1111/add.12393; A. Abbey, "Alcohol's Role in Sexual Violence Perpetration: Theoretical Explanations, Existing Evidence and Future Directions," *Drugs and Alcohol Review* 30, no. 5 (2011): 481–85; J. M. Boden, D. M. Fergusen, and L. J. Horwood, "Alcohol Misuse and Violent Behavior: Findings from a 30-Year Longitudinal Study," *Drugs and Alcohol Dependence* 122 (2012): 135–41; United Nations Office on Drugs and Crime, "World Drug Report," 2013, http://www.unodc.org/unodc/secured/wdr/wdr2013/World_Drug_Report_2013.pdf; A. Sanderlund, K. O'Brian, and P. Kremer, et al. "The Association between Sports Participation, Alcohol Use and Aggression and Violence: A Systematic Review," *Journal of Science and Medicine in Sport* 17, no. 1 (2014): 2–7.
15. P. H. Smith et al., "Intimate Partner Violence and Specific Substance Use Disorders: Findings from the National Epidemiologic Survey on Alcohol and Related Conditions," *Psychology of Addictive Behaviors* 26, no. 2 (2012): 236–45.
16. A. Abbey, "Alcohol's Role in Sexual Violence Perpetration," 2011.
17. Ibid.
18. Mary McMurran, ed., *Alcohol-Related Violence Prevention and Treatment* (West Sussex, U.K.: John Wiley and Sons, 2013); K. Graham et al., "Alcohol-Related Negative Consequences among Drinkers Around the World," *Addiction* 106, no. 8 (2011): 1391–1405; A. Abbey, "Alcohol's Role in Sexual Violence Perpetration," 2011; J. M. Boden, D. M. Fergusson, and L. J. Horwood, "Alcohol Misuse and Violent Behavior," 2012.
19. W. Gunter and K. Daley, "Causal or Spurious? Using Propensity Score Matching to Detangle the Relationship between Violent Video Games and Violent Behavior," *Computers in Human Behavior* 4, no. 28 (2012): 1348–55.
20. T. Niederkrotenthaler et al., "Changes in Suicide Rates Following Media Reports of Celebrity Suicide: A Meta-Analysis," *Journal of Epidemiology and Community Health* 66, no. 11 (2012): 1037–42, DOI: 10.1136/jech-2011-200707.
21. R. A. Ramos et al., "Comfortably Numb or Just Yet Another Movie? Media Violence Exposure Does NOT Reduce Viewer Empathy for Victims of Real Violence among Primarily Hispanic Viewers," *Psychology of Popular Media Culture* 2, no. 1 (2013): 2–10.
22. ChildStats.Gov, "America's Children in Brief: Key National Indicators of Well-Being, 2012," Accessed June 2014, http://childstats.gov/pdf/ac2012/ac_12.pdf.
23. World Health Organization, *World Report on Violence and Health*, 2002.
24. Centers for Disease Control and Prevention, "Health, United States, 2013," May 2014, www.cdc.gov/nchs/data/hus/hus13.pdf.
25. Centers for Disease Control and Prevention, "Deaths: Preliminary Data for 2013," *National Vital Statistics Reports* 61, no. 6 (2012), Available at www.cdc.gov/nchs/data/nvsr/nvsr61/nvsr61_06.pdf; Centers for Disease Control and Prevention, "Faststats: Assault or Homicide," December 2013, www.cdc.gov/nchs/fastats/homicide.htm.
26. Centers for Disease Control and Prevention, National Center for Injury Prevention and Control, Web-Based Injury Statistics Query and Reporting System (WISQARS), 2011, www.cdc.gov; U.S. Department of Justice, Federal Bureau of Investigation, *Crime in the United States 2011*, 2012, www.fbi.gov.
27. D. Drysdale, W. Modzeleski, and A. Simons, "Campus Attacks: Targeted Violence Affecting Institutions of Higher Learning," Washington DC: United States Secret Service, United States Department of Education, and the Federal Bureau of Investigation,

2010; Brady Campaign to Prevent Gun Violence, "Facts: Gun Violence," Revised 2010, www.bradycampaign.org; S. Lewis, "Concealed Carry on Campus—Guns on Campus—College Campus Carry," *CNN Report*, 2011, www.campuscarry.com.
28. Ibid.
29. Federal Bureau of Investigation, "Hate Crime Statistics, 2012," November 2013, www.fbi.gov/news/stories/2013/november/annual-hate-crime-statistics-show-slight-decease/annual-hate-crime-statistics-show-slight-decrease.
30. Ibid.
31. Bureau of Justice Statistics, "Hate Crime Victimization—2004–2012—Statistical Tables," February 2014, www.bjs.gov/index.cfm?ty=pbdetail&iid=4883.
32. Ibid.
33. P. Lin and J. Gill, "Homicides of Pregnant Women," *Journal of Forensic Medicine and Pathology* (2010), DOI: 10-1097/PAF.obo13e3181d3dc3b.
34. Violence Policy Center, *American Roulette: Murder-Suicide in the United States*, 4th ed. (Washington, DC: Violence Policy Center, 2012), Available at www.vpc.org.
35. M. C. Black et al., *The National Intimate Partner and Sexual Violence Survey (NISVS): 2010 Summary Report* (Atlanta, GA: National Center for Injury Prevention and Control, Centers for Disease Control and Prevention, 2011), Available at www.cdc.gov.
36. L. Walker, *The Battered Woman* (New York, NY: Harper and Row, 1979).
37. L. Walker, *The Battered Woman Syndrome*, 3rd ed. (New York, NY: Springer, 2009).
38. Bureau of Justice Statistics, "Intimate Partner Violence, 1993–2010," November 2012, www.bjs.gov/index.cfm?ty=pbdetail&iid=4536.
39. U.S. Department of Health and Human Services Administration for Children and Families, "Definitions of Child Abuse and Neglect," February 2011, www.childwelfare.gov/systemwide/laws_policies/statutes/define.cfm.
40. Childhelp, National Child Abuse Statistics, "Child Abuse in America–2012," 2012, www.childhelp.org/pages/statistics; National Children's Alliance, "National Statistics on Child Abuse," Accessed June 2014, www.nationalchildrensalliance.org/NCANationalStatistics.
41. M. Stoltenborgh et al., "The Current Prevalence of Child Sexual Abuse Worldwide: A Systematic Review and Meta-Analysis," *International Journal of Public Health* 58, no. 3 (2013): 469–83; L. P. Chen et al., "Sexual Abuse and Lifetime Diagnosis of Psychiatric Disorders: Systematic Review and Meta-Analysis," *Mayo Clinic Proceedings* 85, no. 7 (2010): 618–29; Childhelp, National Child Abuse Statistics, "Child Abuse in America—2012," Accessed June 2014, www.childhelp.org/pages/statistics; U.S. Department of Health and Human Services, Children's Bureau, "Child Maltreatment," February 2013, www.acf.hhs.gov/sites/default/files/cb/cm2012.pdf.
42. Ibid; Childhelp, National Child Abuse Statistics, "Child Abuse in America–2012," Accessed June 2014, www.childhelp.org/pages/statistics.
43. Childhelp, National Child Abuse Statistics, "Child Abuse in America–2012," 2014; L. P. Chen et al., "Sexual Abuse and Lifetime Diagnosis of Psychiatric Disorders," 2010; M. Stoltenborgh et al., "The Current Prevalence of Child Sexual Abuse Worldwide: A Systematic Review and Meta-Analysis," *International Journal of Public Health* 58, no. 3 (2013): 469–83; T. Hilberg, C. Hamilton-Giachrtsis, and L. Dixon, "Review of Meta-Analyses on the Association between Child Sexual Abuse and Adult Mental Health Difficulties: A Systematic Approach." *Trauma, Violence, Abuse* 12, no. 1 (2011): 38–49.
44. Childhelp, National Child Abuse Statistics, "Child Abuse in America–2012," 2014.
45. Centers for Disease Control and Prevention, "Elder Abuse Prevention," June 2014, www.cdc.gov/Features/ElderAbuse/; National Institute on Aging, "Elder Abuse," March 2014, www.nia.nih.gov/health/publication/elder-abuse.
46. J. Grohol, "DSM-5 Changes: PTSD, Trauma and Stress-Related Disorders," *Psych Central-Professional*, May 28, 2013, http://pro.psychcentral.com/dsm-5-changes-ptsd-trauma-stress-related-disorders/004406.html.
47. M. L. Walters, J. Chen, and M. J. Breiding, *The National Intimate Partner and Sexual Violence Survey (NISVS): 2010 Findings on Victimization by Sexual Orientation* (Atlanta, GA: National Center for Injury Prevention and Control, Centers for Disease Control and Prevention, 2013).
48. D. G. Kilpatrick et al., "Drug-Facilitated, Incapacitated, and Forcible Rape: A National Study," July 2007, www.ncjrs.gov/pdffiles1/nij/grants/219181.pdf; White House Task Force to Protect Students from Sexual Assault, "Not Alone: First Report of White House Task Force to Protect Students from Sexual Assault," April 2014. www.whitehouse.gov.
49. National Criminal Justice Reference Service, "School and Campus Crime," *Resource Guide*, Accessed June 2014, www.victimsofcrime.org/docs/ncvrw2013/2013ncvrw_stats_school.pdf?sfvrsn=0.
50. White House Task Force to Protect Students from Sexual Assault, "Not Alone: First Report of White House Task Force to Protect Students from Sexual Assault," April 2014, www.whitehouse.gov.
51. White House Task Force to Protect Students from Sexual Assault, "Not Alone: First Report of White House Task Force to Protect Students from Sexual Assault," 2014.
52. R. Bergen and E. Barnhill, National Online Resource Center on Violence against Women, "Summary: Marital Rape: New Research and Directions," 2011.
53. Ibid.
54. Oregon State University, Sexual Harassment and Sexual Violence, Accessed June 2014, oregonstate.edu/oei/sexual-harassment-and-violence-policy.
55. Centers for Disease Control, "Sexual Violence, Stalking, and Intimate Partner Violence Widespread in the US," NISVS 2010 Summary Report, Press Release, December 2011.
56. Centers for Disease Control and Prevention, "Sexual Violence, Stalking, and Intimate Partner Violence Widespread in the US," NISVS 2010 Summary Report, Press Release, December 2011; NCVRW Resource Guide–2012, "Crime Victimization in the United States: Statistical Overviews," Accessed June 2014, www.ncjrs.gov/ovc_archives/ncvrw/2012/pdf/StatisticalOverviews.pdf.
57. Centers for Disease Control and Prevention, "Sexual Violence, Stalking, and Intimate Partner Violence Widespread in the US," NISVS 2010 Summary Report, Press Release, December 2011; NCVRW Resource Guide–2012, "Crime Victimization in the United States: Statistical Overviews," Accessed June 2014, www.ncjrs.gov/ovc_archives/ncvrw/2012/pdf/StatisticalOverviews.pdf.
58. Centers for Disease Control and Prevention, "Sexual Violence, Stalking, and Intimate Partner Violence Widespread in the US," Accessed December 2011, www.cdc.gov/media/releases/2011/p1214_sexual_violence.html; NCVRW Resource Guide–2012, "Crime Victimization in the United States: Statistical Overviews," Accessed June 2014, Available at www.ncjrs.gov/ovc_archives/ncvrw/2012/pdf/StatisticalOverviews.pdf.
59. U.S. Department of Justice, "Juvenile Justice Fact Sheet-Highlights of the 2011 National Youth Gang Survey," September 2013, www.ojjdp.gov/pubs/242884.pdf; Federal Bureau of Investigation, "2011 National Gang Threat Assessment-Emerging Trends," Accessed June 2014, www.fbi.gov/stats-services/publications/2011-national-gang-threat-assessment.
60. Federal Bureau of Investigation, "2011 National Gang Threat Assessment-Emerging Trends," Accessed June 2014, www.fbi.gov/stats-services/publications/2011-national-gang-threat-assessment.
61. D. McDaniel, "Risk and Protective Factors Associated with Gang Affiliation among High-risk Youth: A Public Health Approach," *Injury Prevention*, January 11, 2012, Available at http://injuryprevention.bmj.com/content/early/2012/01/04/injuryprev-2011-040083.full.pdf+html.
62. U.S. Code of Federal Regulations, Title 28CFR0.85.
63. Adapted from E. Allan and M. Madden, *Hazing in View: College Students at Risk* (Orono, ME: National Collaborative for Hazing Research and Prevention, 2008), Available at www.hazingstudy.org, Reprinted by permission of Elizabeth Allan; Emory Law Journal, "Am I My Brother's Keeper? Reforming Criminal Hazing Laws Based on Assumption of Care," (2014), www.law.emory.edu/fileadmin/journals/elj/63/63.4/Chamberlin.pdf.
64. Ibid.
65. Ibid.
66. National Highway Traffic Safety Administration, "Traffic Safety Facts: 2012 Data," April 2014, www-nrd.nhtsa.dot.gov/Pubs/812016.pdf.
67. National Safety Council, "Motor Vehicle Safety," Accessed May 2014, www.nsc.org/safety_home/MotorVehicleSafety/Pages/MotorVehicleSafety.aspx.
68. Governors Highway Safety Association, *Distracted Driving: What Research Shows and What States Can Do*, Executive Summary, 2011, www.ghsa.org/html/publications/pdf/sfdist11execsum.pdf
69. National Highway Traffic Safety Administration, "What Is Distracted Driving? Key Facts and Statistics," Accessed May 2014, www.distraction.gov/content/get-the-facts/facts-and-statistics.html.
70. U.S. Centers for Disease Control and Prevention, "Distracted Driving," January 2014, www.cdc.gov/Motorvehiclesafety/Distracted_Driving.
71. National Highway Traffic Safety Administration, "What Is Distracted Driving? Key Facts and Statistics," Accessed May 2014, www.distraction.gov/content/get-the-facts/facts-and-statistics.html.
72. Governors Highway Safety Association, "Cell Phone and Texting Laws," Accessed May 2014, www.ghsa.org/html/stateinfo/laws/cellphone_laws.html.
73. National Highway Traffic Safety Administration, "What Is Distracted Driving? Key Facts and Statistics," 2014.
74. National Highway Traffic Safety Administration, "Traffic Safety Facts: 2012 Data," April 2014, www-nrd.nhtsa.dot.gov/Pubs/812016.pdf.
75. Ibid.
76. National Institute on Drug Abuse, "NIDA InfoFacts: Drugged Driving," Revised October 2013, drugabuse.gov/infofacts/driving.html.
77. National Highway Traffic Safety Administration, "Traffic Safety Facts: 2012 Data," 2014, www-nrd.nhtsa.dot.gov/Pubs/812016.pdf.

78. Ibid.
79. Centers for Disease Control and Prevention, "Policy Impact: Seat Belts," Updated January 2014, www.cdc.gov/Motorvehiclesafety/seatbeltbrief.
80. Insurance Institute for Highway Safety, "Vehicle Size and Weight," February 2014, www.iihs.org/iihs/topics/t/vehicle-size-and-weight/qanda.
81. National Highway Traffic Safety Administration, "Traffic Safety Facts: 2012 Data," April 2014, www-nrd.nhtsa.dot.gov/Pubs/812016.pdf
82. Governors Highway Safety Association, "Helmet Laws," May 2014, www.ghsa.org/html/stateinfo/laws/helmet_laws.html
83. National Highway Traffic Safety Administration, "Aggressive Driving," www.nhtsa.gov/Aggressive.
84. National Highway Traffic Safety Administration, "Traffic Safety Facts 2011 Data: Bicyclists and Other Cyclists," April 2013, www.nrd.nhtsa.dot.gov/Pubs/811743.pdf.
85. Ibid.
86. Consumer Product Safety Commission, "CPSC Fact Sheet: Skateboarding Safety," *CPSC Publication* 93 (2012), Available at www.cpsc.gov//PageFiles/122356/093.pdf.
87. Ibid.
88. National Ski Areas Association, "Facts About Skiing/Snowboarding Safety," October 2013, www.nsaa.org/media/175091/Facts_on_Skiing_and_Snowboarding_10_4_13.pdf.
89. Ibid.
90. Centers for Disease Control and Prevention, "Unintentional Drowning: Get the Facts," May 2014, www.cdc.gov/HomeandRecreationalSafety/Water-Safety/waterinjuries-factsheet.html.
91. American Red Cross, "Summer Water Safety Guide," March 2009, http://american.redcross.org/site/DocServer/watersafety0609.pdf?docID=735.
92. Centers for Disease Control and Prevention, "Unintentional Drowning: Get the Facts," May 2014, www.cdc.gov/HomeandRecreationalSafety/Water-Safety/waterinjuries-factsheet.html.
93. U.S. Coast Guard, "Coast Guard News: U.S. Coast Guard Releases 2013 Recreational Boating Statistics Report," May 2014, http://coastguardnews.com/u-s-coast-guard-releases-2013-recreational-boating-statistics-report/2014/05/14/?utm_source=feedburner&utm_medium=feed&utm_campaign=Feed%3A+CoastGuardNews+(Coast+Guard+News).
94. Ibid.
95. Ibid.
96. Ibid.
97. U.S. Coast Guard, "Boating Safety Resource Center: Boating Under the Influence Initiatives," April 2014, www.uscgboating.org/safety/boating_under_the_influence_initiatives.aspx
98. American Boating Association, "Boating Safety—It Could Mean Your Life," 2013, www.americanboating.org/safety.asp.
99. F. R. Lin, J. K. Niparko, and L. Ferrucci, "Hearing Loss Prevalence in the United States," *Archives of Internal Medicine* 171, no. 20 (2011): 1851–53.
100. C. G. LePrell et al., "Evidence of Hearing Loss in a 'Normally-Hearing' College Student Population," *International Journal of Audiology* 50, Suppl 1 (2011): S21–31.
101. K. Hannah et al, "Evaluation of the Olivocochlear Efferent Reflex Strength in the Susceptibility to Temporary Hearing Deterioration After Music Exposure in Young Adults," *Noise Health* 16, no. 69 (2014): 108–15, DOI: 10.4103/1463-1741.132094.
102. National Institute on Deafness and Other Communication Disorders, "Noise-Induced Hearing Loss," April, 2014, www.nidcd.nih.gov/health/hearing/pages/noise.aspx; P. Henry and A. Foots, "Comparison of User Volume Control Settings for Portable Music Players with Three Earphone Configurations in Quiet and Noisy Environments, *Journal of the American Academy of Audiology* 23, no. 3 (2012): 182–91, DOI: 10.3766/jaaa.23.3.5.
103. J. B. Mowry et al., "2012 Annual Report of the American Association of Poison Control Centers' National Poison Data System (NPDS): 30th Annual Report" *Clinical Toxicology* 51, no. 10 (2013): 949–1229, DOI: 10.3109/15563650.2013.863906.
104. American Association of Poison Control Centers, "Prevention," Accessed May 2014, www.aapcc.org/prevention.
105. Centers for Disease Control and Prevention, "Falls among Older Adults: An Overview," September 2013, www.cdc.gov/HomeandRecreationalSafety/Falls/adultfalls.html.
106. Centers for Disease Control and Prevention, "Fire Deaths and Injuries: Fact Sheet," October 2011, www.cdc.gov/HomeandRecreationalSafety/Fire-Prevention/fires-factsheet.html.
107. Ibid.
108. U.S. Bureau of Labor Statistics, "Census of Fatal Occupational Injuries Summary, 2012," August 2013, www.bls.gov/news.release/cfoi.nr0.htm.
109. National Institute of Neurological Disorders and Stroke, "Low Back Pain Fact Sheet," April 2014, www.ninds.nih.gov/disorders/backpain/detail_backpain.htm.
110. American College Health Association, *American College Health Association—National College Health Assessment II: Reference Group Executive Summary, Fall 2013* (Hanover, MD: American College Health Association, 2014), Available at: www.acha-ncha.org/reports_ACHA-NCHAII.html.
111. Mayo Clinic, "Carpal Tunnel Syndrome: Prevention," 2014, www.mayoclinic.org/diseases-conditions/carpal-tunnel-syndrome/basics/prevention/con-20030332.

Pulled Statistics

page 318: D. Drystdale, W. Modzeleski, and A. Simons, Campus Attacks: Targeted Violence Affecting Institutions of Higher Education (Washington, DC: U.S. Secret Service, U.S. Department of Homeland Security, Office of Safe and Drug-Free Schools, U.S. Department of Education, and Federal Bureau of Investigation, U.S. Department of Justice, 2010), Available at www.fbi.gov.

page 324: White House Task Force to Protect Students from Sexual Assault, "Not Alone: First Report of White House Task Force to Protect Students from Sexual Assault," April 2014, www.whitehouse.gov.

page 326: Data are from U.S. Equal Employment Opportunity Commission, "Sexual Harassment," 2013, www.eeoc.gov.

Chapter 14

1. R. Caplan, *Our Earth, Ourselves* (New York, NY: Bantam, 1990), 247.
2. United Nations, "World Population to Reach 10 Billion by 2100 if Fertility in All Countries Converges to Replacement Level," 2012, Available at http://esa.un.org/unpd/wpp/index.htm.
3. R. Engelman, "Fertility Surprise Implies More Populous Future," Worldwatch Institute, July 2013, http://vitalsigns.worldwatch.org/vs-trend/world-population-fertility-surprise-implies-more-populous-future.
4. United Nations, "World Population to Reach 10 Billion by 2100 if Fertility in All Countries Converges to Replacement Level," May 2011, http://esa.un.org/unpd/wpp/Other-Information/Press_Release_WPP2010.pdf.
5. Central Intelligence Agency, "The World Factbook: Country Comparison: Total Fertility Rate," 2013, www.cia.gov/library/publications/the-world-factbook/rankorder/2127rank.html.
6. U.S. Census Bureau, Population Division, "International Data Base Country Rankings," 2010, www.census.gov/idb/ranks.html.
7. Ibid; Global Footprint Network, "Key Findings of the National Footprint Accounts, 2012 ed" (Oakland, CA: Global Footprint Network, 2013) Available at www.footprintnetwork.org/images/article_uploads/National_Footprint_Accounts_2012_Edition_Report.pdf; U.S Census Bureau, "Annual Population Estimates," Revised 2013, www.census.gov/popest/data/national/totals/2012/index.html.
8. World Wildlife Report, *Living Planet Report 2012*, 2012, Available at wwf.panda.org/about_our_earth/all_publications/living_planet_report/2012_lpr/; United Nations, *Global Environmental Outlook*, 2012, www.unep.org/geo/about.asp.
9. United Nations, "UNEP Yearbook: Emerging Issues in our Global Environment, 2013," 2013, www.unep.org.
10. Ibid.
11. United Nations Environmental Program, "New Elephant Poaching and Ivory Smuggling Figures Released," June 2014, www.unep.org.
12. United Nations, *Global Environment Outlook*, 2012.
13. United Nations Environmental Program, "Towards a Green Economy: Pathways to Sustainable Development and Poverty Eradication," 2011, www.unep.org/greeneconomy/greeneconomyreport/tabid/29846/default.aspx; United Nations Environmental Program (UNEP), *Green Economy Report*, 2010, www.unep.org/greeneconomy/greeneconomyreport/tabid/29846/default.aspx.
14. United Nations, "Emerging Issues in our Global Environment, 2012," 2012, www.unep.org/publications/contents/Annual_Reports.asp.
15. Ibid.
16. U.S. Energy Information Administration, "Independent Statistics and Analysis," 2013, www.eia.gov/oiaf/aeo/tablebrowser/#release=IEO2011&subject=1-IEO2011&table=9-IEO2011®ion=0-0&cases=Reference-0504a_1630.
17. U.S. Environmental Protection Agency, "Air Enforcement," 2013, www2.epa.gov/enforcement/air-enforcement.
18. U.S. Environmental Protection Agency, "Overview of Greenhouse Gases: Emissions and Trends: Carbon Dioxide Emissions," Updated April 2014, www.epa.gov/climatechange/ghgemissions/gases/co2.html.
19. S. M Platt et al. "Two-Stroke Scooters Are a Dominant Source of Air Pollution in Many Cities," *Nature Communications* 5, no. 3749 (2014), DOI:10.1038/ncomms4749.
20. Environmental Protection Agency, "Our Nation's Air: Status and Trends through 2010," Updated February 2012, http://www.epa.gov/airtrends/2011/report/fullreport.pdf; American Lung Association, *State of the Air 2014* (Washington, DC: American Lung Association, 2014), Available at www.stateoftheair.org.
21. A. Soos, "Acid Rain Change," Environmental News Network, January 2012, www.enn.com/enn_news/article/43885.
22. Ibid; American Lung Association, "Health Effects of Ozone and Particle Pollution," 2014, www.stateoftheair.org/2014/health-risks.
23. U.S. Environmental Protection Agency, "Reducing Acid Rain," Updated December 2012, www.epa.gov/acidrain/reducing.

24. U.S. Environmental Protection Agency, "Acid Rain: Effects of Acid Rain—Surface Waters and Aquatic Animals," Updated December 2012, www.epa.gov/acidrain/effects/surface_water.html.
25. Ibid.; A. Soos, "Acid Rain Change," Environmental News Network, 2013.
26. U.S. Environmental Protection Agency, "Acid Rain: Effects of Acid Rain—Human Health," Updated December 2012, www.epa.gov/acidrain/effects/health.html.
27. U.S. Energy Information Administration, "Independent Statistics and Analysis," 2012, http://www.eia.gov.
28. U.S. Environmental Protection Agency, "Overview of Greenhouse Gases: Emissions and Trends: Carbon Dioxide," Updated April 2014, www.epa.gov/climatechange/ghgemissions/gases/co2.html; U.S. Global Change Research Group, 3rd National Climate Assessment, "Climate Change Impacts in the United States," May 2014, www.globalchange.gov; U.S. Environmental Protection Agency, "Ozone Layer Depletion: Ozone Science: Brief Questions and Answers on Ozone Depletion," Updated August 2010, www.epa.gov; National Aeronautics and Space Administration, "Ozone Hole Watch," Updated June 2014, http://ozonewatch.gsfc.nasa.gov.
29. U.S. Environmental Protection Agency, "An Introduction to Indoor Air Quality," Updated November 2013, www.epa.gov/iaq/ia-intro.html.
30. Ibid.
31. U.S. Environmental Protection Agency, "Health Effects of Exposure to Secondhand Smoke," Updated November 2011, www.epa.gov/smokefree/healtheffects.html; American Cancer Society, "Secondhand Smoke," Revised February 2014. www.cancer.org/cancer/cancercauses/tobaccocancer/secondhand-smoke.
32. U.S. Environmental Protection Agency, "Indoor Air Quality: Radon: Health Risks," Updated March 2013, www.epa.gov/radon/healthrisks.html.
33. U.S. Environmental Protection Agency, "Why Is Radon the Health Risk That It Is?," Updated January 2014, www.epa.gov/radon/aboutus.html.
34. Centers for Disease Control and Prevention, "Lead," 2013, www.cdc.gov; Centers for Disease Control and Prevention, "Blood Lead Levels in Children Aged 1–5 Years—United States, 1999–2010," *Morbidity and Mortality Weekly Report* 62, no. 13 (2013): 245–48, Available at www.cdc.gov.
35. National Safety Council, "Sick Building Syndrome," Revised April 2009, www.nsc.org/news_resources/Resources/Documents/Sick_Building_Syndrome.pdf.
36. T. Stafford, "A School Input That Matters: Indoor Air Quality and Academic Performance," University of New South Wales, Australian School of Business, School of Economics, 2012; Z. Bako-Biro et al., "Ventilation Rates in Schools and Pupil's Performance," *Building and Environment* 48, no. 1 (2012): 215–23.
37. U.S. Environmental Protection Agency, "IAQ Tools for Schools: Improved Academic Performance: Evidence from Scientific Literature," Updated January 2013, www.epa.gov/iaq/schools/student_performance/evidence.html
38. American Lung Association, "Reduce Asthma Triggers," Accessed June 2014, www.lung.org/lung-disease/asthma/taking-control-of-asthma/reduce-asthma-triggers.html.
39. Centers for Disease Control and Prevention, "FastStats: Asthma," Updated February 2014, www.cdc.gov/nchs/fastats/asthma.htm.
40. White House Press Release, "Remarks by the President on Climate Change-Georgetown University," June 2013, www.whitehouse.gov/the-press-office/2013/06/25/remarks-president-climate-change.
41. Ibid.
42. J. G. L. Olivier et al., *Trends in Global CO_2 Emissions–2013 Report* (The Hague, The Netherlands: PBL Netherland Environmental Assessment Agency, ISPRA: Joint Research Center, 2012), Available at http://edgar.jrc.ec.europa.eu/CO2REPORT2012.pdf.
43. EPA, "Climate Change, Overview of Greenhouse Gases," Updated 2014, www.epa.gov/climatechange/ghgemissions/gases.html.
44. NASA, "Global Climate Change, Evidence of Change: How Do We Know?," Accessed June 2014, http://climate.nasa.gov/evidence; J. G. L. Olivier et al., *Trends in Global CO_2 Emissions–2013 Report*, 2012.
45. U.S. Environmental Protection Agency, "Climate Change: Basic Information," Updated March 2014, http://epa.gov/climatechange/basicinfo.html.
46. NASA, "Global Climate Change, Evidence of Change: How Do We Know?," Accessed June 2014, http://climate.nasa.gov/evidence; J. G. L. Olivier et al., "Trends in Global CO2 Emissions—2013 Report," 2012; NOAA, "State of the Climate Global Analysis, May 2014," 2014, www.ncdc.noaa.gov/sotc/global.
47. J. G. L. Olivier et al., *Trends in Global CO2 Emissions-2013 Report*, 2012; EPA, "National Greenhouse Gas Emissions Data," Updated June 2014, www.epa.gov/climatechange/ghgemissions/usinventoryreport.html.
48. United Nations Framework Convention on Climate Change, "Kyoto Protocol," Accessed June 2014, http://unfccc.int/kyoto_protocol/items/2830.php.
49. D. Malakoff and E. M. Williams, "Q & A: An Examination of the Kyoto Protocol," NPR, June 2007, www.npr.org/templates/story/story.php?storyId=5042766.
50. World Commission on Environment and Development, *Our Common Future* (Oxford, U.K.: Oxford University Press, 1987): 27.
51. J. G. L. Olivier et al., *Trends in Global CO2 Emissions—2013 Report*, 2012.
52. Ibid.
53. U.S. Geological Survey, "Where Is Earth's Water?," Modified March 2014, http://ga.water.usgs.gov/edu/earthwherewater.html.
54. Department of National Intelligence, "Global Water Security," ICA 2012-08, 2012, www.dni.gov/files/documents/Newsroom/Press%20Releases/ICA_Global%20Water%20Security.pdf.
55. World Economic Forum, "Global Council of Water Security 2012–2014," 2014, www.weforum.org/content/global-agenda-council-water-security-2012-2014.
56. Department of National Intelligence, "Global Water Security," 2012; World Economic Forum, "Global Council of Water Security 2012–2014," 2014.
57. EPA, "Drinking Water Contaminants," Updated June 2013, http://water.epa.gov/drink/contaminants; U.S. Geological Survey, "Emerging Contaminants in the Environment," Modified June 2014, http://toxics.usgs.gov/regional/emc/; U.S. Environmental Protection Agency, "Pharmaceuticals and Personal Care Products (PPCPs)," Updated February 2012, www.epa.gov/ppcp.
58. M. Kostich, A. Batt, and J. Lazorcheck, "Concentrations of Prioritized Pharmaceuticals in Effluents from 50 Large Wastewater Treatment Plants in the U.S. and Implications for Risk Estimation," *Environmental Pollution* 184 (2014): 354–59; J. Donn et al., "AP Probe Finds Drugs in Drinking Water," Associated Press, March 8, 2008.
59. Environmental Protection Agency, Office of Underground Storage Tanks, "FY 2011 Annual Report on the Underground Storage Tank Program," 2012, www.epa.gov/oust.
60. Agency for Toxic Substances and Disease Registry (ATSDR), "Toxic Substances Portal: Polychlorinated Biphenyls (PCBs)," Updated March 2011, www.atsdr.cdc.gov/substances/toxsubstance.asp?toxid=26.
61. U.S. Environmental Protection Agency, Pesticides: Topical & Chemical Fact Sheets, "The EPA and Food Security," Updated November 2013, www.epa.gov/pesticides/factsheets/securty.htm.
62. EPA, "Natural Gas Extraction: Hydraulic Fracturing," Updated June 2014, www.epa.gov/hydraulicfracture; U.S. Energy Information Administration (EIA), "What Is Shale Gas and Why Is It Important?," Updated December 2012, www.eia.gov/energy_in_brief/about_shale_gas.cfm.
63. Ibid.
64. B. Walsh, "The Seismic Link between Fracking and Earthquakes," *Time*, May 1, 2014. http://time.com/84225/fracking-and-earthquake-link.
65. U.S. Environmental Protection Agency, *Municipal Solid Waste Generation, Recycling, and Disposal in the United States: Facts and Figures for 2012*, EPA-530-F-14-001 (Washington, DC: U.S. Environmental Protection Agency, 2012), Available at www.epa.gov/osw/nonhaz/municipal/pubs/msw_2012_rcv_factsheet.pdf.
66. Ibid.
67. Ibid.
68. Institute of Mechanical Engineers, "Global Food: Waste Not, Want Not," 2013, Available at www.imeche.org; J. Bloom, *American Wasteland* (Cambridge, MA: DeCapo Press, 2010); National Resource Defense Council, "Food Facts: Your Scraps Add Up," March 2013, www.nrdc.org.
69. Ibid.
70. U.S. Environmental Protection Agency, "Superfund: Superfund National Accomplishments Summary, Fiscal Year 2013," Updated January 2014, www.epa.gov/superfund/accomp/pdfs/FY_2013_SF_EOY_accomp_sum_FINAL.pdf.
71. U.S. Environmental Protection Agency, "Frequent Questions, Hazardous Waste," Updated June 2014, http://waste.supportportal.com/link/portal/23002/23023/ArticleFolder/612/Hazardous-Waste.
72. National Cancer Institute, Factsheet, "Cell Phones and Cancer Risk," Accessed June 2014, www.cancer.gov; M. P. Little et al., "Mobile Phone Use and Glioma Risk: Comparison of Epidemiological Study Results with Incidence Trends in the United States," *British Medical Journal* 344 (2012): e1147, DOI: 10.1136/bmj.e1147; D. Aydin et al., "Mobile Phone Use and Brain Tumors in Children and Adolescents: A Multicenter Case-Control study," *Journal of the National Cancer Institute* 103, no. 16 (2011): 1264–76, DOI: 10.1093/jnci/djr244.
73. U.S. Nuclear Regulatory Commission, "Radiation Basics," 2011, Available at http://nrc.gov/about-nrc/radiation/health-effects/radiation-basics.html.
74. National Council on Radiation Protection and Measurements, "NCRP Report No. 160" www.ncrponline.org/Publications/160_Pie_Charts/160_Pie_charts.html.
75. R. Balmforth, "Factbox: Key Facts on Chernobyl Nuclear Accident," Reuters, March 15, 2011, www.reuters.com/article/2011/03/15/us-nuclear-chernobyl-facts-idUSTRE72E42U20110315.
76. "Japan's Nuclear Emergency," *Washington Post*, 2011, www.washingtonpost.com/wp-srv/special/world/japan-nuclear-reactors-and-seismic-activity/; "Earthquake, Tsunami, and Nuclear

Crisis," *New York Times*, 2011, http://topics.nytimes.com/top/news/international/countriesandterritories/japan/index.html.
77. M. Penny and M. Selden, "The Severity of the Fukushima Daiichi Nuclear Disaster: Comparing Chernobyl and Fukushima," Global Research, March 2013, www.globalresearch.ca/PrintArticle.php?articleId=24949.
78. U.S. Energy Information Administration, "Independent Statistics and Analysis," 2012.
79. K. Eagan et al., *The American Freshman: National Norms Fall 2013* (Los Angeles, CA: Higher Education Research Institute, UCLA, 2013) 2013, Available at www.heri.ucla.edu/monographs/TheAmericanFreshman2013.pdf.
80. Energy Star, "Computers," Accessed June 2014, www.energystar.gov/certified-products/detail/computers.
81. R. Vartabedian, "Cable TV Boxes Become 2nd Biggest Energy Users in Many Homes," *LA Times*, June 19, 2014.
82. American Lung Association, *State of the Air 2014* (Washington, DC: American Lung Association, 2014), Available at www.stateoftheair.org.
83. Sierra Club, "Infographic: Green College Trends," August 2013, http://sierraclub.typepad.com/greenlife/2013/08/infographic-whats-trending-at-americas-greenest-colleges.html.

Pulled Statistics

page 348, U.S. Environmental Protection Agency, "Health Effects of Exposure to Secondhand Smoke," 2011, www.epa.gov/smokefree/healtheffects.html; American Cancer Society, "Health Effects of Secondhand Smoke," March 2014, www.cdc.gov/tobacco/data_statistics/fact_sheets/secondhand_smoke/health_effects.

page 355, International Bottled Water Association, "U.S. Consumption of Bottled Water Shows Continued Growth, increasing 6.2 percent in 2012; Sales up 6.7 percent," 2013, www.bottledwater.org/us-consumption-bottled-water-shows-continued-growth-increasing-62-percent-2012-sales-67-percent.

Chapter 15

1. L. Colloca and C. Grillon, "Understanding Placebo and Nocebo Responses for Pain Management," *Current Pain and Headache Reports* 18, no. 6 (2014): 419, DOI: 10.1007/s11916-014-0419-2.
2. A. Keitel et al., "Expectation Modulates the Effect of Deep Brain Stimulation on Motor and Cognitive Function in Tremor-Dominant Parkinson's Disease," *PLoS One* 8, no. 12 (2013): e81878, DOI: 10.1371/journal.pone.0081878.
3. J. Sarris, M. Fava, I. Schweitzer, and D. Mischoulon, "St John's Wort (Hypericum perforatum) versus Sertraline and Placebo in Major Depressive Disorder: Continuation Data from a 26-Week RCT," *Pharmacopsychiatry* 45, no. 7 (2012): 275–8, DOI: 10.1055/s-0032-1306348; R. A. Litten et al., "The Placebo Effect in Clinical Trials for Alcohol Dependence: An Exploratory Analysis of 51 Naltrexone and Acamprosate Studies," *Alcoholism, Clinical and Experimental Research* 37, no. 12 (2013): 2128–37, DOI: 10.1111/acer.12197; G. L. Petersen et al., "The Magnitude of Nocebo Effects in Pain: A Meta-Analysis," *Pain* (2014), pii: S0304-3959(14)00195-X, DOI: 10.1016/j.pain.2014.04.016. (E-pub ahead of publication.)
4. M. A. Hillen et al., " How Can Communication by Oncologists Enhance Patients' Trust? An Experimental Study," *Annals of Oncology* 25, no. 4 (2014): 896–901.
5. J. Commins, "Defensive Medicine," *Health Leaders Media*, April 13, 2012, www.healthleadersmedia.com/page-4/MAG-278899/Defensive-Medicine.
6. A. T. Chien and M. B. Rosenthal, "Waste Not, Want Not: Promoting Efficient Use of Health Care Resources," *Annals of Internal Medicine* 158, no. 1 (2013): 67–68.
7. Consumer Health, "Patient Rights: Informed Consent," March 2013, www.emedicinehealth.com/patient_rights/article_em.htm#patient_rights.
8. Centers for Disease Control and Prevention, "Therapeutic Drug Use," May 2014, www.cdc.gov/nchs/fastats/drug-use-therapeutic.htm.
9. W. Zhong et al., "Age and Sex Patterns of Drug Prescribing in a Defined American Population," *Mayo Clinic Proceedings* 88, no. 7 (2013): 697–707.
10. L. Gallelli et al., "Safety and Efficacy of Generic Drugs with Respect to Brand Formulation," *Journal of Pharmacology and Pharmacotherapeutics* 4, Supplement 1 (2013): S110–14.
11. U.S. Food and Drug Administration, "The Possible Dangers of Buying Medicine over the Internet," 2014, www.fda.gov/forconsumers/consumerupdates/ucm048396.htm.
12. National Center for Complementary and Alternative Medicine, "Complementary, Alternative, or Integrative Health: What's in a Name?," May 2013, http://nccam.nih.gov/health/whatiscam.
13. Ibid.
14. National Center for Complementary and Alternative Medicine, "Health Topics A to Z," 2014, http://nccam.nih.gov/health/atoz.htm.
15. National Center for Complementary and Alternative Medicine, "Traditional Chinese Medicine: An Introduction," October 2013, http://nccam.nih.gov/health/whatiscam/chinesemed.htm.
16. National Center for Complementary and Alternative Medicine, "Ayurvedic Medicine: An Introduction," NCCAM Publication no. D287, August 2013, http://nccam.nih.gov/health/ayurveda/introduction.htm.
17. Ibid.
18. National Center for Complementary and Alternative Medicine, "Homeopathy: An Introduction," May 2013, http://nccam.nih.gov/health/homeopathy.
19. Ibid.
20. National Center for Complementary and Alternative Medicine, "Chiropractic: An Introduction," NCCAM Publication no. D403, Modified February 2012. http://nccam.nih.gov/health/chiropractic/introduction.htm.
21. Ibid.
22. Bureau of Labor Statistics, U.S. Department of Labor, "Chiropractors," *Occupational Outlook Handbook, 2012–2013 Edition*, March 29, 2012. http://www.bls.gov/ooh/healthcare/chiropractors.htm.
23. Bureau of Labor Statistics, U.S. Department of Labor, "Massage Therapists," *Occupational Outlook Handbook, 2012–2013 Edition*, January 2014, www.bls.gov/ooh/Healthcare/Massage-therapists.htm.
24. Ibid.
25. National Center for Complementary and Alternative Medicine, "Complementary, Alternative, or Integrative Health: What's in a Name?," May 2013, http://nccam.nih.gov/health/whatiscam.
26. National Center for Complementary and Alternative Medicine, "Acupuncture: An Introduction," September 2012, http://nccam.nih.gov/health/acupuncture/introduction.htm.
27. A. J. Vickers et al., "Acupuncture for Chronic Pain: Individual Patient Data Meta-Analysis," *Archives of Internal Medicine* 172, no. 19 (2012): 1444–53.
28. National Center for Complementary and Alternative Medicine, "Acupuncture: An Introduction," 2012.
29. R. Jahnke et al., "A Comprehensive Review of Health Benefits of Qigong and Tai Chi," *American Journal of Health Promotion* 24, no. 6 (2010): e1–e25.
30. D. L. Fazzino et al., "Energy Healing and Pain: A Review of the Literature," *Holistic Nursing Practice* 24, no. 2 (2010): 79–88; National Center for Complementary and Alternative Medicine, "Reiki: An Introduction," April 2013, http://nccam.nih.gov/health/reiki/introduction.htm.
31. Psychoneuroimmunology Research Society, "Mission Statement," November 17, 2010, www.pnirs.org/society/index.cfm.
32. E. Broadbent and H. E. Koschwanez, "The Psychology of Wound Healing," *Current Opinions in Psychiatry* 25, no 2 (2012): 135–40.
33. M. R. Irwin and R. Olmstead, "Mitigating Cellular Inflammation in Older Adults: A Randomized Controlled Trial of Tai Chi," *American Journal of Geriatric Psychiatry* 20, no. 9 (2012): 764–72.
34. Academy of Nutrition and Dietetics, "Position of the Academy of Nutrition and Dietetics: Functional Foods," *Journal of the Academy of Nutrition and Dietetics* 113, no. 8 (2013): 1096–1103.
35. K. Ried et al., "Effect of Cocoa on Blood Pressure," *Cochrane Database of Systematic Reviews* 8, no. CD008893 (2012), DOI: 10.1002/14651858.CD008893.pub2.
36. National Center for Complementary and Alternative Medicine, "Oral Probiotics: An Introduction," December 2012, http://nccam.nih.gov/health/probiotics/introduction.htm
37. National Center for Complementary and Alternative Medicine, "Kava," April 2012, http://nccam.nih.gov/health/kava.
38. Mayo Clinic Staff, "Herbal Supplements: What to Know before You Buy," November 2011, www.mayoclinic.com/health/herbal-supplements/SA00044.
39. U.S. Pharmacopeial Convention, "USP & Patients/Consumers," 2012, www.usp.org/usp-consumers.
40. K. G. Carman and C. Eibner, "Survey Estimates Net Gain of 9.3 Million American Adults with Health Insurance," April 8, 2014, www.rand.org/blog/2014/04/survey-estimates-net-gain-of-9-3-million-american-adults.html.
41. American College Health Association. *American College Health Association–National College Health Assessment II: Reference Group Executive Summary, Fall 2013* (Hanover, MD: American College Health Association, 2014).
42. U.S. Centers for Disease Control and Prevention/National Center for Health Statistics, "Health Insurance Coverage, January–June, 2012," Updated November, 2012, www.cdc.gov/nchs/health_policy/health_insurance_selected_characteristics_jan_jun_2012.htm.
43. Kaiser Family Foundation, "Total HMO Enrollment, July 2012," May 2014, http://kff.org/other/state-indicator/total-hmo-enrollment.
44. Centers for Medicare & Medicaid Services, "National Health Expenditure Projections 2012–2022: Forecast Summary," November, 2013, www.cms.gov/Research-Statistics-Data-and-Systems/Statistics-Trends-and-Reports/NationalHealthExpendData/Downloads/proj2012.pdf.
45. Ibid.
46. Bureau of Labor Statistics, U.S. Department of Labor, "Physicians and Surgeons," *Occupational Outlook Handbook, 2014–2015*, Modified January 2014, www.bls.gov/ooh/healthcare/physicians-and-surgeons.htm.

47. American Hospital Association, "Fast Facts on U.S. Hospitals," January 2014, www.aha.org/research/rc/stat-studies/fast-facts.shtml.
48. O. W. Brawley, *How We Do Harm: A Doctor Breaks Ranks about Being Sick in America* (New York, NY: St. Martin's Press, 2011).
49. Centers for Medicare and Medicaid Services, "National Health Expenditure Projections 2012–2022: Forecast Summary," 2013.
50. Ibid.
51. America's Health Insurance Plans, "Fast Check: Administrative Costs," November 2012, www.ahip.org/ACA-Toolbox/Documents/Communications-Toolkit/Fact-Check–Administrative-Costs.aspx.
52. P. Krugman, "The Medicaid Cure," January 10, 2014, *The New York Times*; Right to Health Care ProCon.org, "Should All Americans Have the Right (Be Entitled) to Health Care?" Updated January 2014, http://healthcare.procon.org.
53. United Nations, "The Universal Declaration of Human Rights," 1948, www.un.org/en/documents/udhr.
54. P. Krugman, "The Medicaid Cure," 2014.
55. Department of Health and Human Services, "Report to Congress: National Strategy for Quality Improvement in Health Care," 2011, www.ahrq.gov/workingforquality/nqs/nqs2011annlrpt.htm.

Pulled Statistics

page 368, Centers for Disease Control and Prevention, "Therapeutic Drug Use," May 2014, www.cdc.gov/nchs/fastats/drug-use-therapeutic.htm.
page 370, P. M. Barnes, B. Bloom, and R. L. Nahin, "Complementary and Alternative Medicine Use among Adults and Children: United States, 2007," *National Health Statistics Reports*, no. 12 (Hyattsville, MD: National Center for Health Statistics, 2008), Available at www.cdc.gov.
page 380, Robert Wood Johnson Foundation, "Survey: Physicians Are Aware that Many Medical Tests and Procedures Are Unnecessary, See Themselves as Solution," May 2014, www.rwjf.org/en/about-rwjf/newsroom/newsroom-content/2014/04/survey--physicians-are-aware-that-many-medical-tests-and-procedu.html.

Photo Credits

Chapter 1 1: Fancy Collection/Superstock; 2: Getty Images; 3: Alamy; 4: Alamy; 4: Getty Images; 4: Yeko Photo Studio/Shutterstock; 5: Getty Images; 6: Alamy; 10: ML Harris/Getty Images; 12: Getty Images; 13: Steve Lindridge/Alamy; 15: JGI/Jamie Grill/Blend Images/Getty Images; 17: Yuri/Getty Images; 18: Getty Images; 19: Tommaso lizzul/Shutterstock

Chapter 2 21: Ocean/Corbis; 23: Blend Images/Terry Vine/Getty Images; 23: Stockbyte/Thinkstock/Getty Images; 25: Stockbyte/Exactostock/Superstock; 26: Pascal Broze/AGE Fotostock; 28: DmitriMaruta/Shutterstock; 30: Chris Ammann/Baltimore Examiner/AP Images; 31: Keren Su/China Span/Alamy; 31: Neal & Molly Jansen/Superstock; 33: Stockbyte/Exactostock/Superstock; 35: Getty Images; 36: Stockbyte/Comstock/Getty Images; 38: Chris Rout/Bubbles Photolibrary/Alamy; 39: Plush Studios/Blend Images/Getty Images; 40: Simon Rawley/Alamy

Chapter 3 45: 68 altrendo images/Ocean/Corbis; 46: Creatista/Shutterstock; 47: Ariel Skelley/Blend Images/Getty images; 47: Pendygraft/John/St. Petersburg Times/PSG/Newscom; 47: Scott Griessel/Getty Images; 49: Oliver Furrer/Alamy; 50: Getty Images; 51: Getty images; 52: Gladskikh Tatiana/Shutterstock; 53: Radius Images/Getty Images; 54: Radius Images/Corbis; 55: Robert Churchill/Getty Images; 56: Imagerymajestic/Alamy; 57: Kate Sept 2004/E+/Getty Images; 58: Susan Montgomery/Fotolia; 60: SuperStock; 61: Getty Images; 62: DK Images; 63: Uniquely india/Getty Images; 64: iStock/Getty images; 65: Getty Images

Chapter 4 67: Blue Jean Images/Corbis; 68: Monkey Business Image/Kalium/Age Fotostock; 70: Masterfile USA Corporation; 72: Wavebreakmedia ltd/Shutterstock; 73: Jim Purdum/Getty Images; 74: Mangostock/Fotolia; 75: Chris Schmidt/Getty Images; 76: abfotolv/Fotolia; 77: Wavebreakmedia Micro/Fotolia; 79: Ryan McVay/Photodisc/Getty Images; 80: PhotoAlto/John Dowland/Getty Images; 80: PhotoAlto/John Dowland/PhotoAlto Agency RF Collections/Getty Images; 82: Echo/Cultura/Getty Images; 82: Getty images; 83: FS2 Wenn Photos/Newscom; 83: Hannibal Hanschke/dpa/picture-alliance/Newscom; 86: David J. Green - lifestyle themes/Alamy; 86: David J. Green/lifestyle themes/Alamy; 89: Mango Stock/Shutterstock; 89: Tom Merton/OJO+/Getty Images; 90: Frederic Cirou/PhotoAlto/Alamy; 90: Frederic Cirou/PhotoAlto / Alamy; 91: BananaStock/Jupiter Images; 91: Getty Images; 92: Allison Michael Orenstein/Photodisc/Getty Images; 93: YanC/iStockphoto.com; 93: Yanik Chauvin/Getty Images

Chapter 5 95: Blend Images/Superstock; 97: Keith Brofsky/Photodisc/Getty Images; 98: Pearson Education; 98: SIU BioMed Comm/Custom Medical Stock/Photo/Newscom; 99: Jules Selmes and Debi Treloar/DK Images; 101: Sean Justice/AGE Fotostock; 102: Magdalena Zurawska; 102: Magdalena Zurawska/Fotolia; 103: Phanie/Science Source; 103: Vario images GmbH & Co.KG/Alamy; 104: Saturn Stills/Science Source; 104: Saturn Stills/Science Source; 105: Pearson Education; 108: Getty Images; 109: David J. Green/Lifestyle Themes/Alamy; 112: Helder Almeida/Fotolia; 113: Getty Images; 115: Hart Photography/Fotolia; 116: Moncherie/Getty Images; 119: Plush Studios/Blend Images/Getty Images; 120: Donna Coleman/Getty Images; 121: Vally/Fotolia; 121: winterling/Getty Images

Chapter 6 123: BSIP SA/Alamy; 125: Allstar Picture Library/Alamy; 126: Adam Brown/UpperCut Images/Alamy; 127: Denis Pepin/Getty Images; 127: Jupiterimages/Photos.com; 129: Ian Hooton/Science Photo Library/Alamy; 129: Ian Hooton/SPL/Science Photo Library/Alamy; 130: Thomas M Perkins/Shutterstock; 132: jannoon028/Shutterstock.com; 132: Charles Tatlock; 132: James Brey/E+/Getty Images; 134: RayArt Graphics/Alamy; 135: Karen Mower/Getty Images; 136: Gregor/Shutterstock; 137: David Hoffman Photo Library/Alamy; 138: Martyn Vickery/Alamy; 139: ACE Stock Limited/Alamy; 139: Ace Stock Limited/Alamy; 139: Bob Cheung/Shutterstock; 140: Janine Wiedel Photolibrary/Alamy; 140: Janine Wiedel Photolibrary/Alamy; 141: Lionel Bonaventure/AFP/Getty Images/Newscom; 142: Ghislain & Marie David de Lossy/Cultura Creative (RF) / Alamy; 142: Design Pics/Getty Images; 144: Jupiter Images/Stockbyte/Getty Images; 145: Tomm L/Getty Images

Chapter 7 147: Michele Constantini/ PhotoAlto/Corbis; 150: DK Images; 150: Steve Gorton/DK Images; 151: D.C. Hughes/ZUMAPRESS/Newscom; 153: Getty Images; 154: Science Source; 154: Martin M. Rotker/Science Source; 155: PhotoLibrary/Getty Images; 156: Joerg Lange/Vario Images/Alamy; 158: Phanie/SuperStock; 160: Elizabeth Weinberg/Getty Images; 161: Helen H. Richardson/Denver Post/Getty Images; 162: matrix76/Getty Images; 163: Oral Health America; 165: Biophoto Associates/Science Source; 165: AllOver images/Alamy; 165: TPH special/allOver photography/Alamy; 166: IS-200510 /Image Source/Alamy; 167: U.S. Food and Drug Administration; 169: Comstock Images/Stockbyte/Getty Images; 170: Stanislav Fadyukhin/Getty Images; 171: Milosluz/iStockphoto/Getty Images; Oral Health America

Chapter 8 173: Golden Pixels LLC/Alamy; 174: webphotographeer/Getty Images; 175: Flashon Studio/iStockphoto/Getty Images; 175: JR Trice/Shutterstock; 175: Westmacott Photograph/Shutterstock; 176: George Muresan/Shutterstock; 177: Shutterstock; 178: Mike Flippo/Shutterstock; 178: Pearson Learning Photo Studio; 181: David R. Frazier Photolibrary, Inc./Alamy; 182: Barry Gregg/keepsake/Corbis; 182: Barry Gregg/Spirit/Corbis; 183: Barry Gregg/keepsake/Corbis; 183: Barry Gregg/Spirit/Corbis; 183: C Squared Studios/Photodisc/Getty Images; 183: VL@D/Fotolia; 184: Bluefern/Fotolia; 184: Brand Pictures/ AGE Fotostock; 184: Martin Darley /Shutterstock; 185: Barry Gregg/keepsake/Corbis; 185: Barry Gregg/Spirit/Corbis; 186: Matka_Wariatka/iStock/360/Getty Images; 189: Pearson Education; 190: Stockbyte/Getty Images; 192: Brian Hagiwara/Photolibrary/Getty Images; 193: ML Harris/Getty Images; 195: MorePixels/iStock / 360/Getty Images; 196: Vladimir Voronin/Fotolia; 198: Dkapp12/iStock/360/Getty Images; 199: Alxpin/E+/Getty Images

Chapter 9 201: Ted Foxx/Alamy; 203: Big Cheese Photo LLC / Alamy; 204: Wavebreakmedia/Shutterstock; 205: Brand X Pictures/Getty Image; 205: Brand X Pictures/Getty Images; 205: Brand X Pictures/Stockbyte/Getty Images; 206: John Anthony Rizzo/Getty Images; 209: David Madison/Photographer's Choice/Getty Images; 209: JGI/Jamie Grill/Blend Images/Getty Images; 209: Julie Brown/Custom Medical Stock; 209: Life Measurement, Inc.; 209: May/Science Source; 209: Phanie/Science Source; 211: David C. Rehner/Shutterstock; 212: Luis Louro/Shutterstock; 213: Asia Images Group Pte Ltd / Alamy; 214: Bobby Bank/Getty Images; 215: Howard Shooter/DK Images; 216: Custom Medical Stock Photo/Alamy; 216: Sakala/Shutterstock; 218: Brand X Pictures/Stockbyte/Getty Images; 218: Li Kim Goh/E+/Getty Images; 219: Favakeh/Custom Medical Stock Photo/Newscom; 220: Barry Gregg/keepsake/Corbis; 221: Nicholas Monu/Getty Images; 221: Photodisc/Getty Images; 222: LeventeGyori/Shutterstock; 223: WavebreakmediaMicro/Fotolia; 224: Micha Klootwijk/Shutterstock; 225: Gustavo Andrade/Gos Photo Design/Getty Images

Chapter 10 227: Image Source/Alamy; 229: Anton Gvozdikov/Getty Images; 229: Graham Mitchell/Exactostock/Superstock; 229: Pearson Education; 229: Photodisc/Getty Images; 229: Teo Lannie/PhotoAlto Agency RF Collections/Getty Images; 229: Teo Lannie/PhotoAlto Agency/Getty Images; 231: Miroslav Georgijevic/Vetta/Getty Images; 233: Rolf Adlercreutz/Alamy; 234: Ali Ender Birer/iStock / 360/Getty Images; 234: Ali Ender Birer/Shutterstock; 234: Bob Jacobson/keepsake/Corbis; 234: Craig Veltri/iStock / 360/Getty Images; 234: Dandanian/Getty Images; 234: Deymos/Shutterstock; 234: GVictoria/Shutterstock; 234: Kirsty Pargeter/iStock/360/Getty Images; 234: PaulMaguire/iStock/360/Getty Images; 234: Rod Ferris/Shutterstock; 234: Stephen VanHorn/Alamy; 234: Tatuasha/Shutterstock; 234: Walter Cruz/MCT/Newscom; 235: Dan Dalton/Digital Vision/Getty Images; 235: Daniel Grill/Alamy; 235: MIXA/Getty Images; 236: Karl Weatherly/Photodisc/Getty Images; 236: Pearson Education; 237: Moodboard/Corbis; 238: Wavebreakmedia Ltd/Getty Images; 239: Blue Jean Images/Alamy; 239: Pearson Education; 240: Pearson Education; 242: Nenad Aksic/E+/Getty Images; 242: Nenad Aksic/Getty Images; 243: Mark Cowan/UPI/Newscom; 244: Alamy; 244: Pearson Education; 244: Pearson Education; 244: Thomas Smith Photography/Alamy; 246: Daniel Hurst/Getty Images; 246: Daniel Hurst/iStock/360/Getty Images; 246: windu/Shutterstock; 247: Dennis Welsh/AGE Fotostock; 247: Dennis Welsh/UpperCut Image/AGE Fotostock; 248: Image Source/Getty Images; 249: Index Stock Imagery/PhotoLibrary/Getty Images; 250: Aleksandr Lobanov/Getty Images; 250: Aleksandr Lobanov/iStock/360/Getty Images; 250: Pearson Education; 250: Pearson Education

Chapter 11 253: B Boissonnet/ Ramble/Corbis; 256: Irina Iglina/Getty Images; 256: Irina Iglina/iStock/360/Getty Images; 261: Radius Images/Alamy; 263: Jupiterimages/Brand X Pictures/Thinkstock/Getty Images; 263: Moodboard/Alamy; 264: Moodboard/Getty Images; 265: Levent Konuk/Shutterstock; 268: Index Stock/Getty Images; 268: PhotoLibrary/Index Stock/Science Source; 269: Dawn Poland/E+/Getty Images; 269: Dawn Poland/Getty Images; 270: dnberty/Getty Images; 271: AfriPics.com/Alamy; 272: Darryl Bush/Modesto Bee/ZumaPress.com/ZUMA Wire Service/Alamy; 274: Digital Vision/Getty Images; 275: Dr. P. Marazzi / Science Source; 275: Dr. P. Marazzi/Science Source; 275: Dr. P. Marazzi/Science Source; 275: James Stevenson/Science Source; 275: James Stevenson/Science Source; 280: Kamdyn R Switzer/Cal Sport Media/Newscom; 282: William Perugini/Shutterstock; 286: Ioana Drutu/Getty Images; 286: Loana Drutu/iStock/360/Getty Images; 287: Getty Images; 287: Sebastian Kaulitzki/Getty Images; 287: vm/Getty Images; 289: Martin Shields/Alamy

Chapter 12 291: Tetra Images/Superstock; 292: Ocean/Corbis; 293: Eric Raptosh/Blend Images/Getty Images; 296: Lezh/iStockphoto; 297: Dr. Gary Gaugler/Science Source; 297: Dr. Linda M. Stannard, University of Cape Town/Science Source; 297: Eye of Science/Science Source; 297: Mediscan/Medical on Line/Alamy; 297: Steve Gschmeissner/Science Source; 298: ZUMA Press, Inc./Alamy; 299: Sidea Revuz /Science Source; 302: Antagain/iStockphoto; 303: Michael Krinke/iStockphoto/Getty Images; 304: Gabriel Moisa/iStock; 305: Peter Bernik/Shutterstock; 306: Kevin Foy/Alamy; 308: Western Ophthalmic Hospital/Science Source; 309: Centers for Disease Control and Prevention; 310: Science Source; 311: Mediscan/Alamy Limited; 312: Dr. P. Marazzi / Science Source; 313: Eye of Science/Science Source; 314: arturbo/iStockphoto/Getty Images; 314: Tomaz Levstek/iStockphoto/Getty Images; 315: Brandon Brown/iStock/Getty Images; 315: Simon Valentine/iStockphoto/Getty Images; lexx72/Fotolia

Chapter 13 317: Seb Oliver/Image Source/Corbis; 318: Jochen Tack/Alamy; 319: D. Hurst/Alamy; 320: Dean Millar/Getty Images; 321: Africa Studio/Shutterstock; 321: Robyn Beck/AFP/Getty Images/Newscom; 322: Janine Wiedel / Janine Wiedel Photolibrary/Alamy; 324: AP Photo/The Sentinel, Jason Malmont; 325: Bill Aron/PhotoEdit; 326: Roy McMahon/Corbis/Glow Images; 327: Anthony Dunn/Alamy; 328: Charles Sturge/Alamy; 330: Olivier Douliery/ABACAUSA.COM; 332: Adrin Shamsudin/Fotolia; 333: Paul Conklin/PhotoEdit; 334: Kristin Piljay/Pearson Science; 335: Erik Isakson/Getty Images; 337: Jeff Greenberg/PhotoEdit; 338: Science Photo Library/Alamy; 340: Dmitry Melnikov/Shutterstock; 340: Kruglov_Orda/Shutterstock; 341: Jeremy Trew/Trewimage/Alamy; 341: Kunal Mehta/Shutterstock

Chapter 14 343: Wavebreak Media LTD/ Alloy/Corbis; 345: Brianindia/Alamy; 346: Science Source; 347: Justin Sullivan/Staff/Getty Images; 348: Auborddulac/123RF; 349: moodboard/Alamy; 350: Dave King/DK Images; 353: Qa photos/Alamy; 355: Alterfalter/Shutterstock; 356: John Henley/Blend Images/Alamy; 357: AP Images; 357: Chine Nouvelle/SIPA/Newscom; 358: Ari Joseph/Middlebury College; 359: Ilene MacDonald/Alamy; 360: Christopher Conrad/Getty Images; 361: Thinkstock/Getty Images

Chapter 15 363: ableimages/Alamy; 364: Adrian Sherratt/Alamy; 365: Tatiana Popova/Shutterstock; 367: Jiang Jin/SuperStock; 368: Steve Snowden/Shutterstock; 371: Design Pics Inc/Alamy; 372: Thomas Boehm/Alamy; 373: Monkey Business Images/Shutterstock; 374: Illie Hill, Jr./The Image Works; 375: Jeffrey Blackler/Alamy; 376: eAlisa/Shutterstock; 376: Elena Elisseeva/Shutterstock; 376: joanna wnuk/Shutterstock; 376: Shapiso/Shutterstock; 376: WEKWEK/iStock/Getty Images; 378: Jochen Tack/Alamy; 379: Blend Images/Alamy; **380:**; 382: DNY59/iStockphoto/Getty Images; 382: jo unruh/iStockphoto/Getty Images

Cover Tetra Images/Corbis

Index

Note: Page references followed by *fig* indicate an illustrated figure; by *t* a table; and by *p* a photograph.

A

B

C

D

E

F

G

J

K

L

M

N

O

P

Q

R

S

T

Web Links for Health and Wellness

Chapter 1 Healthy Change

- **CDC Wonder.** A clearinghouse for information from the Centers for Disease Control and Prevention. http://wonder.cdc.gov
- **Mayo Clinic.** A reputable resource for information about health topics, diseases, and treatment options. www.mayoclinic.com
- **National Center for Health Statistics.** Information about health status in the United States, including key reports and national survey information. www.cdc.gov/nchs
- **healthfinder.gov.** A resource for consumer information about health. www.healthfinder.gov
- **World Health Organization.** A resource on global health; provides information on illness and disease statistics, trends, and outbreak alerts. www.who.int/en

Chapter 2 Psychological Health

- **American Foundation for Suicide Prevention.** Resources for suicide prevention; support for family and friends of those who have committed suicide. www.afsp.org
- **American Psychological Association Help Center.** Information on psychology at work, the mind-body connection, psychological responses to war, and other topics. www.apa.org/helpcenter
- **National Alliance on Mental Illness.** Support and advocacy for families and friends of people with severe mental illnesses. www.nami.org
- **National Institute of Mental Health (NIMH).** An overview of mental health information and research. www.nimh.nih.gov
- **Helpguide.** Resources for improving mental and emotional health, plus information on topics such as self-injury, sleep, depressive disorders, and anxiety disorders. www.helpguide.org
- **National Suicide Prevention Lifeline.** Help 24 hours a day for people in crisis via online chat, text, or phone. www.suicidepreventionlifeline.org or 1-800-273-8255.

Chapter 3 Stress

- **American College Health Association.** This site provides information and data from the National College Health Assessment survey. www.acha.org
- **Higher Education Research Institute.** This organization provides annual surveys of first-year and senior college students that cover academic, financial, and health-related issues. www.heri.ucla.edu
- **American College Counseling Association.** The website of the professional organization for college counselors offers useful links and articles. www.collegecounseling.org

Chapter 4 Relationships and Sexuality

- **American Association of Sexuality Educators, Counselors, and Therapists (AASECT).** Professional organization providing standards of practice for treating sexual issues and disorders. www.aasect.org
- **Go Ask Alice!** An interactive question-and-answer resource from the Columbia University Health Services. www.goaskalice.columbia.edu
- **Sexuality Information and Education Council of the United States (SIECUS).** Information, guidelines, and materials for advancement of healthy and proper sex education. www.siecus.org
- **The Human Rights Campaign.** Advocacy and resources about LGBT issues by the largest civil rights organization for lesbian, gay, bisexual, and transgender Americans. www.hrc.org
- **Advocates for Youth.** Current news, policy updates, research, and other resources about the sexual health of and choices particular to high school and college-aged students. www.advocatesforyouth.org

Chapter 5 Reproductive Choices

- **Guttmacher Institute.** This nonprofit organization is focused on sexual and reproductive health research, policy analysis, and public education. www.guttmacher.org
- **Association of Reproductive Health Professionals.** This independent organization, originally the educational arm of Planned Parenthood, provides education for health care professionals and the general public. It includes an interactive tool to help you choose a birth control method that will work for you. www.arhp.org
- **The American Pregnancy Association.** A wealth of resources to promote reproductive and pregnancy wellness. www.americanpregnancy.org
- **Planned Parenthood.** A range of up-to-date information on issues such as birth control, the decision of when and whether to have a child, STIs, and safer sex. www.plannedparenthood.org

Chapter 6 Addiction and Drug Abuse

- **National Council on Problem Gambling.** Information and help for people with gambling problems and their families. www.ncpgambling.org
- **National Institute on Drug Abuse (NIDA).** Information on the latest statistics and findings in drug research. www.nida.nih.gov
- **Substance Abuse and Mental Health Services Administration (SAMHSA).** An outstanding resource for information about national surveys, ongoing research, and national drug interventions. www.samhsa.gov

Chapter 7 Alcohol and Tobacco

- **Alcoholics Anonymous (AA).** General information about AA and the 12-step program. www.aa.org
- **College Drinking: Changing the Culture.** This resource center targets the student population as a whole, the college and its surrounding